DERMATOPATHOLOGY COMPASS

Vladimir Vincek, MD, PhD

Professor and former founding Chairman
Department of Dermatology
University of Florida

Notice

Medicine is an ever-changing science. Discoveries through new research and clinical experiences broaden our knowledge and may necessitate changes to recommended treatment and drug therapy over time. Practitioners and researchers must always rely on their own experiences and knowledge in evaluating and potentially using any information or recommendations described herein. When using the information, they should be mindful of their own safety and the safety of others, including those parties for whom they have a professional responsibility.

In their efforts to provide information that is complete and generally accepted in the medical community at the time of publication, the author and publisher of this work have researched and checked with sources believed to be reliable and reputable. With regard to any drug or pharmaceutical product identified herein, readers are advised to check the most current information available from the manufacturer of each product to be administered and any other current analysis or research available to verify the recommended dosage or formula, the method and duration of administration, and/or any contraindications. It is incumbent on all practitioners, relying on their own experience and knowledge of their patients, to make diagnoses, to determine dosages and the best treatment for each individual patient, and to take all safety precautions. Readers are encouraged to confirm the information contained herein with other sources, including, but not limited to consulting the product information sheet included in the package of each drug they plan to administer, to be certain that the information contained herein is current and accurate and that changes have not been made in the recommended dose or in the contraindications for administration.

Neither the publisher nor the author(s), contributor(s), or editors(s) assume any liability for any injury and/or damage to any persons or property as a matter of products liability, negligence, or any other legal theory or doctrine, or from any use or operation of any methods, products, instructions, or ideas contained in the material herein.

ISBN: 978-0-578-83674-4

Dedication

This book is dedicated to my granddaughter Mila,
my sunshine

Acknowledgment

I am immensely thankful to Dr. Paula Beers, an extremely bright young dermatologist, who was kind enough to read an original draft of this book. At the time she was our senior dermatology resident preparing for her board exam and I just wanted her general opinion. However, Paula dissected my draft in great detail and came back with numerous recommendations on how to improve the book so that it is practical and useful as a textbook and board exam review book for residents. Her suggestions made the book so much better and I am extremely thankful to Paula for all of her help.

I also want to thank Dr. Kiran Motaparthi for kindly sharing images of some rarely encountered diagnoses.

Preface

This book is intended for residents of dermatology and pathology. The sheer number of different skin diseases makes the field of dermatopathology very hard to master. For a novice in the field, it is easy to get lost in the myriad of names and patterns that are often so similar but still different. Many years ago, as a new resident studying the field of dermatopathology, I remember many times where I felt like I was lost in the woods.

Therefore, my goal for this book was to serve as a compass to residents to orients themselves in their dermatopathology journey.

The chapters are organized so that the text description and photos are on the same page. I tried to provide low and high magnification photos for each disease as that is the way slides are examined under the microscope. I also tried to describe two diseases with similar histopathology on the same page so that they can be compared. Toward the end of each chapter, after describing all entities, I provided a summary page with recommendations for how to approach the diseases described in that chapter. Every chapter ends with composite photos of all diseases in that chapter for a quick overview. Some diseases are intentionally described in multiple chapters because of their overlapping histology.

My hope is that Dermatopathology Compass will help all readers to navigate through the maze of dermatopathology more easily.

Contents

Chapter 1

BASIC SKIN HISTOLOGY AND DERMATOPATHOLOGY TERMS

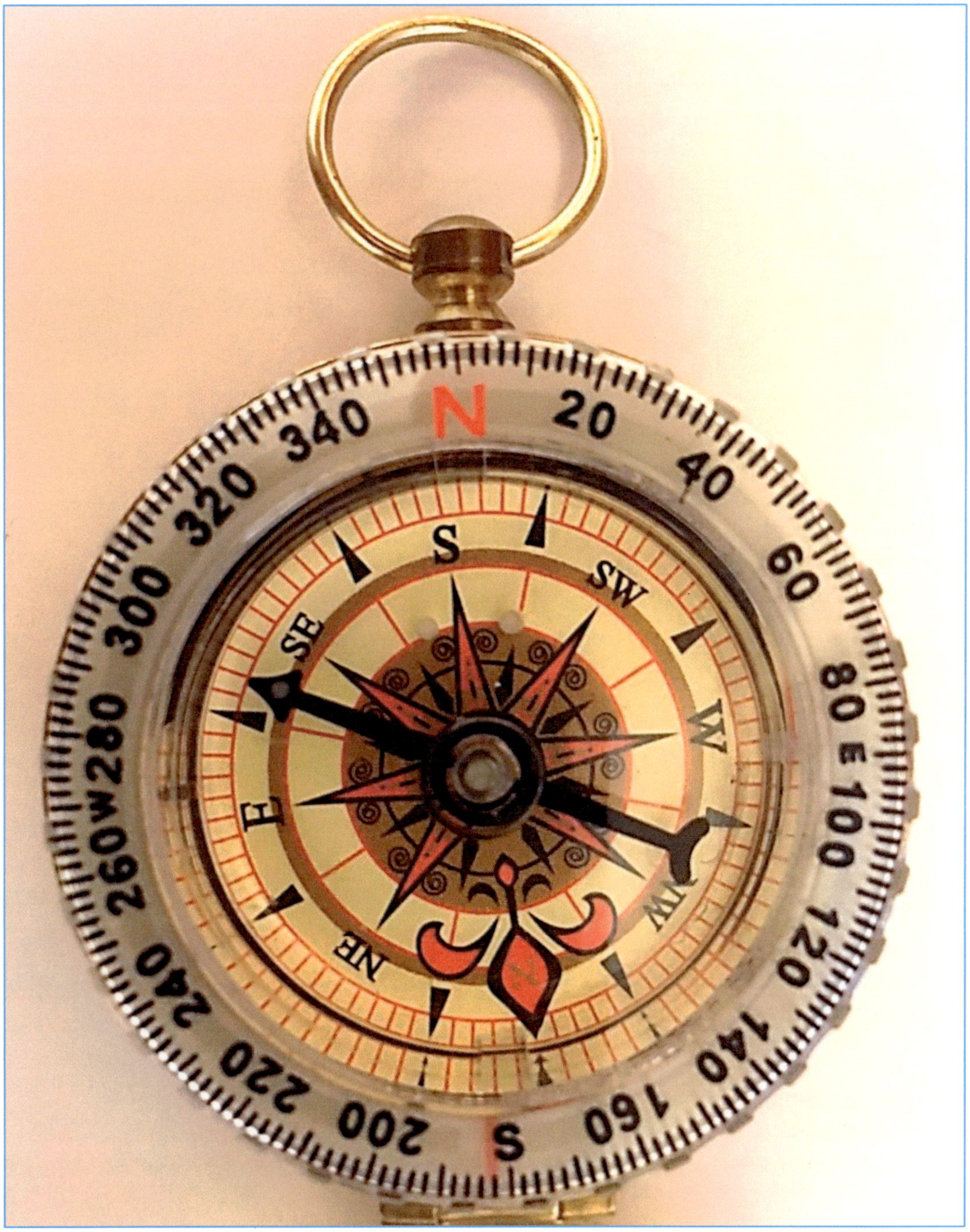

Basic skin histology and dermatopathology terms

BASIC HISTOLOGY FOR STUDENTS OF DERMATOPATHOLOGY

SKIN (CUTIS) consists of

EPIDERMIS →

DERMIS →

Beneath cutis is

SUBCUTIS →
(HYPODERMIS)

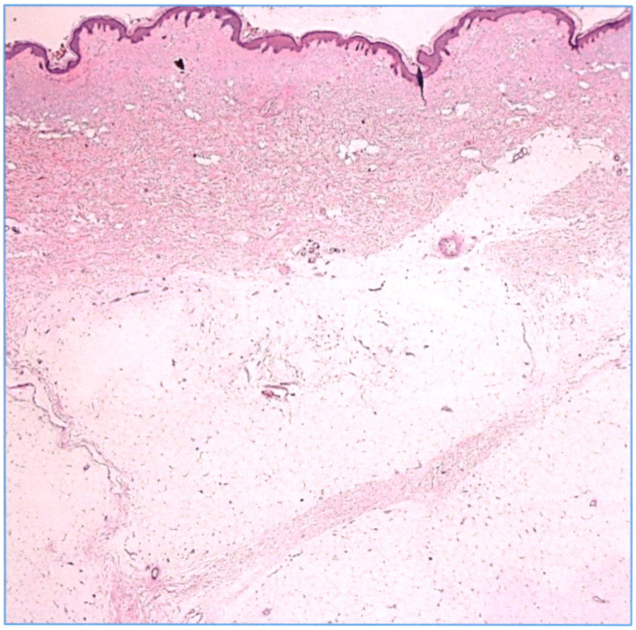

DERMIS consists of

PAPILLARY DERMIS →
-thin area underneath epidermis
-haphazard thin collagen fibers

RETICULAR DERMIS →
-thick zone extending to subcutis
-orthogonal thick bundles of collagen

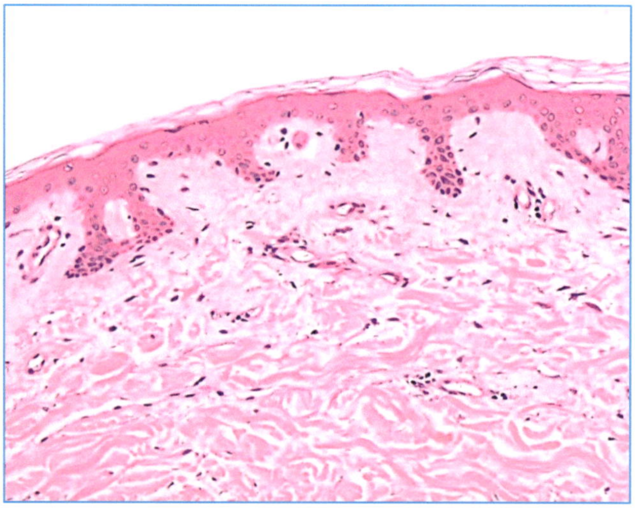

SUBCUTIS consists of

LOBULES →
-mature adipose tissue
-a few scattered capillaries

SEPTA →
-thin collagen fibers with scattered fibroblasts that separate lobules
-arteries and veins are within septa

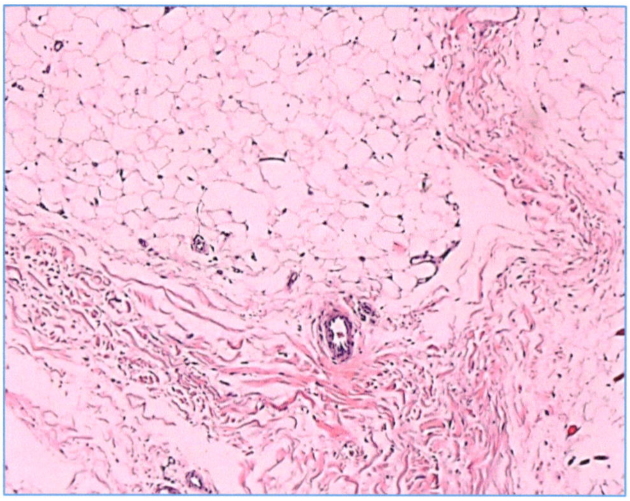

Chapter 1

EPIDERMIS

-made mostly of KERATINOCYTES
-MELANOCYTES with dark nuclei and clear cytoplasm are found along basal layer (see arrows below)
-melanocytes number between 1 per 5 (face and genitalia) to 1 per 10 basal layer keratinocytes
-LANGERHANS CELLS and MERKEL CELLS are not seen on H&E stain slides

ARCHITECTURALLY EPIDERMIS CAN BE

-flat or mildly wavy (non-acral sites)
with thin "basket-weave" stratum corneum (see in the middle of the page)

-thick and undulated (acral sites)
with compact stratum corneum (see at the bottom of the page)

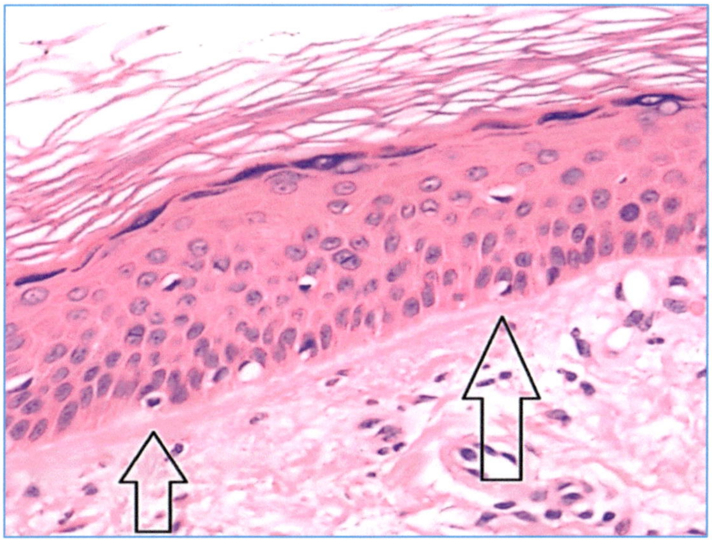

EPIDERMIS consists of five strata:

STRATUM CORNEUM →
-made of keratin with no nuclei

STRATUM LUCIDUM
-with pale keratin (ONLY at acral sites) →

STRATUM GRANULOSUM →
-with dark keratohyalin granules

STRATUM SPINOSUM →
-"spiny" cells connected by desmosomes
-shape of nuclei changes from round to oval with upward maturation

STRATUM BASALE
-single layer of keratinocytes lying on the top of basement membrane
-connected to basement membrane by hemidesmosomes →

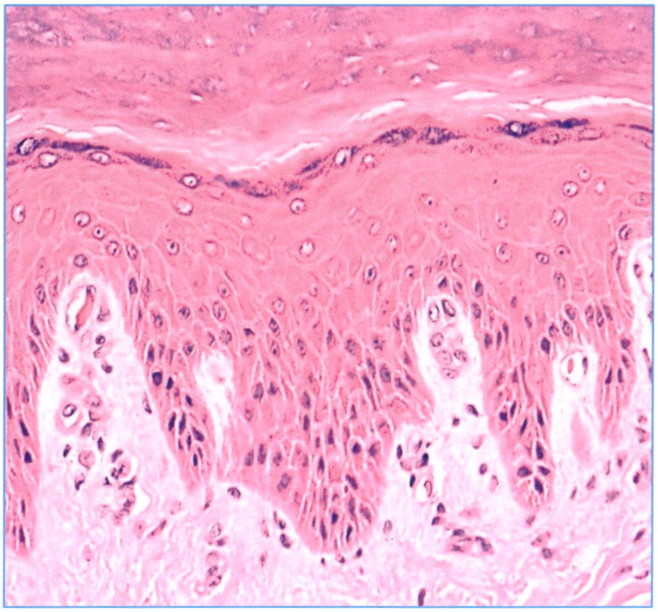

Basic skin histology and dermatopathology terms

PAPILLARY DERMIS

-made of pale eosinophilic collagen fibers
-it contains:
  -free nerve endings
  -Meissner corpuscles (tactile receptor) particularly on hands, feet, lips
  -capillaries
-inferior edge is bounded by superficial vascular elements

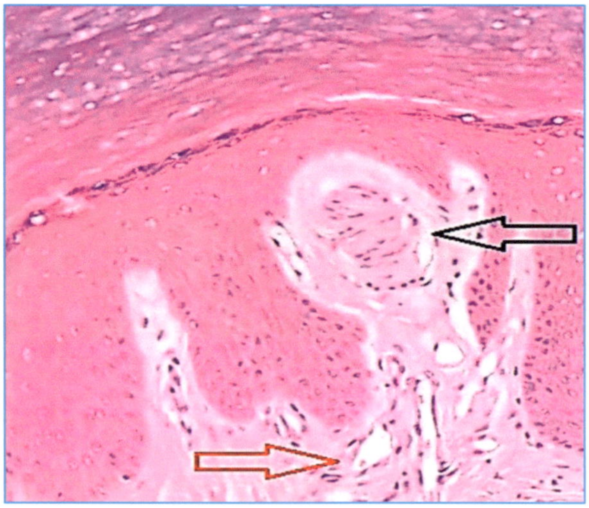

Meissner corpuscle (black arrow) and *vascular elements* (red arrow)

RETICULAR DERMIS

-made of thick bundles of collagen with admixed elastic fibers and scattered spindle fibroblasts
-it contains:
  -smaller and larger vessels
  -nerve bundles
  -can contain Pacinian corpuscles (vibration and pressure receptor)
  -glomus bodies
  -pilar muscle
  -adnexal structures (hair follicles, sebaceous glands, sweat glands)

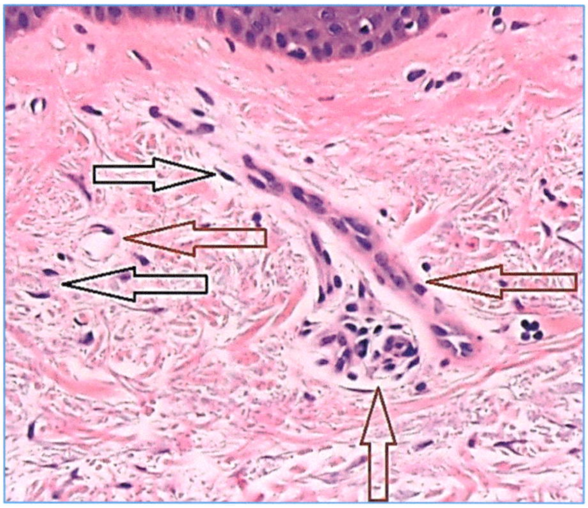

Dermal capillaries lined with endothelial cells. Endothelial cells (red arrows) can resemble fibroblasts (black arrows) or histiocytes.

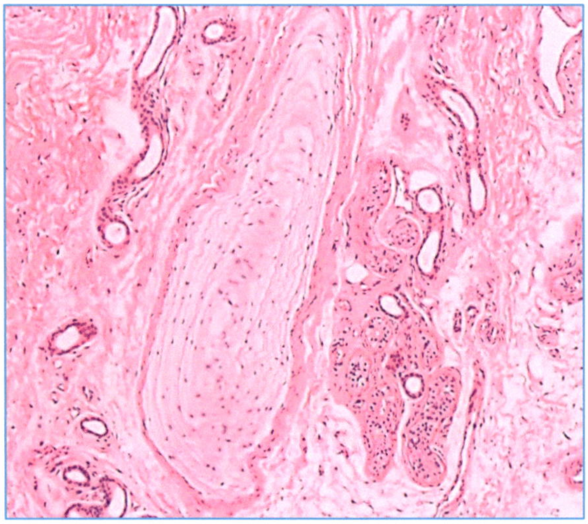

Pacinian corpuscle surrounded by sweat glands and ducts

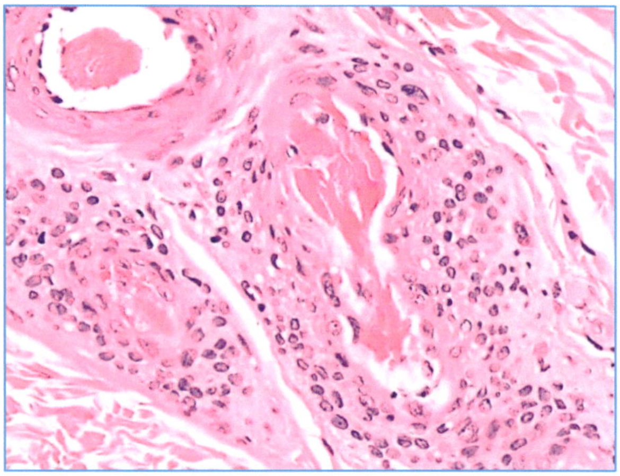

Medium size vessel (upper left) and two *glomus bodies* (lower) made of vessels surrounded by uniform glomus cells

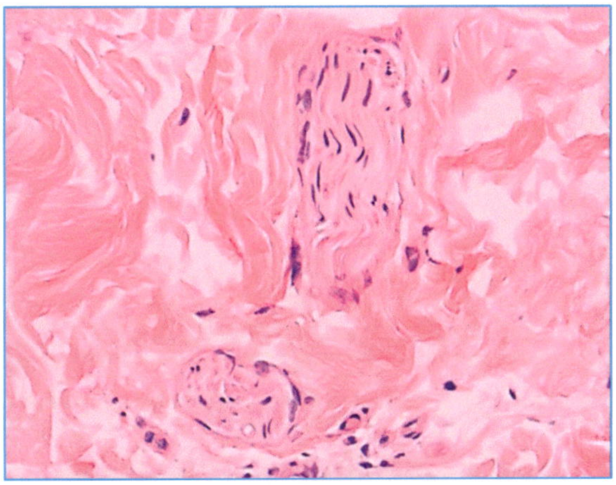

Nerves made of curly light pink spindle cells with wavy nuclei with pointed ends

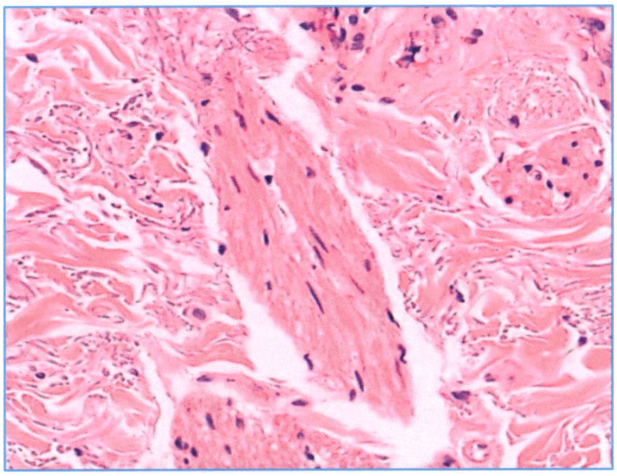

Muscle bundle made of cells with dark pink cytoplasm and elongated nuclei with blunt ends ("Cuban cigar" shape)

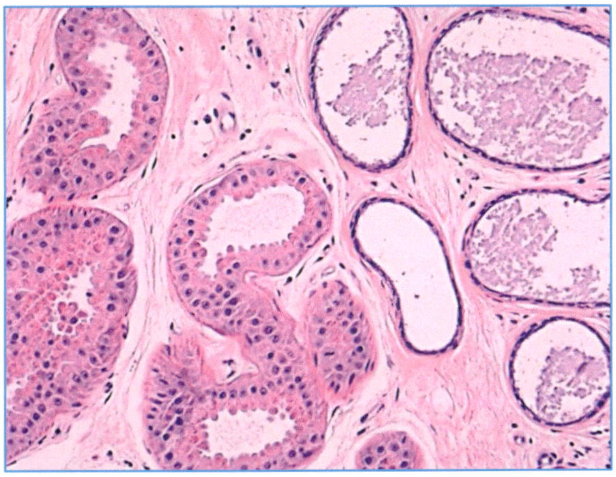

Apocrine sweat glands (found in axilla, anogenital area, areola, eyelid) with characteristic apocrine snouts (left) and ducts (right) that open into follicular infundibulum near skin surface

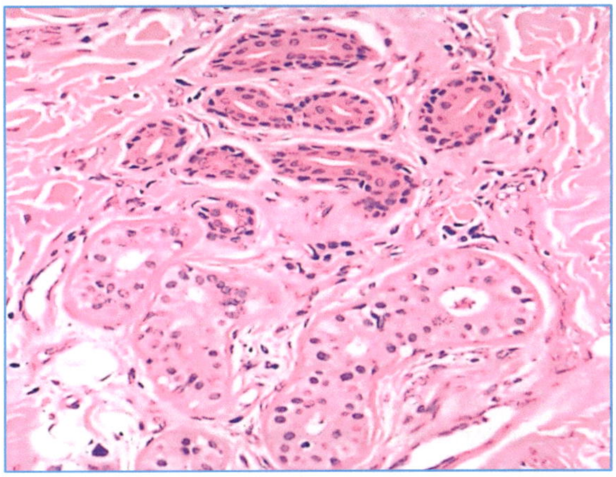

Eccrine sweat glands (bottom) made of a single layer of cuboidal cells with underlying myoepithelial cells. *Eccrine sweat ducts* (above) made of 2 layers of cuboidal cells that open directly to epidermal surface

Terminal hair in anagen stage consists of four segments:

Infundibulum- between attachment of sebaceous gland and epidermal surface
-resembles normal epidermis with granular layer

Isthmus- between the attachment of pilar muscle and the attachment of sebaceous gland
-inner root sheath disappears
-external root sheath start to cornify without granular layer
-bulge containing stem cells is present at the insertion of pilar muscle

Stem- between Adamson's fringe (place where Huxley layer is keratinized above the Henle's layer) and attachment of pilar muscle

Bulb- in subcutis or deep dermis
-made of dermal papilla surrounded by basophilic hair matrix
-ends superficially at Adamson's fringe

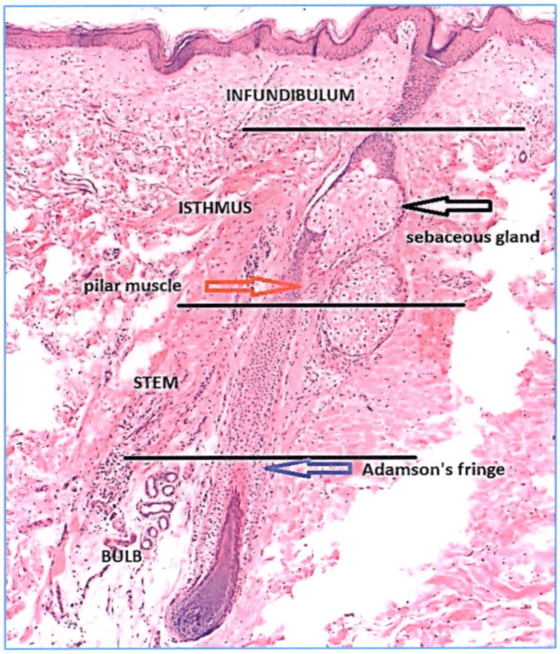

Basic skin histology and dermatopathology terms

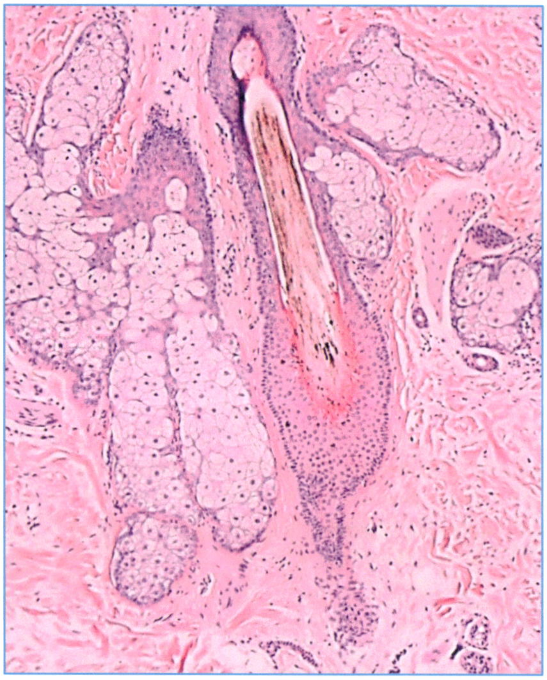

Terminal hair in telogen stage

- -consist of only upper hair segments (infundibulum and isthmus)
- -below isthmus there are a few scattered fibrocytes representing a remnant of follicular papilla
- -root is surrounded by red-staining trichilemmal keratin

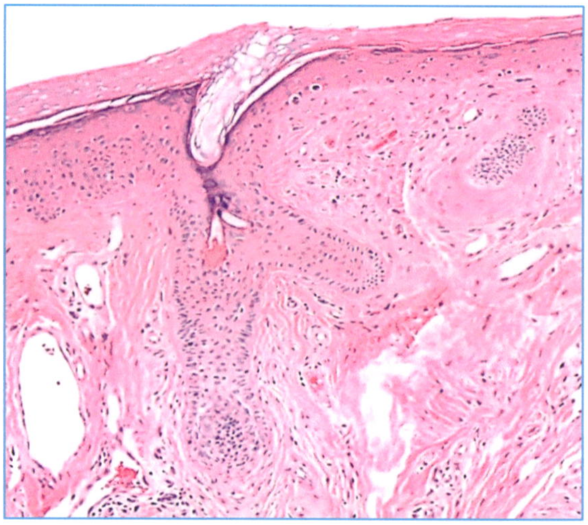

Vellus hair

- -present everywhere with the exception of lips, palms, soles, and back of the ear
- -replaced by terminal hair on many body parts during puberty
- -remain as vellus hair particularly on the face, ears, eyelids
- -looks like miniaturized terminal hair
- -bulb is located in the superficial dermis unlike bulb of terminal hair

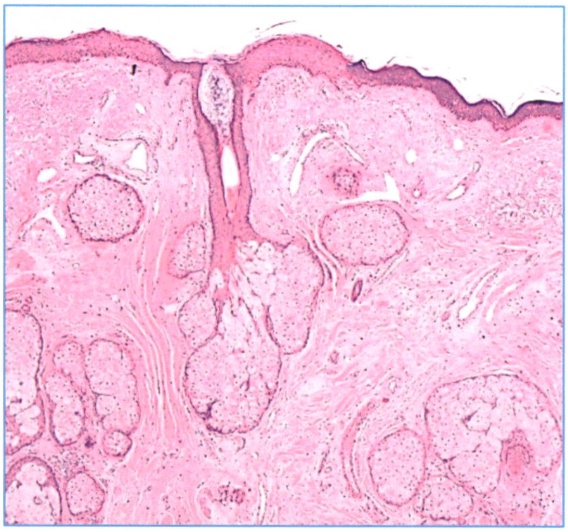

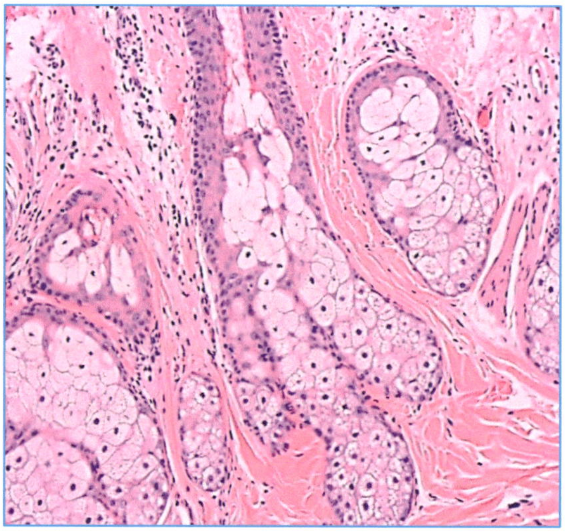

Sebaceous glands

- -found throughout all areas of skin
- -exceptions are the palms of the hands and the soles of the feet
- -consist of several lobules connected to the hair follicle
- -each lobule consists of external thin layer (1-2 cells thick) of cuboidal or flattened basaloid cells and inner group of vacuolated lipid-laden cells

TYPES OF INFLAMMATORY CELLS

-even clinically unremarkable skin will have a few perivascular lymphocytes and occasional mast cells or histiocytes in dermis
-the presence of more than a few lymphocytes/mast cells/ histiocytes and any neutrophils, eosinophils, giant cells, or plasma cells is an indication of a dermal inflammatory disorder

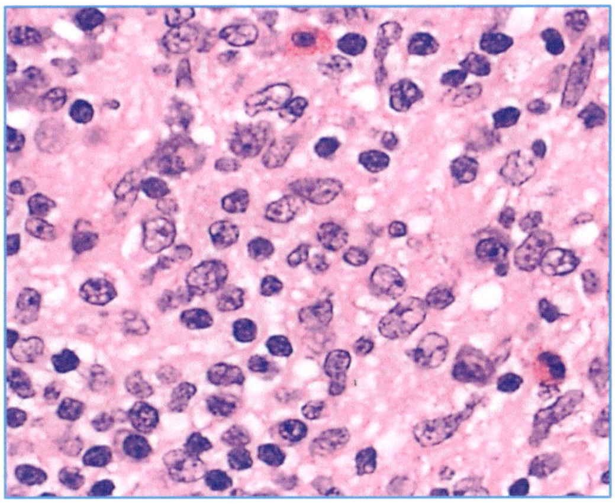

Lymphocytes **(dark round nuclei) are admixed with *histiocytes* (larger pale nuclei/abundant cytoplasm) and *eosinophils (*red granules)**

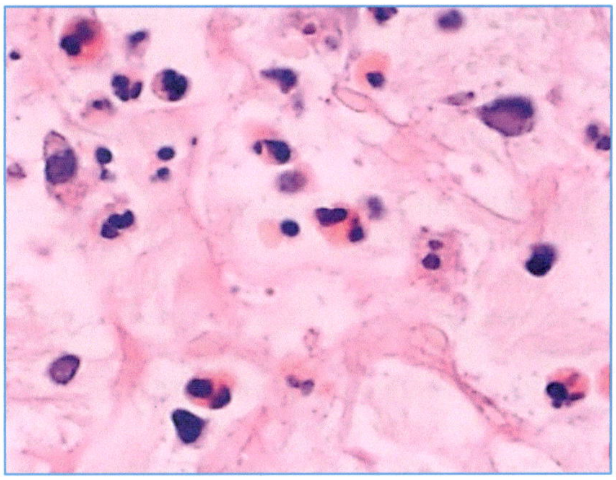

Neutrophils **with multilobulated nucleus and pink cytoplasm admixed with *eosinophils* with similar nucleus with red granular cytoplasm**

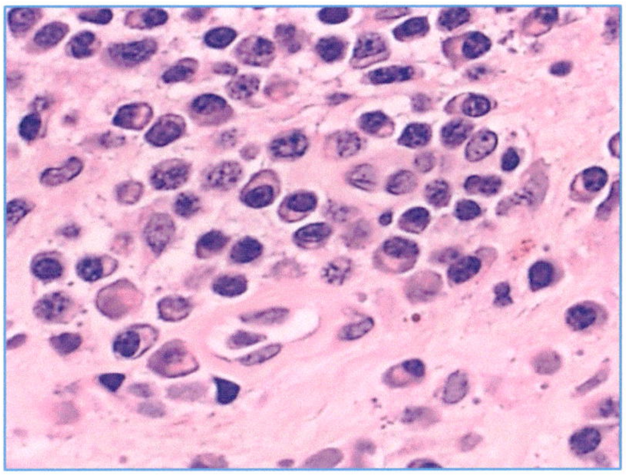

Plasma cells **with eccentric nucleus with coarse chromatin and "cartwheel" pattern. Admixed *histiocytes* are present.**

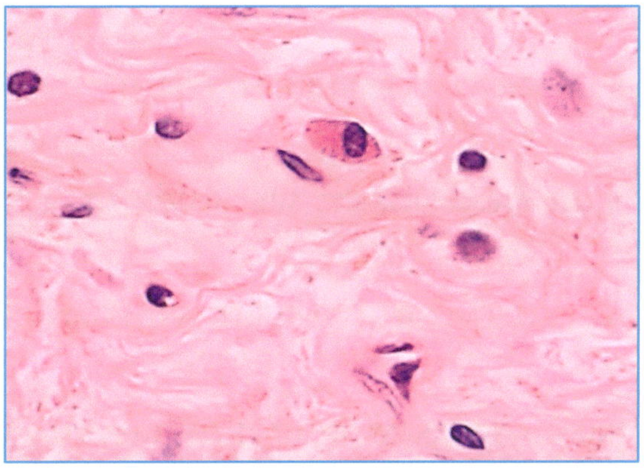

Mast cell **with pink cytoplasm and "fried egg" appearance. Admixed *lymphocytes* (dark nuclei), histiocytes (pale round nuclei) and *endothelial cells* (spindled irregular nuclei)**

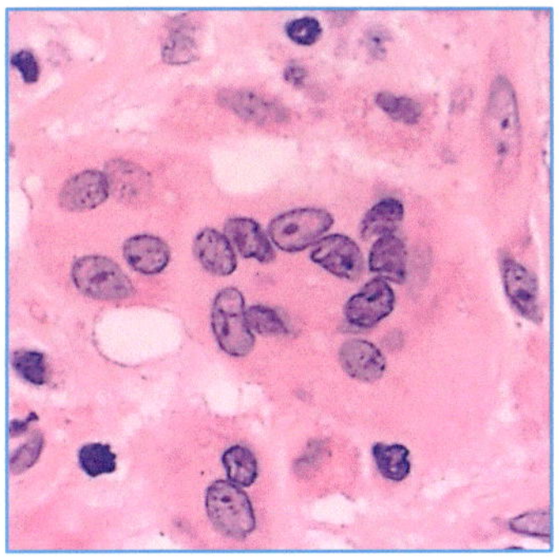

Foreign body giant cell with multiple randomly distributed nuclei

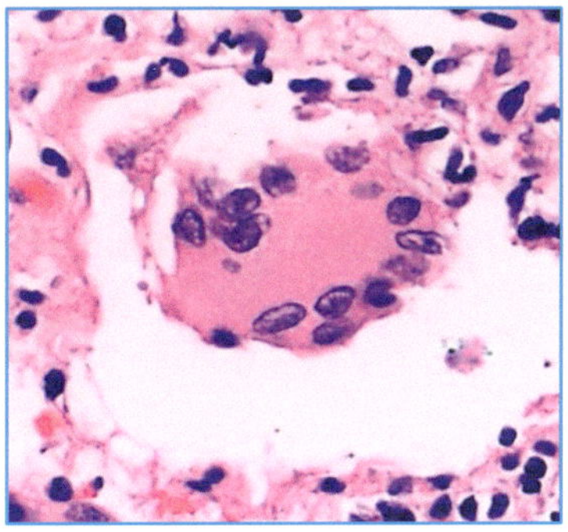

Langerhans giant cell with peripheral "horse-shoe" nuclei

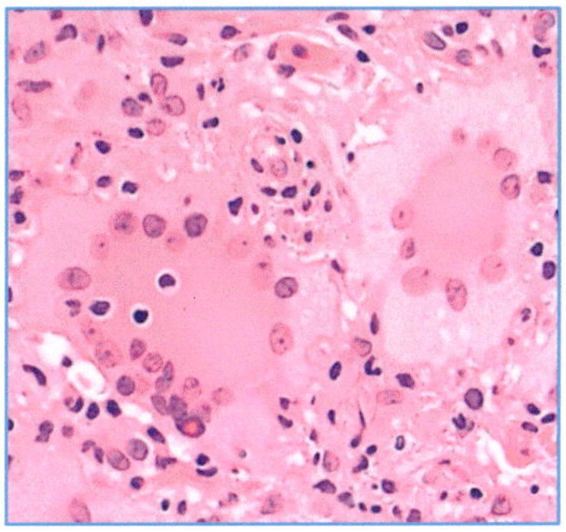

Touton giant cells with central, darker cytoplasm, "wreath" of nuclei, and peripheral lighter cytoplasm

Basic skin histology and dermatopathology terms

NORMAL SKIN VARIATION BY LOCATION

-variations in skin histology reflect different function
-many parts of the body have similar histology of skin

HOW TO DETERMINE SKIN LOCATION

IF NUMEROUS MUSCLE BUNDLES ARE PRESENT

-nipples	corrugated epidermis + sebaceous glands + mammary ducts
-scrotum	corrugated epidermis + no glands or ducts
-clitoris	wavy epidermis + numerous vessels and nerves

IF VELLUS HAIRS ARE PRESENT

-nose and cheek	vellus hairs and dilated follicles + sebaceous glands
-ear	mostly vellus follicles + atrophic sebaceous glands
-eyelid	dermal edema + thin muscle bundles

IF STRATUM CORNEUM IS PROMINENT
-palmoplantar skin

IF APOCRINE GLANDS ARE PRESENT
-axilla, anogenital area, nipple

IF NUMEROUS TERMINAL HAIRS ARE PRESENT
-scalp

IF UNDERLYING CARTILAGE IS PRESENT
-ear, nose

IF DERMAL CAPILLARIES ARE PROMINENT
-shin

IF GRANULAR LAYER IS PRESENT AND IS MISSING IN ADJACENT EPIDERMIS
-lips, perianal and perivulvar area

TRUNK AND EXREMITIES HAVE SIMILAR HISTOLOGY AND IT IS DIFFICULT TO SEPARATE THEM

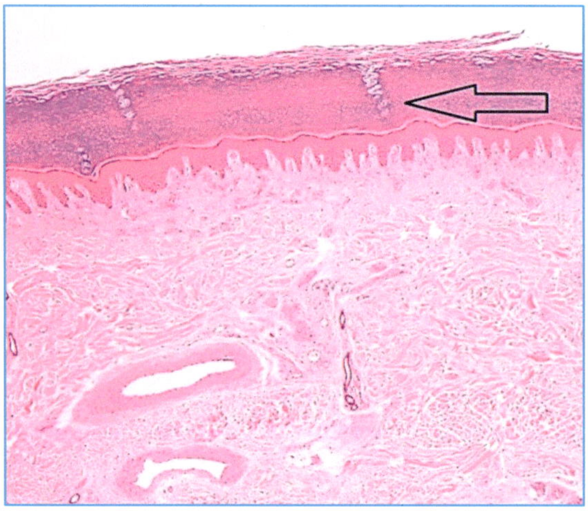

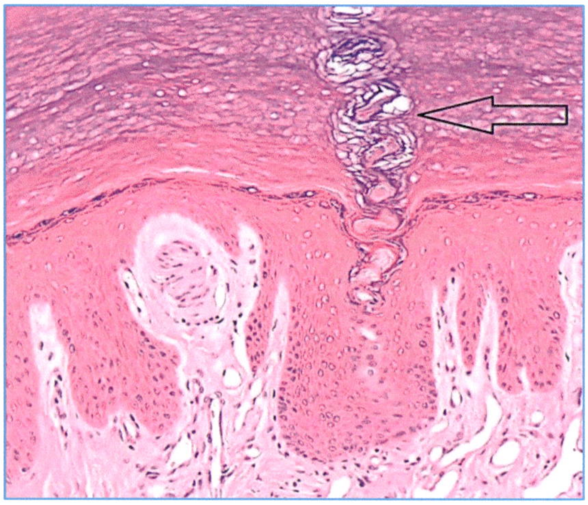

Thumb **skin with thick, compact stratum corneum and thick dermis.**
Acrosyringium **(intraepidermal portion of eccrine duct) is easily detected; see arrows.**

Chapter 1

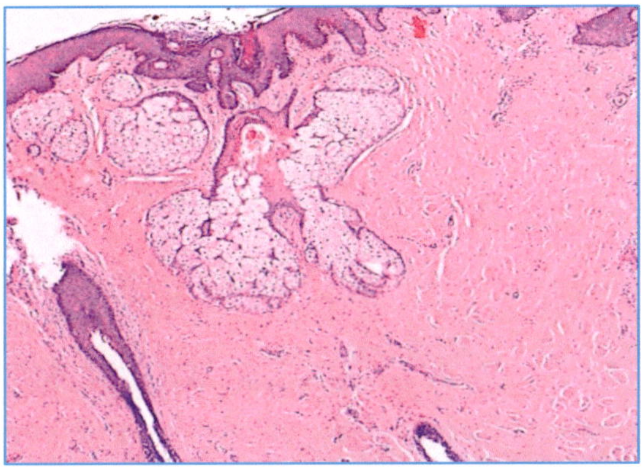
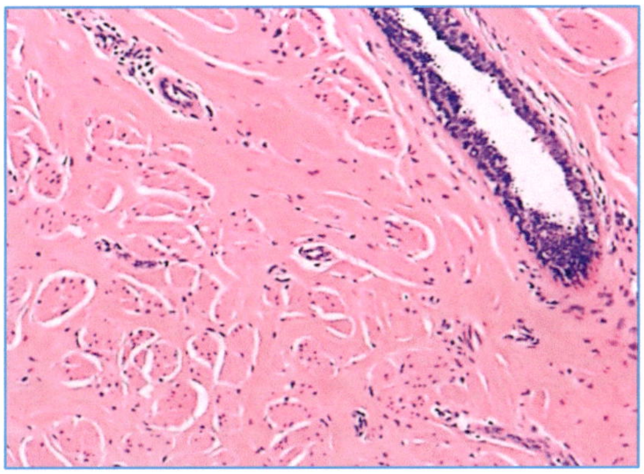

Nipple **skin with papillomatous epidermis and sebaceous glands. Mammary duct and numerous muscle bundles are present.**

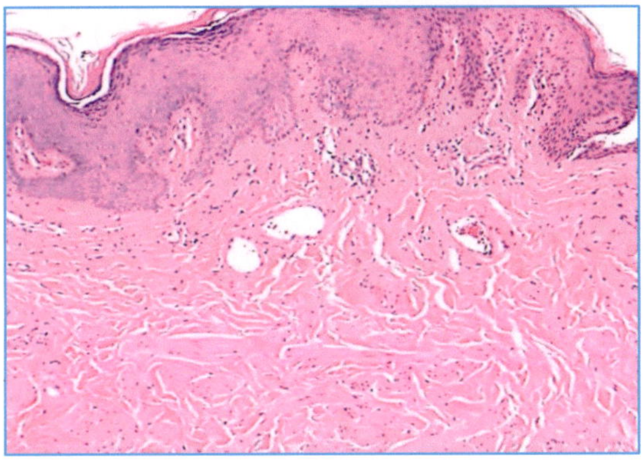
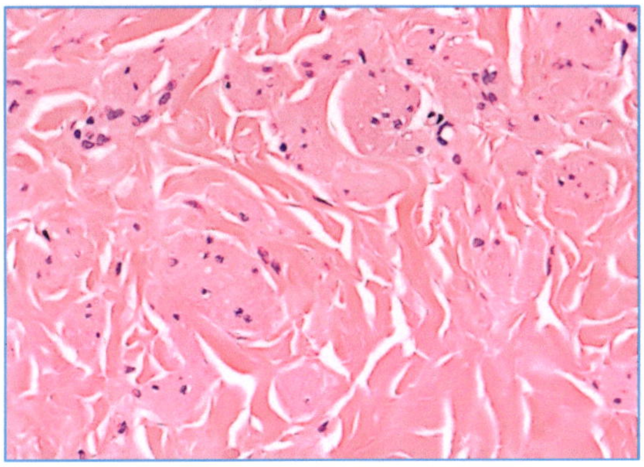

Scrotal **skin with papillomatous pigmented epidermis and numerous muscle bundles**

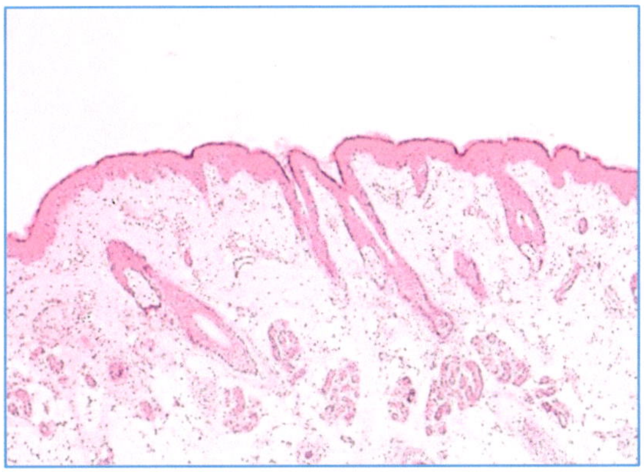
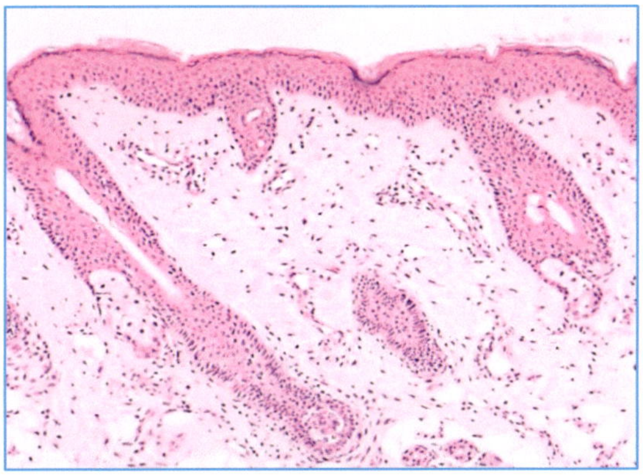

Ear **skin with wavy epidermis, multiple vellus hairs and atrophic sebaceous glands**

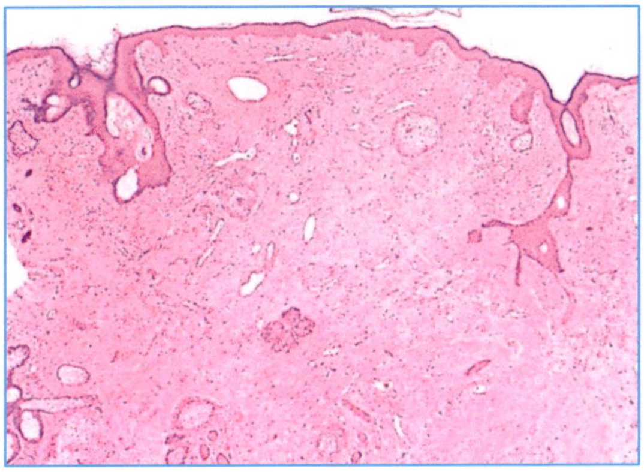
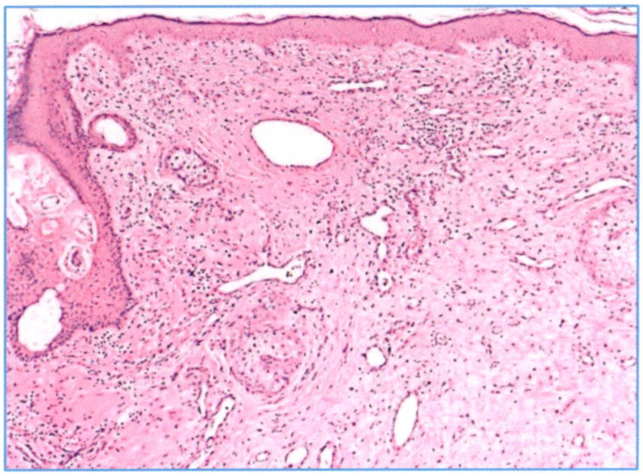

Nose **skin with short, distorted follicles with dilated ostia and multiple sebaceous glands**

Basic skin histology and dermatopathology terms

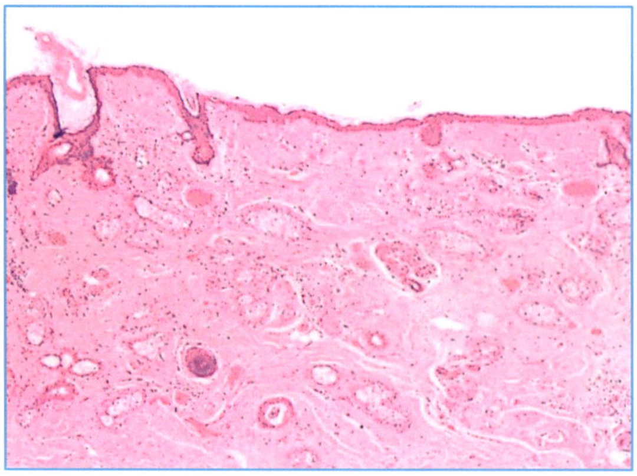

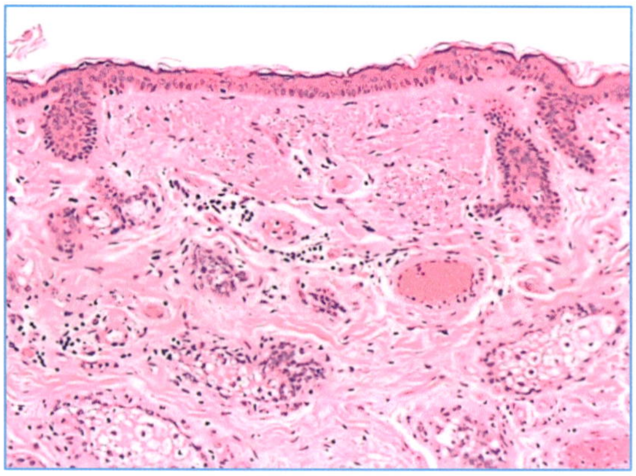

Cheek **skin with short, distorted follicles with dilated ostia and multiple sebaceous glands**

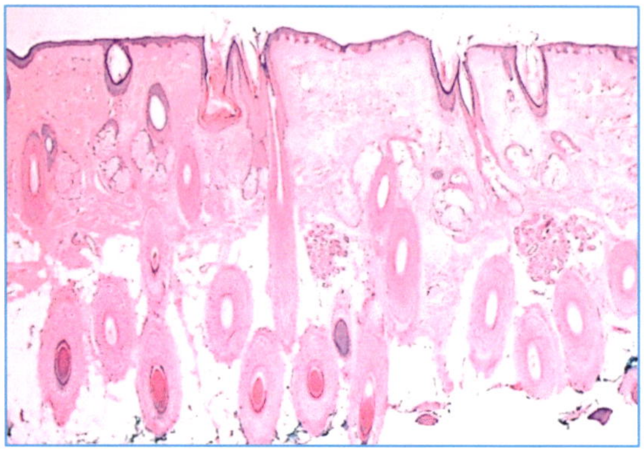

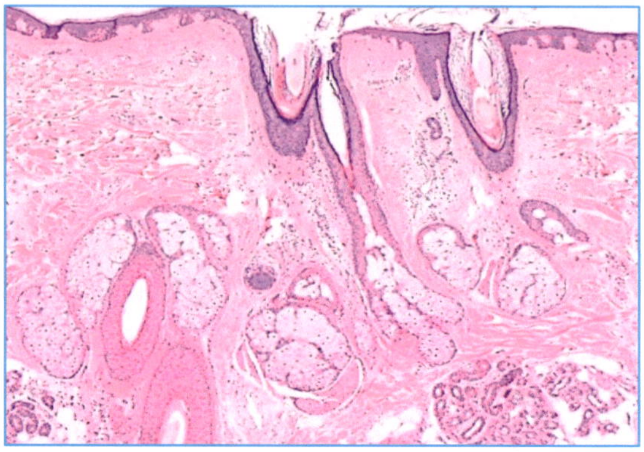

Scalp **skin with numerous terminal hairs in anagen stage**

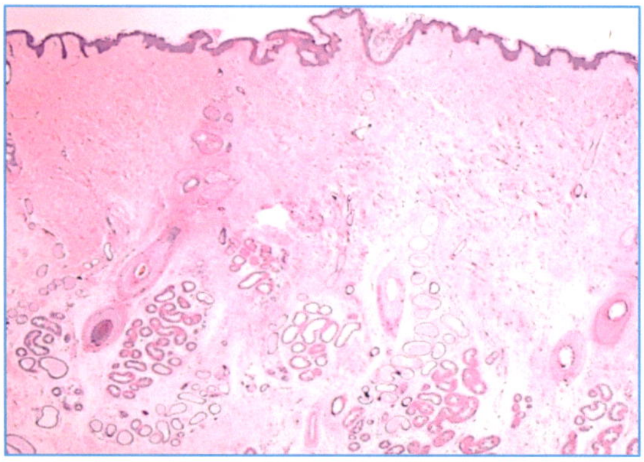

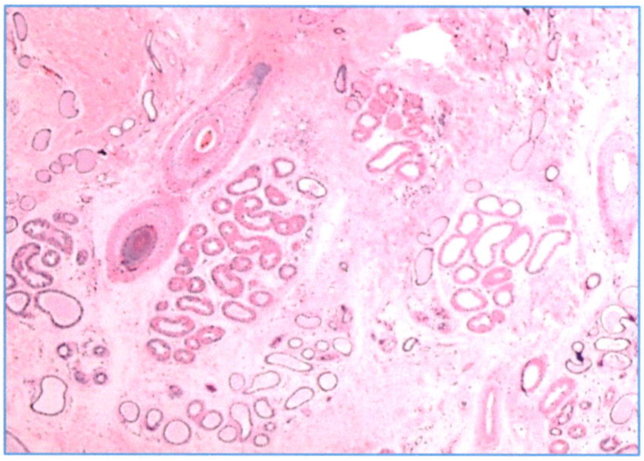

Axillary **skin with numerous apocrine glands and ducts**

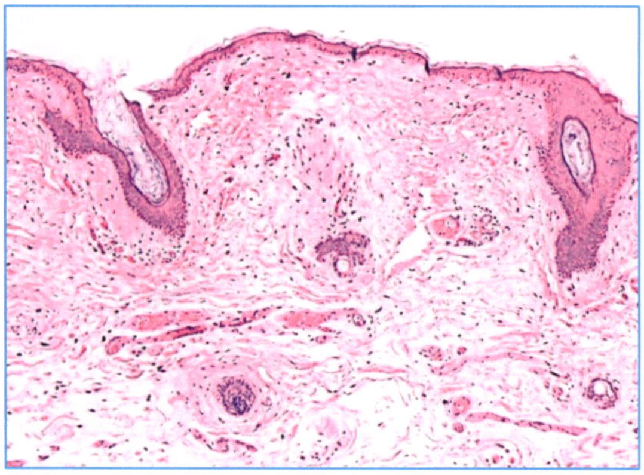

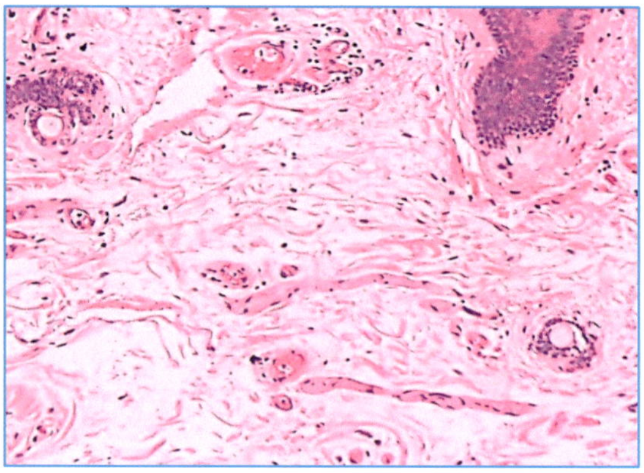

Eyelid **skin with thin epidermis, dermal edema, and slender dermal muscles**

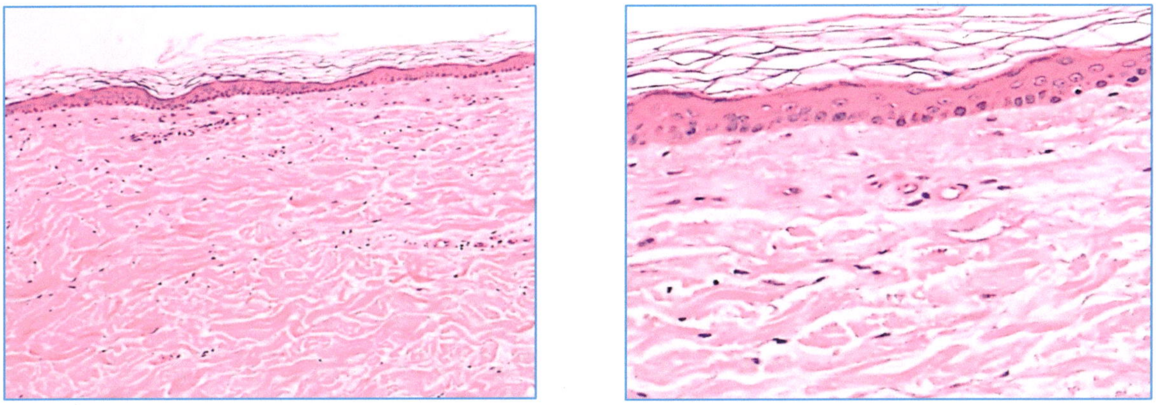

Shin **skin with thin, flat epidermis and sclerotic, thick dermis with proliferation of superficial dermal capillaries**

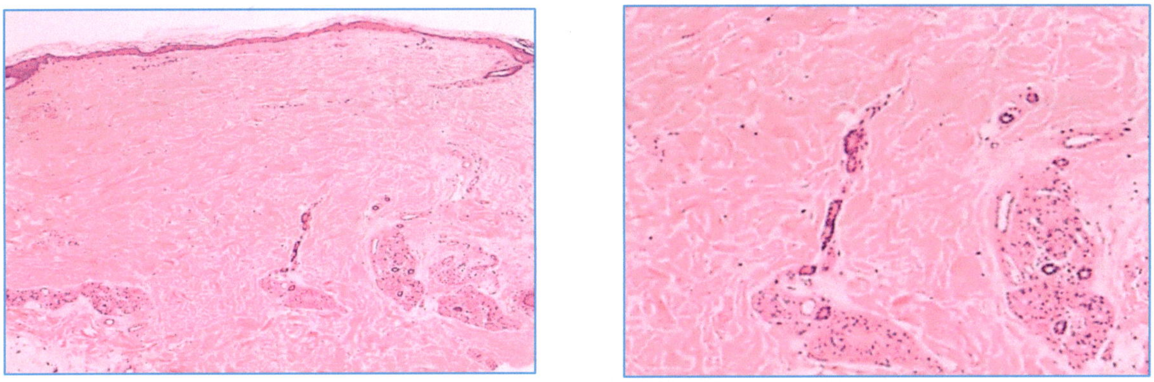

Back **(above) and** ***abdominal*** **skin (below) have similar appearance with thin, flat epidermis and thick reticular dermis**

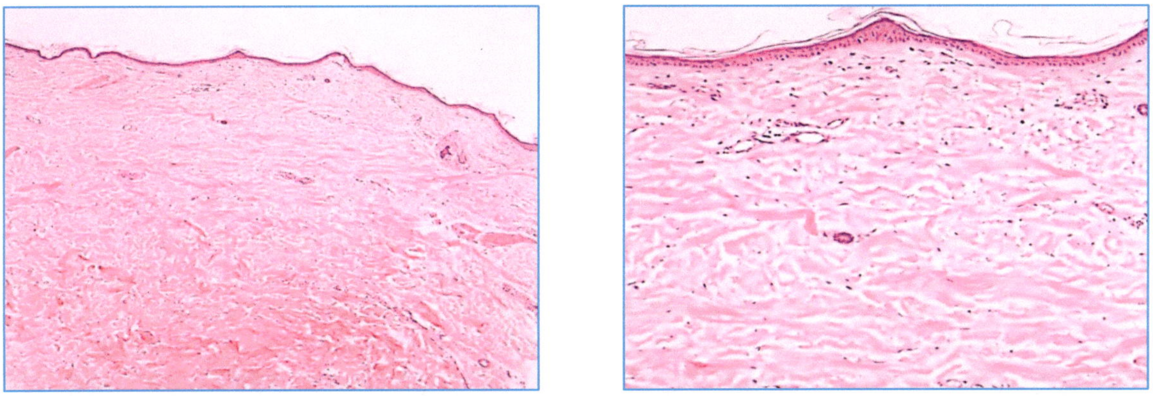

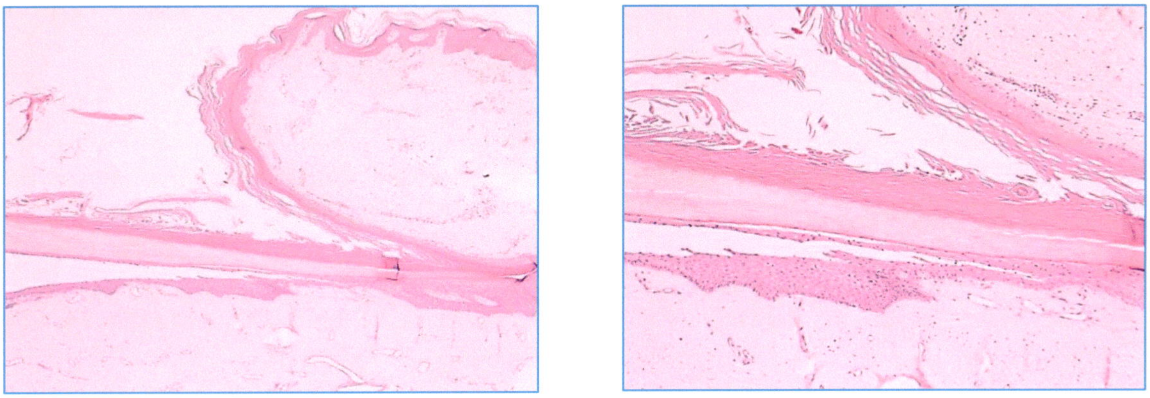

Nail **with nail bed that has absent granular layer**

TERMS COMMONLY USED TO DESCRIBE SKIN PATHOLOGY

HOW TO DESCRIBE CELLS

BASALOID- dark purple/blue cells resembling keratinocytes of epidermal basal layer. Basal cell carcinoma, Merkel cell carcinoma, and follicular tumors are good examples.

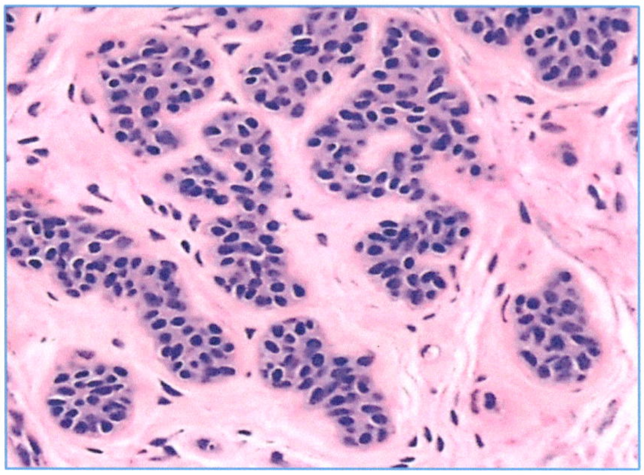

Basal cell carcinoma

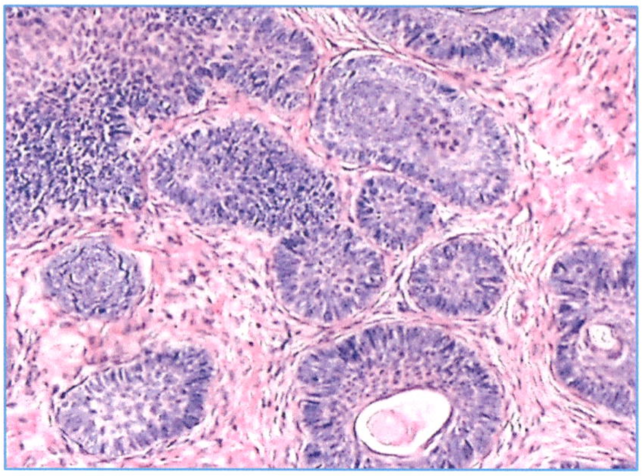

Trichoepithelioma

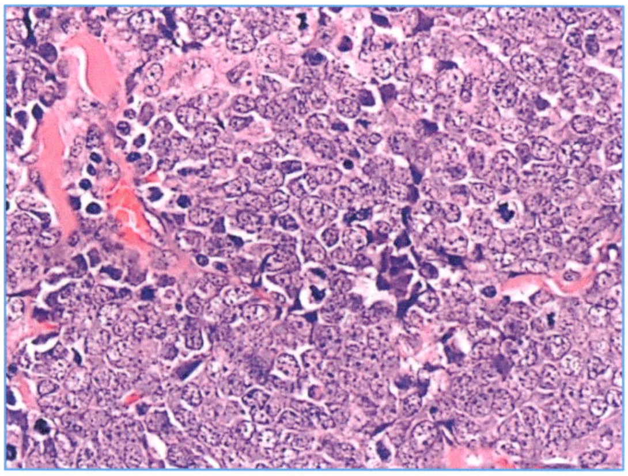

Merkel cell carcinoma

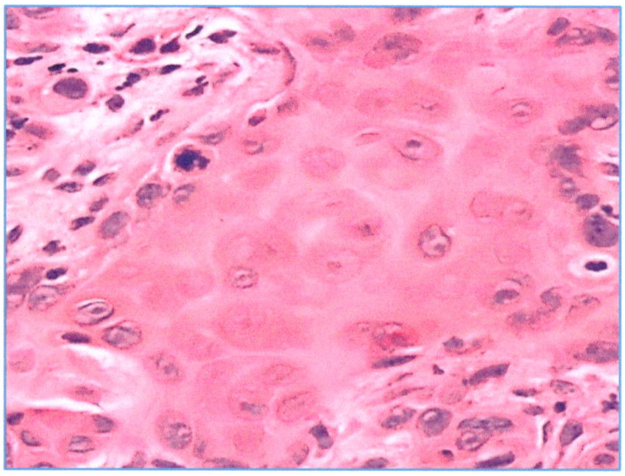

Squamous cell carcinoma

EPITHELIOID- pale pink cells resembling keratinocytes of epidermal stratum spinosum. Squamous cell carcinoma, Spitz nevus cells, histiocytes in sarcoidosis are good examples.

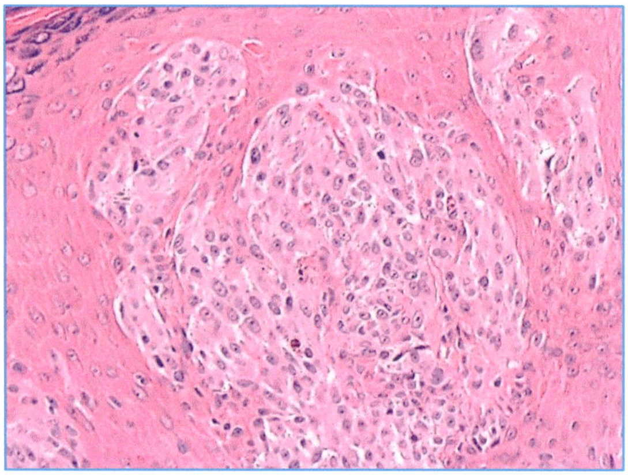

Spitz nevus

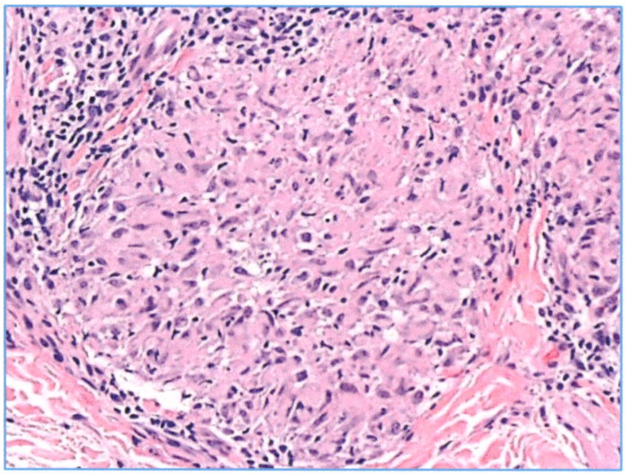

Sarcoidosis

Chapter 1

HOW TO DESCRIBE EPIDERMIS

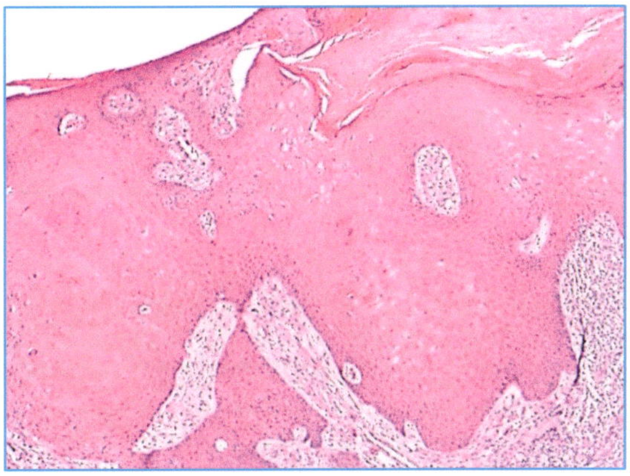

Pseudoepitheliomatous hyperplasia

ACANTHOSIS a.k.a. EPIDERMAL HYPERPLASIA

-increased thickness of epidermal stratum spinosum
-pseudoepitheliomatous hyperplasia, psoriasis, prurigo nodularis are good examples

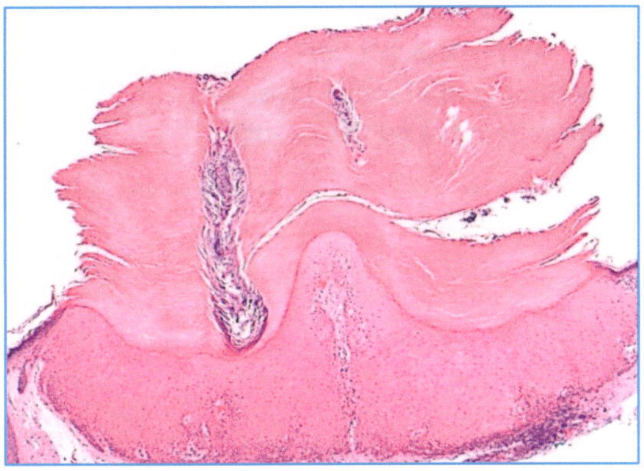

Actinic keratosis with cutaneous horn

HYPERKERATOSIS
-thickened epidermal stratum corneum
-cutaneous horn, lichen simple chronicus, prurigo nodularis are good examples

HYPERKERATOSIS can be classified as ORTHOKERATOSIS and PARAKERATOSIS

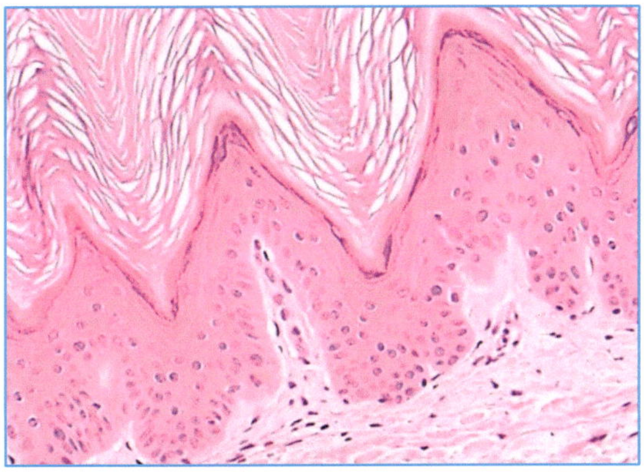

Stucco keratosis

ORTHOKERATOSIS
-hyperkeratosis in which nuclei are not present in the stratum corneum
-ichthyosis vulgaris, stucco keratosis are good examples

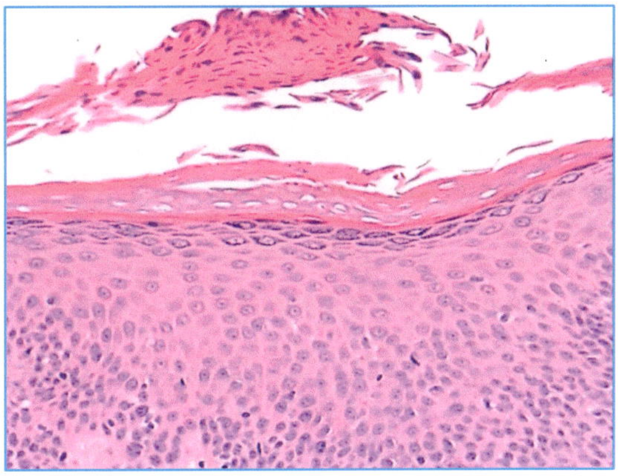

Pityriasis rubra pilaris

PARAKERATOSIS
-hyperkeratosis in which nuclei are retained in the stratum corneum
-psoriasis, seborrheic dermatitis, pityriasis rosea, pityriasis rubra pilaris are good examples

Basic skin histology and dermatopathology terms

HYPERGRANULOSIS
-increased thickness of granular layer
-lichen planus and lichen simplex chronicus are good examples

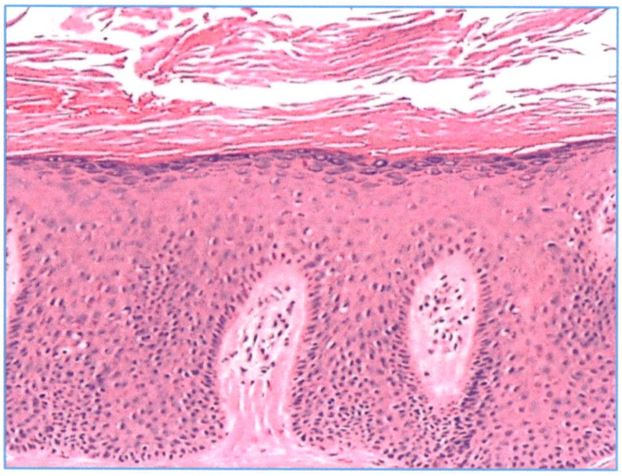

Lichen simplex chronicus

HYPOGRANULOSIS
-thinning of granular layer
-psoriasis is a good example

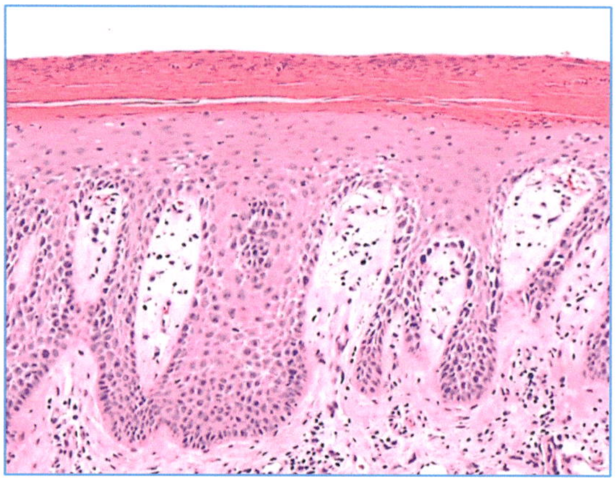

Psoriasis

PAPILLOMATOSIS
-because of epidermal thickening and elongation of rete ridges dermal papillae are elevated above adjacent epidermis
-acanthosis nigricans and epidermal nevus are good examples

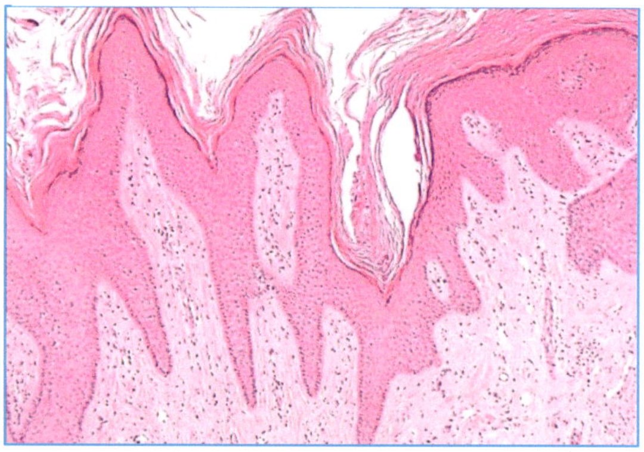

Epidermal nevus

ACANTHOLYSIS
-loss of attachment between individual keratinocytes
-seen in blistering disorders but also in squamous cell carcinoma

DYSKERATOSIS
-spinous layer keratinocytes prematurely cornify and die
-they have dark pyknotic nuclei and pink cytoplasm

-Grover's and Darier's disease are good examples of acantholysis and dyskeratosis

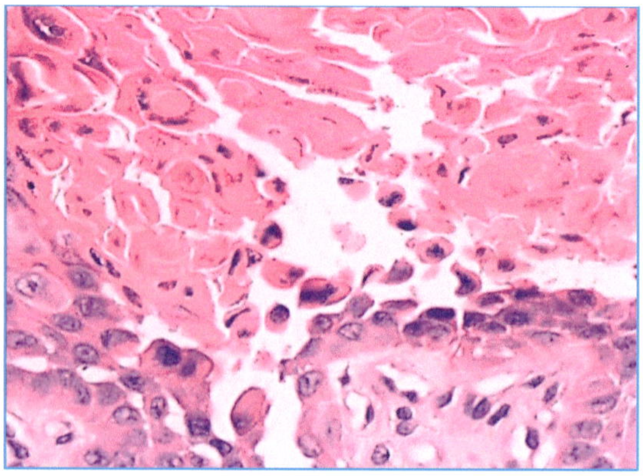

Grover's disease

HOW TO DESCRIBE DERMIS

FIBROSIS
-increase in number of fibroblasts and collagen
-the best example is a dermal scar

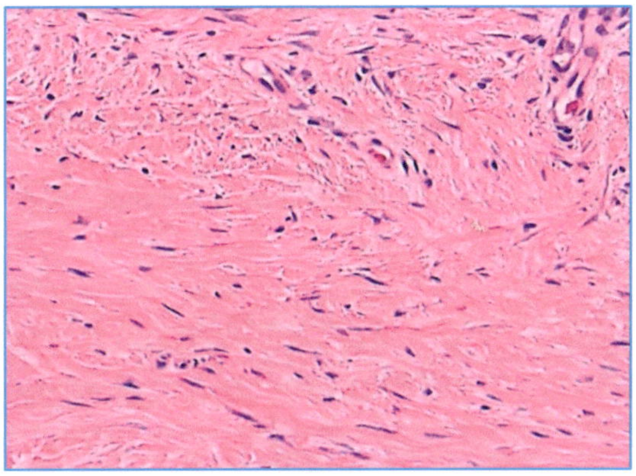

Scar

SCLEROSIS
-homogenized collagen with a decreased number of fibroblasts
-the best example is lichen sclerosus et atrophicus

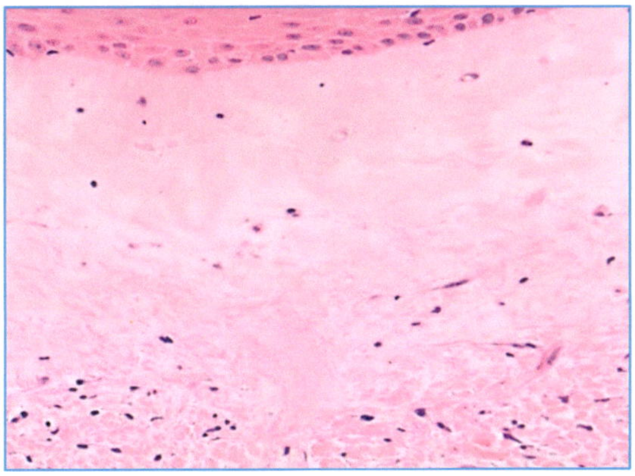

Lichen sclerosus et atrophicus

NECROSIS
-death of cells caused by trauma, malignancy, infection, vascular insufficiency
-in complete dermal necrosis tissue appears smudged with loss of cellular contours

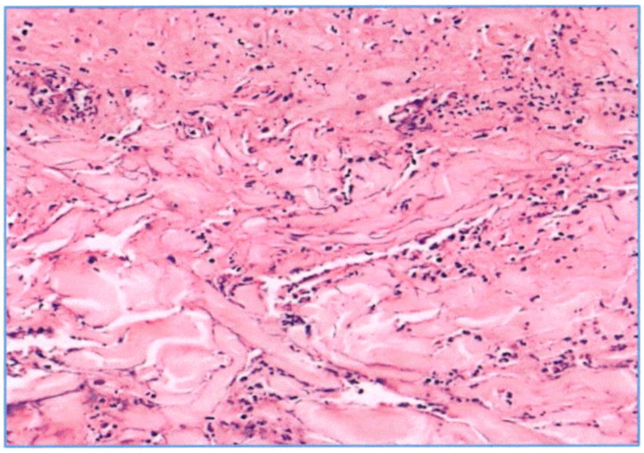

Necrosis

EDEMA
-swelling caused by excess fluid trapped in dermis
-fluid separates individual cells and fibers producing pale appearing stroma
-pernio, PMLE, and Sweet's syndrome are good examples

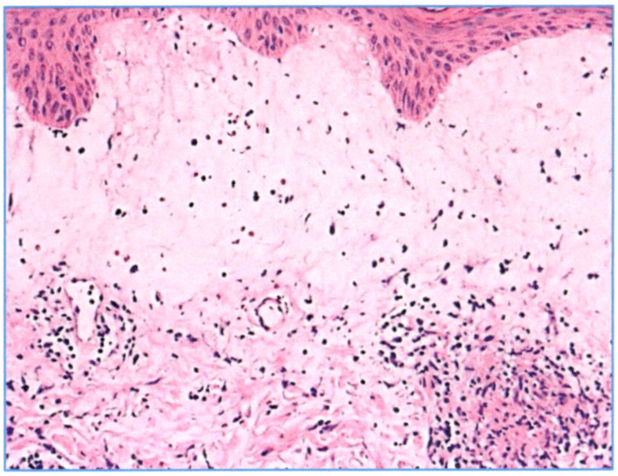

Sweet's syndrome

Basic skin histology and dermatopathology terms

ABSCESS
- dermal or subcutaneous collection of intact and disintegrated neutrophils (KARYORRHEXIS) in necrotic tissue forming pus
- usually in response to infection or foreign body

PUSTULE
- intraepidermal accumulation of neutrophils
- pustular psoriasis and impetigo are good examples

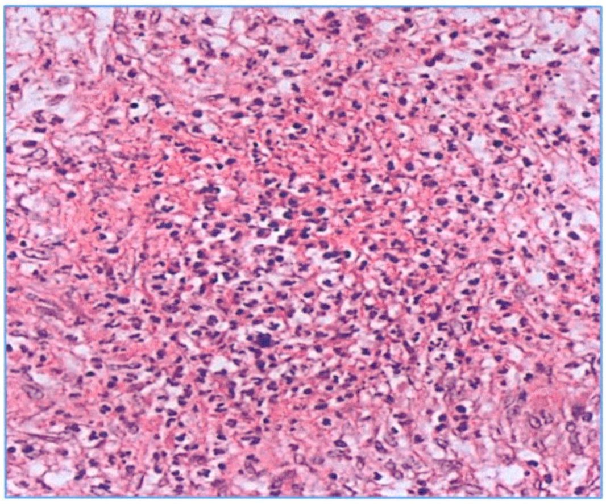

Abscess

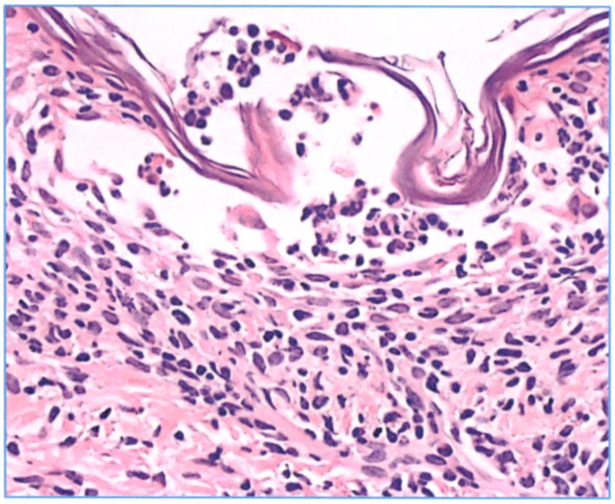

Impetigo

GRANULOMA
- an organized collection of histiocytes
- divided into non-caseating granuloma without central necrosis (e.g. sarcoidosis)
- caseating granuloma with central necrosis (e.g. TB granuloma)

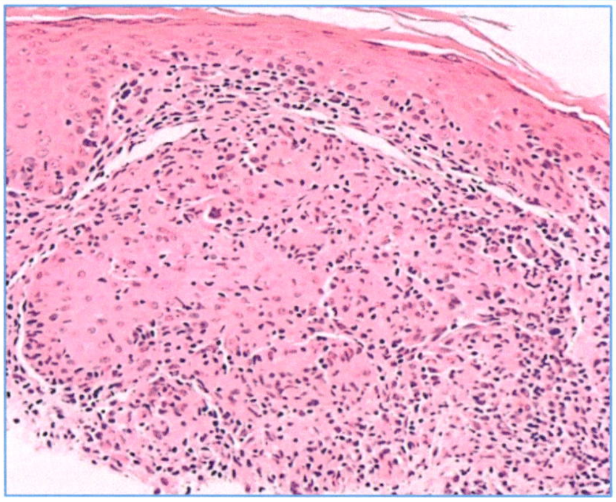

Sarcoidosis

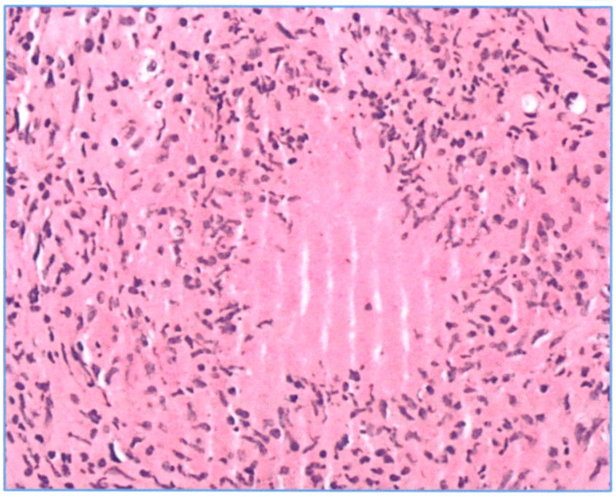

Tuberculosis

NECROBIOSIS
- not an accurate term
- it indicates degenerated collagen, in conjunction mostly with mucin, as part of necrobiotic granuloma
- the best example of necrobiosis is seen in granuloma annulare

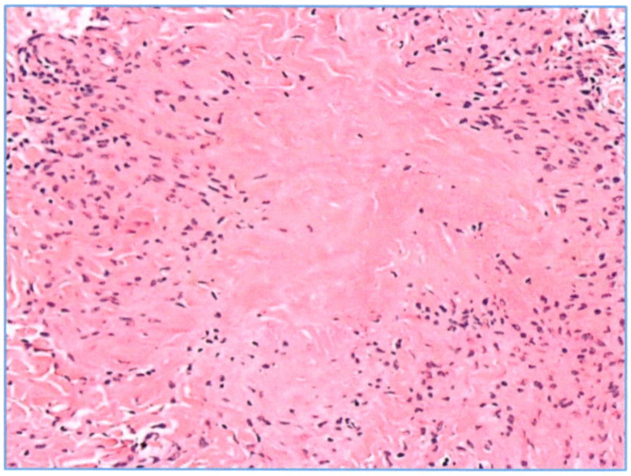

Granuloma annulare

Chapter 2

SPONGIOTIC DERMATITIS

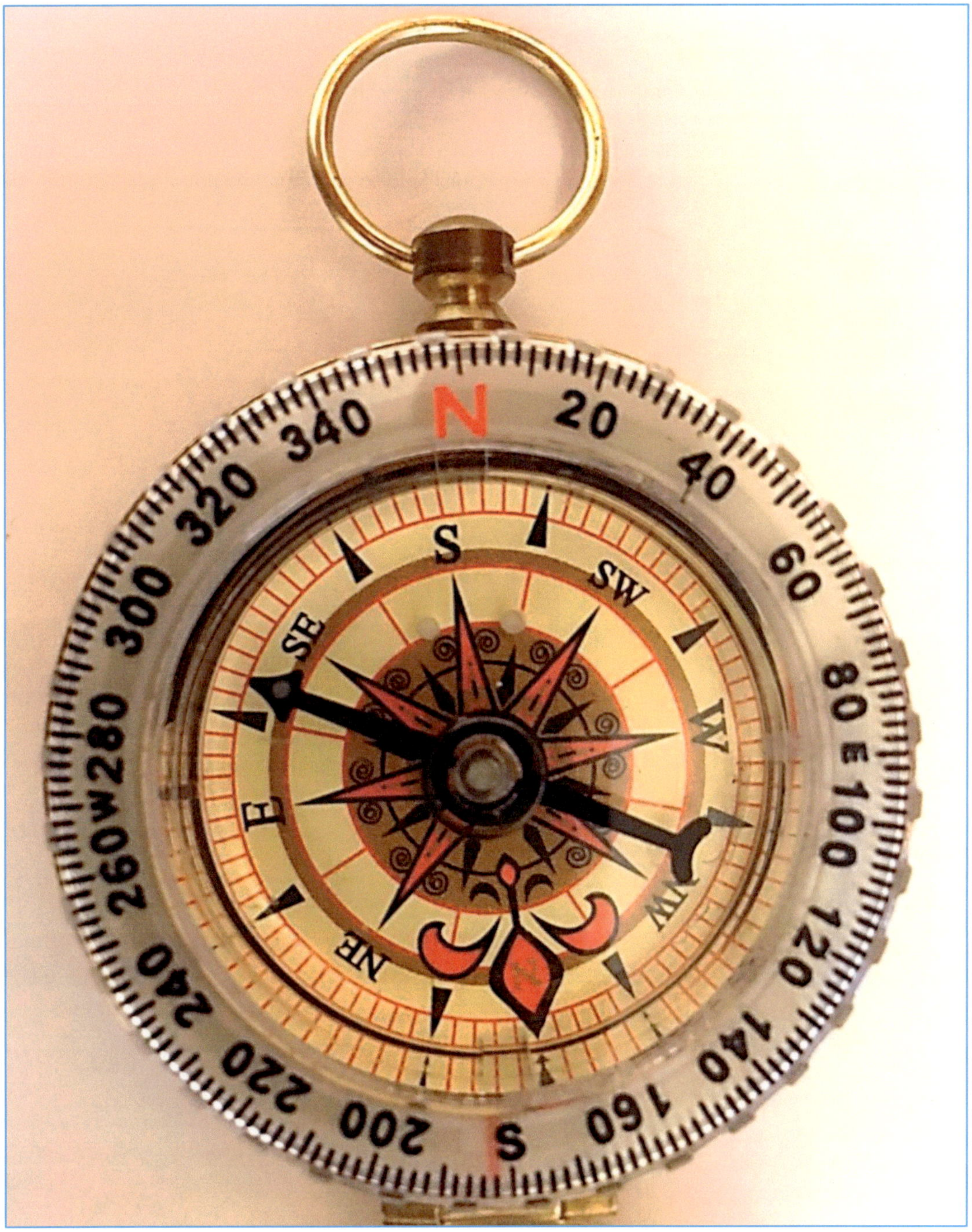

Spongiotic dermatitis

SPONGIOTIC DERMATITIS ranges from mild to acute, subacute, and chronic

Mild: epidermis of normal thickness with prominent **stretched desmosomes (spongiosis)**

Acute: diffuse epidermal spongiosis with **prominent intraepidermal macrovesicles**

Subacute: diffuse epidermal spongiosis with **intraepidermal microvesicles.**
More prominent epidermal acanthosis and parakeratosis.

Chronic: epidermal acanthosis, hyperkeratosis with **minimal spongiosis** and **rare to no microvesicles**

All phases have dermal lymphocytic inflammation.
Presence of epidermal and dermal eosinophils and neutrophils help to separate individual spongiotic diseases.

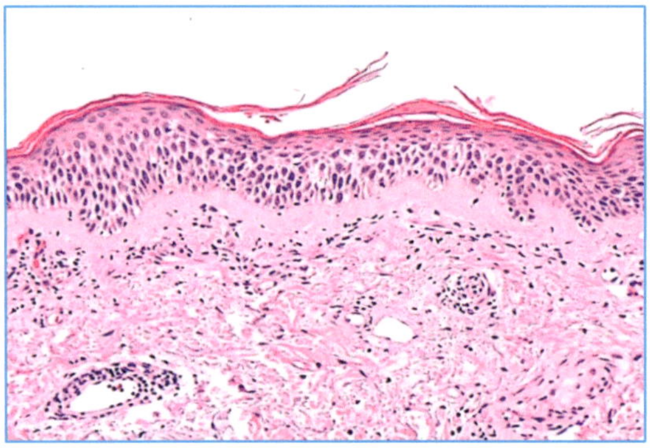
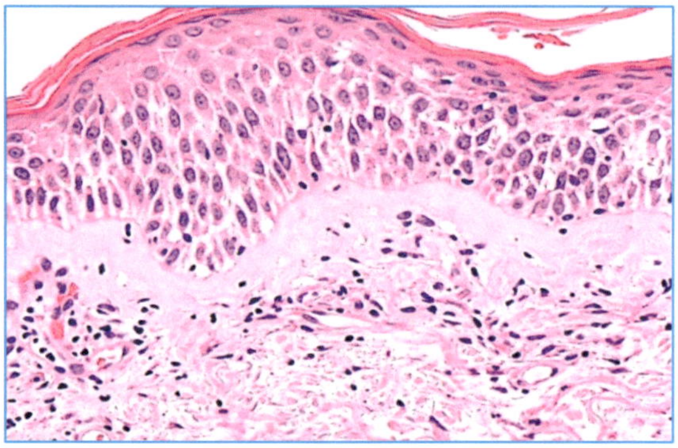

Early mild spongiotic dermatitis with prominent desmosomes forming white network

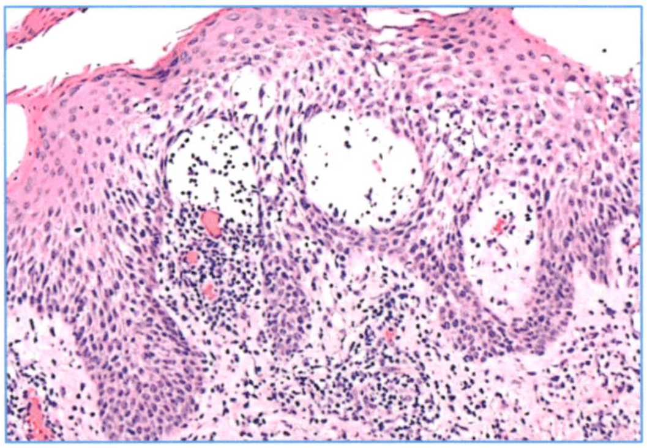
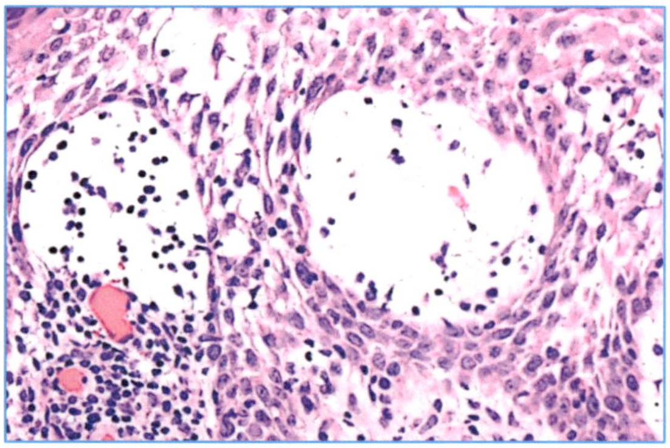

Acute spongiotic dermatitis with prominent epidermal macrovesicles

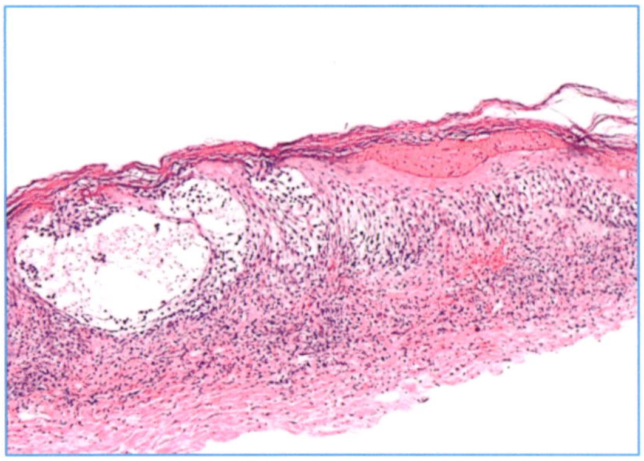
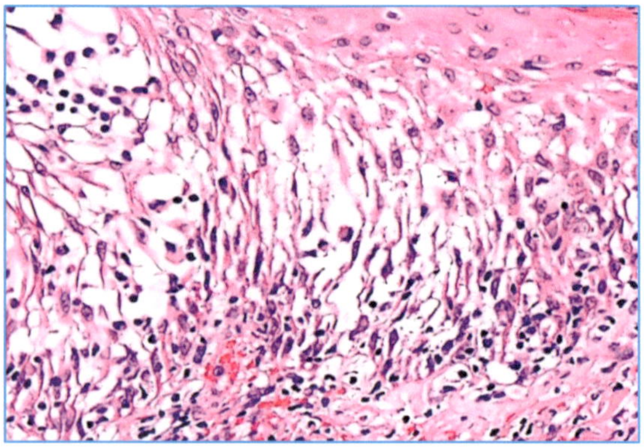

Acute spongiotic dermatitis with epidermal and dermal inflammatory cells

Chapter 2

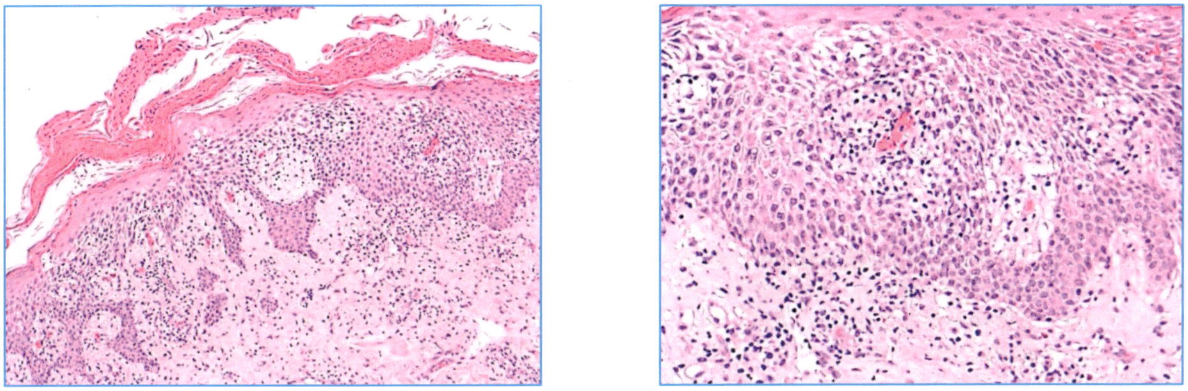

Subacute spongiotic dermatitis with thickened epidermis and diffuse epidermal spongiosis

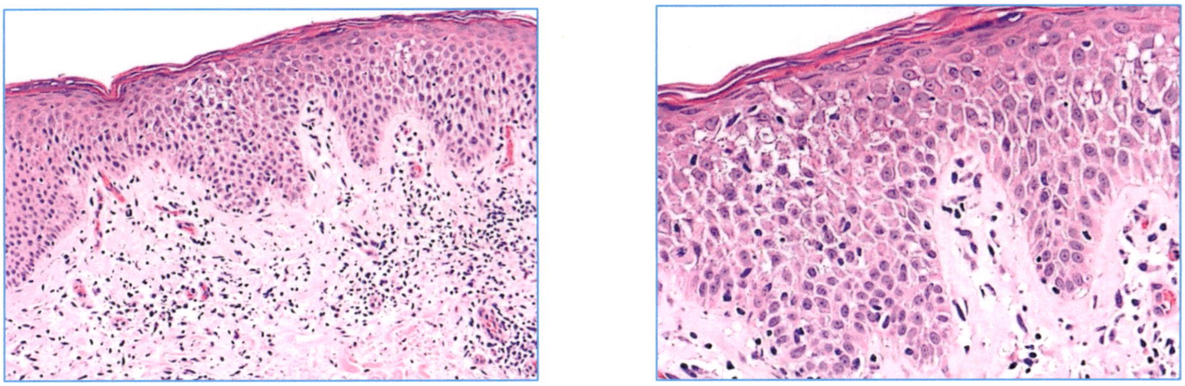

Subacute spongiotic dermatitis with diffuse dermal spongiosis and an attempt to form small microvesicles

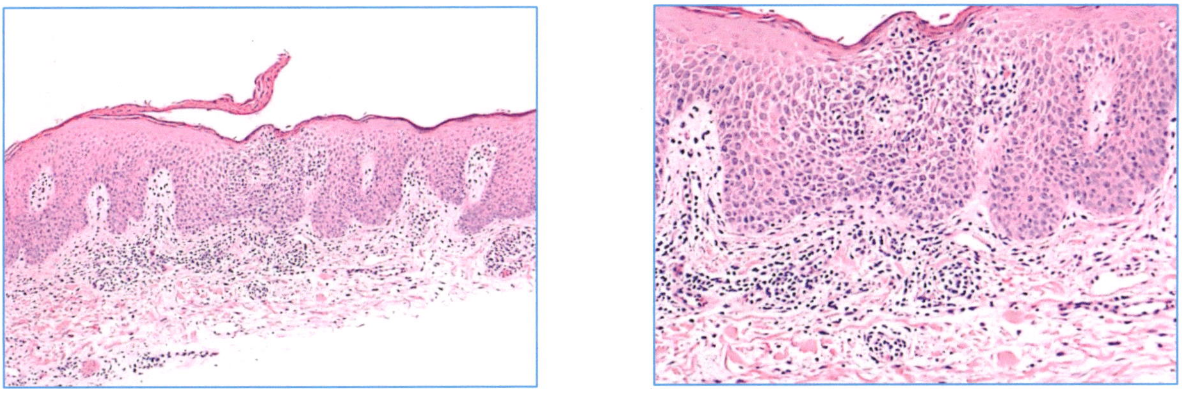

Chronic spongiotic dermatitis with thickened wavy epidermis with minimal spongiosis

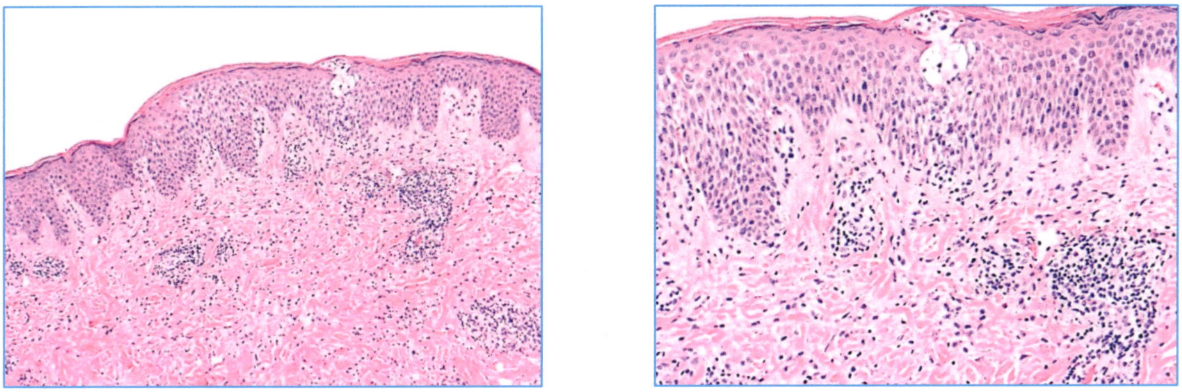

Chronic spongiotic dermatitis with only focal spongiosis and Langerhans cells microabscess

Spongiotic dermatitis

ALLERGIC CONTACT DERMATITIS

-type IV hypersensitivity reaction with nickel and poison ivy as the two most common antigens
-distribution is patterned based on the nature of contact
-acute presentation (days to weeks of exposure) present with erythema, papules, vesicles, bulla
-chronic presentation (months to years of exposure) presents with lichenified plaques, excoriations

Histopathology

acute form- epidermal spongiosis and **large** intraepidermal **vesicles** containing **eosinophils** and variable number of lymphocytes and neutrophils
-mild to moderate dermal perivascular lymphocytic infiltrate with **eosinophils**
subacute form- epidermal hyperplasia with spongiosis, **smaller vesicles** and scattered **epidermal eosinophils**
-mild to moderate dermal perivascular lymphocytic infiltrate with **eosinophils**
chronic form- acanthosis, hyperkeratosis and **minimal spongiosis**
-dermal fibrosis, mild dermal perivascular lymphocytic infiltrate, and **few eosinophils**
-epidermal **Langerhans cell microabscesses** can be found in all stages but not in all cases (it is common in this entity but not entirely specific)

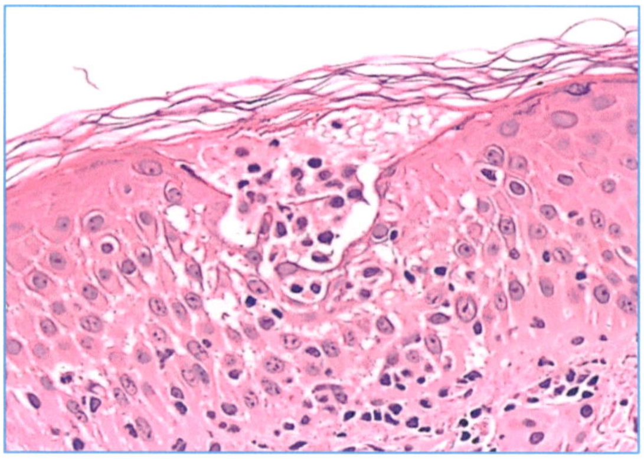

Langerhans cells microabscess

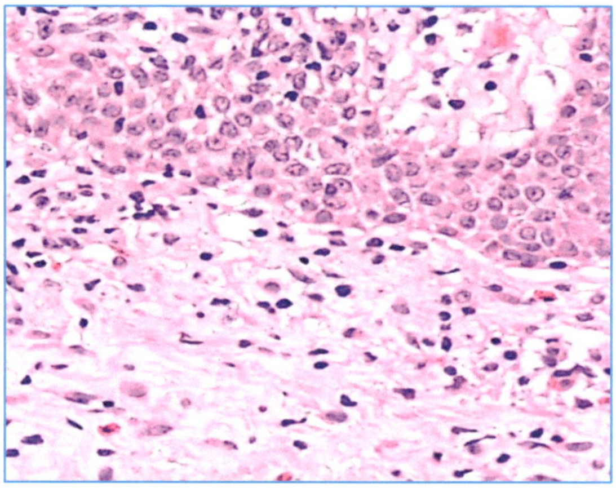

Subacute allergic contact dermatitis with epidermal spongiosis and scattered dermal eosinophils

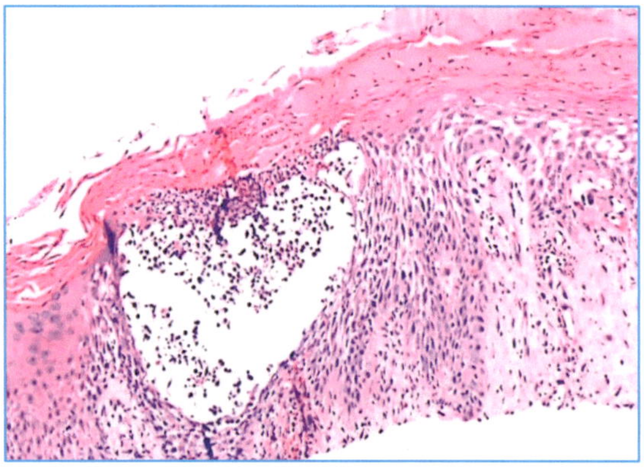

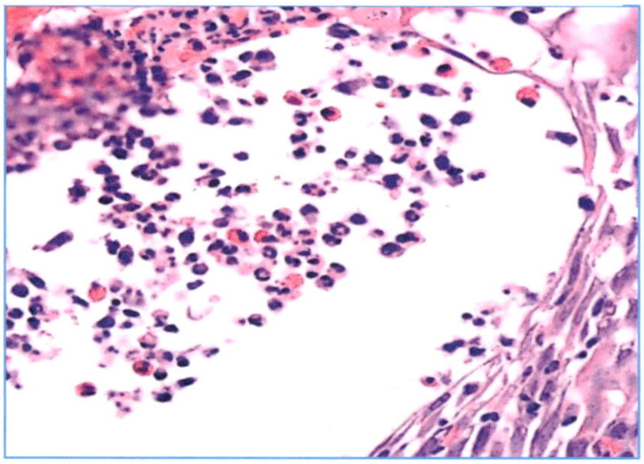

Acute allergic contact dermatitis with intraepidermal vesicles filled with eosinophils and neutrophils

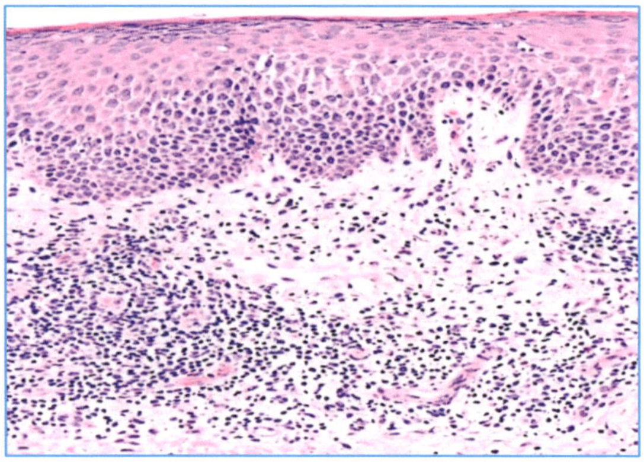

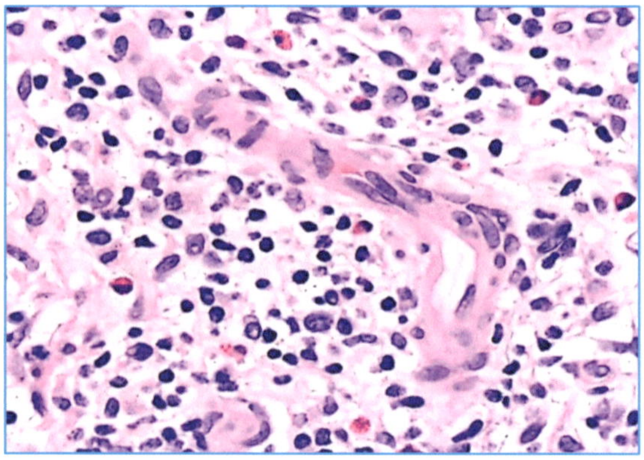

Chronic allergic contact dermatitis with dermal eosinophils

IRRITANT CONTACT DERMATITIS

-the most common occupational skin disease caused by direct damage to skin by a chemical irritant (**not immune mediated**)
-infants, elderly, and patients with atopic dermatitis are at higher risk
-hands and face are the most common sites
-acute lesions, confined to exposure site, present with erythema that progress to vesicles which erode and become crusted
-burning sensation is more common than itchiness
-chronic lesions are less well-defined and consist of papules, plaques with fissures, scales

Histopathology

acute form- large intraepidermal **vesicles** with lymphocytes and **neutrophils**
-dermal lymphocytic infiltrate with **neutrophils**
subacute form- acanthosis, diffuse spongiosis and few epidermal neutrophils
-dermal lymphocytic infiltrate with **neutrophils**
chronic form- acanthosis, hyperkeratosis and minimal spongiosis
-dermal fibrosis, mild lymphocytic infiltrate, and **occasional neutrophils**

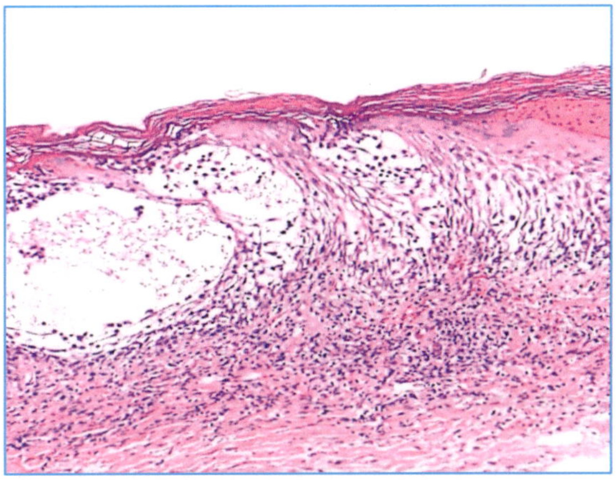

Acute irritant contact dermatitis with large vesicles with lymphocytes and neutrophils

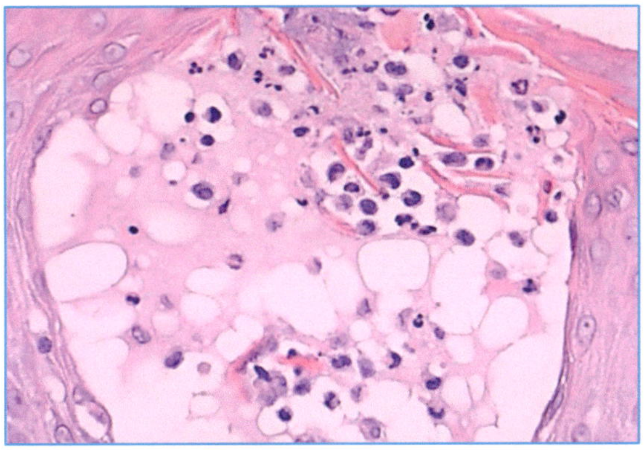

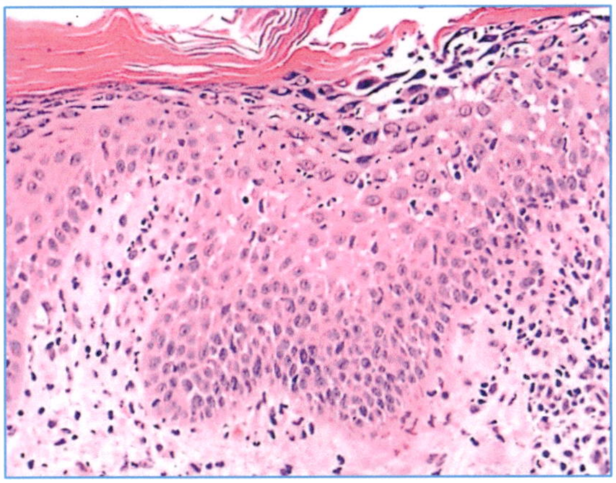

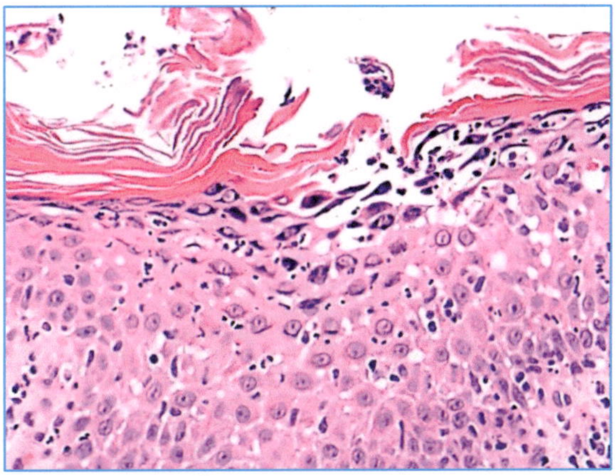

Subacute irritant contact dermatitis with epidermal spongiosis and epidermal and dermal neutrophils

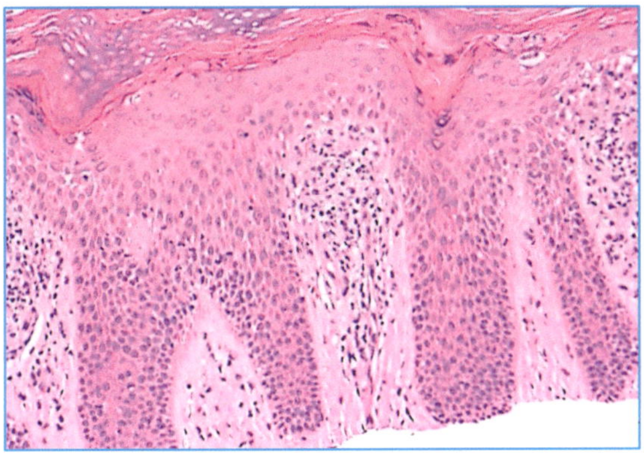

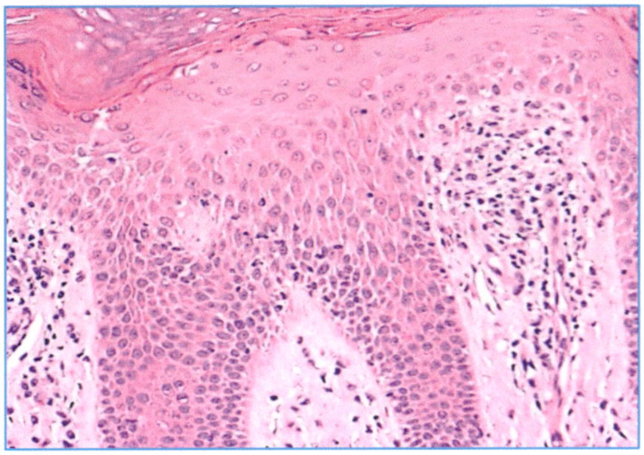

Chronic irritant contact dermatitis with minimal spongiosis, lymphocytes, and only occasional neutrophils

Spongiotic dermatitis

PHOTOALLERGIC CONTACT DERMATITIS

- type IV hypersensitivity reaction to topical drugs (e.g. oxybenzones, local anesthetics) or reaction to systemic drugs (e.g. NSAIDs, sulphonamides, quinine)
- clinically present as erythema and vesicles with honey colored crust on sun exposed area

Histopathology

- presents as acute, subacute, or chronic spongiotic dermatitis with epidermal and dermal **eosinophils**
- histology is almost identical to allergic contact dermatitis but with the additional presence of **necrotic keratinocytes** in the upper portion of the epidermis

PHOTOTOXIC DERMATITIS

- non-immunologically mediated phototoxic reaction to photosensitizing drugs (e.g. tetracycline, NSAIDs, fluoroquinolones, psoralens)
- presents as exuberant sun burn on sun exposed skin

PHYTOPHOTODERMATITIS

- phototoxic reaction resulting from contact with plants containing furocoumarins followed by sun exposure
- common culprits are celery, parsley, hogweeds, citrus, and fig trees
- present with erythema, edema, blisters

Histopathology of phototoxic and phytophotodermatitis is identical

- presents as acute, subacute, or chronic spongiotic dermatitis with epidermal and dermal **neutrophils**
- histology is almost identical to irritant contact dermatitis but with the additional presence of **necrotic keratinocytes** in the upper portion of the epidermis

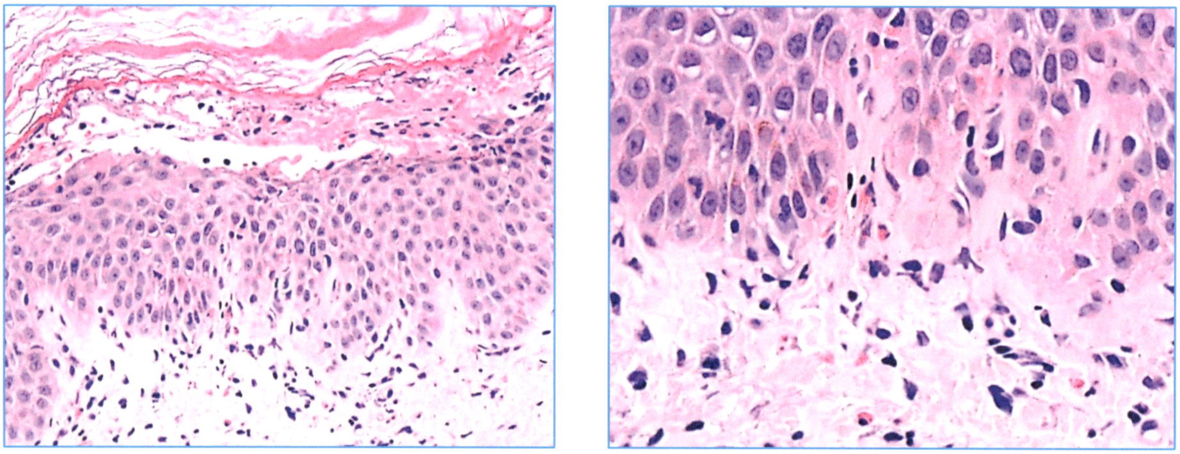

Photoallergic dermatitis with superficial necrotic keratinocytes and epidermal and dermal eosinophils

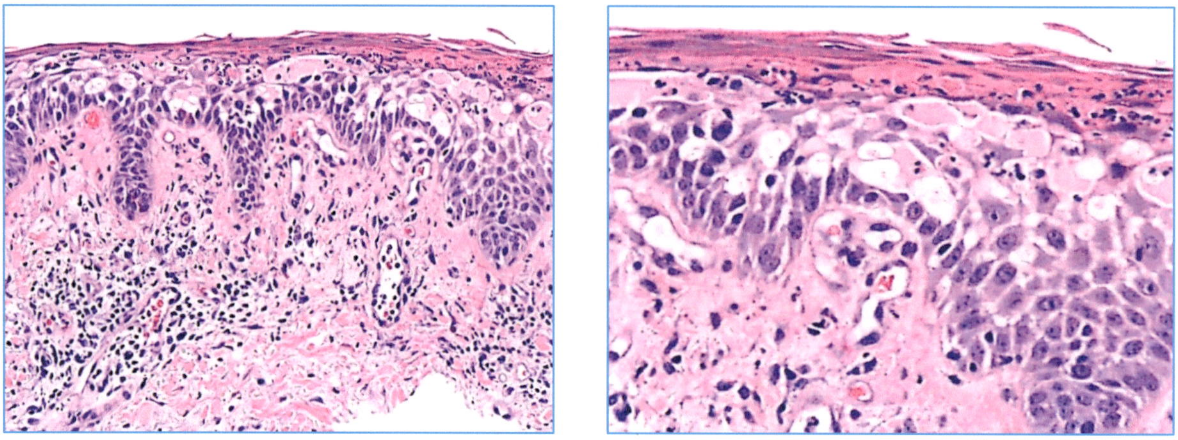

Phototoxic dermatitis with necrotic keratinocytes in superficial epidermis and epidermal and dermal neutrophils

ATOPIC DERMATITIS (ECZEMA)

-most common chronic and relapsing dermatitis
-commonly the first manifestation of atopic march followed by allergic rhinitis and asthma
-majority of patients (over 70%) have positive family history of atopy
-associated with null mutation in *fillagrin* gene
-patients are susceptible to colonization and recurrent infections of *S. aureus*
-in infants pruritic eczematous patches with xerosis that involves face, scalp, and extensor surfaces of extremities
-in childhood erythematous patches, papules, and plaques favoring flexural folds of extremities
-in adults it affects flexural areas, neck, face, feet with erythema, xerosis, and lichenification

Histopathology
-although it can present as acute, subacute or chronic, **subacute,** and **chronic** forms are **usually biopsied**
-in all forms **dermal eosinophils** are present in **mild to moderate numbers**

DYSHIDROTIC DERMATITIS (POMPHOLYX)

-type of eczematous dermatitis affecting hands and feet
-sudden onset of numerous, deep-seated, very pruritic vesicles
-older lesions show scaling, fissures, and lichenification

Histopathology
-can present as acute, subacute, and chronic spongiotic dermatitis
-acute form is **the most common**
-acral skin with thick stratum corneum
-epidermal spongiosis with **large intraepidermal vesicles**
-vesicles contain some lymphocytes and occasional neutrophils/eosinophils
-mild to moderate dermal perivascular lymphocytic infiltrate with **scattered eosinophils**

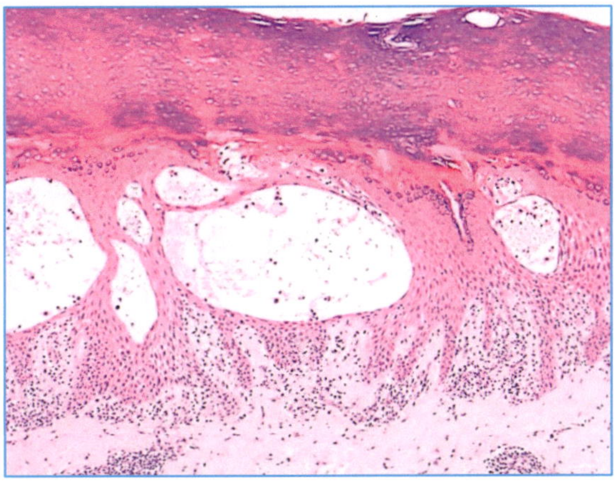
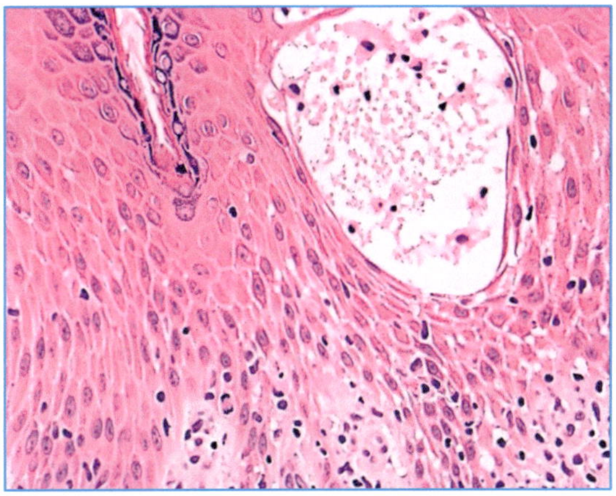

Acute dyshidrotic dermatitis of acral skin with large vesicles with lymphocytes and few neutrophils

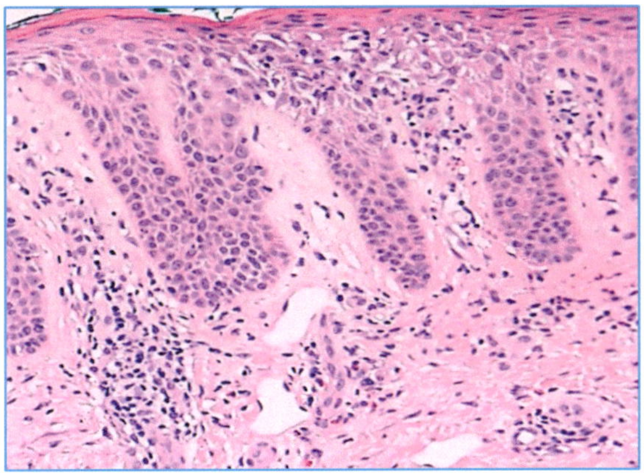
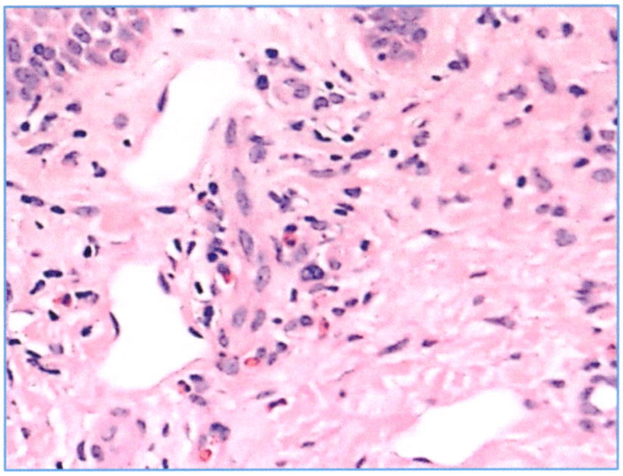

Subacute atopic dermatitis with scattered dermal eosinophils

Spongiotic dermatitis

ID REACTION (AUTOECZEMATIZATION)

-type IV hypersensitivity reaction in response to a skin infection or rash at another site
-contact dermatitis, stasis dermatitis, and tinea are the most common inducing diseases
-lesions appear days to weeks after primary rash
-presents as symmetrically distributed itchy papules

Histopathology
-**not specific, clinical history is paramount**
-usually presents as acute or subacute spongiotic dermatitis
-**mostly** perivascular **lymphocytic** infiltrate
-**few eosinophils may be present**

NUMMULAR DERMATITIS

-generally considered a subtype of eczema
-small papules that coalesce into pruritic "coin-shaped" (nummular) pink to dull red plaques
-lower extremity are favored sites

Histopathology
-biopsy typically shows subacute spongiotic dermatitis
-if biopsied early, it would show acute spongiotic dermatitis
-**not very specific findings**
-**mostly** perivascular **lymphocytic** infiltrate
-**few eosinophils may be present**

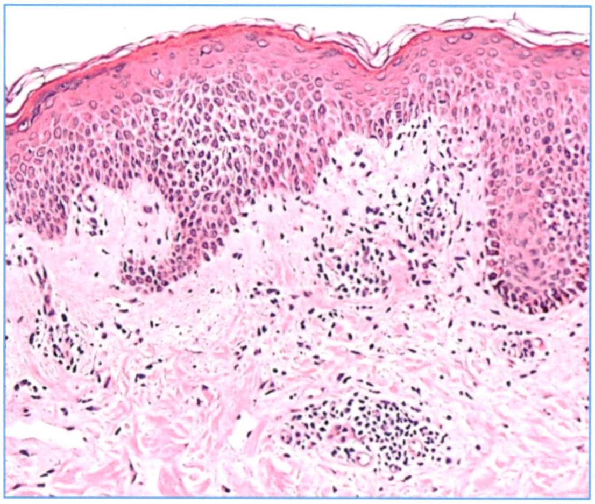

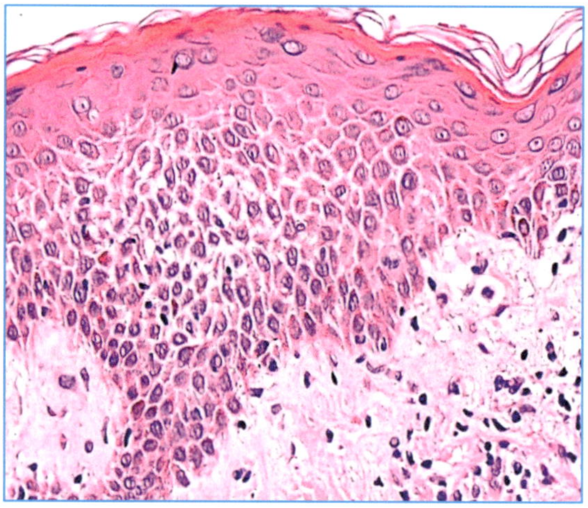

Subacute ID reaction with epidermal spongiosis, dermal lymphocytes, and rare eosinophils

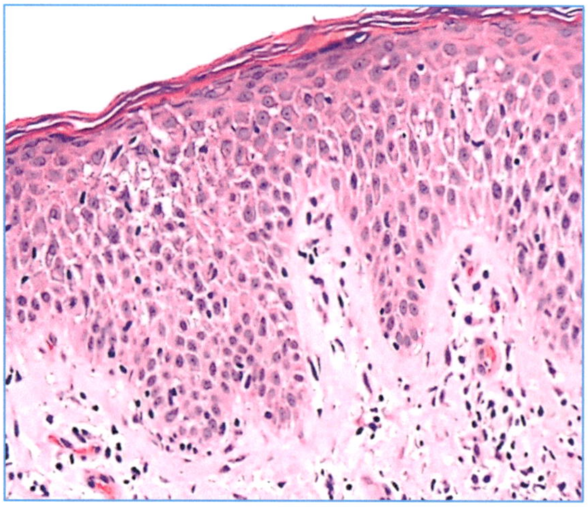

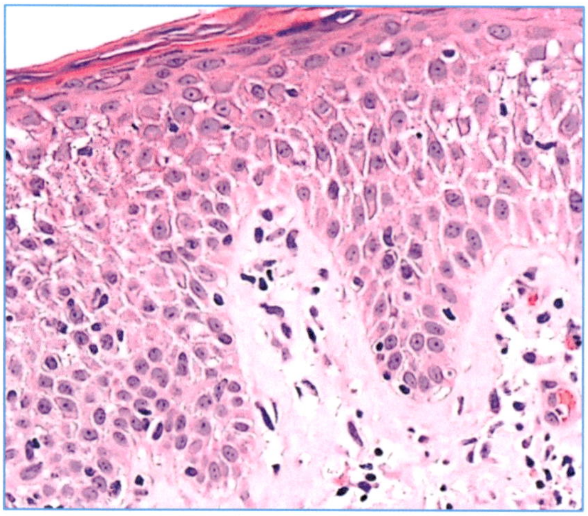

Subacute nummular dermatitis with epidermal spongiosis, dermal lymphocytes and occasional eosinophils

ASTEATOTIC ECZEMA (ECZEMA CRAQUELE, WINTER ITCH)

-most common in elderly patients on lower extremities
-skin is very dry, pruritic, with fine scales and cracks resembling a **"dry riverbed"**

Histopathology

-usually chronic spongiotic dermatitis
-epidermal **hyperkeratosis and hypergranulosis**
-focal epidermal lymphocytic exocytosis

STASIS DERMATITIS

-consequence of long-standing venous insufficiency
-more common in elderly and obese individuals
-affects lower legs and feet
-presents with edema, hyperpigmentation, and dry scales
-can also present more acutely with weepy, eczematous changes
-chronic stasis can lead to lipodermatosclerosis with "inverted wine bottle" presentation (discussed in the panniculitis chapter)

Histopathology

-subacute or chronic spongiotic dermatitis
-**proliferation of small dermal vessels in lobular pattern**
-vessels have round lumina and plump endothelial cells
-common dermal red blood cell extravasation

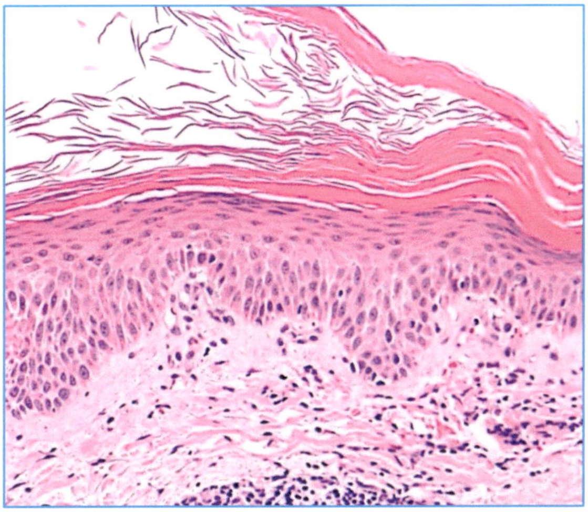

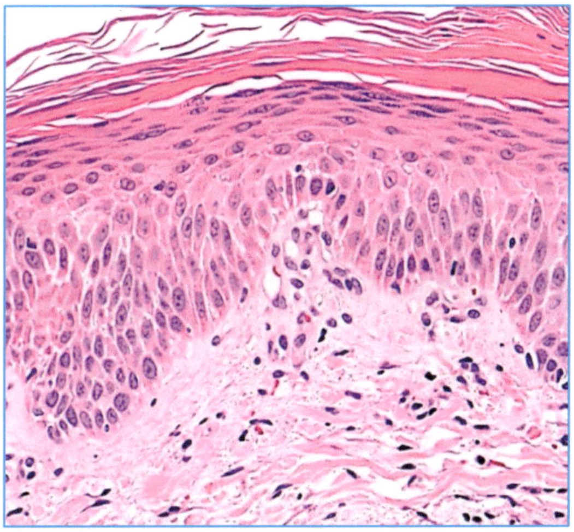

Asteatotic dermatitis with hyperkeratosis and hypergranulosis

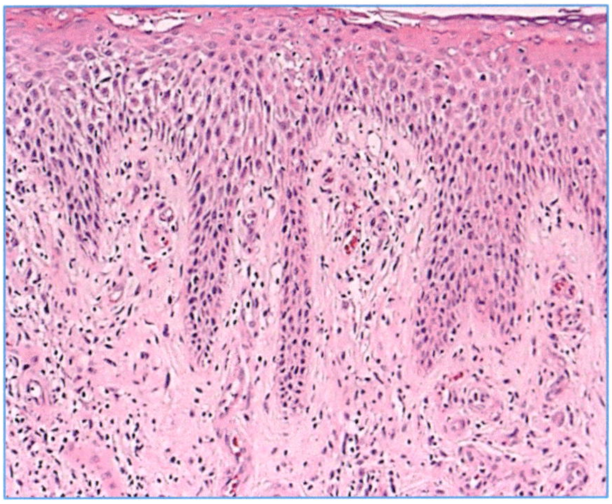

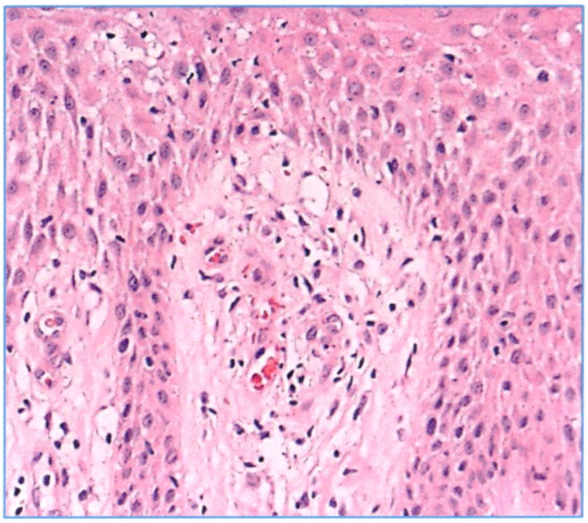

Stasis dermatitis with subacute spongiotic dermatitis and proliferation of dermal vessels

Spongiotic dermatitis

PITYRIASIS ROSEA

-more common in spring and fall
-more frequent among young women
-starts with **"herald patch",** oval red slightly raised plaque with fine collarette scale
-1 to 2 weeks later, exanthema follows with fine papules and plaques with collarette scale
-lesions follow skin cleavage lines (**"Christmas tree" distribution**) with trunk and proximal part of extremities favored
-rule out secondary syphilis; "when you think PR check on RPR"
-inverse pityriasis rosea favors intertriginous areas and extremities

Histopathology
-mild epidermal spongiosis
-focal **"mounds" of parakeratosis**
-attenuated underlying granular layer
-perivascular lymphocytic inflammation with **dermal red blood cell extravasation**

SEBORRHEIC DERMATITIS

-affects "seborrheic" areas (scalp, face, postauricular, presternal, intertriginous areas)
-pediatric presentation is erythematous, scaly rash with "cradle cap" in infants
-adult presentation is with well-defined pink patches with greasy scales
-disease is more severe and more frequent in patients with HIV and Parkinson's disease
-dandruff (*pityriasis sicca*) is a type of seborrheic dermatitis

Histopathology is **ambiguous** with **psoriasiform** and **spongiotic** features
-newer lesion are more spongiotic and older are more psoriasiform
-usually **irregular** wavy (mildly psoriasiform) **epidermis** with **variable** epidermal **spongiosis**
-epidermal **parakeratosis** with neutrophils especially **around follicular ostia**
-**granular layer is usually diminished**

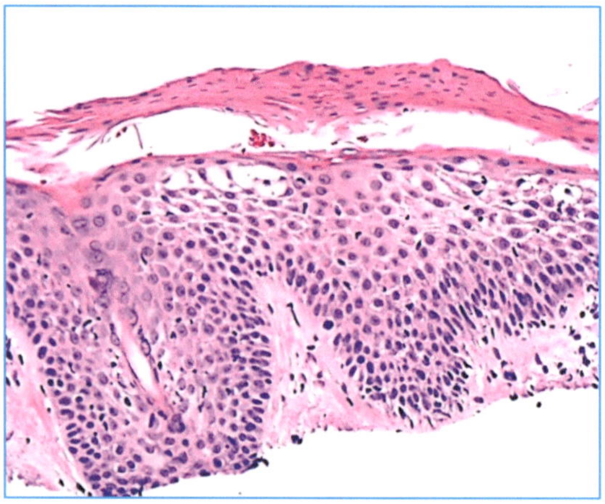

More spongiotic variant of seborrheic dermatitis with parakeratosis and diminished granular layer

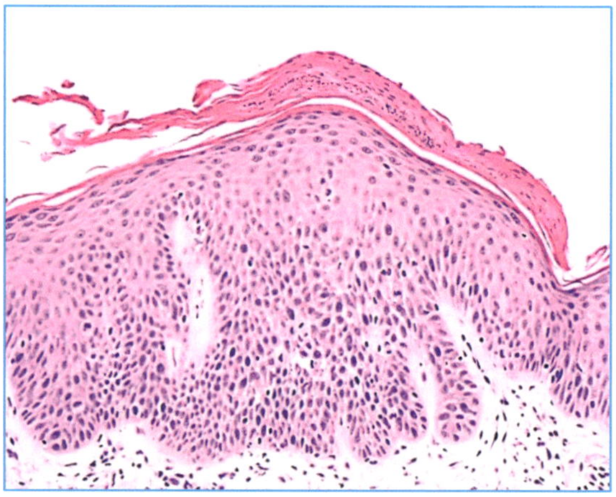

More psoriasiform variant of seborrheic dermatitis with parakeratosis and diminished granular layer

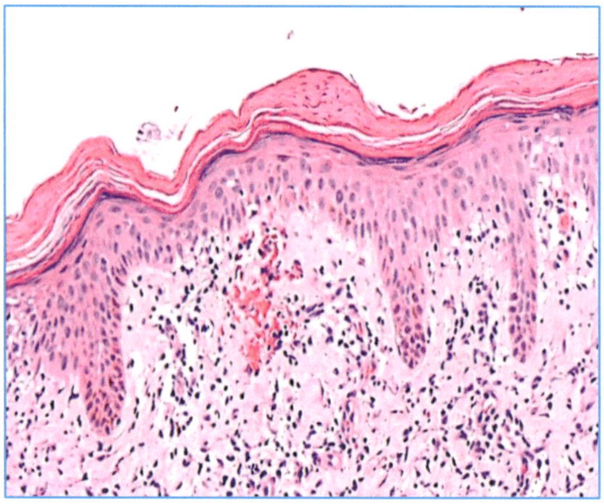

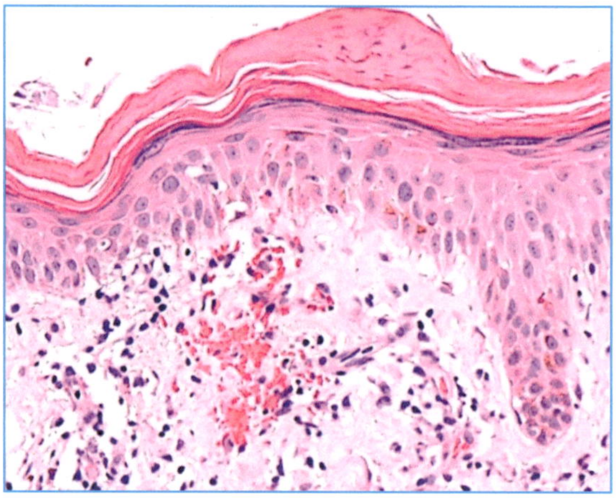

Pityriasis rosea with mound of parakeratosis, mild epidermal spongiosis, and red blood cell extravasation

ARTHROPOD BITE

-itchy single or grouped papules and vesicles with erythema
-discussed in more details in the chapter on exogenous skin insults

Histopathology
-**epidermis** is commonly **excoriated** and filled with serum crust
-epidermis abutting excoriation is variably spongiotic
-**V-shaped,** superficial and deep perivascular lymphohistiocytic infiltrate
-perivascular and interstitial **eosinophils and neutrophils** are present
-dermal edema and focal dermal necrosis commonly present

INCONTINENTIA PIGMENTI

-X-linked, dominant genodermatosis
-four phases with only the first one being spongiotic
-**first vesicular phase** (birth to 2-3 weeks) with coalescing vesicles on erythematous base on trunk and extremities
-**second verrucous phase** (2-6 weeks) with hyperkeratotic verrucous papules on extremities
-**third hyperpigmented phase** (2-6 months) with linear area of hyperpigmentation often distributed in a linear manner along Blaschko's lines
-**forth hypopigmented phase** (puberty) with atrophic linear hypopigmented skin

Histopathology
-**1st phase**- spongiosis with **vesicles** filled with **eosinophils**
-**2nd phase**- hyperkeratotic, acanthotic epidermis, **focal necrotic keratinocytes** and **few eosinophils**
-**3rd phase**- focal interface vacuolar changes with **dermal pigment incontinence**
-**4th phase**- apoptotic keratinocytes with **atrophic hair follicles and absence of arrector pili**

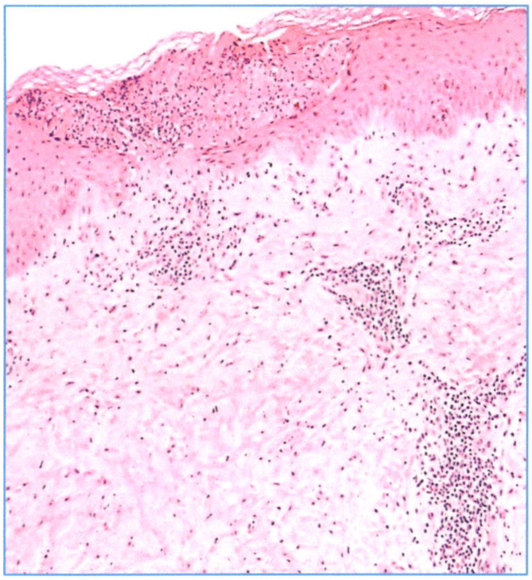
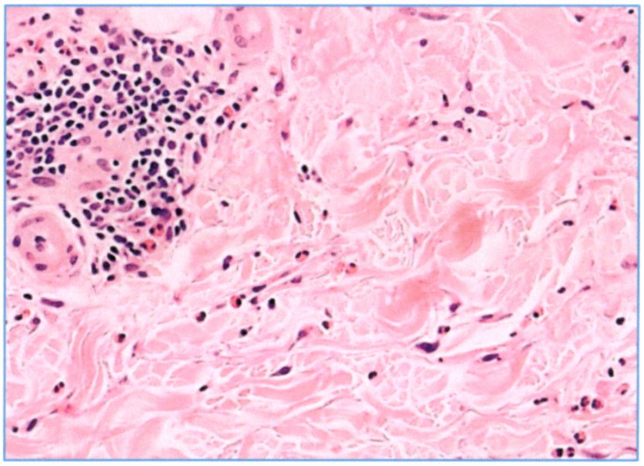

Arthropod bite with excoriated epidermis and underlying V-shaped inflammation with eosinophils

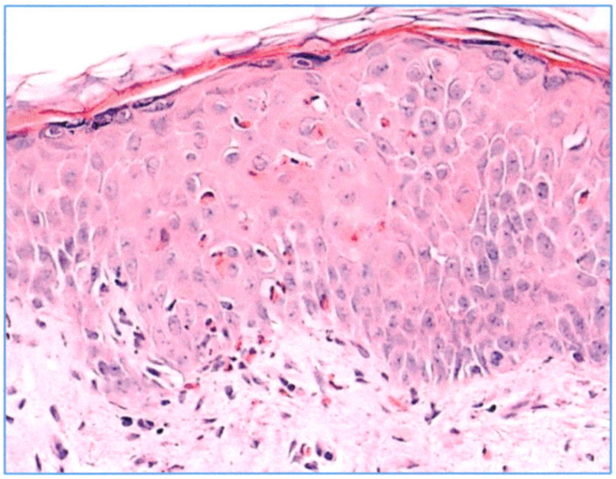
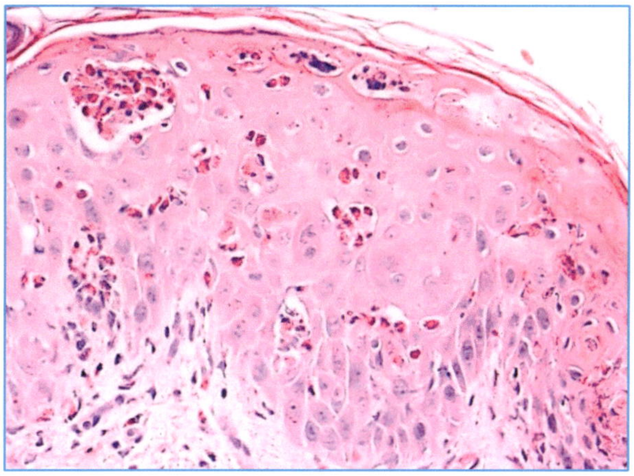

Incontinentia pigmenti with scattered epidermal eosinophils (left) forming intraepidermal vesicles filled with eosinophils (right)

Spongiotic dermatitis

MORBILLIFORM (EXANTHEMATOUS) DRUG ERUPTION

-most common type of drug reaction
-discussed in more details in the drug reactions chapter
-the most common culprits are penicillin, carbamazepin, allopurinol, NSAID, sulfonamide, chloramphenicol
-maculopapular diffuse rash that usually appears on the trunk first and then spread

PRURITIC URTICARIAL PAPULES AND PLAQUES OF PREGNANCY (POLYMORPHIC ERUPTION OF PREGNANCY, TOXIC ERYTHEMA OF PREGNANCY)

-occurs in the third trimester of about 1% of pregnancies
-demonstrates pruritic urticarial papules, plaques that mostly develop in and around the abdominal striae before spreading to the abdomen
-usually spares periumbilical area (in contrast to herpes gestationis)
-resolves spontaneously after delivery

These two diseases are histologically identical

Histopathology
-mild epidermal spongiosis
-perivascular lymphocytic infiltrate
-variable number of perivascular and interstitial **dermal eosinophils**
-variable urticarial **dermal edema**
Clinical information separates these two entities

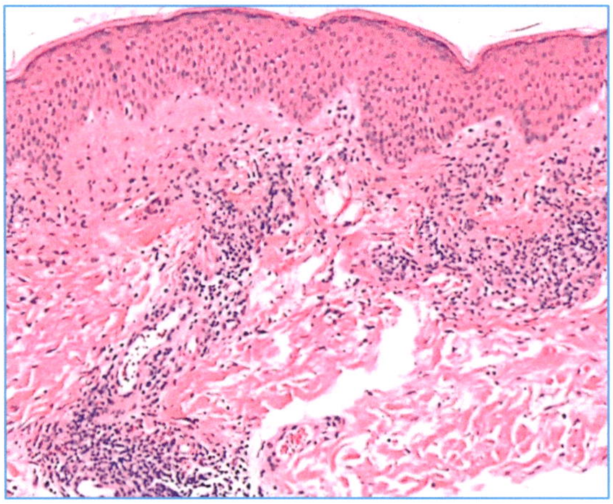
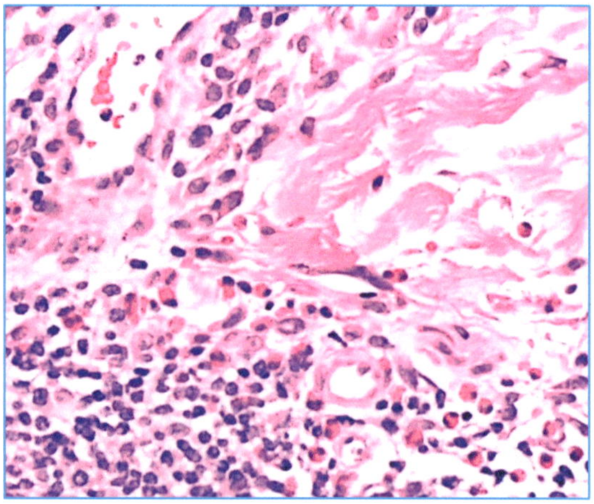

Morbilliform drug reaction with numerous eosinophils

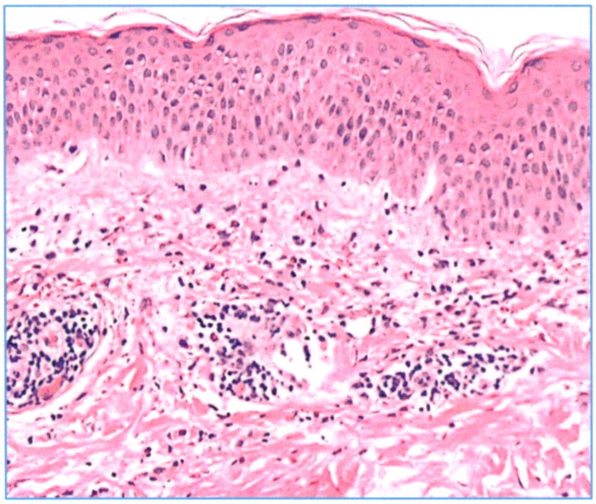
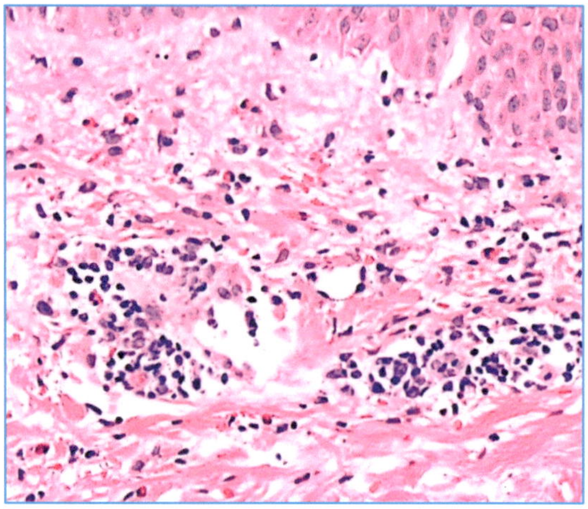

Pruritic urticarial papules and plaques of pregnancy with dermal eosinophils and mild edema

TINEA and VIRAL EXANTHEMA (depending on the type) have multiple clinical and histological presentations and are discussed in more details in the chapters on viral and fungal infections.
However, because histologically **they might present as spongiotic dermatitis** they are discussed here for comparison with other spongiotic disorders.

Viral exanthema (of unknown origin) is **very unspecific**
-usually present with mild epidermal spongiosis
-mild to moderate perivascular lymphocytic inflammation

Tinea
-mild epidermal spongiosis with more **compact stratum corneum**
-common focal parakeratosis alternating with orthokeratosis, so called **"sandwich" sign**
-fungal elements in stratum corneum

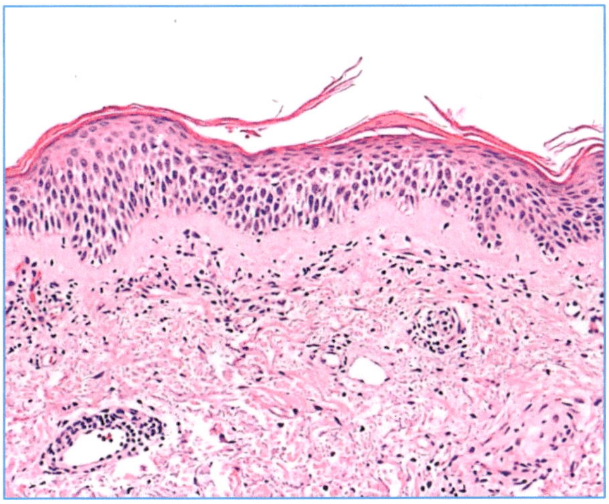

Viral exanthema presenting as mild spongiotic dermatitis

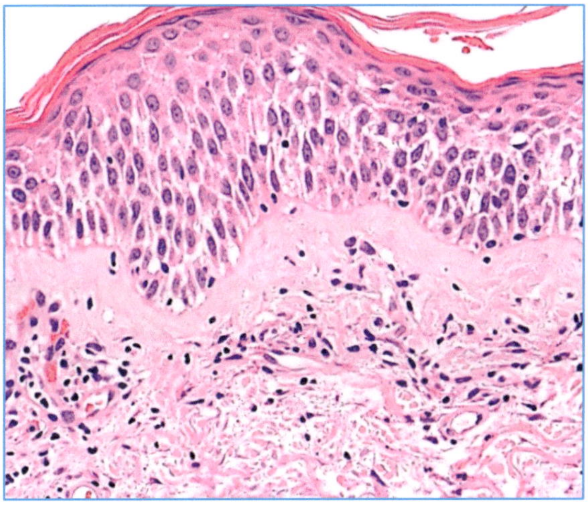

Stretched epidermal desmosomes with no vesicles and mild perivascular lymphocytic inflammation

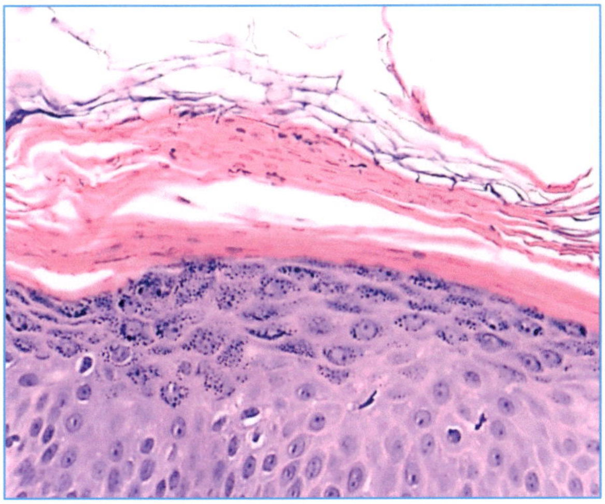

Tinea within alternating para and orthokeratosis, "sandwich" sign

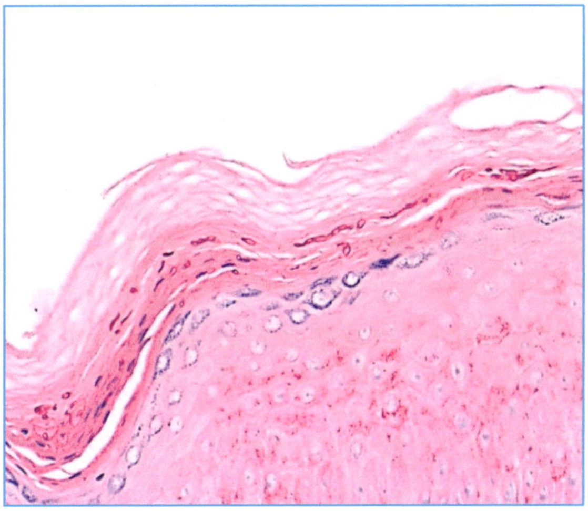

PAS stain outlines fungal elements in the stratum corneum

Spongiotic dermatitis

HOW TO APPROACH SPONGIOTIC DERMATITIS

All entities can present as **acute, subacute, or chronic** spongiotic dermatitis **with the exception** of **pityrisis rosea and seborrheic dermatitis** that present as **mild** spongiotic dermatitis

IF YOU SEE EPIDERMAL EOSINOPHILS

-allergic contact dermatitis	no necrotic keratinocytes + Langerhans cells microabscess
-photoallergic dermatitis	necrotic keratinocytes "sunburn cells"
-incontinentia pigmenti	disease of newborn (whereas allergic contact is not)

IF YOU SEE EPIDERMAL NEUTROPHILS

-irritant contact dermatitis	does not have necrotic keratinocytes
-phototoxic dermatitis	necrotic keratinocytes "sunburn cells"
-tinea	parakeratosis and "sandwich" sign

IF YOU SEE FOCAL EPIDERMAL PARAKERATOSIS

-pityriasis rosea	mild focal spongiosis + dermal red blood cells
-seborrheic dermatitis	psoriasiform and spongiotic epidermal changes
-tinea	"sandwich" sign + neutrophils

IF YOU SEE DERMAL EOSINOPHILS (seen in many entities but differ quantitatively)

A LOT OF DERMAL EOSINOPHILS

-allergic contact dermatitis	eosinophils also in epidermis
-photoallergic dermatitis	eosinophils also in epidermis + necrotic keratinocytes
-drug reaction	diffuse rash unlike patterned lesions in ACD
-pigmented urticarial papules and plaques of pregnancy	only in pregnancy

MILD TO MODERATE NUMBER OF DERMAL EOSINOPHILS

-atopic dermatitis	skin flexures + atopic history
-dyshidrotic dermatitis	hand, feet, fingers, toes

FEW EOSINOPHILS

-nummular dermatitis	coin-shaped patch/plaque
-ID reaction	multiple papules at site distant from previous dermatitis

PRESENCE OF DERMAL EOSINOPHILS AND NEUTROPHILS

-arthropod bite	**s**ingle or multiple lesions in localized area + ulcerated epidermis
-drug reactions	diffuse rash

IF YOU SEE MOSTLY DERMAL LYMPHOCYTES AND NO NEUTROPHILS OR EOSINOPHILS

-**asteatotic dermatitis**	shins of elderly but no vascular proliferation
-**stasis dermatitis**	lower legs with vascular proliferation of capillaries
-**pityriasis rosea**	mounds of parakeratosis and RBC extravasation
-**seborrheic dermatitis**	psoriasiform appearance with focal parakeratosis
-**viral exanthem**	usually diffuse morbilliform rash

THE RULE THAT SUPERCEDES ALL RULES IS THAT *THERE IS NO ABSOLUTE RULE*. WHEN IT COMES TO SPONGIOTIC DERMATITES, HISTOLOGICAL AND CLINICAL CORRELATION IS *PARAMOUNT.*

Chapter 2

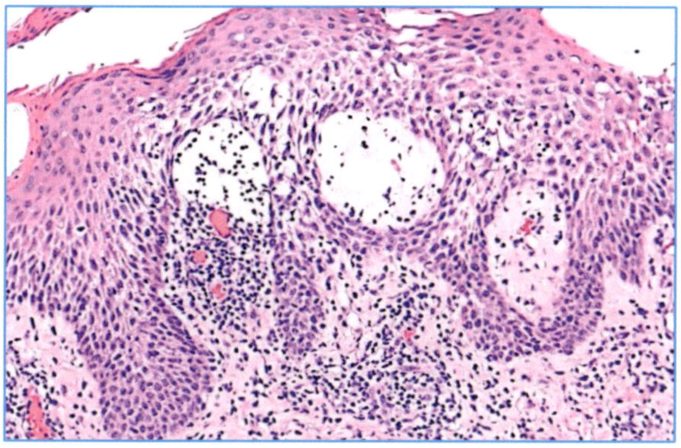

Acute spongiotic dermatitis with large vesicles

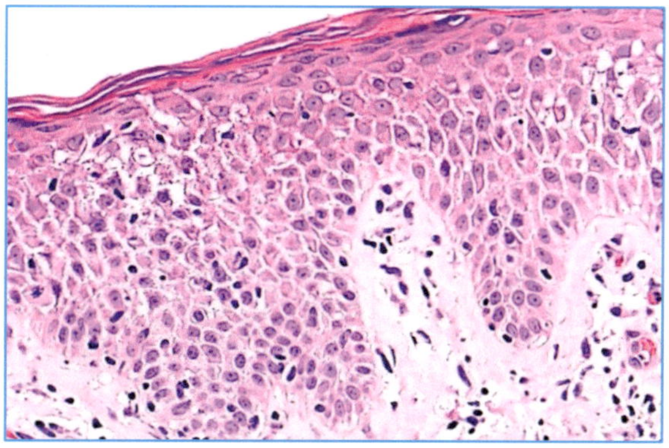

Subacute spongiotic dermatitis with diffuse spongiosis and an attempt to make a vesicle

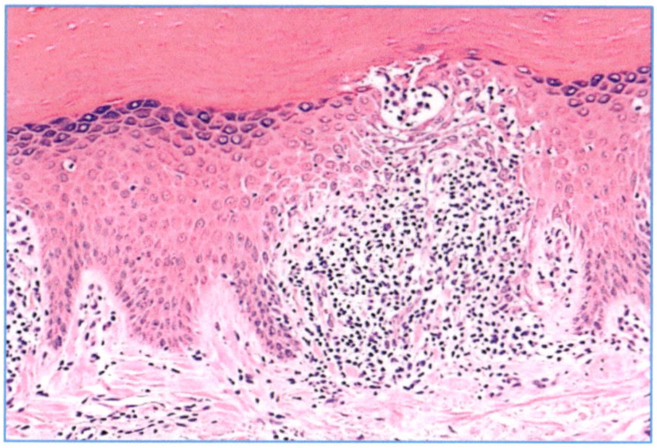

Chronic spongiotic epidermis with only focal spongiosis

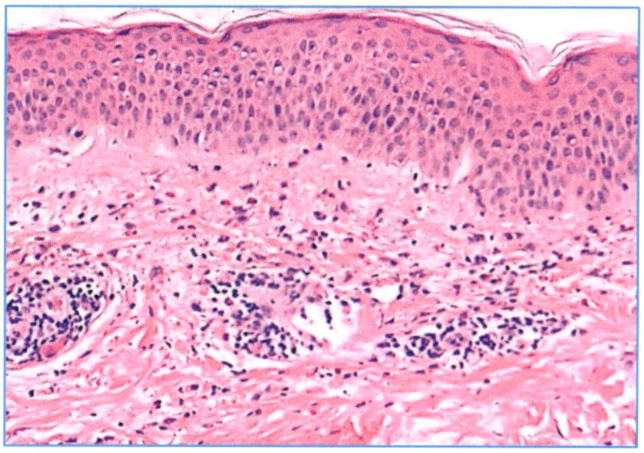

Mild spongiotic dermatitis with eosinophils

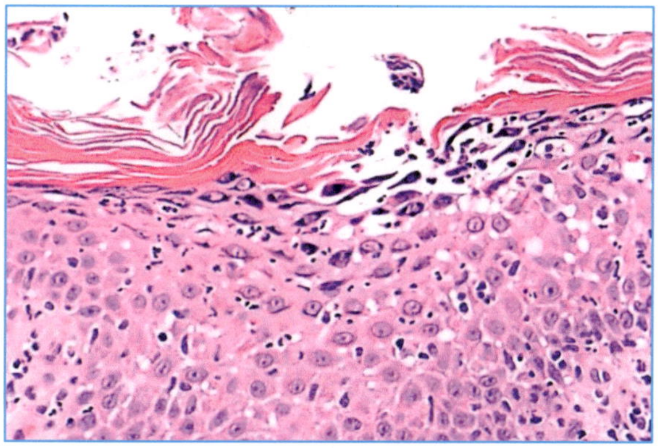

Subacute spongiotic dermatitis with neutrophils

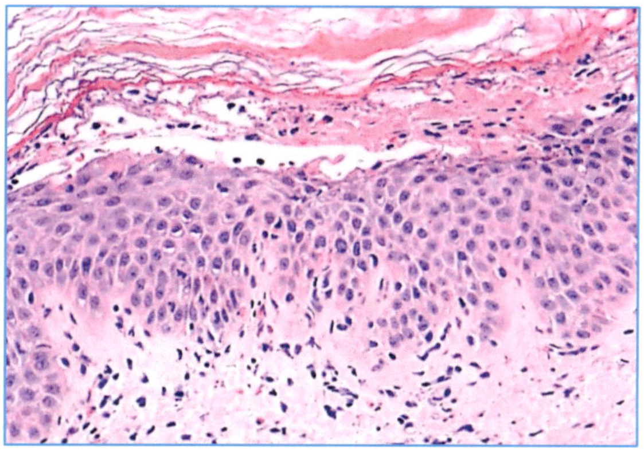

Spongiotic dermatitis with necrotic keratinocytes

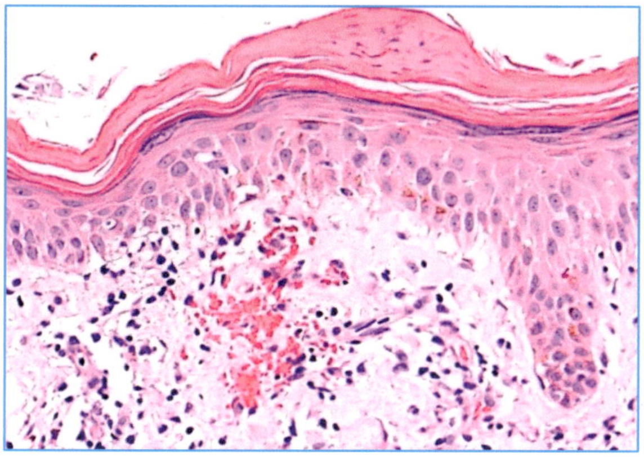

Pityriasis rosea with focal parakeratosis and dermal RBCs

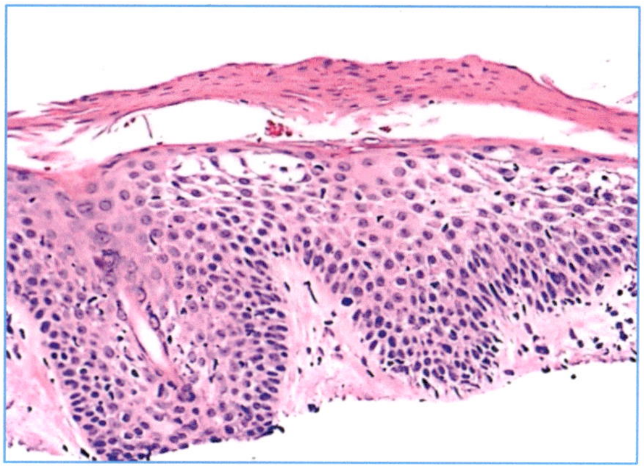

Seborrheic dermatitis with psoriasiform epidermis and parakeratosis adjacent to hair follicle

Spongiotic dermatitis

Chapter 3

PSORIASIFORM DERMATITIS

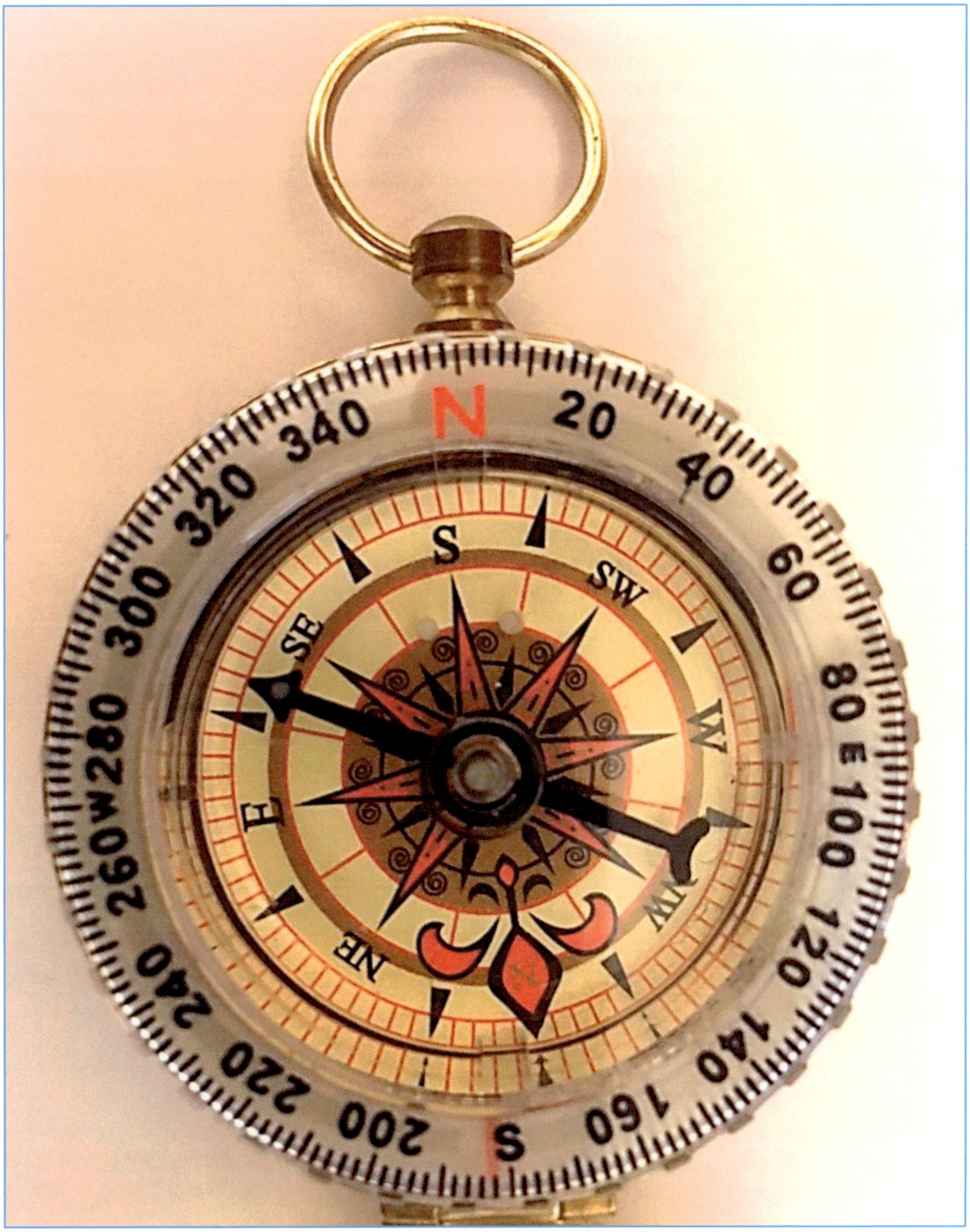

Psoriasiform dermatitis

PSORIASIS

There are three main clinical variants that can be further subdivided:

Psoriasis vulgaris (plaque psoriasis)
-most common type of psoriasis
-well-defined "salmon pink" plaques with silvery scale
-plaques can be round-oval, polycyclic, and/or linear
-removal of scale results in minute bleeding (Auspitz sign)
-elbows, knees, scalp, hands, feet, genitalia, and intertriginous areas are favored
-nail changes are common (pitting, onycholysis, oil spots)
-can progress to psoriasiform erythroderma with generalized redness and scale involving ≥ 90% BSA, typically due to poor clinical management

Guttate psoriasis
-more common in children and young adults
-may occur several weeks after *group A Strep*. infection
-"drop-like", "salmon pink" papules with overlying scale
-more generalized symmetrical distribution on the trunk and extremities
-usually resolves but causes higher risk for plaque psoriasis later

Pustular psoriasis

Pustular psoriasis of von Zumbusch
-life-threatening disease with an abrupt onset
-skin is sore and red with generalized, tiny, yellow pustules occurring in waves and resolving with collarette scale
-associated with hypocalcemia

Impetigo Herpetiformis
-pregnancy-associated generalized pustular psoriasis
-pustules start in flexures and then spread

Palmoplantar pustulosis
-sterile pustules and yellow brown macules on the palms and soles

Acrodermatitis continua of Hallopeau
-painful sterile pustules affecting the distal tips of one or more digits
-may lead to nail dystrophy

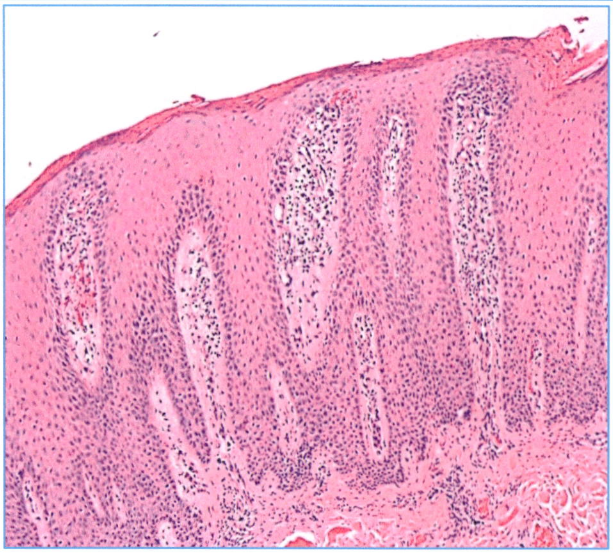
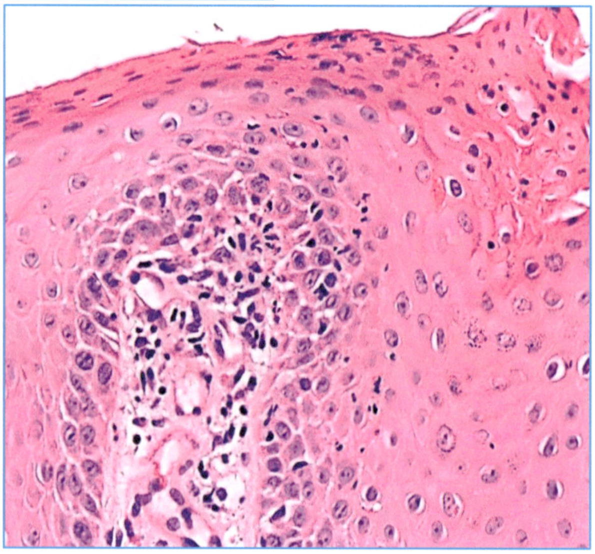

Psoriasis vulgaris with elongated rete ridges, thin suprapapillary epidermal plate, parakeratosis, and loss of granular layer

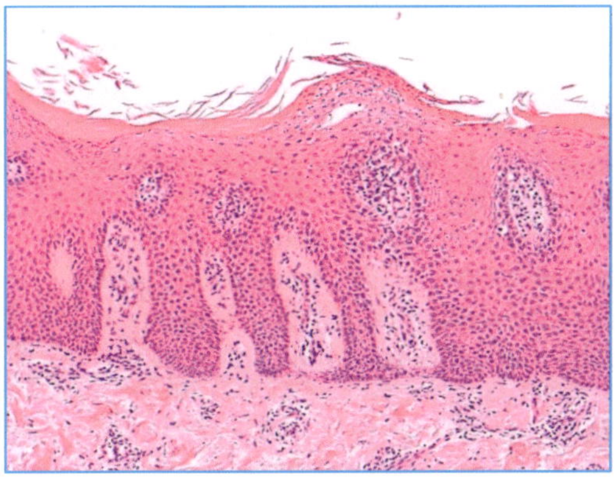

Psoriasis vulgaris

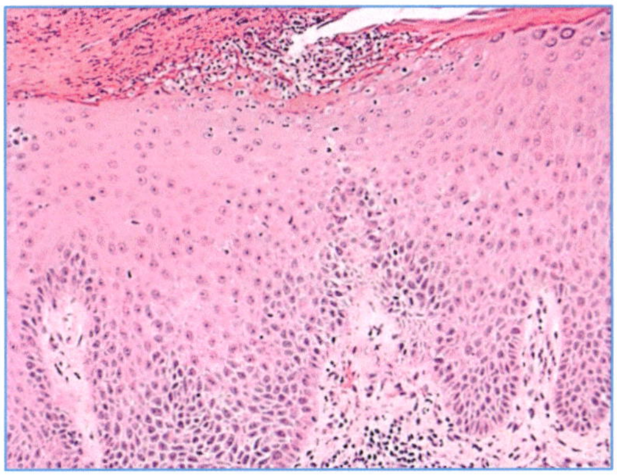

Generalized pustular psoriasis

Histopathology

Psoriasis vulgaris

-**epidermal hyperplasia with uniform elongation of the rete ridges (psoriasiform hyperplasia)**

-hyperkeratosis with mounds of **parakeratosis** (in early lesions) or confluent parakeratosis (in established lesions)

-**absence of the granular layer**

-thinning of the suprapapillary epidermis

-Munro's microabscesses (neutrophils in stratum corneum) and Kogoj's pustules (neutrophils in stratum spinosum) are seen

-dilated capillaries within the papillary dermis

-superficial perivascular lymphocytic infiltrate

Guttate psoriasis

-very subtle psoriasiform hyperplasia

-**epidermis is more wavy** and mildly spongiotic and less psoriasiform

-**"mounds" of parakeratosis with adherent neutrophils**

Pustular psoriasis

-acral or non-acral skin, depending on the clinical type

-prominent **intraepidermal pustules of Kogoj**

-pustules in early lesions are surrounded by a **spongiotic epidermis with minimal psoriasiform hyperplasia**

-pustules in older lesions are surrounded by psoriasiform hyperplasia with parakeratosis and **hypogranulosis**

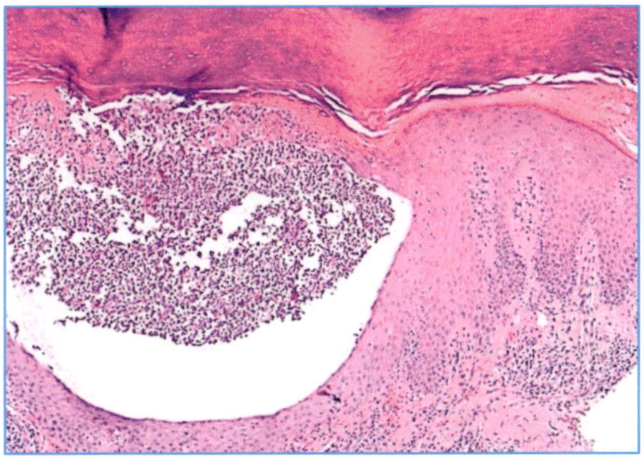

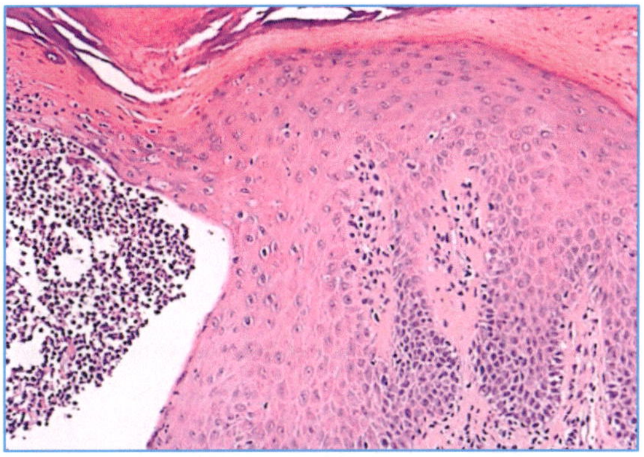

Acral pustular psoriasis with intraepidermal pustule of Kogoj and adjacent psoriasiform epidermis with hypogranulosis

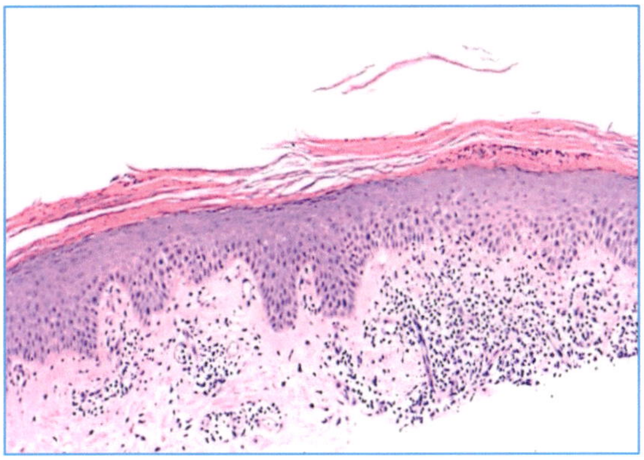

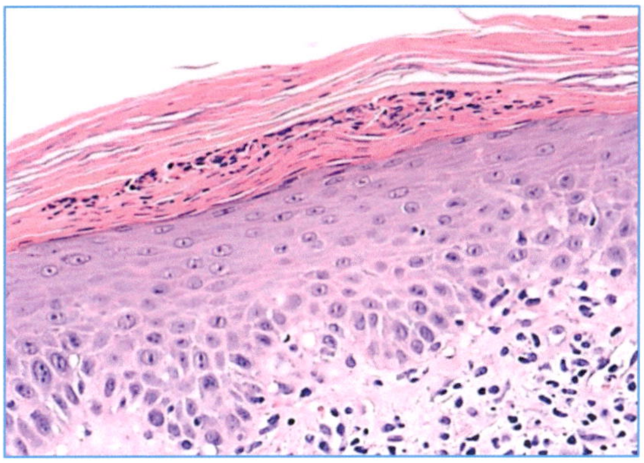

Guttate psoriasis with wavy epidermis and mound of parakeratosis with admixed neutrophils

Psoriasiform dermatitis

LICHEN SIMPLEX CHRONICUS

-thickening of the skin caused by chronic scratching due to an underlying trigger (e.g. atopy, contact, stasis, bite)
-well demarcated, pruritic, hyperpigmented plaques with marked accentuation of the skin creases (lichenification)
-located in areas that can be easily scratched (e.g. the nape of the neck, hand, elbow, ankle, or genitalia)

Histopathology

-**bottom flat,** more regular psoriasiform **epidermis with uniform rete**
-epidermal hyperkeratosis, **hypergranulosis,** and acanthosis
-papillary **dermis appears fibrotic**

PRURIGO NODULARIS (PICKER'S NODULE)

-firm, dome-shaped, itchy, often visibly excoriated papules and nodules resulting from prolonged picking/scratching
-papules and nodules are commonly grouped
-may be seen on any area of body that is easily accessible for scratching
-spares the mid upper back ("butterfly sign")

Histopathology

-nodular "**dome-shaped"** silhouette
-**irregular** psoriasiform hyperplasia
-hyperkaratotic, acanthotic epidermis with **hypergranulosis**
-papillary dermal fibrosis
-mild perivascular lymphocytic infiltrate

Lichen simplex chronicus (LSC) and prurigo nodularis (PN) are within the spectrum of the same disease. If the lesion is clinically and histologically flat it is LSC and if it is nodular that it is PN.

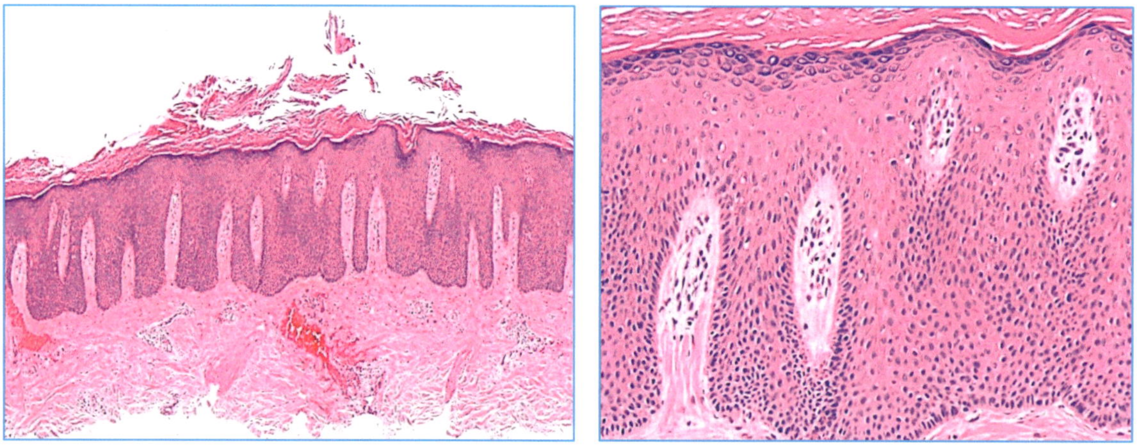

Lichen simplex chronicus with regular psoriasiform epidermis with prominent granular layer

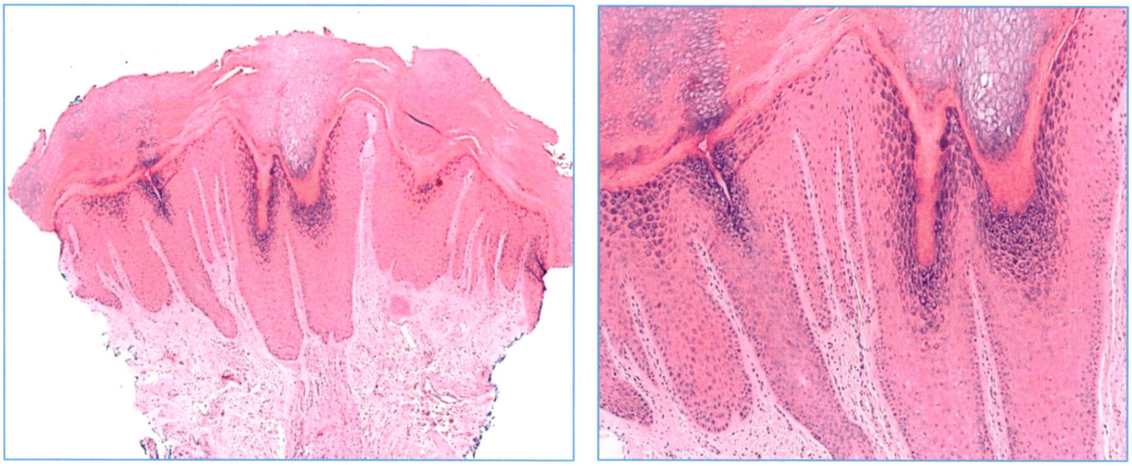

Prurigo nodularis with irregular, "dome-shaped" psoriasiform proliferation and hypergranulosis

INFLAMMATORY LINEAR VERRUCOUS EPIDERMAL NEVUS (ILVEN)

-variant of epidermal nevus discussed in detail in the chapter on epidermal tumors
-usually presents in infants and children
-multiple discrete papules that coalesce into a linear plaque and follow Blaschko lines
-leg, thigh, and buttock are favorite sites

Histopathology
-psoriasiform epidermis with **diminished or absent granular layer**
-**alternating broad bands of ortho and parakeratosis**
-variable perivascular lymphocytic infiltrate

PITYRIASIS RUBRA PILARIS (PRP)

-uncommon idiopathic inflammatory skin condition
-has bimodal age of onset (first and sixth decades)
-classically starts on the head/neck and progresses caudally
-itchy, rapidly evolving disease
-characterized by orange-red scaly papules/plaques that spread all over the body often creating erythroderma
-follicular plugging ("nutmeg grater papules") and islands of spared skin are characteristic
-common palmoplantar, orange-red, waxy keratoderma ("sandal-like")
-nail changes with longitudinal ridges, subungual hyperkeratosis

Histopathology
-**wavy, barely psoriasiform epidermis** with broad rete ridge
-**granular layer is present**
-**vertically and horizontally alternating orthokeratosis and parakeratosis (checkerboard pattern)**
-**follicular shoulder parakeratosis and follicular plugging**
-mild dermal lymphocytic inflammation

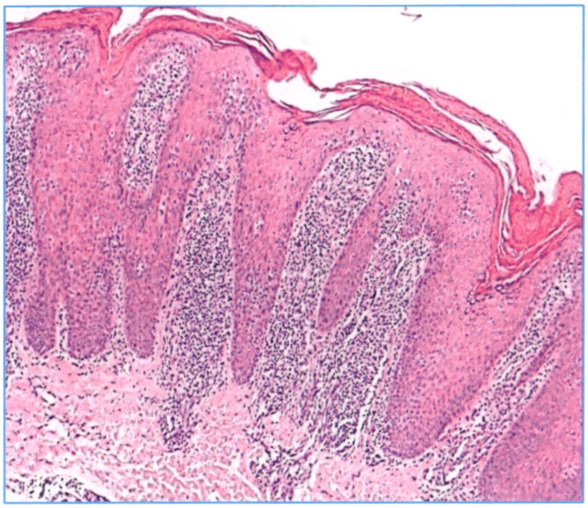

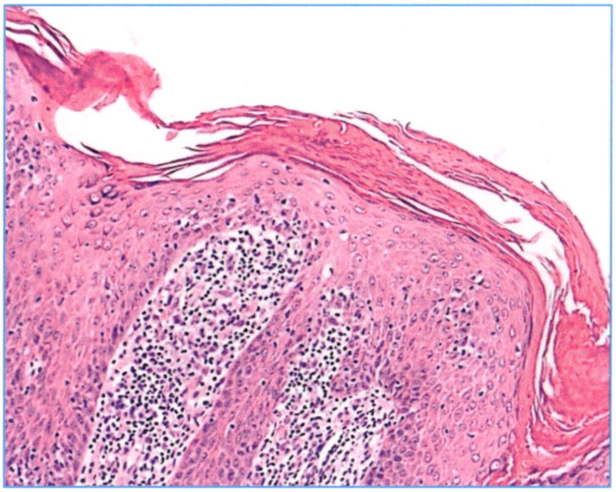

ILVEN with irregular psoriasiform epidermis with alternating parakeratosis and absent granular layer

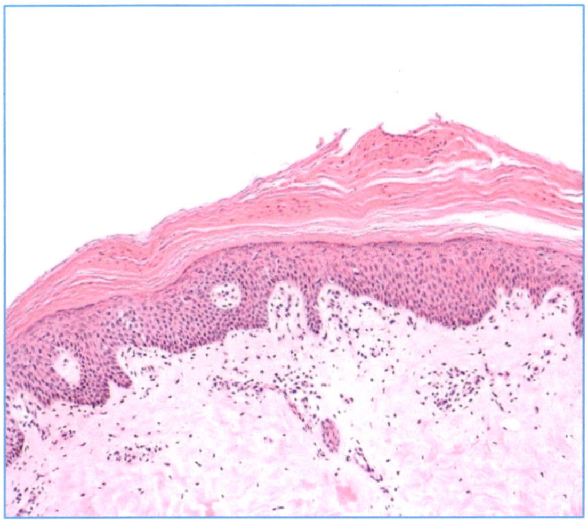

PRP with wavy epidermis and alternating parakeratosis

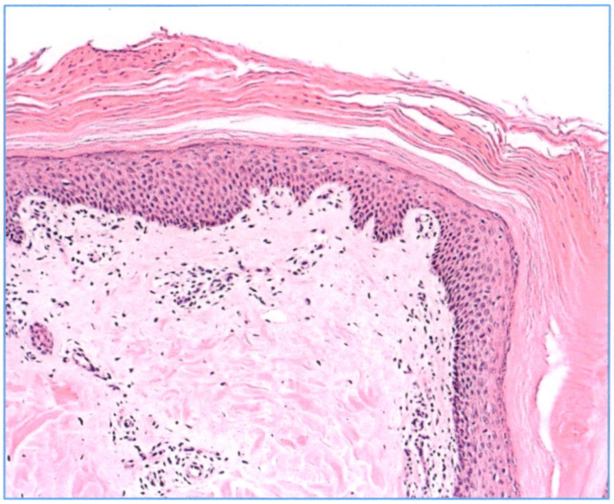

PRP with follicular shoulder parakeratosis

Psoriasiform dermatitis

CHRONIC ACTINIC DERMATITIS (ACTINIC RETICULOID)

-rare condition characterized by itchy, pink-red, lichenified, eczematous plaques and papules
-usually in elderly men in areas of chronically sun-damaged skin
-frequently there is a history of another kind of dermatitis (contact, atopic) in preceding years

Histopathology
-**irregular** psoriasiform epidermis
-**preserved granular layer**
-**lymphocytic epidermal exocytosis** in **spongiotic vesicles** (unlike MF)
-dermal lymphocytic infiltrate with some atypical cells
-dermal fibrosis

SEBORRHEIC DERMATITIS

-common inflammatory dermatitis possibly related to overgrowth of/overreaction to *Malassezia furfur* yeast
-affects "seborrheic" (oily) areas (scalp, face, postauricular, presternal, intertriginous areas)
-infants can present with "cradle cap"
-adult presentation with ill-defined, pink-red patches with greasy scales
-more severe and more frequent in patients with HIV and Parkinson's disease
-dandruff (***pityriasis sicca***) is a type of seborrheic dermatitis

Histopathology
-ambiguous with psoriasiform and spongiotic features
-newer lesions show more chronic spongiotic dermatitis and older lesions are more psoriasiform
-**irregular** wavy **psoriasiform epidermis** with **hypogranulosis** and **variable** epidermal **spongiosis**
-epidermal **parakeratosis** with neutrophils
-parakeratosis commonly around follicular ostia

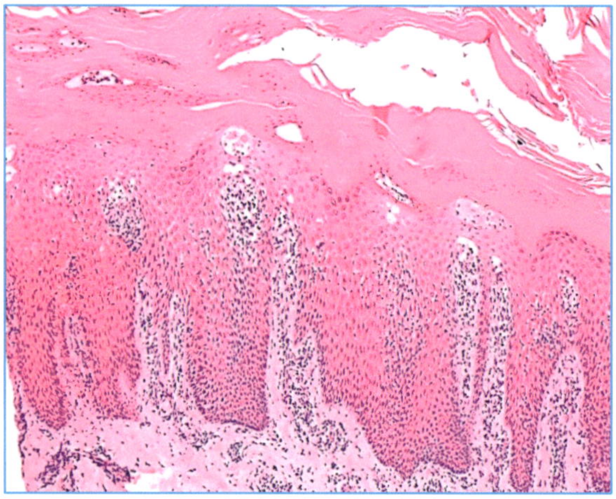

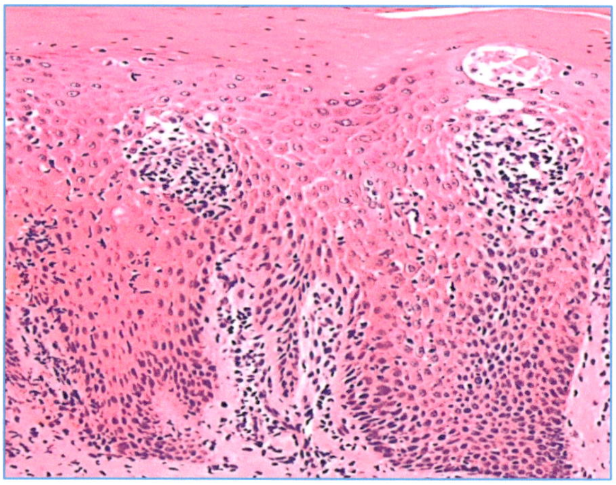

Actinic prurigo with irregular psoriasiform epidermis and epidermal lymphocytes within spongiotic vesicles

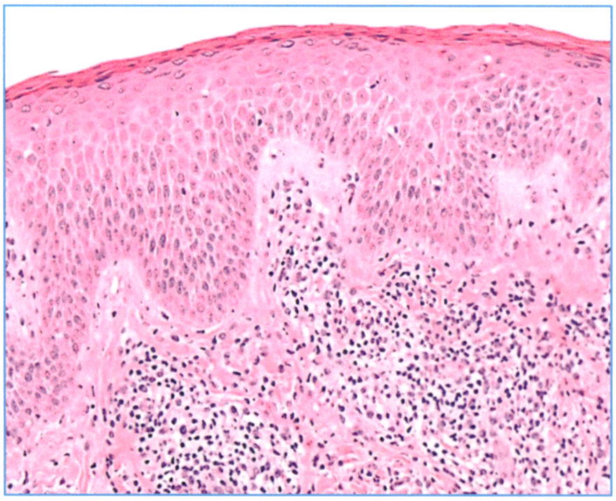

Seborrheic dermatitis with chronic spongiosis, parakeratosis, and diminished granular layer

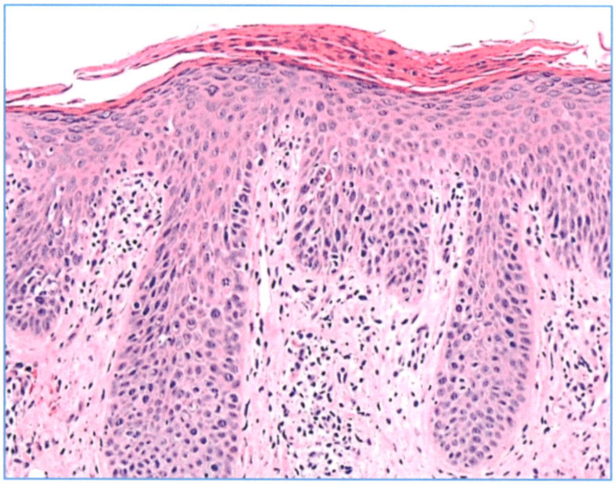

Seborrheic dermatitis with psoriasiform epidermis, parakeratosis, and hypogranulosis

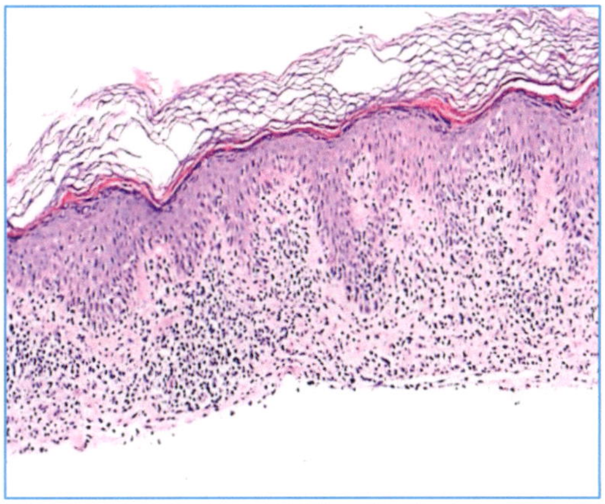

Large plaque parapsoriasis with epidermal lymphocytes

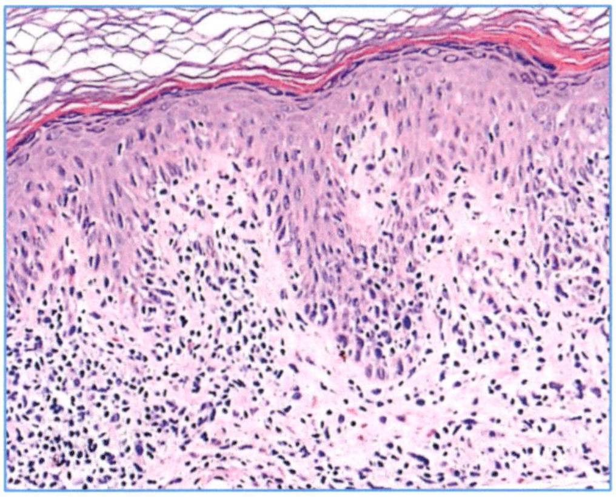

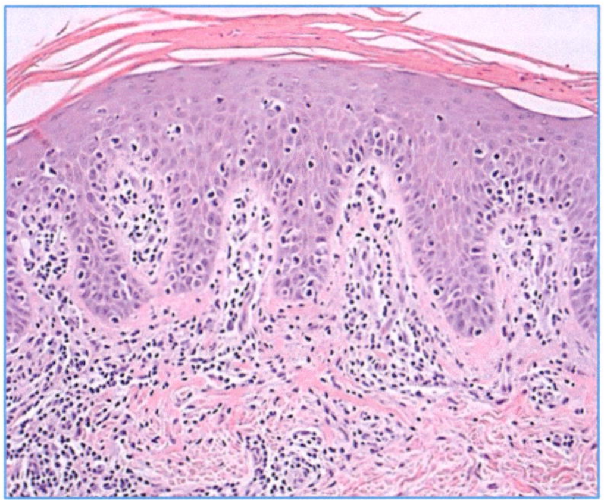

MF with prominent epidermal lymphocytes

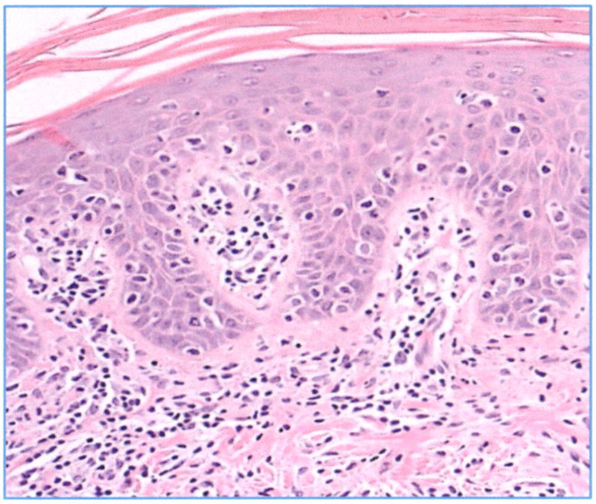

PARAPSORIASIS

Small plaque parapsoriasis
-umbrella term for debated entity which refers to a group of conditions characterized by chronic, pink, faintly scaly plaques (<5cm in diameter)
-lasts several months to years and can spontaneously resolve
-trunk, buttocks, and lower extremities (sun-protected area) are favorable locations
-benign condition that rarely if ever progresses into mycosis fungoides

Large plaque parapsoriasis (poikiloderma atrophicans vasculare)
-irregularly-shaped, scaly, large (>5cm), salmon-colored, thin plaques
-favor sun-protected skin areas
-considered a generally premalignant condition with an indolent chronic course that may progress into mycosis fungoides
-does not resolve without treatment

Histopathology

Small plaque parapsoriasis
-non-specific histology
-mild spongiotic dermatitis with sparse perivascular lymphocytic infiltrates

Large plaque parapsoriasis
-resembles early mycosis fungoides
-mild **psoriasiform hyperplasia** with focal parakeratosis
-**focal epidermal exocytosis of lymphocytes**
-variable dermal perivascular or "band-like" lymphocytic infiltrate

MYCOSIS FUNGOIDES

-described in more detail under the chapter on lymphoproliferative disorders, but is discussed here as it can have a psoriasiform pattern
-clinically presents as ill-defined, large patches (>3cm) of varying hue with fine scaling
-later may become thickened, forming red to violaceous plaques or nodules

Histopathology
-in patch and plaque stage of MF the epidermis may appear psoriasiform
-**lymphocytes** surrounded by a clear halo are aligned **along the epidermo-dermal junction**
-lymphocytic aggregates (**Pautrier's microabscesses**) can be present in the epidermis
-in plaque stage there is a denser dermal infiltrate

Psoriasiform dermatitis

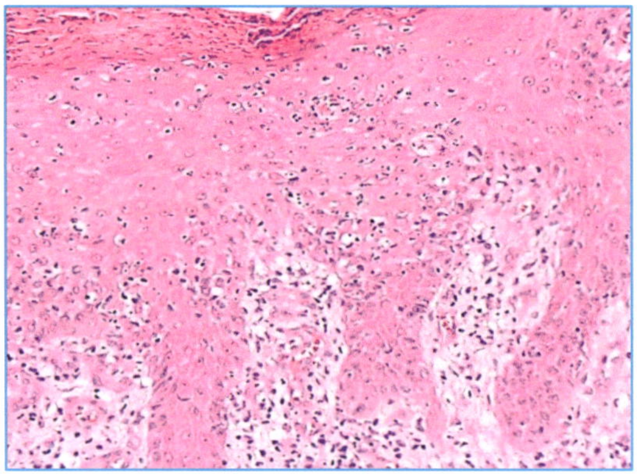

Condyloma lata with epidermal neutrophils and dermal plasma cells

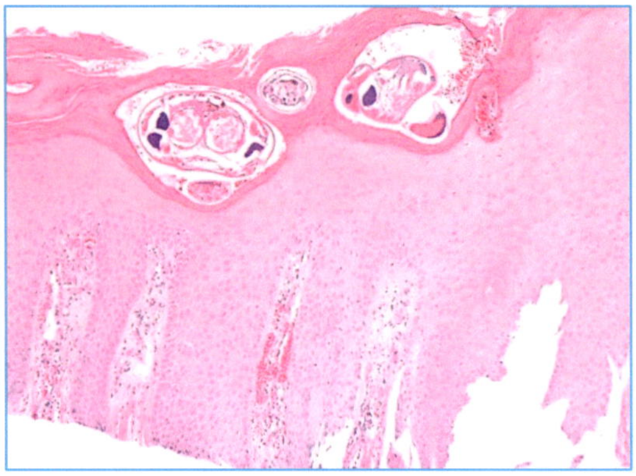

Norwegian scabies mites in the stratum corneum

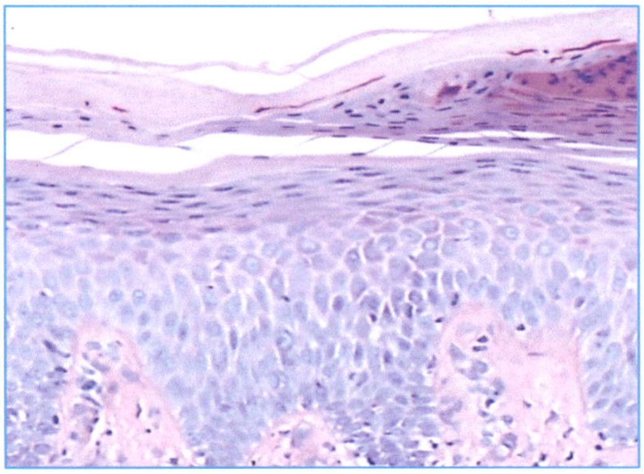

Tinea with PAS stain outlining fungal elements

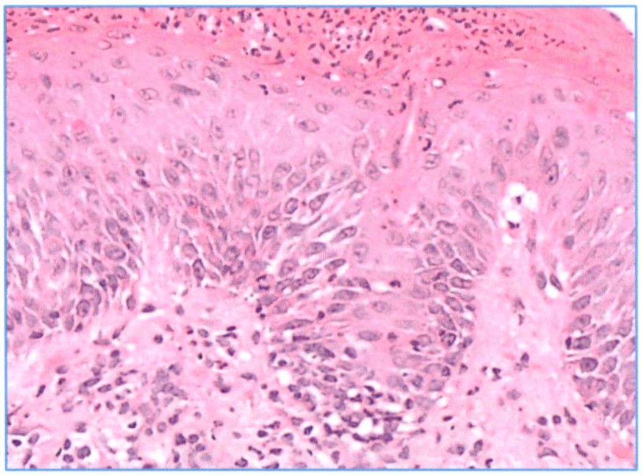

" Guttate-like" psoriasiform GvHD with interface vacuolar changes

Secondary syphilis, scabies, tinea, and GvHD have multiple clinical and histological presentations and are discussed in more details in the infectious diseases and the vacuolar interface dermatitis chapters.

However, because histologically **they might present as psoriasiform dermatitis,** they are discussed here for comparison with other psoriasiform disorders.

CONDYLOMA LATA

-variant of secondary syphilis
-presents as moist, flesh-colored papules with a verrucous surface resembling genital wart

Histopathology

-irregular psoriasiform epidermis
-characteristic **intracorneal neutrophilic pustules**
-prominent **dermal plasmocytic inflammation**

SCABIES

Two clinical variants with a psoriasiform appearance:

Nodular scabies

-red-pink or brown nodules that persist after scabies treatment
-usually in children

Crusted or Norwegian scabies

-marked hyperkeratosis with scaling and crusting due to severe infection with large number of scabies mites

Histopathology

-irregular hyperkeratotic psoriasiform epidermis with mild spongiosis
-intraepidermal burrow with **scabies mite or egg remnants,** similar to **"pig tails"**
-dermal lymphocytes with numerous eosinophils

TINEA CORPORIS

-dermatophyte infection in intertriginous skin area commonly demonstrate psoriasiform dermatitis

Histopathology

-irregular psoriasiform epidermis with adjacent epidermal spongiosis
-focal parakeratosis and intracorneal neutrophils
-**fungal hyphae in stratum corneum**

PSORIASIFORM GvHD

-rare form of chronic GvHD
-typically seen 60 or more days after transplantation
-clinically resembles guttate psoriasis

Histopathology

-**vague psoriasiform epidermis** with **intracorneal neutrophils** ("guttate-like")
-**interface vacuolar changes** underlying intracorneal pustule

Chapter 3

HOW TO APPROACH PSORIASIFORM DERMATITIS

IF EPIDERMIS IS GENUINELY PSORIASIFORM

GRANULAR LAYER IS

ABSENT	
-psoriasis vulgaris	focal neutrophils in stratum corneum
-pustular psoriasis	intraepidermal neutrophilic pustule
DIMINISHED	
-ILVEN	alternating parakeratosis
-condyloma lata	epidermal neutrophils + dermal plasma cells
-psoriasiform drug reaction	dermal eosinophils
-seborrheic dermatitis	spongiosis + focal parakeratosis
INCREASED	
-lichen simplex chronicus	uniform epidermal papillomatosis
-prurigo nodule	irregular epidermal papillomatosis
NORMAL	
-actinic reticuloid	spongiosis + epidermal lymphocytes
-tinea	epidermal neutrophils + hyphae
-scabies	mites

IF EPIDERMIS IS PSEUDOPSORIASIFORM AND UNDULATED

-guttate psoriasis	mounds of parakeratosis with neutrophils
-GvHD	mounds of parakeratosis with neutrophils; hx. of transplant
-pityriasis rubra pilaris	alternating and shoulder parakeratosis
-mycosis fungoides	prominent epidermal lymphocytes
-parapsoriasis	epidermal lymphocytes

Psoriasiform dermatitis

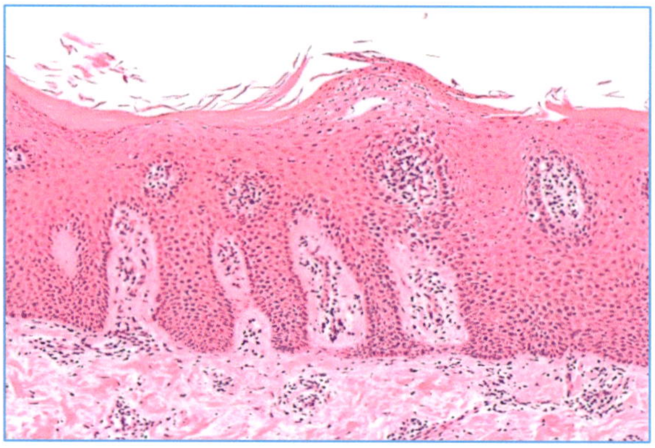

Psoriasis with no granular layer

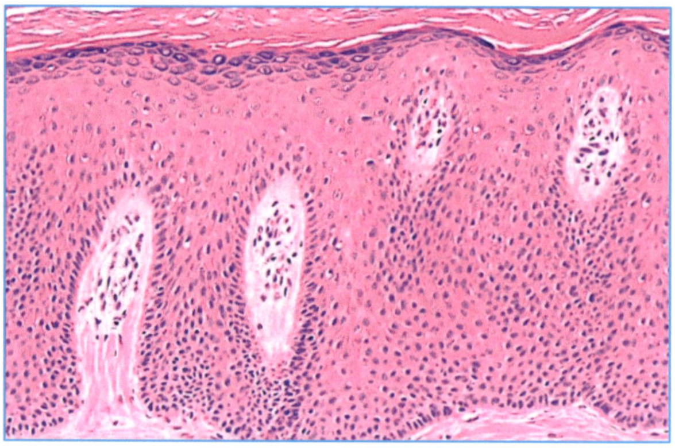

LSC with prominent granular layer

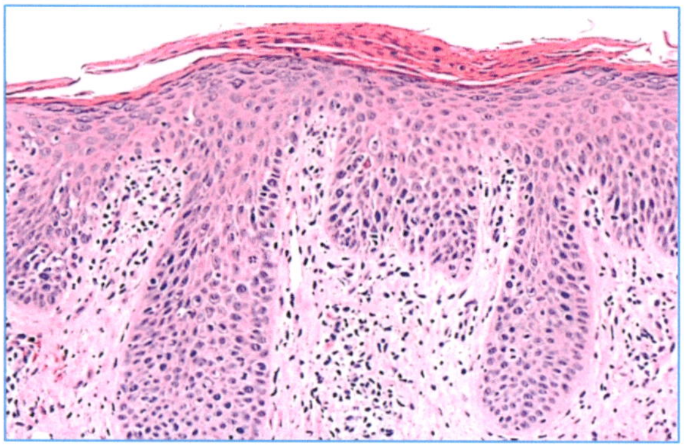

Seborrheic dermatitis with parakeratosis and diminished granular layer

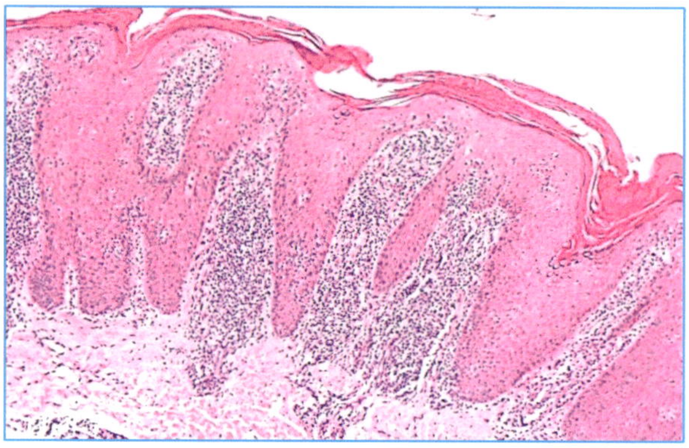

ILVEN with alternating parakeratosis and diminished granular layer

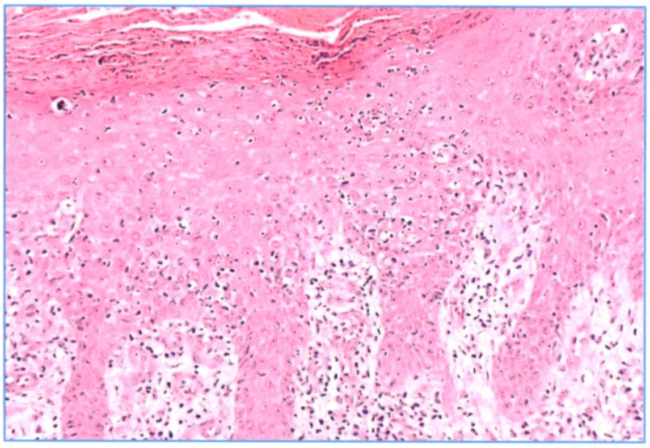

Condyloma lata with intraepidermal neutrophils and dermal plasma cells

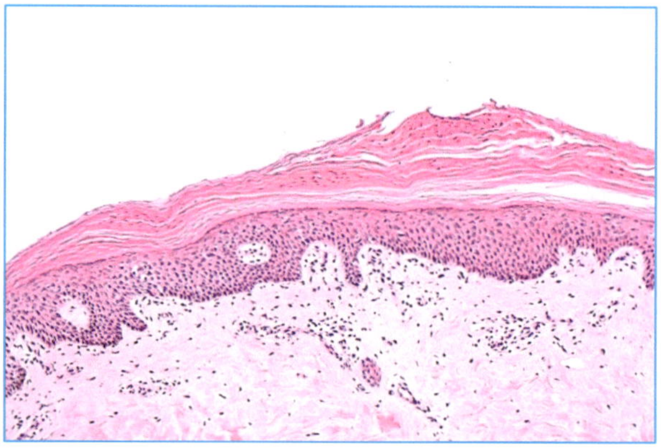

PRP with wavy epidermis and alternating parakeratosis

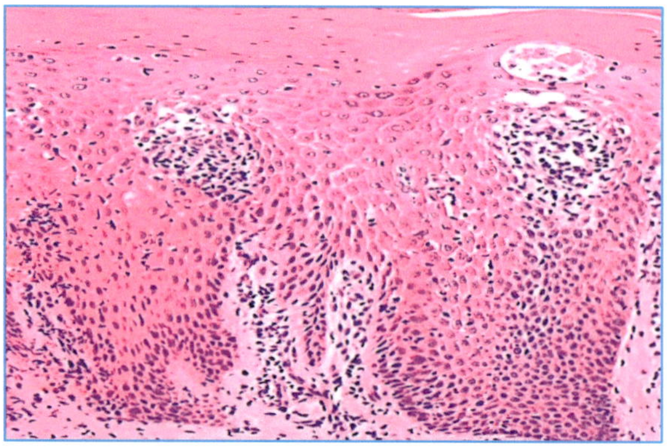

Chronic actinic dermatitis with irregular psoriasifom epidermis, spongiosis and epidermal lymphocytes within vesicles

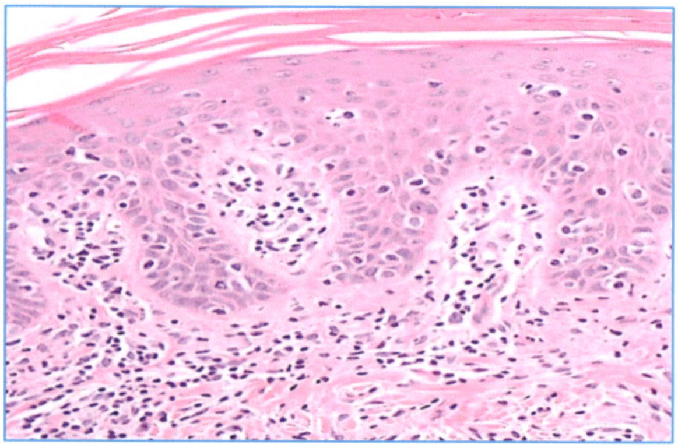

MF with prominent epidermal lymphocytes

Chapter 4

LICHENOID INTERFACE DERMATITIS

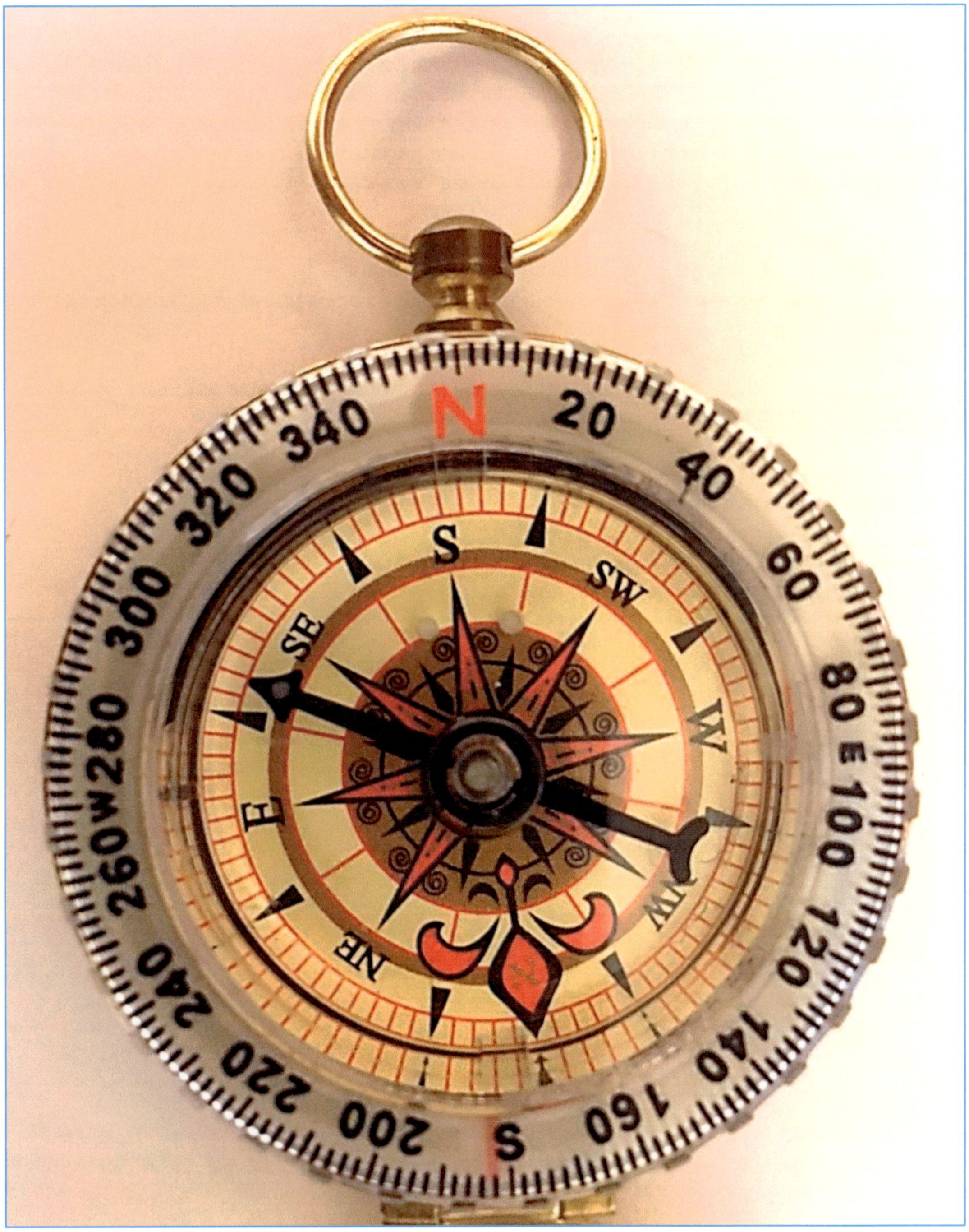

Lichenoid interface dermatitis

LICHEN PLANUS

-common pruritic, mucocutaneous disorder of middle-aged adults
-flat topped, violaceous, shiny papules with overlying lacy white pattern (**Wickham's striae**)
-**P**ruritic, **P**urple, **P**olygonal **P**apules (**PPPP**)
-lesions tend to be symmetrical with predilection for wrists, hands, forearms, ankles, and genitalia
-oral involvement in 70% of patients

Clinical variants

Hypertrophic- well-defined thickened purple plaques on the shin; more common in African American
Actinic (atrophic) lichen planus- UVB induced atrophic papules on sun exposed areas, particularly dorsal hands and arms
Bullous- blisters on lower legs which arise in sites of existing lichen planus
Lichen planopilaris- keratotic follicular papules leading to scaring alopecia
Oral lichen planus- milky white papules in **"lace-like"** pattern

Histopathology

-lichen planus is the epitome of lichenoid interface dermatitis
-**linear "band-like" dermal lymphocytic** infiltrate that **abuts epidermo-dermal junction**
-hyperkeratotic **epidermis without parakeratosis**
-**V-shaped hypergranulosis** and "**saw teeth**" pattern of **rete ridges**
-**interface vacuolar** changes and individual necrotic keratinocytes **(Civatte bodies)**
-dermal pigment incontinence usually seen

Variants

Hypertrophic type- LP with hyperkeratosis and acanthosis
Actinic type- LP with atrophic epidermis
Bullous type- LP with subepidermal blister
Lichen planopilaris- is discussed in the alopecia chapter
Oral LP- LP but **with parakeratosis** and no granular layer

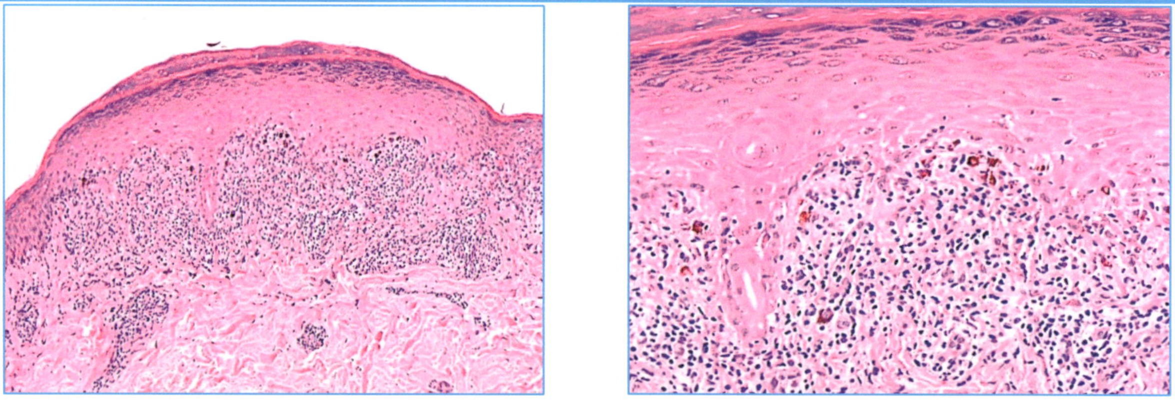

Hypertrophic lichen planus with V-shaped hypergranulosis and "saw teeth" pattern of rete ridges

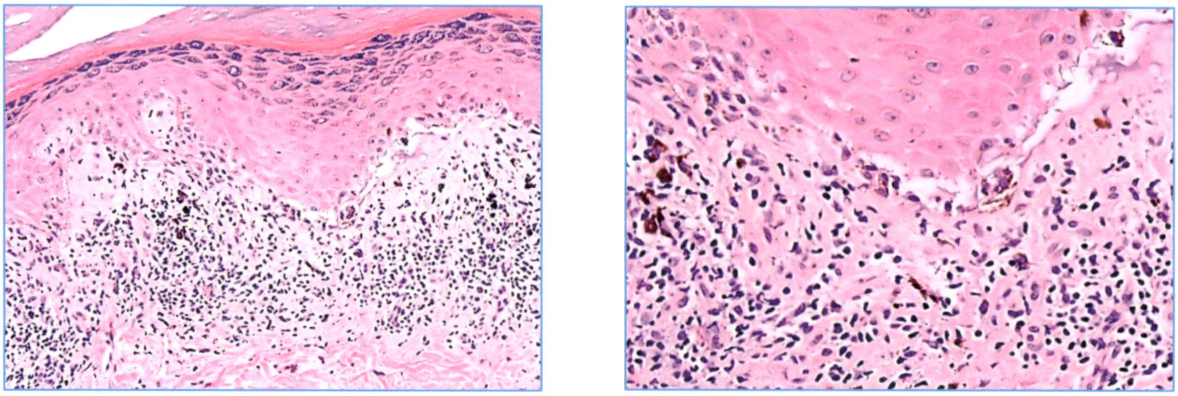

Lichen planus with characteristic granular layer, "band-like" lymphocytes, and interface vacuolar changes

Chapter 4

LICHEN PLANUS-LIKE KERATOSIS (LICHENOID KERATOSIS)

-favors chest and back of middle-aged adults
-solitary, discrete mildly pruritic violaceous or pigmented papule
-usually biopsied to rule out basal cell carcinoma or squamous cell carcinoma and not lichen planus

Histopathology

-almost identical to lichen planus
-**adjacent solar lentigo** is commonly seen
-presence of **parakeratosis**, dermal red blood cells and occasional eosinophils favor LPLK over LP

LICHENOID GvHD

-chronic form of chronic GvHD usually 100 or more days after transplant
-slowly progressive rash on periorbital skin, ears, palms, and soles resembling lichen planus
-histopathology is **identical to lichen planus**

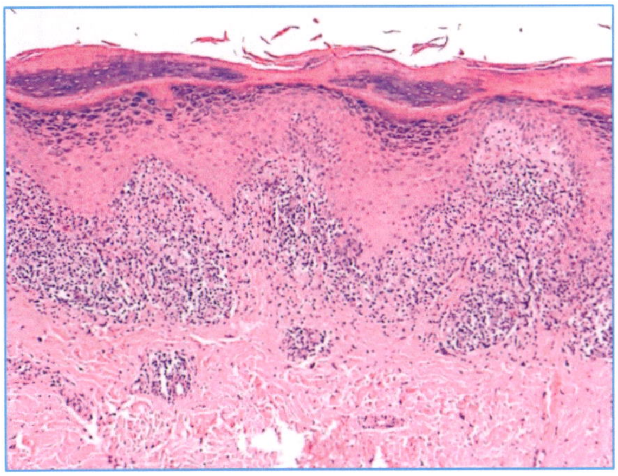

Lichenoid GvHD is identical to lichen planus

ZOON'S BALANITIS

-middle-aged to elderly individuals
-sharply defined orange-red plaque/patch
-penis is most common site (*Zoon's balanitis)*
-vulvar lesions are extremely rare (*Zoon's vulvitis*)
-lips can occasionally be involved (*Zoon's cheilitis*)

Histopathology

-mildly spongiotic epidermis with few neutrophils
-dense, lichenoid, "band-like" infiltrate made of **plasma cells** with admixed lymphocytes

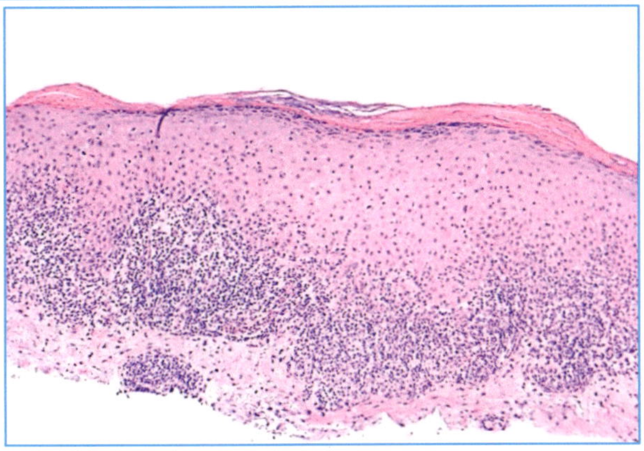

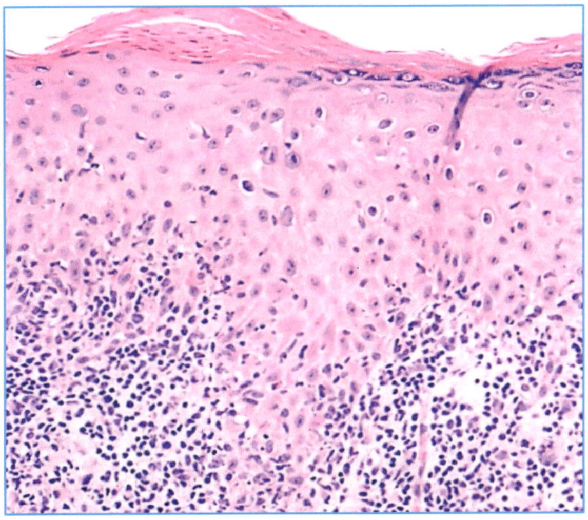

LPLK with lichenoid dermal infiltrate and focal parakeratosis

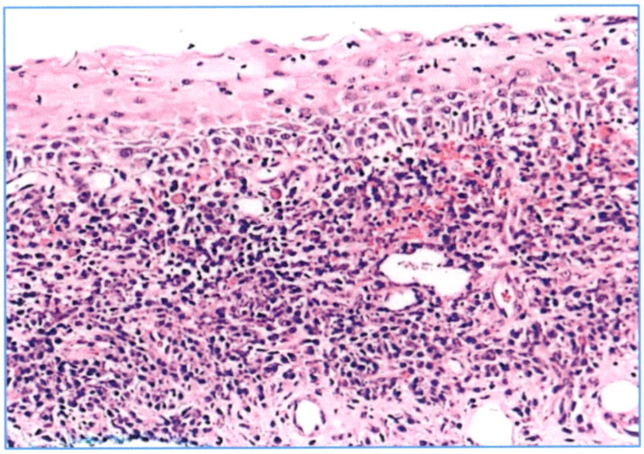

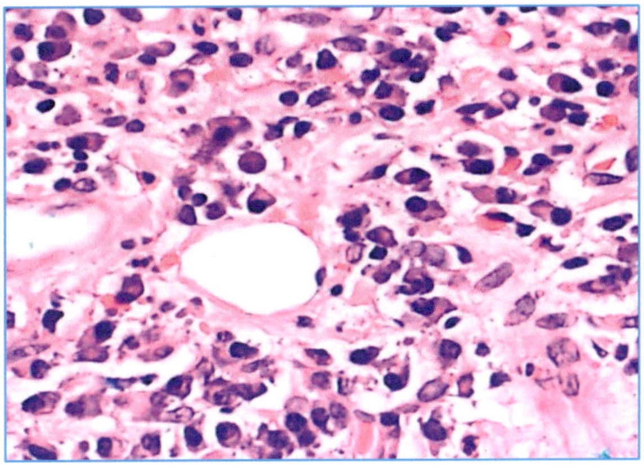

Zoon's balanitis with numerous plasma cells

Lichenoid interface dermatitis

LICHEN NITIDUS

-mostly in children and young adult males
-multiple, grouped, small, flat-topped or umbilicated skin-colored papules
-usually hypopigmented in dark skinned individuals
-predilection for genitalia, lower abdomen, dorsal hands, wrists

Histopathology

-thin epidermis with **"claw-like"** epidermal collarette around dermal inflammatory **ball,** so-called **"ball and claws" appearance**
-dermal inflammation consists of **more histiocytes** then lymphocytes

LICHEN STRIATUS

-favors extremities of young girls (average 4 years of age) with atopic dermatitis
-more common in spring and summer
-lichenoid mildly pruritic papules in linear Blaschkoid distribution
-spontaneously resolves (3-24 months)
-postinflammatory hypopigmentation is common

Histopathology

-superficial part is **similar to lichen planus**
-infiltrate is usually less dense than in lichen planus
-epidermis usually has less dyskeratotic keratinocytes compared to lichen planus
-additional **deep perieccrine/perivascular lymphocytic infiltrate**

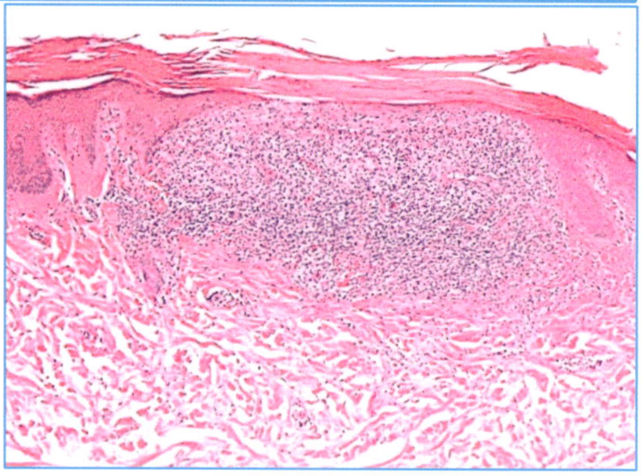

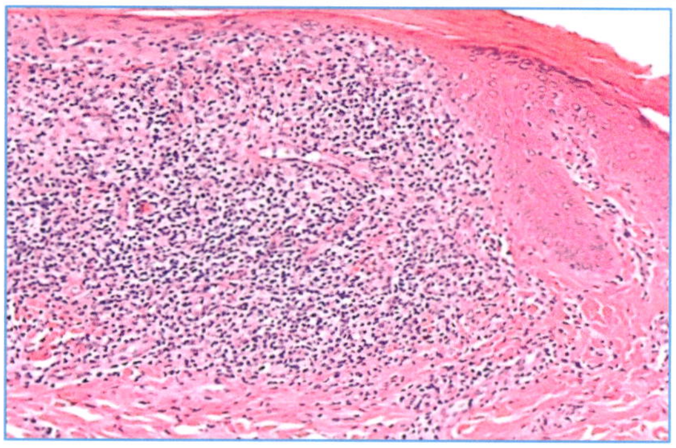

Lichen nitidus with "ball and claws"

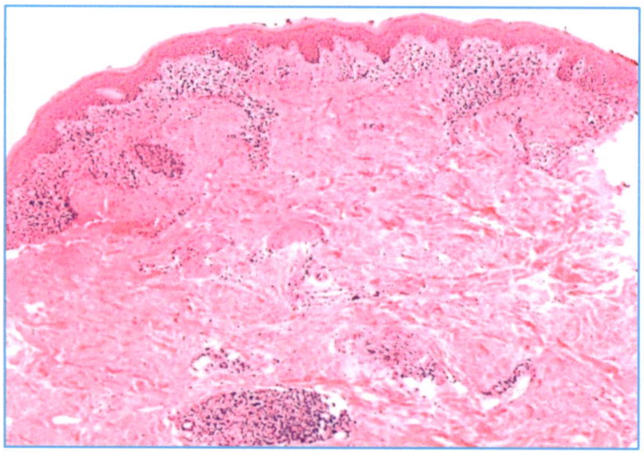

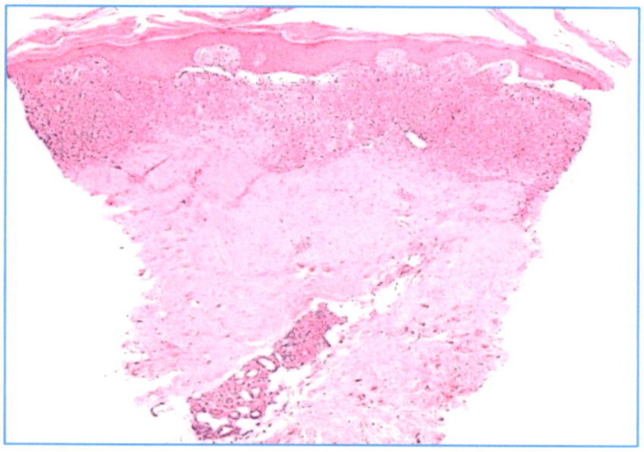

Lichen striatus with hyperkeratotic epidermis and "band-like" lymphocytic inflammation resembling lichen planus

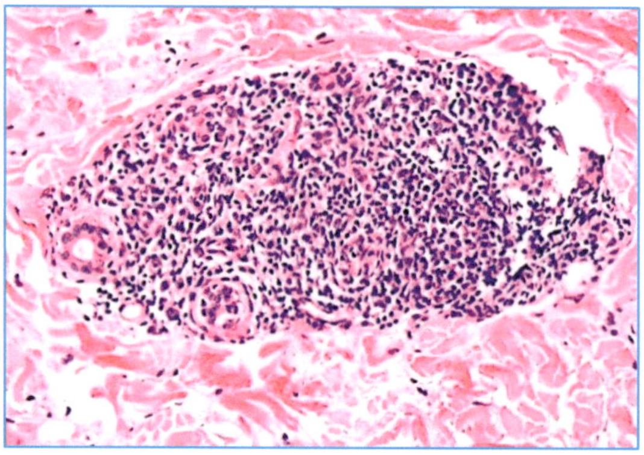

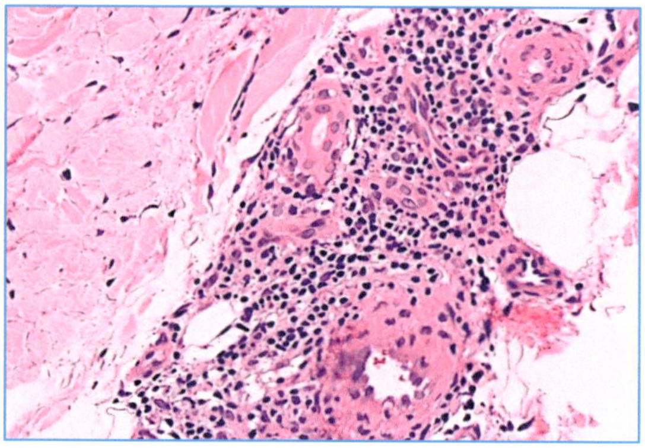

Lichen striatus has deep perieccrine and perivascular lymphocytic inflammation

LICHEN AUREUS

-uncommon, chronic type of pigmented purpuric dermatitis
-localized rust-colored macule, papules or plaques resembling a bruise with lichenoid papules
-slightly raised petechiae are common
-predilection for feet and lower legs of younger individuals or children

Histopathology

-normal epidermis with dermal lichenoid lymphocytic infiltrate
-usually the **Grenz zone** separates epidermis from lymphocytic infiltrate
-dermal **RBC extravasation**
-hemosiderin in older lesions

Note: Histopathology is the same as in pigmented purpuric dermatosis of **Gougerot and Blum** (see the vasculitis chapter). Differentiate them clinically.

LICHEN SCLEROSUS ET ATROPHICUS

-chronic, atrophic mucocutaneous disorder
-affects anogenital area (90%) but not exclusively (trunk, neck)
-sharply-demarcated, white, atrophic papules and plaques
-occasional follicular plugging and petechia/purpura
-pruritus and soreness are common
-most common in post-menopausal women
-also common in prepubertal girls
-less common in men (*balanitis xerotica obliterans*) where can cause phimosis

Histopathology

-**atrophic epidermis** with hyperkeratosis
-subepidermal edema with **sclerosis**
-subepidermal split occasionally present
-**vague lichenoid or patchy lymphocytic infiltrate** underneath dermal sclerosis
-it is called **red-white -blue** lesion although under microscope it is **purple-pink-blue**

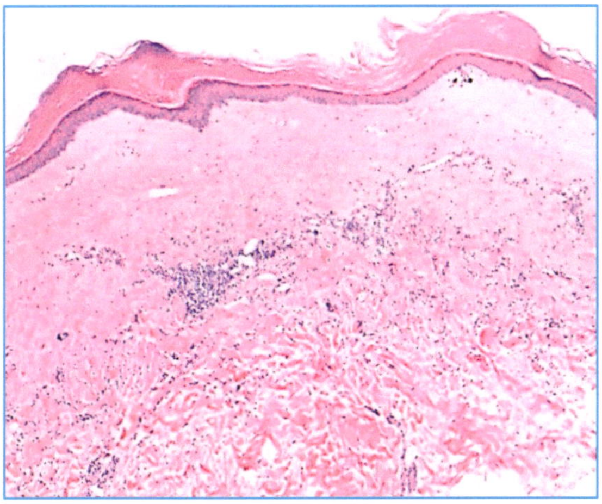
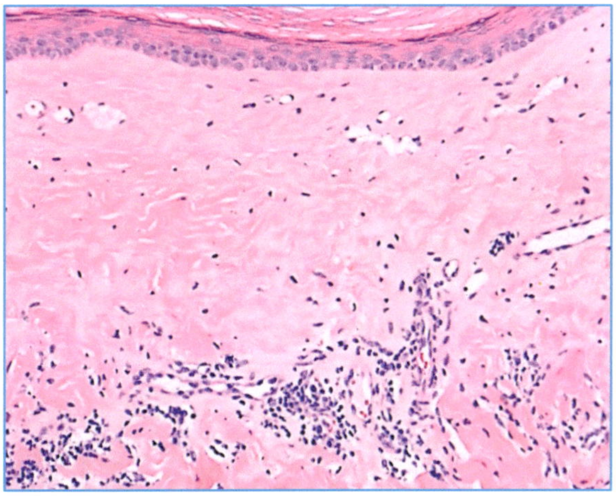

Lichen sclerosus at atrophicus with 3 layers in different colors

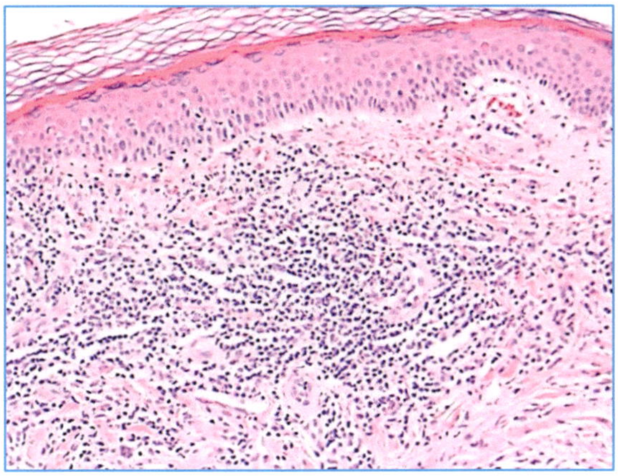
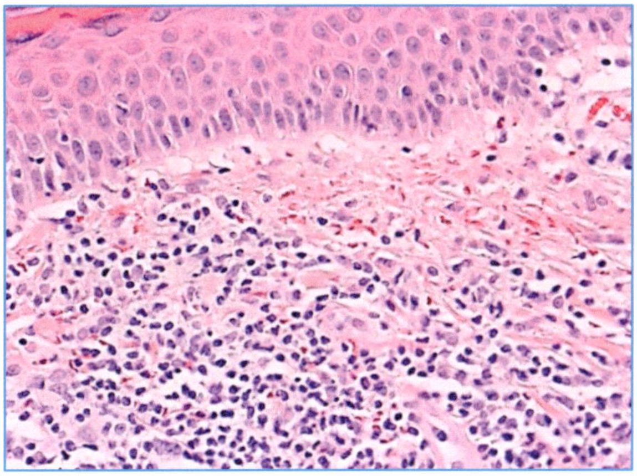

Lichen aureous with perivascular lymphocytes and RBCs

Lichenoid interface dermatitis

PITYRIASIS LICHENOIDES ET VARIOLIFORMIS ACUTA	PITYRIASIS LICHENOIDES CHRONICA

PLEVA and PLC are probably **two ends of the same disease.**
PLEVA is at the **acute** end and **PLC** on the **chronic end of the spectrum**.

PITYRIASIS LICHENOIDES ET VARIOLIFORMIS ACUTA

-recurrent self-resolving lesions
-acute onset favoring younger adults
-crop of vesicles and pustules that become hemorrhagic and necrotic
-resolves over several weeks with varioliform pitting scars resembling chicken pox
-widespread distribution (trunk, buttock, proximal extremities)

Histopathology
-epidermis with focal **parakeratosis**, variable number of **necrotic keratinocytes** and lymphocytic exocytosis
-variable "**V-shaped**" linear superficial and tapering deep perivascular **lymphocytic infiltrate**
-**interface vacuolar changes**
-dermal **red blood cell extravasation**

PITYRIASIS LICHENOIDES CHRONICA

-chronic disease that persists for years
-usually in children and young adults
-inner aspects of the limbs are favored sites
-purple macules that become red brown papules and plaques with adherent scale
-resolves with hypopigmentation

Histopathology
-**mild variant of PLEVA**
-**lymphocytic infiltrate is less dense**, more superficial and **patchy**
-**interface vacuolar changes**
-lymphocytic exocytosis is minimal and **only occasional necrotic keratinocytes** are present
-**minimal or no red blood cell extravasation**

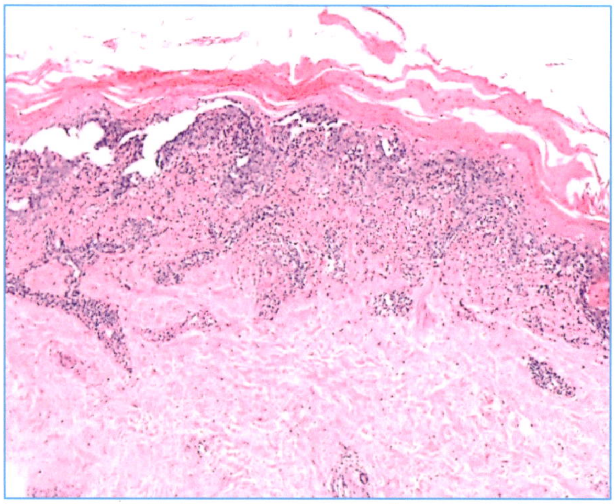
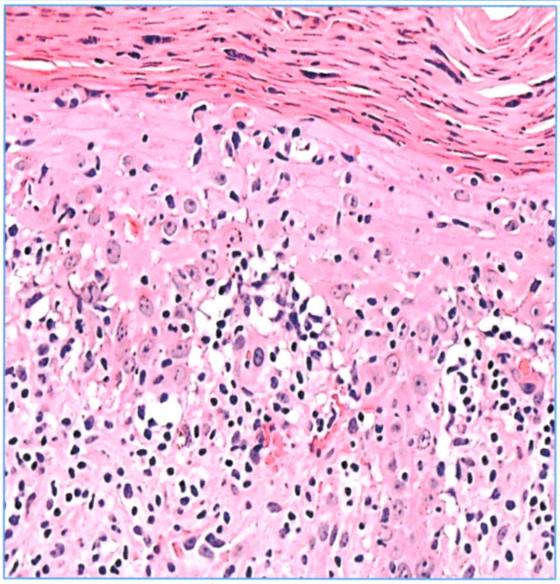

PLEVA with parakeratosis, scattered necrotic keratinocytes, interface vacuoles, V-shaped inflammation, and dermal RBCs

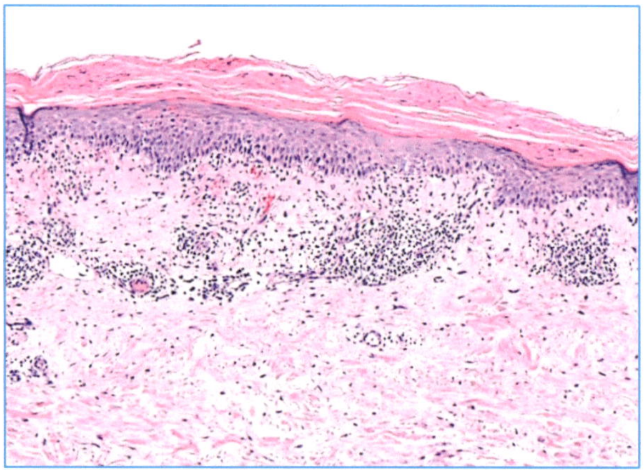
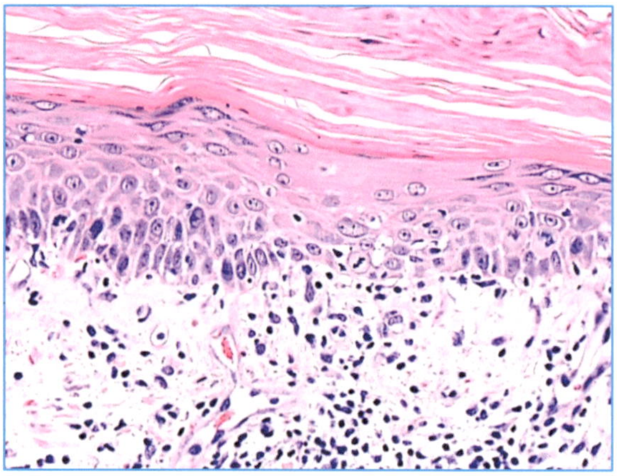

PLC with focal parakeratosis, patchy inflammation, and mild interface vacuolar changes

Chapter 4

HOW TO APPROACH LICHENOID DERMATITIS

LINE OR BALL OF DERMAL LYMPHOCYTES WILL GET YOUR ATTENTION FIRST
DERMAL VACUOLAR CHANGES ARE PRESENT BUT ARE SUBTLE

IF YOU SEE SUBEPIDERAL BALL OF LYMPHOCYTES

-lichen nitidus	epidermal claws surround the ball of lymphocytes "ball and claws"

IF YOU SEE "BAND-LIKE" LYMPHOCYTES + DEEP PERIECCRINE LYMPHOCYTES

-lichen striatus

IF YOU SEE "BAND-LIKE" LYMPHOCYTES + DERMAL RBCS

-lichen aureous

IF YOU SEE "BAND-LIKE" LYMPHOCYTES + DERMAL EOSINOPHILS

-lichenoid drug reaction

IF YOU SEE "BAND-LIKE" LYMPHOCYES WITH NUMEROUS PLASMA CELLS

-Zoon's balanitis	clinically will be located on penis

IF YOU SEE DERMAL "WEDGE-SHAPED" LYMPHOCYTES
+ DERMAL RBCS + NECROTIC KERATINOCYTES

-PLEVA-PLC	lymphocytic infiltrate is more "V-shaped" in PLEVA and patchy in PLC

IF YOU SEE SCLEROTIC DERMIS WITH DEEPER DERMAL LYMPHOCYTIC BAND

-LSeA	3 colors "red, white, blue" atrophic epidermis sclerotic dermis lymphocytic band

IF YOU SEE "BAND-LIKE" LYMPHOCYTIC INFILTRATE, NOS
DIFFERENTIATE THEM CLINICALLY

-lichen planus	multiple itchy lesions
-LPLK	single lesion; typically biopsied to rule out NCSC
-GvHD	3-6 months after transplant

Lichenoid interface dermatitis

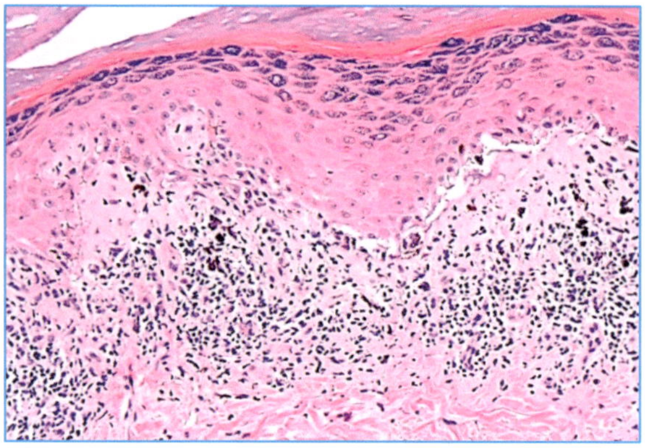

Lichen planus with wavy hypergranulosis

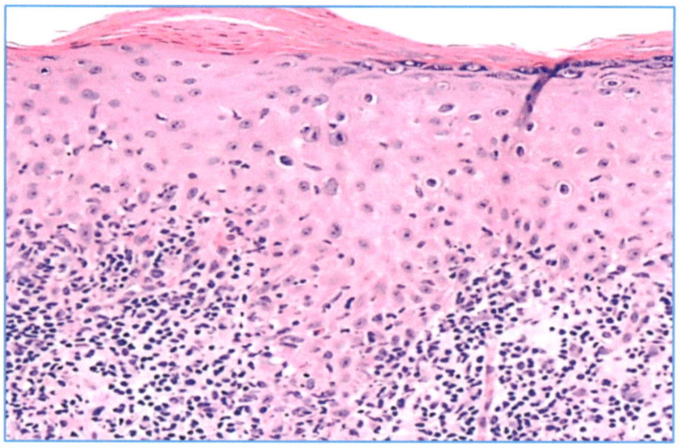

LPLK with focal parakeratosis

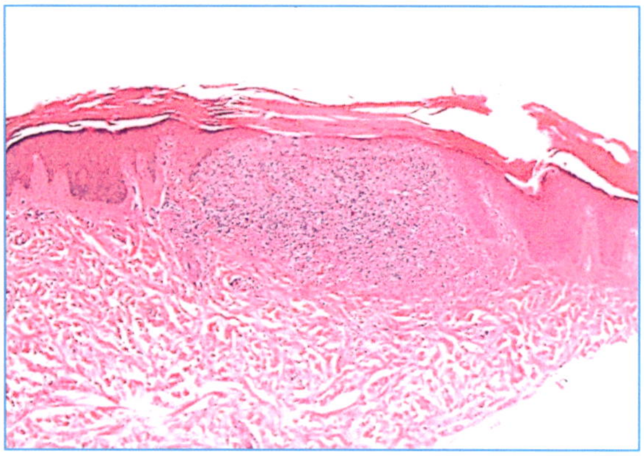

Lichen nitidus with dermal ball of lymphocytes

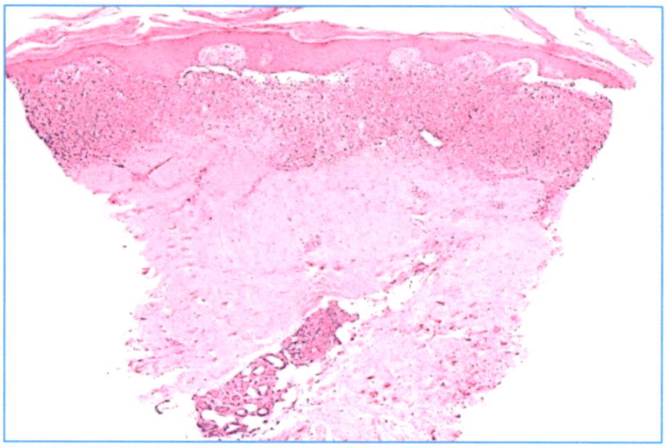

Lichen striatus with deep perieccrine inflammation

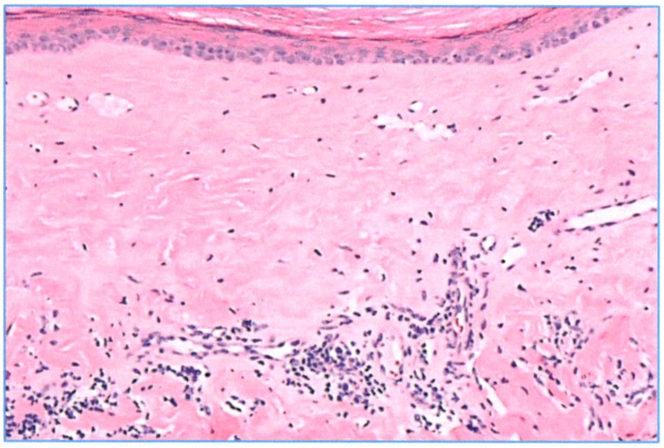

LSeA with horizontal layers in 3 colors

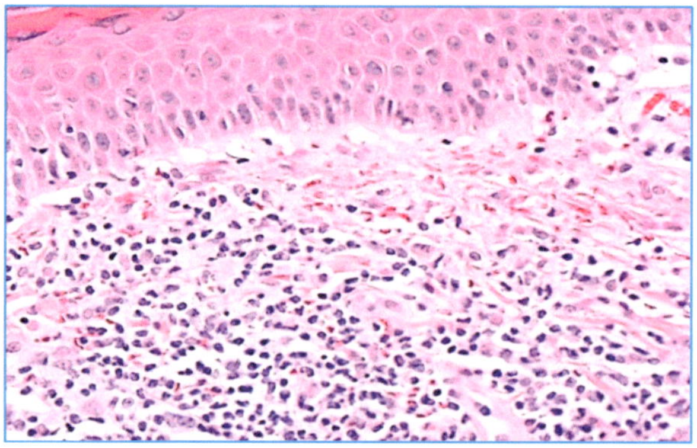

Lichen aureous with dermal red blood cells

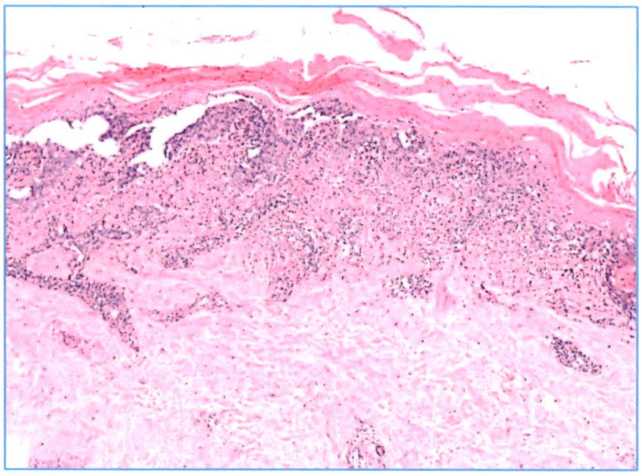

PLEVA with "V-shaped" inflammation

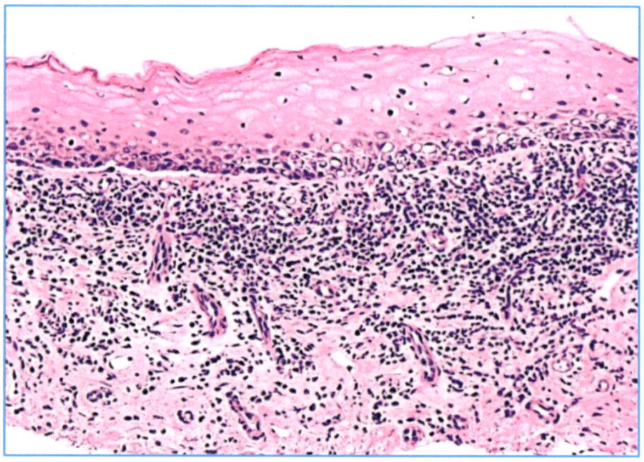

Zoon's balanitis with linear infiltrate of plasma cells

Chapter 5

VACUOLAR INTERFACE DERMATITIS

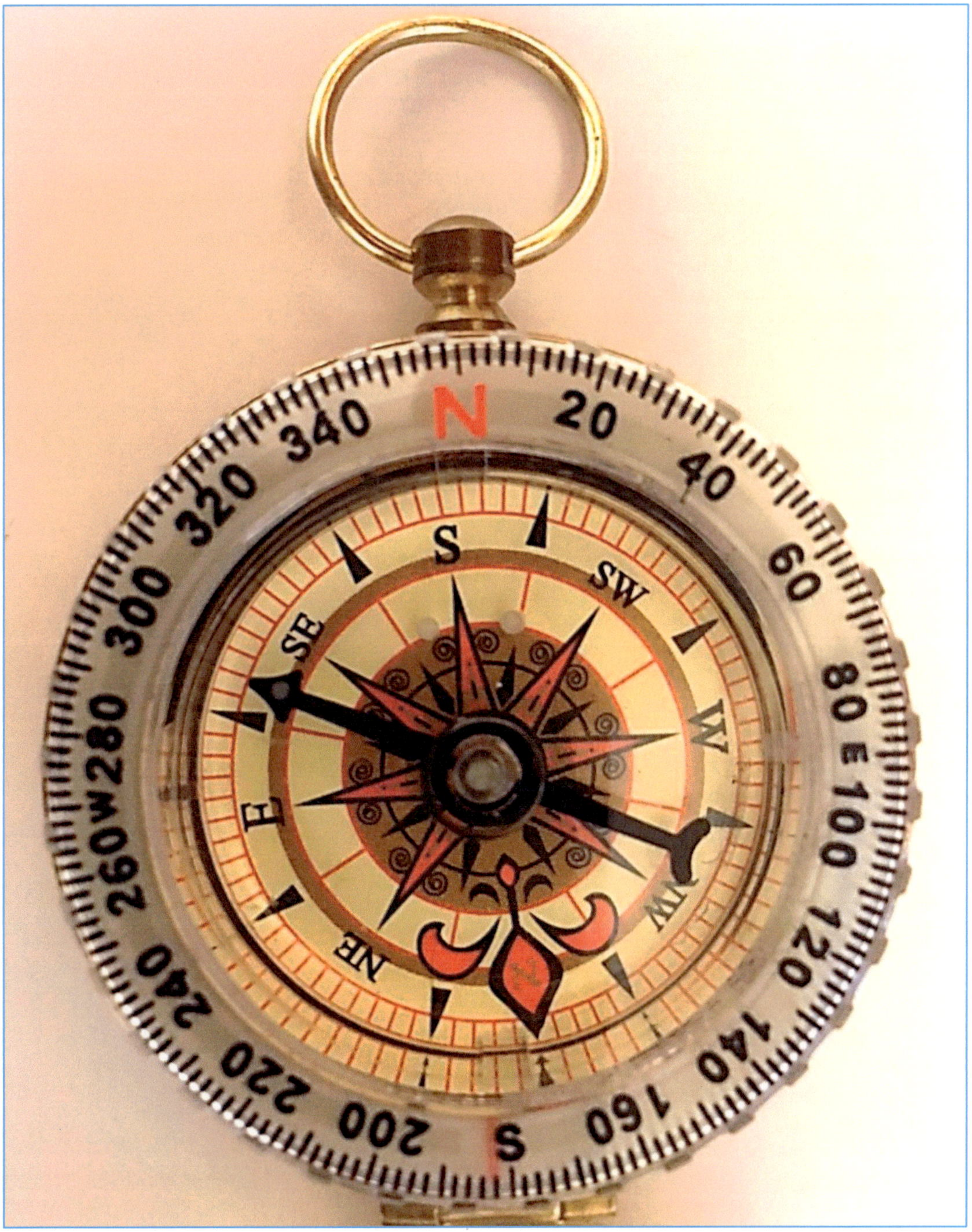

Vacuolar interface dermatitis

LUPUS ERYTHEMATOSUS

-chronic, autoimmune condition which can be systemic or skin-limited
-usually more common in women and African Americans

Acute cutaneous lupus erythematosus

-cutaneous form **most associated** with **systemic lupus erythematosus** (musculoskeletal, renal, pulmonary, CNS, and/or cardiovascular involvement)
-"butterfly-shaped", bright red erythema on nasal bridge and cheeks sparing the **melolabial folds** (in contrast to dermatomyositis)
-papules, scale and erosions may develop

Subacute cutaneous lupus erythematosus

-less than half of the patients have systemic disease
-annular or psoriasiform well-demarcated plaques with central clearing
-tendency for lesions to coalesce and form retiform pattern
-usually on lateral face (sparing central part), "V" of the chest, back, upper extremities

Chronic cutaneous lupus erythematosus with several variants

Discoid lupus erythematosus (most common chronic type)

-rare systemic involvement (5-20% of patients)
-sharply marginated, scaly, atrophic red plaques on sun exposed areas (scalp, nose, cheeks, ears, lower lip)
-follicular plugging is present

Tumid lupus

-indurated annular plaques favoring trunk and face
-overlying epidermis is normal

Chilblain lupus erythematosus

-chronic, cold precipitated papules and plaques on fingertips, tips of ears, heels

Lupus panniculitis (lupus profundus)

-deep, non-tender subcutaneous nodules discussed in the panniculitis chapter
-upper trunk, upper arm, face are common locations

Histopathology

-lupus erythematosus is the **epitome of vacuolar interface dermatitis**
-**vacuolar interface "bubbly" changes, focal necrotic keratinocytes,** mild or patchy dermal lymphocytic inflammation, and mildy increased dermal mucin are hallmarks

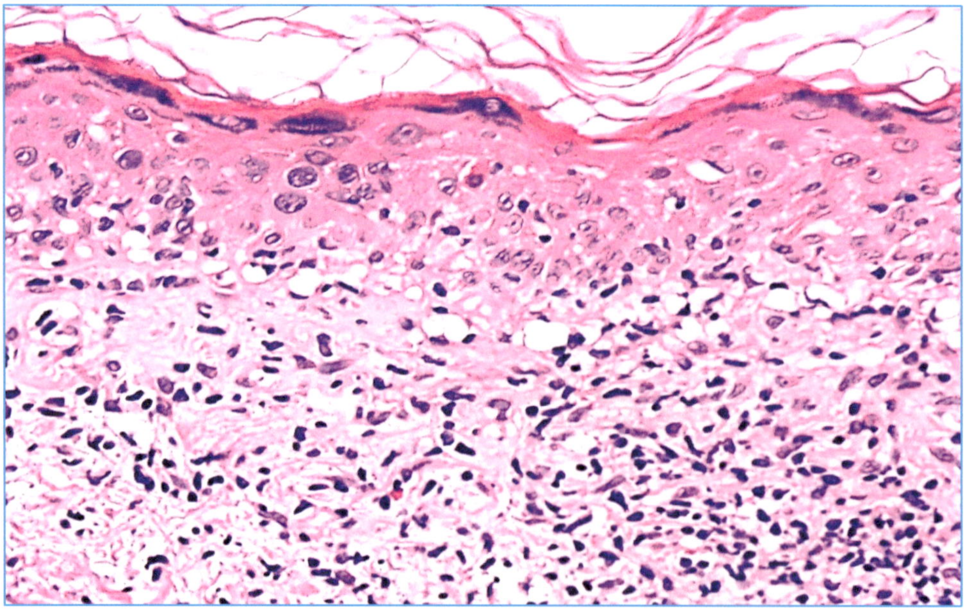

Interface vacuolar changes and focal necrotic keratinocytes

ACUTE CUTANEOUS LUPUS ERYTHEMATOSUS (ACLE)
SUBACUTE CUTANEOUS LUPUS ERYTHEMATOSUS (SCLE)

Histopathology is almost identical and clinical correlation is necessary

-changes in ACLE are more subtle than in SCLE
-atrophic epidermis with **focal interface vacuolar changes** (more in SCLE)
-**occasional necrotic keratinocytes** (more in SCLE)
-increased **dermal mucin** (more in SCLE)
-mild patchy perivascular and interstitial lymphocytic infiltrate (more in SCLE)

ACLE ↓ **SCLE ↓**

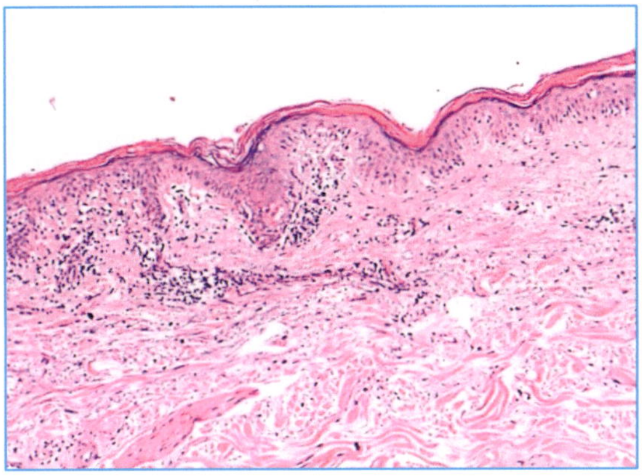
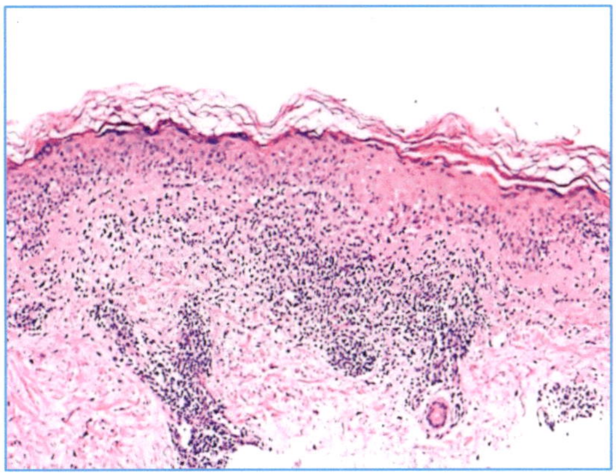

Vacuolar interface changes are suggestive at low magnification

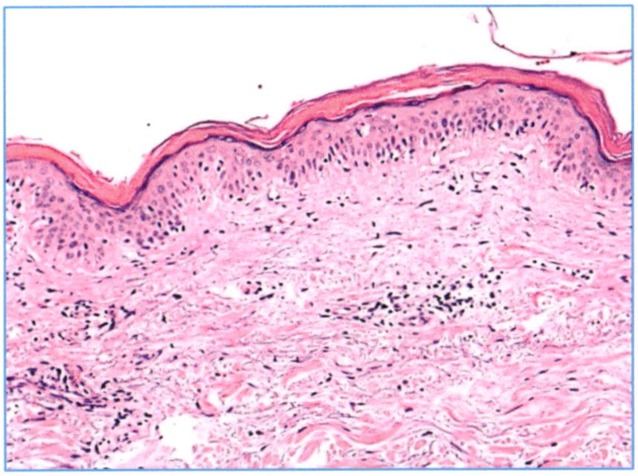
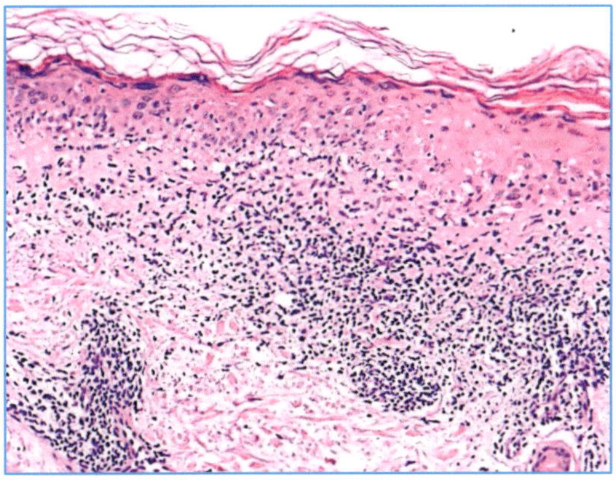

Dermal mucin and lymphocytic inflammation can be appreciated at medium magnification

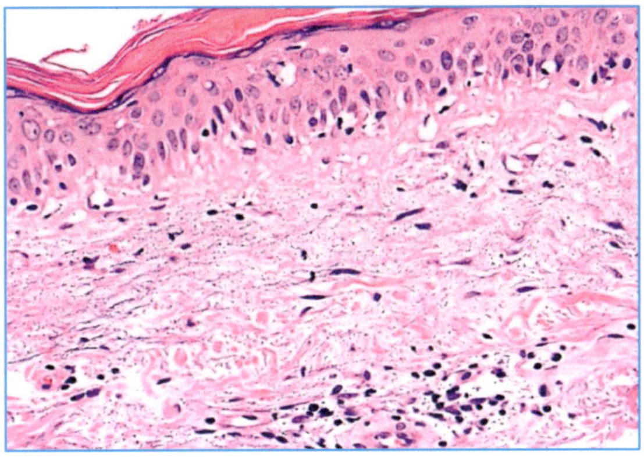
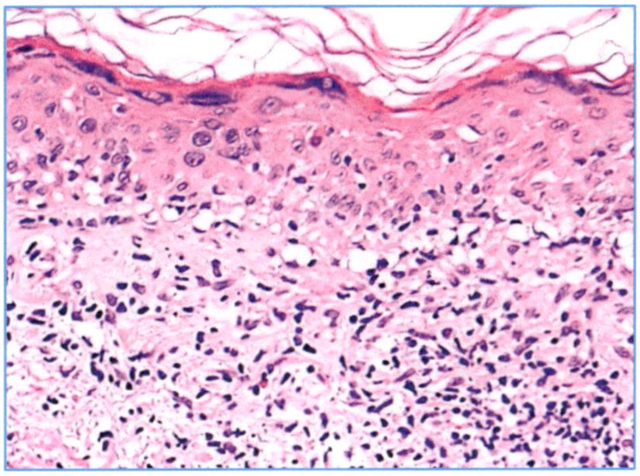

Interface vacuoles and occasional necrotic keratinocytes are appreciated at high magnification

Vacuolar interface dermatitis

DISCOID LUPUS ERYTHEMATOSUS

-hyperkeratotic but atrophic epidermis with **dilated keratin-plugged follicles**
-**interface vacuolar** changes with focal necrotic keratinocytes
-thickened basement membrane
-**increased dermal mucin**
-superficial and deep **patchy** perivascular and periadnexal **lymphocytic infiltrate** with a tendency to concentrate around hair follicles

TUMID LUPUS

-**no epidermal changes**
-**patchy** perivascular and periadnexal lymphocytic infiltrate
-**prominent dermal and subcutaneous mucin**

DLE ↓

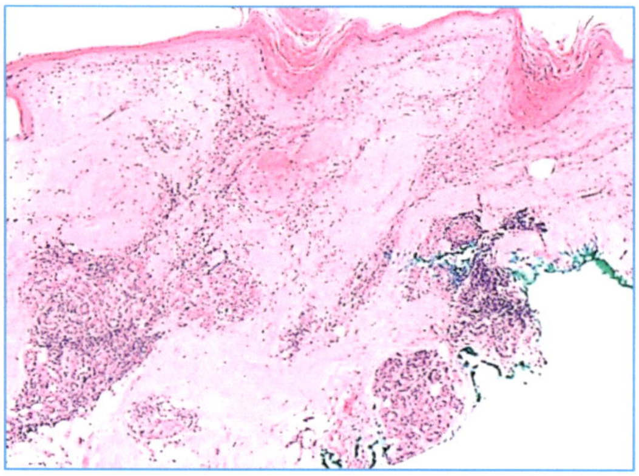

Hyperkeratotic epidermis and patchy inflammation

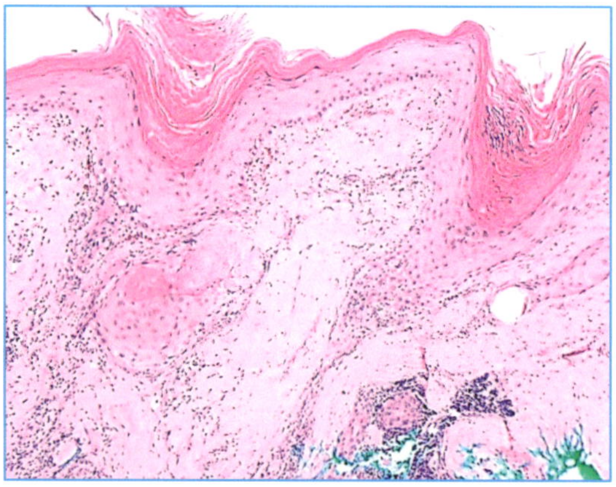

Keratin filled dilated follicles

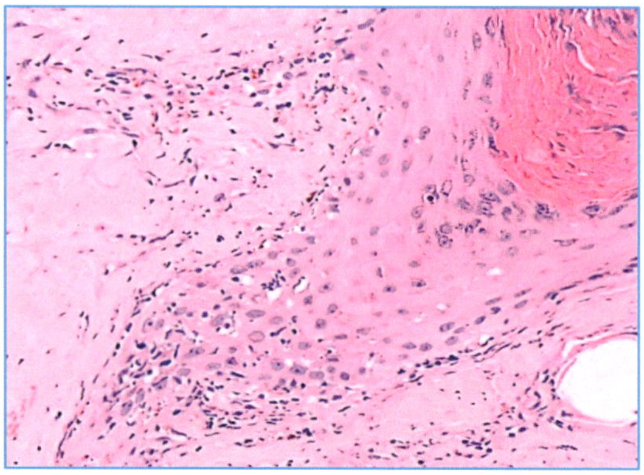

Interface vacuolar changes

TUMID LUPUS ↓

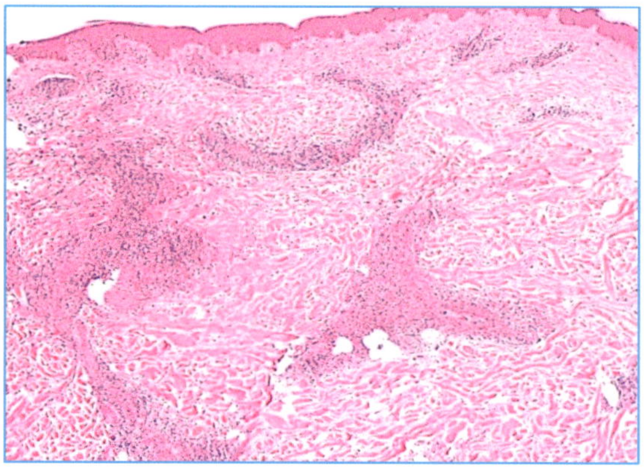

Normal epidermis and patchy inflammation

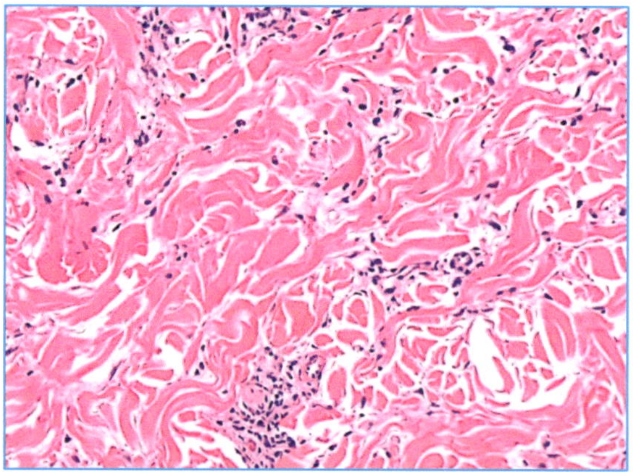

Dermal mucin separates collagen bundles

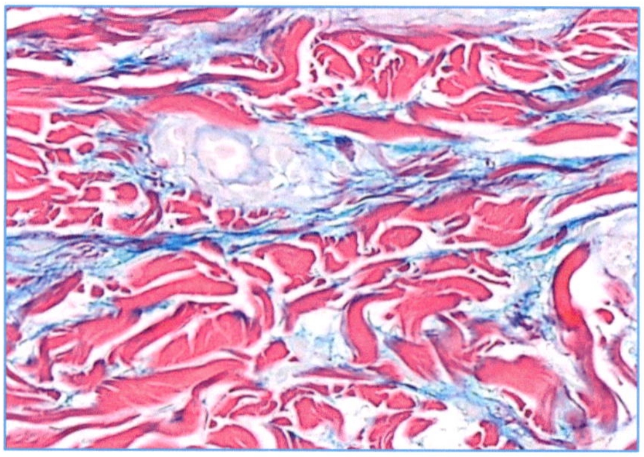

Colloidal Iron stain (blue) outlines dermal mucin

DERMATOMYOSITIS

-bimodal occurrence (5-15 and 45-65 years of age)
-may be virally induced in children
-may be paraneoplastic or drug-induced in adults
-most common drug is hydroxyurea
-violaceous (**heliotrope**) periorbital erythema
-erythema of face (**unlike lupus involves the melolabial folds**), chest and back (**with "shawl" or "V-sign"**)
-flat-topped violaceous papules over knuckles (**Gottron's papules**)
-**"ragged" cuticles** and periungual erythema

Histopathology
-subtle changes, very **similar to SCLE**
-atrophic epidermis with mild interface vacuolar changes
-focal apoptotic keratinocytes
-mild perivascular lymphocytic infiltrate
-increased **dermal mucin (more than in SCLE)**

Gottron's papule
-features of psoriasiform and interface dermatitis
-psoriasiform epidermis with interface vacuolar changes of dermatomyositis with dermal mucin

FIXED DRUG ERUPTION

-adverse skin reaction to an ingested drug
-usually 1-2 weeks after the first drug administration
-more rapid if previously exposed
-most common drugs are sulfonamide, naproxen, tetracycline, barbiturates
-usually lesion is solitary but can be multiple
-most common sites are oral and genital mucosa
-presents as dusky red, violaceous macule or plaque that resolves in 1-2 weeks with hyperpigmentation

Histopathology
-interface vacuolar changes with focal **necrotic keratinocytes**
-variable perivascular lymphocytic infiltrate
-dermal **eosinophils**, neutrophils can be seen
-**dermal pigment incontinence** is characteristic

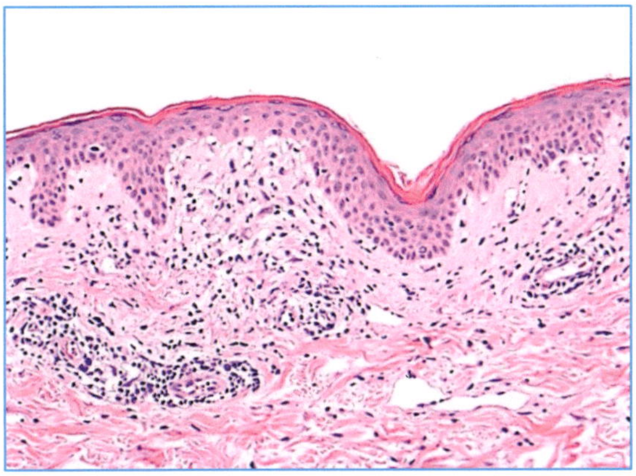
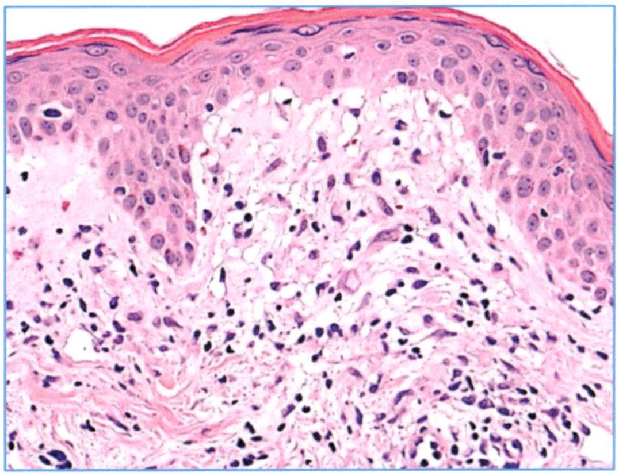

Dermatomyositis with interface vacuolar changes and dermal mucin

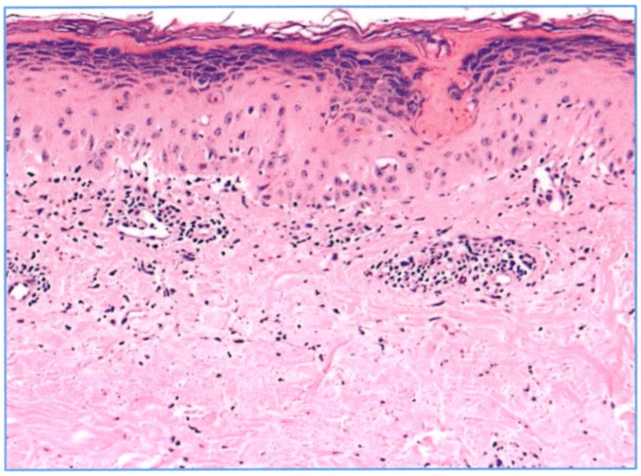
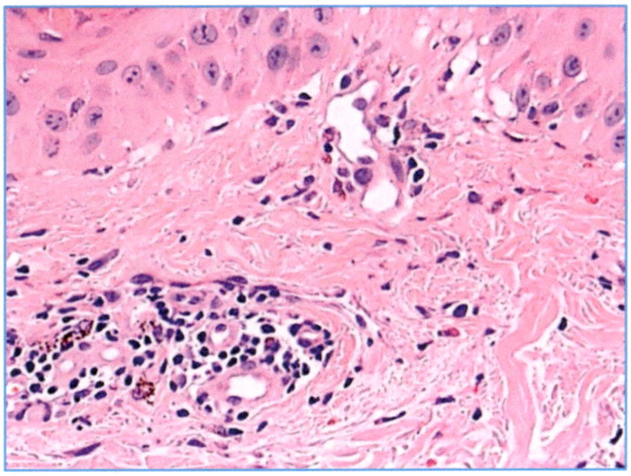

Fixed drug eruption with interface vacuolar changes, dermal pigment, and few eosinophils

Vacuolar interface dermatitis

ERYTHEMA MULTIFORME

-more common in **young** adults
-abrupt onset of **classic targetoid** lesions with **three zones** (outer ring of erythema, middle elevated, pale ring, and darker vesicular or necrotic center)
-or **palpable papular atypical targets** with **two zones and ill-defined borders**
-distribution often bilateral/symmetric
-hands, palms, soles, face, or generalized

EM major

-major cause is *Mycoplasma pneumoniae*
-targetoid lesions with **mucosal involvement** and **systemic symptoms**

EM minor

-majority triggered by *HSV* infection
-targetoid lesions **without or with minimal mucosal involvement** and **no systemic symptoms**

Histopathology

-individual **scattered necrotic keratinocytes at all levels of the epidermis**
-**interface vacuolization** of mildly spongiotic epidermis
-mild perivascular lymphocytic infiltrate and **usually no eosinophils**

TOXIC EPIDERMAL NECROLYSIS/ STEVENS-JOHNSON SYNDROME

-more common in elderly and is life-threatening
-one of the few real emergencies in dermatology
-thousand-fold increased risk in AIDS patients
-always drug induced and usually starts 1-2 weeks after taking medication
-most common culprits are allopurinol, NSAIDs, anticonvulsants, antibiotic (sulfonamides)
-degree of epidermal detachment determines the name
  -**SJS** <10 % detachment
  -**SJS-TEN overlap** has **10-30%**
  -**TEN** >30%
-all three forms have mucosal involvement with erosions and erythema
-usually starts on trunk and spreads to extremities, face, and neck
-diffuse erythematous macules and patches with purpuric center
-become confluent followed by formation of flaccid bullae and denudation
-denuded surface is red, raw, oozing, and tender

Histopathology

-**full thickness epidermal necrosis**
-**negligible dermal inflammation**
-common subepidermal split

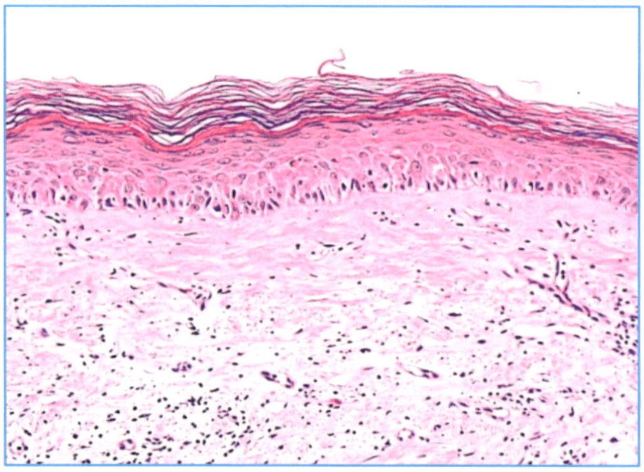
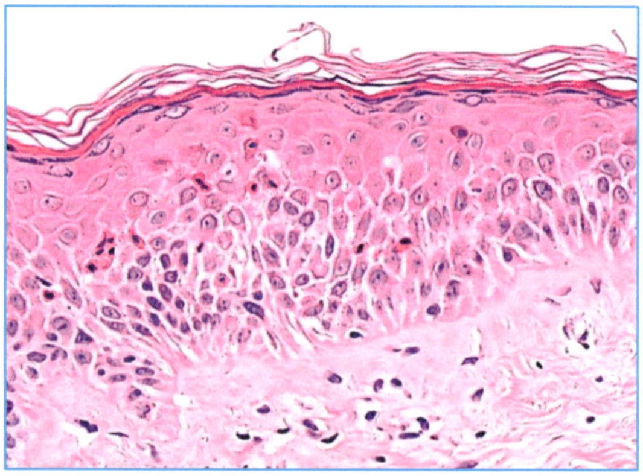

Erythema multiforme with mild spongiosis and scattered necrotic keratinocytes

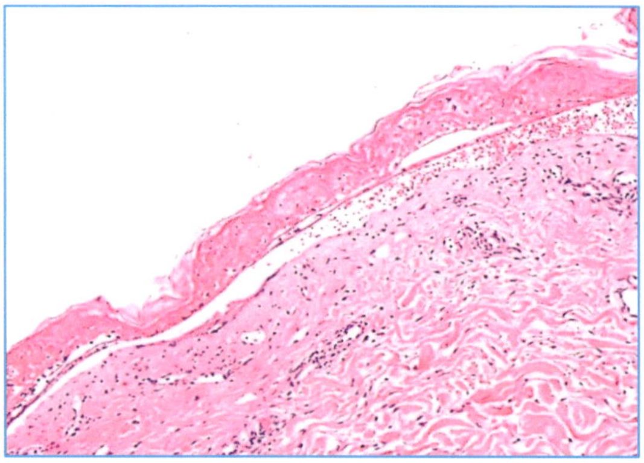
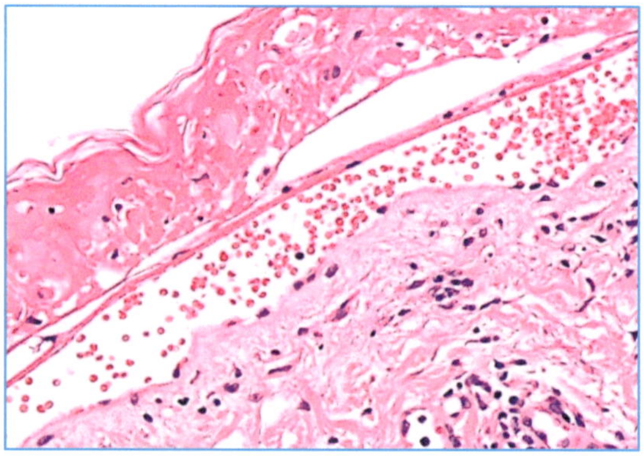

Toxic epidermal necrolysis with full thickness epidermal necrosis

GRAFT-VERSUS-HOST DISEASE (GvHD)

-can occur in any transplant patient but most frequently in allogeneic hematopoietic stem cell transplantation

Acute

-classically within first 100 days post-transplant with the peak at day 30
-presents as *morbilliform rash* on acral sites and upper trunk
-may progress to *erythema multiforme* to *SJS/TEN* presentation

Chronic

-classically after 100 days, and is proceeded by acute form in 50% of patients
-*lichenoid form*- slowly progressive rash on periorbital skin, ears, palms, and soles that progresses to lesions resembling lichen planus
-*sclerodermatous form*- patchy, "morphea-like" changes and less frequently progressive, "scleroderma-like" changes
-*psoriasiform form*- rare presentation that clinically resembles guttate psoriasis

Histopathology correlate with clinical presentation

Acute

-*morbilliform rash*- **mild spongiotic dermatitis** with dermal lymphocytes
-*"EM-like" presentation*- interface vacuolar changes and **scattered necrotic keratinocytes**
-*"SJS/TEN-like" presentation*- **full thickness epidermal necrosis**

Chronic

-*lichenoid form*- band-like **dermal lymphocytic infiltrate** and focal interface vacuoles
-*sclerodermatous form*- **dermal and subcutaneous fibrosis** and absent adnexal structures
-*psoriasiform form*- **"guttate psoriasis-like"** changes and focal interface changes

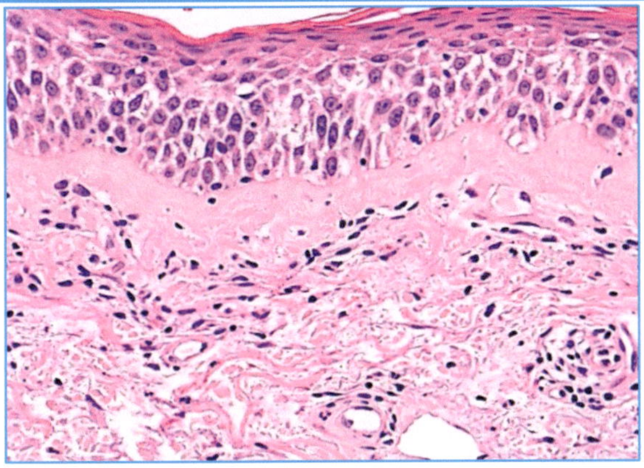

Acute morbilliform GvHD

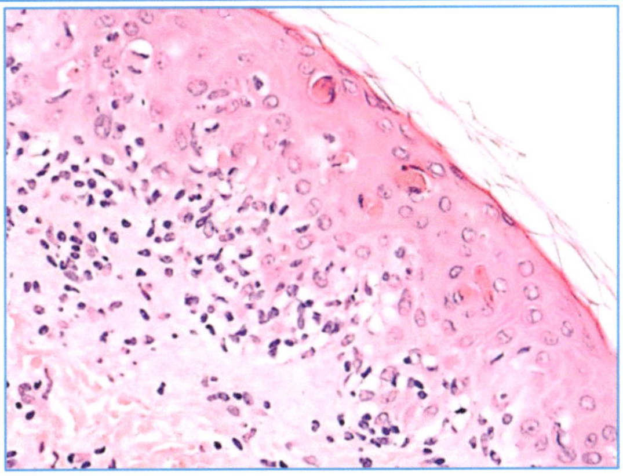

Acute "EM-like" GvHD

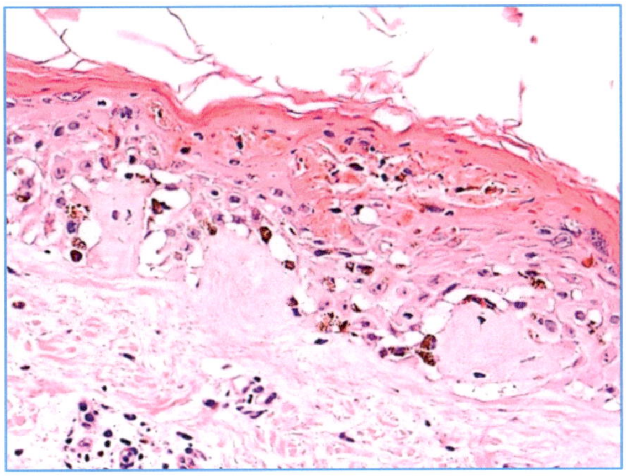

Acute "TEN-like" GvHD

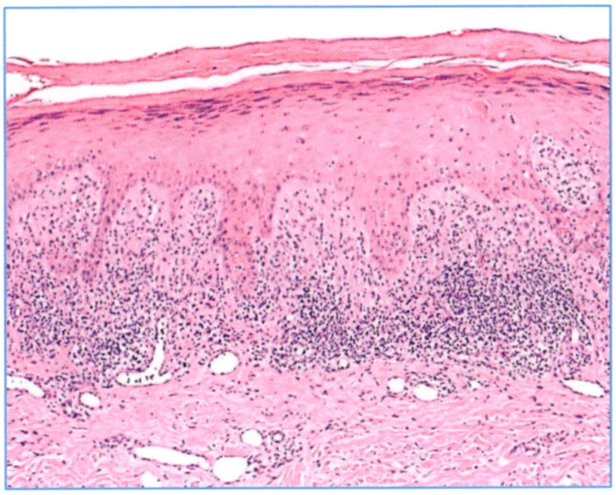

Chronic lichenoid GvHD

Vacuolar interface dermatitis

HOW TO APPROACH INTERFACE VACUOLAR DERMATITIS

DERMAL LYMPHOCYTES ARE PRESENT BUT ARE SUBTLE

IF YOU SEE VACUOLES IN THE BASAL LAYER OF EPIDERMIS FIRST
then you see occasional necrotic keratinocytes
and then hopefully you see some dermal mucin

-acute (ACLE) and subacute (SCLE) cutaneous lupus erythematosus
histology is almost identical for both
SCLE has slightly more vacuoles, necrotic keratinocytes, and mucin

-dermatomyositis
histology resembles ACLE or SCLE but with more mucin

-fixed drug reaction
dermal pigment incontinence and occasional eosinophils

IF YOU SEE NECROTIC KERATINOCYTES FIRST
and then vacuolar changes of the epidermis

-erythema multiforme	numerous necrotic keratinocytes many in small clusters but not full thickness necrosis
-GvHD	same as EM but with history of recent transplant
-TEN	full thickness epidermal necrosis

IF YOU SEE DILATED PLUGGED HAIR FOLLICLES FIRST
then periadnexal lymphocytic inflammation
and then vacuolar changes of follicular epidermis and dermal mucin

-discoid lupus erythematosus

Chapter 5

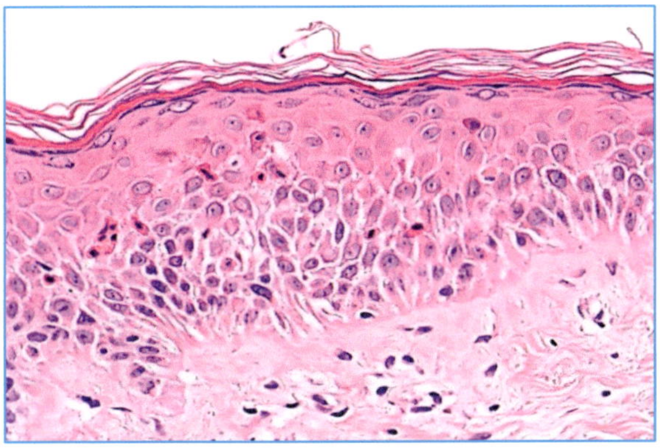

Erythema multiforme with scattered necrotic keratinocytes

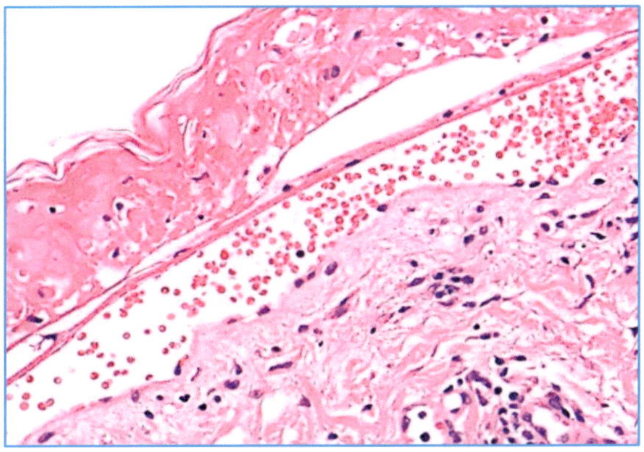

TEN with full thickness epidermal necrosis

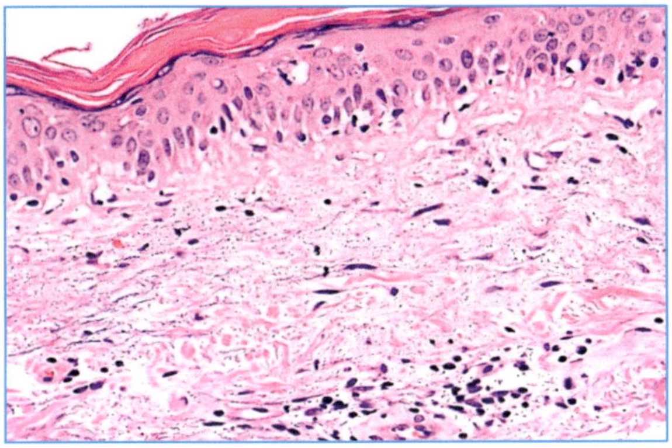

ACLE with very subtle interface vacuolar changes

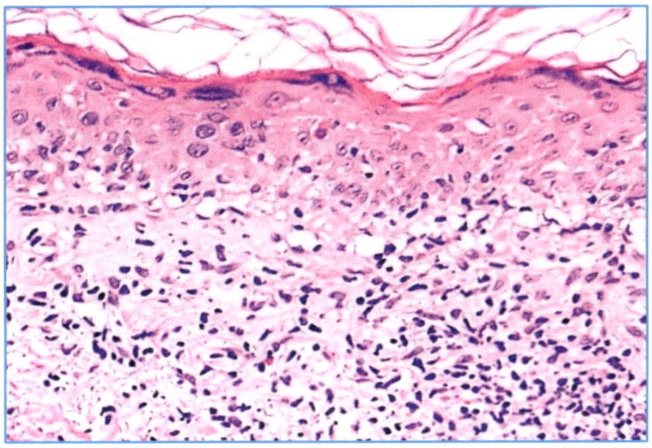

SCLE compared to ACLE has more vacuoles and inflammation

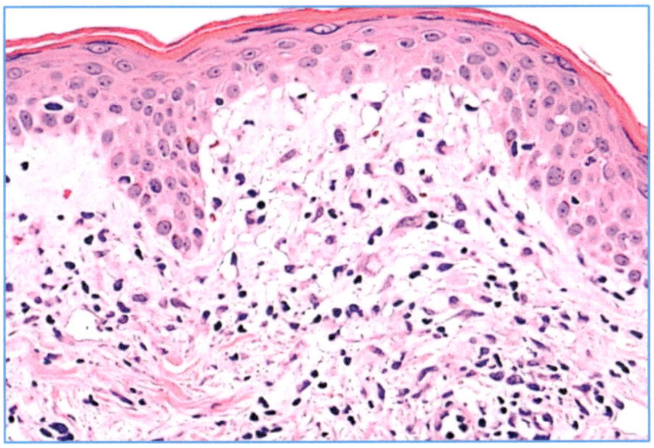

Dermatomyositis with prominent dermal mucin

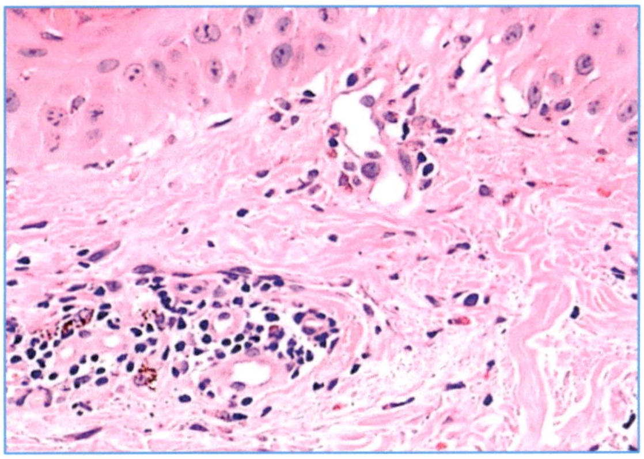

Fixed drug with dermal pigment incontinence and eosinophils

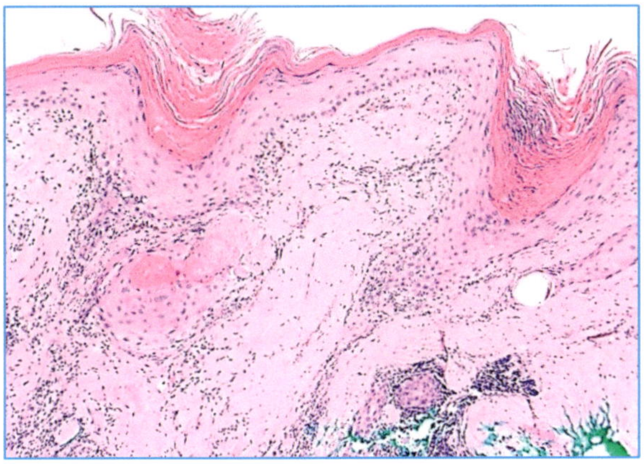

DLE with dilated keratin plugged hair follicles

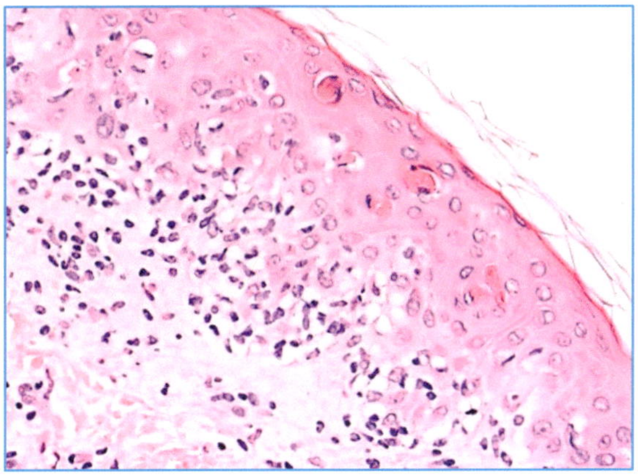

Acute GvHD with necrotic keratinocytes identical to EM

Vacuolar interface dermatitis

Chapter 6

DERMAL INFLAMMATORY DISORDERS

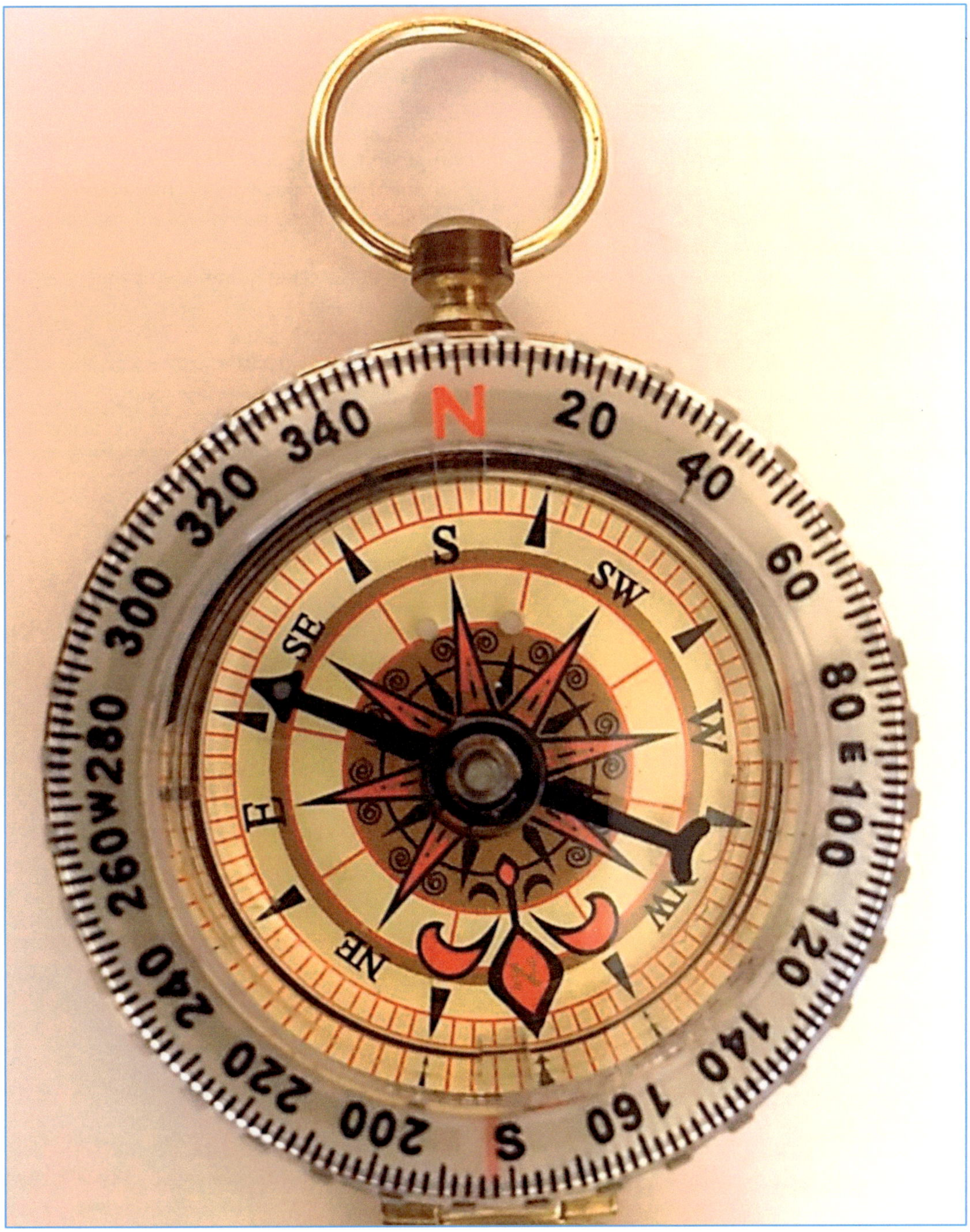

Dermal inflammatory disorders

POLYMORPHOUS LIGHT ERUPTION (PMLE)

-most common light-induced dermatosis
-confluent, very pruritic papules and vesicles on sun exposed areas that appears minutes to hours after sun exposure
-typically presents in early spring and diminishes with continued sun exposure over the summer months

Histopathology
-normal or mildly spongiotic epidermis
-prominent "band-like" superficial **dermal edema** that can lead to blister formation
-**dermal perivascular lymphocytic inflammation**
-in early lesions, inflammation is more superficial
-in older lesions, it is superficial and deep
-admixed eosinophils and neutrophils can be seen

PERNIOSIS (CHILBLAINS)

-localized inflammatory lesions of extremities induced by cold, damp conditions
-presents as crops of tender dusky red to purple papules after cold exposure
-acral skin, ears, and nose are favorite sites
-more frequent in patient with lupus erythematosus

Histopathology
-normal or mildly spongiotic epidermis
-prominent **linear** papillary **dermal edema**
-superficial and deep perivascular **lymphocytic infiltrate**
-common **perieccrine lymphocytes** and reactive endothelial cells
-occasional microthrombi

These two entities are histologically very similar and clinical correlation is necessary.
If perieccrine lymphocytes are present perniosis is favored.

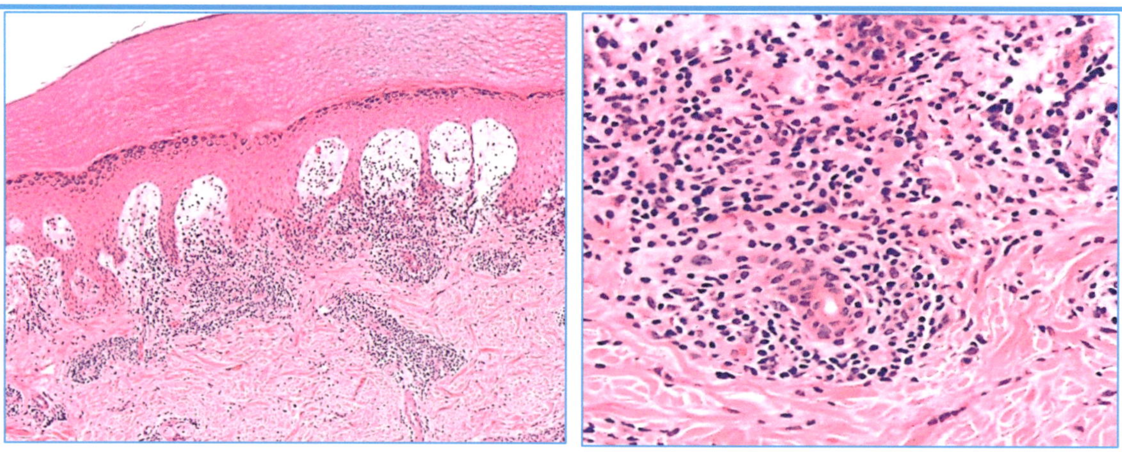

Perniosis with linear dermal edema and perivascular and perieccrine lymphocytes

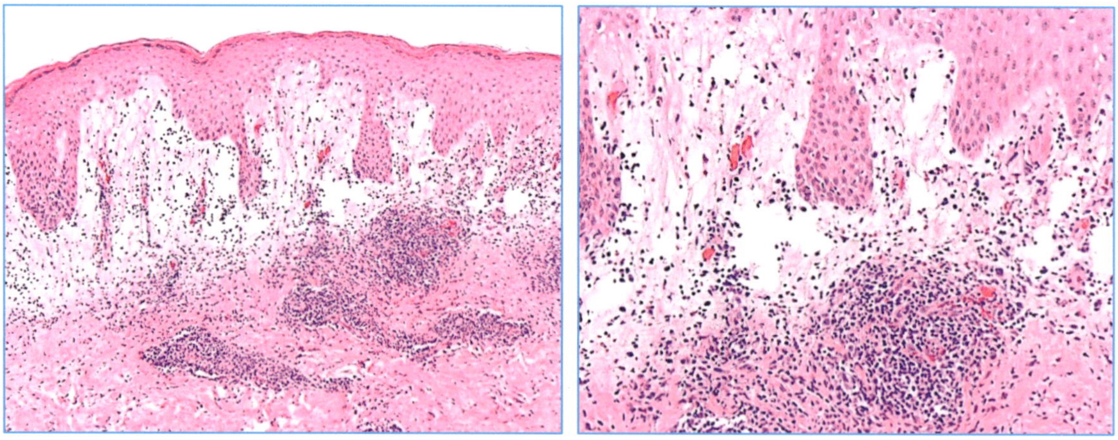

PMLE with linear dermal edema and superficial and deep perivascular lymphocytic inflammation

SWEET'S SYNDROME

-reactive neutrophilic dermatosis more common in women
-over 60% of cases are idiopathic, but can be associated with malignancy, inflammatory disease (RA, IBD), pregnancy, or drug use
-rapid onset of tender, single or multiple, edematous, erythematous papules, plaques
-coalesces to form irregular plaques in a symmetrical distribution
-face, neck, upper extremities are favored

Histiocytoid variant

-associated with hematologic malignancies
-presents as erythematous edematous papules on the neck, chest, abdomen, and upper extremities

Subcutaneous variant

-deep and tender red nodules on extremities

Histopathology

-normal epidermis and **massive dermal edema**
-dense dermal **neutrophilic infiltrate**
-some eosinophils can be present
-focal leukocytoclasia and vascular damage

Histiocytoid variant

-additional immature "histiocyte-like" myeloid cells

Subcutaneous variant

-neutrophilic panniculitis (see the panniculitis chapter)

PRURITIC URTICARIAL PAPULES AND PLAQUES OF PREGNANCY (POLYMORPHOUS ERUPTION OF PREGNANCY)

-occurs in the third trimester in about 1% of pregnancies, with no risk to fetus
-pruritic, urticarial papules and plaques that classically develop **in and around the abdominal striae** before spreading
-usually **spares the periumbilical area** (in contrast to herpes gestationis)
-resolves spontaneously after delivery

Histopathology

-mild epidermal spongiosis and mild dermal edema
-perivascular lymphocytic infiltrate
-easily detected perivascular and interstitial **dermal eosinophils**

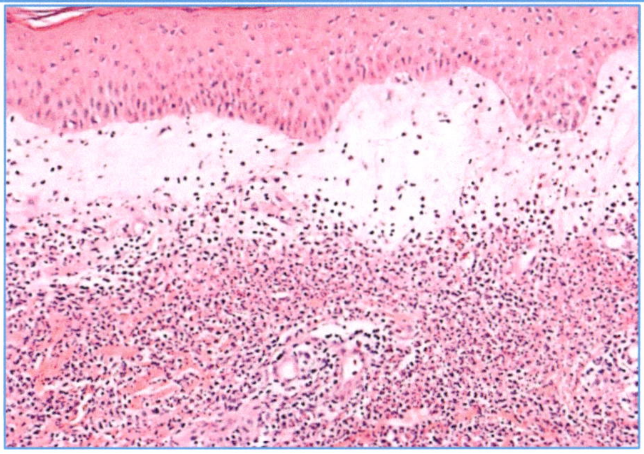
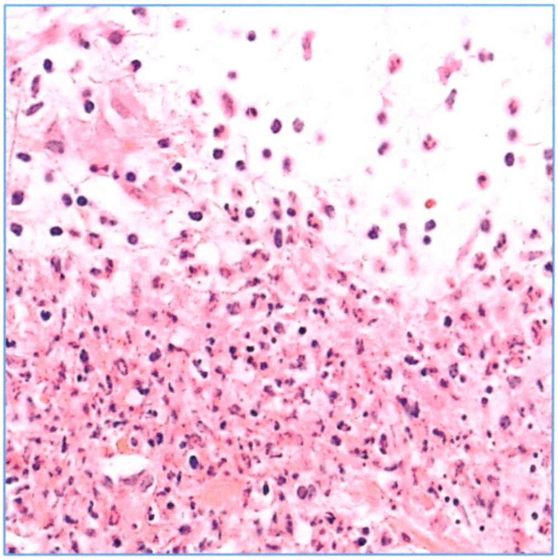

Sweet's syndrome with linear dermal edema and numerous dermal neutrophils

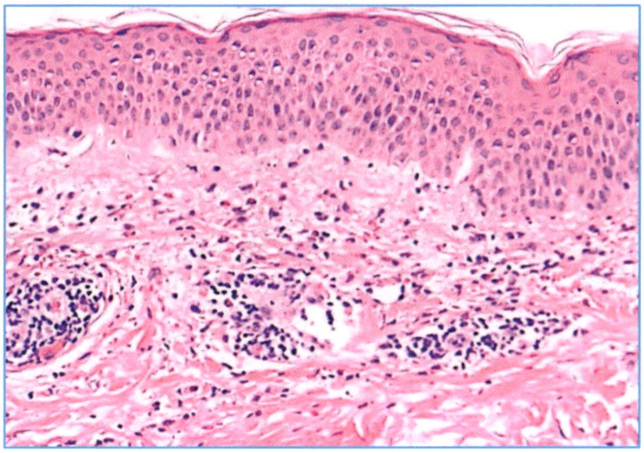
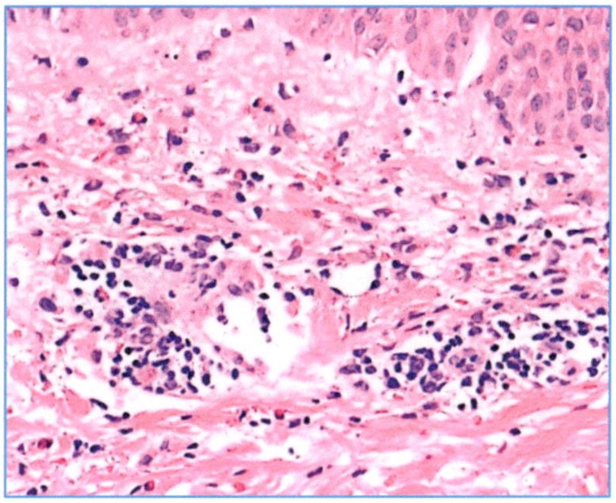

PUPPP with mild epidermal spongiosis and numerous dermal eosinophils

Dermal inflammatory disorders

LEUKOCYTOCLASTIC VASCULITIS (LCV)

-heterogenous group of vasculitides
-associated with hypersensitivity to an antigen which can vary from infectious agents (hepatitis B, hepatitis C, *Streptococcus*, *Staphylococcus*), to drugs (sulfonamide, penicillin), to endogenous sources (neoplasms, autoimmune disorders, cryoglobulinemia)
-presents as palpable purpura ranging in size from pinpoint to a few centimeters
-predilection for lower legs, ankles, buttocks, and arm
-usually resolves in several weeks with resulting hyperpigmentation

Histopathology

-vascular damage of capillaries with endothelial swelling and **fibrinoid necrosis**
-intravascular and perivascular **neutrophilic infiltrate**
-**leukocytoclasia** (degeneration and breaking apart of neutrophils resulting in nuclear dust)
-variable thrombi and red blood cell extravasation

Numerous diseases can present in the skin as leukocytoclastic vasculitis:

-Henoch-Schönlein purpura
-acute hemorrhagic edema of infancy
-meningococcemia
-gonococcemia
-Rocky Mountain spotted fever
-Behçet's disease
-cryoglobulinemia type II and III
-microscopic polyarteritis nodosa
-erythema elevatum diutinum
-eosinophilic granulomatosis with polyangiitis
-granulomatosis with polyangiitis

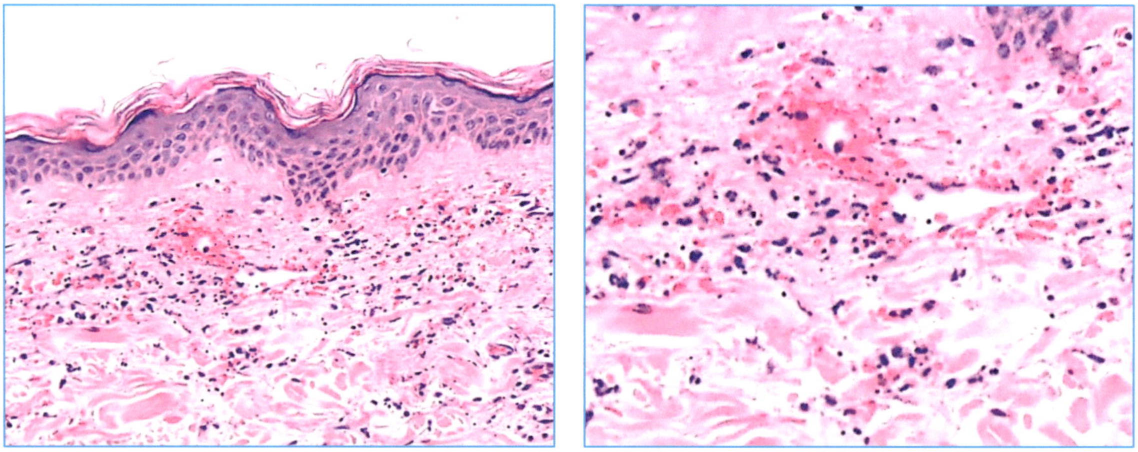

LCV with damaged dermal capillaries and dermal neutrophils many of which are fragmented

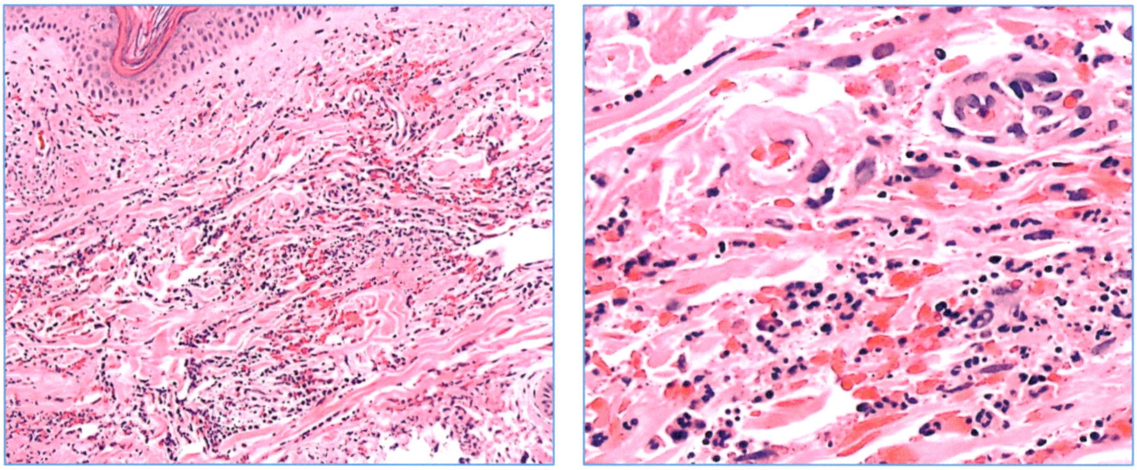

LCV with fibrin within vessel walls, dermal neutrophilic nuclear dust, and red blood cell extravasation

URTICARIAL VASCULITIS

-resembles urticaria with wheals that persists for more than 24 hours (unlike urticaria)
-recurrent episodes last months to years
-lesions burn or are painful rather than itchy as in urticaria
-resolves with hyperpigmentation or purpura
-favors trunk and lower extremities
-75% are normocomplemententemic
-they are idiopathic or association with medications, viral infections (hepatitis B/C, EBV), or malignancy (leukemia/lymphoma)
-25% are associate with hypocomplementemia in patients with collagen vascular diseases and are more common in women

Histopathology
-**mild dermal edema** (less than in urticaria)
-there is a **continuum** of inflammatory changes
-range from mild to moderate perivascular lymphocytic and neutrophilic infiltrate with **few intravascular intact neutrophils**
-to **LCV** presentation with **numerous fragmented intravascular and perivascular neutrophils**, fibrinoid vascular deposits
-severe LCV form is more common in type with hypocomplementemia
-**scattered dermal eosinophils are present**

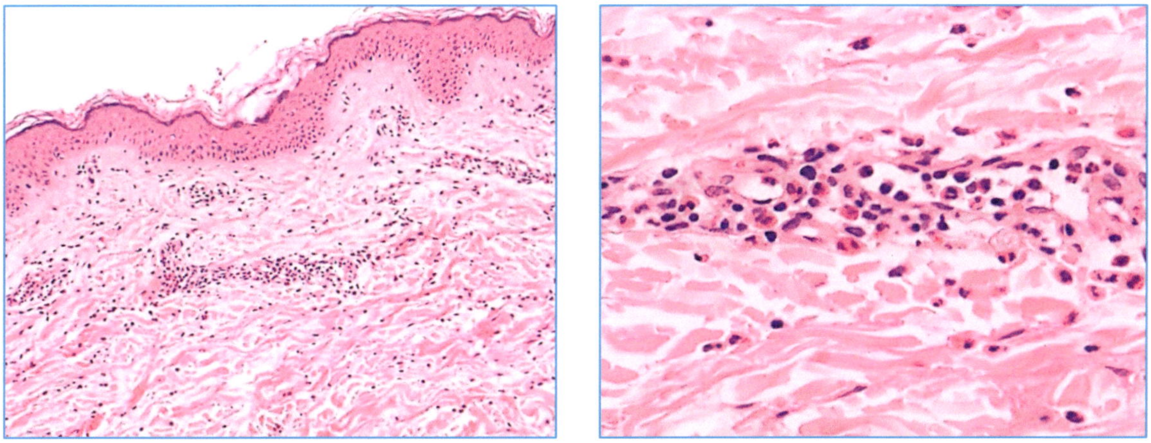

Mild urticarial vasculitis with dermal edema and perivascular and intravascular mostly intact neutrophils. Dermal eosinophils are present.

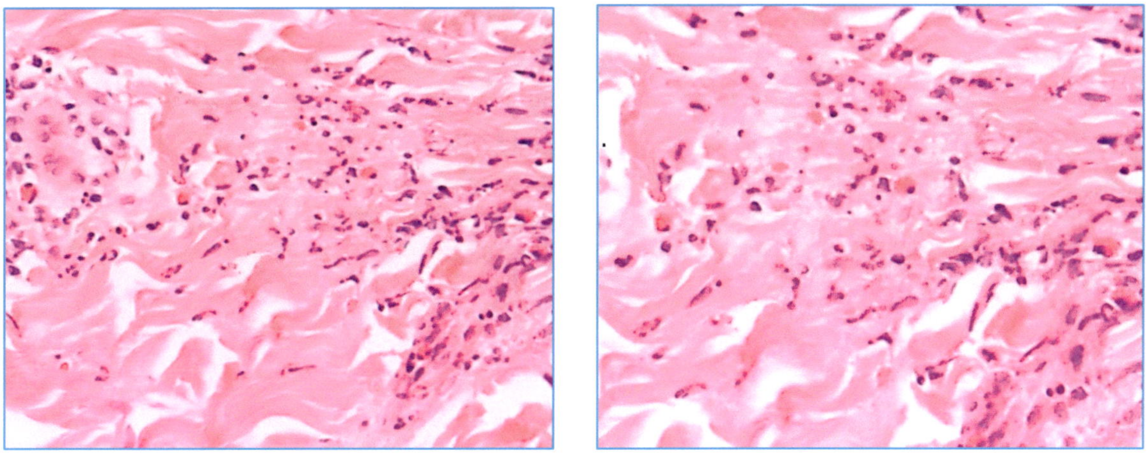

Urticarial vasculitis with leukocytoclastic vasculitis and dermal eosinophils

Dermal inflammatory disorders

URTICARIA/ANGIOEDEMA

-20% of people will be affected at some point in their lifetime
-acute urticaria usually lasts less than 6 weeks with higher chance of specific etiology being found (drugs, food, pressure, heat, cold, cholinergic)
-chronic urticaria lasts more than 6 weeks and may last for years
-it is mostly idiopathic or less frequently caused by exogenous physical stimulus
-acute and chronic urticaria presents with transient **itchy wheals** (smooth edematous dermal papules and plaques)
-lesions can vary in size and shape
-individual wheals **last <24 hours**

Angioedema

-can be hereditary or acquired resulting from absolute or relative deficiency of C1 esterase inhibitor
-presents like urticaria but process extends to the deep dermis and subcutis
-manifests as **swelling of eyelids, tongue, lips**
-can affect the upper airways, making it potentially fatal

Histopathology

-**subtle** findings with **dermal edema**
-**dilated dermal vessels** with sparse perivascular lymphocytic infiltrate and **scattered dermal eosinophils** and occasional neutrophils
-in **very early urticaria** (1 hour into process) **neutrophils** and sometimes eosinophils are present **in the lumen** of small vessels (**resembles mild urticarial vasculitis**)

Neutrophilic urticaria

-variant with dermal neutrophils without eosinophils

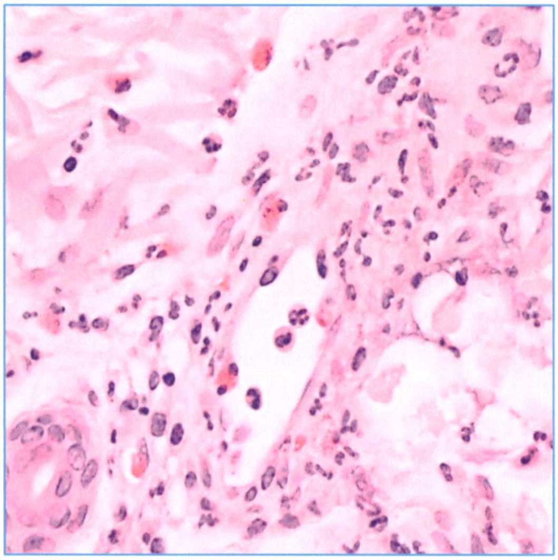

Early urticaria can have neutrophils in the capillary lumen and dermal eosinophils

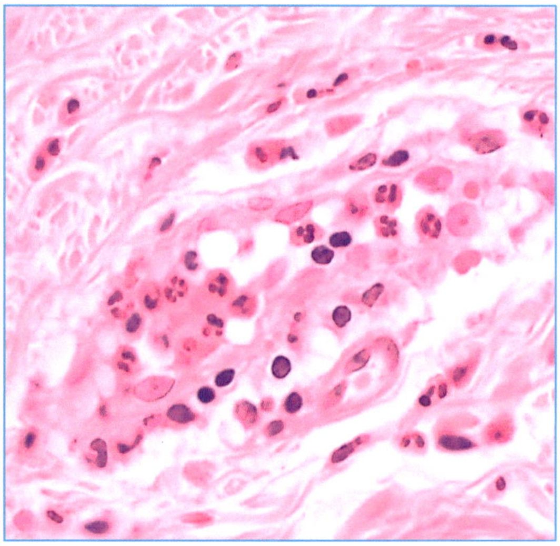

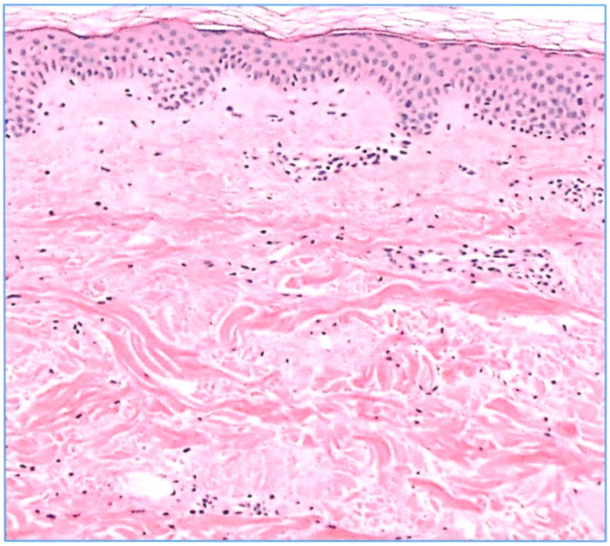

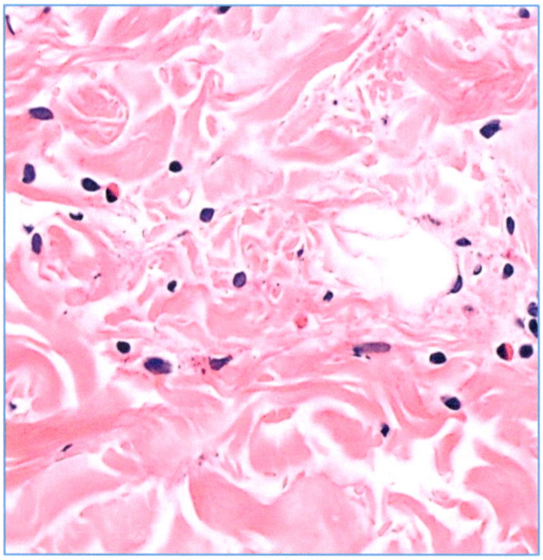

Urticaria with dermal edema, dilated capillaries, and scattered dermal eosinophils

WELL'S SYNDROME (EOSINOPHILIC CELLULITIS)

-reactive process associated with insect bites, parasite infection, drug reactions, and myeloproliferative disorders
-many cases are idiopathic
-characterized by indurated "cellulitis-like" plaques
-blister formation is common
-upper back and extremities are favored sites
-lesions resolve as "morphea-like" indurated plaques within 1-2 months

Histopathology

-diffuse dermal eosinophilic infiltrate
-infiltrate often extends into subcutis
-characteristic **"flame figures"** (pink collagen bundles coated with granules of degranulated eosinophils)
-subepidermal blister may form

ARTHROPOD BITE

-skin reaction depends on the kind of insect (see the chapter on exogenous skin insults)
-usually single or grouped itchy pink-red papules and vesicles

Histopathology

-histology is variable and depends on the age of the lesion and kind of insect

New lesions

-spongiotic epidermis with **central ulceration** and serum crust
-superficial and deep, **"V-shaped"** lymphohistiocytic infiltrate with perivascular and interstitial **eosinophils** and **neutrophils**
-**dermal edema** with focal dermal necrosis and abscess formation can be present

Older lesions

-epidermis is healed but mildly spongiotic
-dermal edema can be prominent with blister formation
-**inflammation is more diffuse** (not so "V-shaped") and more **mixed** with less **eosinophils and neutrophils**

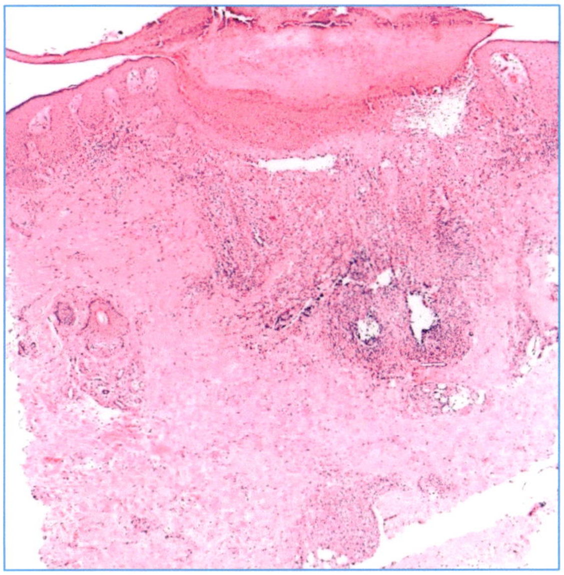

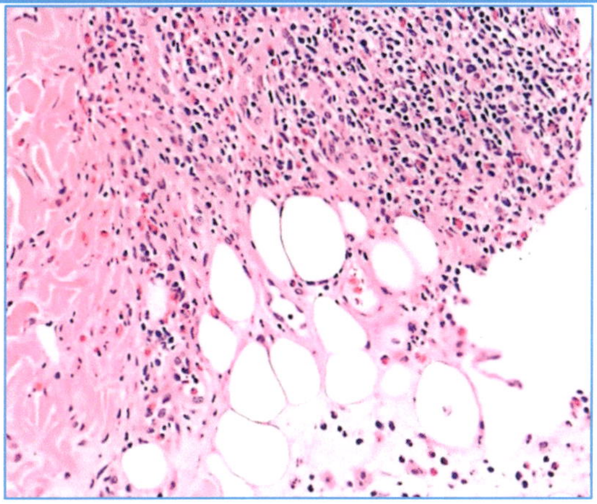

Recent arthropod bite with ulcerated epidermis and "V-shaped" inflammation with neutrophils and numerous eosinophils

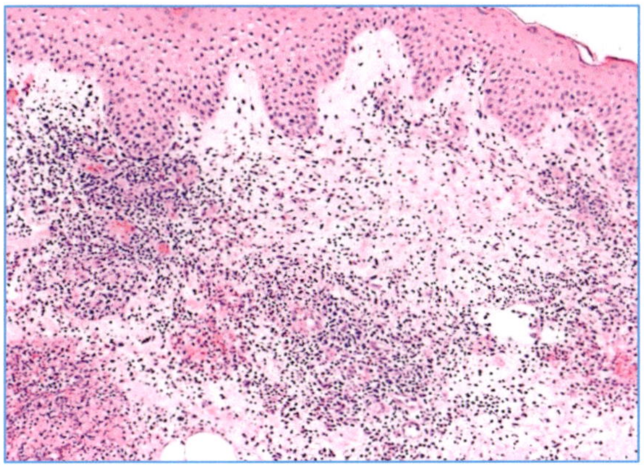

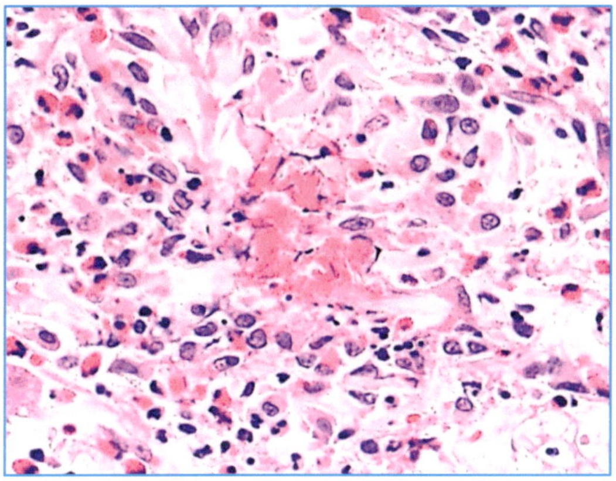

Well's syndrome with dermal edema and numerous eosinophils forming "flame figure"

Dermal inflammatory disorders

ERYTHEMA ANNULARE CENTRIFUGUM (GYRATE ERYTHEMA)

-erythematous, solitary or multiple annular lesions that expand outward
-fine trailing scale inside the advancing edge is common
-predilection for proximal part of extremities (thighs/hips)
-pathogenesis is unknown but it is associated with infections, drugs, connective tissue disorders

Histopathology

Superficial EAC

-mild epidermal spongiosis
-superficial dermal perivascular lymphocytic inflammation **"tightly cuffed"** around capillaries ("**coat-sleeve"** appearance)
-**minimal interstitial inflammation**

Deep EAC

-the same as the superficial variant with additional "tightly cuffed" lymphocytic inflammation around deep dermal vessels

ERYTHEMA MARGINATUM

-seen in children not treated for group A Streptococcus infection of the throat in the setting of rheumatic fever
-occurs 2-5 weeks after infection
-expanding annular erythematous patches/plaques
-trunk, axilla, proximal extremities are favored sites
-lesions resolve in a few weeks

Histopathology

-mild epidermal spongiosis
-superficial dermal **perivascular neutrophils and lymphocytes**
-**no leukocytoclasia** (degeneration of neutrophils with formation of nuclear dust) **or vascular damage**

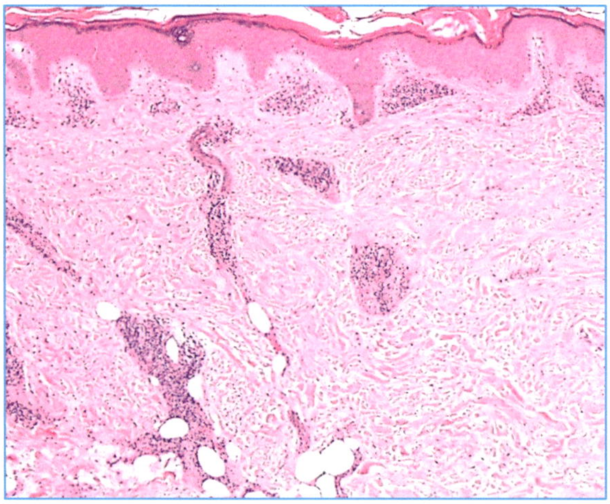
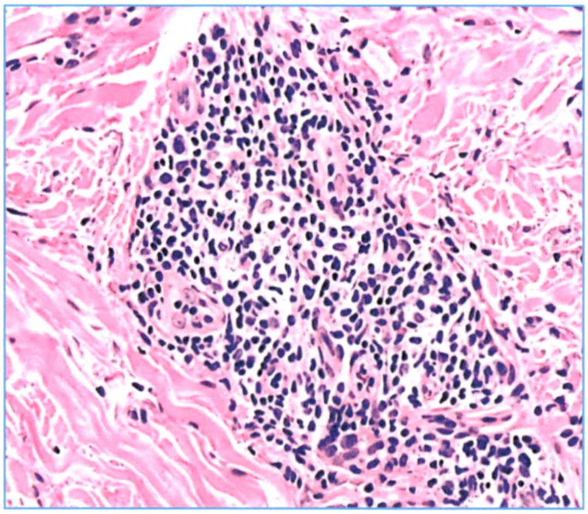

EAC with lymphocytes tightly grouped around dermal vessels and no lymphocytes in between vessels

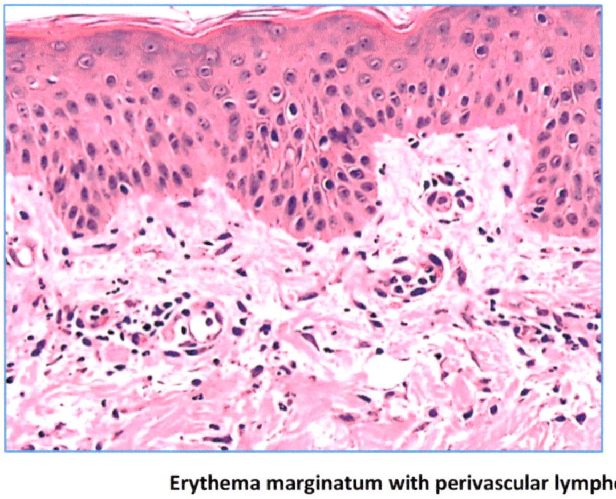
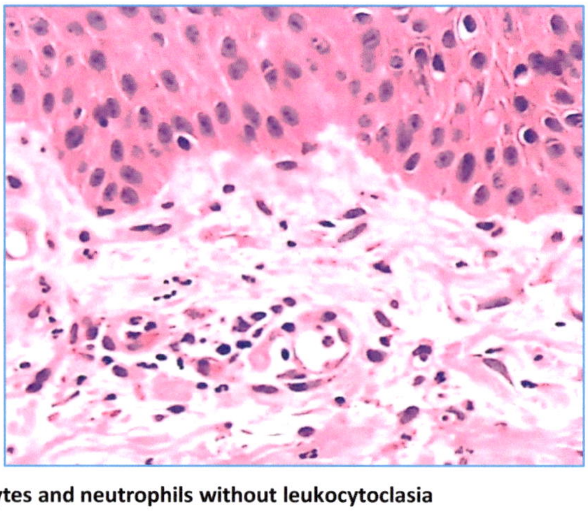

Erythema marginatum with perivascular lymphocytes and neutrophils without leukocytoclasia

ERYTHEMA CHRONICUM MIGRANS

-initial cutaneous manifestation of Lyme disease (see more in the chapter on bacterial infections)
-enlarging "**bull's eye**" **like macule/patch** at the site of a bite
-within days macule obtains distinct red border and partially cleared center
-days to weeks after primary lesion, up to half of patients, develop disseminated erythema migrans lesions that are smaller than the original lesion
-if left untreated, lesions self-resolve in 6 weeks but with long term risk for arthritis, neurological abnormalities, and cardiac complications

Histopathology
-normal or mildly spongiotic epidermis
-superficial and deep mild perivascular lymphocytic inflammation
-**loss of pilosebaceous elements**
-**perivascular plasma cells** and **subtle focal mucin**

SECONDARY SYPHILIS

-manifests 6-8 weeks after primary syphilis infection (see more in the chapter on bacterial infections)
-lesions show great clinical variability **("the great mimicker")**
-usually starts as "ham-colored" erythematous macules on the head, face and neck, which then generalize and classically involve the palms and soles
-left untreated, secondary syphilis resolves within 2-10 weeks

Histopathology
-similar to clinical presentation, histology can be variable
-mild epidermal spongiosis
-perivascular lymphocytic inflammation with **numerous plasma cells**

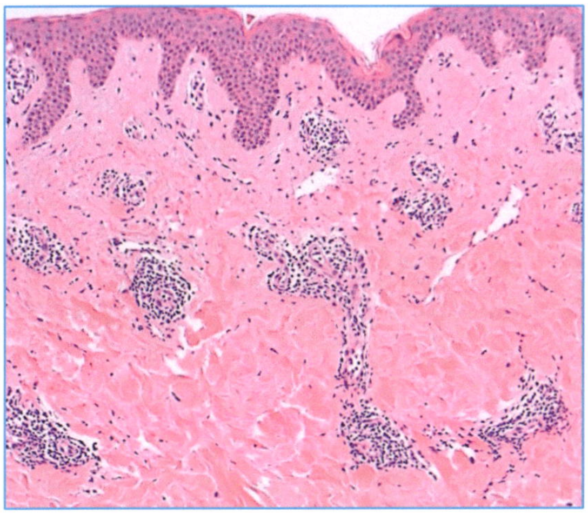
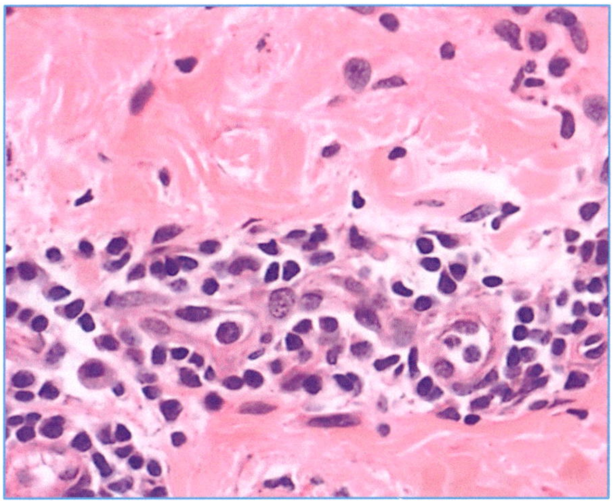

Erythema chronicum migrans with lack of pilosebaceous structures and perivascular lymphocytes and plasma cells

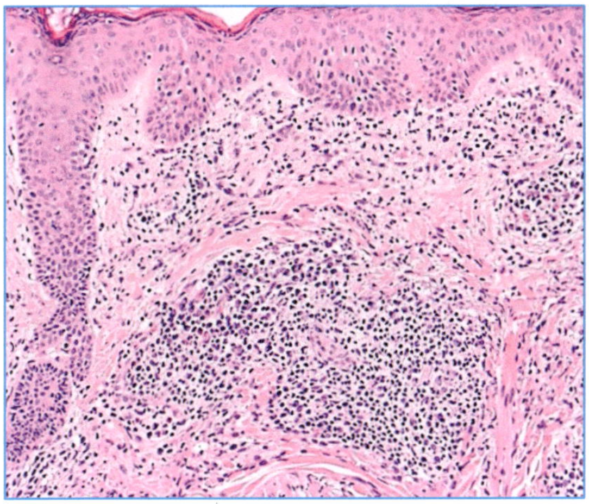
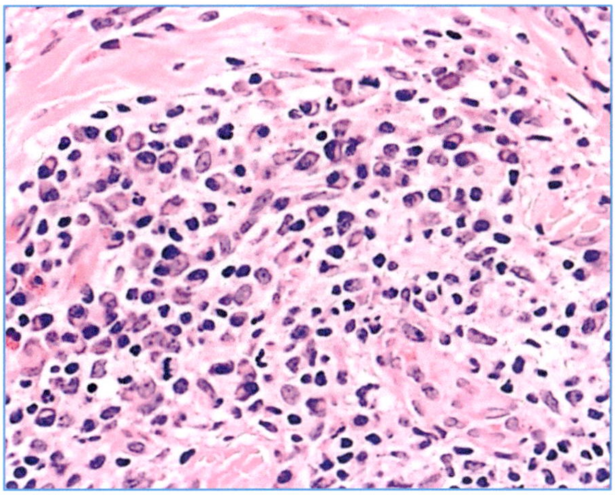

Secondary syphilis with mildly spongiotic epidermis and numerous dermal plasma cells

Dermal inflammatory disorders

NEUTROPHILIC ECCRINE HIDRADENITIS

-self-limiting, reactive neutrophilic dermatosis in patients receiving chemotherapy
-red purple plaques, located on the extremities, trunk, face, and palms
-unilateral or bilateral periorbital erythematous edema is common
-most commonly associated drugs are cytarabine, bleomycin, and mitoxantrone in patients with acute myeloid leukemia

Histopathology

-**neutrophilic infiltrate around eccrine glands** and secretory coils
-**necrosis of eccrine epithelial cells**
-squamous syringometaplasia may be present

PYODERMA GANGRENOSUM

-chronic, destructive neutrophilic skin disease
-50% associated with Crohn's disease, ulcerative colitis, leukemia, myeloma, Behcet's disease, rheumatoid arthritis, or hepatitis
-early lesion is a painful, solitary, deep-seated nodule
-it evolves to purulent ulcer with irregular, undermined "gunmetal grey" border
-heals with atrophic irregular scar

Histopathology

-variable; a diagnosis of exclusion
-non-ulcerated lesions show perifollicular inflammation with abscess formation
-ulcerated, established lesions show necrosis of epidermis and superficial dermis
-dermal and subcutaneous inflammatory response with leukocytoclasia and abscess
-**dermal neutrophilic infiltrate extends beyond ulcer edges**
-vascular damage is secondary

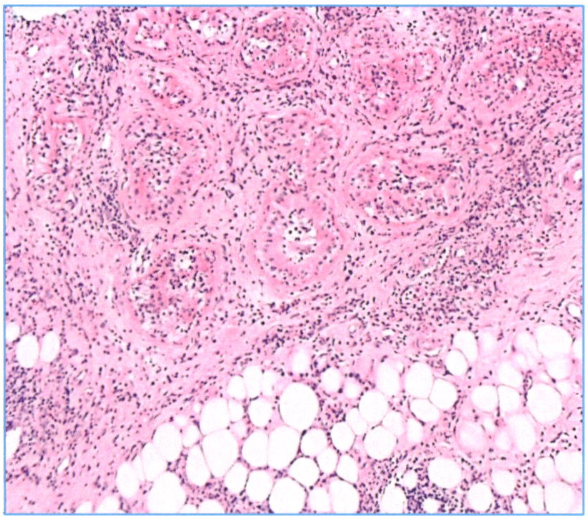
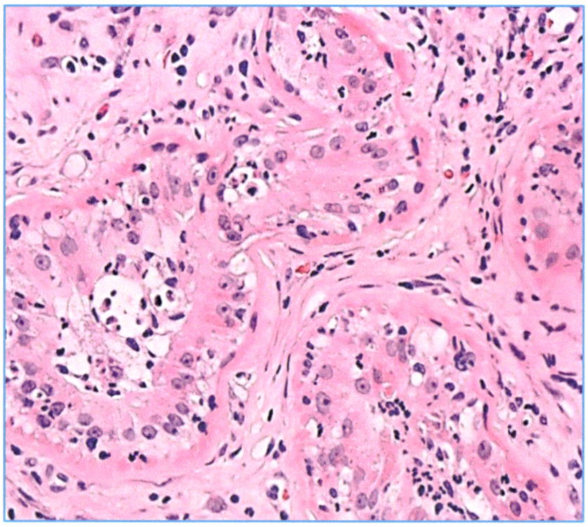

Neutrophilic eccrine hidradenitis with neutrophils in and around damaged eccrine glands and ducts

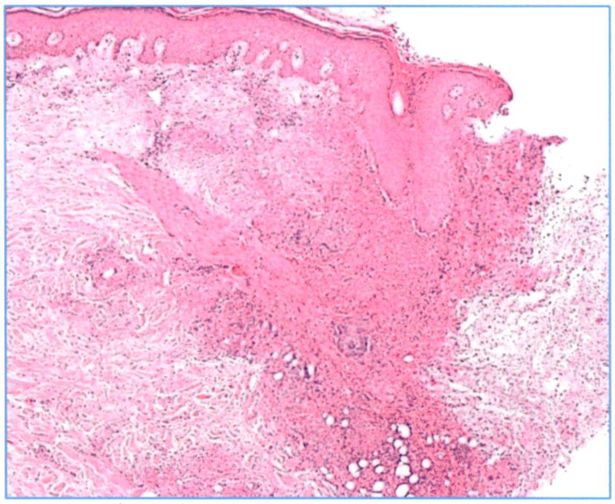
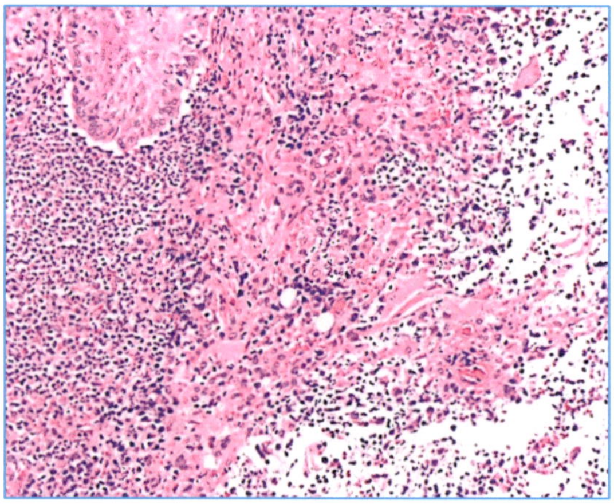

Pyodermal gangrenosum with dermal neutrophilic infiltrate extending beyond ulcer edge

TUMID LUPUS

-variant of chronic cutaneous lupus erythematosus (see more in the vacuolar interface chapter)
-indurated annular plaques favoring upper trunk and proximal extremities
-overlying epidermis is normal

Histopathology
-no epidermal changes
-**patchy,** superficial, and deep **perivascula**r and **periadnexal** lymphocytic infiltrate
-**prominent** dermal and subcutaneous **mucin** seen even without special stains

PIGMENTED PURPURIC DERMATOSES

-group of disorders with overlapping clinical presentation and histomorphology
-see more in the vasculitis chapter
-generally, purpuric lesions with variable pigmentation and predilection for the lower extremities
-can be itchy or not depending on the type (see the chapter on vasculitis)

Histopathology
-normal or mildly spongiotic epidermis
-**perivascular lymphocytic** infiltrate
-dermal **red blood cell extravasation**

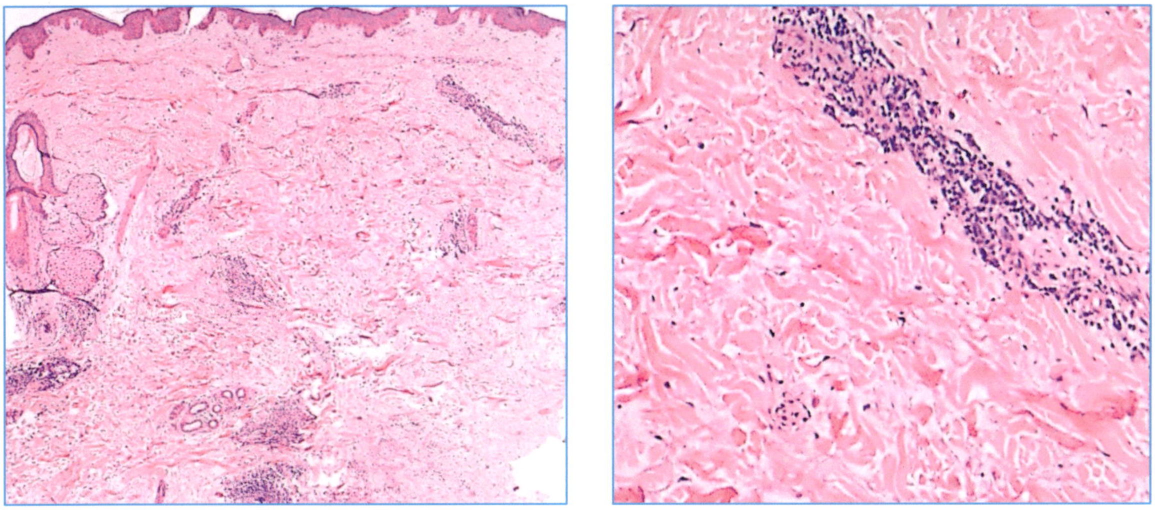

Tumid lupus with patchy dermal lymphocytic inflammation and prominent dermal mucin

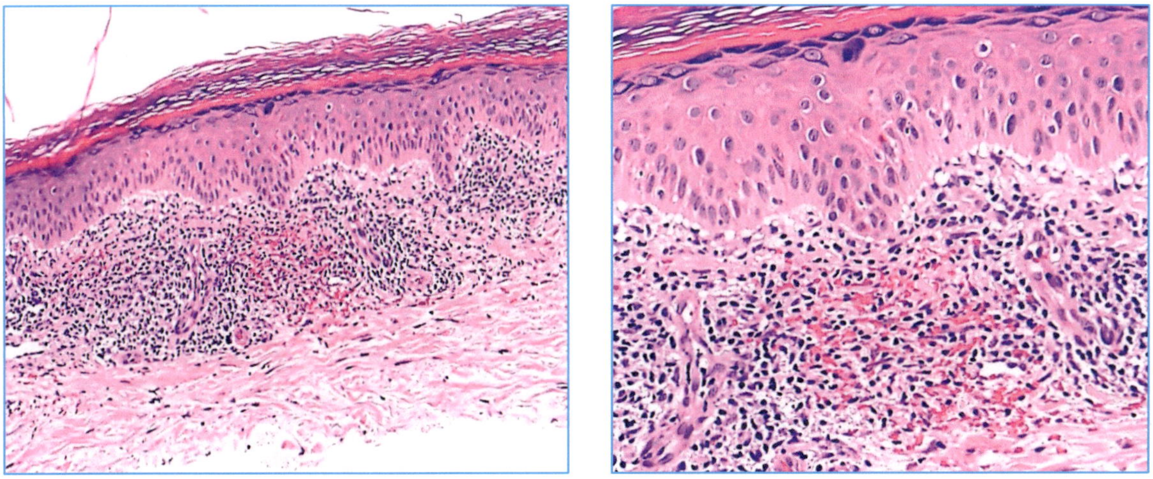

Pigmented purpuric dermatosis with dermal perivascular lymphocytes and extensive red blood cell extravasation

Dermal inflammatory disorders

RETICULATED ERYTHEMATOUS MUCINOSIS (REM)

-rare, chronic, indolent disease of women in 3rd-4th decade of life
-commonly starts after intense sun exposure
-erythematous reticulated plaques and patches favoring midline chest and back

Histopathology

-**perivascular lymphocytic** infiltrate with mildly separated collagen and variable amount of **dermal mucin**

TELANGIECTASIA MACULARIS ERUPTIVA PERSTANS (TMEP)

-a form of cutaneous mastocytosis
-widespread itchy rash with telangiectatic macules on erythematous base
-can occur at any age but favors young adults

Histopathology

-**dermal telangiectasias**
-increased number of perivascular **mast cells** (>10 in high power field)
-mast cells stain with CD119, mast tryptase, Giemsa and toluidine blue

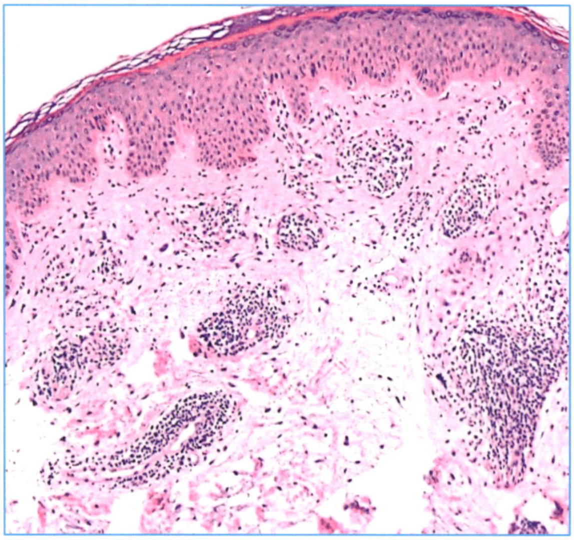

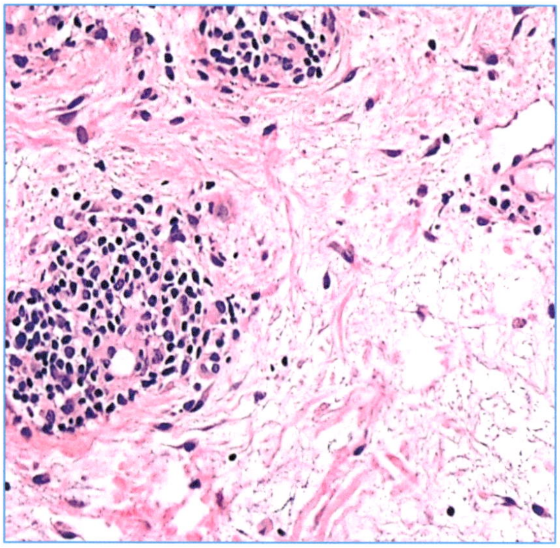

REM with perivascular lymphocytes and dermal mucin

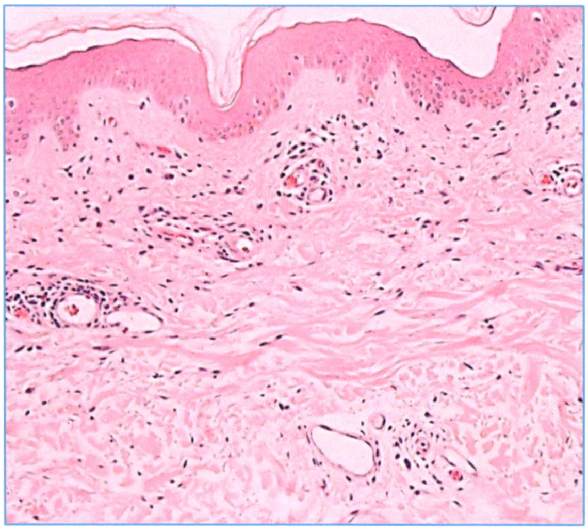

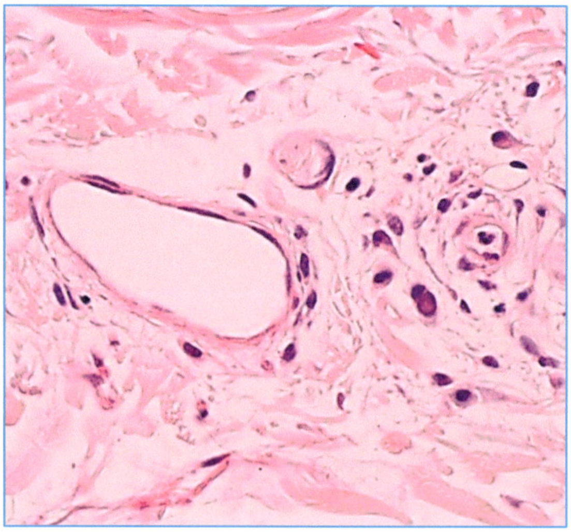

TMEP with telangiectasias and mast cells

Chapter 6

TINEA

-superficial fungal infection of the skin
-described in more details in the chapter on fungal infections
-small to large scaly, erythematous annular plaques with central clearing

Histopathology

-many times, referred to as "**invisible dermatosis**" as **findings** can be **subtle**
-normal-appearing epidermis with compact stratum corneum and focal parakeratosis
-"**sandwich sign"** with hyphae "sandwiched" between upper normal stratum corneum and lower parakeratosis or compact orthokeratosis
-mild perivascular lymphocytic inflammation

ERYTHRASMA

-superficial bacterial infection by *Corynebacterium minutissimum*
-red-brown slightly wrinkled patches in moist intertriginous areas
-coral pink-red fluorescence with Wood's lamp

Histopathology

-an example of "**invisible dermatosis**"
-**bacteria in the stratum corneum**
-epidermal hyperkeratosis and focal parakeratosis
-minimal to mild perivascular lymphocytic inflammation

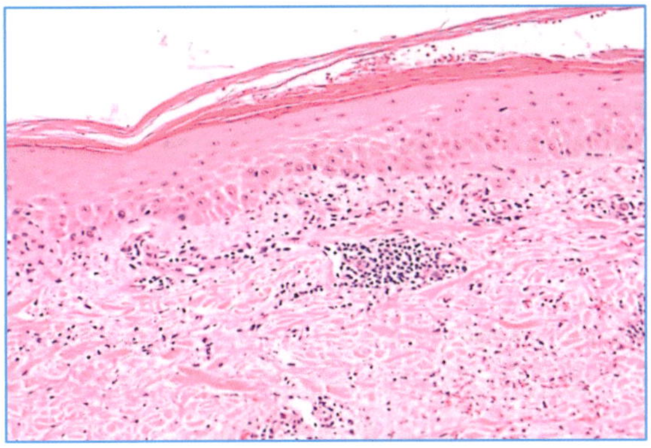

Invisible dermatosis of tinea

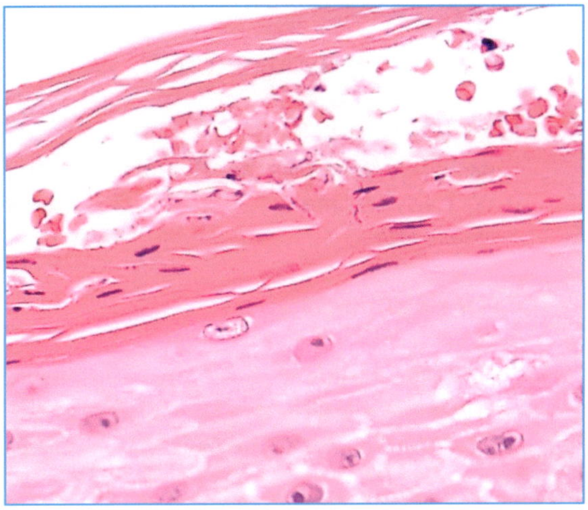

Tinea with "sandwich sign"

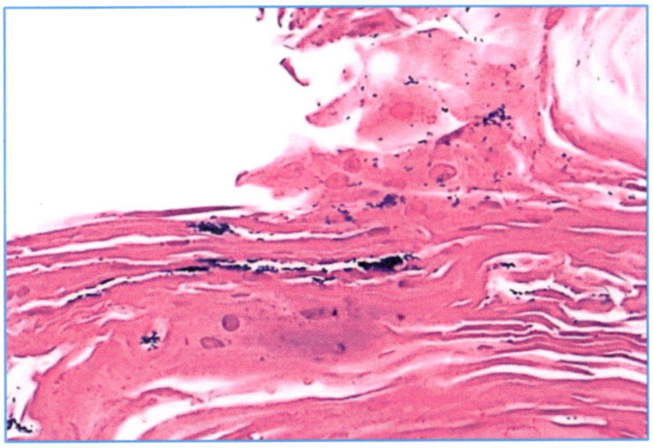

Erythrasma with Gram stain detecting bacteria

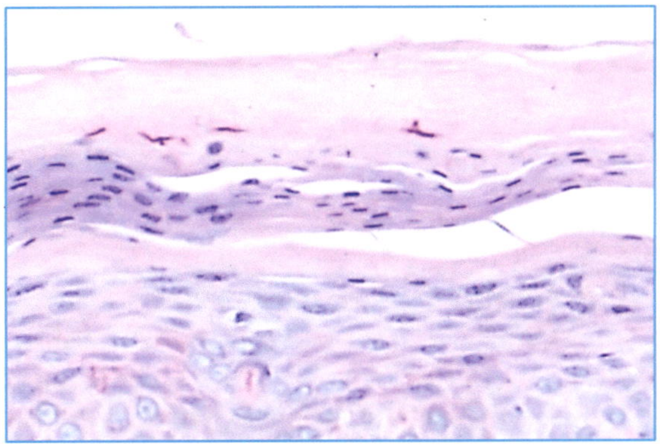

Tinea with PAS stain outlining fungal elements

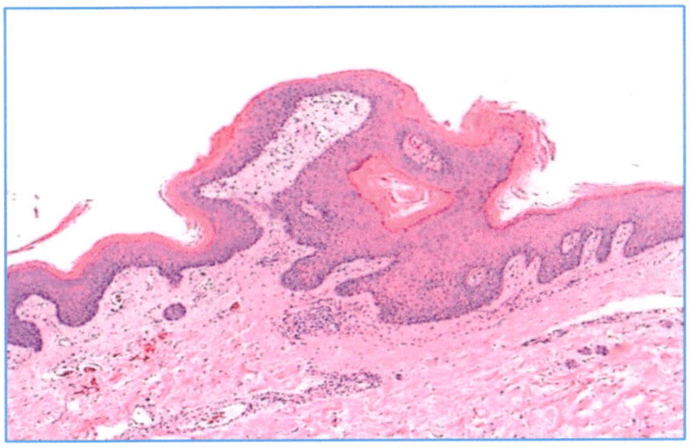

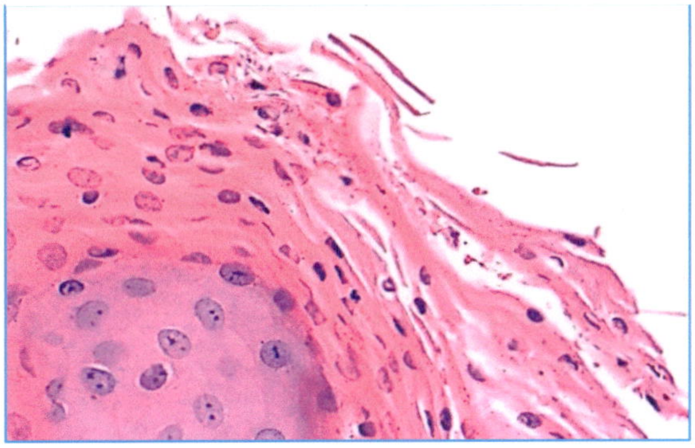

Erythrasma with mild hyperkeratosis and focal parakeratosis

Dermal inflammatory disorders

HOW TO APPROACH DERMAL INFLAMMATIONS

CHECK FOR DERMAL EDEMA

IF OBVIOUS "BAND-LIKE" DERMAL EDEMA IS PRESENT

-PMLE	dermal perivascular lymphocytes
-pernio	dermal perivascular lymphocytes + perieccrine lymphocytes
-Sweet's	dermal neutrophils

IF EDEMA IS SUBTLE AND DIFFUSE:

-urticaria	lasting <24 hours
-PUPPP	3rd trimester of pregnancy
-morbilliform drug	history of medication use

all 3 entities have similar histology with scattered dermal eosinophils and clinical correlation is needed

INFLAMATORY CELLS PREDOMINATE

LOTS OF EOSINOPHILES

-exclude 3 diagnosis mentioned above plus

-Well's syndrome	numerous eosinophils "flame" figures
-insect bite	eosinophils + neutrophils + "V-shaped" inflammation + excoriation

LOTS OF NEUTROPHILS

-LCV	neutrophilic leukocytoclasia
-urticarial vasculitis	variable neutrophylic leukocytoclasia + eosinophils
-erythema marginatum	intact neutrophils + lymphocytes
-neutrophilic eccrine hidradenitis	deep perieccrine neutrophils + eccrine gland necrosis

LOTS OF LYMPHOCYTES

IN SUPERFICIAL DERMIS

-EAC	"tightly cuffed" perivascular lymphocytes and no interstitial lymphocytes
-pigmented purpuric dermatosis	RBC extravasation
-REM	perivascular lymphocytes + dermal mucin
-TMEP	perivascular lymphocytes + mast cells
-2nd syphilis	perivascular lymphocytes + numerous plasma cells

IN SUPERFICIAL AND DEEP DERMIS

-EAC	"tightly cuffed" perivascular lymphocytes and no interstitial lymphocytes
-erythema chronicum migrans	perivascular lymphocytes, + plasma cells + focal mucin
-tumid lupus	patchy perivascular + periadnexal lymphocyte + diffuse mucin

IF MINIMAL OR VERY SUBTLE LYMPHOCYTIC INFLAMMATION IS PRESENT

-tinea	"sandwich" sign hyphae
-erythrasma	bacteria in stratum corneum

IF SKIN IS ULCERATED

-insect bite	"V-shaped" deep inflammation + neutrophils + eosinophils
-pyoderma gangrenosum	necrosis + mixed inflammation with neutrophils predominating

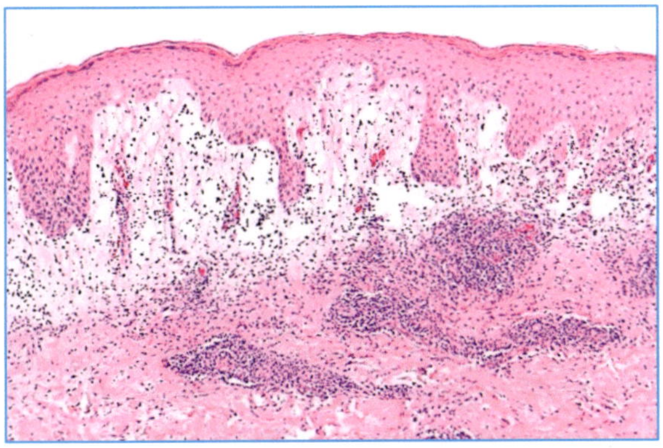

PMLE with dermal edema and perivascular lymphocytic inflammation

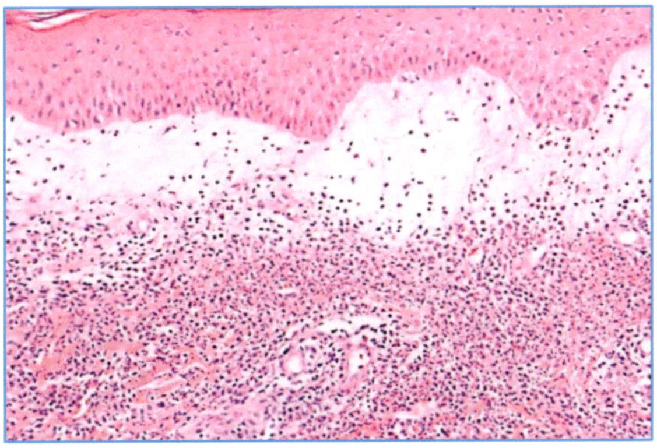

Sweet's syndrome with dermal edema and neutrophils

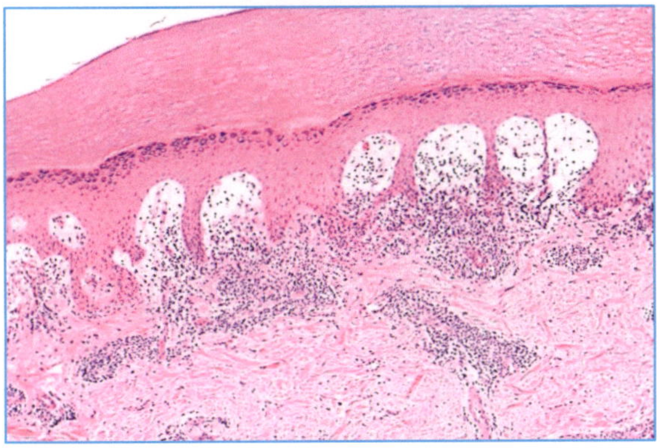

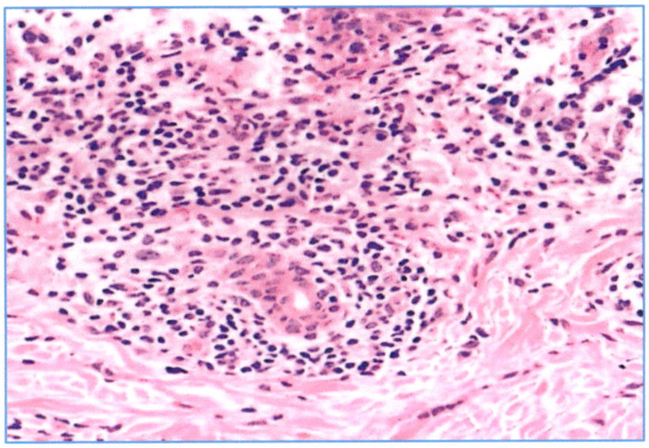

Pernio with dermal edema and perivascular and perieccrine lymphocytic inflammation

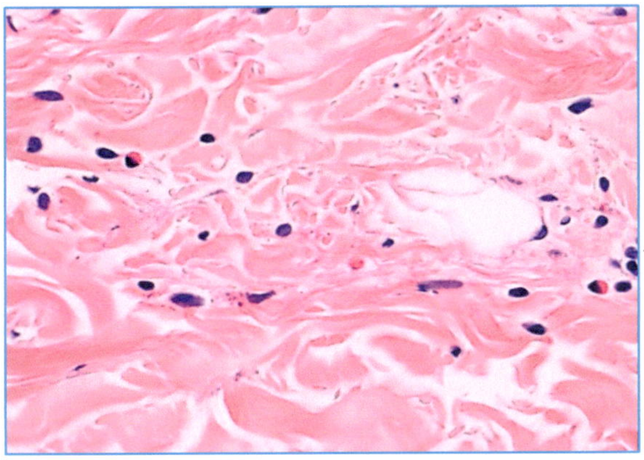

Urticaria with dermal edema and scattered eosinophils

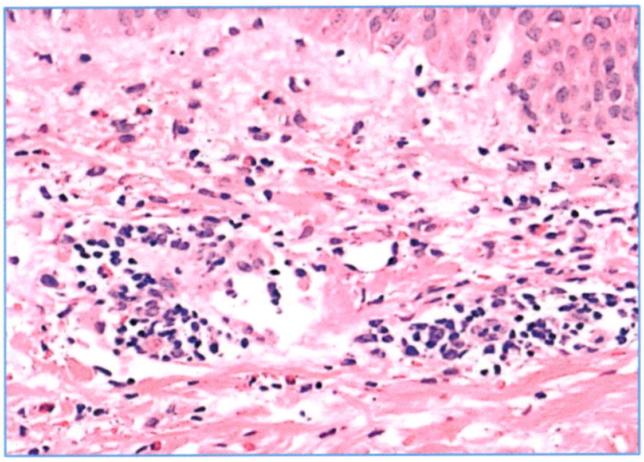

PUPPP with epidermal spongiosis and dermal eosinophils

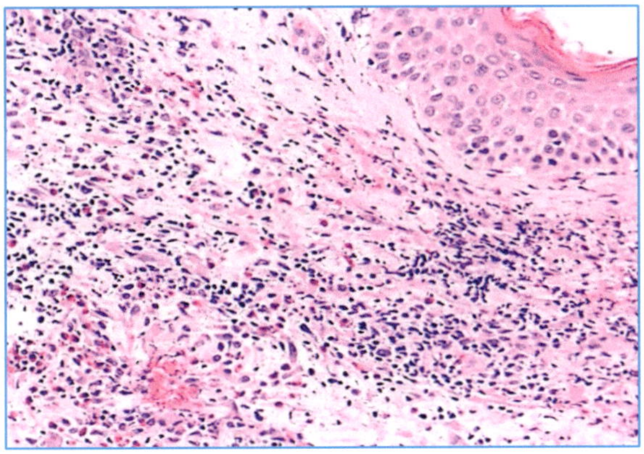

Well's syndrome with dermal eosinophils and "flame" figure

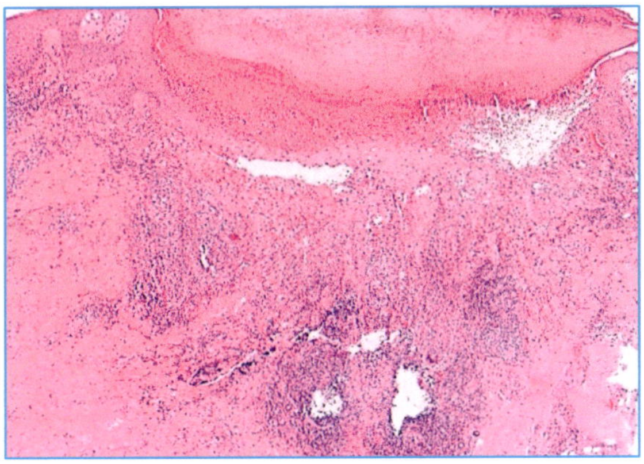

Bite with excoriated epidermis and "V-shaped" mixed inflammation

Dermal inflammatory disorders

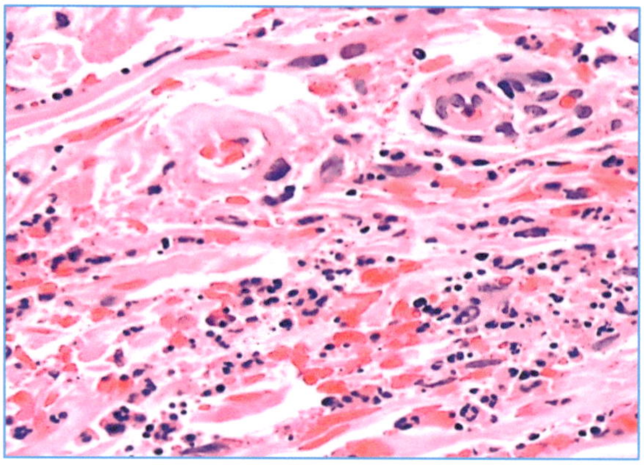

LCV with neutrophils and leukocytoclasia

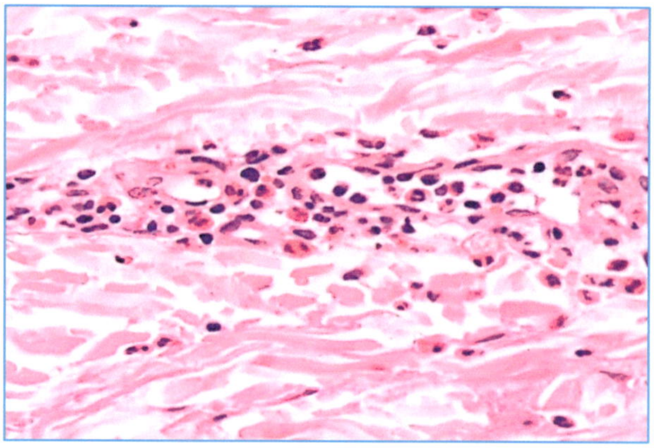

Urticarial vasculitis with many intact neutrophils in and around the vessel and numerous dermal eosinophils

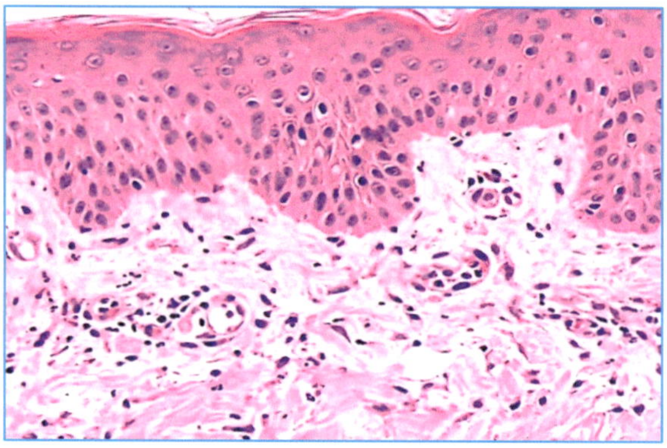

Erythema marginatum with perivascular neutrophils and lymphocyte and no leukocytoclasia

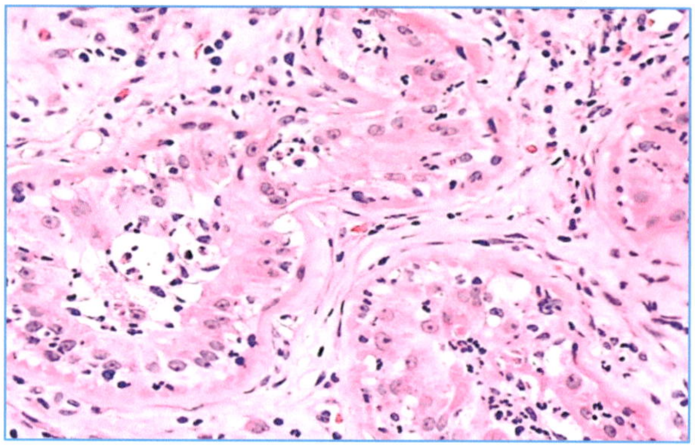

Neutrophilic eccrine hidradenitis with perieccrine neutrophils and necrosis of sweat glands

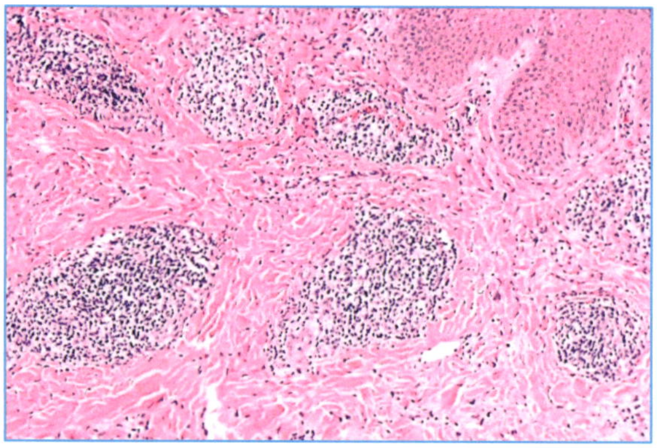

EAC with tightly cuffed perivascular lymphocytes

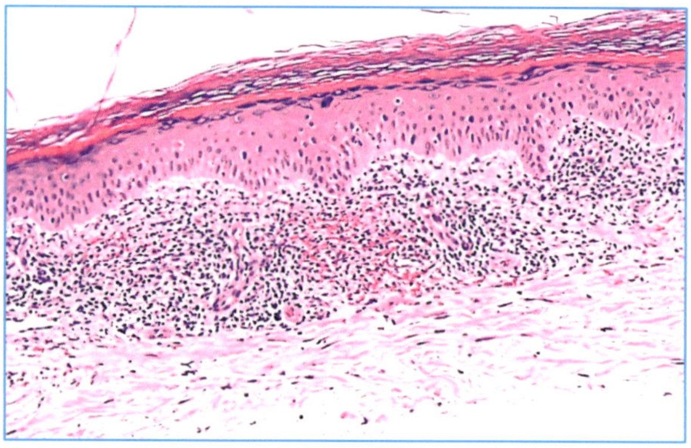

Pigmented purpura with perivascular lymphocytes and RBCs

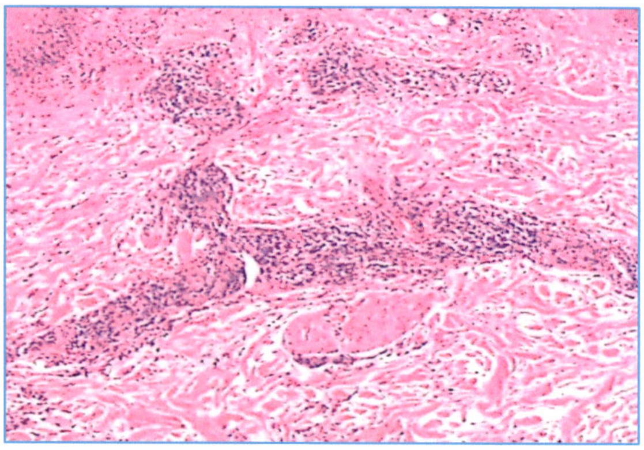

Tumid lupus with perivascular lymphocytes and dermal mucin

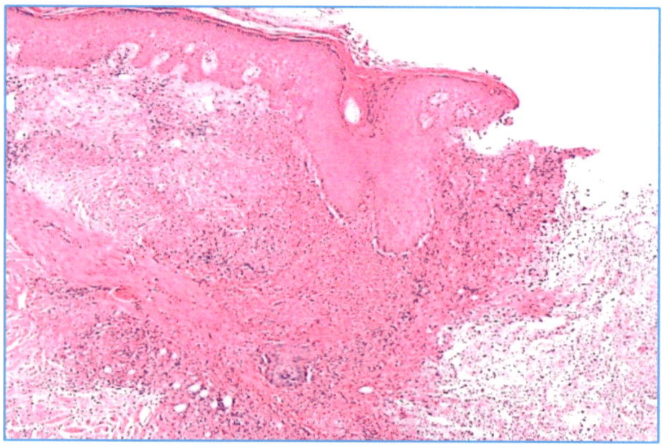

Pyoderma gangrenosum with follicular based ulcer, dermal abscess, and necrosis

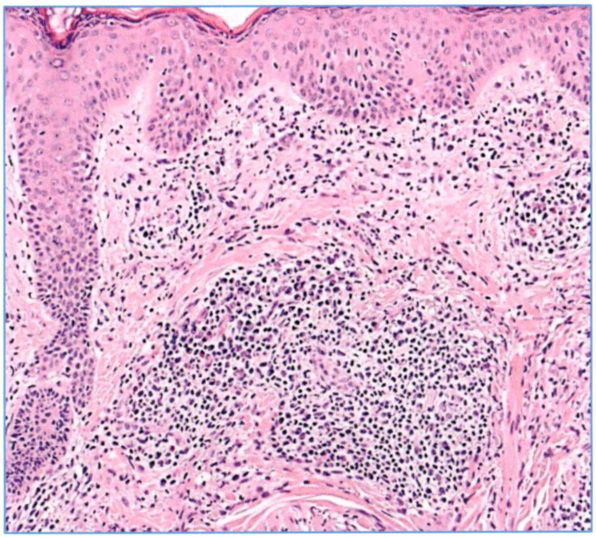

Secondary syphilis with perivascular lymphocyte and numerous plasma cells

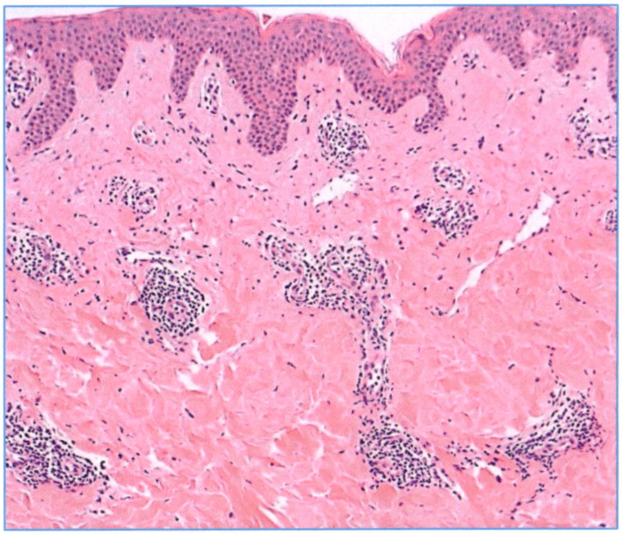

Erythema chronicum migrans with perivascular plasma cells and focal mucin

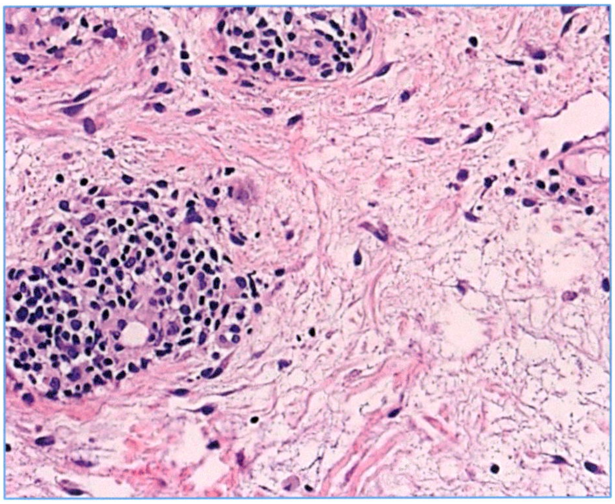

REM with perivascular lymphocytes and dermal mucin

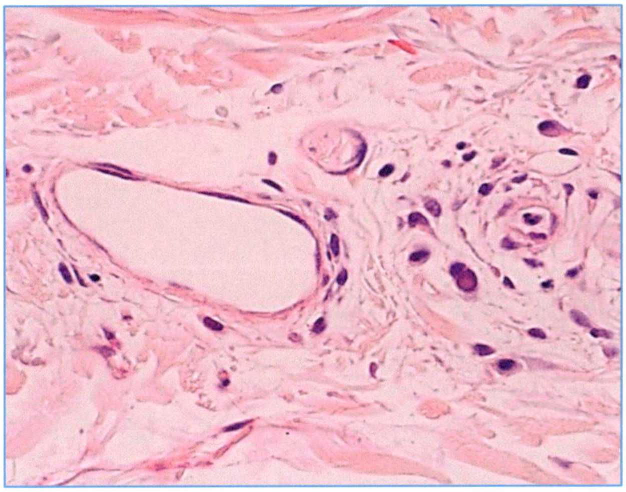

TMEP with telangiectasia and mast cells

Dermal inflammatory disorders

Chapter 7

DISORDERS OF STRATUM CORNEUM

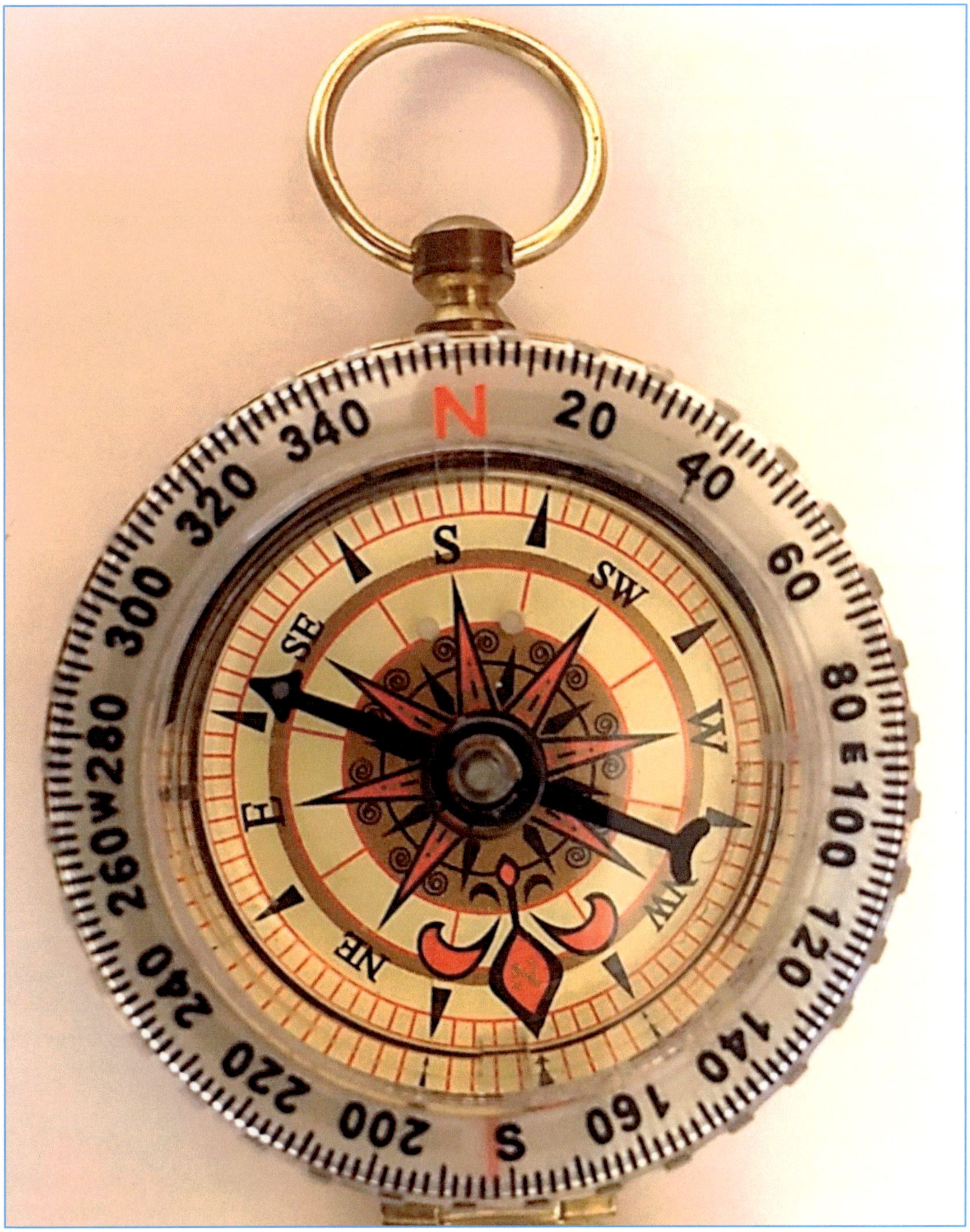

Disorders of stratum corneum

ICHTHYOSES

-group of hereditary disorders characterized by excessive keratinization
-severity varies among different clinical subtypes
-many are part of syndromes and are extremely rare
-keratoderma is the term used for ichthyosis involving the palm and soles

Three most common types are:

Ichthyosis vulgaris

-autosomal semidominant condition due to a mutation in the *filaggrin* gene
-presents in early childhood
-associated with keratosis pilaris and atopy
-fine, "fish scale-like" hyperkeratosis on extremities with sparing of flexures
-larger scales on lower extremities

Histopathology

-mild to moderate hyperkeratosis
-**diminished or absent granular layer**
-normal epidermal thickness
-absent or diminished filaggrin immunostaining

X-linked recessive ichthyosis

-X-linked recessive condition due to mutation in the *steroid sulfatase* gene
-presents in infancy
-fine to large, dirty brown scales involving the entire body, sparing the palms/soles and flexures
-associated with corneal opacities, cryptorchidism, and prolonged labor with affected child

Histopathology

-epidermal acanthosis and hyperkeratosis
-**thickened granular layer**
-retained corneodesmosomes within stratum corneum on electron microscopy

Lamellar ichthyosis

-presents at birth as autosomal recessive condition
-90% due to *TGM1* gene mutation
-born with ectropion and shiny, waxy layer of skin (collodion membrane) that sheds during the first two weeks
-the skin beneath develops thick "plate-like" brown scales with variable erythroderma
-general distribution with flexural involvement
-associated with hypohidrosis, heat intolerance, scarring alopecia, dystrophic nails

Histopathology

-**epidermal acanthosis**
-**compact hyperkeratosis**
-**widened granular layer**

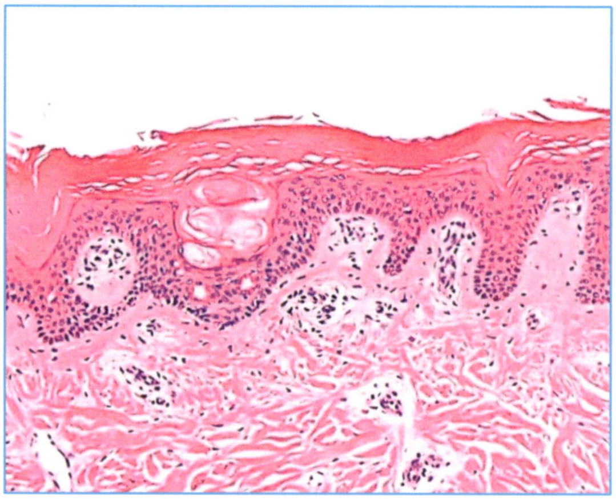

Ichthyosis vulgaris with absent granular layer

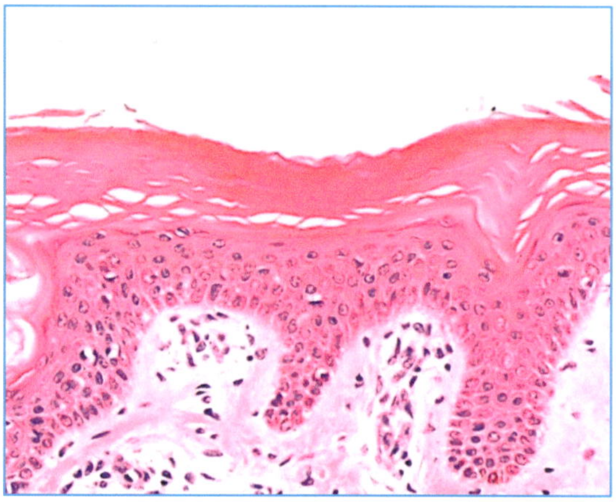

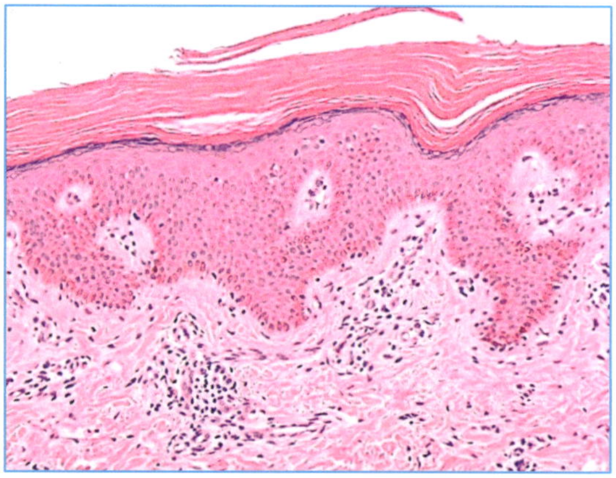

X-linked ichthyosis with prominent granular layer

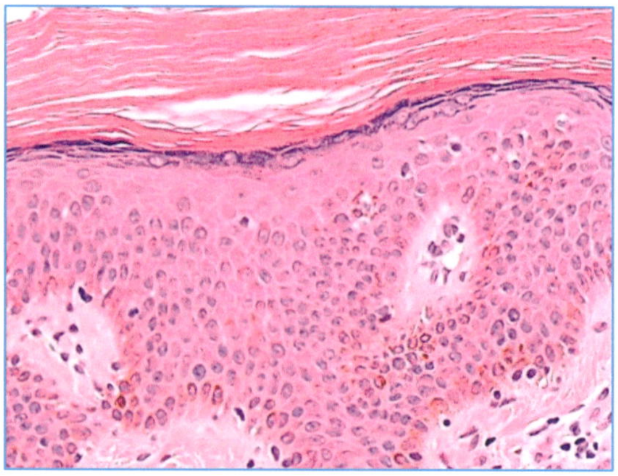

Histologically, most disorders of keratinization can be divided into 4 groups based on presence or absence of a granular layer and presence of prominent parakeratosis and epidermolysis

Group 1
Orthokeratosis with **prominent granular layer** includes:

-**X-linked recessive ichthyosis**
-**Lamellar ichthyosis**
-**Erythrokeratodermia variabilis**
-**IFAP syndrome**
-**KID syndrome**
-**Palmoplantar keratoderma**
-**Sjögren Larsson syndrome**

Group 2
Orthokeratosis with **reduced or absent granular layer** includes:

-**Ichthyosis vulgaris**
-**X-Linked dominant ichthyosis**
-**Harlequin ichthyosis**
-**Refsum syndrome** (can also be in group 1)
-**Tay syndrome**

Group 3
Variable granular layer with **prominent parakeratosis** includes:

-**Netherton syndrome** (vaguely psoriasiform epidermis)
-**CHILD syndrome** (granular layer is normal or thinned)

Group 4
Orthokeratosis with **epidermolytic acantholysis** (coarse purple blue keratohyaline granules) includes:

-**Epidermolytic ichtyosis** also known as **bullous congenital ichthyosiform erythroderma**
-**Ichthyosis hystrix**
-**Ichthyosis bullosa of Siemens**
-**Palmoplantar keratoderma, Vorner type**
-**Nevus unis lateralis**
-**Epidermolytic leukoplakia**
-**Epidermolytic acanthoma**

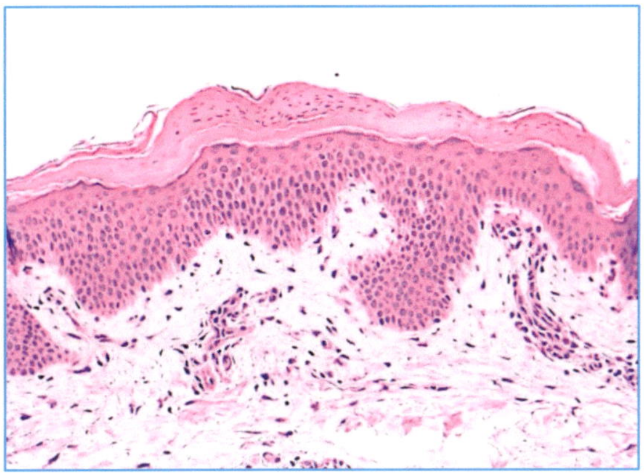

Netherton syndrome with prominent parakeratosis

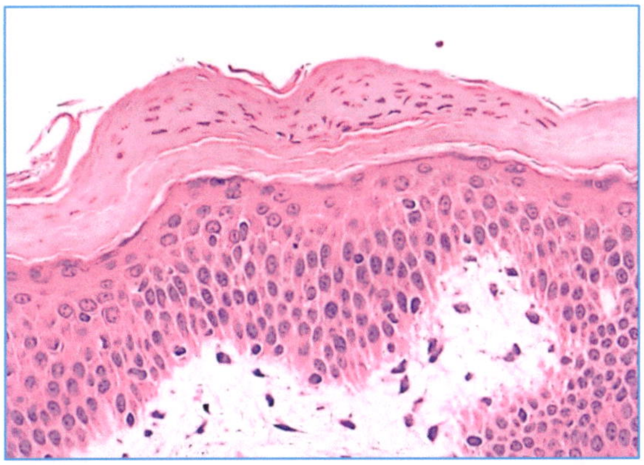

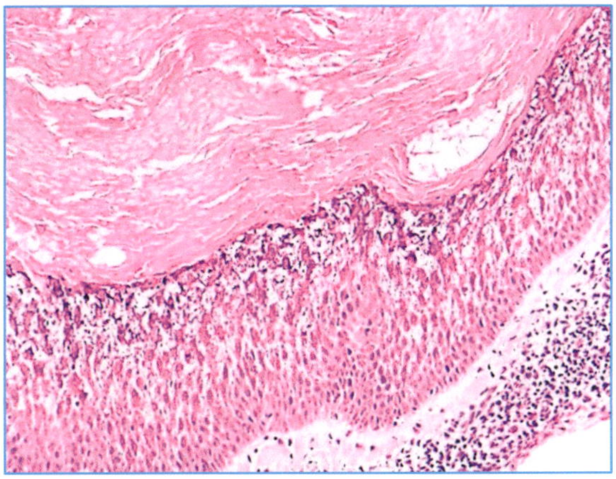

Epidermolytic ichtyosis with coarse, purple-blue keratohyaline granules

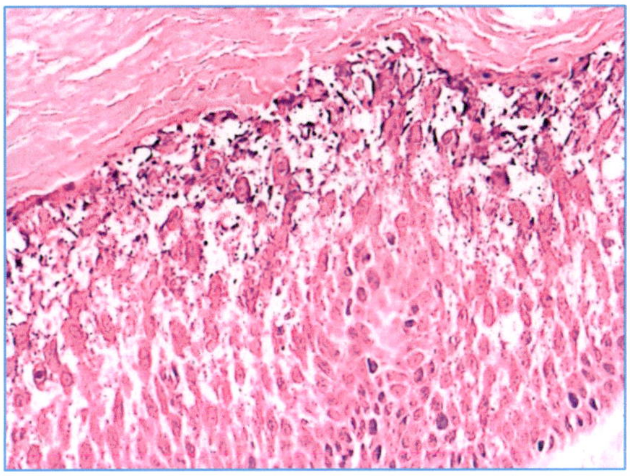

Disorders of stratum corneum

EPIDERMODYSPLASIA VERRUCIFORMIS

-rare autosomal recessive disorder due to mutation in *EVER1* or *EVER2* genes
-characterized by abnormal susceptibility to *HPV*, particularly types 5 and 8
-presents with widespread flat "wart-like" papules that can turn into "horn-like" lesions
-highly susceptible to development of squamous cell carcinoma

Histopathology
-epidermal architecture varies from verrucous (like verruca vulgaris) to undulated (like in flat wart)
-large clustered pale cells with **blue-gray or pink-gray cytoplasm** in upper and middle part of epidermis
-individual cells have **clear intranuclear spaces and perinuclear halos**
-coarse keratohyaline granules are present in keratinocytes

POROKERATOSIS

-heterogenous group of benign epidermal neoplasms with similar histomorphology
-the two most common types are:

Disseminated superficial actinic porokeratosis
-more common in middle-aged women
-numerous, red-brown, small annular lesions with slightly raised keratotic rim
-predilection for sun exposed areas, particularly shin and arms

Porokeratosis of Mibelli
-present in childhood as annular plaque with atrophic center and keratotic margins
-predilection for extremities

Histopathology
-pathognomonic sign in all forms is the **"cornoid lamella"**, a leaning column of parakeratosis
-the granular layer underneath the cornoid lamellae is diminished and keratinocytes are mildly atypical and dyskeratotic
-if the lesion is biopsied in toto, two cornoid lamellae leaning toward each other are detected

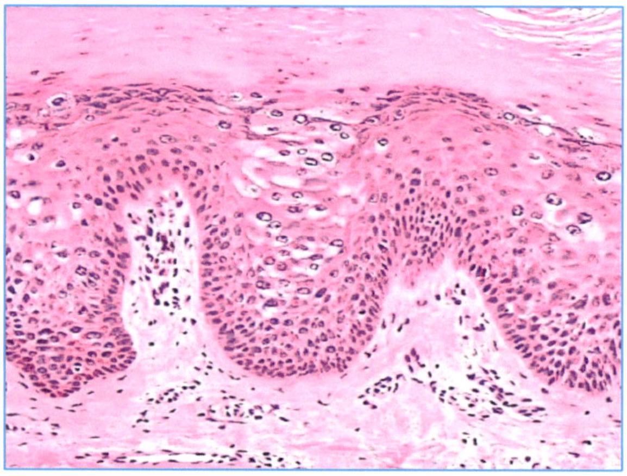

Epidermodysplasia verruciformis with clusters of swollen pale keratinocytes

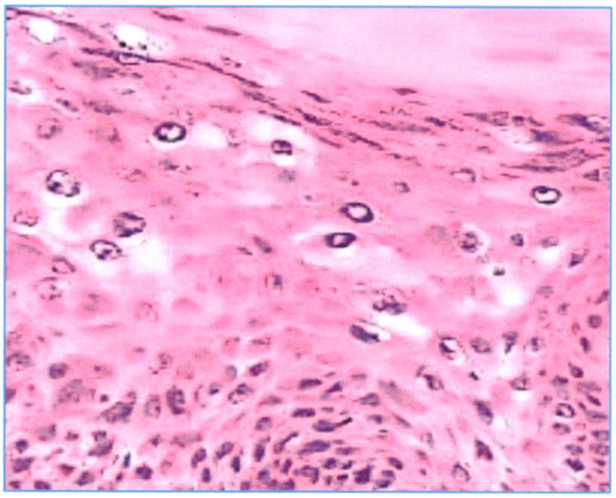

Epidermodysplasia verruciformis with intranuclear clear spaces and perinuclear halo

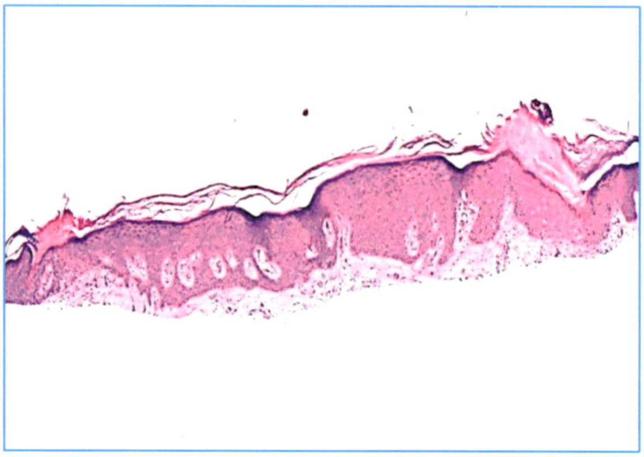

Porokeratosis with two cornoid lamellae facing each other

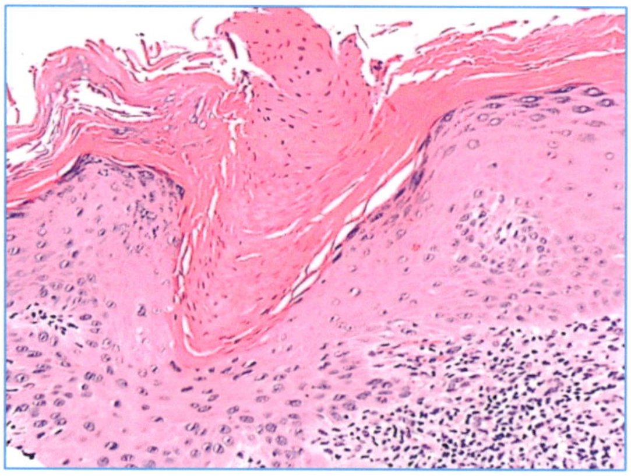

Porokeratosis with leaning column of parakeratosis

GRANULAR PARAKERATOSIS (INTERTRIGINOUS/AXILLARY)

-more common in adult women
-pruritic hyperpigmented papules and plaques
-favors axillae and less commonly inguinal and inframammary areas
-possible association with contact reaction to antiperspirant and *filaggrin* defect

Histopathology
-irregular wavy epidermis
-epidermal hyperkeratosis with **bordeaux red stratum corneum**
-stratum corneum with **thick parakeratosis** with **retained keratohyaline granules**

PITTED KERATOLYSIS

-bacterial infection most commonly due to *Kytococcus sedentarius,* a corynebacterium
-presents with shallow pits and malodor of the soles, particularly the weight-bearing areas
-palms can also be affected but less frequently

Histopathology
-rarely biopsied
-acral hyperkeratotic epidermis
-shallow epidermal indentations filled with keratin (narrower than in callus or clavus)
-bacteria are present in the pits
-no dermal inflammation

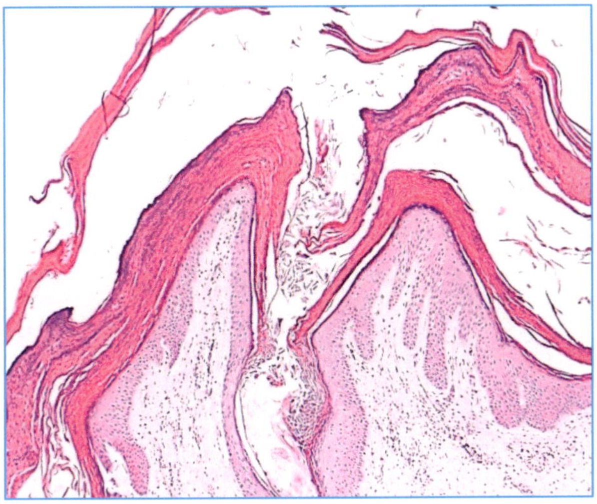
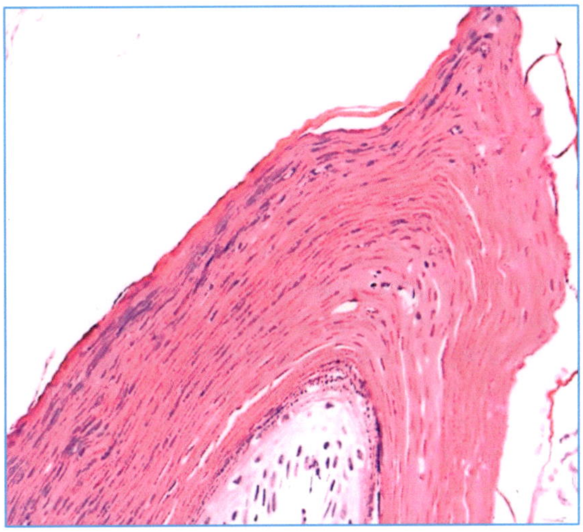

Granular parakeratosis with irregular, wavy epidermis with bordeaux red stratum corneum

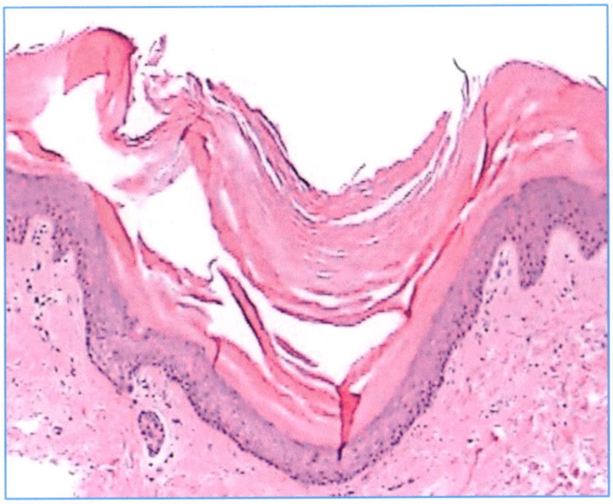

Pitted keratolysis with shallow epidermal pit filled with keratin

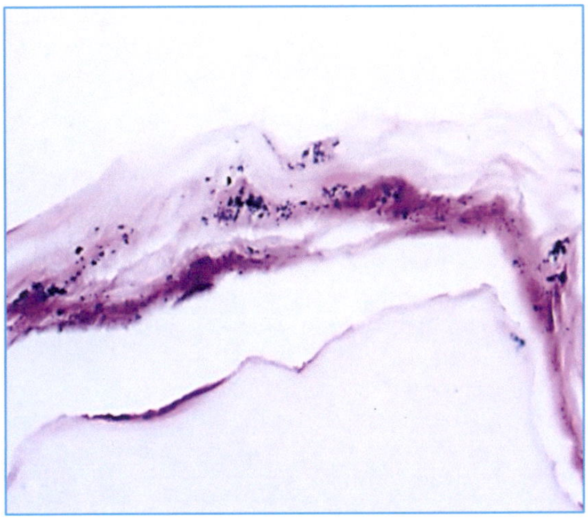

Pitted keratolysis with bacteria in the stratum corneum (Gram stain)

Disorders of stratum corneum

ACRODERMATITIS ENTEROPATHICA/ NECROLYTIC MYGRATORY ERYTHEMA (ERYTHEMA FIGURATUM)/ PELLAGRA

Acrodermatitis enteropathica

-defect in dietary zinc absorption results in growth retardation, impaired immune function, and diarrhea
-primary form is rare autosomal recessive disease due to *SLC39A4* gene mutation
-secondary form due to low zinc intake (alcoholics, anorexia) or zinc malabsorption
-present as eczematous, scaly plaque on perioral and acral skin along with alopecia and diarrhea

Necrolytic migratory erythema

-occur in glucagon producing pancreatic tumor (glucagonoma)
-presents as red, figurate erythema with papules, vesicles, and erosions
-most often affects the genital and anal region, the buttocks, groins, and lower legs
-associated glossitis and nail ridging

Pellagra

-deficiency of niacin (vitamin B_3)
-3D; diarrhea, dementia, dermatitis
-erythema, scaling, and thickening of sun-exposed skin

Histopathology

-all entities demonstrate similar histology
-starts with epidermal **hyperkeratosis, absence of granular layer and pallor and ballooning of keratinocytes in the upper epidermis**
-**in older lesions pallor disappear** and epidermis is psoriasiform
-**parakeratosis is present and granular layer is missing**
-focal necrotic keratinocytes are present

TALON NOIR

-known as "black heel"
-post-traumatic intraepidermal hemorrhage
-unilateral brown-black or blue-black petechiae
-coalesce to hyperpigmented macule or patch
-usually horizontally oriented on the posterior aspect of the heel, just superior to the hyperkeratotic edge of the plantar surface
-can occur on other traumatized acral sites like toe ("tennis toe"), thumb ("play station thumb")

Histopathology

-hyperkeratotic stratum corneum consistent with an acral site
-**within the stratum corneum there is collection of blood at various stages of hemolysis**
-extravasated red blood cells can sometimes be seen in papillary dermis and intracorneal portion of the eccrine sweat ducts

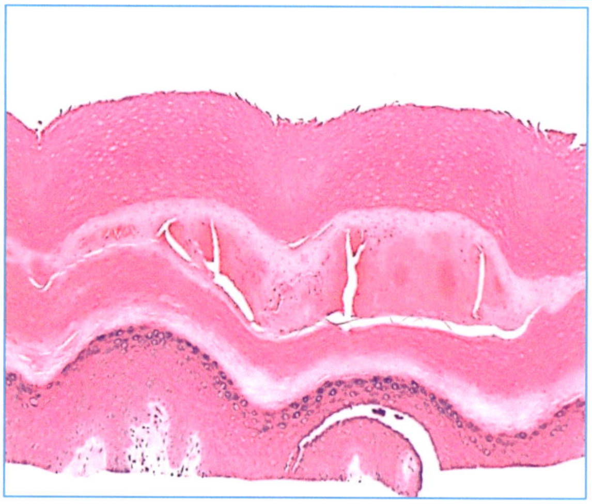

Talon noir of acral skin with intracorneal RBCs

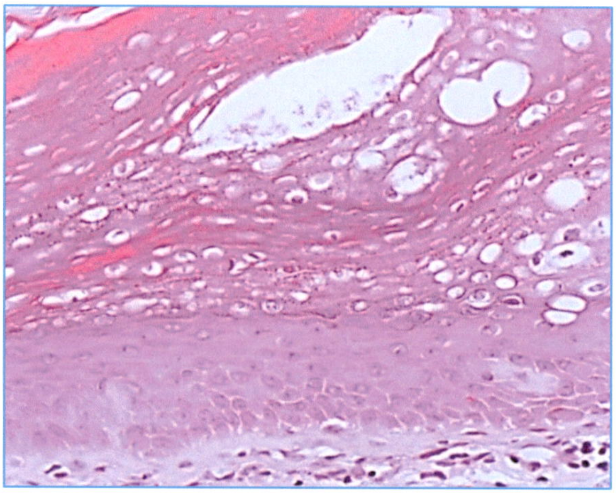

Early lesion of necrolytic migratory erythema (NME) with pale, ballooned keratinocytes

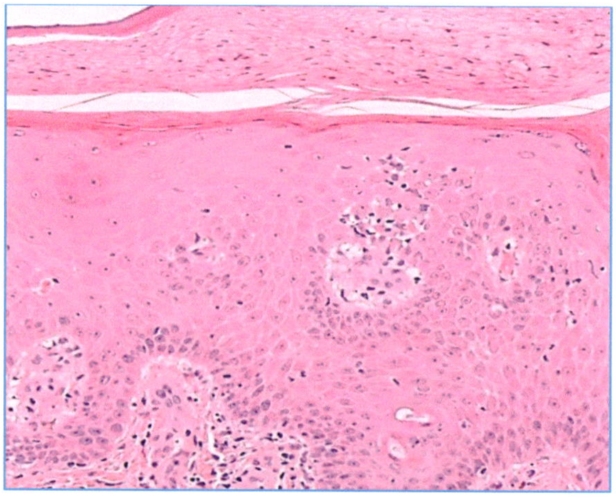

Late psoriasiform lesion of NME with parakeratosis and absent granular layer

CALLUS/ CLAVUS

Callus

-thickening of epidermis caused by chronic friction or pressure
-mainly located on soles but also palms
-circumscribed, hyperkeratotic lesion
-non-painful with pressure

Clavus (corn)

-localized skin thickening which develops a central keratotic plug
-results from chronic pressure or friction
-develop on the feet
-painful with pressure

Histopathology

-both are "cup-shaped" and well-circumscribed
-the difference is presence of **hypergranulosis in callus and hypogranulosis in clavus**

KNUCKLE PAD (GARROD PAD)

-thick skin-colored plaques
-overlays the extensor aspect of the interphalangeal and metacarpophalangeal joints
-usually multiple and develops rapidly
-may be part of a hereditary syndrome or develop sporadically related to chronic trauma
-considered a form of fibromatosis but some consider it a condition associated with fibromatosis

Histopathology

-epidermal acanthosis with **extensive hyperkeratosis**
-mild to moderate dermal fibrosis

CIRCUMSCRIBED ACRAL HYPOKERATOSIS

-idiopathic, acquired condition
-presents as solitary, asymptomatic, depressed, flat-based deformity, with a slightly raised border on the palm or, rarely, the sole

Histopathology

-abrupt cleft at the transition point from normal acral epidermis to hypokeratotic epidermis

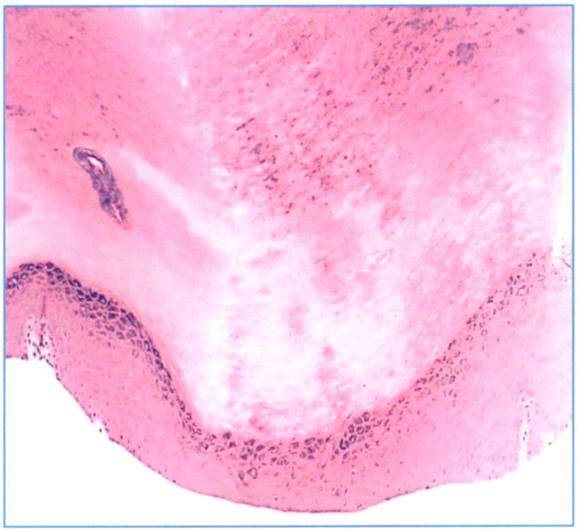

Callus with prominent granular layer

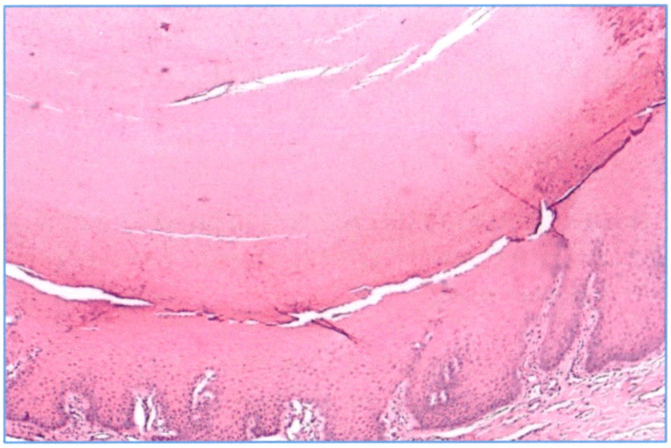

Clavus with loss of granular layer

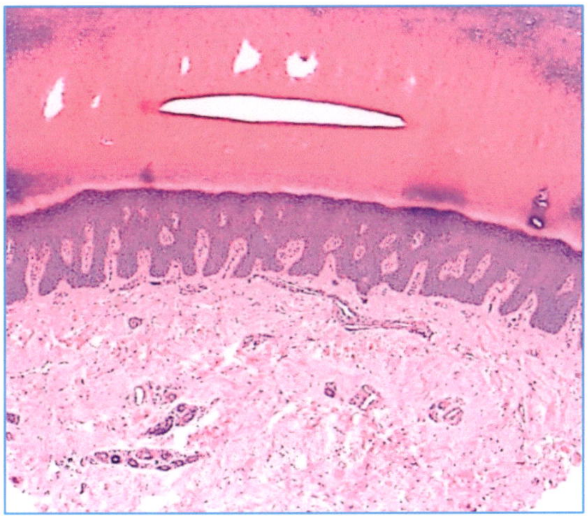

Knuckle pad with prominent epidermal hyperkeratosis and moderate dermal fibrosis

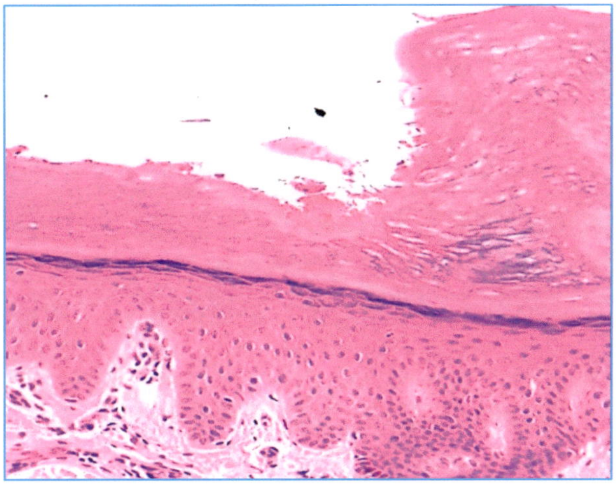

Circumscribed acral hypokeratosis with sharp delineation between normal and hypokeratotic acral skin

Disorders of stratum corneum

HOW TO APPROACH WHEN EPIDERMIS IS NOT INFLAMED BUT NOT NORMAL

EXCLUDE BENIGN OR MALIGNANT EPIDERMAL TUMORS (NON-MELANOMA SKIN CANCERS AND VERRUCAE)

EPIDERMIS IS ICHTHYOTIC AND PATIENT IS A CHILD	
-X-linked recessive ichthyosis	prominent granular layer
-ichthyosis vulgaris	reduced granular layer
-Netherton syndrome	prominent parakeratosis
EPIDERMOLYTIC HYPERKERATOSIS IS PRESENT	
-epidermolytic ichthyosis	child
-epidermolytic acanthoma	adult
STRATUM CORNEUM IS BORDEAUX RED WITH PROMINENY GRANULES	
-granular parakeratosis	axilla
PALE, BALLON-LIKE KERATINOCYTES ARE PRESENT	
-nutritional deficiencies, glucagonoma	
"PIT-LIKE" EPIDERMAL INVAGINATION IS PRESENT	
-pitted keratolysis	bacteria present
BLOOD IS PRESENT IN THE STRATUM CORNEUM	
-talon noir	heel
"CUP SHAPED" EPIDERMAL INVAGINATION PRESENT ON FEET	
-callus	prominent granular layer
-clavus	no granular layer
EPIDERMIS LOOKS LIKE ACTINIC KERATOSIS BUT NOT QUITE, LOOK FOR CORNOID LAMELLAE AND IF PRESENT	
-porokeratosis	leaning parakeratosis
EPIDERMIS LOOKS LIKE AN UNUSUAL WART	
-epidermodysplasia verruciformis	pale cells with gray-blue cytoplasm

Chapter 7

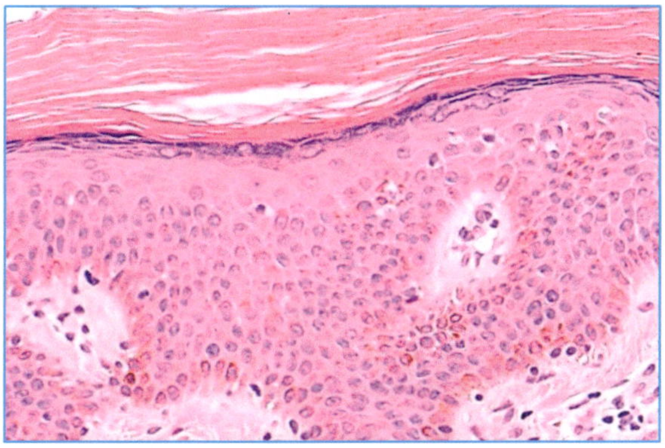

X-linked ichthyosis with hypergranulosis

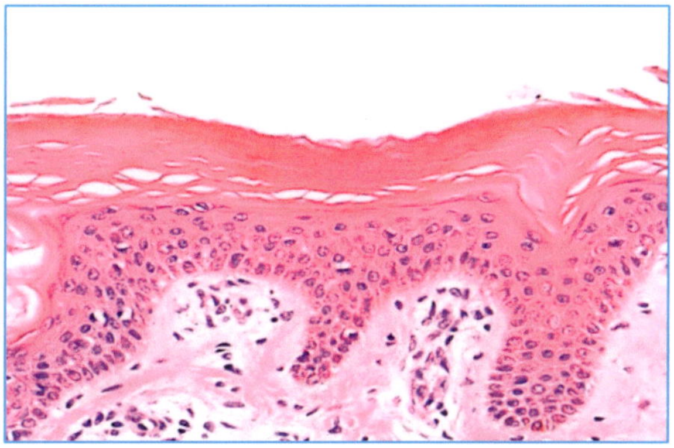

Ichthyosis vulgaris with absent granular layer

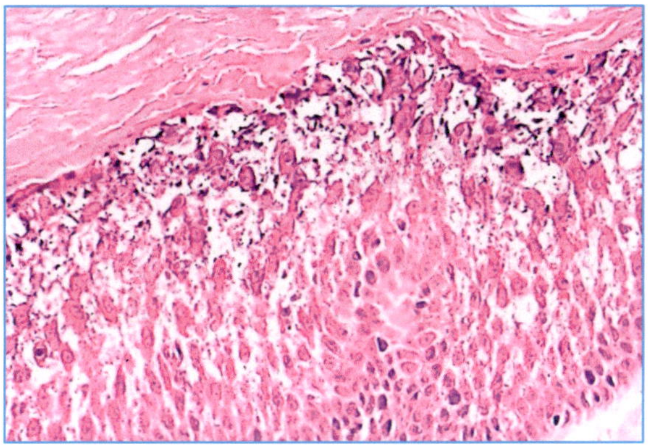

Epidermolytic ichthyosis with coarse, basophilic and eosinophilic granules

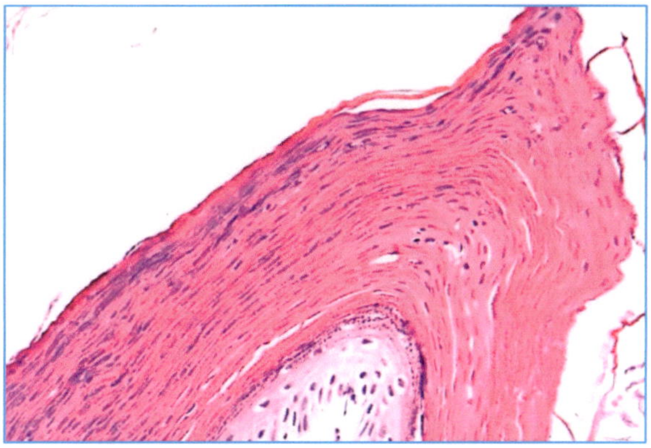

Granular parakeratosis with bordeaux red stratum corneum and compact parakeratosis

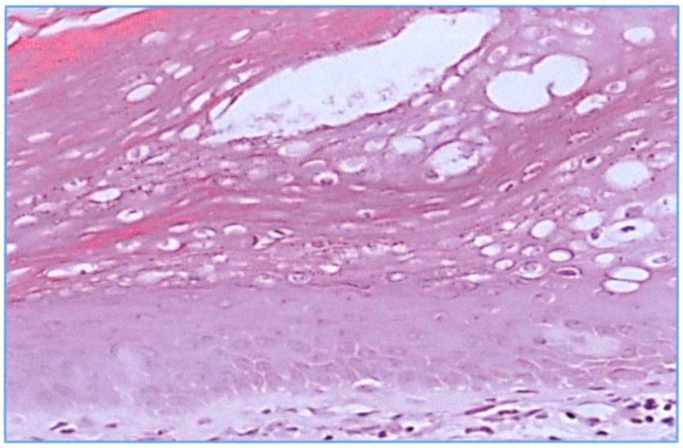

Acrodermatitis enteropathica with pale keratinocytes in superficial epidermis

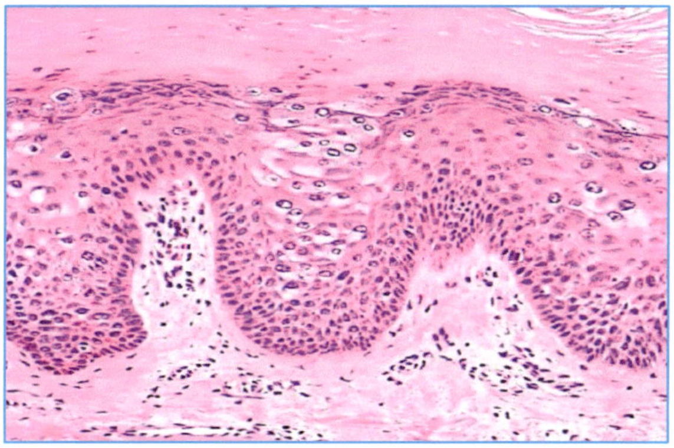

Epidermodysplasia verruciformis with large, clustered, gray-pink, pale cells

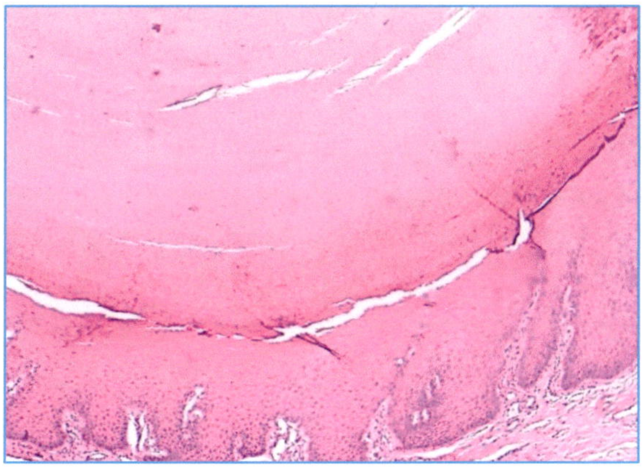

Cup shaped clavus with epidermal hypogranulosis

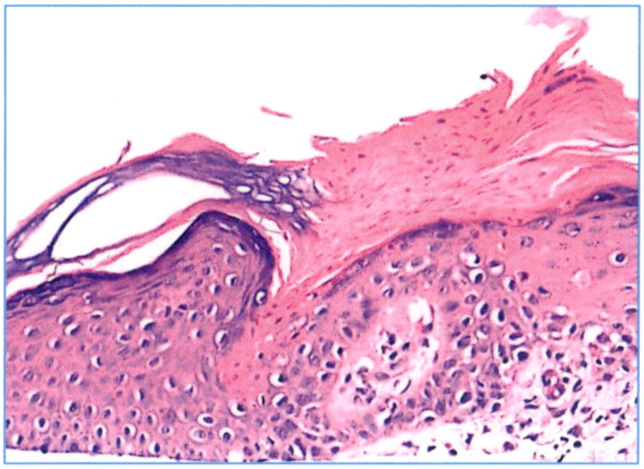

Porokeratosis with leaning column of parakeratosis

Disorders of stratum corneum

Chapter 8

INTRAEPIDERMAL VESICULAR AND BLISTERING DISORDERS

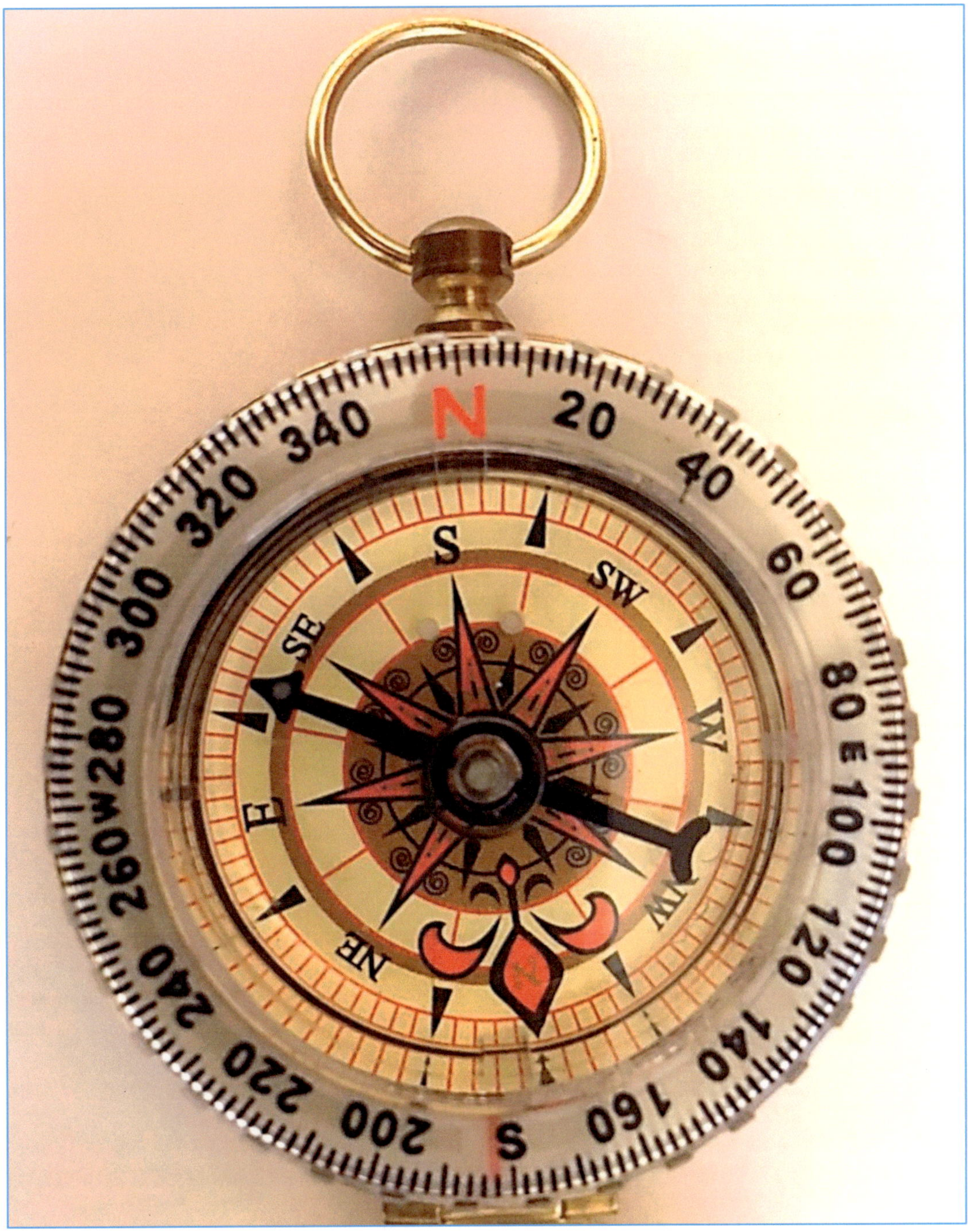

Intraepidermal vesicular and blistering disorders

PEMPHIGUS VULGARIS (PV)

-severe blistering autoimmune disease due to IgG antibodies to *desmoglein 3* (mucosal dominant pemphigus) and *Dsg1* and *Dsg3* (mucocutaneous pemphigus)
-favors middle-aged adults and is more common in Jewish population
-painful erosions in the mouth with or without flaccid skin vesicles and bullae, with positive Nikolsky's sign
-lesions slowly heal without scarring
-skin lesions are randomly distributed and any part of the skin can be affected

Histopathology
-**eosinophilic spongiosis** in early lesions followed by **"cell poor" intraepidermal blister with suprabasal acantholysis**
-basal layer keratinocytes stay attached to the basement membrane (**"tombstones")**
-**individual acantholytic keratinocytes within the blister**
-**hair follicles** are involved by **acantholysis**
-superficial dermal perivascular lymphocytic infiltrate with frequent eosinophils
-DIF shows intercellular **"chicken-wire like" staining** with IgG+/-C3, **stronger in the lower part of the epidermis**
-IIF positive for circulating IgG autoantibodies using monkey esophagus as the substrate

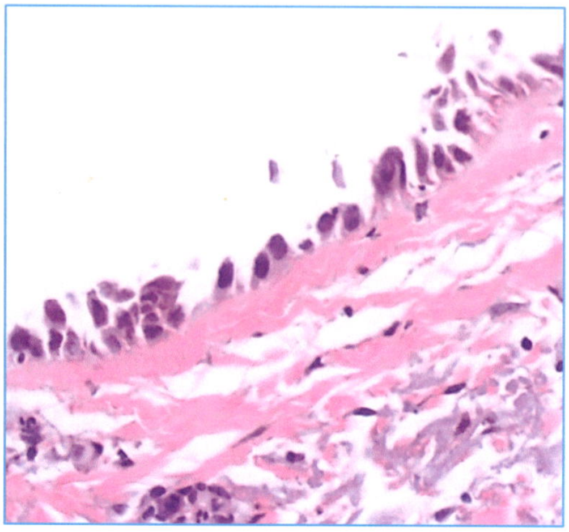

"Tombstones" of pemphigus vulgaris preserved basal layer keratinocytes

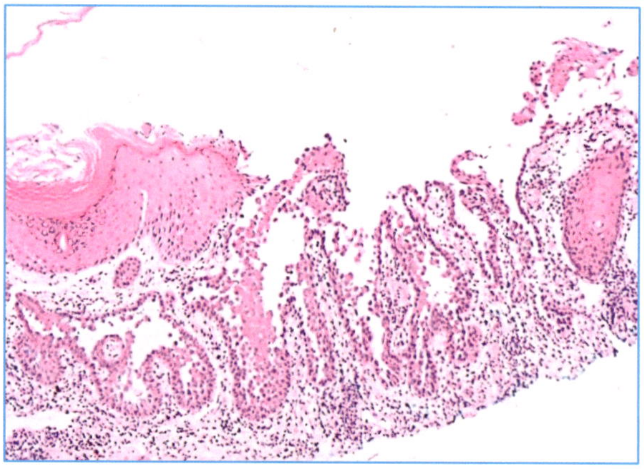

PV with suprabasal acantholysis

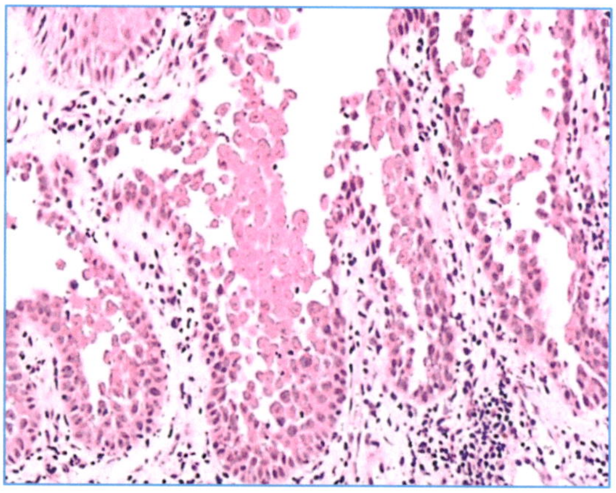

PV with intraepidermal blister without inflammatory cells

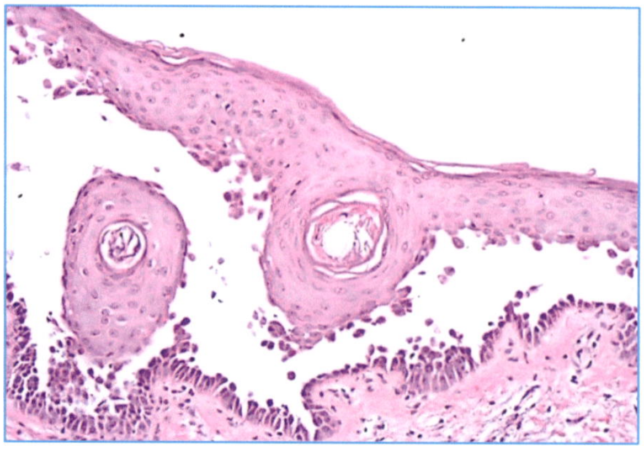

PV with acantholysis involving hair follicles

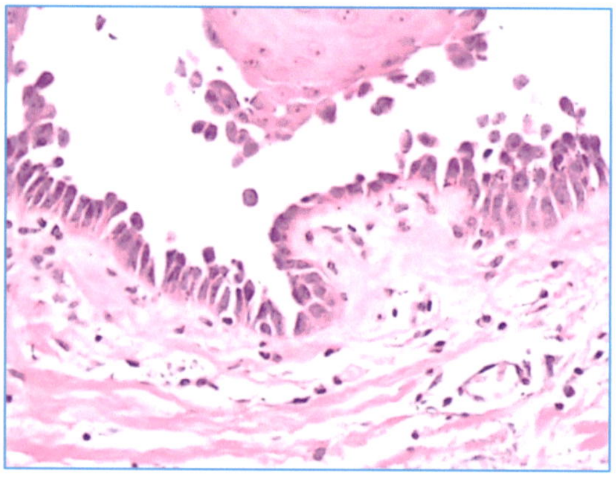

PV with individual acantholytic keratinocytes within the blister

Chapter 8

PEMPHIGUS FOLIACEUS (PF)

-less severe variant of pemphigus due to IgG autoantibodies to *desmoglein 1*
-erythematous patches and erosions covered with "cornflake" scales that typically favor seborrheic distribution
-flaccid bullae rarely present and Nikolsky's sign is positive
-lacks mucosal involvement

Clinical variants:

Fogo selvagem

-endemic form in children and young adults in rural Brazil (identical clinically and histologically to PF)

Pemphigus erythematosus (Senear-Usher syndrome)

-clinical and histological overlap between PF and lupus

Histopathology

-starts with variable spongiosis and focal **subcorneal/ intragranular acantholysis** with neutrophils and eosinophils in serum crust
-in older lesions, **the blister roof is absent, denuded of stratum corneum**
-**scattered neutrophils are present in epidermis**
-dermis is edematous with mild mixed inflammation
-DIF shows intercellular **"chicken-wire like"** staining with IgG+/-C3, as in PV, but **upper epidermis stains more intensely**
-IIF has the same appearance as in PV with guinea pig esophagus as best substrate

PEMPHIGUS VEGETANS

-localized variant of pemphigus vulgaris
-usually confined to intertriginous areas and less frequently scalp and face
-early on, flaccid blisters and bullae that break easily
-as these heal, warty vegetative purulent plaques are formed

Histopathology

-**early lesions show suprabasal acantholysis** with intraepidermal blister (same as in pemphigus vulgaris)
-**established lesions** demonstrate **verrucous epidermal hyperplasia** with eosinophilic spongiosis and **intraepidermal eosinophilic pustules**
-DIF shows intercellular **"chicken-wire like"** staining with IgG+/-C3 as in pemphigus vulgaris

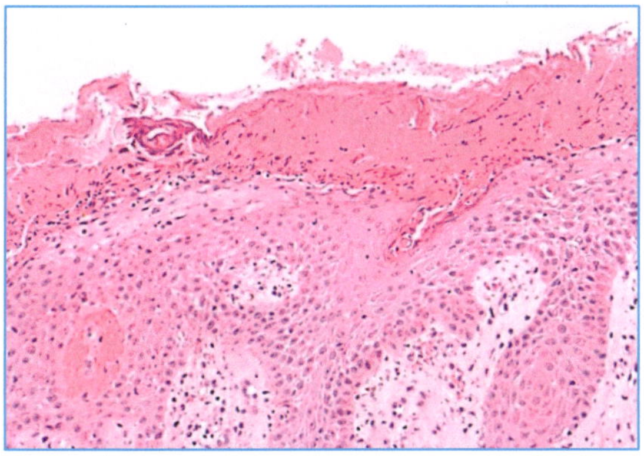

Early PF with subcorneal acantholysis with neutrophils in serum crust

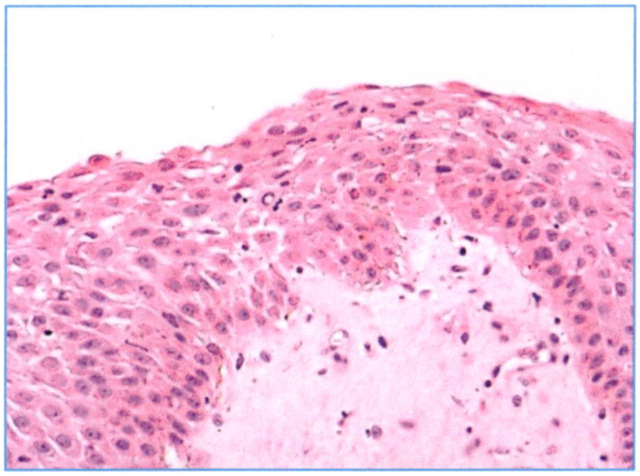

Established PF with absent stratum corneum and scattered intraepidermal neutrophils

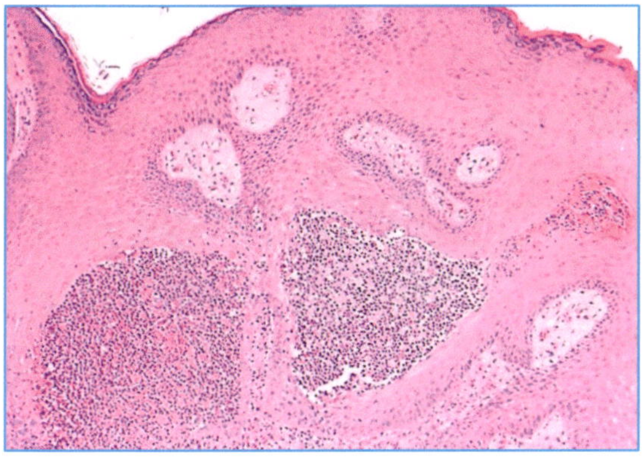

P. vegetans with epidermal hyperplasia

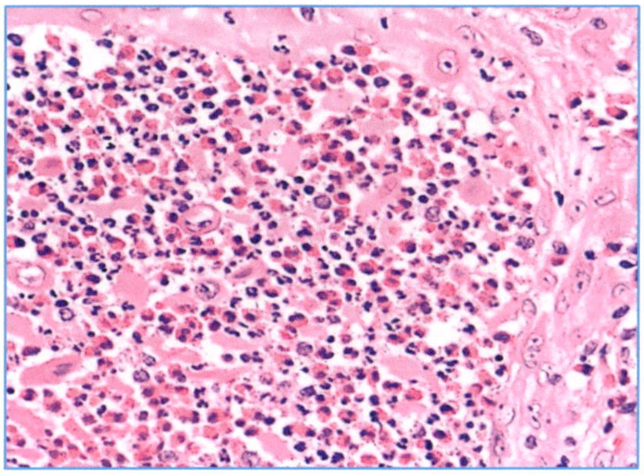

P. vegetans with intraepidermal eosinophilic pustule

Intraepidermal vesicular and blistering disorders

IgA PEMPHIGUS

-variant of pemphigus vulgaris
-middle-aged or the elderly individuals
-characteristically has pruritic flaccid vesicles/pustules in an annular/circinate pattern with central crusting
-favors flexural areas (axilla, groin), although it can affect any area
-may be associated with IgA gammopathy

Histopathology

-two types with subcorneal or intraepidermal (suprabasal) neutrophilic pustules
-**subcorneal pustular dermatosis (SPD) type** with subcorneal neutrophilic pustule is indistinguishable from Sneddon-Wilkinson disease
-target antigen is *desmocolin 1*
-**intraepidermal neutrophilic (IEN) type** with neutrophilic pustule in lower part of the epidermis
-target antigens are *desmogleins 1 and 3*
-in both types, there is a mixed inflammatory infiltrate in the underlying dermis
-DIF reveals IgA deposits in cell membrane of epidermal keratinocytes

PARANEOPLASTIC PEMPHIGUS

-paraneoplastic variant of pemphigus associated with underlying malignancy (most commonly non-Hodgkin's lymphoma, CLL, or Castleman's disease)
-due to IgG antibodies to members of *plakin* family and *desmogleins*
-characteristic severe oral ulcerations
-skin lesions are polymorphous ("pemphigus-like" blisters, lichenoid papules and/or "erythema multiforme-like" macules)
-high mortality rate

Histopathology

-variable histomorphology reflecting polymorphic clinical presentation
-suprabasal acantholysis with minimal inflammation in "pemphigus-like" blisters
-lichenoid dermal infiltrate with focal interface changes in lichenoid papules
-interface vacuolar changes with some necrotic keratinocytes in "EM-like" lesions
-DIF shows staining with IgG and C3 in intercellular **"chicken-wire like"** and **linearly along basement membrane**
-IIF shows same pattern using rat bladder

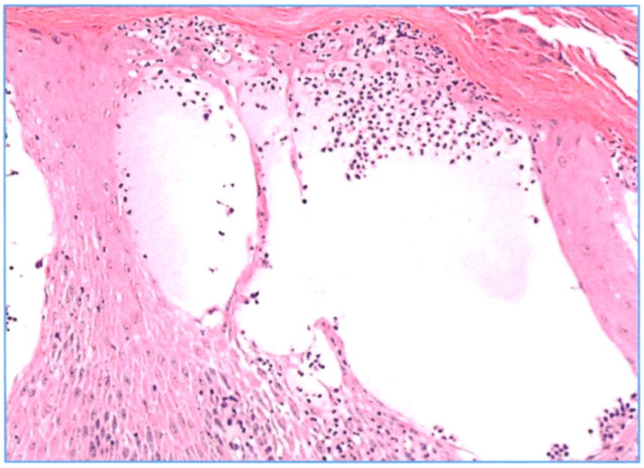
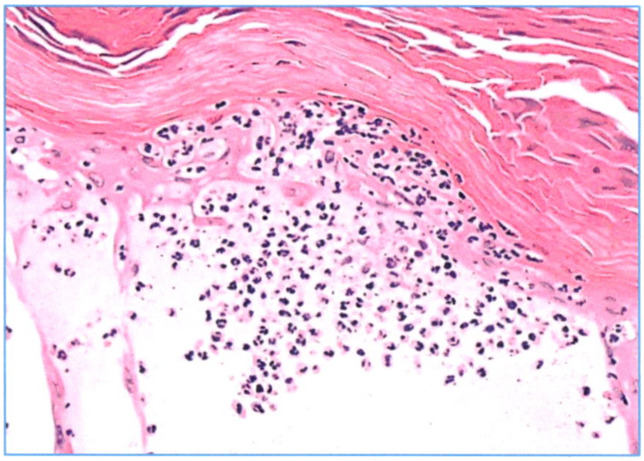

IgA pemphigus with subcorneal neutrophilic pustule similar to subcorneal pustular dermatosis

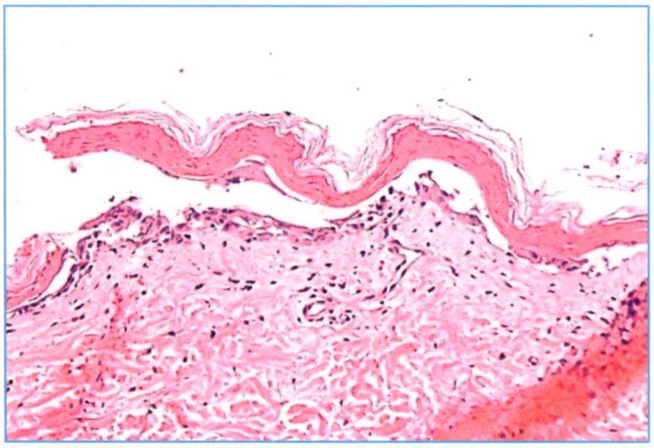
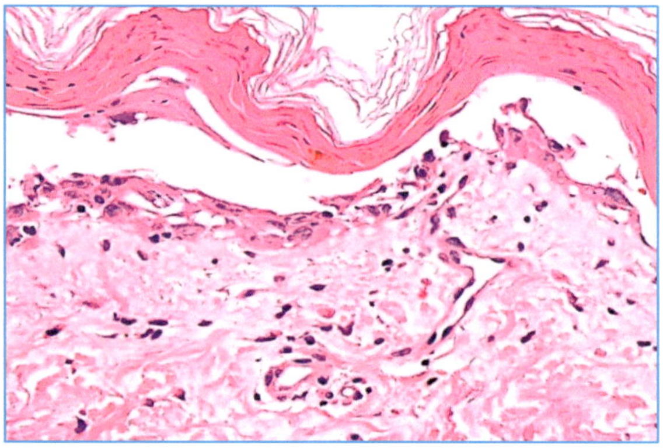

Paraneoplastic pemphigus with suprabasal blister

INCONTINENTIA PIGMENTI

-X-linked dominant genodermatosis with four cutaneous phases classically presenting in timelines outlined below, but may vary

Vesicular phase

-birth to 3 weeks

-coalescing vesicles on an erythematous base on the trunk and extremities

Verrucous phase

-2-6 weeks but can be seen up to 2 years of age

-hyperkeratotic verrucous papules on the extremities

Hyperpigmented phase

-2-6 months but can be seen up to adolescence

-linear hyperpigmentation distributed along Blaschko's lines

Hypopigmented phase

-in puberty, but can persist through adulthood

-linear atrophic, hypopigmented and hairless lesions

Histopathology

Vesicular- mild epidermal spongiosis with numerous **intraepidermal eosinophils forming vesicles**

Verrucous- hyperkeratotic, acanthotic epidermis with **dyskeratotic cells and scattered eosinophils**

Hyperpigmented- focal interface vacuolar changes with **dermal pigment incontinence**

Hypopigmented- apoptotic keratinocytes with **atrophic hair follicles and absence of arrector pili**

TRANSIENT NEONATAL PUSTULAR MELANOSIS

-benign pustular dermatosis that often presents at birth or rarely develops on the first day of life

-more common in African American infants

-clustered flaccid vesicles and sterile pustules that can occur anywhere

-resolves with desquamation and hyperpigmentation that gradually fades

-rarely biopsied

Histopathology

-**intracorneal or subcorneal neutrophilic aggregation**

-**smear of pustular content reveals neutrophils**

-few eosinophils can be present

-mild dermal inflammation

-**no dermal melanin**, despite the name

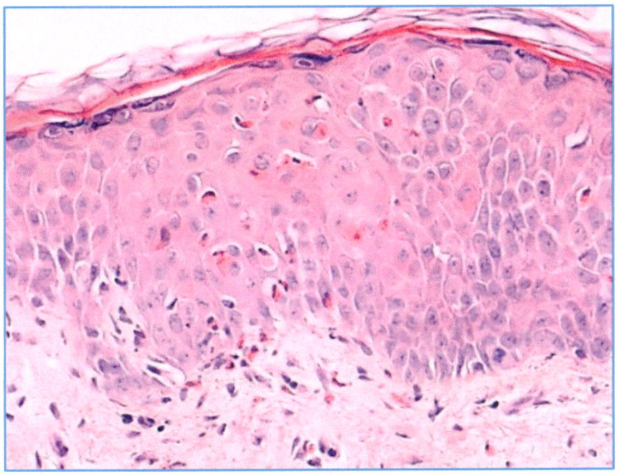
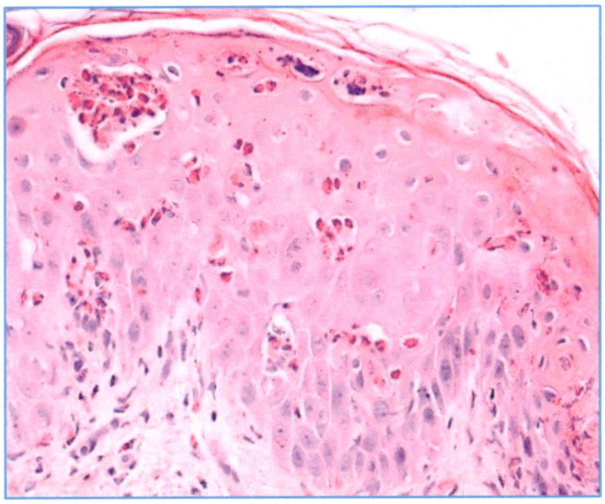

Vesicular phase of incontinentia pigmenti with intraepidermal eosinophils and eosinophilic vesicles

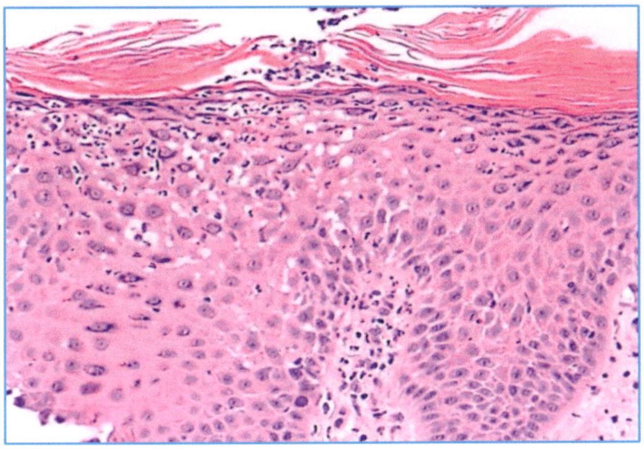
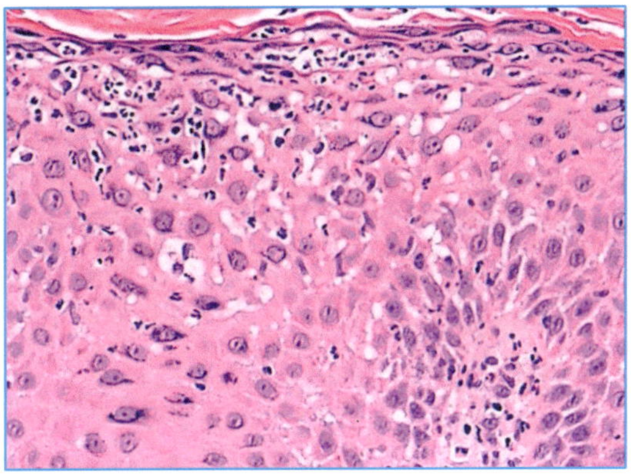

Transient neonatal pustular melanosis with intracorneal neutrophilic aggregate

Intraepidermal vesicular and blistering disorders

ERYTHEMA TOXICUM NEONATORUM (TOXIC ERYTHEMA OF THE NEWBORN)

-benign pustular eruption in one quarter to one third of full-term neonates
-rarely biopsied
-characterized by erythematous macules with small pustules
-usually appears on the **second or third day** of life and disappears in about two weeks
-predilection for face, trunk, and proximal extremities

Histopathology

-**intraepidermal pustules** near opening of follicular infundibulum
-**pustules made of predominantly eosinophils** and some neutrophils
-**eosinophils seen on smear of a pustule**
-adjacent epidermis is mildly spongiotic
-mild dermal edema and **dermal eosinophils**

ACROPUSTULOSIS OF INFANCY (INFANTILE ACROPUSTULOSIS)

-condition characterized by recurrent crops of intensely pruritic vesicles and pustules
-classically occurs between birth and 2 years of age
-most common in African American children
-predilection for edges of the hands and feet
-many cases are postscabietic
-resolves spontaneously by 3 years of age

Histopathology

-**acral skin**
-**subcorneal/intraepidermal blister** with **neutrophils**
-variable number of eosinophils

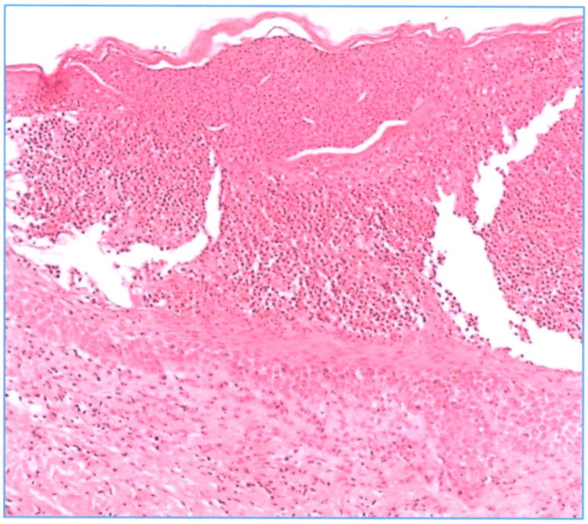
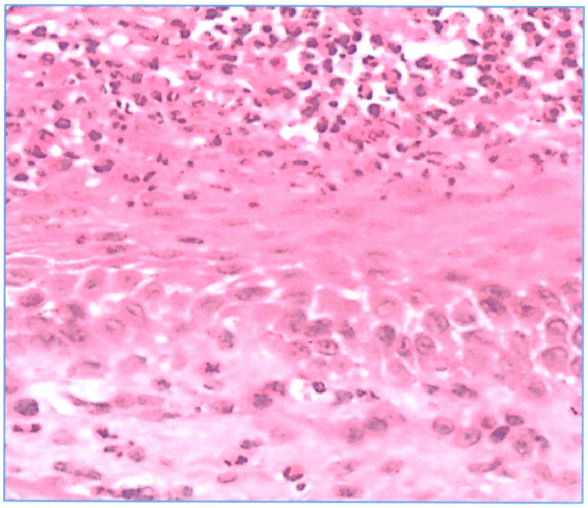

Erythema toxicum neonatorum with dermal eosinophils and intraepidermal vesicle with eosinophils

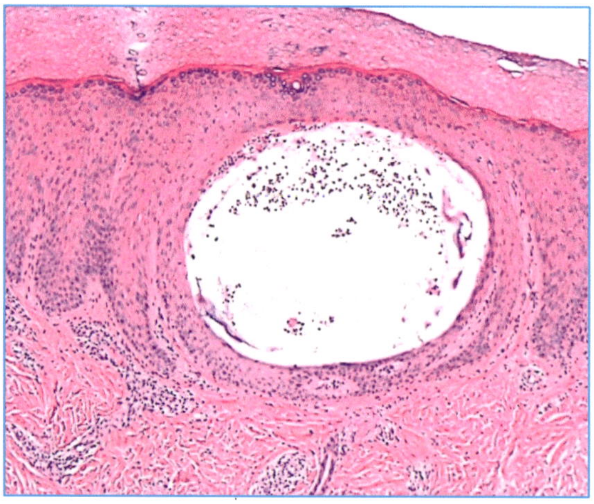
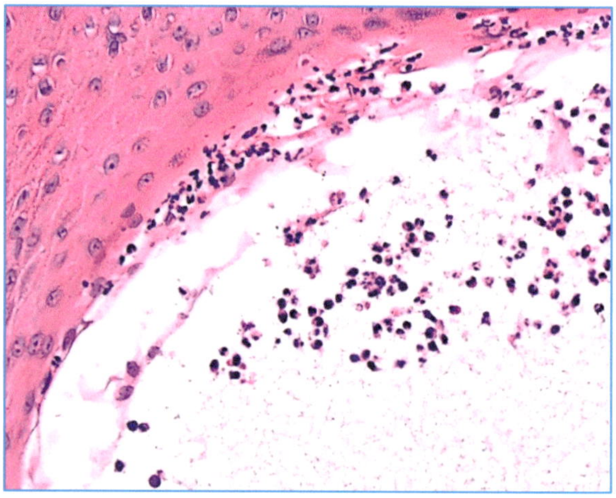

Acropustulosis of infancy of acral skin with intraepidermal vesicle with neutrophils

FRICTION BLISTER

-blister formed at the site of rubbing
-mainly on the soles, palms, heels

Histopathology
-intraepidermal blister with **split in the stratum spinosum**
-occasional necrotic keratinocytes in the blister's roof
-common intravesicular serum and some hemorrhage
-minimal dermal inflammation

TALON NOIR (BLACK HEEL)

-epidermal hemorrhage caused by trauma
-present as minute, black, punctate macules
-most often on plantar surface of one or both heels

Histopathology
-acral skin with pools of red blood cells within the stratum corneum
-intraepidemal **blister is not present**

STAPHYLOCOCCAL SCALDED SKIN SYNDROME (SSSS, LYELL'S DISEASE, RITTER'S DISEASE)

-desquamating skin eruption due to epidermolytic exotoxin from group 2 *Staphylococcus* infection at a distant site
-classically seen in infants and children under the age of 5 or adults with renal failure or malignancy
-starts with fever and redness in the intertriginous area (neck, groin, axilla)
-rapidly evolves to skin sloughing and spreads to involve another areas of body (typically sparing palms and soles)
-cultures from bullae are negative (mediated by exotoxin in blood)

Histopathology
-**subcorneal separation** with split in the granular layer
-**below the split epidermis is normal**
-**no or minimal inflammation**

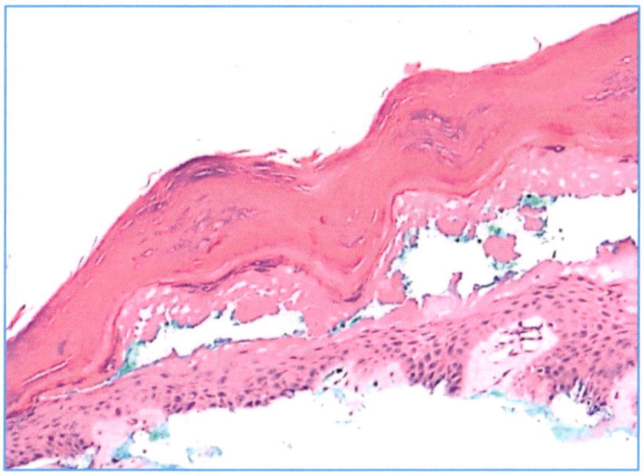
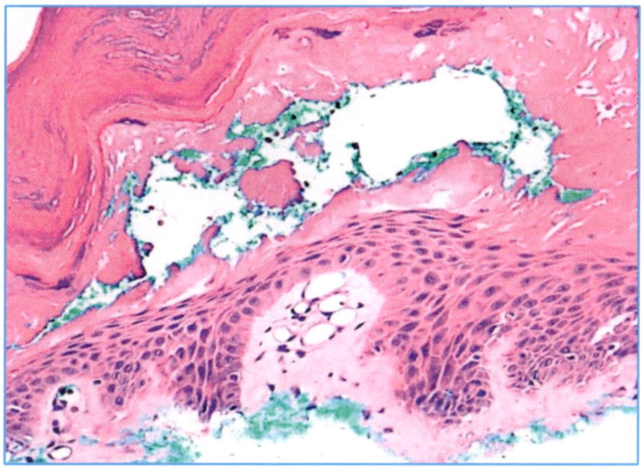

Friction blister with split within stratum spinosum and no inflammation

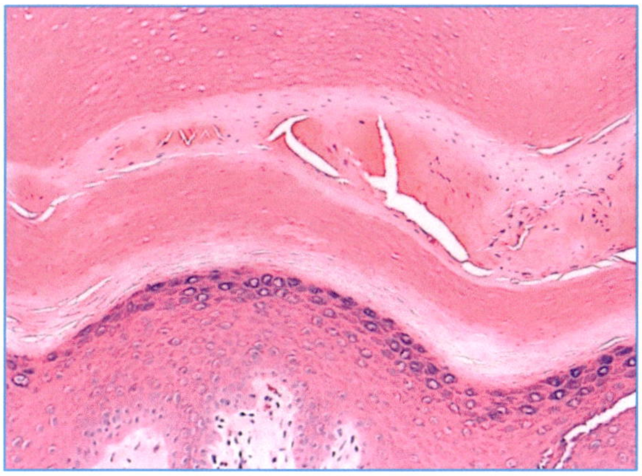

Talon noir with hemorrhage in the stratum corneum

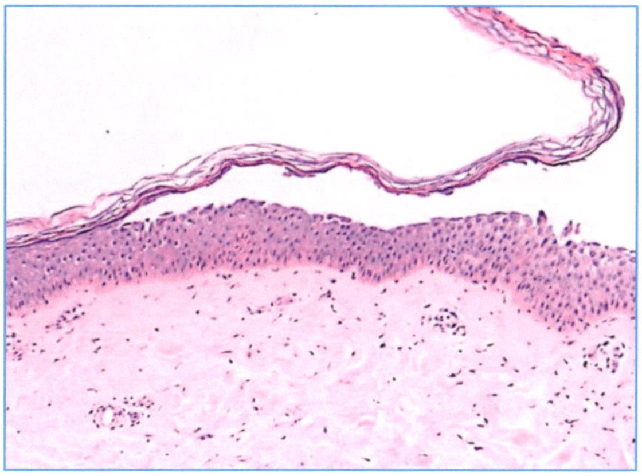

SSSS with subcorneal separation and no inflammation

Intraepidermal vesicular and blistering disorders

DARIER'S DISEASE (KERATOSIS FOLLICULARIS)

-autosomal dominant condition with variable expressivity due to mutation in *ATP2A2* gene
-usually starts in adolescence
-presents with malodorous, symmetrical, small, red-brown, warty papules and plaques in a seborrheic distribution (face, scalp, upper chest, back)
-half of patients have oral (usually palate) mucosal "cobble stoning"
-keratotic palmoplantar pits and longitudinal red/white nail streaks with "V-shaped" nicking are characteristic

Histopathology
-acanthotic, hyperkeratotic epidermis with **narrow suprabasal acantholysis** of keratinocytes
-epidermal clefts in the upper epidermis with **prominent dyskeratotic cells, corp ronds, and corp grains**
-corp ronds are keratinocytes with **dark, shrunken nuclei and** clear **paranuclear halo**
-**corps grains** are compressed keratinocytes with **elongated large dark nuclei** and **pink cytoplasm**

HAILEY-HAILEY DISEASE (FAMILIAL BENIGN PEMPHIGUS)

-uncommon autosomal dominant disease with variable expressivity due to *ATP2C1* mutation
-recurrent vesicles and flaccid blisters that evolve into eroded plaques
-predilection for intertriginous sites (neck, axilla, and groin area)
-lesions can be induced by trauma, heat, light, perspiration, infection
-no mucosal lesions (unlike Darier's disease)

Histopathology
-acanthotic epidermis with **broad** epidermal **acantholysis**
-epidermal appearance of **"dilapidated brick wall"** (keratinocytes falling apart)
-hair follicles are not involved
-occasional dyskeratosis with corp ronds and grains but not prominent

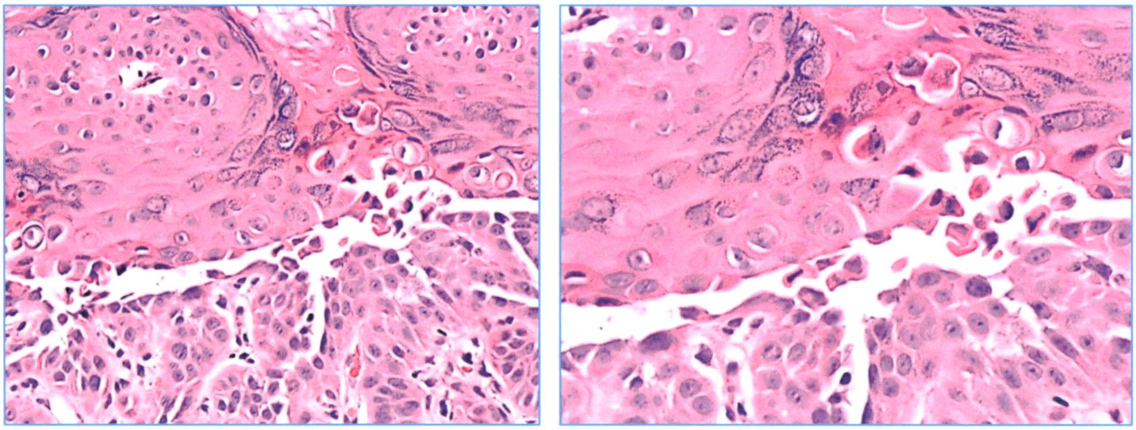

Narrow acantholytic lesion of Darier's disease with corp ronds and corp grains in the upper portion of the epidermis

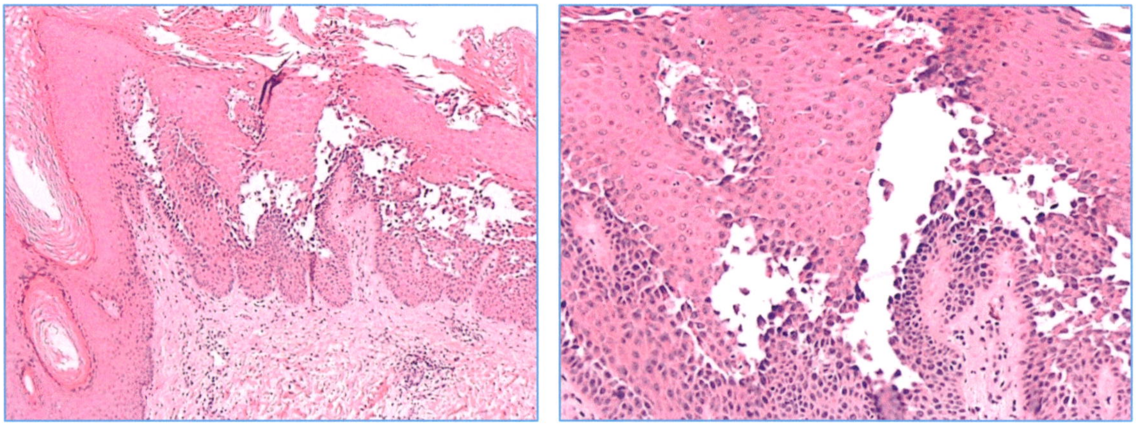

Broad acantholytic lesion of Hailey-Hailey disease with "dilapidated brick wall" pattern

GROVER'S DISEASE (TRANSIENT ACANTHOLYTIC DERMATOSIS)

-usually transient (but not always) pruritic skin disease more common in males over 50 years of age
-abrupt onset of discrete pink papules and vesicles that rapidly turn into crusted erosions
-predilection for chest and upper back
-can be induced by heat exposure (heavy exercise, sun exposure, or high fever)

Histopathology

Five histological patterns (more than one of these histological patterns may be present)

"**Darier's- like**" pattern (most common variant)
-focal epidermal acantholysis with suprabasal split and **corp ronds and grains**

"**Hailey-Hailey-like**" pattern- **"dilapidated brick wall"** appearance

"**Pemphigus vulgaris-like**" pattern- suprabasal acantholysis with **"tombstones"**

"**Pemphigus foliaceous-like**" pattern
-subcorneal/ intragranular blister with sparse acantholytic keratinocytes

Spongiotic dermatitis- epidermal spongiosis and focal microvesicles

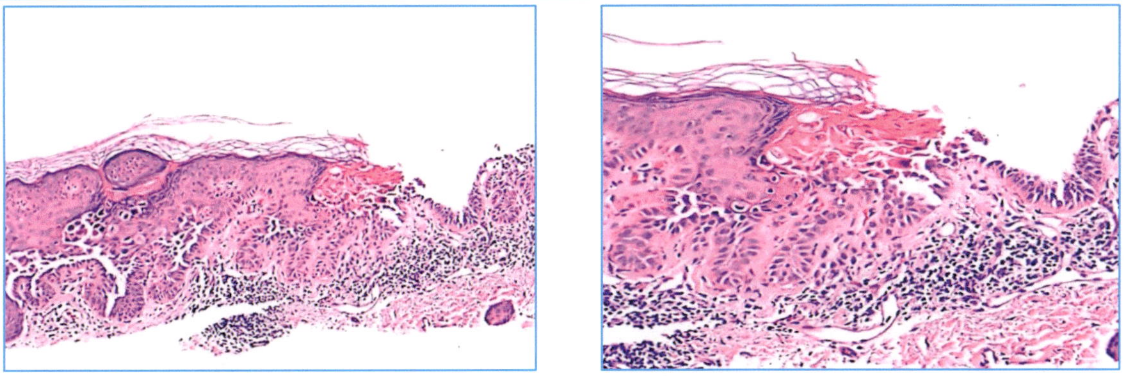

Grover's disease with "Darier's-like" pattern on the left and "pemphigus vulgaris-like" pattern on the right part of the biopsy

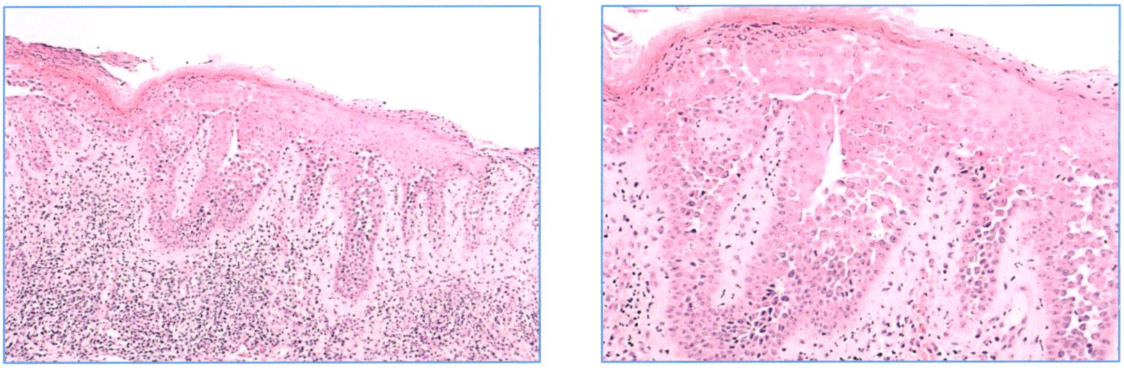

"Hailey-Hailey-like" Grover's disease with "dilapidated brick wall" appearance

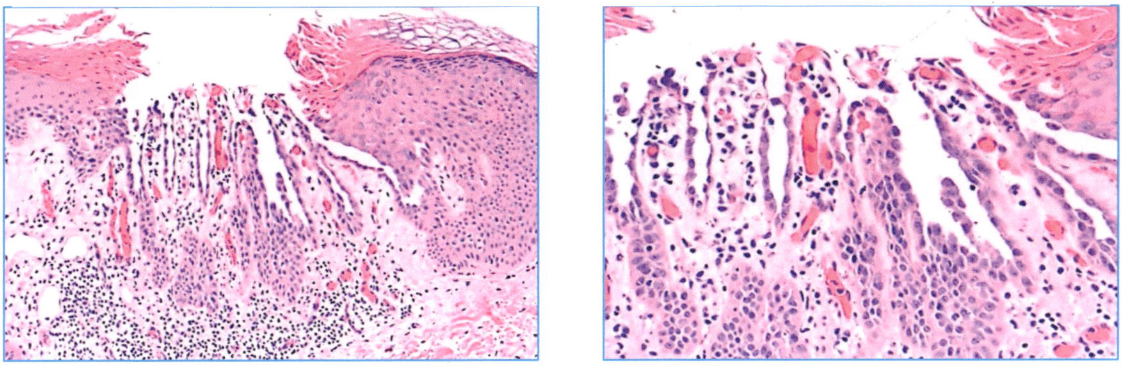

"Pemphigus vulgaris-like" Grover's disease with suprabasal acantholysis and basal layer "tombstones"

MILIARIA

-benign pinpoint papules resulting from sweat gland obstruction
-usually in neonates and children (*m. crystallina* and *m. rubra*) who did not fully develop eccrine glands
-may also occur in adults in humid climate (*m. rubra, m. pustulosa and m. profunda*)

Miliaria crystallina

-small **non-pruritic,** discrete "dew-drop" vesicles
-lesions rupture spontaneously with clear fluid (sweat)
-trunk is the favored site

Miliaria rubra

-numerous uniform pink papules and some small pustules ***(m. pustulosa*)** that can be intensely **pruritic**
-more common in friction areas covered with clothing

Miliaria profunda

-small number of small **non-pruritic** flesh-colored papules only seen in tropics
-preceded by multiple bouts of miliaria rubra

Histopathology

Miliaria crystallina

-**"cell-poor" vesicle** in the granular layer **associated with an adjacent sweat duct**
-mild spongiosis and mild perivascular lymphocytic infiltrate around acrosyringium

Miliaria rubra

-same as m. crystalline with **vesicle within the stratum spinosum**

Miliaria pustulosa

-considered a variant of miliaria rubra with **neutrophilic pustule involving acrosyringium**

Miliaria profunda

-**subepidermal vesicle** associated with **adjacent sweat duct**

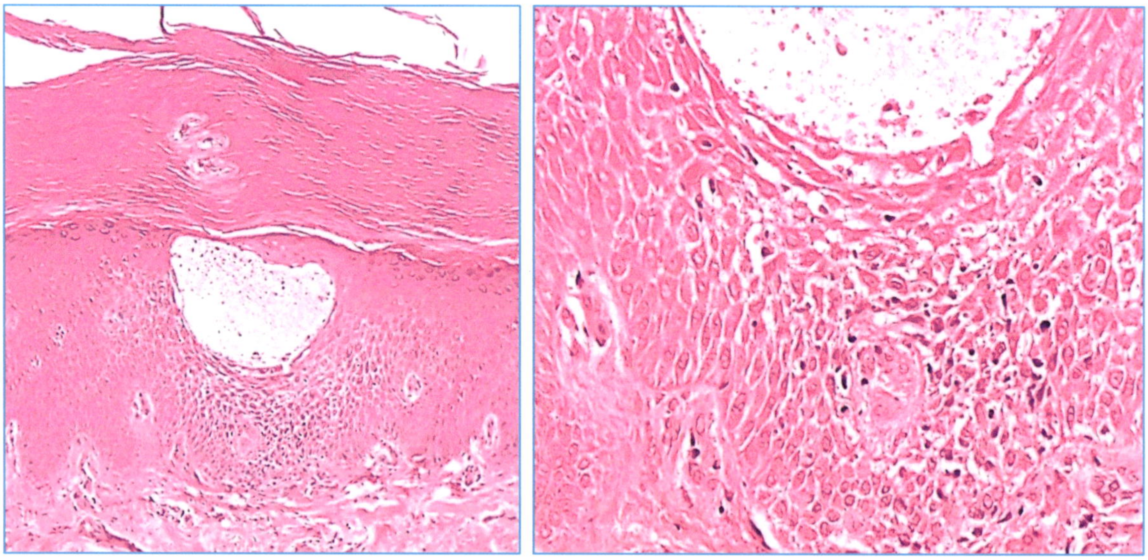

M. crystallina with "cell-poor" vesicle in granular layer at the site of sweat duct

ACUTE GENERALIZED EXANTHEMATOUS PUSTULOSIS (AGEP)

-rapid onset eruption with high fever
-90% are drug induced (β lactams, macrolides, antimalarials)
-small pustules on erythematous skin starting on the face and flexural folds
-rapidly spreads all over the body
-spontaneously resolves with desquamation

Histopathology
-subacute **epidermal spongiosis**
-**subcorneal** or **intraepidermal neutrophilic pustules varying from small to large**
-mild dermal edema with dermal mixed inflammation and **rare eosinophils**

SUBCORNEAL PUSTULAR DERMATOSIS (SNEDDON-WILKINSON DISEASE)

-chronic pustular disease in middle-aged women
-"half and half" pustules (clear fluid overlying sterile pus)
-pustules symmetrically arranged in annular and serpiginous pattern
-predilection for abdomen, axilla, groins
-resolves with mild hyperpigmentation
-associated with IgA paraproteinemia, pyoderma gangrenosum, inflammatory bowel disease, rheumatoid arthritis

Histopathology
-**subcorneal** neutrophilic pustule (usually **wider** than in AGEP) in **unremarkable or minimally spongiotic epidermis**
-mild mixed dermal inflammation

These two entities can have very similar histopathology and clinical correlation is necessary to separate them. **IgA pemphigus and bullous impetigo** share similar histology and should be included **in differential diagnosis**.

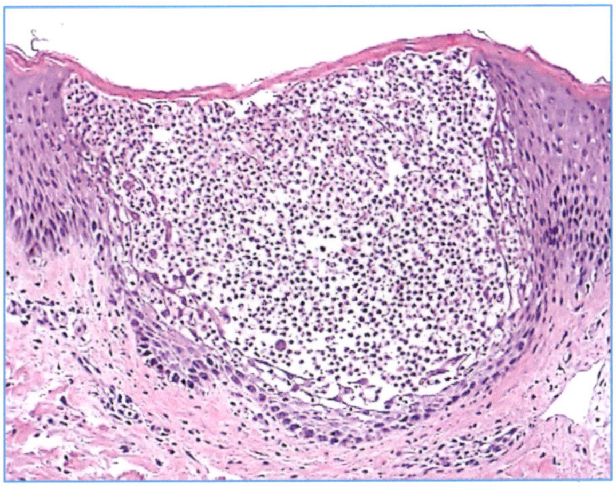

AGEP with larger, rounded, intraepidermal neutrophilic pustule

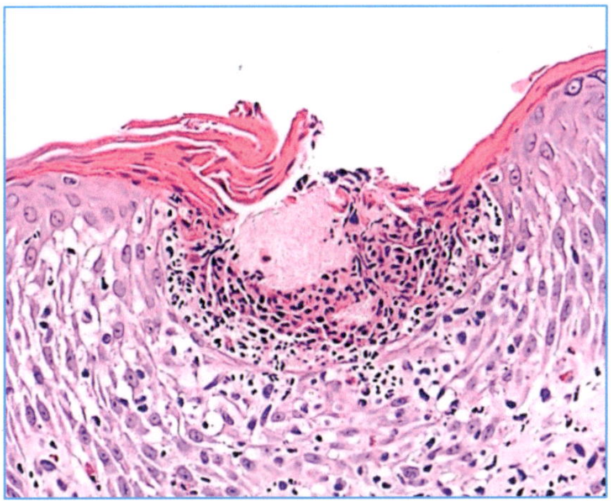

AGEP with smaller neutrophilic pustule in spongiotic epidermis

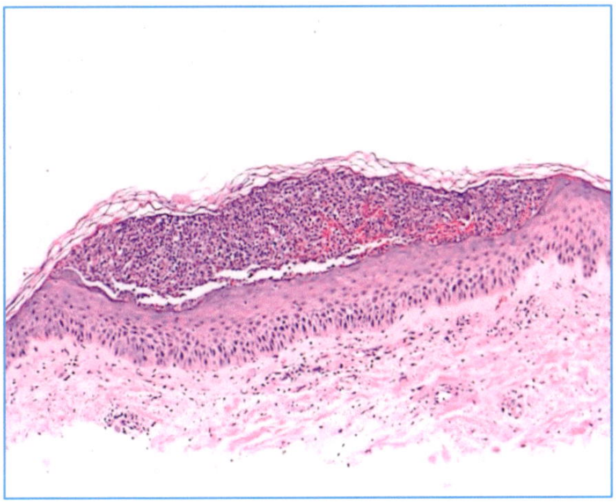

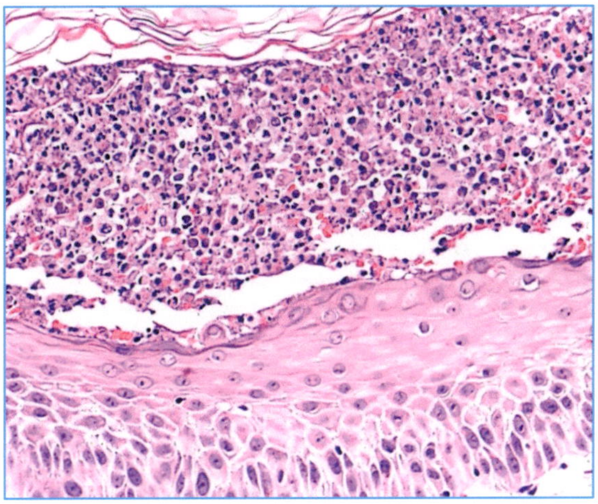

Subcorneal pustular dermatosis with wider subcorneal neutrophilic pustule

Intraepidermal vesicular and blistering disorders

BULLOUS IMPETIGO

-impetigo is the most common bacterial infection in children due to *Staph. aureus*
-it can present as non-bullous (more frequent and described in the chapter on bacterial infections) and bullous form (less frequent)
-bullous impetigo is the most common in children 2-5 years of age but can occur in adults too
-affects intact skin with more generalized distribution but favored sites are diaper area, axillae, neck, face
-presents with flaccid bullae with collarette of scale and minimal surrounding edema

Histopathology

-**subcorneal pustule filled with neutrophils**
-Gram (+) cocci are present but not always

BULLOUS TINEA

-cutaneous dermatophyte infection with bullae formation
-caused by *Trichophyton rubrum* or *T. mentagrophytes*
-feet are favored sites and commonly both are affected
-presents as pruritic papules/vesicles that can turn into bullae
-see more in the chapter on fungal infections

Histopathology

-acanthotic epidermis of **acral site** with **spongiosis** or **intraepidermal vesicle**
-focal parakeratosis and intracorneal **neutrophilic pustule**
-**fungal elements in the stratum corneum (PAS+)**

PUSTULAR PSORIASIS

-multiple clinical variants
-presents as generalized or acral plaques of yellow-white pustules
-see more in the chapter on psoriatic dermatitis

Histopathology

-acral or non-acral site depending on the clinical type
-intraepidermal neutrophilic pustules of Kogoj within upper spinous layer
-pustules in early lesions are surrounded with spongiotic epidermis with minimal psoriasiform hyperplasia
-**pustules** in older lesions are surrounded by **psoriasiform hyperplasia** with parakeratosis and hypogranulosis

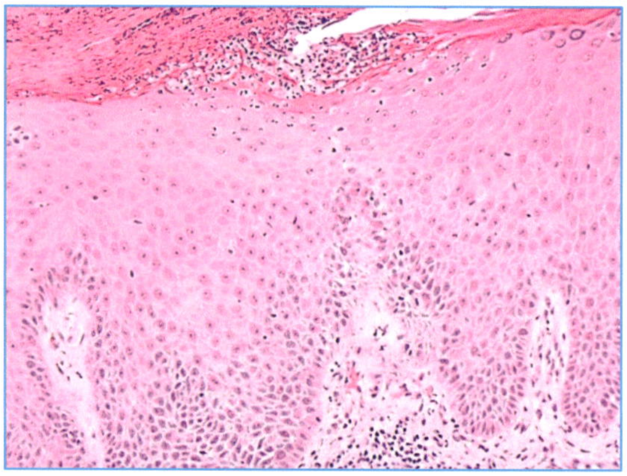

Pustular psoriasis with neutrophilic pustule in psoriasiform epidermis

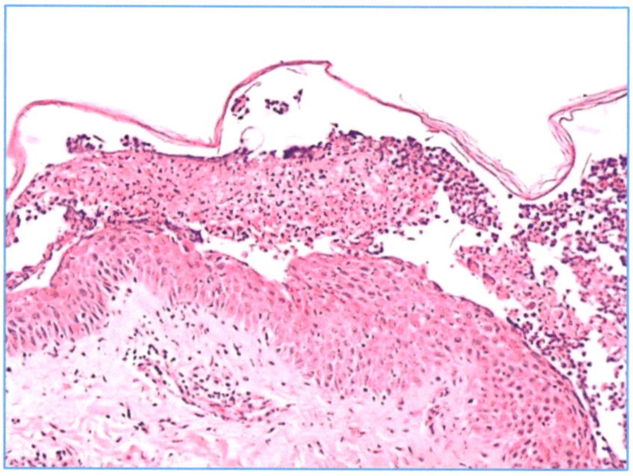

Bullous impetigo with subcorneal neutrophilic pustule

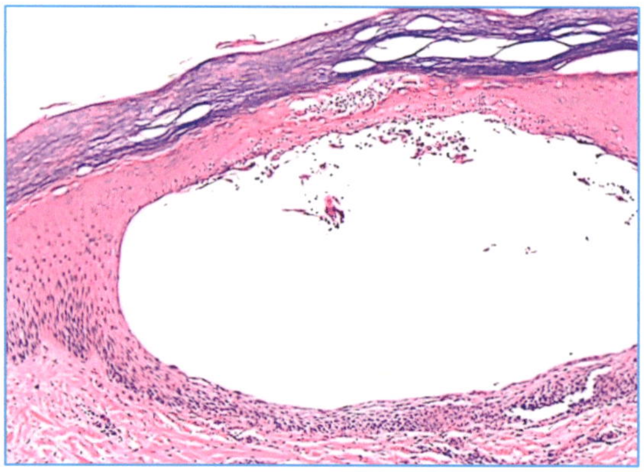

Bullous tinea with vesicle of acral skin

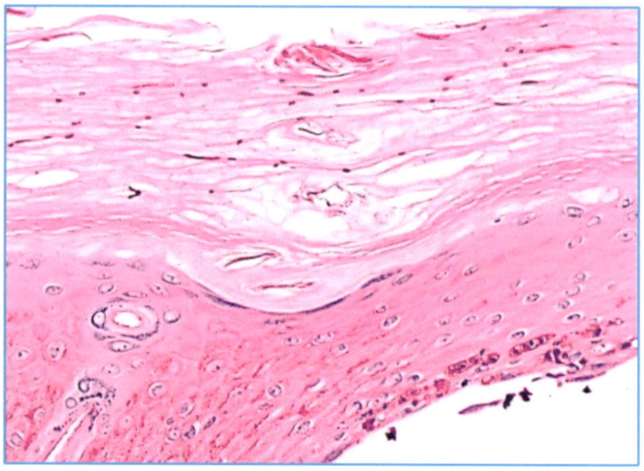

Bullous tinea with hyphae in stratum corneum (PAS stain)

Chapter 8

HOW TO APPROACH INTRAEPIDERMAL BLISTERS

DETERMINE PATIENT'S AGE

CHILDREN

-transient neonatal pustular melanosis	at birth	neutrophils	
-incontinencia pigmenti	birth-4 weeks	eosinophils	tiny vesicles
-erythema toxicum neonatorum	2-3 days	eosinophils	larger vesicles
-acropustulosis of infancy	birth-2 years	neutrophils	acral site
-miliaria crystallina/rubra	childhood	"cell-poor" vesicle associated with sweat duct	

ADULTS AND CHILDREN

-staphylococcal scalded skin syndrome	children under 5 years of age and adults with kidney failure "cell poor" subcorneal separation
-friction blister	intraepidermal split filled with serum, hemorrhage

ADULTS ONLY

DETERMINE NATURE OF THE INFLAMMATION

NO INTRAEPIDERMAL INFLAMMATION

-Darier's disease	seborrheic distribution	"corp ronds and grains"	DIF-
-Hailey-Hailey	intertriginous area	"dilapidated brick wall"	DIF-
-pemphigus vulgaris	any area + mucosa	"tomb stones"	DIF+
-Grover's disease	chest	spongiosis and multiple patterns including all above	

EOSINOPHILS

-pemphigus vegetans	verruciform epidermis	intraepidermal eosinophils	DIF+

NEUTROPHILS

-IgA pemphigus	flexural areas	more neutrophils	DIF IgA+
-pemphigus foliaceus	seborrheic areas	less neutrophils	DIF IgG+
-bullous impetigo	children	face	*Staph. aureous*
-bullous tinea		feet	*Trichophyton rubrum*
-pustular psoriasis	surrounding epidermis is psoriasiform		
-AGEP	drug history, fever	multiple (clinical and microscopic) small pustules with few eosinophils	
-subcorneal pustular dermatosis	chronic pustulosis	diagnosis of exclusion	
-miliaria pustulosa	acrosyringial pustule	intraepidermal	
-miliaria profunda	acrosyringial pustule	subepidermal	

DO NOT FORGET PARANEOPLASTIC PEMPHIGUS

-it can present like pemphigus vulgaris
-it can show an "erythema multiforme-like" pattern with necrotic keratinocytes
-it can demonstrate a lichenoid pattern with epidermal vacuolar changes

Intraepidermal vesicular and blistering disorders

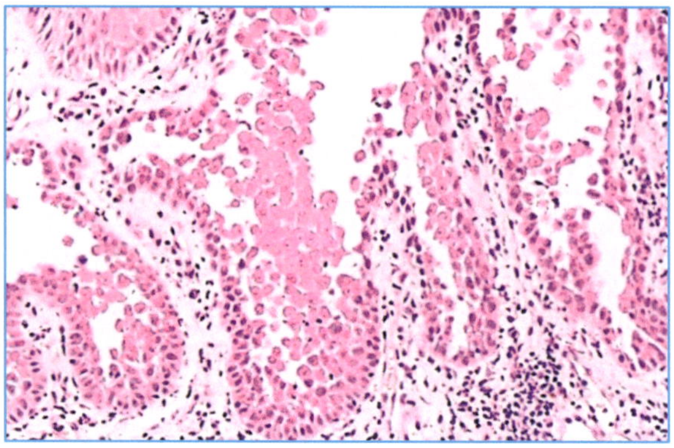

Pemphigus vulgaris with suprabasal split and "tombstones"

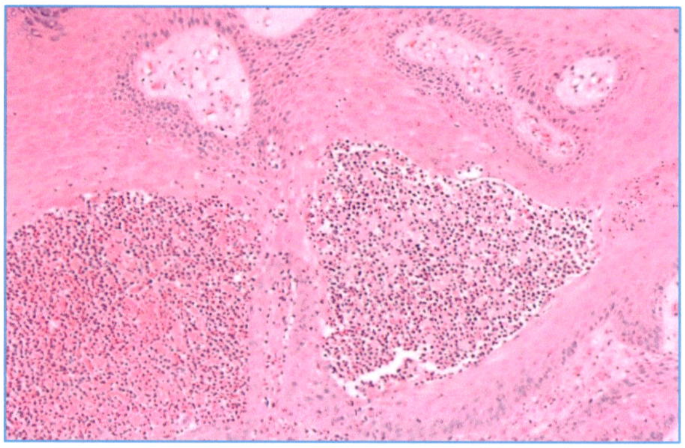

Pemphigus vegetans with intraepidermal eosinophils

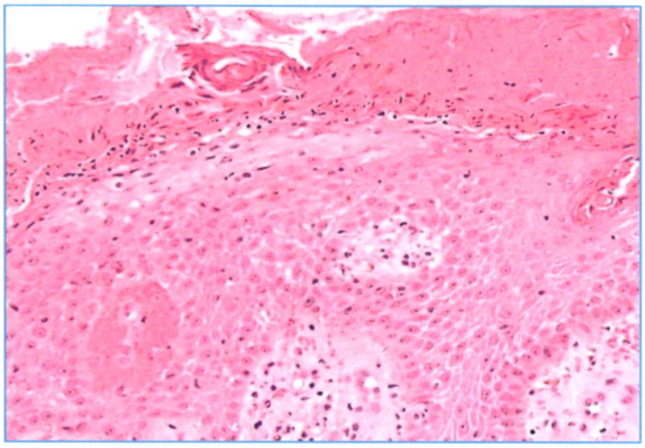

Pemphigus foliaceous with intragranular acantholysis and neutrophils

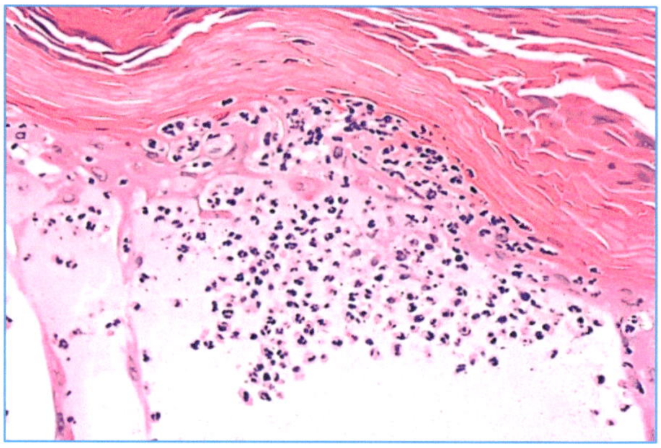

IgA pemphigus with subcorneal neutrophilic pustule

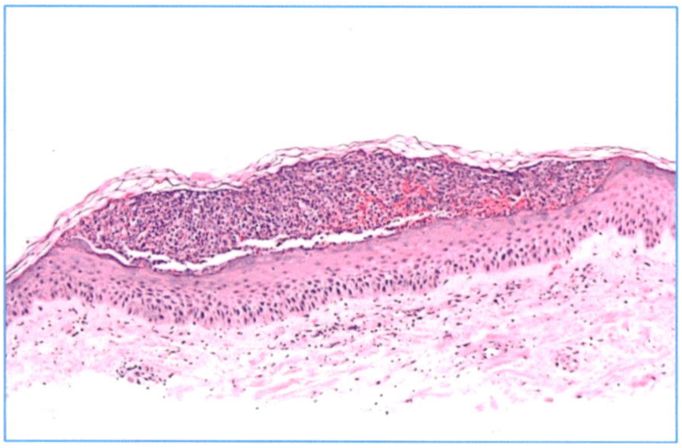

Subcorneal pustular dermatosis requires clinical correlation

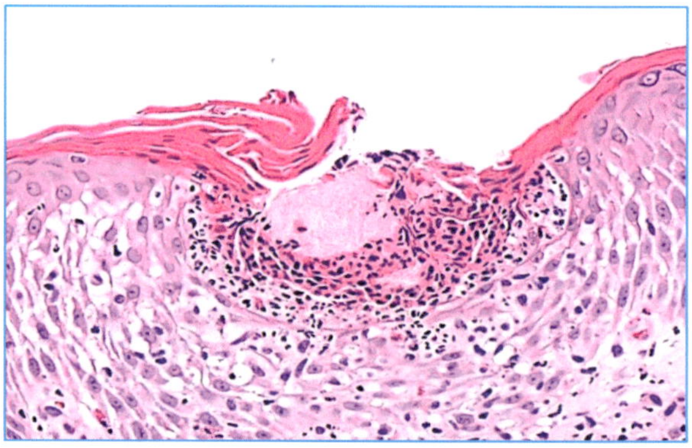

AGEP with intracorneal neutrophilic pustule

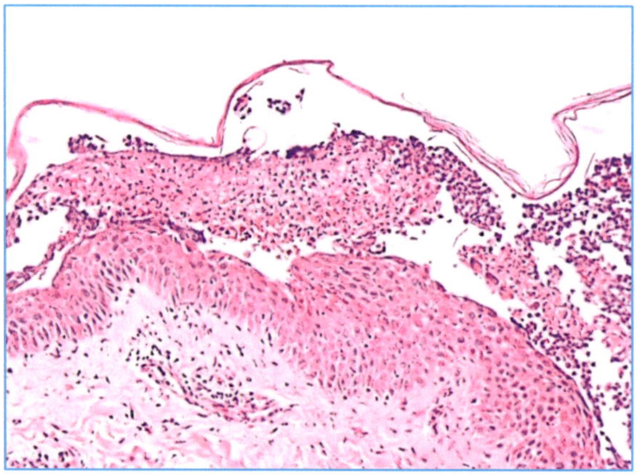

Impetigo with intracorneal neutrophilic pustule

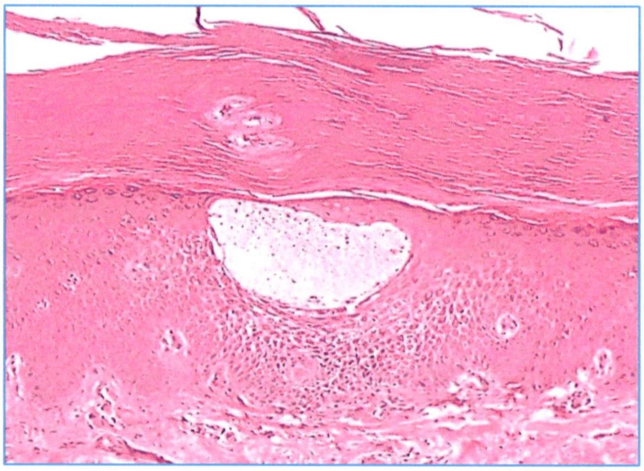

M. crystallina with epidermal, sweat duct associated, "cell-poor" vesicle

Chapter 8

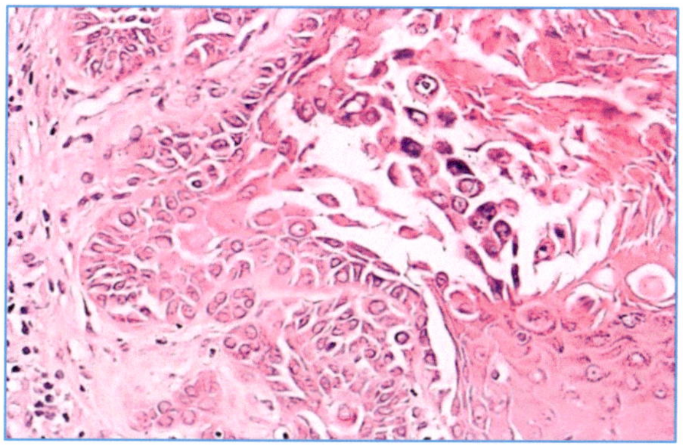

Darier's disease with corp ronds and corp grains

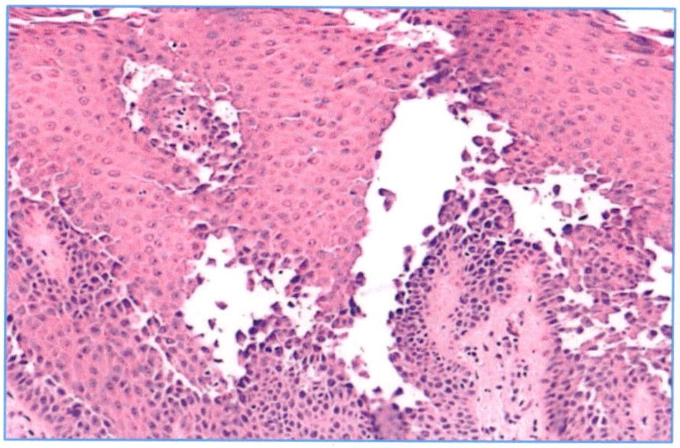

Hailey-Hailey disease with "dilapidated brick wall"

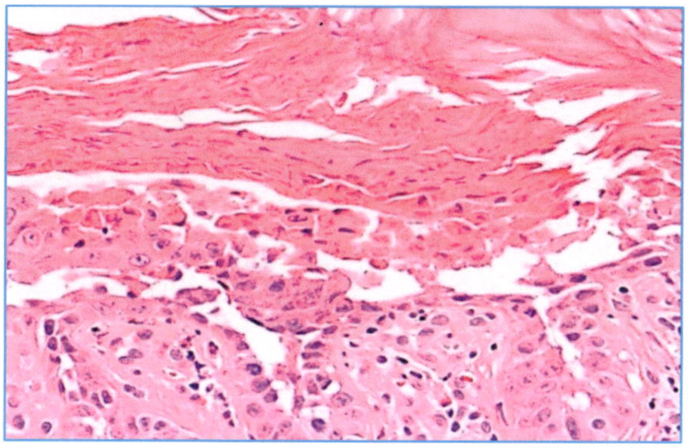

Darier's type of Grover's disease

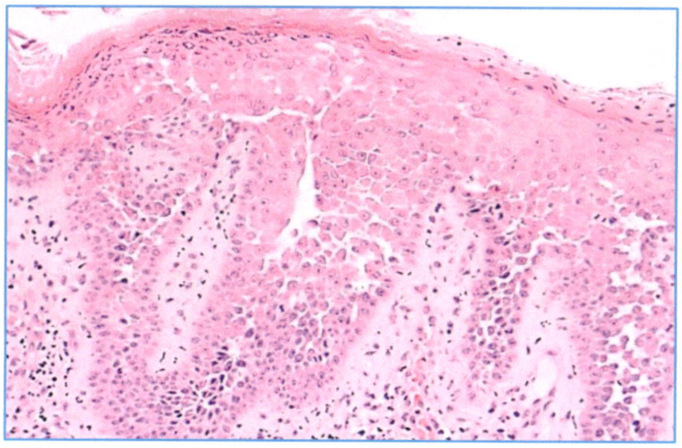

Hailey-Hailey's type of Grover's disease

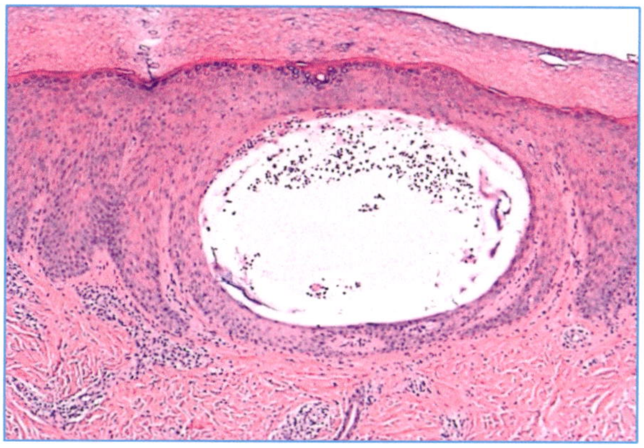

Infantile acropustulosis with
intraepidermal neutrophilic pustule

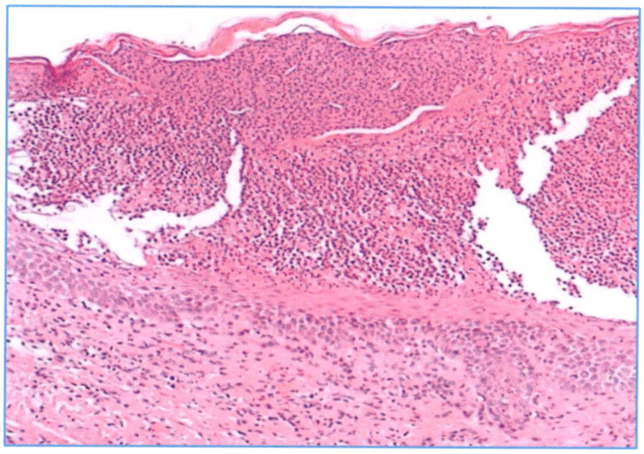

Erythema toxicum neonatorum with
intraepidermal pustule with eosinophils

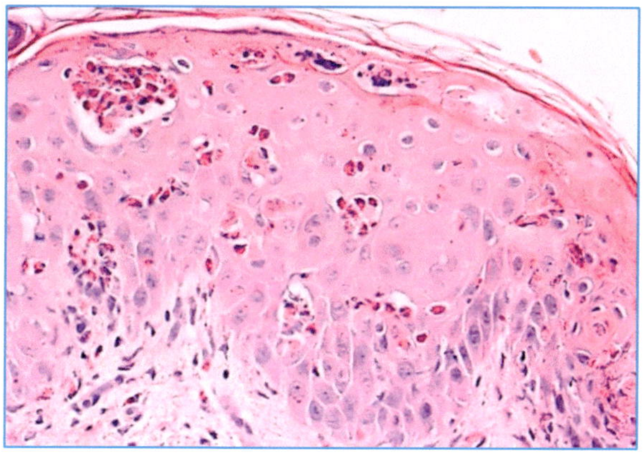

Incontinentia pigment with intraepidermal eosinophils

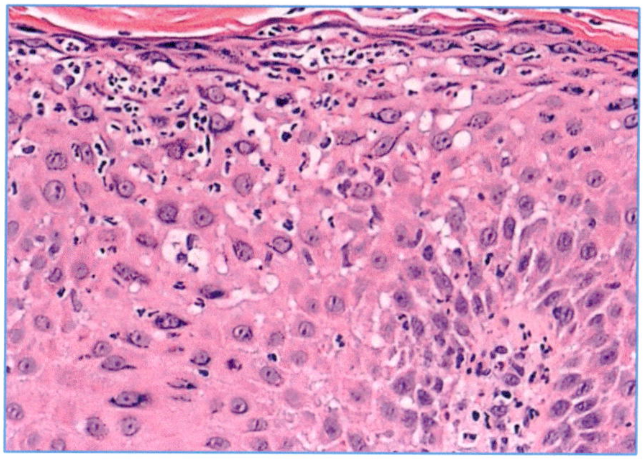

Transient neonatal pustular melanosis with subcorneal neutrophils

Intraepidermal vesicular and blistering disorders

Chapter 9

SUBEPIDERMAL BLISTERING DISORDERS

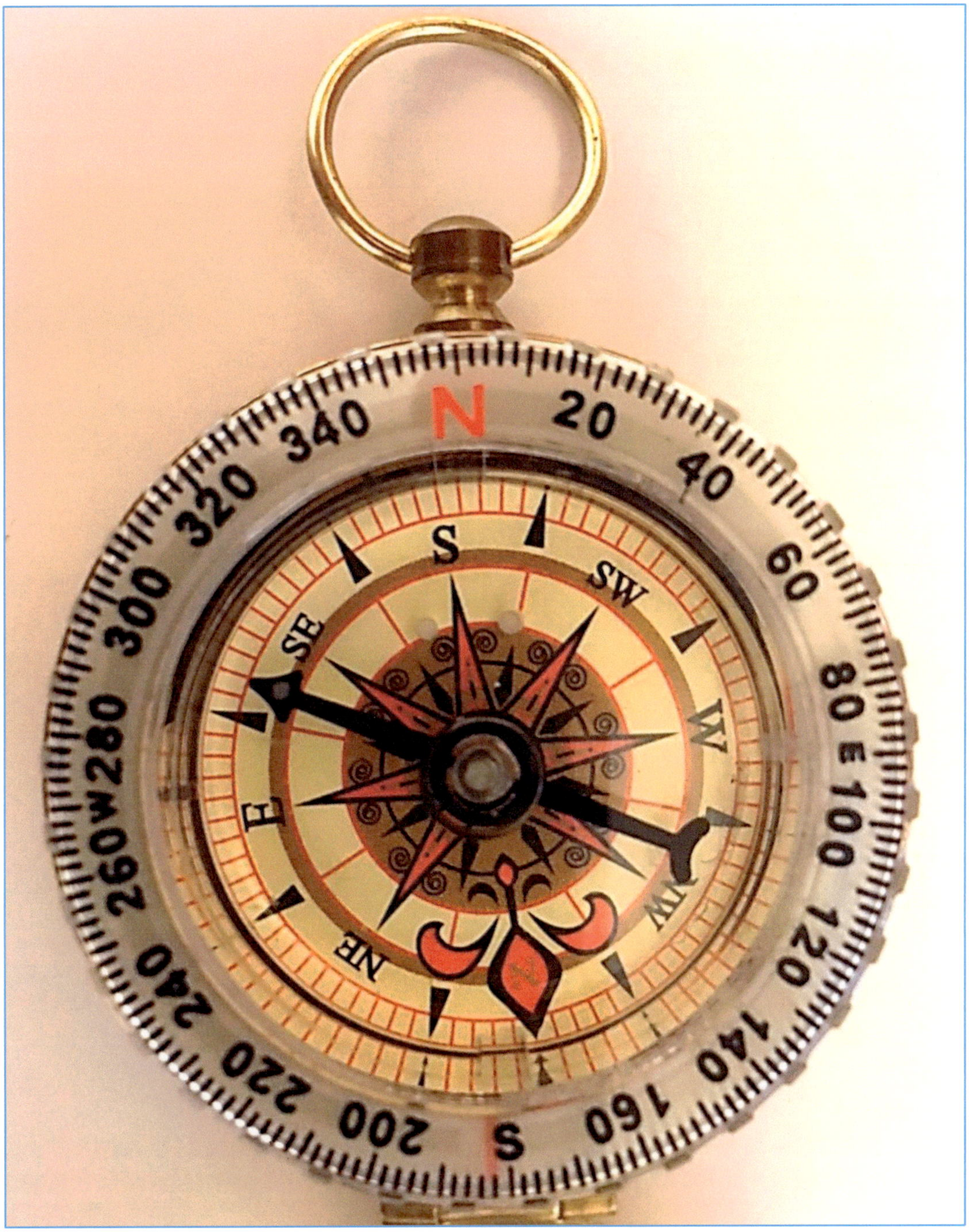

Subepidermal blistering disorders

BULLOUS PEMPHIGOID

-most common autoimmune blistering disease
-affects elderly patients

Urticarial stage

-annular urticarial plaques usually on trunk, abdomen, and flexural extremities

Bullous stage

-pruritic, large, tense bullae arising on normal or erythematous skin
-bullae rupture and leave erosions
-mucosal surfaces can be involved, but less commonly than in pemphigus vulgaris

Histopathology

Urticarial stage

-**dermal edema** with **numerous** dermal **eosinophils**

Bullous stage

-**subepidermal blister** with **numerous eosinophils** in the blister
-dermal lymphocytic inflammation with numerous eosinophils
-DIF: **linear C3 and IgG** along dermo-epidermal junction

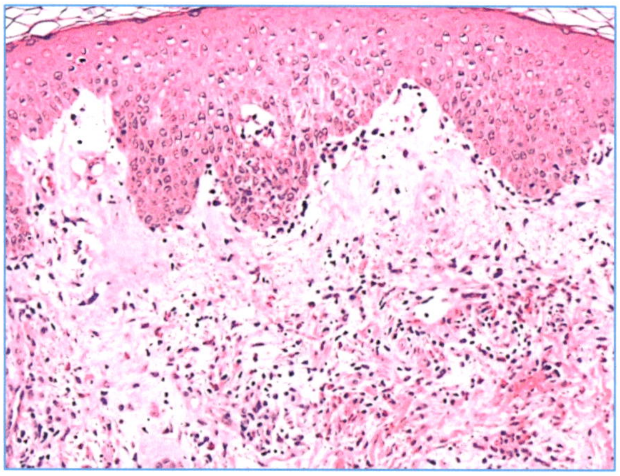
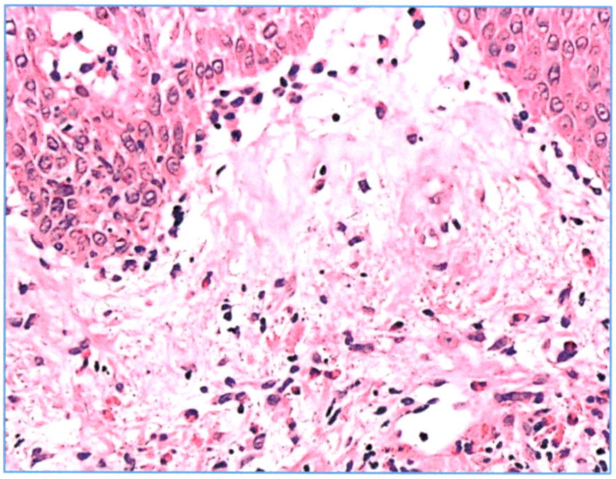

Urticarial stage of bullous pemphigoid with dermal edema and numerous dermal eosinophils

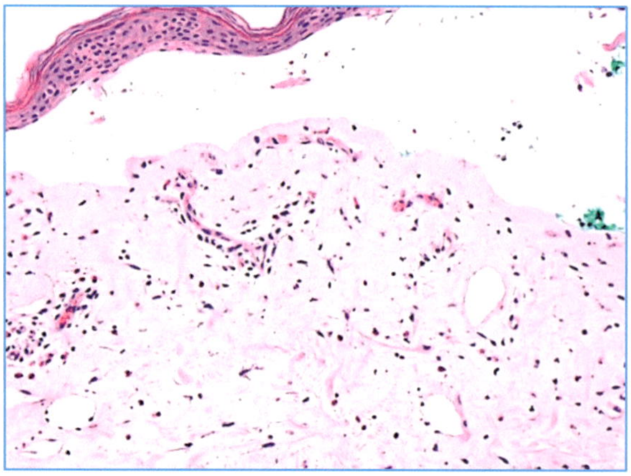
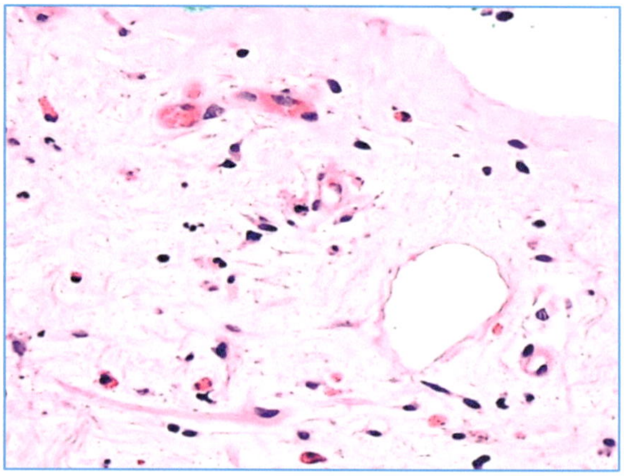

Bullous stage of bullous pemphigoid with subepidermal blister and eosinophils in the blister and in the dermis

PEMPHIGOID GESTATIONIS (HERPES GESTATIONIS)

-rare autoimmune blistering disease associated with pregnancy
-usually in second or third trimester of pregnancy
-may recur in subsequent pregnancies and postpartum when precipitated by menses and the use of oral contraceptives
-associated with premature delivery, Hashimoto thyroiditis, Graves' disease, and pernicious anemia
-extremely pruritic papulovesicular eruption, "herpes-like", on the abdomen and lateral sides of the trunk, classically involving umbilicus
-within days, spreads over the entire body
-mucosal surfaces are spared
-5-10% of babies develop a blistering rash following delivery lasting up to 6 weeks

Histopathology

-**subepidermal clefting** with blister formation
-blister and dermis contain **eosinophils** admixed with lymphocytes, histiocytes, and some neutrophils
-DIF: **linear C3 (100%)** and sometimes linear IgG (25%) pattern along the basement membrane

CICATRICIAL PEMPHIGOID

-uncommon chronic immunobullous disease of the elderly
-also called mucous membrane pemphigoid
-80% of patients present with oral lesions and only 20% with cutaneous lesions (scalp, face, neck)
-after oral mucosa, conjunctiva is the second most common site
-presents with vesiculobullous lesions that erode and cause extensive scarring

Histopathology

-most commonly on mucosal surface
-**submucosal or subepidermal blister with mixed dermal inflammation**
-dermal fibrosis and scarring
-DIF: positive in 85% of cases with **linear IgG, IgA** and/or C3 at basement membrane

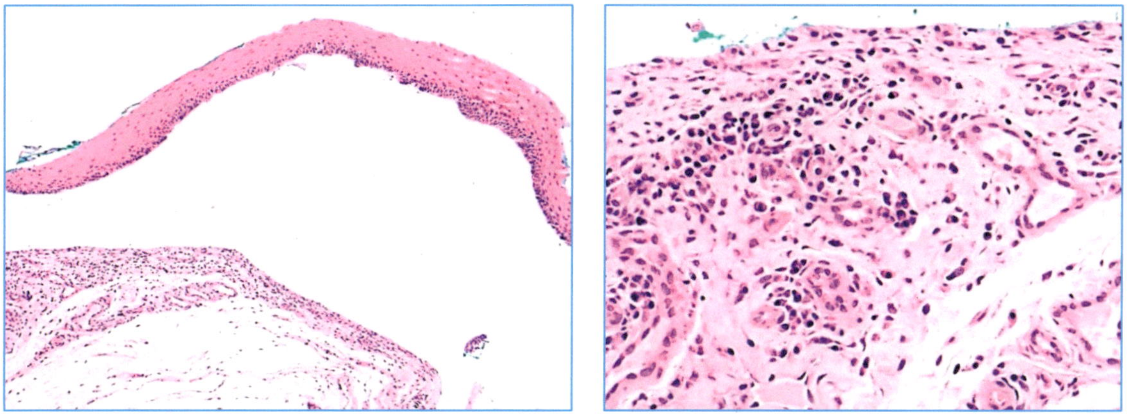

Cicatricial pemphigoid with submucosal blister and mixed dermal inflammation

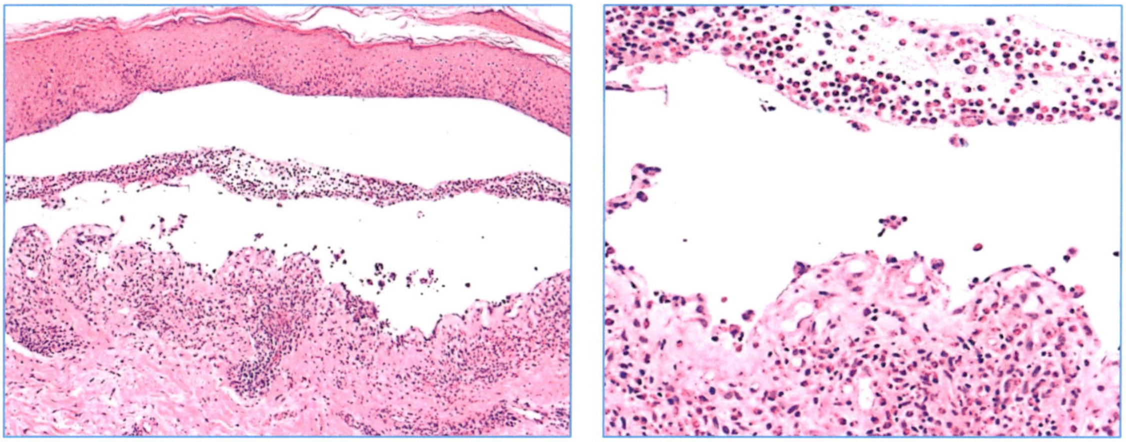

Pemphigoid gestationis with subepidermal blister and mixed inflammation with numerous eosinophils

Subepidermal blistering disorders

PORPHYRIA

Heterogeneous group of genetic diseases.
Four forms cause cutaneous changes.

Porphyria cutanea tarda
-most common cutaneous porphyria
-AD; starts in adult life
-fragile skin that breaks at the slightest trauma and blisters in the sun
-erosions heal with **milia and scars**
-patients also have hyperpigmentation and **hypertrichosis**

Erythropoietic protoporphyria (EPP)
-the second most common porphyria with onset in childhood with AD and AR forms
-stinging burning skin almost immediately after sun exposure
-typically followed by erythema, mild edema, and petechiae a few hours later
-pitted linear scars can subsequently appear

Variegate porphyria (VP)
-rare, serious AD disease that starts after puberty
-cutaneous changes identical to PCT, plus neuropsychiatric and abdominal symptoms

Congenital erythropoietic porphyria (CEP)
-AR or XLR; starts in childhood
-**mutilating** photosensitivity with blisters, ulceration, scarring, and deformation

PSEUDOPORPHYRIA

-a bullous photosensitive disorder that clinically and histologically mimics PCT
-**no abnormalities in urine or serum porphyrin** are noted, unlike in PCT
-can be induced by a wide range of medications (naproxen, estrogen), excessive UVA exposure (tanning booths), alcohol, and hemodialysis
-**hypertrichosis, milia, scars** and hyperpigmentation typical of PCT are usually **not seen**

EPIDERMOLYSIS BULLOSA

Inherited
-multiple variants with different severity
-caused by inhereted mutations in structural molecules of the epidermal basement membrane
-shortly after birth, patients develop blisters, erosions, and ulcers at sites of friction
-extent of lesions depends on subtype
Simplex AD -mutations in *keratin 5, 14*
Junctional AR -mutations in *laminin 332, type XVII collagen* or *integrin*
Dystrophic AR or AD- mutation in *type VII collagen*

Acquisita
-rare, acquired bullous disease of middle-aged adults with higher incidence in Asian and African American patients
-due to IgG antibodies against NC1 domain of *type VII collagen*
-associated with Crohn's disease, multiple myeloma
-non-inflamatory bullae and erosions on trauma-prone sites (e.g.elbow, knees, hands)
-heals with atrophic scars and milia
-DIF: **linear IgG band** along basement membrane

Histopathology

-**similar in all forms of epidermolysis bullosa, porphyria, and pseudoporphyria**
-**subepidermal "cell-poor" blister** with no or minimal inflammation
-wavy dermal papillae **("festooning")**
-common **caterpillar bodies** (eosinophilic linear material overlying blister base)

Differences
-in EBA, DIF shows **linear IgG and C3** at epidermal-dermal junction
-in porphyria and pseudoporpyria, dermal **solar elastosis** and **"festooning" is more prominent**

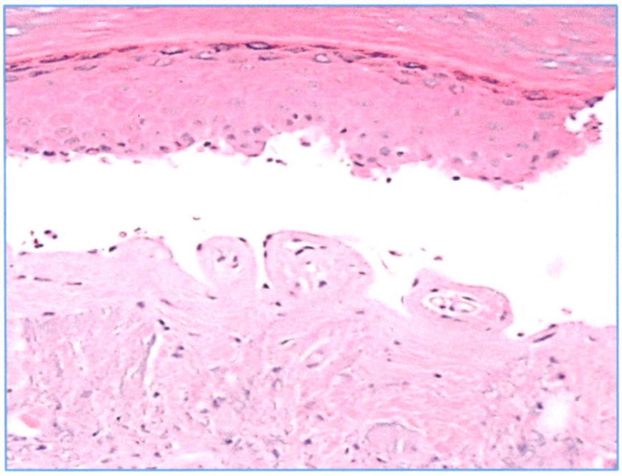

PCT with dermal solar elastosis and "festooning"

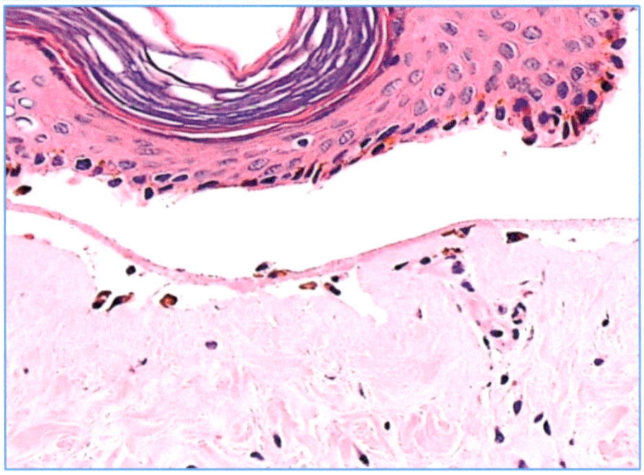

EB with caterpillar body and less solar elastosis

DERMATITIS HERPETIFORMIS

-chronic, relapsing severely pruritic disease of adults (30-40 years of age) associated with gluten sensitivity
-gluten induces flares of disease
-only 20% of patients have celiac disease but more than 90% of patient's GI biopsies have some degree of gluten enteropathy
-symmetric, grouped ("herpetiform") vesicles and papules
-lesions are so itchy that most patients present with excoriated papules only
-elbows, knees, and buttocks are classic sites of predilection

Histopathology

-**clusters of neutrophils within dermal papillae**
-progresses to subepidermal blister with neutrophils
-mild perivascular lymphocytic infiltrate
-DIF: **granular deposits of IgA** in the **dermal papillae**

LINEAR IgA BULLOUS DERMATOSIS/ CHRONIC BULLOUS DISEASE OF CHILDHOOD

-chronic bullous disease of childhood is rare blistering disorder in young children (first decade of life)
-in the majority of cases the cause is idiopathic
-linear IgA bullous dermatosis is disease of the elder individuals and is frequently drug-induced (vancomycin)
-both are due to IgA autoantibodies to *desmocollin 1*
-presents as large tense bullae on an erythematous base
-classically with annular grouping "**crown of jewels**"
-sites of predilection are perioral area, genital area, lower abdomen, and thighs
-mucosal involvement in up to 50% of patients but less common in adults

Histopathology

-focal subepidermal split
-**linear neutrophilic infiltrate in papillary dermis**
-DIF: **linear IgA** at epidermo-dermal junction

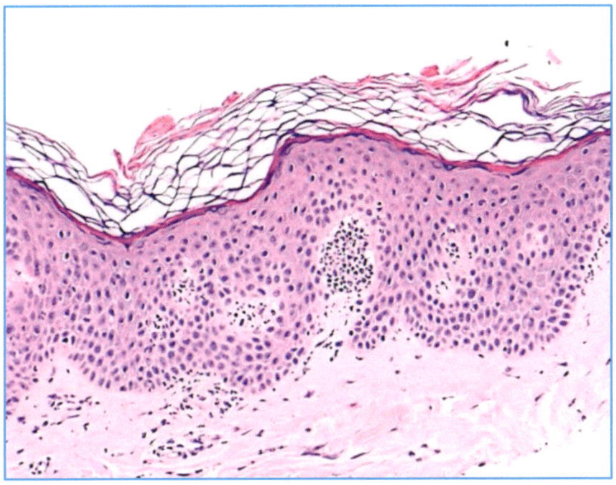
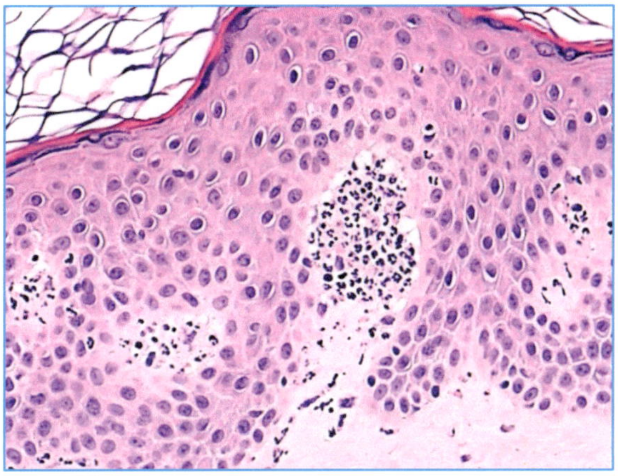

Dermatitis herpetiformis with neutrophilic abscess in dermal papilla

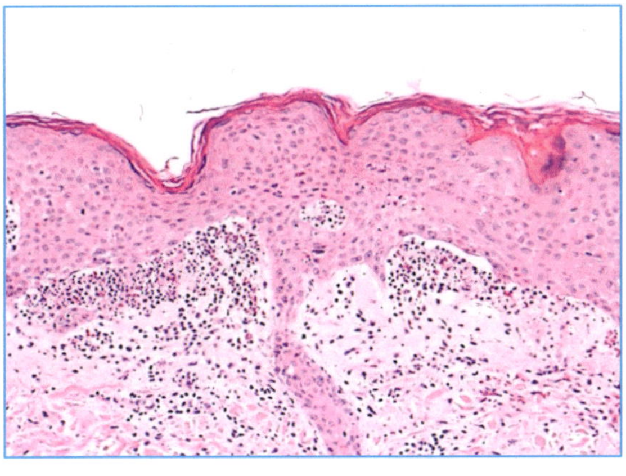
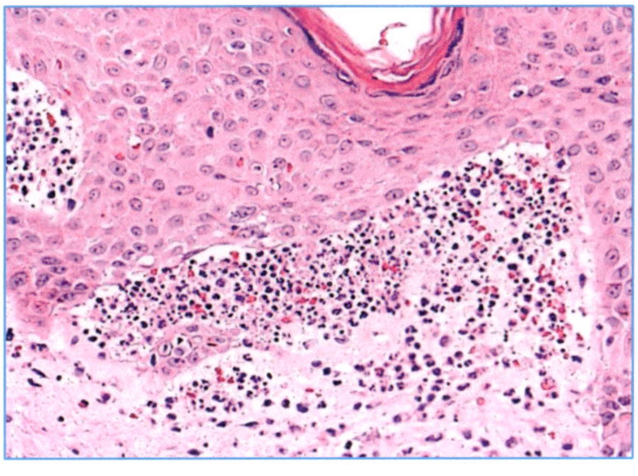

Linear IgA bullous dermatosis with linear dermal neutrophilic infiltrate underneath the epidermis

Subepidermal blistering disorders

BULLOSIS DIABETICORUM

-bullous disorder in patients with poorly controlled diabetes
-non-inflammatory, tense, painless bullae usually confined to the extremities
-heals spontaneously in 2-4 weeks

Histopathology

-**subepidermal blister** with minimal perivascular dermal lymphocytic inflammation **("cell-poor")**
-**necrotic keratinocytes in the blister roof**
-dermal vessels can show thickening
-bottom of the blister can re-epithelized forming an intraepidermal blister

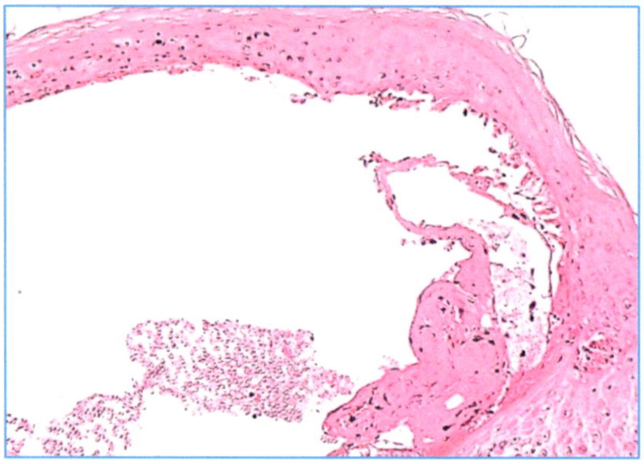

Bullosis diabeticorum with epidermal necrosis above blister

TOXIC EPIDERMAL NECROLYSIS/ STEVEN JOHNSON SYNDROME

-clinical presentation is described in detail in the chapter on vacuolar interface dermatitis
-most commonly induced by drugs and is life-threatening
-starts on trunk and spreads to periphery
-initially, diffuse erythematous macules and patches that turn into flaccid bullae and desquamate
-mucosal surfaces are involved

Histopathology

-**full thickness dirty epidermal necrosis, minimal inflammation, and subepidermal separation**

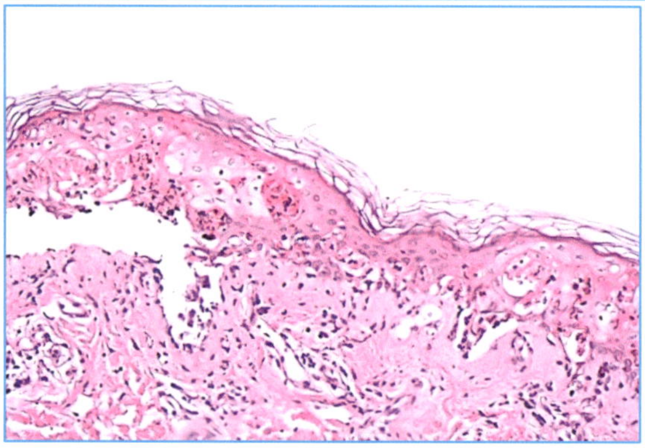

TEN with full thickness "dirty" epidermal necrosis

BULLOUS LUPUS ERYTHEMATOSUS

-bullous variant of cutaneous lupus seen in patients with systemic lupus erythematosus
-detailed clinical presentation is described in chapter on the vacuolar interface dermatitis

Histopathology

-**interface vacuolar changes** and increased number of **necrotic keratinocytes** with **subepidermal "cell-poor" blister**
-dermal lymphocytes and mucin are present
-DIF: continues granular IgG, IgM, IgA, C3 staining along the basement membrane

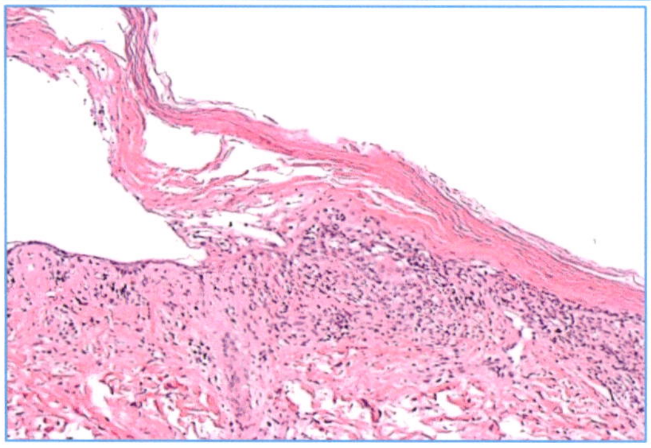

Bullous LE with interface vacuolar changes

COMA BLISTER

-48–72 hrs. after the onset of unconsciousness
-multiple tense hemorrhagic blisters
-heals spontaneously over 1 or 2 weeks

Histopathology

-subepidermal blister with variable lymphocytic dermal inflammation
-focal necrosis of epidermis is common
-**sweat duct necrosis** is the most remarkable and significant change

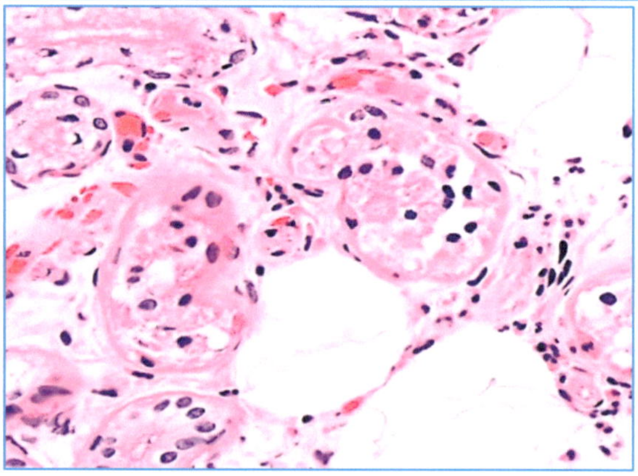

Coma blister with necrosis of eccrine glands

Chapter 9

HOW TO APPROACH SUBEPIDERMAL BLISTERS

DETERMINE IF BLISTER IS "CELL POOR" OR CONTAINS INFLAMATION

"CELL-POOR" (NO OR MINIMAL INFLAMMATION)

-epidermolysis bullosa	inherited	children	- DIF	no photosensitivity
	acquired	adult	+ DIF-linear IgG	no photosensitivity

-porphyria urine/serum porphyrin pos. hypertrichosis milia photosensitivity

-pseudoporphyria urine/serum porphyrin neg. no hypertrichosis, no milia photosensitivity

-TEN acutely ill necrotic epidermis above blister, adjacent epidermis EM-like

-bullosis diabeticorum painless necrotic epidermis above blister, adjacent epidermis normal

NEUTROPHILS

-dermatitis herpetiformis adult neutrophils in dermal papillae + DIF-IgA in papillae

-chronic bullous disease of childhood children linear dermal neutrophils + DIF-linear IgA

-linear IgA bullous dermatitis adult drug induced linear dermal neutrophils + DIF-linear IgA

EOSINOPHILS

-bullous pemphigoid elderly + DIF-linear C3 and IgG

LYMPHOCYTES

-bullous lupus interface changes of lupus + DIF-granular pattern along BMZ IgG, IgA, IgM, C3

-coma blister necrotic eccrine glands - DIF

MIXED (lymphocytes, neutrophils, eosinophils)

-pemphigoid gestationis pregnancy eosinophils predominate + DIF-linear C3 along BMZ

-cicatricial pemphigoid elderly mucosa lymphocytes predominate + DIF-linear IgG, IgA along BMZ

-insect bite ulceration common focal dermal necrosis - DIF

Subepidermal blistering disorders

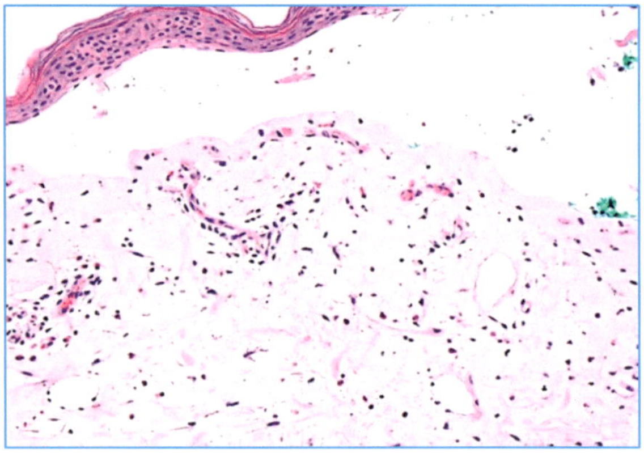

BP with subepidermal blister and eosinophils

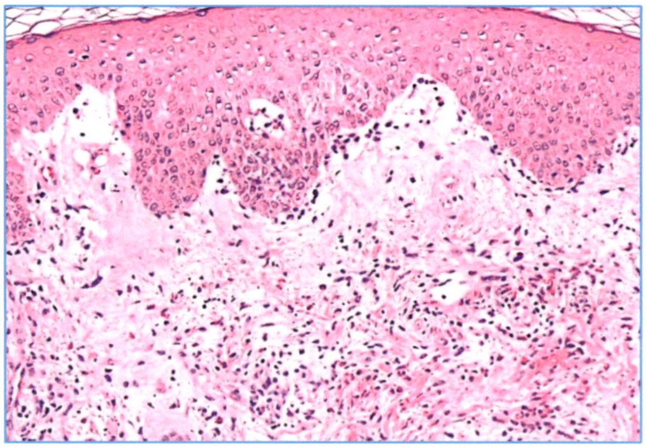

Urticarial BP with dermal edema and eosinophils

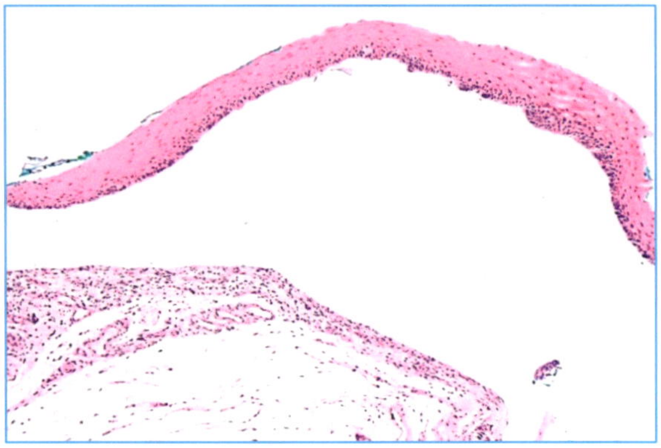

Cicatricial pemphigous with submucosal blister with mixed submucosal inflammation

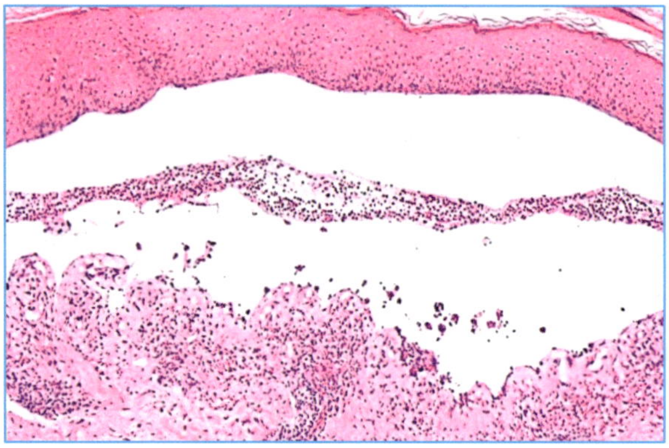

Pemphigoid gestationis blister with mostly eosinophils and some lymphocytes and neutrophils

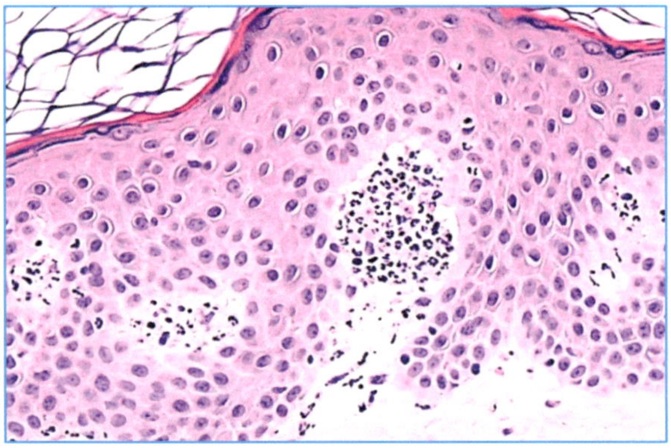

Dermatitis herpetiformis with neutrophils in dermal papilla

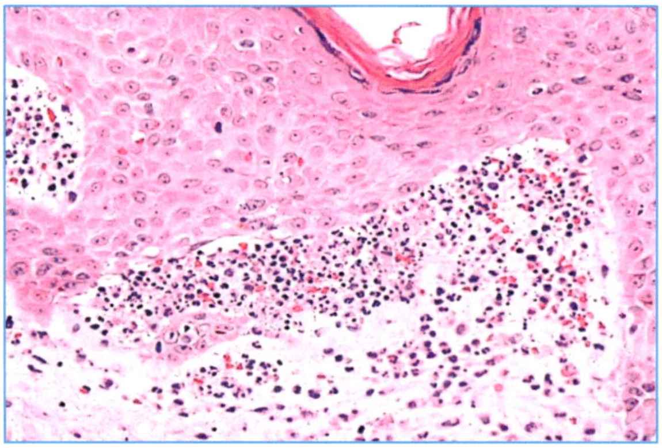

Linear IgA bullous dermatosis with linear neutrophils

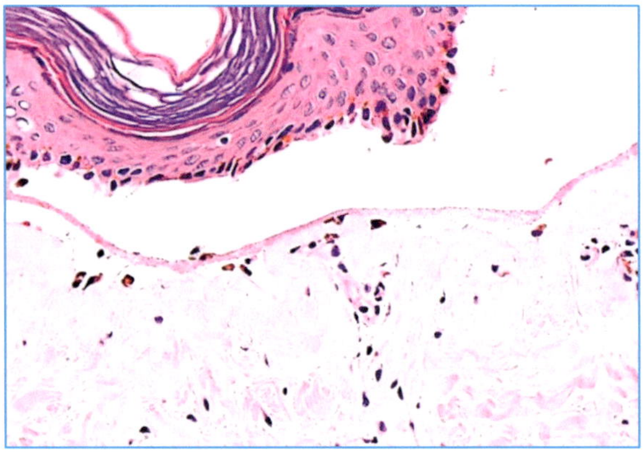

Epidermolysis bullosa with "cell-poor" blister

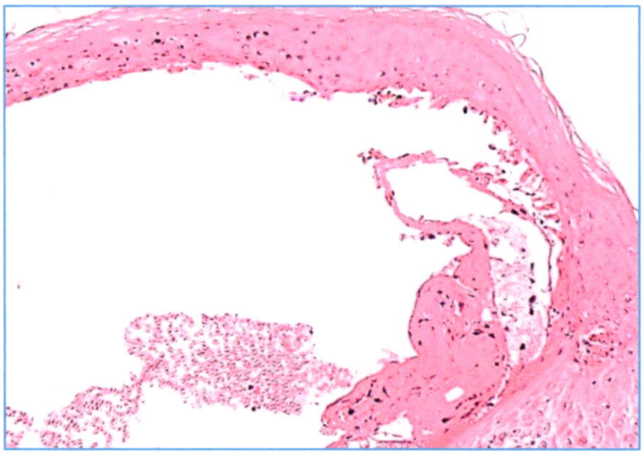

Bullosis diabeticorum with necrotic epidermis above blister

NON-INFECTIOUS GRANULOMATOUS DISORDERS

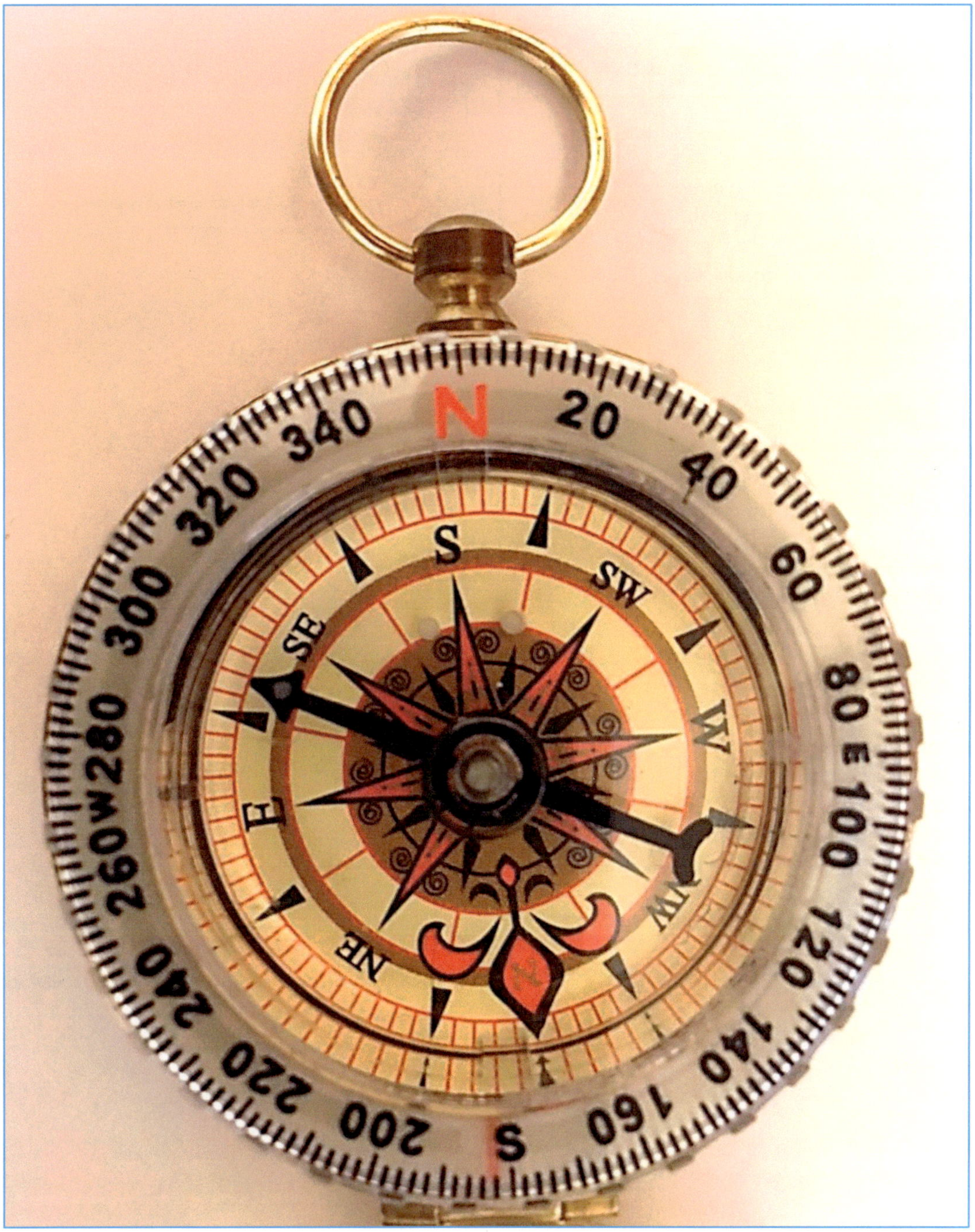

Granulomatous dermatitis

GRANULOMA ANNULARE

-idiopathic granulomatous dermatitis
-favors children, young adults, and women

Localized form (most common)
-smooth, shiny, skin-colored to violaceous annular plaques with central clearing and no scales
-favors acral sites (dorsal hand and arms)

Generalized form
-rare, usually in older patients
-numerous, small, red-purple papules coalescing into small annular plaques
-favor upper trunk and upper extremities

Subcutaneous form
-subcutaneous nodules on dorsal feet (#1), hands, shin, buttocks, scalp of **children**

Perforating form
-very rare favoring dorsal hands and fingers
-small papules with central keratin plug

Histopathology

Interstitial form (70% of cases)
-lymphocytes and histiocytes arranged between collagen fibers with **dermal mucin**
-no obvious necrobiosis of collagen
-**vaguely granulomatous** appearance

Palisaded form (25% of cases)
-palisaded granulomatous dermatitis
-rim of lymphocytes and histiocytes **(palisade)** arranged loosely perpendicular to central degenerated collagen with mucin **(necrobiosis)**

Subcutaneous form
-appears as exuberant palisaded form with deep location

Perforating form
-typical GA findings with transepidermal extrusion of degenerated collagen

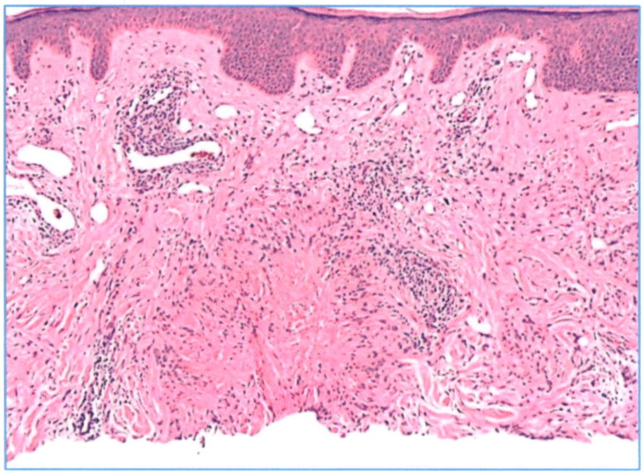

Palisaded GA with central necrobiosis

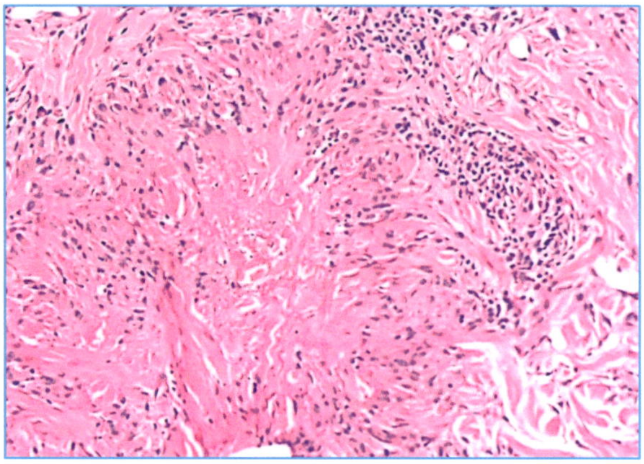

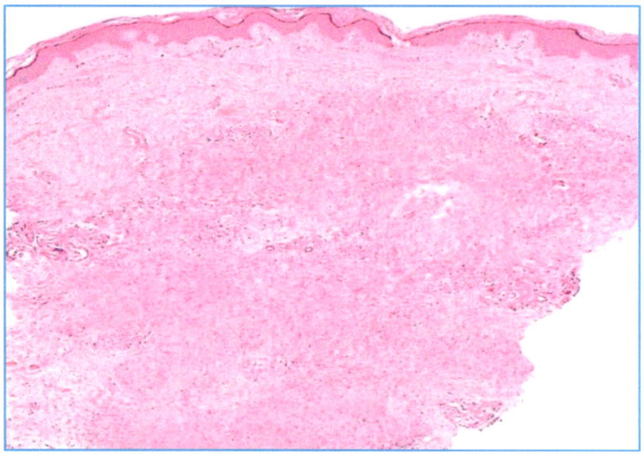

Subcutaneous GA with deep necrobiotic granulomas

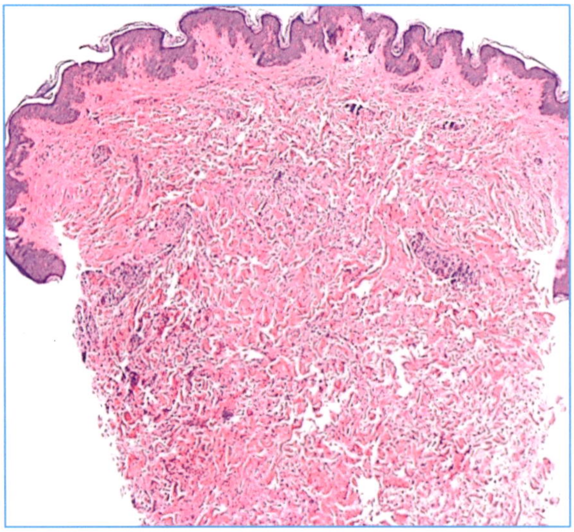

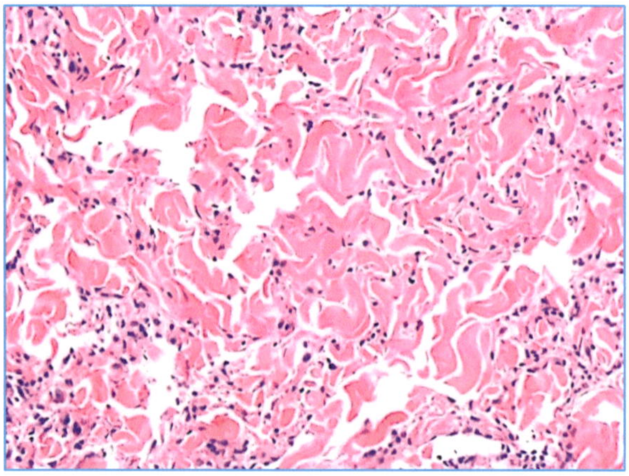

Interstitial form of GA with histiocytes and lymphocytes infiltrating in between collagen bundles and mucin

Chapter 10

ACTINIC GRANULOMA/ANNULAR ELASTOLYTIC GIANT CELL GRANULOMA OF O'BRIAN

-on chronically sun exposed areas
-similar presentation as granuloma annulare
-pink papules coalescing into an annual plaque

Histopathology

-extensive **solar elastosis** with damaged elastic fibers
-scattered histiocytes in between collagen bundles or forming palisading granulomas
-multinucleated **giant cells** engulfing **broken elastic fibers**
-dermal **mucin is not increased** (unlike in GA)

NECROBIOSIS LIPOIDICA

-favors young to middle age women
-**associated with diabetes** (a quarter of patients have or will develop diabetes)
-anterior or lateral aspect of the lower legs
-sharply circumscribed, multicolored (yellow red orange) plaques
-epidermis appears atrophic with telangiectasias and common ulceration
-heals with depressed scar

Histopathology

-usually slightly atrophic epidermis
-horizontally organized lesion with **"layered cake" square sign**
-alternating **darker** layers of inflammation consisting of lymphocytes and histiocytes and **pale** layers of degenerating hypocellular collagen
-deep perivascular lymphocytic infiltrate with **numerous plasma cells is characteristic**
-dermal **mucin** is not present (unlike in GA)

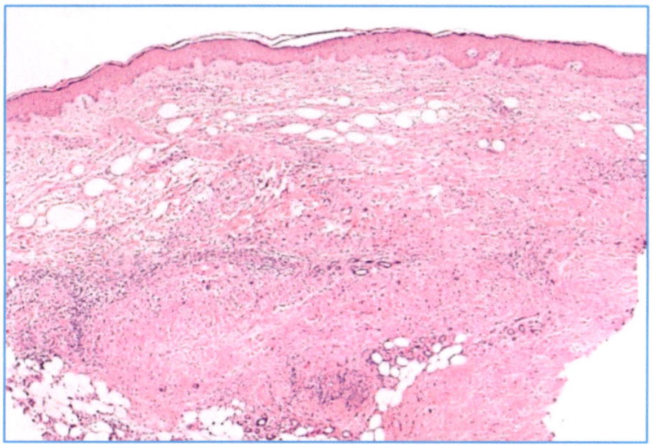

NLD with "layered cake" appearance

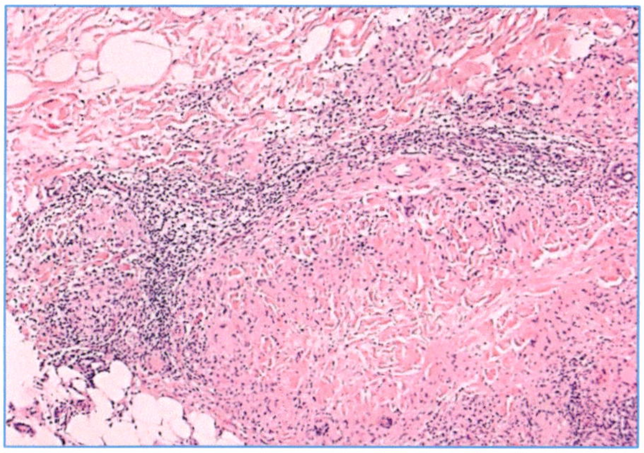

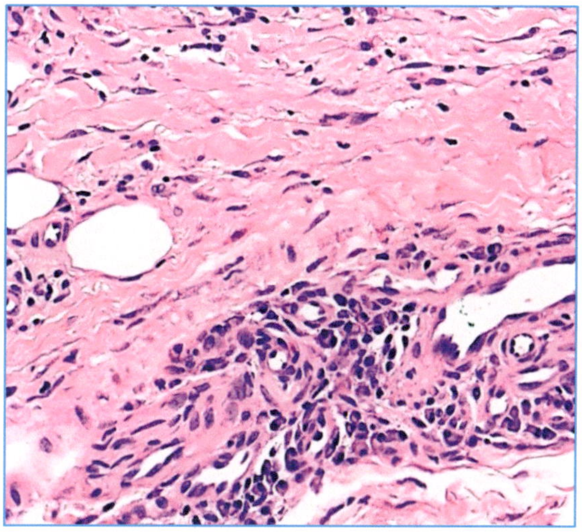

NLD with deep plasma cells

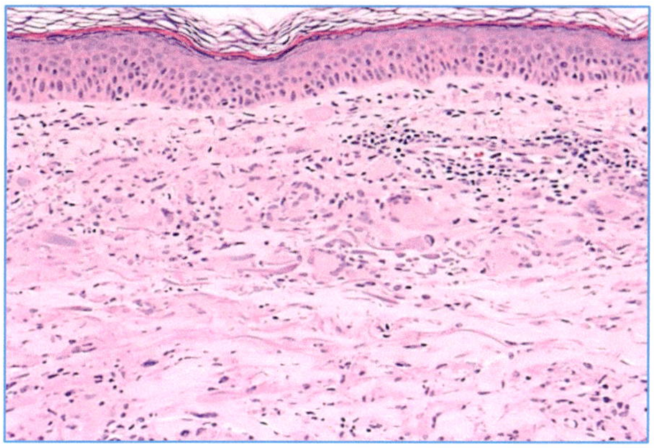

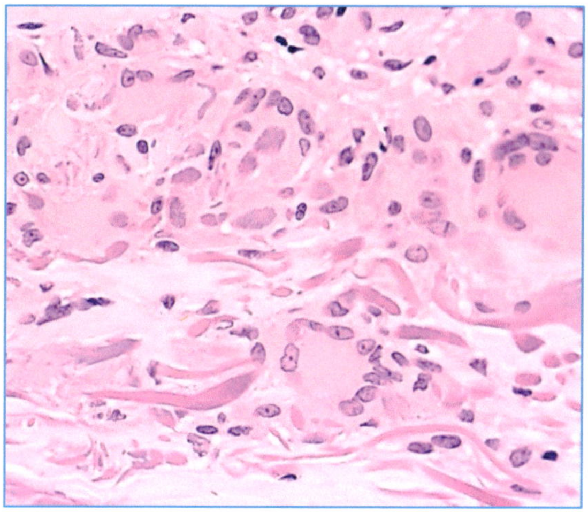

Actinic granuloma with multinucleated giant cells containing broken fragments of elastic fibers

Granulomatous dermatitis

RHEUMATOID NODULE

- firm, non-tender subcutaneous nodules found in 20% of patients with severe rheumatoid arthritis
- most common over bony prominences (elbow, hands, knee)
- persists for months to years

Histopathology

- large, dermal and subcutaneous palisaded granulomas with **irregular shape**
- tends to be deep
- central, **pink-red** degenerated collagen with fibrinoid necrosis
- peripheral histiocytic infiltrate with some lymphocytes and variable number of giant cells
- **mucin is not present** in necrobiotic area (unlike GA)

SARCOIDOSIS

- chronic systemic granulomatous disease
- 1/3rd of patients with sarcoidosis develop skin lesions
- skin may be only site involved (30%)
- purple, single or multiple, brownish papules, plaques, nodules
- predilection for face, limbs, trunk
- often arise in preexisting scars, tattoos, piercing
- one of the **"great mimicker"** of other diseases

Histopathology

- superficial and deep dermal **"naked"** granulomas (histiocytic granulomas lacking significant lymphocytic rimming)
- **asteroid bodies** (star-shaped eosinophilic intracytoplasmic inclusion) and **Schaumann bodies** (laminated calcium collection) present in only minority of cases
- variable number of giant cells
- no necrosis or neutrophilic inflammation
- diagnosis of exclusion

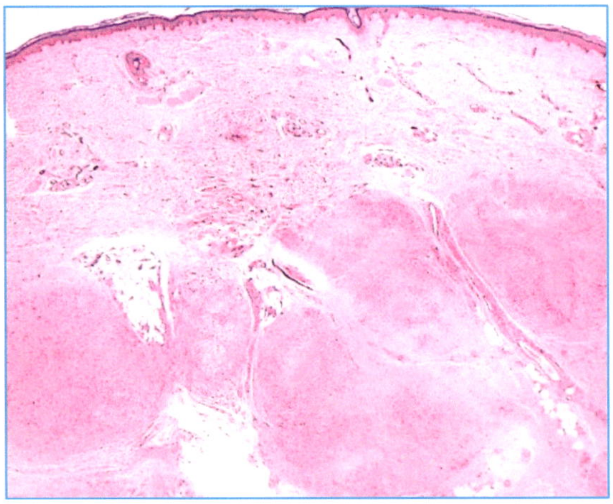
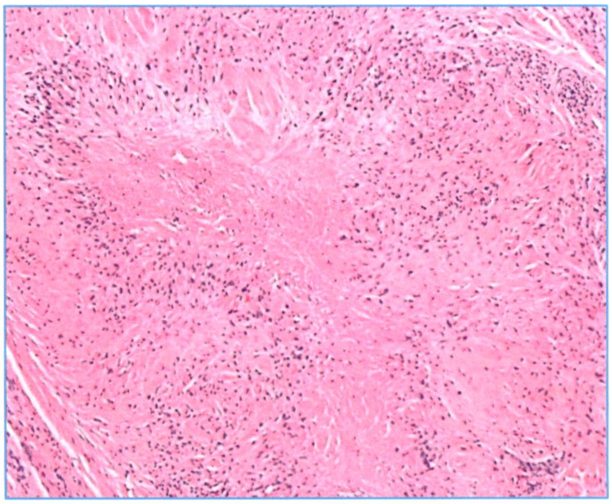

Rheumatoid nodule with pink-red central necrosis

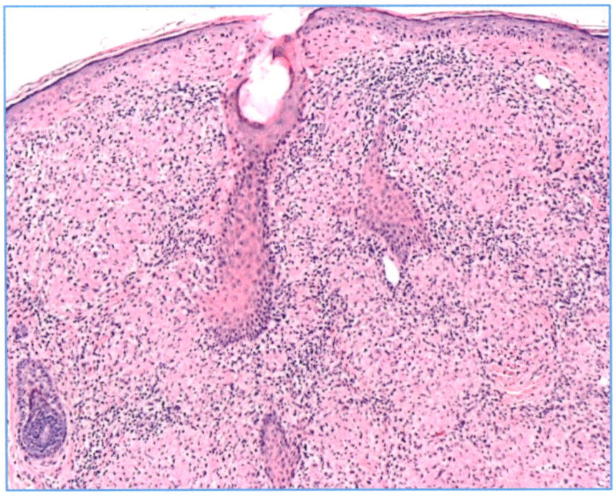
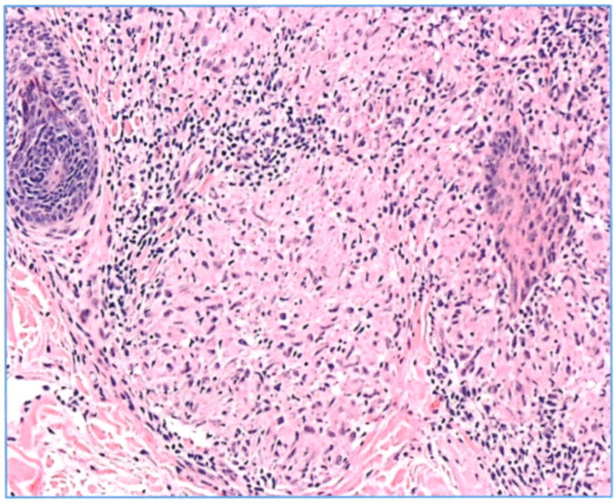

Sarcoidosis with "naked" granulomas without central necrosis

NECROBIOTIC XANTHOGRANULOMA

-multicentric histiocytic disease of the elderly
-multiple, violaceous, yellowish nodules and plaques that often ulcerate and leave scar
-periorbital face area is favored site
-50% have ophthalmic complications
-associated with IgG kappa monoclonal gammopathy

Histopathology
-diffuse, dermal and subcutaneous infiltration of lymphocytes and foamy histiocytes
-central area of necrobiosis with **cholesterol clefts**
-common Touton and foreign body giant cells around necrobiotic area

PALISADED NEUTROPHILIC GRANULOMATOUS DERMATITIS/INTERSTITIAL GRANULOMATOUS DERMATITIS AND ARTHRITIS

-probably a spectrum of the same disease
-both are associated with SLE, RA, inflammatory bowel disease, and lymphoproliferative disorders
-skin colored or erythematous papules
-favors extremities, especially elbows
-2/3rd resolves within months to years
-1/3rd becomes chronic

Histopathology
-variable presentation
-neutrophilic infiltrate with **karyorrhectic debris** (necrotic fragmented neutrophils)
-necrosis with collagen degeneration surrounded by mixed inflammation and giant cells
-irregular, poorly defined granulomas
-LCV in 1/5 of the cases

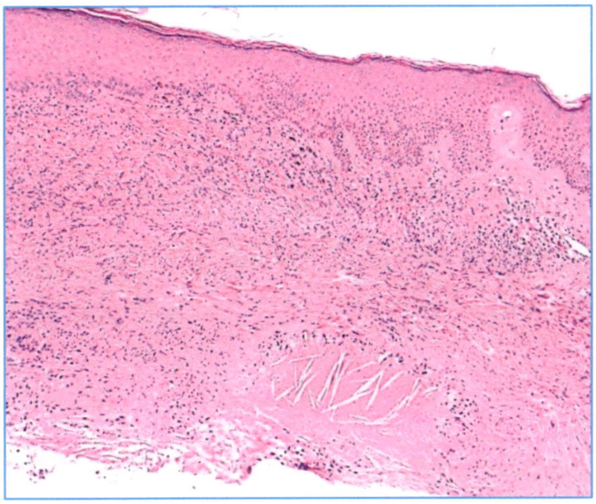
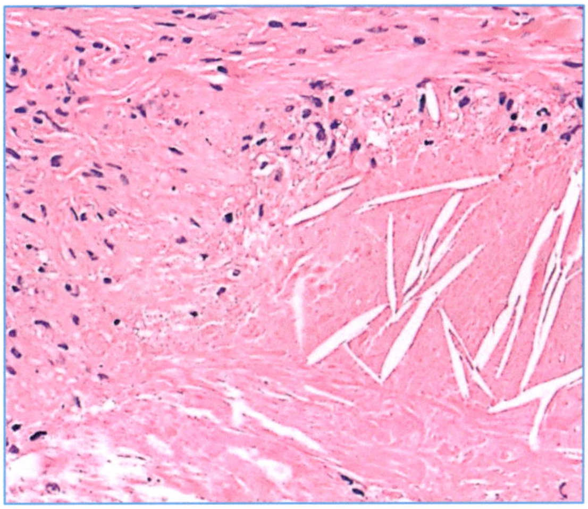

Necrobiotic xanthogranuloma with cholesterol clefts

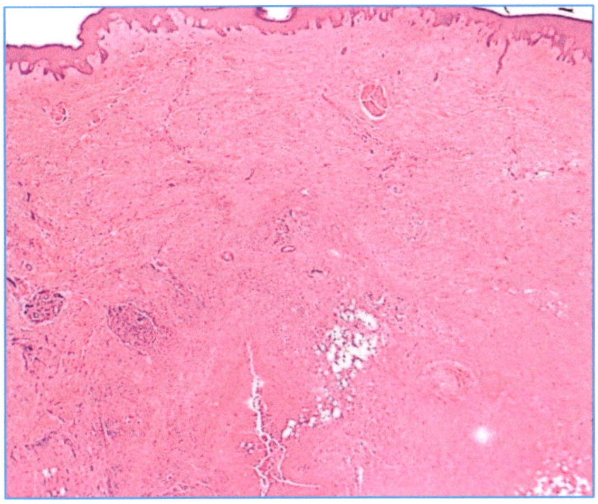
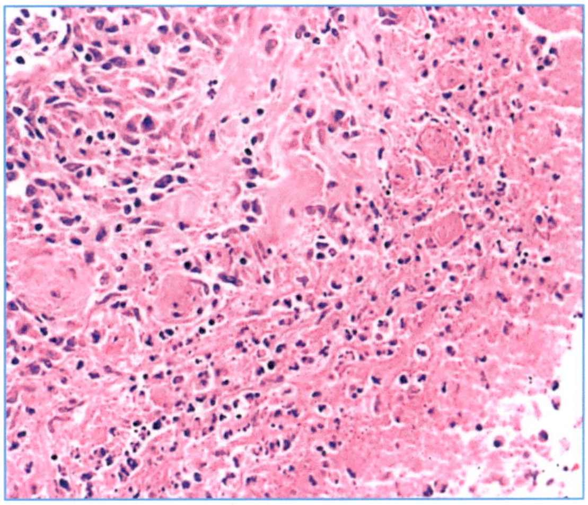

Palisaded neutrophilic granulomatous dermatitis with karyorrhexis and necrosis surrounded with giant cells

Granulomatous dermatitis

CHALAZION

-painless, gradually enlarging eyelid nodule
-mostly due to **blocked Meibomian glands**
-less frequently blocked gland of Zeis

Histopathology
-foreign body granuloma in reaction to lipids from ruptured glands
-non-caseating, **poorly defined granulomas around empty lipid vacuoles**
-usually mostly lymphohistiocytic inflammation with few giant cells

CUTANEOUS CROHN'S DISEASE

-rare manifestation of Crohn's disease
-it can present as an extension of intestinal Crohn's disease
-perianal, perioral, scrotal, or vulvar location
-**genital swelling and "knife-like" fissures**
-rarely presents as metastatic Crohn's disease
-present as patches or plaques found on the trunk, arms, and leg

Histopathology
-diffuse dermal and subcutaneous mixed inflammation
-**small, inconspicuous, non-caseating granulomas**

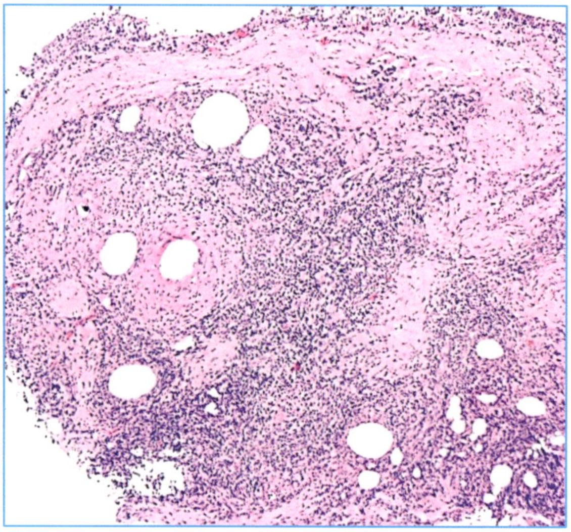
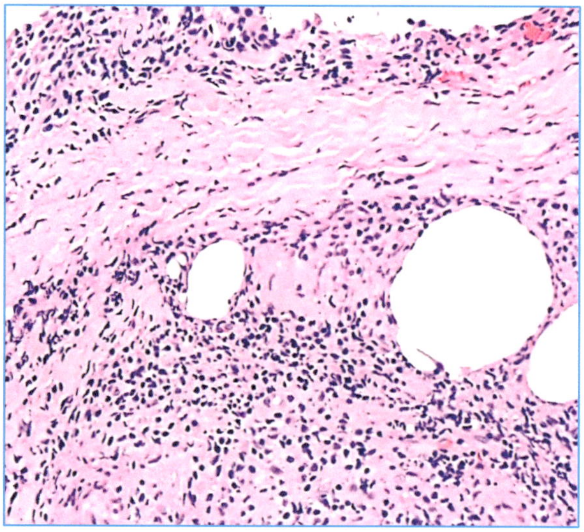

Chalazion with granulomas around empty round spaces (washed out lipids)

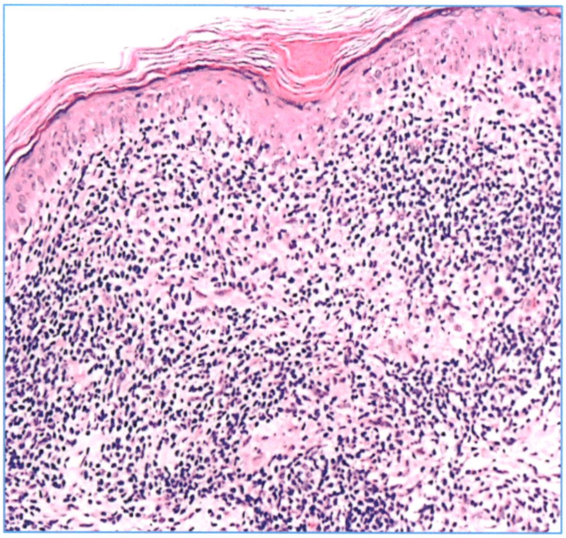
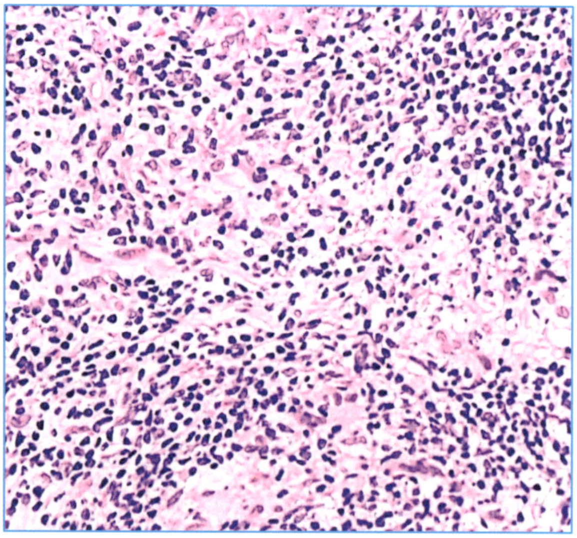

Cutaneous Crohn's disease with vague dermal granulomas surrounded by dense lymphocytic inflammation

GRANULOMA FACIALE

-red brownish papules, plaques, or nodules
-solitary lesion in 2/3rd of cases
-follicular openings are prominent
-can cause burning sensation
-involves face, particularly nose
-more common in middle age males

Histopathology

-**Grenz zone** (narrow area of uninvolved superficial dermis) separates **dense mixed inflammation** of **neutrophils, eosinophils, lymphocytes, histiocytes, and plasma cells** from epidermis
-variable vascular damage and **leukocytoclasia** (nuclear debris of neutrophils)
-**no granulomas, despite the name**

FOREIGN BODY REACTION (GRANULOMA)

-indurated papules and nodules at the site of inoculation of a foreign material

Exogenous materials

-tattoo, talc, silicon, suture, bovine collagen, wood splinter, etc.

Endogenous materials

-keratin, hair, calcium

Histopathology

-reaction differs depending on nature of foreign body and host response
-usually **granulomatous** dermatitis with lymphocytes, histiocytes, and giant cells
-plant material causes extensive **neutrophilic** reaction/abscess
-some fillers and tattoo dyes cause **lymphohistiocytic** response
-gelfoam and gauze are surrounded by **granulation tissue**

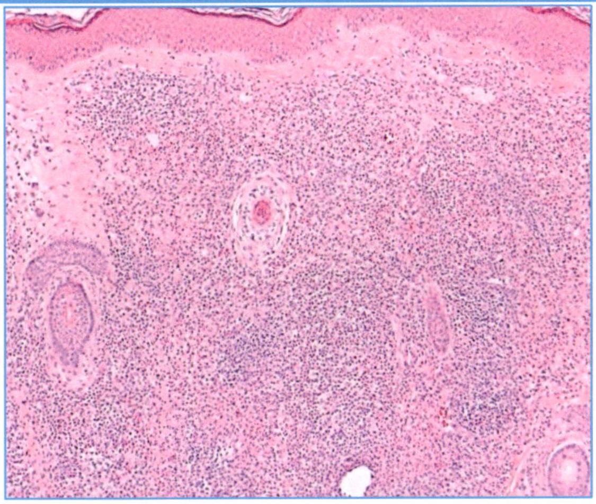

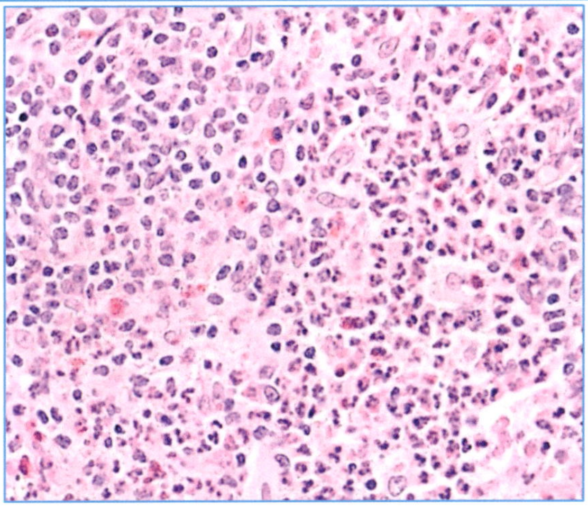

Granuloma faciale with Grenz zone and mixed, dense, dermal inflammation

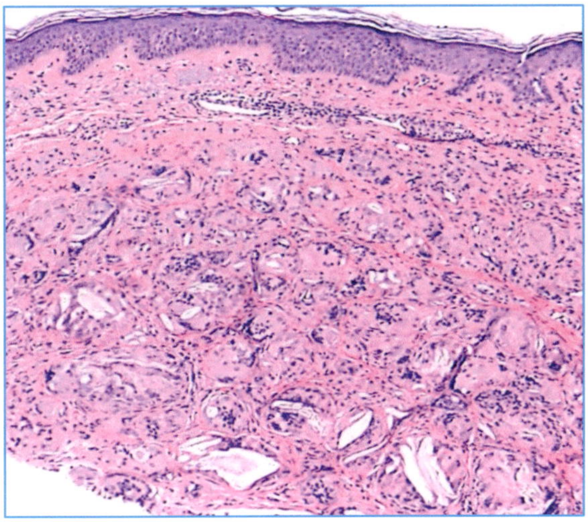

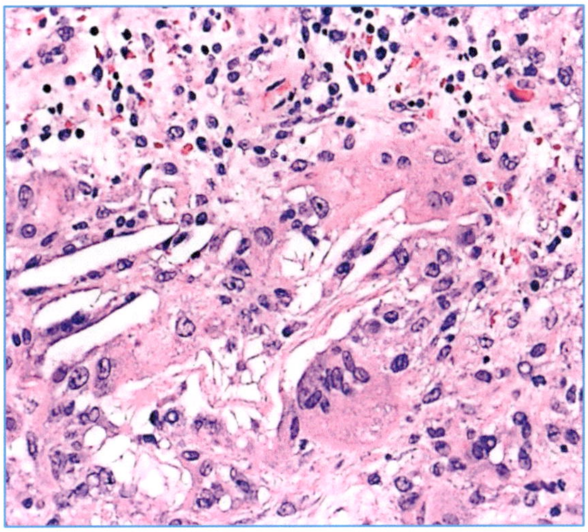

Keratin granuloma with keratin flakes within giant cells

Granulomatous dermatitis

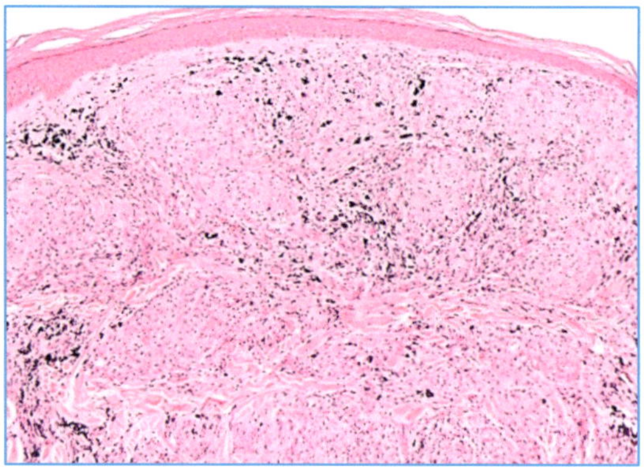
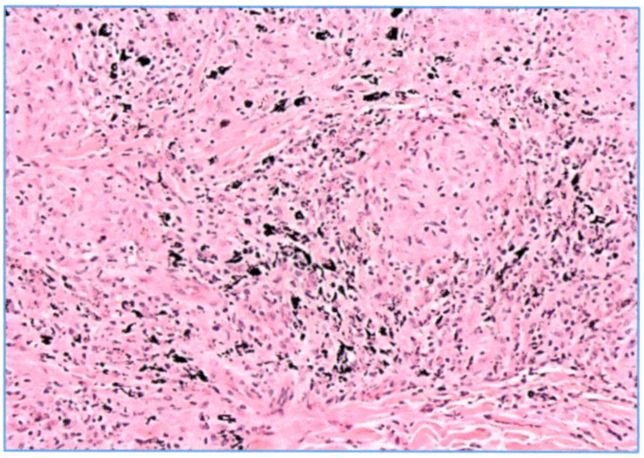

Tattoo with pigmented material inducing granulomatous reaction

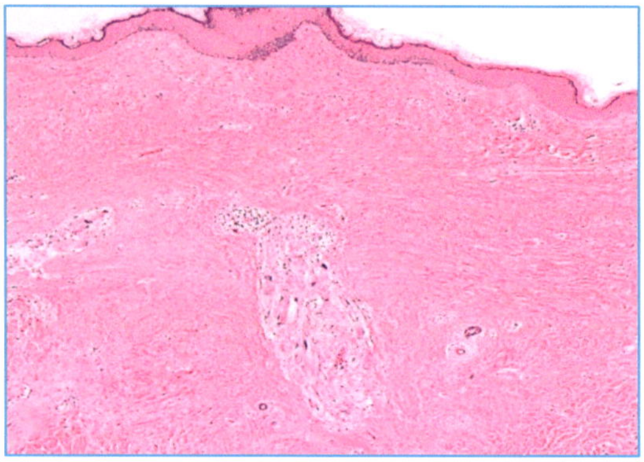
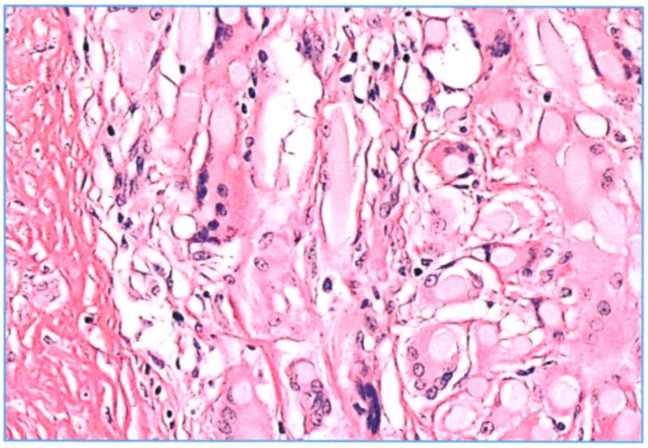

Suture granuloma with suture material surrounded by scar

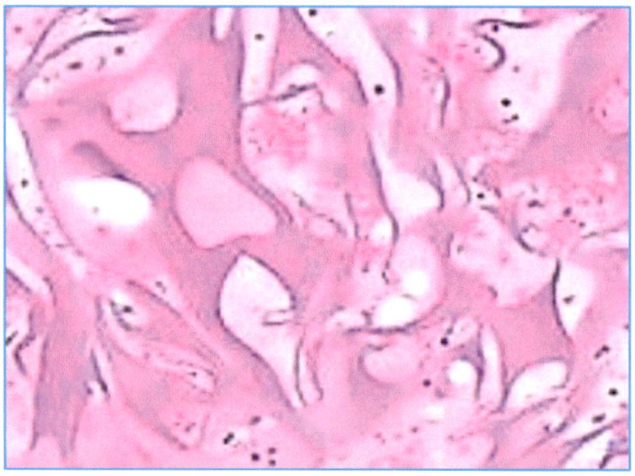

Gelfoam with dark purple "ghost" fragments

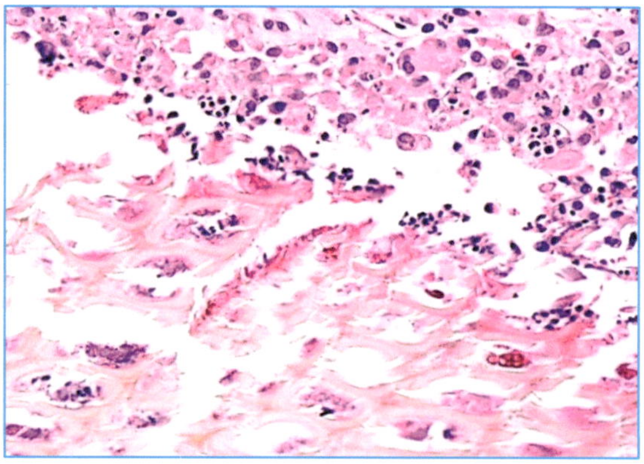

Splinter with pigmented plant material and acute inflammation

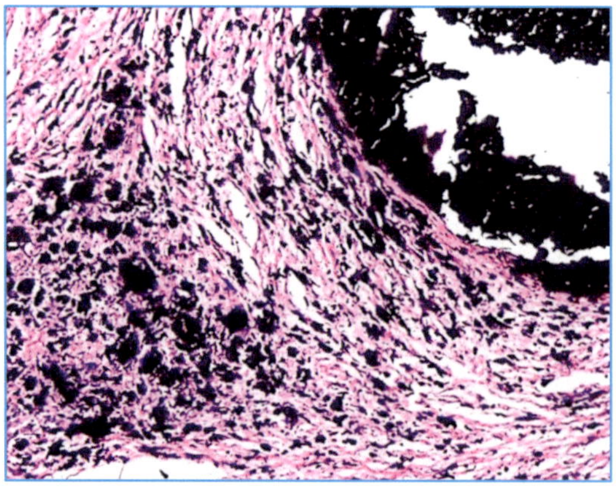

Foreign body reaction to black pencil graphite

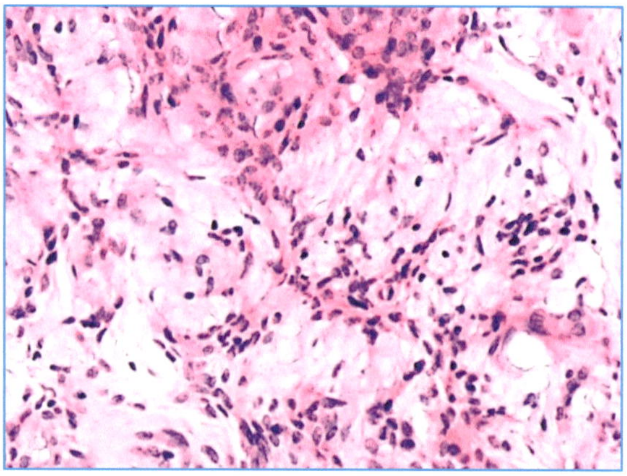

Juvéderm (hyaluronic acid) foreign body reaction

ROSACEA

-chronic, evolving disorder in adults (peaks at 30-40 years)
-more common in skin type I and II
-primarily limited to central face with multiple types:

Erythematotelangiectatic type- symmetrical, persistent facial erythema with telangiectasias
Papulopustular type- erythema and telangiectasias plus papules and tiny pustules
Granulomatous type- similar to papulopustular type with additional deeper nodules
Rhinophyma- mostly in men with hyperplasia of nose, cheeks, forehead tissue

Histopathology

Erythematotelangiectatic type

-perivascular and perifollicular lymphoplasmocytic infiltrate with **dermal telangiectasias**
-findings are non-specific

Papulopustular type

-denser perivascular and perifollicular lymphoplasmocytic infiltrate
-occasional foci of **neutrophilic pustules** within hair follicles

Granulomatous type

-similar to papulopustular type with **perifollicular, vague, non-caseating granuloma** and mild sebaceous hyperplasia
-Demodex mites commonly present within dilated hair follicles

Rhinophyma

-variable **sebaceous hyperplasia**
-diffuse dermal fibrosis with dermal telangiectasias
-dilated hair follicles with formation of "**comedo-like" cysts**

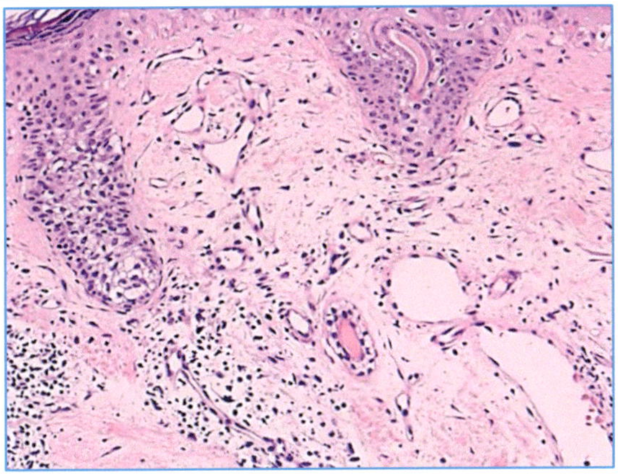

Rosacea with prominent telangiectasias

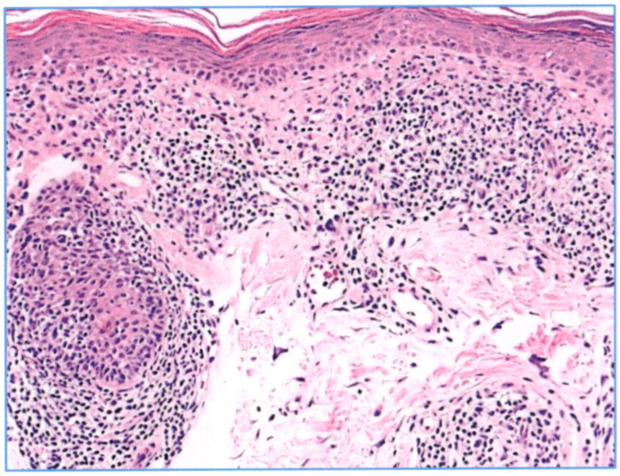

Papulopustular rosacea with perifollicular inflammation

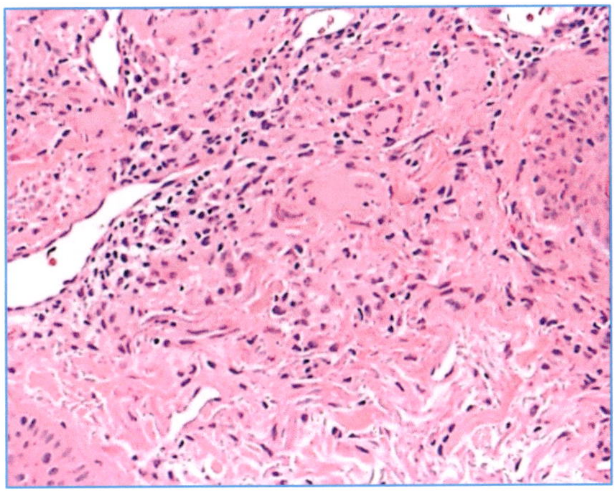

Rosacea with perifollicular granuloma

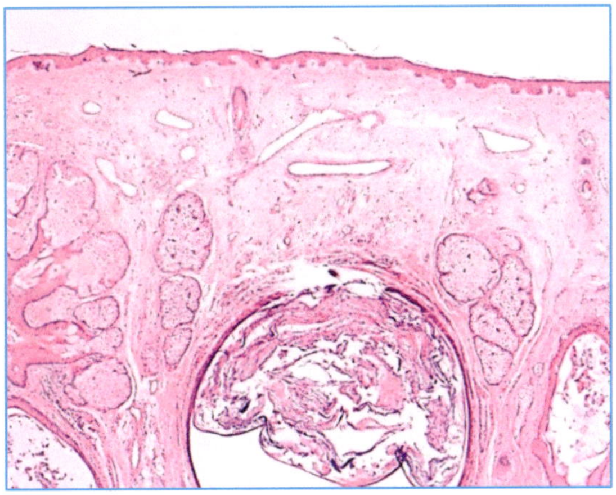

Rhinophyma with sebaceous hyperplasia and dilated "comedo-like" follicles

Granulomatous dermatitis

ROSACEA VARIANTS

Perioral dermatitis
-young women with small papules/pustules
-perioral distribution with **clear zone around the vermillion border**
Histopathology
-is identical to granulomatous rosacea
-perivascular and perifollicular lymphoplasmocytic infiltrate
-**perifollicular non-caseating granulomas**

Pyoderma faciale (rosacea fulminans)
-rapidly developing disease in young women
-darkly erythematous skin with nodules and cysts that drain pus
-**scarring** very common
Histopathology
-ulcerated epidermis with exuberant dermal mixed inflammation with numerous neutrophils
-**follicular abscess** formation

Lupus miliaris disseminatus faciei (acne agminata)
-still debated if it is a variant of rosacea or form of sarcoidosis
-more common in young Asian patients
-reddish to yellow-brown papules in malar **"butterfly"** distribution that resolves with **scarring**
-eyelids are also commonly involved
Histopathology
-usually **perifollicular, sarcoidal granuloma** that can become necrotic (tuberculoid appearance)
-surrounding chronic inflammation

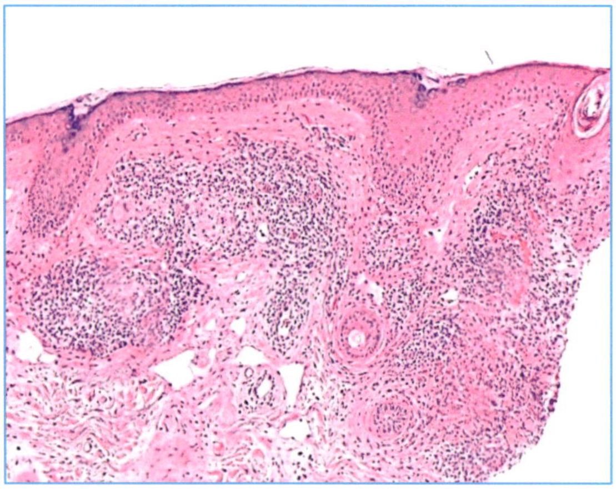
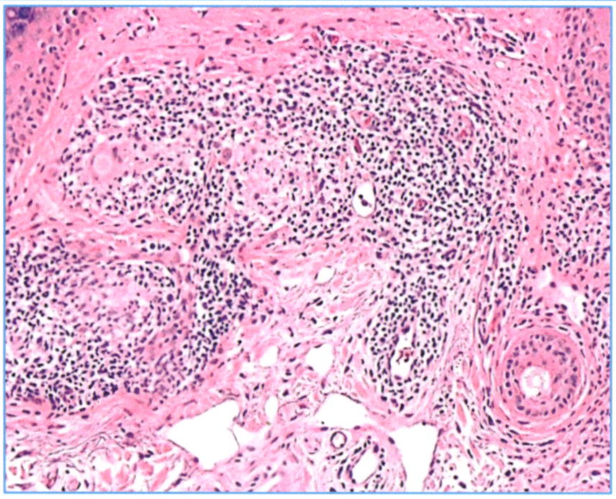

Perioral dermatitis with perifollicular noncaseating granulomas

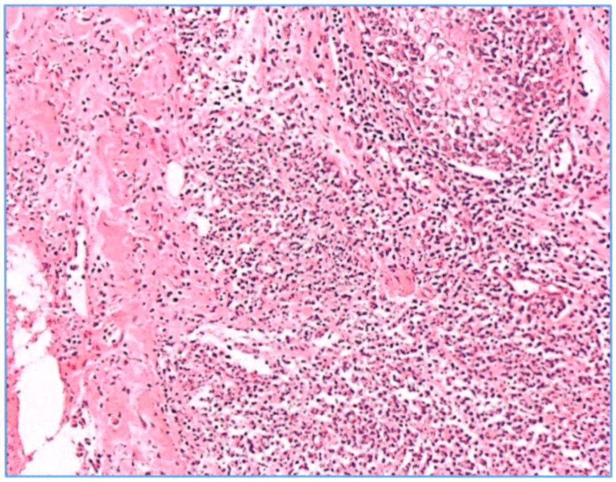

Pyoderma faciale with abscess formation

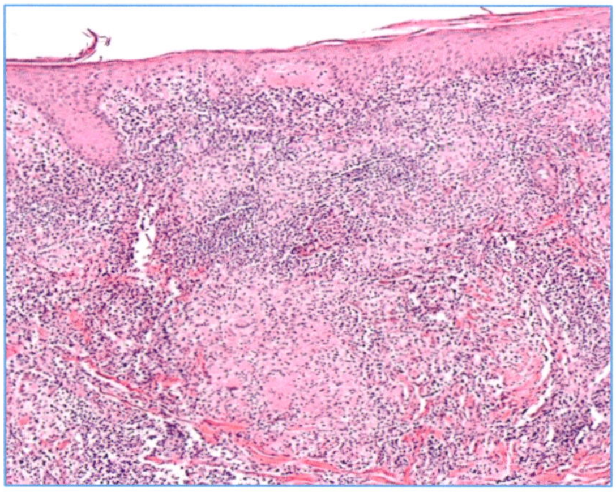

Lupus miliaris disseminates faciei with sarcoidal granulomas

Chapter 10

HOW TO APPROACH NON-INFECTIOUS GRANULOMATOUS DERMATITIS

IF YOU SEE NECROSIS AND NEUTROPHILS
ALWAYS THINK ABOUT AND EXCLUDE INFECTION

THEN

CHECK LOCATION

-granuloma faciale	**nose**	Grenz zone + mixed inflammation + no granuloma
-chalazion	**eyelid**	vague granuloma + empty lipid holes
-Crohn's	**perianal/perioral**	subtle granuloma + mixed inflammation
-rosacea	**face/perioral**	perifollicular granuloma + telangiectasias +sebaceous hyperplasia

CHECK FOR FOREIGN BODY MATERIAL

-foreign body granulomas (tattoo, splinter, suture, keratin, etc.)

CHECK FOR NECROBIOSIS/NECROSIS

NECROBIOSIS

-granuloma annulare	central necrobiosis	mucin
-rheumatoid nodule	central necrobiosis	no mucin
-necrobiosis lipoidica	layered necrobiosis	no mucin + plasma cells
-necrobiotic xanthogranuloma	cholesterol clefts	

NO NECROBIOSIS/NECROSIS

-sarcoidosis	"naked" granulomas with only few lymphocytes
-actinic granuloma	vague granulomas with broken elastic fibers many engulfed within giant cells

IF YOU SEE EXUBERANT SUPERFICIAL AND DEEP MIXED INFLAMMATION
WITH VAGUE GRANULOMAS

-necrobiotic xanthogranuloma	cholesterol clefts	
-palisaded neutrophilic granulomatous dermatitis	necrosis	karyorrhexis

IF YOU SEE ROUND AREAS OF BLUISH DERMAL MUCIN
WITH INTERCALATED HISTIOCYTES

-interstitial granuloma annulare

Granulomatous dermatitis

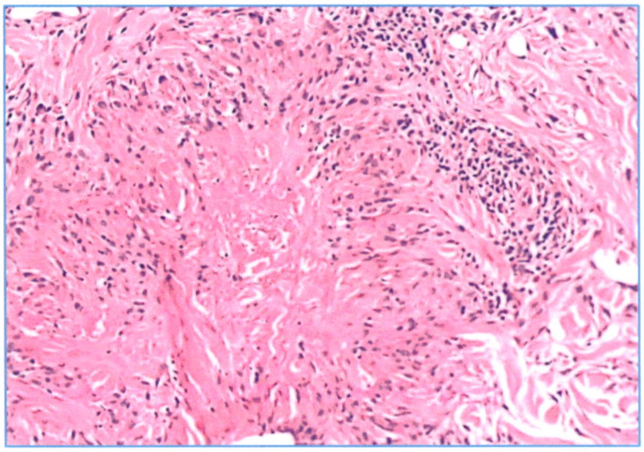

Palisaded GA with histiocytic palisade around central mucin

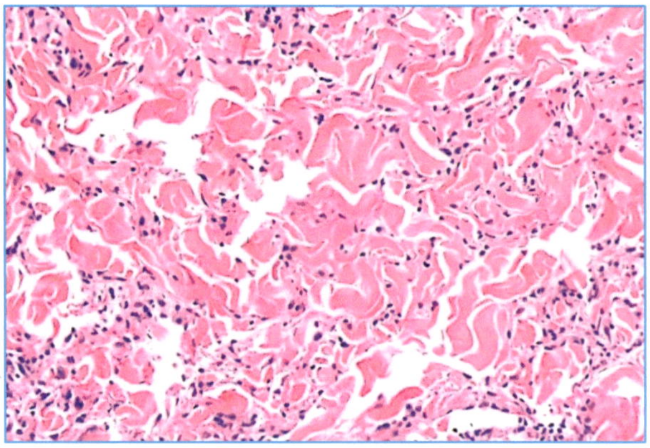

Interstitial GA with histiocytes between collagen bundles and increased dermal mucin

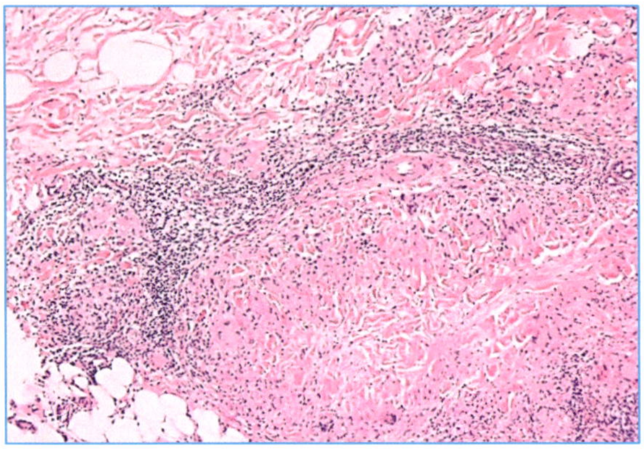

NLD with layered appearance with plasma cells and no mucin

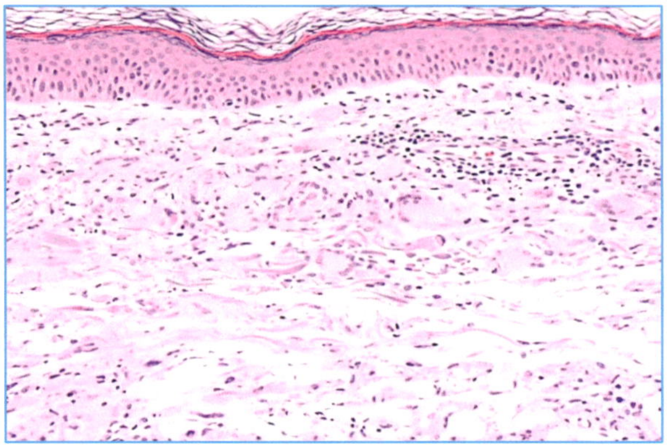

Actinic granuloma with fragmented elastic fibers in giant cells

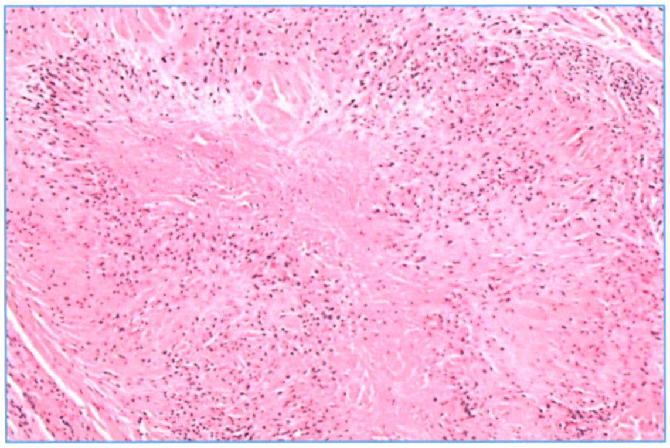

Rheumatoid nodule with red granuloma with no mucin

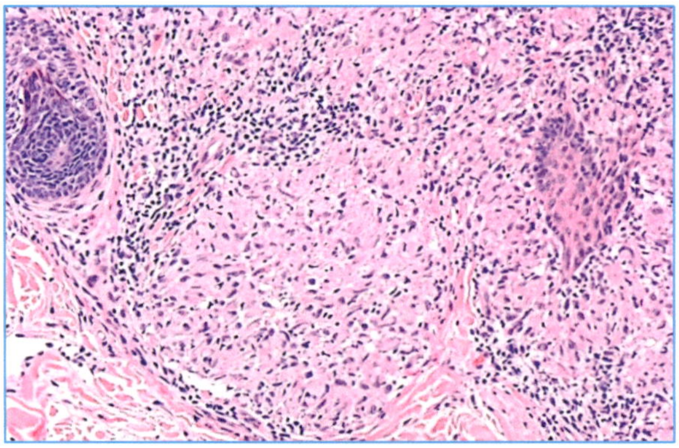

Sarcoidosis with ball of histiocytes with few lymphocytes, so-called "naked granuloma"

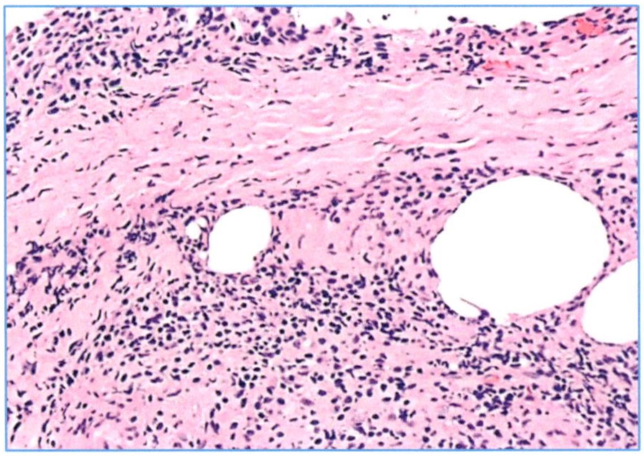

Chalazion with empty lipid vacuoles

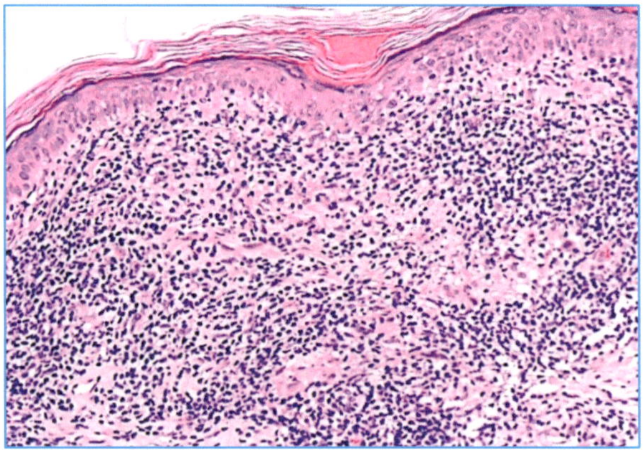

Crohn's disease with inconspicuous non-caseating granuloma

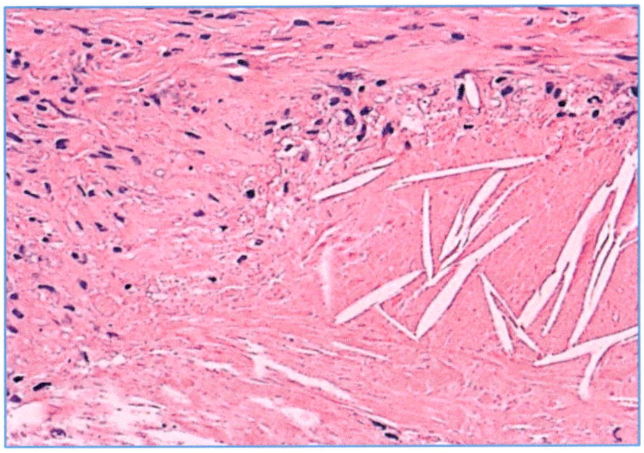

NXG with necrobiosis and cholesterol clefts

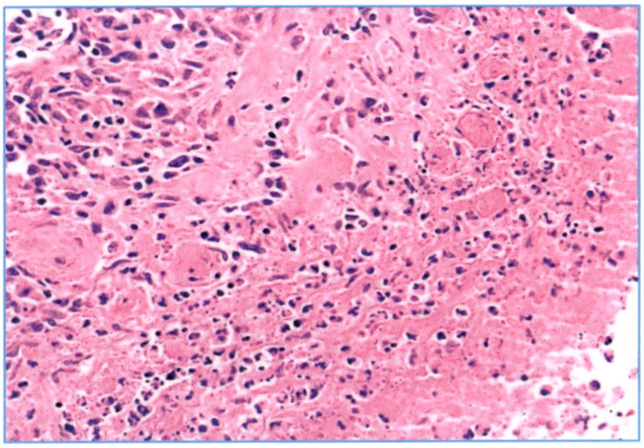

PNG with necrosis and degenerated neutrophils

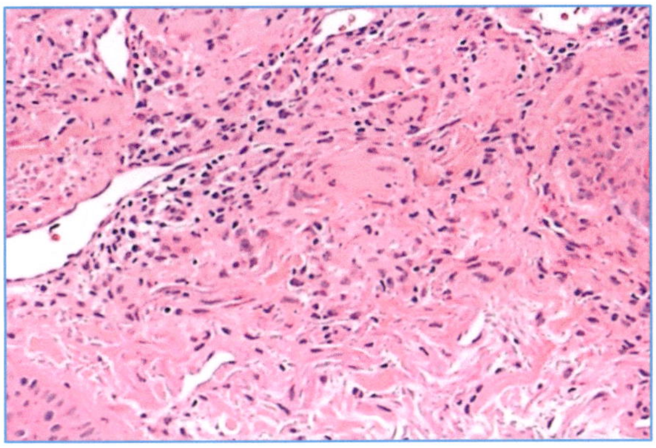

Rosacea with telangiectasias and vague granuloma

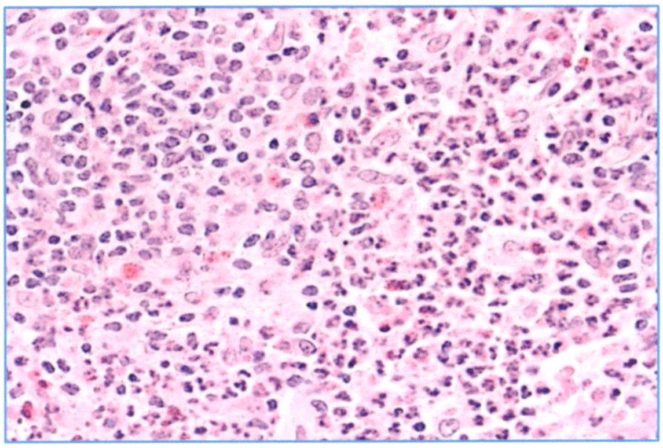

Granuloma faciale with mixed inflammation with eosinophils and no granuloma

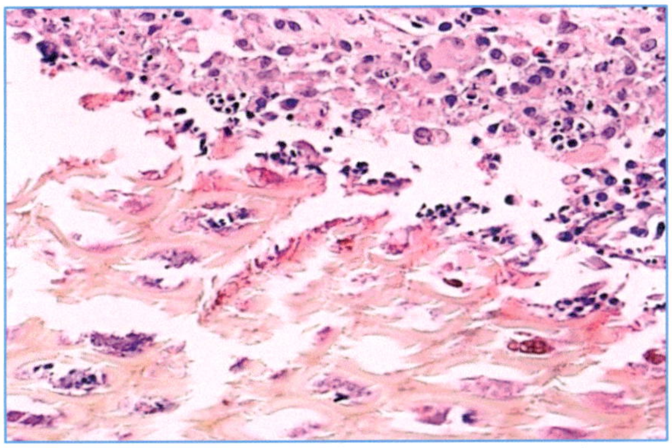

Splinter granuloma with pigmented plant material surrounded by acute inflammation

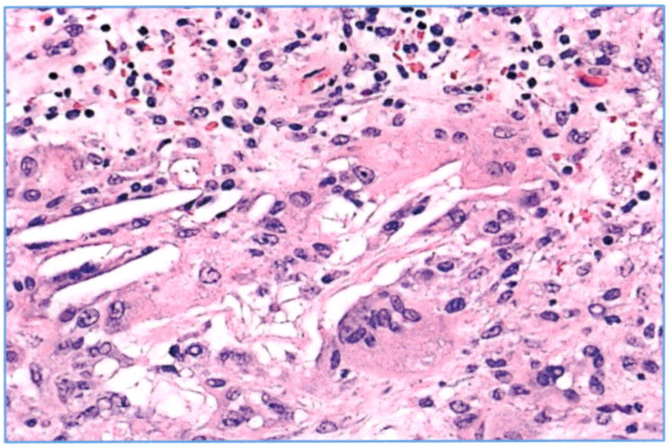

Keratin granuloma with flakes of keratin in giant cells

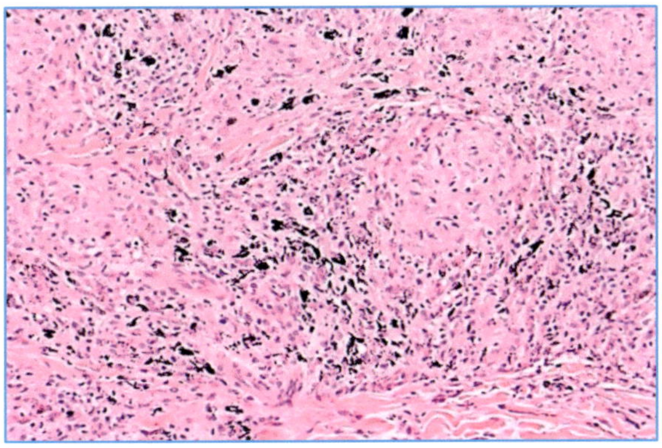

Tattoo granuloma with pigmented material in and around non-necrotizing granulomas

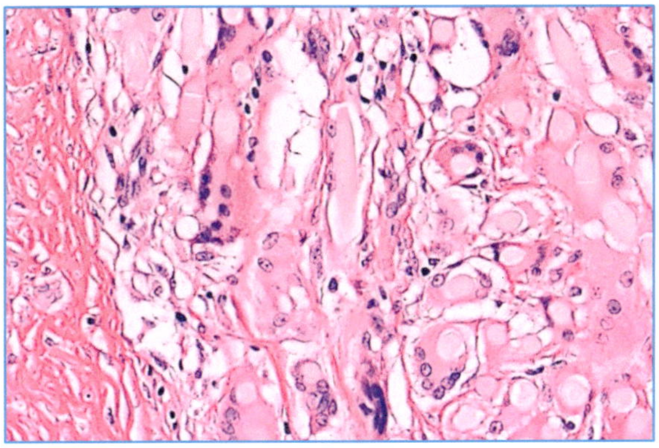

Suture granuloma with suture fragments surrounded by histiocytes

Granulomatous dermatitis

Chapter 11

INFLAMMATORY VASCULAR DISORDERS AND MIMICKERS

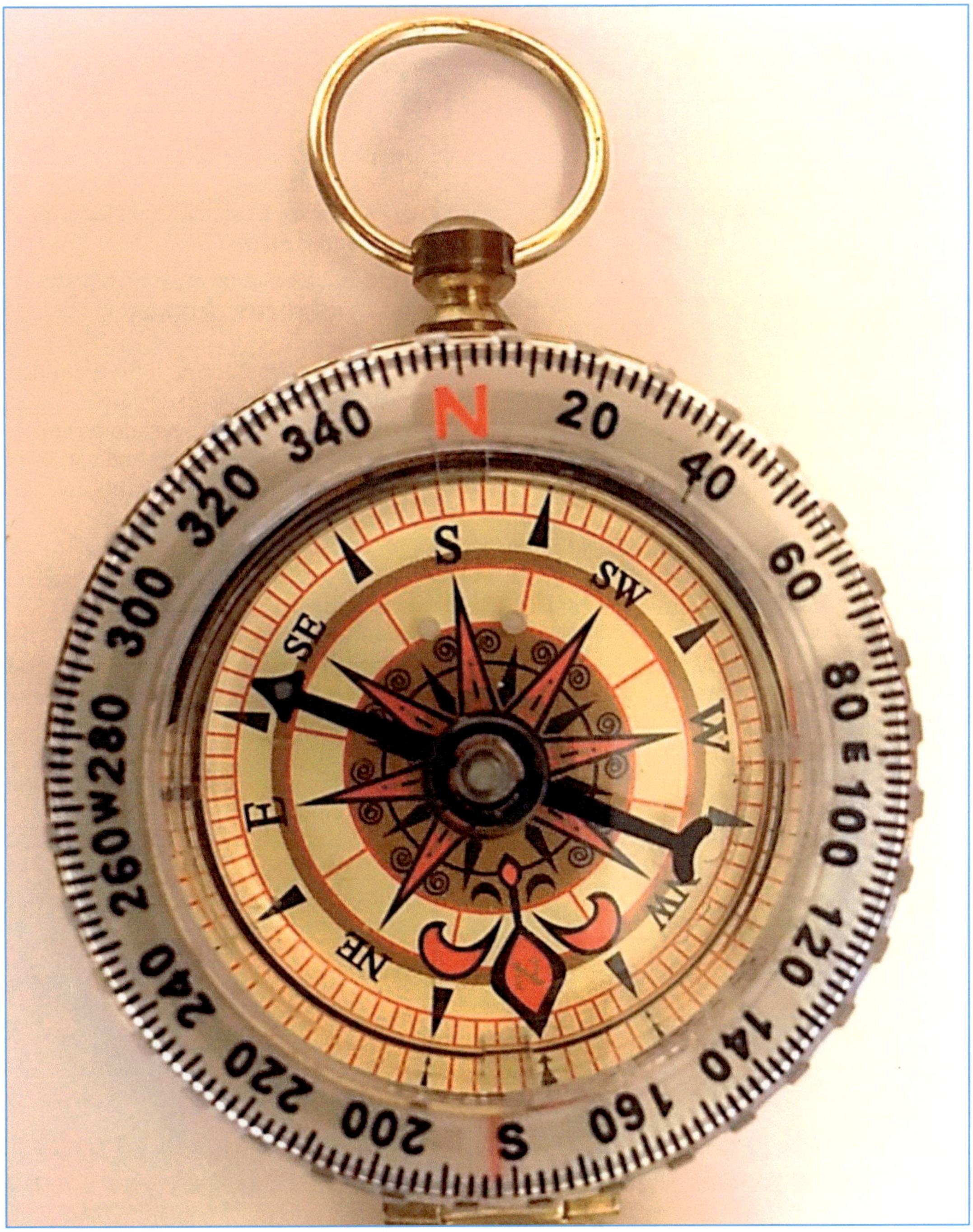

Inflammatory vascular disorders and mimickers

LEUKOCYTOCLASTIC VASCULITIS (LCV)

-histological term for a heterogenous group of conditions causing inflammation of the small dermal vessels
-associated with hypersensitivity to an antigen
-antigens vary from infectious agents (hepatitis B, hepatitis C, *Streptococcus*, *Staphylococcus,* gonococcemia, Rocky Mountain spotted fever), to drugs (sulfonamide, penicillin), to endogenous sources (neoplasms, autoimmune disorders)
-present as palpable purpura with lesions ranging in size from pinpoint to a few centimeters
-predilection for lower legs and buttocks
-usually resolves in several weeks, with occasional hyperpigmentation

Histopathology

-endothelial swelling and **fibrinoid necrosis** of capillaries
-**intravascular and perivascular neutrophilic infiltrate**
-breaking apart of neutrophils **(leukocytoclasia)** with formation of **nuclear dust**
-variable red blood cell extravasation

HENOCH-SCHÖNLEIN PURPURA (IgA VASCULITIS)

-subtype of LCV due to IgA immune complex depositions
-viral infections and *Strep* pharyngitis are triggers
-mostly in children (peak between 2-8 years of age)
-triad of pulpable purpura, arthralgia, and abdominal pain
-may also have renal insufficiency (IgA glomerulonephritis)
-purpura has predisposition for lower extremities and buttocks; spontaneously resolves in several months

Histopathology

-indistinguishable from other forms of LCV on H&E
-DIF will show **IgA deposition** in capillaries

ACUTE HEMORRHAGIC EDEMA OF INFANCY

-small vessel vasculitis of children (classically younger than 2 year of age)
-may be triggered by preceding infection or medication
-presents as large targetoid or annular purpuric bruise-like plaques on face and extremities
-characteristic acral tender edema
-child appears well although can have low fever
-self-limited disease with spontaneous recovery in 2-3 weeks

Histopathology

-leukocytoclastic vasculitis that **lacks IgA depositions on DIF**

MENINGOCOCCEMIA

-bloodstream infection with the gram-negative bacterium, *Neisseria meningitidis*
-usually young children and adolescents
-patients develop petechiae and purpura that may progress to ecchymosis, bullae, and finally necrosis, as purpura fulminans
-predilection for trunk and lower extremities
-patients are severely ill with fever, chills, hypotension, and meningitis

Histopathology

-LCV with prominent **necrosis of capillaries and small veins** in the dermis and subcutaneous tissue
-fibrin thrombi and hemorrhage
-***Meningococci* are present** within endothelium and thrombi

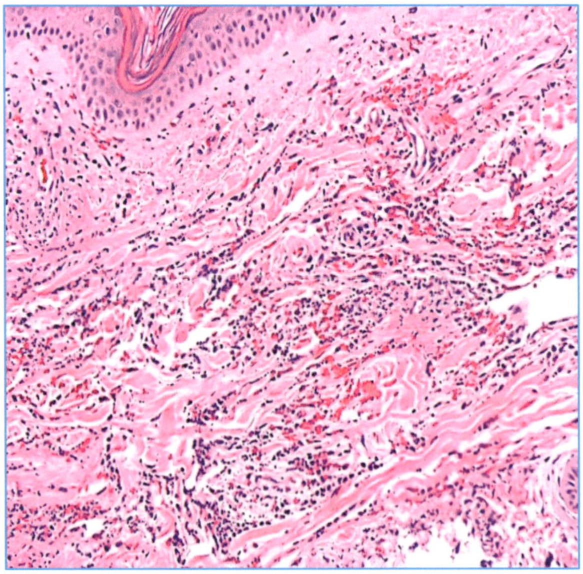
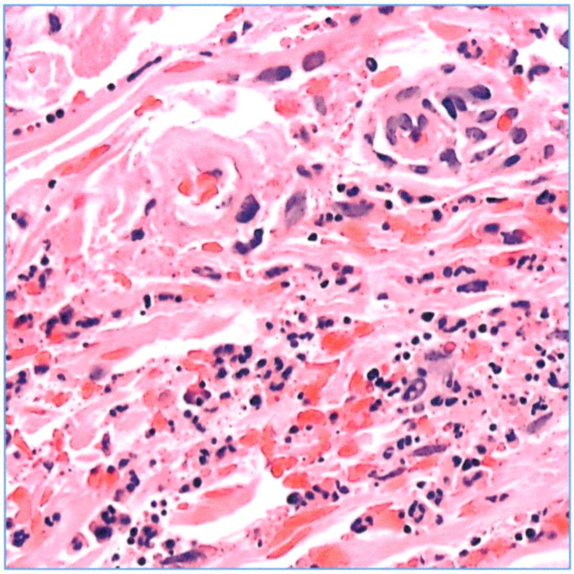

LCV with fibrinoid necrosis of capillaries, neutrophilic inflammation, nuclear dust, and red blood cell extravasation

ERYTHEMA ELEVATUM DIUTINUM

-rare, chronic disease involving fibrosis from repeated bouts of inflammation and immune complex deposition
-associated with HIV, multiple myeloma, and autoimmune diseases
-chronic red purple violaceous papules, plaques, and nodules
-initially soft and later become firm
-predisposition for skin over joints and extensor surfaces

Histopathology

Early lesions
-capillaries with **prominent endothelial cells** and **leukocytoclastic vasculitis**

Established lesions
-extensive **sclerosis of dermis** and subcutis with **cleft formation** around vessels (**"onion skin" fibrosis**, resembles sclerotic fibroma)
-neutrophilic **nuclear debris** between collagen

URTICARIAL VASCULITIS

-resembles urticaria with wheals that persists for more than 24 hours (unlike urticaria)
-recurrent episodes last months to years
-lesions burn or are painful rather than itchy
-favors trunk and lower extremities
-resolves with hyperpigmentation or purpura
-75% are normocomplementemic
-they are idiopathic or association with medications, viral infections, or malignancy
-25% are associate with hypocomplementemia in patients with collagen vascular diseases

Histopathology

-**mild dermal edema** (less than in urticaria)
-there is a **continuum** of inflammatory changes
-range from mild to moderate perivascular lymphocytic and neutrophilic infiltrate with **few intravascular intact neutrophils**
-to **LCV** presentation with **numerous fragmented intravascular and perivascular neutrophils**
-**scattered dermal eosinophils are present**

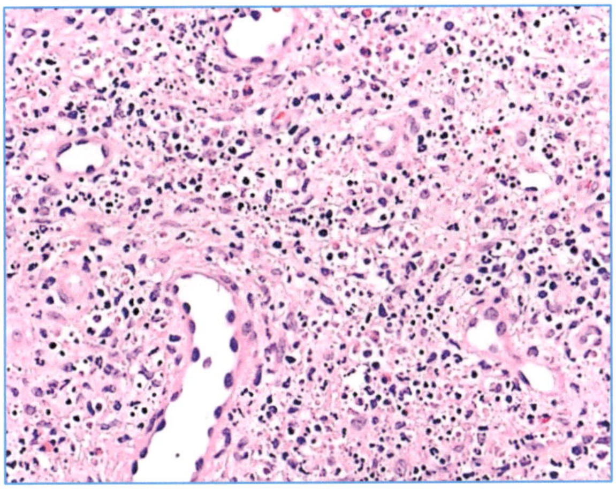

Early EED with prominent endothelial cells and perivascular neutrophilic inflammation with nuclear dust

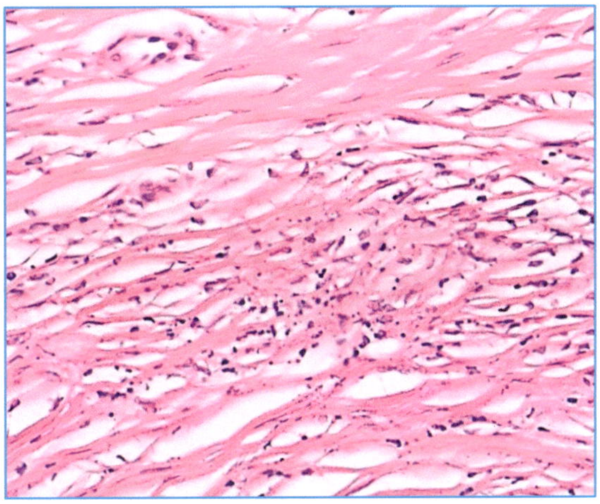

Late EED with "onion skin" fibrosis and nuclear dust

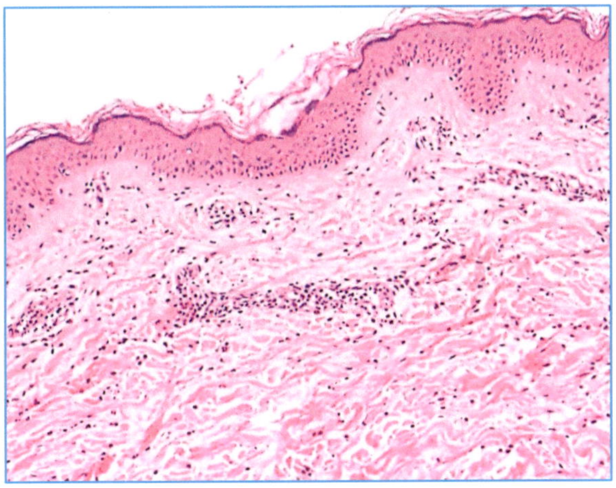

Urticarial vasculitis with mild dermal edema

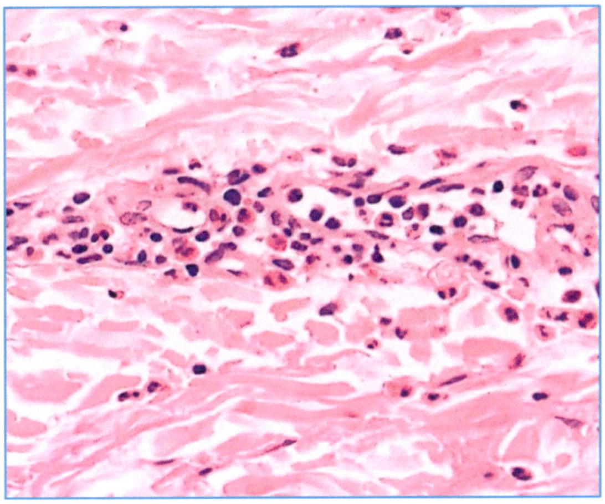

Intravascular neutrophils and perivascular dermal neutrophils and eosinophils

Inflammatory vascular disorders and mimickers

BEHÇET'S DISEASE

-multisystemic disease more common in Middle Eastern, Mediterranean, and Japanese population
-diagnosis is based on **one major** criteria: recurrent oral aphthae, and **two minor** criteria: recurrent genital aphthae, posterior uveitis, skin lesions

Aphthae

-presents as punched out ulcer with red rim, overhanging border, and necrotic base

Skin lesions are variable:

-most commonly facial/acral papules, pustules, and purpura ("LCV-like" changes)
-less commonly "erythema nodosum-like" lesions, "Sweet's syndrome-like" lesions, or "pyoderma gangrenosum-like" ulcer

Histopathology

-non-specific findings

Aphthae

-**mucosal ulcer** with mixed lymphohistiocytic and neutrophilic infiltrate

Cutaneous lesions

-ulcerated skin with mixed inflammation and **necrotizing LCV**

CRYOGLOBULINEMIA

-group of vasculitis and vasculopathic conditions due to immunoglobulins precipitated at cold temperature

Type I

-monoclonal (typically IgM) which cause vascular occlusion and vasculopathy
-Raynaud's phenomenon, cold induced acrocyanosis
-purpura, livedo reticularis, and ulceration
-presents in setting of underlying leukemia, lymphoma, or multiple myeloma

Type II and III (account for 80% of cases)

-monoclonal (type II) or polyclonal (type III) antibody complex that results in vasculitis
-present as palpable purpura and urticarial lesions after cold exposure
-systemic findings are common (arthralgia, myalgia, glomerulonephritis)
-associated with connective tissue diseases and hepatitis C infection

Histopathology

Type I: dermal **capillaries filled with homogeneous, eosinophilic material** (PAS+)

Type II and **III**: indistinguishable from other forms of **leukocytoclastic vasculitis**

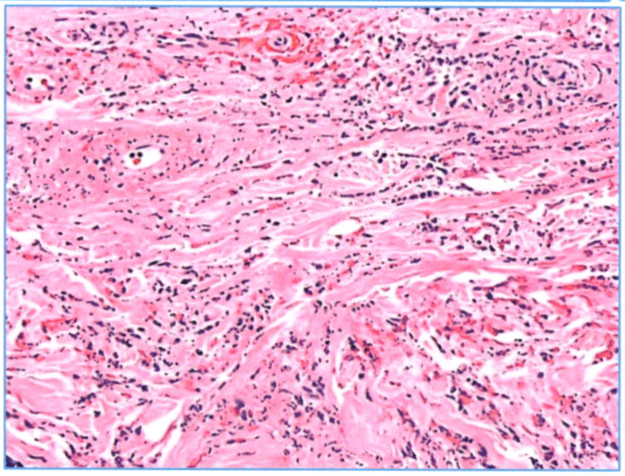
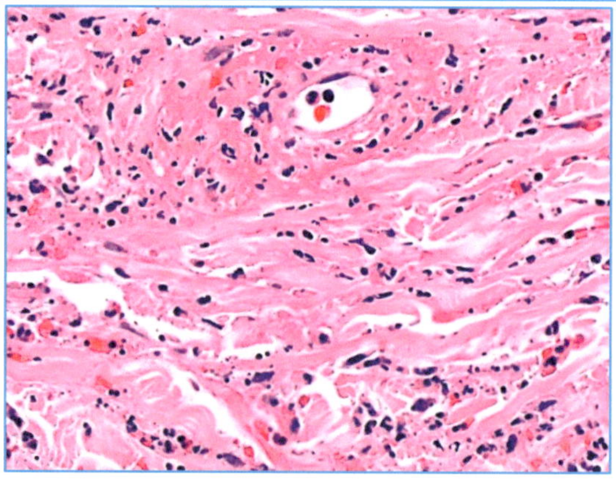

Behçet's disease with vascular fibrinoid necrosis, neutrophilic inflammation, nuclear dust, and RBC extravasation

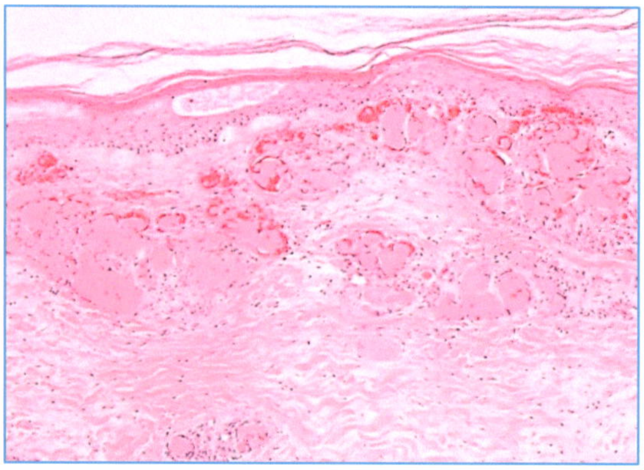
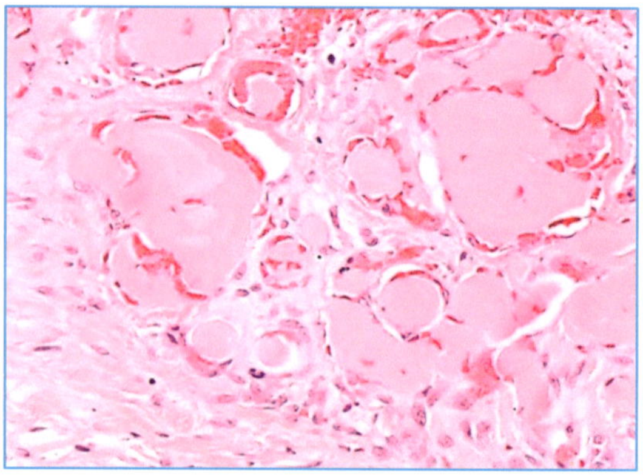

Cryoglobulinemia, type I, with dermal capillaries filled with homogenous, pink material and no inflammation

MICROSCOPIC POLYARTERITIS NODOSA

-rare ANCA+ small-medium vessels vasculitis
-favors elderly men and starts with flu-like prodromes with systemic symptoms (fever, weight loss, myalgia)
-majority of patients have systemic involvement including renal (focal segmental necrotizing glomerulonephritis), pulmonary (alveolar hemorrhage), and neurological (mononeuritis multiplex)
-cutaneous lesions seen in only 30-50% of patients, presenting as pulpable purpura, livedo reticularis, or ulcerations
-serum p-ANCA+ in 60% and c-ANCA in 30% of patients

Histopathology
-**presents as dermal leukocytoclastic vasculitis**
-nuclear dust, fibrinoid depositions in vessels and red blood cell extravasation
-no granulomas unlike in eosinophilic granulomatosis with polyangiitis
-**small to medium-sized vessels in deeper dermis are inflamed**

SOLAR PURPURA (ACTINIC PURPURA)

-easy bruising on the hands and arms of elderly patients due to blood vessels' fragility from aging/sun damage
-purple brown ecchymotic patches ("bruise-like") in the background of sun damaged skin

Histopathology
-atrophic epidermis with exuberant dermal **solar elastosis**
-extensive dermal and subcutaneous **red blood cell extravasation**
-no dermal inflammation

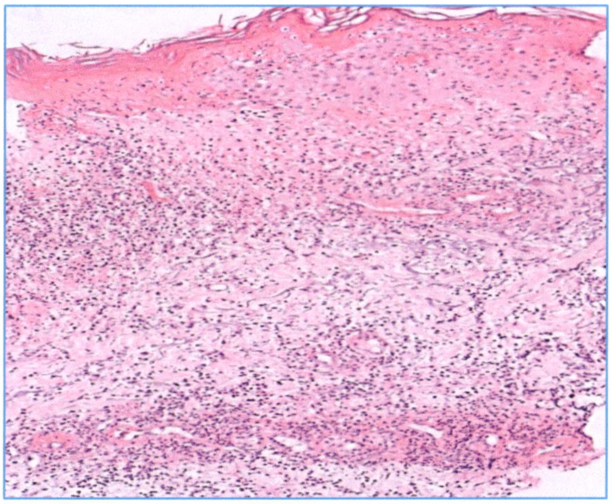

MPN with dermal leukocytoclastic vasculitis

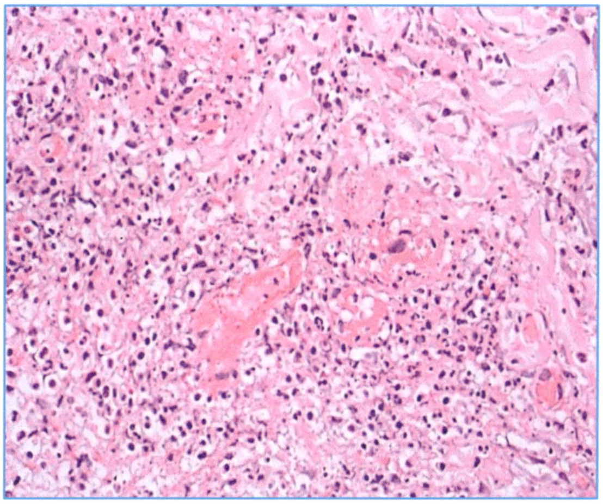

MPN with inflamed medium-sized vessel in deeper dermis

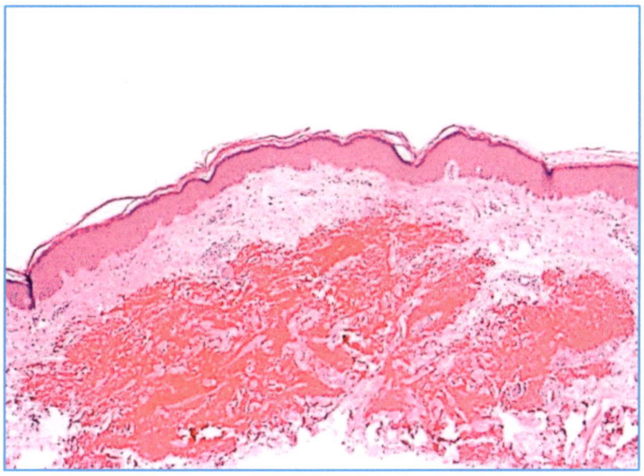

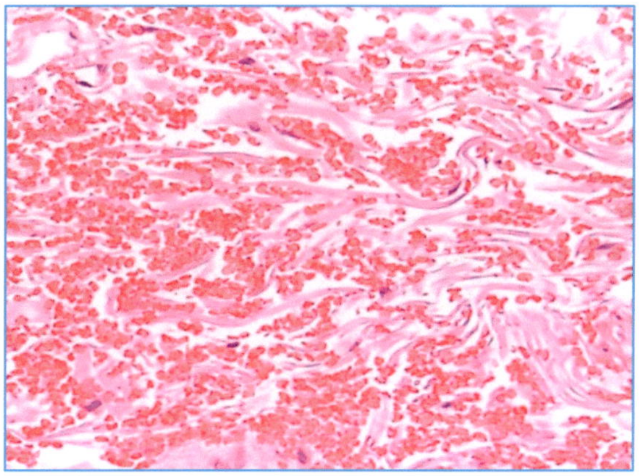

Solar purpura with extensive solar elastosis and red blood cell extravasation

Inflammatory vascular disorders and mimickers

EOSINOPHILIC GRANULOMATOSIS WITH POLYANGIITIS (CHURG-STRAUSS SYNDROME)

-systemic p-ANCA+ small-medium vessel vasculitis and hypereosinophilia
-stage 1: asthma, nasal polyps, allergic rhinitis
-stage 2: pneumonia and gastroenteritis with minimal renal involvement unlike GPA and MPA
-stage 3: systemic necrotizing vasculitis that can involve any organ
-2/3rd of patients will have skin lesions
-pulpable purpura and painful subcutaneous nodules on the extensor surfaces of the extremities and the scalp
-commonly serum p-ANCA+ with eosinophilia

Histopathology

-**leukocytoclastic vasculitis with eosinophils**
-dermal and subcutaneous granulomas **"red granulomas"** may be present
-granulomas are made of central degenerated collagen surrounded by neutrophils, histiocytes and some eosinophils

GRANULOMATOSIS WITH POLYANGIITIS (WEGENER'S GRANULOMATOSIS)

-systemic idiopathic c-ANCA mediated small to medium vessels vasculitis
-characterized by necrotizing granulomas of the respiratory tract, focal necrotizing glomerulonephritis, and peripheral neuropathy
-30-50% of patients have cutaneous lesions
-classically presents with palpable purpura and nodules in dependent areas that ulcerate, resembling pyoderma gangrenosum
-characteristic gingival hyperplasia ("strawberry gums"), mucosal ulceration, and "saddle nose"
-commonly serum c-ANCA positive

Histopathology

-majority of biopsies demonstrate **nonspecific leukocytoclastic vasculitis**
-about 20% of cases will also have subtle **necrotizing granuloma** (usually **in nasal mucosa**)

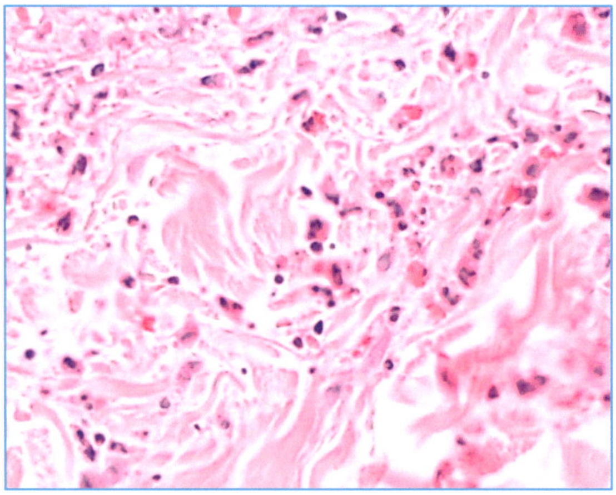

EGPA with leukocytoclastic vasculitis and dermal eosinophils

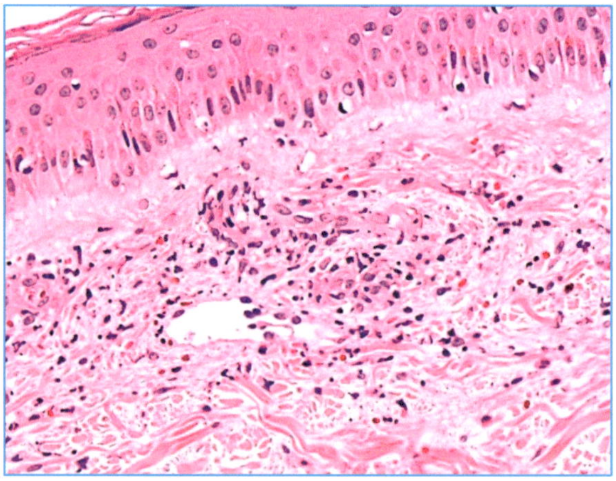

GPA with non-specific leukocytoclastic vasculitis

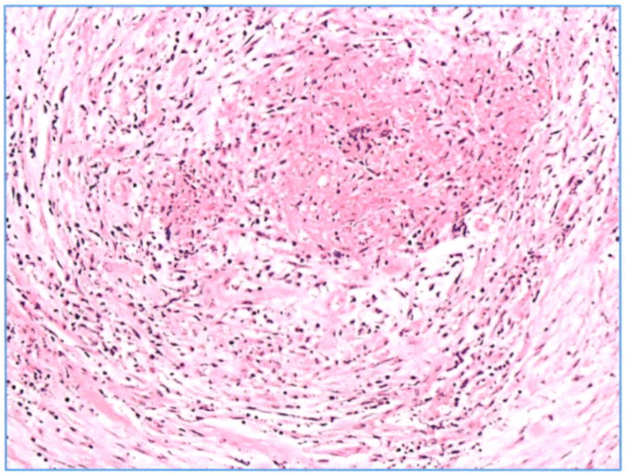

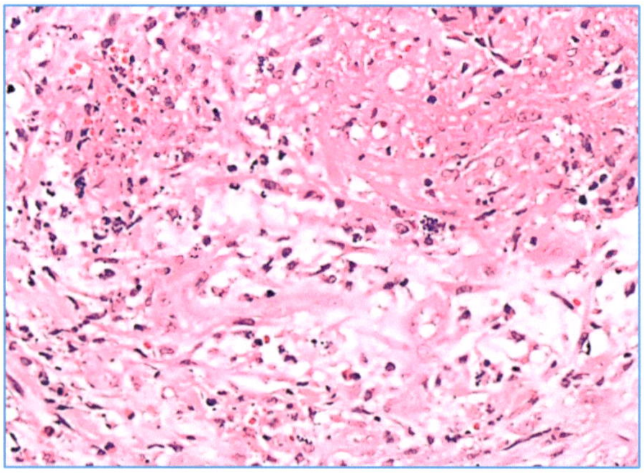

EGPA with characteristic "red granulomas"

LIVEDOID VASCULOPATHY (ATROPHIE BLANCHE)

-reticulated purpuric papules and plaques that progress to small painful ulcers
-ulcers heal with "porcelain white scar" (atrophie blanche) and surface telangiectasias
-seen in middle-aged and elderly women on the lower legs
-typically worse in summer
-associated with autoimmune diseases and hypercoagulability

Histopathology

-**epidermis gets atrophic and necrotic** as lesion progress
-fibrinoid material in the wall of dermal vessels **"pink-red crayons"**
-**microthrombi** are present in the lumen
-variable dermal lymphocytic inflammation
-extravasated RBCs
-older lesions show prominent scarring with hyalinized blood vessels

LIVEDO RETICULARIS

-mottled arborizing bluish (livid) discoloration due to vasospasm and decreased blood flow to and within skin
-forms symmetric "net-like" pattern on the arms, legs, and/or buttock
-idiopathic or secondary to vasculitis
-worsens with cold which exacerbates vasospasm

Histopathology

-very subtle changes
-thickened capillaries with **prominent endothelial cells**
-occasional microthrombi
-minimal perivascular lymphocytic inflammation

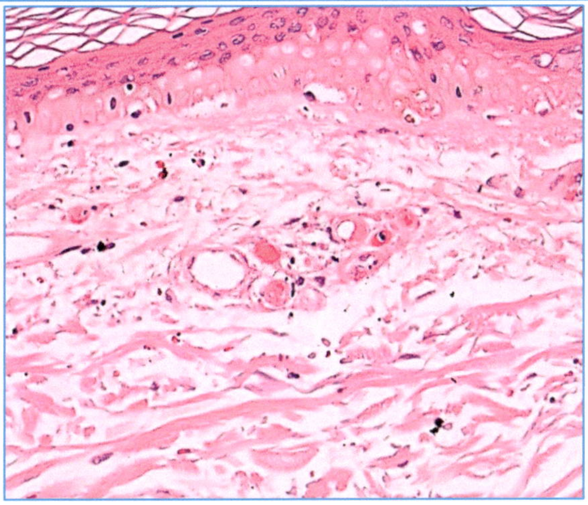

Livedoid vasculopathy with partially necrotic epidermis

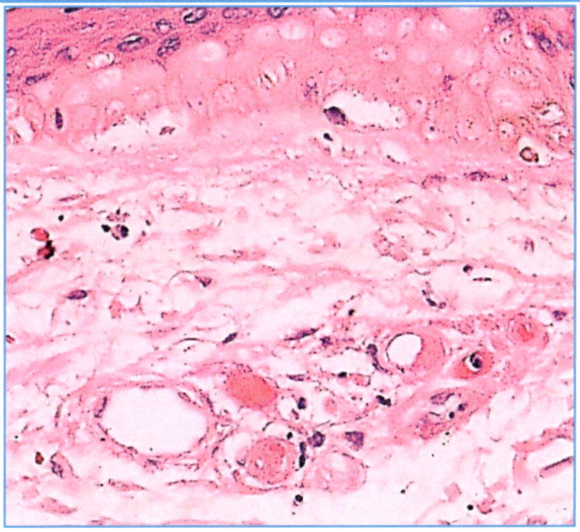

Microthrombi and fibrinoid material in vessel's wall

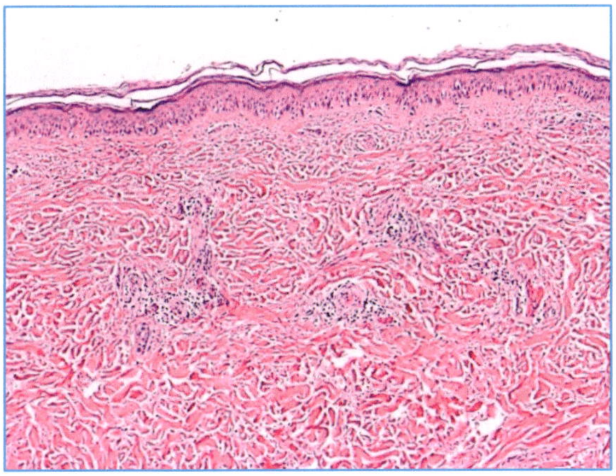

Livedo reticularis with subtle dermal changes

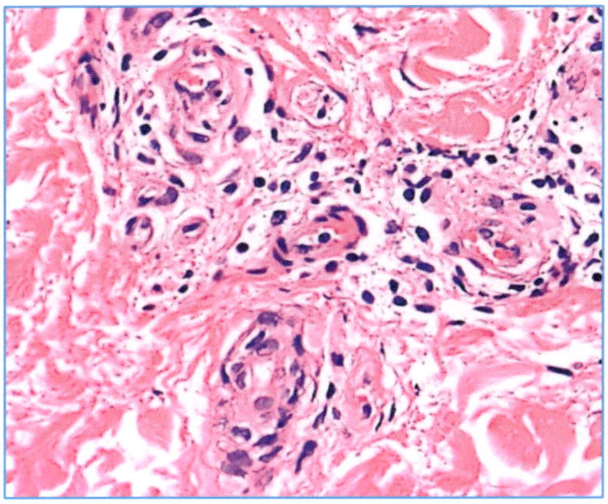

Capillaries with prominent endothelial cells

VASCULOPATHIES

-conditions in which small blood vessels become occluded
-it includes several different entities
-all entities have similar clinical pattern with "net-like" (reticulate) pattern of livedo reticularis or retiform purpura

Idiopathic thrombocytopenic purpura (ITP)
-immune mediated thrombocytopenia with antiplatelet antibodies
-occasionally forerunner of SLE
-patients do not appear sick

Thrombotic thrombocytopenic purpura (TTP)
-deficiency of *ADAMTS16* activity (congenital or idiopathic with autoantibodies)
-hemolytic anemia, neurologic, and renal symptoms are common

Hemolytic uremic syndrome (HUS)
-was considered a type of TTP but is now separate
-triggered by infection and caused by endothelial damage by a bacterial toxin and subsequent complement activation
-mostly in children and causes acute renal failure
-most common cause of renal transplant in children

Disseminated intravascular coagulation (DIC)
-life-threatening, widespread intravascular coagulation in setting of severe inflammatory response/infection

Protein C or S deficiency
-genetic or idiopathic deficiency in coagulation cascade resulting in hypercoagulable state

DIC, protein C or S deficiency, and infectious vasculopathy can progress into purpura fulminans

Purpura fulminans
-rapidly progressing, often fatal disease
-characterized by sudden onset of large ecchymotic areas progressing to necrosis on the extremities

Histopathology
-**vascular occlusion** and damage with **variable inflammation**
-endothelial cells are plump and reactive
-**thrombi** present in dermal small vessels
-**red blood cell extravasation** is variably present
-**in purpura fulminans, neutrophils and necrosis are additionally seen**

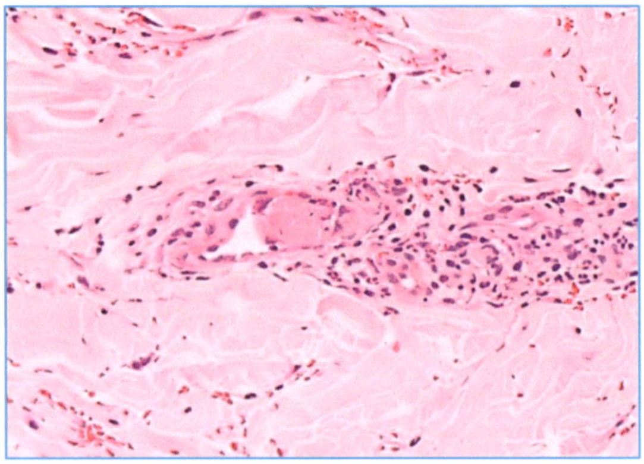

ITP with intravascular thrombi, scattered dermal RBCs, and few perivascular lymphocytes

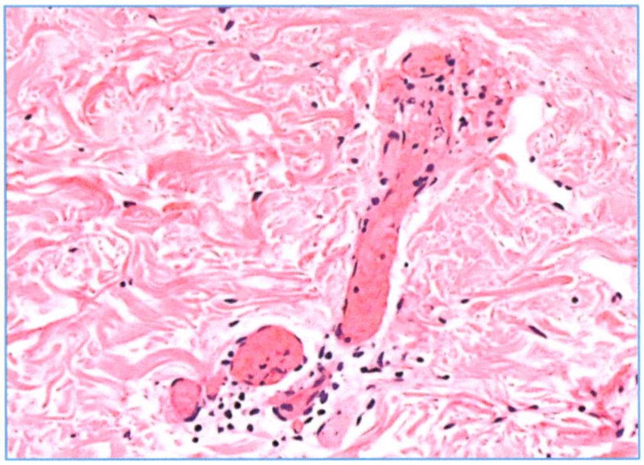

TTP with microthrombi and minimal inflammation

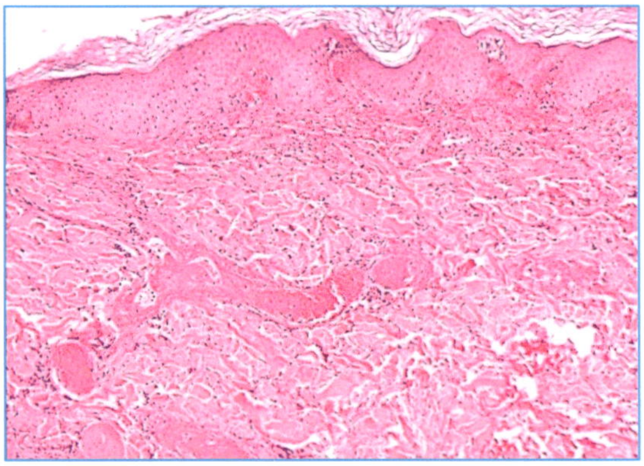

Purpura fulminans with extensive capillary thrombosis

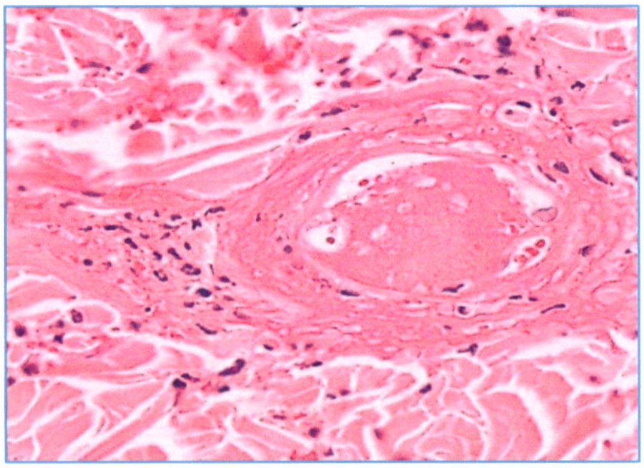

Purpura fulminans with vascular necrosis, neutrophils, and red blood cell extravasation

PIGMENTED PURPURIC DERMATOSES

-group of disorders characterized by inflammation of dermal capillaries and subsequent extravasation of erythrocytes into surrounding tissue
-overlapping clinical presentation and histomorphology
-presents as purpuric lesions with variable hyperpigmentation and predilection for the lower extremities

Schamberg's disease (progressive pigmentary dermatosis)
-the most common variant
-chronic, asymptomatic, red-brown macules/patches made of tiny petechiae ("cayenne pepper" spots)
-usually on lower legs of older adults

Majocchi's disease (purpura annularis telangiectodes of Majocchi)
-1-3 cm annular patches with telangiectasias and petechiae
-peripheral extension with central involution forming "target-like" lesions
-classically on lower leg or trunk of women

Lichenoid dermatitis of Gougerot-Blum (pigmented purpuric lichenoid dermatosis)
-presentation and distribution is similar to Schamberg's disease but with superimposed lichenoid papules
-lesions have darker color and are indurated, unlike Schamberg's disease

Eczematid-like purpura of Doucas and Kapetanakis
-presentation and distribution is similar to Schamberg's disease but with scaly eczematous appearance
-short-lived itching purpura (unlike Schamberg's disease)

Lichen aureus
-solitary patch rust-colored patch
-may occur on any part of body but more common on the feet and lower legs

Histopathology

Schamberg's disease
-normal epidermis with **perivascular lymphocytic infiltrate**
-dermal red blood cell extravasation
-dermal hemosiderin depositions in older lesions

Majocchi's disease
-similar histopathology as Schamberg's disease with additional **telangiectasias**

Lichenoid dermatitis of Gougerot-Blum
-similar histopathology as Schamberg's disease but lymphocytic inflammation is denser and **lichenoid** ("band like")

Eczematid-like purpura of Doucas and Kapetanakis
-similar to Schamberg's disease but with more **epidermal spongiosis**

Lichen aureus
-similar histopathology **as lichenoid dermatitis of Gougerot-Blum**
-separate based on clinical presentation

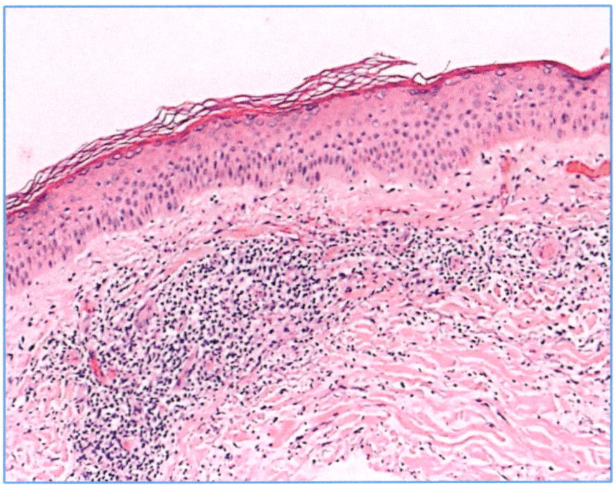

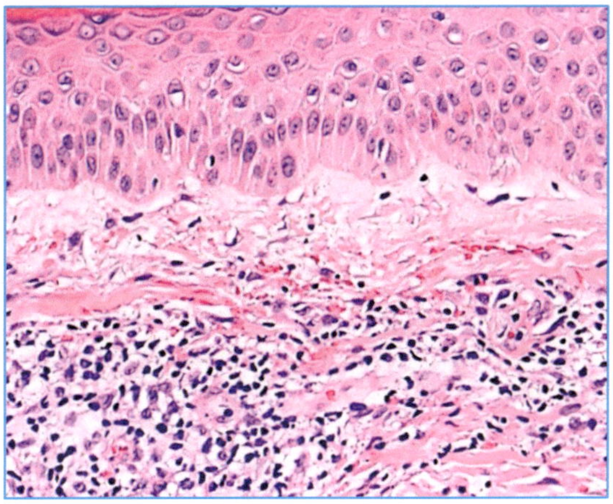

Schamberg's disease with perivascular lymphocytes and dermal red blood cells

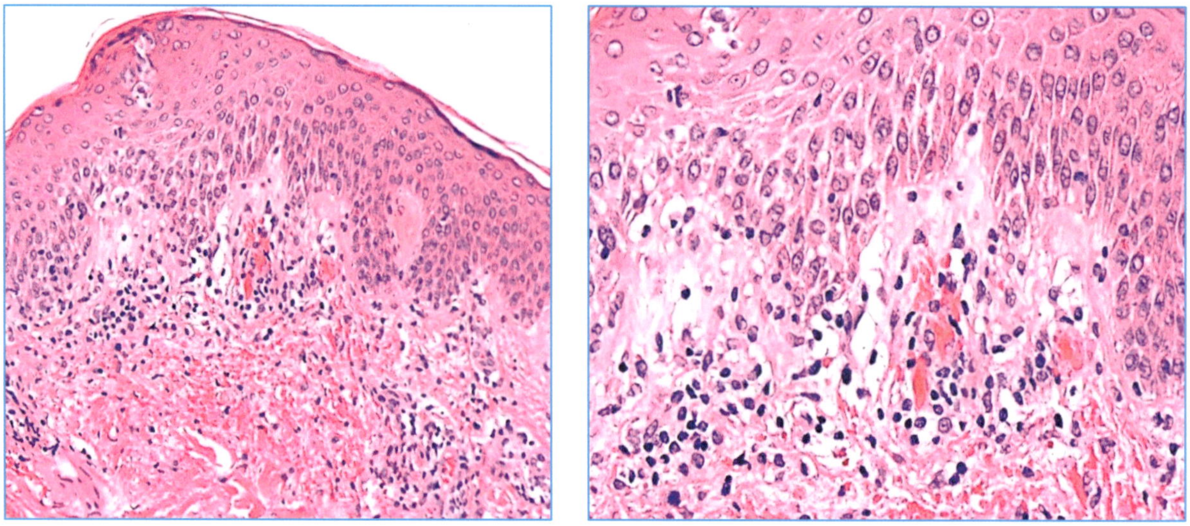

Eczematid-like purpura of Doucas and Kapetanakis with epidermal spongiosis

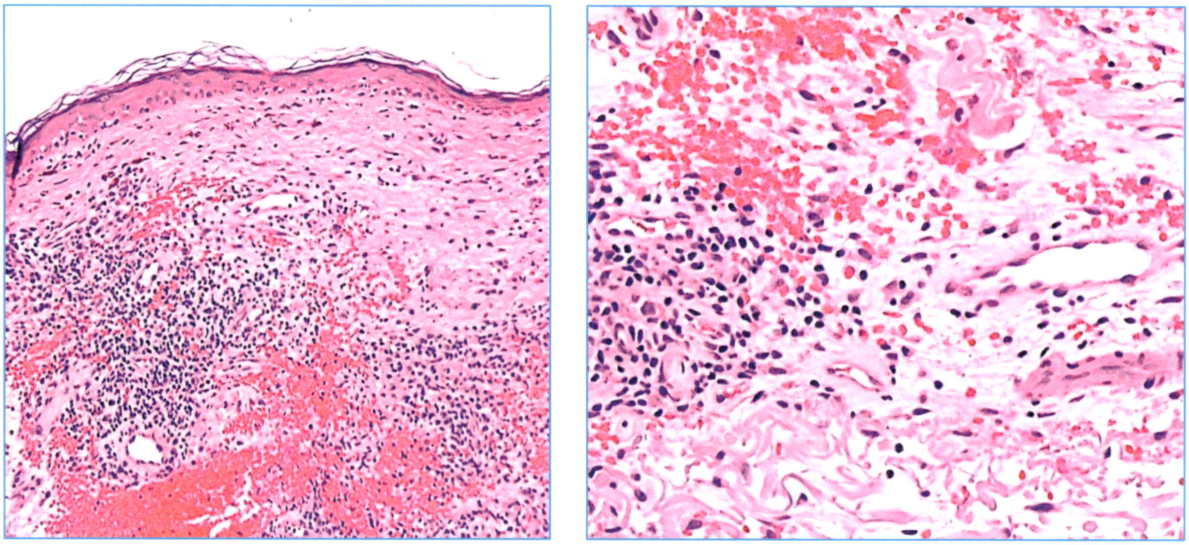

Majocchi's disease with dermal telangiectasias

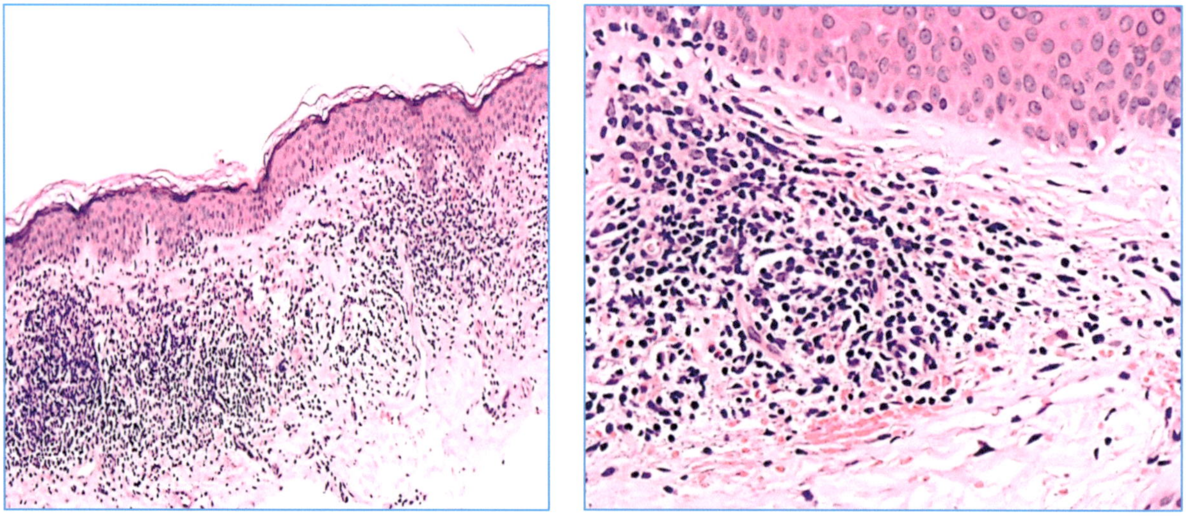

Lichen aureus with "band-like" lymphocytic inflammation

DEGOS DISEASE (MALIGNANT ATROPHIC PAPULOSIS)

-rare condition characterized by crops of pinkish papules on the trunk that develop atrophic, porcelain-white centers
-lesions heal with scarring (similar to atrophie blanche)
-potentially fatal but many have a long benign course
-more common in men
-associated with ischemic infarcts of the gastrointestinal system

Histopathology
-vascular endothelial swelling with fibrin **micro thrombi** and increased dermal **mucin** in early lesions
-**V-shaped dermal ischemia** with necrosis and edema in older lesions

POLYARTERITIS NODOSA

-systemic vasculitis of **medium-sized vessels**
-**generalized form** (more common in middle aged men) is a multi-system vasculitis involving the kidneys, liver, heart, adrenals, and joints and 50% have skin lesions
-**cutaneous form** (at any age) has no or limited systemic symptoms
-presents with painful subcutaneous nodules on the lower extremities, livedo reticularis, pulpable purpura, or digital infarction
-nodules may ulcerate and heal with scarring
-associated with multiple triggers including infection (Hep B, Hep C, Strep), autoimmune diseases (IBD, SLE) and malignancy (hairy cell leukemia)
-common systemic symptoms including weight loss and fever

Histopathology
-**necrotizing vasculitis of medium-sized arteries** in deeper dermis and subcutis (frequently cause microaneurysms seen on angiography)
-destruction of vessel wall with **neutrophilic infiltrate in the vessel wall** and around it
-**fibrinoid deposition in the vessel wall** with variable thrombi
-no involvement of fat lobules

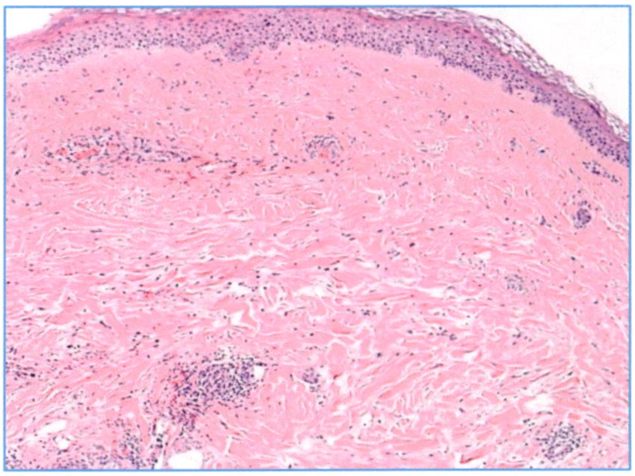

Degos disease with V-shaped ischemia

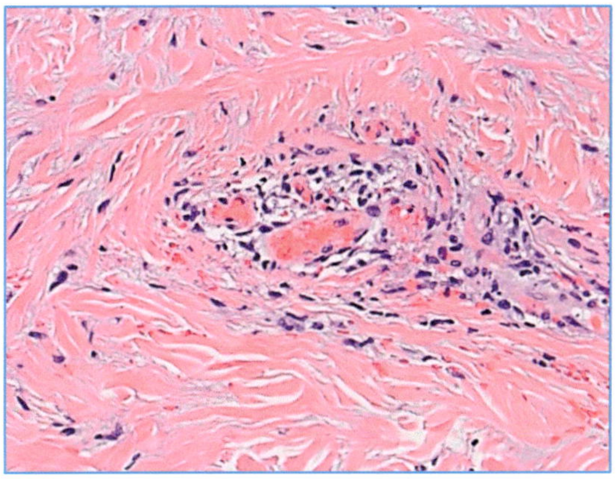

Degos disease with microthrombi and dermal mucin

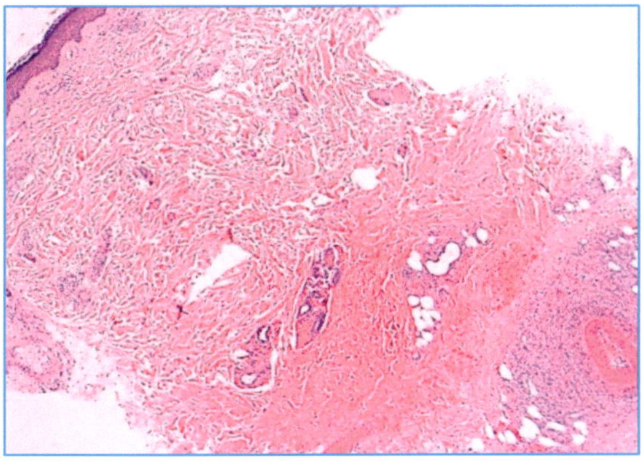

PN with vasculitis in subcutis

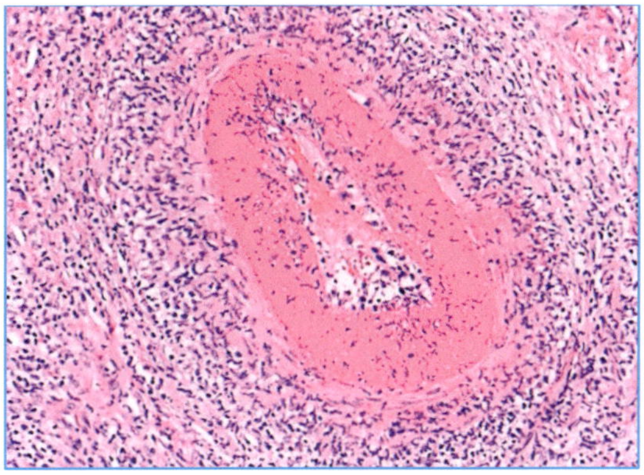

PN with fibrinoid deposition and inflammation of medium-sized artery

Inflammatory vascular disorders and mimickers

TAKAYASU'S ARTERITIS

-large vessel vasculitis of the aorta and its main branches
-favors young Asian women
-causes occlusions of large vessels
-associated skin lesions are seen in half of patients, but are not specific (purpura, "erythema nodosum-like" nodules, or "pyoderma gangrenosum-like" ulcers)

Histopathology

-**large vessel vasculitis** with full thickness vessel necrosis, mixed inflammation and intravascular thrombus
-**never seen in dermatopathology** due to nature of vessels involved (aorta and main branches)
-cutaneous lesions are non-pathognomonic ("pyoderma gangrenosum-like" ulcer or mixed panniculitis)

TEMPORAL ARTERITIS (GIANT CELL ARTERITIS)

-granulomatous vasculitis of large-sized arteries in elderly individuals
-predilection for temporal and ophthalmic arteries with characteristic loss of temporal pulse
-patients experience headache and visual and neurological disturbances
-cutaneous manifestations are uncommon; most frequent are erythema and edema of overlying skin with necrosis and ulceration

Histopathology

-transmural lymphohistiocytic inflammation (sometimes granulomatous) of **medium/large-sized vessels**
-destruction of the internal elastic lamina
-common thrombus formation
-giant cells are usually present but not mandatory for diagnosis
-in late stages there is less inflammation and more fibrosis
-**never seen in dermatopathology** due to deep nature of vessel involved (temporal artery)

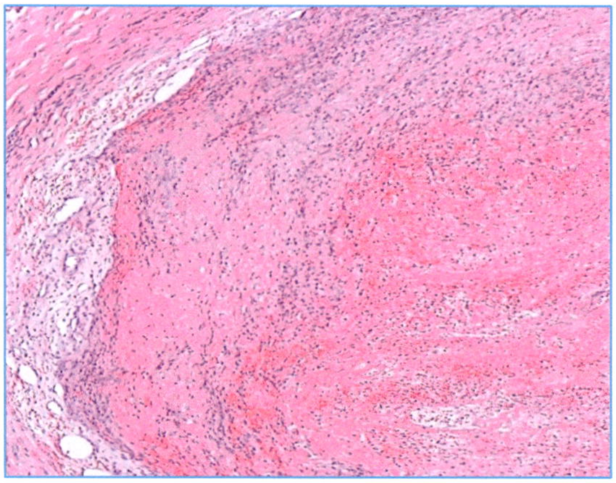

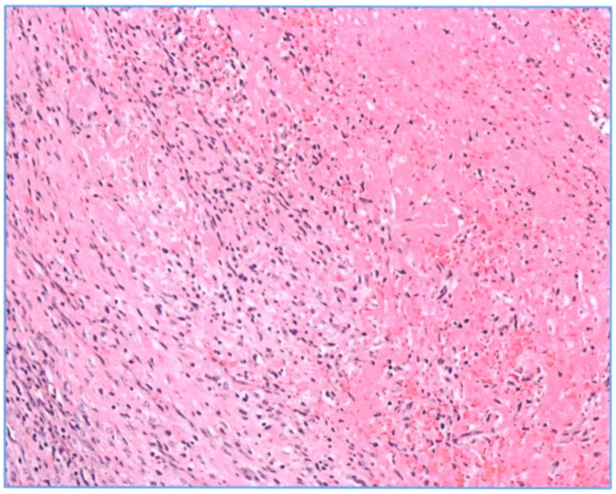

Takayasu's arteritis with full thickness necrosis of vessel wall and intravascular thrombus

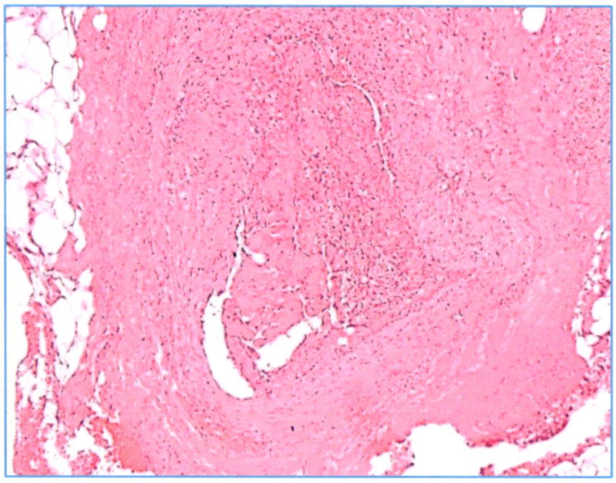

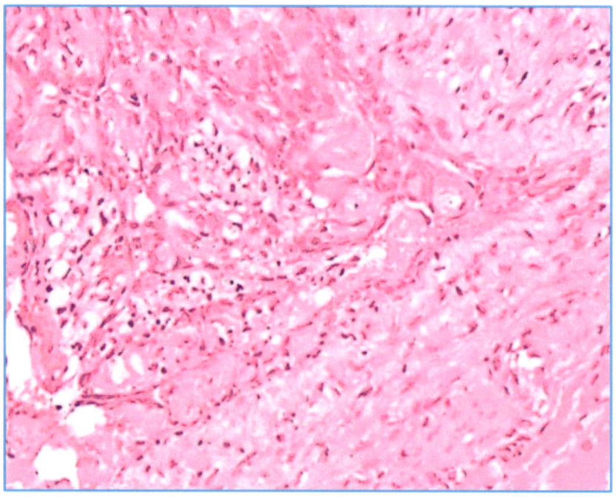

Temporal arteritis with transmural lymphohistiocytic inflammation and few giant cells

Chapter 11

THROMBOANGIITIS OBLITERANS (BUERGER'S DISEASE)

-recurring progressive inflammatory vascular disease with ischemic symptoms
-strongly associated with smoking
-usually in middle-aged men
-thrombosis of **arteries** (unfrequently veins) at periphery of extremities
-results in cutaneous ischemia, ulceration, and gangrene

Histopathology

-**thrombosis** of medium and large sized **arteries** and sometimes veins
-**microabscess** formation within thrombi
-attempt at thrombus recanalization can be seen
-mixed inflammatory response (some giant cells can be present) in vessel wall

THROMBOPHLEBITIS

-inflammation and thrombosis of the veins of the lower extremities or chest wall (Mondor's disease)
-firm, tender "cord-like" induration of the skin over a superficial vein
-associated with varicose veins, pregnancy, Behçet's disease, Buerger's disease, and cancer

Histopathology

-**organizing thrombus** in subcutaneous medium to large-sized **veins**
-in early lesions, there is a thrombus with a neutrophilic infiltrate present in the vessel wall
-in late lesions, there is an organizing thrombus (a blood clot that holds fibrous tissue that can be organized into layers)
-**lymphohistiocytic infiltrate** is present in the vessel wall

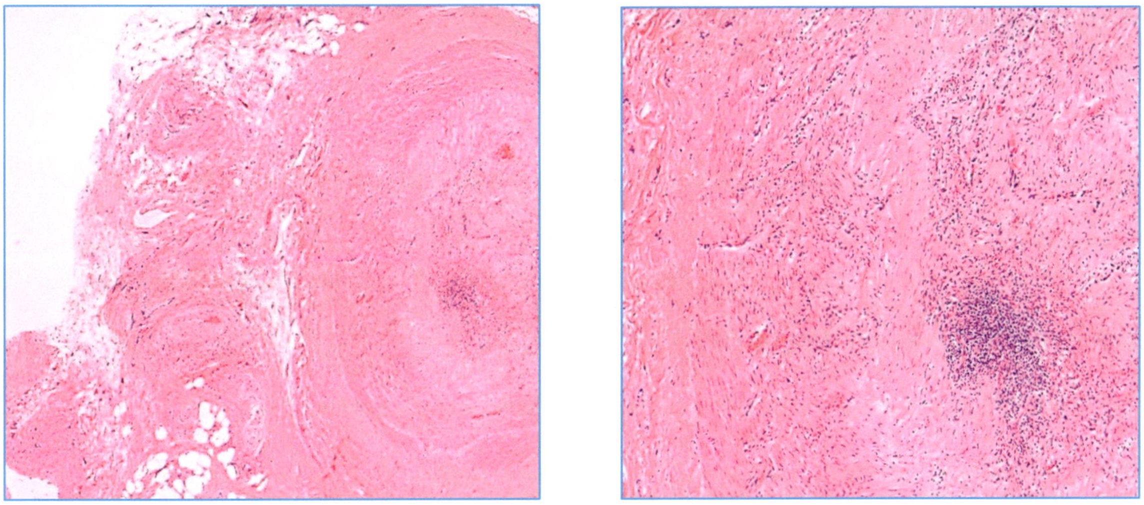

Thromboangiitis obliterans with arterial thrombus and microabscess within the thrombus

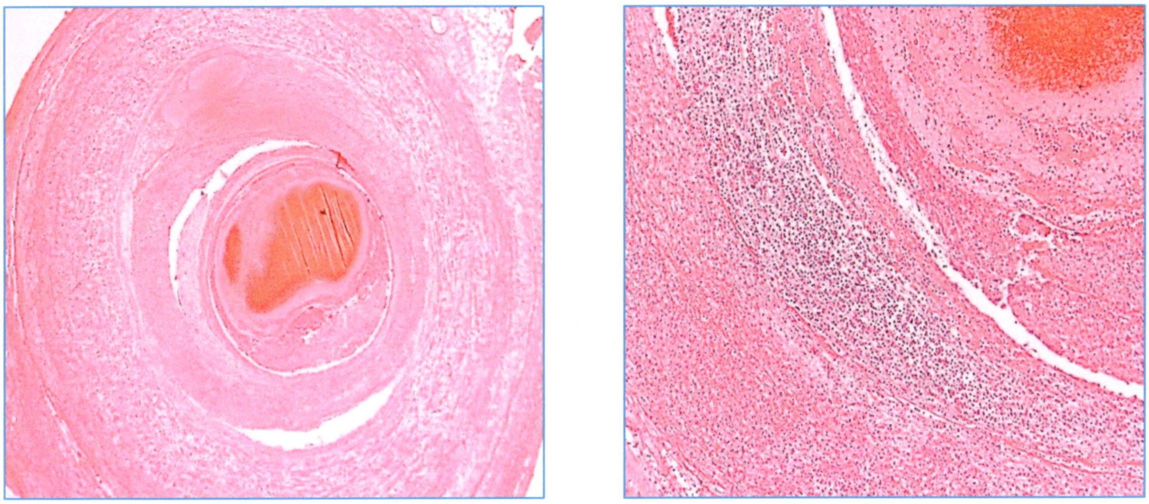

Thrombophlebitis with organized (layered) thrombus in vein and lymphocytic inflammation in the vessel wall

Inflammatory vascular disorders and mimickers

HOW TO APPROACH VASCULITIS AND MIMICKERS

VASCULITIS OF SMALL VESSELS (CAPILLARIES)

IF LEUKOCYTOCLASTIC VASCULITIS (LCV) IS PRESENT
(neutrophilic inflammation of dermal capillaries with broken neutrophils forming nuclear dust)
REMEMBER LEUKOCYTOCLASTIC VASCULITIS OF ALL CAUSES LOOK ALIKE

AGE AND HISTORY WILL HELP

CHILDREN

-Henoch-Schönlein purpura	2-8 years old	systemic symptoms (GI, renal)	DIF positive
-acute hemor. edema of infancy	<2years of age	no systemic symptoms	DIF negative
-meningococcemia	older children, adolescents		LCV with prominent vessel necrosis

ADULT

-Beçhet's disease	oral aphthae	
-cryoglobulinemia type II+III	cold induced	cryoglobulin in blood
-microscopic polyangiitis	kidney disease	serum p-ANCA > c-ANCA
-granul. with polyangiitis	respiratory and kidney disease	serum c-ANCA
-eosin. granul. with polyangiitis	asthma, rhinitis, no kidney disease	p-ANCA LCV with eosinophils
-erytema elevatum diutinum		LCV with plump capillaries

IF IT LOOKS LIKE LCV (neutrophils around capillaries) BUT THERE IS NO OR MINIMAL LEUKOCYTOCLASIA

-urticarial vasculitis intact neutrophils and eosinophils

Remember that urticarial vasculitis can also look like regular LCV

MIMICKERS OF CAPILLARY VASCULITIS

IF THROMBI ARE PRESENT IN CAPILLARIES WITH NO OR MINIMAL INFLAMMATION

-vasculopathies (TTP, ITP, DIC, protein C or S deficiency)				thrombi diffusely present
-livedo reticularis	mottled	not painful	worse in winter	thrombi focally present
-atrophie blanche	ulcer	painful	worse in summer	thrombi focally present
-Degos disease			V-shaped necrosis above deep thrombi	

IF ONLY LYMPHOCYTES AND RBCs ARE PRESENT AROUND DERMAL CAPILLARIES
-pigmented purpuric dermatoses

IF ONLY RED BLOOD CELL EXTRAVASATION IS SEEN IN DERMIS
-solar purpura solar elastosis

VASCULITIS OF MEDIUM SIZED VESSELS
-polyartheritis nodosa vessel wall is inflamed, necrotized with fibrinoid deposit in the wall

VASCULITIS OF LARGE VESSELS IN SUBCUTIS

-Takayasu arteritis	affects aorta and its branches with thrombus formation
-temporal arteritis	affects temporal and ophthalmic artery with thrombus formation
-thromboangiitis obliterans	affects arteries of lower legs with thrombus formation
-thrombophlebitis	affects veins of lower legs with thrombus formation

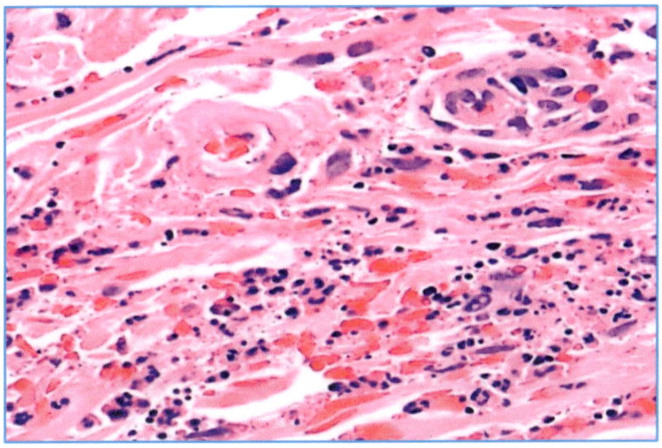

LCV with perivascular neutrophils, nuclear dust, and RBCs

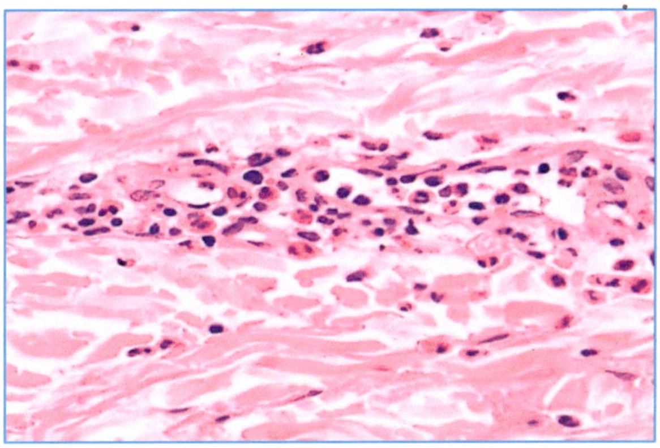

Urticarial vasculitis with intact neutrophils in the vessels and numerous eosinophils

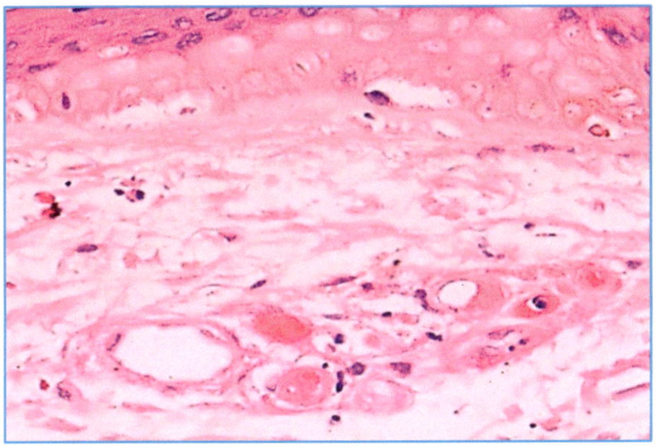

Atrophie blanche with epidermal necrosis and microthrombi

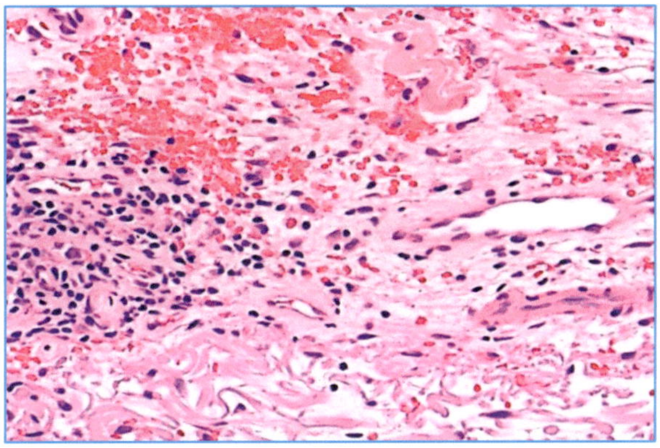

Pigmented purpura with perivascular lymphocytes and RBCs

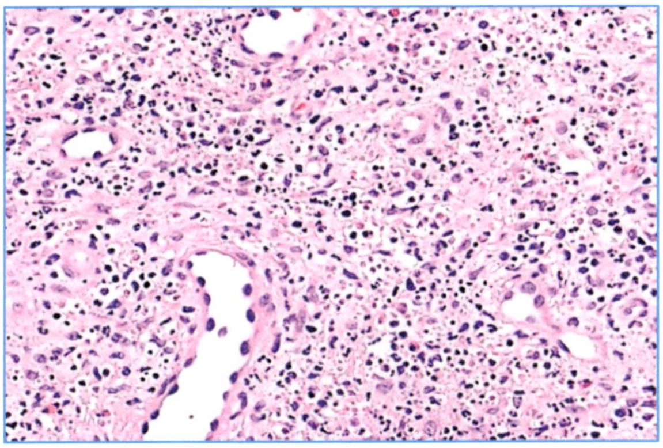

EED with LCV changes and prominent endothelial cells

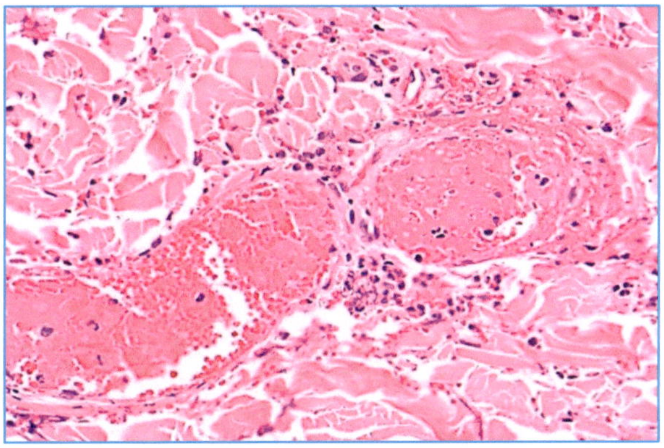

Vasculopathy with numerous thrombi and minimal inflammation

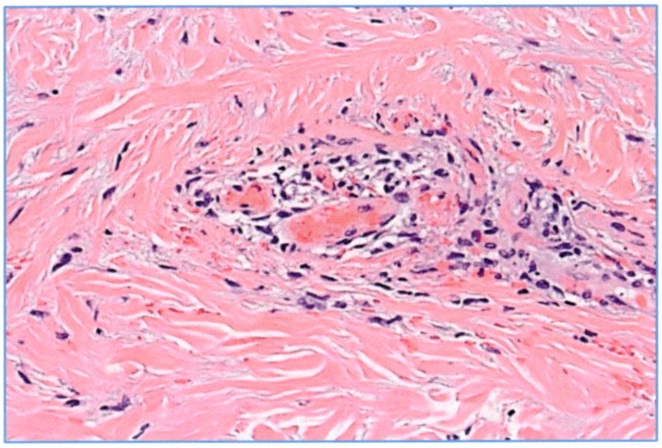

Degos disease with microthrombi in deep vessels and increased dermal mucin

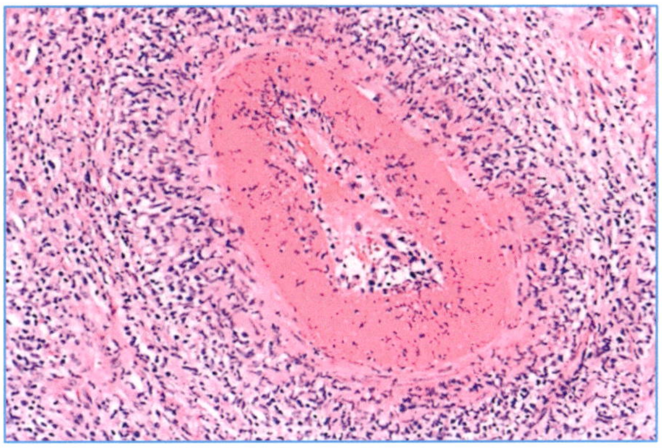

Polyarteritis nodosa with fibrinoid necrosis of medium-sized vessel

Inflammatory vascular disorders and mimickers

Chapter 12

PANNICULITIS

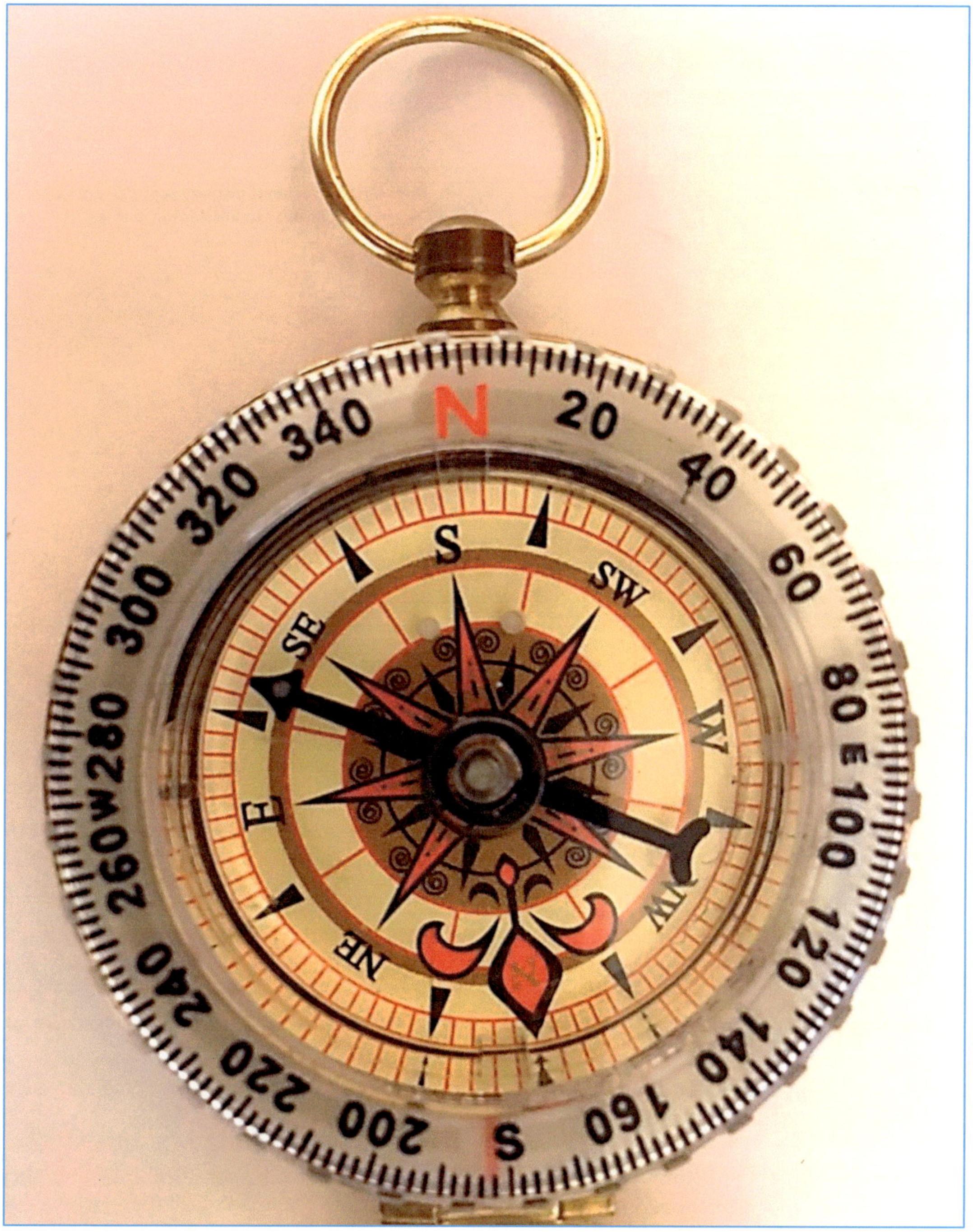

Panniculitis

ERYTHEMA NODOSUM

-**most common panniculitis**
-more common in **women**
-usually idiopathic but can be associated with multiple triggers: infection (*Strep,* tuberculosis) drugs (estrogen, sulfonamides, NSAIDs), and inflammatory/autoimmune conditions (sarcoidosis, inflammatory bowel disease)
-presents as painful, tender, deep-seated nodule(s) **on the shin**
-overlying erythema but **no ulceration**

Histopathology
-prototypic **septal panniculitis**
-presentation varies with the age of the lesion
-early lesions (usually never biopsied) show septal edema and mixed inflammation with neutrophils
-established lesions show **widened, fibrotic septa containing** lymphocytes, histiocytes, and giant cells
-characteristic **Miescher's granulomas** made of a cluster of histiocytes and giant cells around small vessels or "slit-like" spaces
-eosinophils are frequently seen
-eventually, there is spillover of inflammation into lobular fat causing a mixed panniculitis

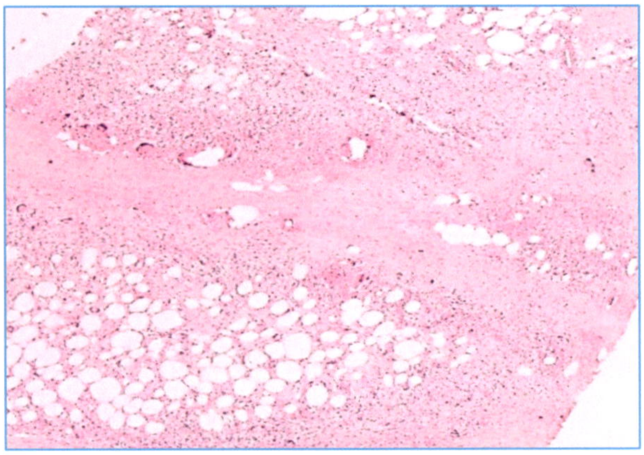

Erythema nodosum is primary septal panniculitis that spills over to lobules in older lesions

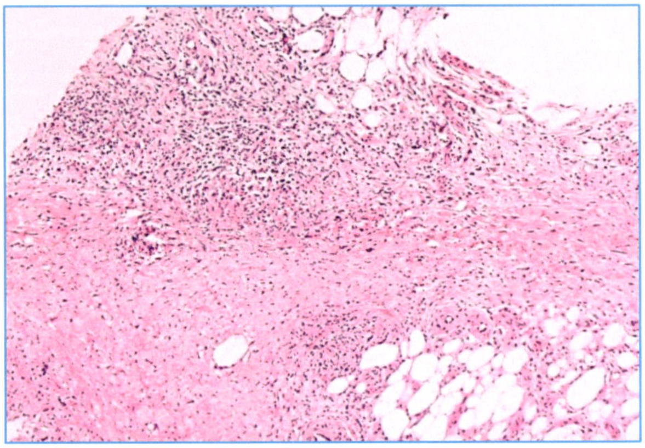

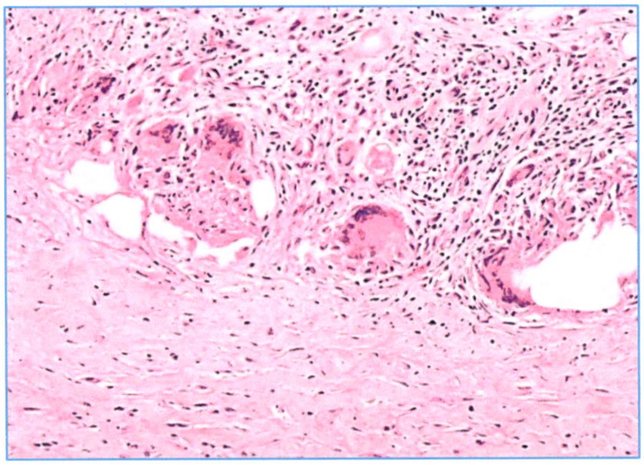

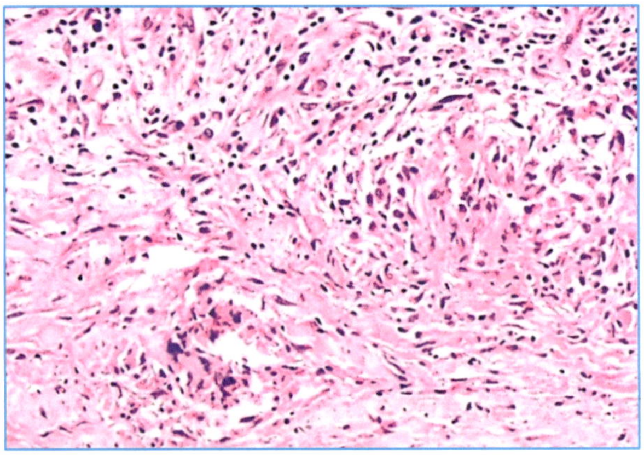

Erythema nodosum with widened, fibrotic septa and aggregates of histiocytes and giant cells forming Miescher's granulomas

Note: Do not confuse erythema nodosum with ERYTHEMA NODOSUM LEPROSUM

-it is type 2 leprosy treatment reaction
-erythematous nodules appear on previously unaffected skin
-mixed inflammation of deep dermis and subcutis with foamy histiocytes
-perineural inflammation is characteristic
-see the bacterial chapter for detailed description

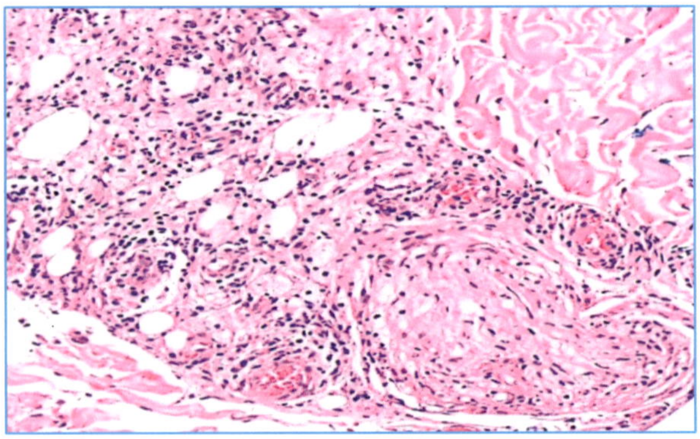

Erythema nodosum leprosum

PANCREATIC PANNICULITIS

-in patients with acute panniculitis or less commonly, pancreatic carcinoma
-pancreatic enzymes hydrolyze fat
-erythematous tender nodules that may ulcerate and release **oily discharge**
-**lower extremities** are favored site
-**clinically mimic erythema nodosum** (but EN does not ulcerate)

Histopathology
-**lobular panniculitis** with enzymatic fat necrosis
-**"saponification"** (blue gray calcifications of necrotic adipose tissue) with fat **"ghost" cells**
-**neutrophils** are usually present surrounding the saponified area

TRAUMATIC FAT NECROSIS

-follows trauma that is many times not remembered
-predilection for breast and thigh (e.g. **equestrian panniculitis** on lateral thighs)
-some cases are factitious in nature

Histopathology
-**necrotic fat** surrounded by lymphocytes, foamy macrophages, and often giant cells
-**adipocytes vary in size**
-necrotic degeneration of adipose tissue results in **fat microcysts**
-red blood extravasation and hemosiderin can be present
-fibrosis and dystrophic **calcification common** in long standing lesions

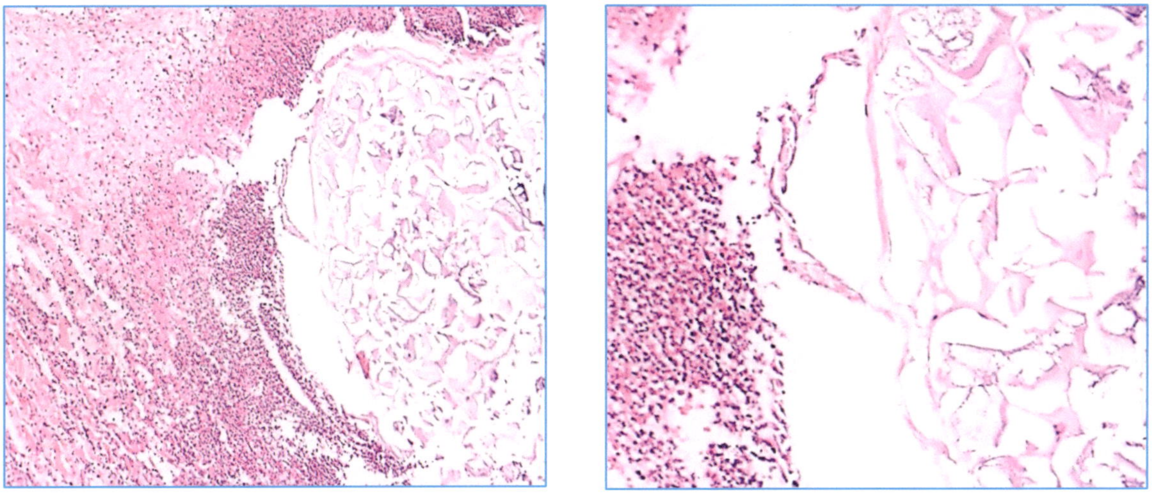

Pancreatic panniculitis with neutrophils on the left side and saponification with "ghost" cells on the right side of the image

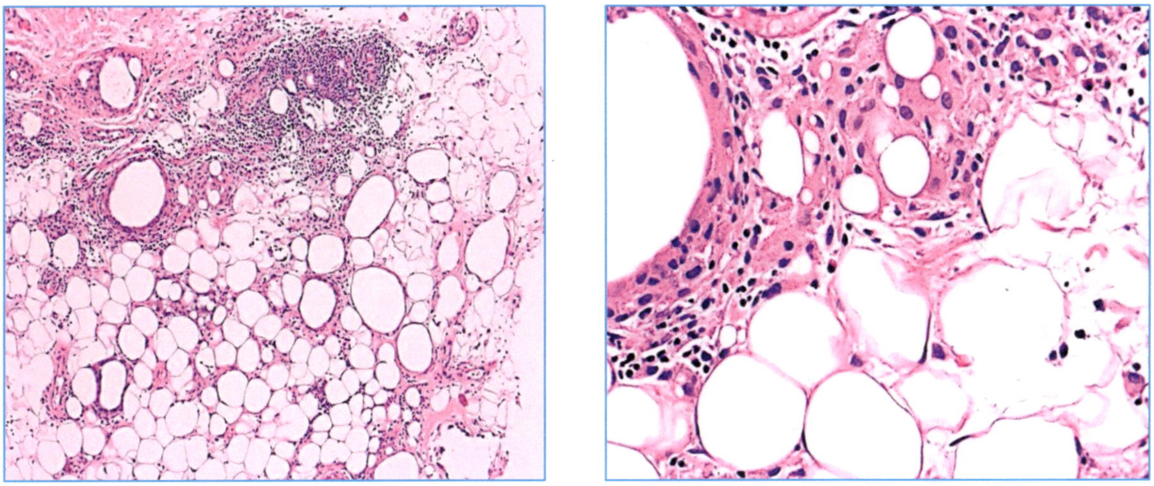

Traumatic fat necrosis with adipocytes of variable size, fat microcysts, and inflammation

Panniculitis

EOSINOPHILIC FASCIITIS (SHULMAN SYNDROME)

-classically presents in a middle-aged female with recent history of strenuous physical activity
-associated with eosinophilia, hypergammaglobulinemia, and arthralgia
-rapidly developing symmetrical edema and induration of forearms and legs
-eventually result in woody fibrosis
-spares hands and feet
-Raynaud's phenomenon is not present (unlike scleroderma)
-responds well to corticosteroid (unlike morphea profunda)

Histopathology
-thickening and **sclerosis of subcutis and fascia**
-variable number of lymphocytes and plasma cells with **scattered eosinophils**
-in more extensive cases, fibrosis extends into dermis

EOSINOPHILIC PANNICULITIS

-reactive process associated with drug reaction, insect bite, atopy, lymphomas, or infections (*Boreliosis*, parasites)
-presents as single or multiple deep nodules
-commonly associated with vesicles and pustules (in cases of insect bite)

Histopathology
-**mixed** lobular and septal **panniculitis**
-**numerous eosinophils** and occasional **"flame" figures** (degranulated eosinophils attached to collagen bundles)
-minimal fat necrosis
-no fibrosis (unlike eosinophilic fasciitis)
-epidermal changes vary depending on the cause

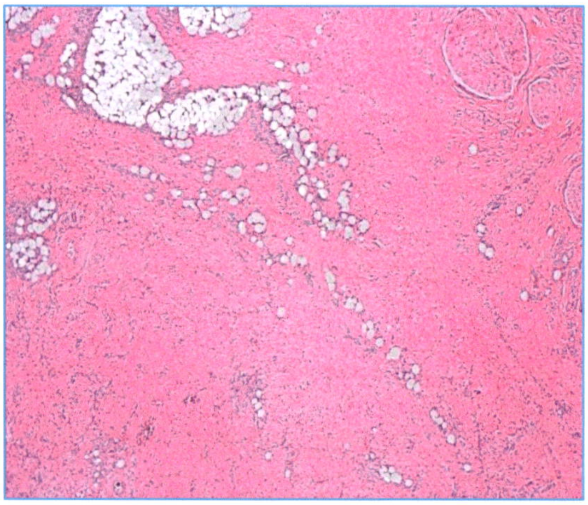
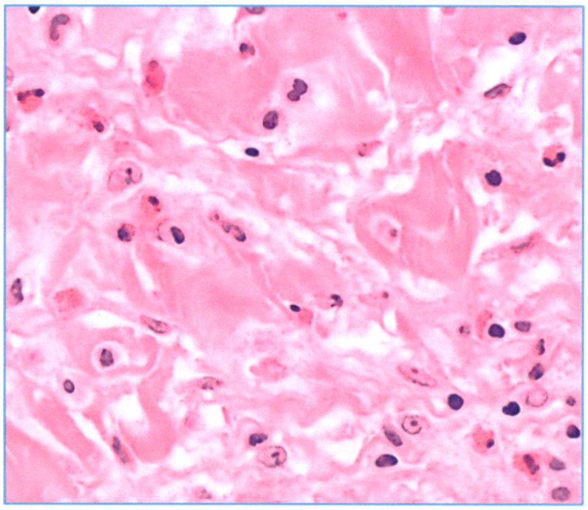

Eosinophilic fasciitis with sclerotic subcutis and fascia and scattered eosinophils

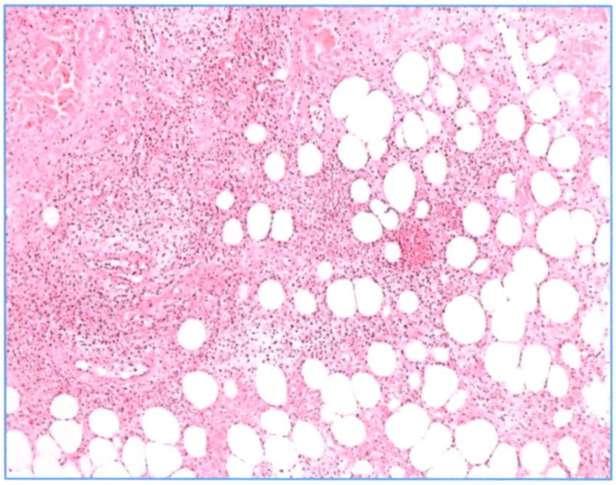
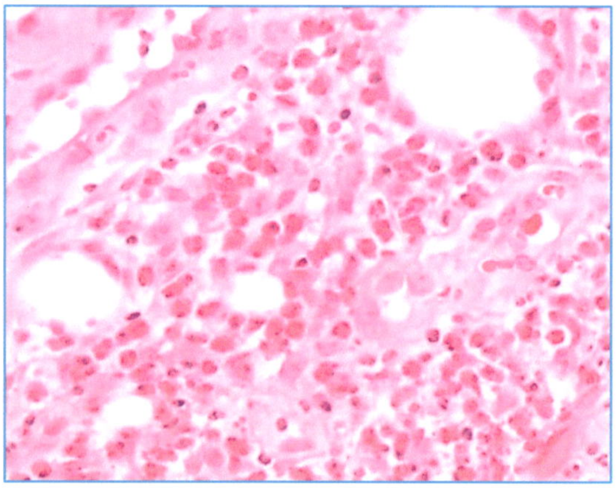

Eosinophilic panniculitis is not sclerotic and has numerous eosinophils

Chapter 12

ALPHA-1-ANTITRYPSIN DEFICIENCY PANNICULITIS

-genetic disorder with deficiency of alpha 1-antytripsin enzyme, produced by the liver
-males and females of any age are equally affected
-rarely presents in children
-it may be preceded by trauma because an injury causes increased protease activation
-low serum levels of alpha-1-antitrypsin
-patients can develop emphysema, pancreatitis, hepatitis, glomerulonephritis, and panniculitis
-panniculitis presents as “bruise-like”, tender, indurated nodules favoring **trunk and proximal extremities**
-lesions ulcerate with **oily discharge**
-heals with scarring and atrophy

Histopathology
-acute **lobular or mixed** panniculitis
-starts as neutrophilic inflammation in deep dermis
-later develops into mixed **neutrophilic panniculitis**

CYTOPHAGIC HISTIOCYTIC PANNICULITIS

-chronic, recurring, frequently fatal panniculitis that is part of a multisystem disease
-associated with lymphoma, leukemia, viral infections, and connective tissue disease
-erythematous, painful subcutaneous nodules typically on extremities
-nodules may ulcerate
-systemic symptoms are fever, lymphadenopathy, and hemorrhagic diathesis

Histopathology
-**lobular panniculitis** with **red blood cell extravasation** and mixed inflammation
-characteristic findings are histiocytes with phagocytosed red and white blood cells and nuclear debris, so called “**bean bag” cells**

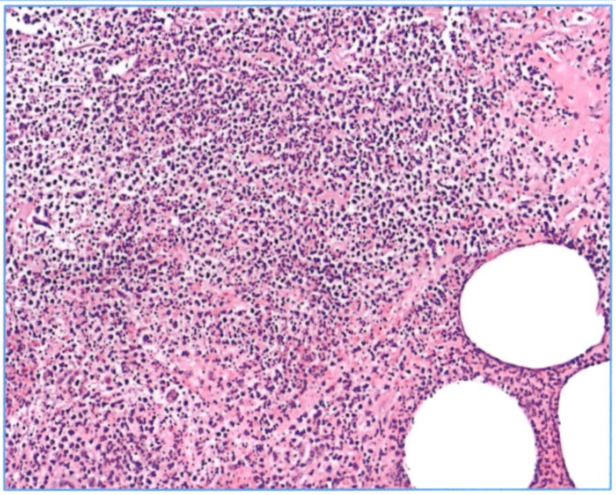
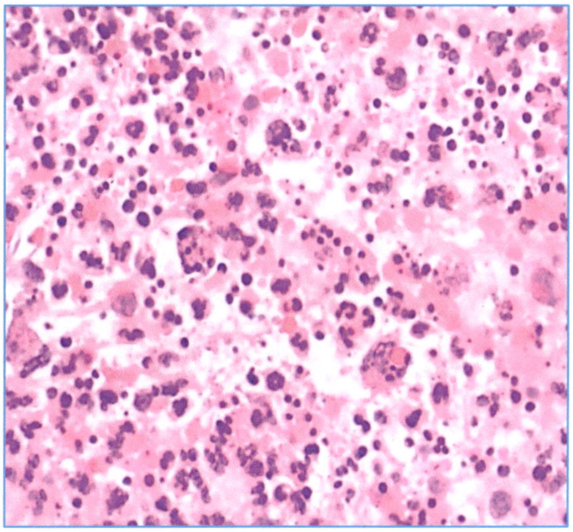

Cytophagic histiocytic panniculitis is lobular with mixed inflammation and characteristic “bean bag” cells

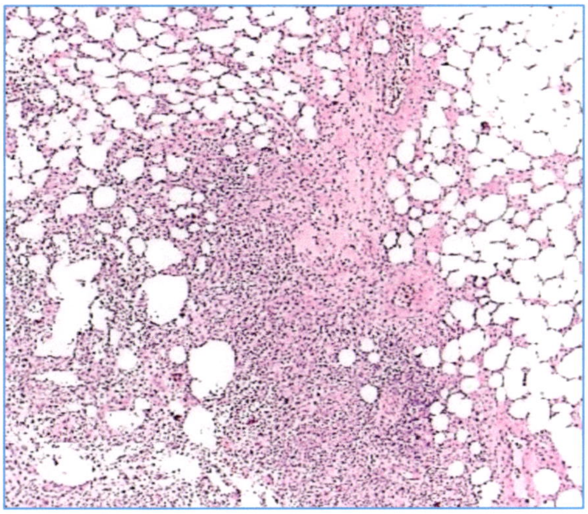
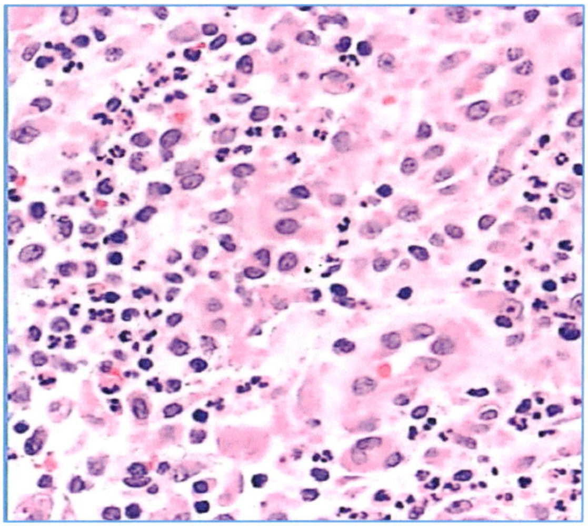

Alpha-1-antitrypsin deficiency with septal and lobular neutrophilic panniculitis

Panniculitis

ERYTHEMA INDURATUM/NODULAR VASCULITIS

-more common in middle-aged women
-idiopathic or reaction to tuberculosis infection (type IV reaction), but tissue culture for TB is usually negative
-tender, reddish plaques and nodules usually on calves
-may ulcerate and scar

Histopathology
-mixed lobular and septal panniculitis
-mixed inflammation with many histiocytes
-**ill-defined epithelioid granulomas and giant cells** are common
-**neutrophilic vasculitis with fibrinoid changes**
-the term **erythema induratum** is used if **granulomas predominate**
-the term **nodular vasculitis** is used if **vascular changes** predominate

SUBCUTANEOUS SWEET'S SYNDROME

-rare subtype of Sweet's syndrome
-similar triggers to classical Sweet's
-tender, erythematous papules and nodules with predilection for legs

Histopathology
-predominantly **neutrophilic infiltrate** exclusively or predominantly in the subcutis
-mixed septal and lobular panniculitis
-histiocytes and lymphocytes are also present
-**lacks dermal edema of classic Sweet's syndrome**

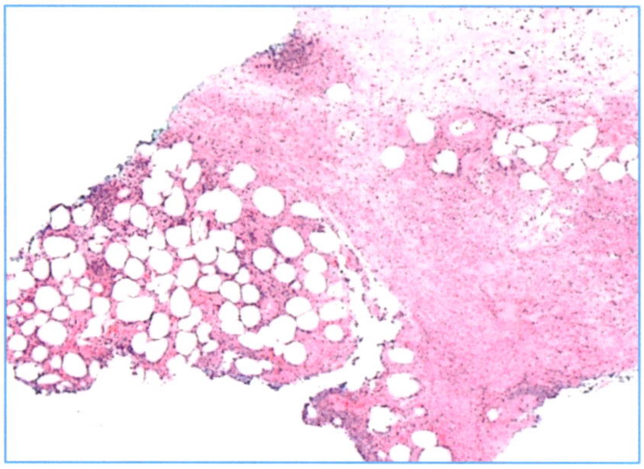

Erythema induratum / Nodular vasculitis

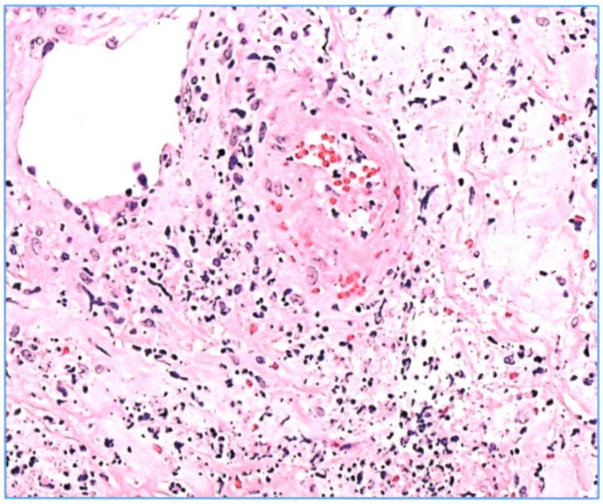

Nodular vasculitis with fibrinoid vascular changes

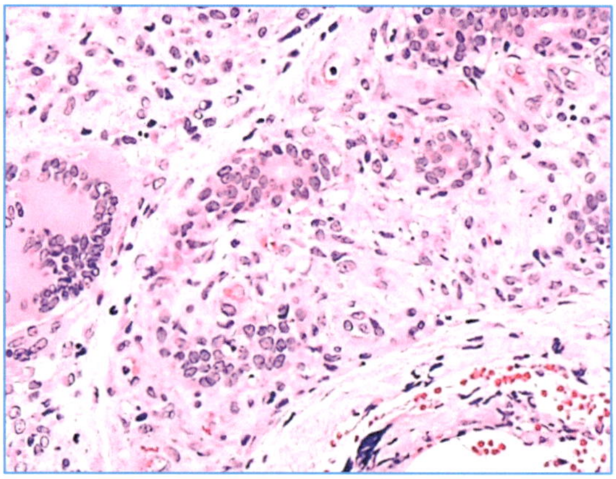

Erythema induratum with giant cells and granulomas

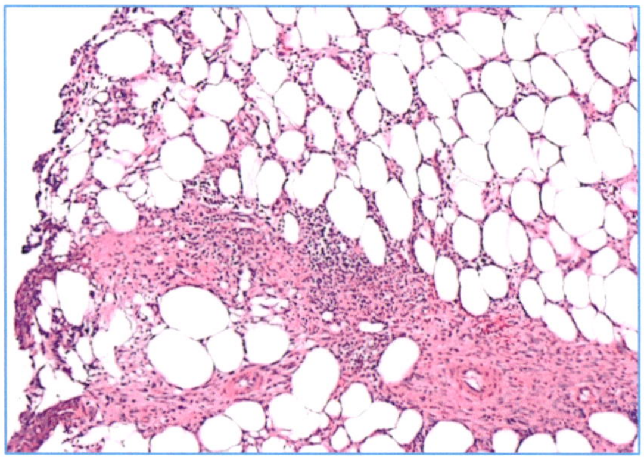

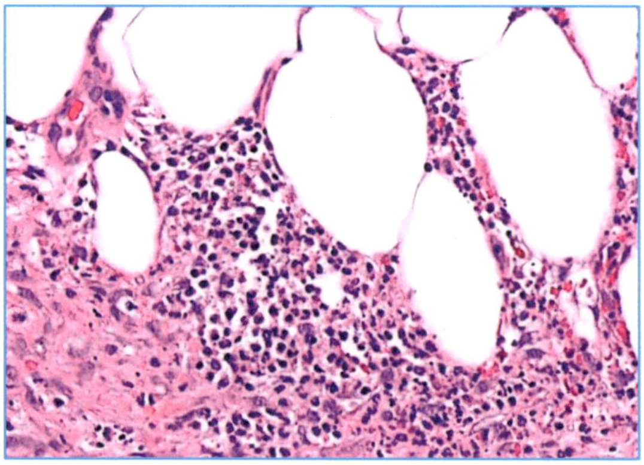

Subcutaneous Sweet's syndrome with neutrophils in lobules and septae

Chapter 12

LUPUS PANNICULITIS/ LUPUS PROFUNDUS

-deep non-tender subcutaneous nodules
-overlying epidermis is either normal (lupus panniculitis) or can have "DLE-like" changes (lupus profundus)
-upper trunk, upper arm, and face are common locations

Histopathology
-if epidermal changes of DLE are present, disease is referred to as lupus profundus
-if there are no epidermal changes present, disease is referred to as lupus panniculitis
-lobular panniculitis with prominent **patchy lymphocytic infiltrate**
-characteristic presence of **paraseptal lymphoid aggregates,** so called **"lymphoid bombs"**
-**plasma cells** can be abundant
-**hyalinized necrosis ("pink wax")** of adipocytes with septal sclerosis

SUBCUTANEOUS PANICULITIS-LIKE T CELL LYMPHOMA

-subcutaneous painless nodules favoring legs and trunk
-rarely ulcerate
-usually middle-aged adults but can occur at any age
-excellent prognosis

Histopathology
-**diffuse,** mostly lobular, **lymphocytic infiltrate** of adipose tissue
-lymphocytes surround adipocytes, so called **"rimming"**
-lack of patchy germinal centers
-lymphocytes are CD3+ and mostly CD4-/CD8+

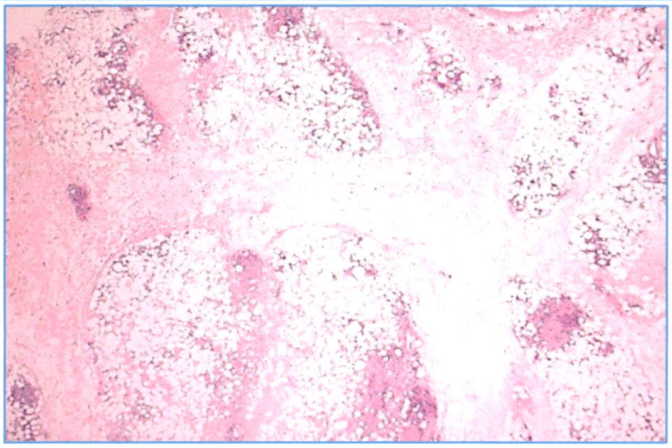

Lupus panniculitis with patchy lymphocytic infiltrate and septal sclerosis

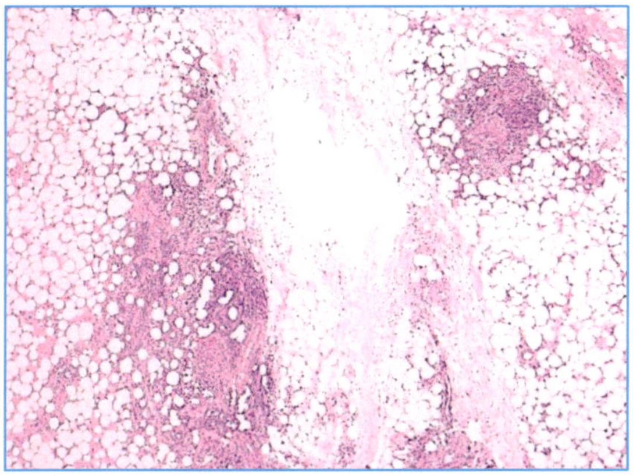

Lupus panniculitis with paraseptal "lymphoid bombs"

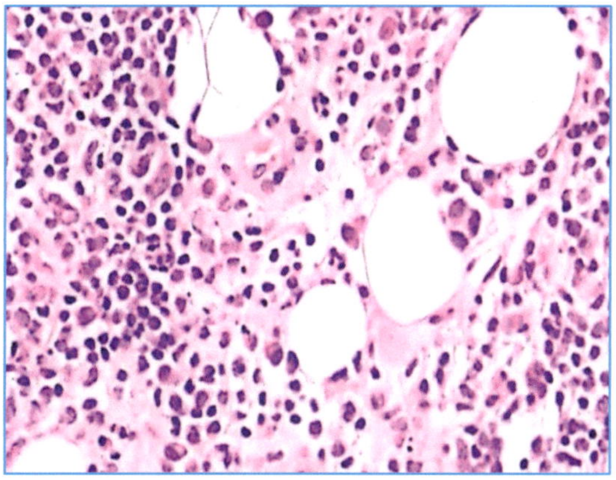

Lupus panniculitis with lymphocytes and plasma cells

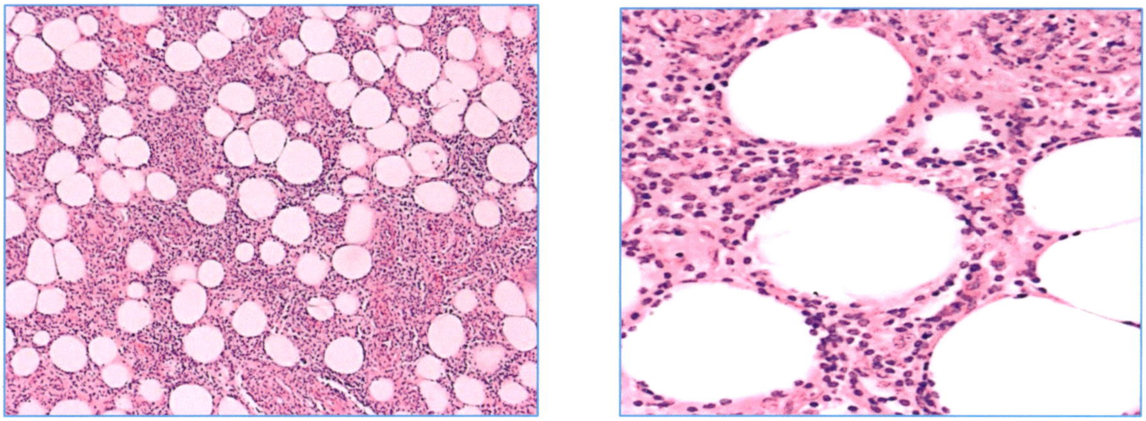

Subcutaneous panniculitis-like T cell lymphoma with diffuse lymphocytic infiltrate and rimming around adipocytes

Panniculitis

LIPODERMATOSCLEROSIS

-sclerosing panniculitis resulting from chronic venous insufficiency
-more common in women, the elderly, and obese patients
-acutely presents with inflammation and redness, progressing to induration, hyperpigmentation, and an **"inverted champagne bottle appearance"** of the lower leg (edema above and sclerosis below)

Histopathology
-dermal stasis with fibrosis
-septal fibrosis and thickening with lobular fat necrosis with **"feathery" lipomembranous** changes, also called **"frost on windowpane"**

LOBULAR PANNICULITIS OF UNKNOWN ETIOLOGY (IDIOPATHIC LOBULAR PANNICULITIS/WEBER CHRISTIAN DISEASE)

-many consider this a non-specific, wastebasket category for lobular panniculitis not otherwise classified
-erythematous painful nodules usually on the limbs and torso
-common systemic symptoms (fever, fatigue)

Histopathology
-lobular panniculitis with neutrophils and liponecrosis in acute form
-lymphohistiocytic infiltrate with lipophages and giant cells in chronic form

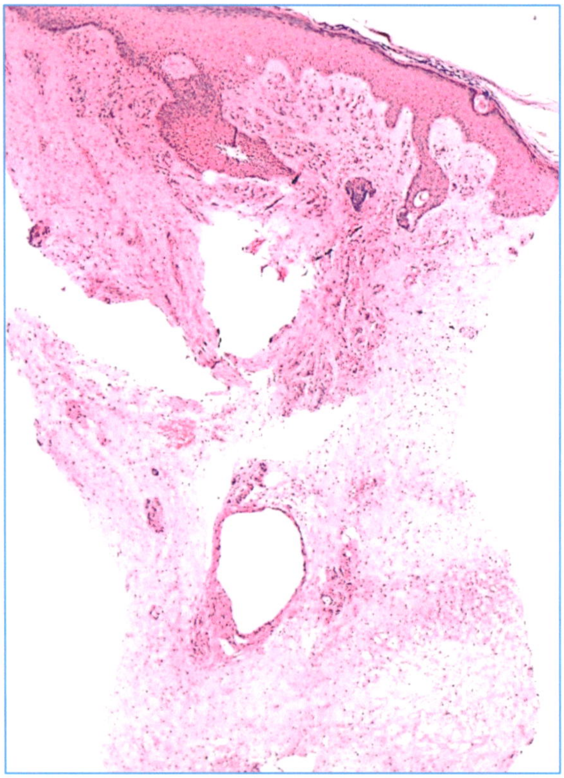

Lipodermatosclerosis

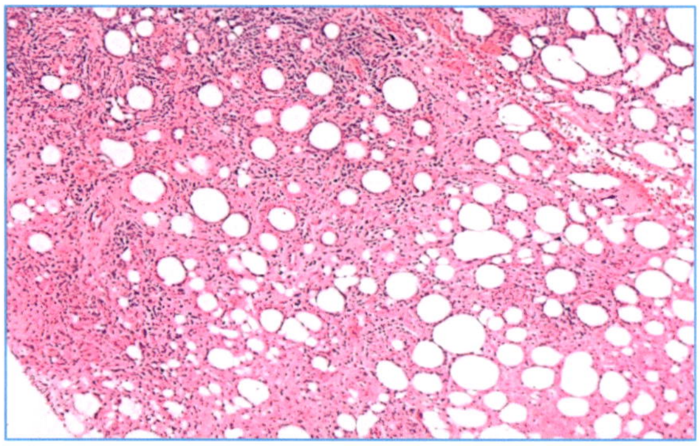

Idiopathic lobular panniculitis with lipophages and giant cells

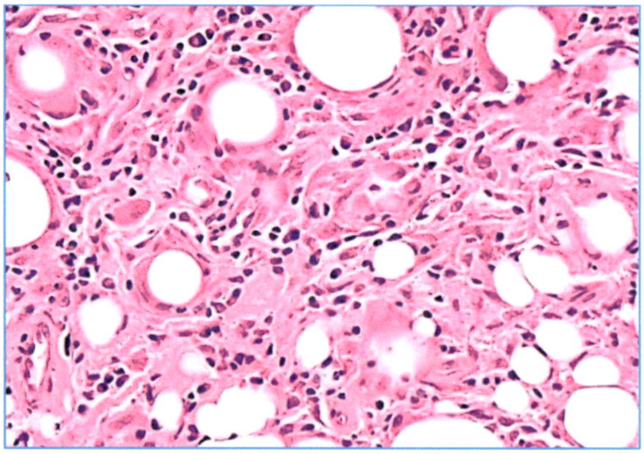

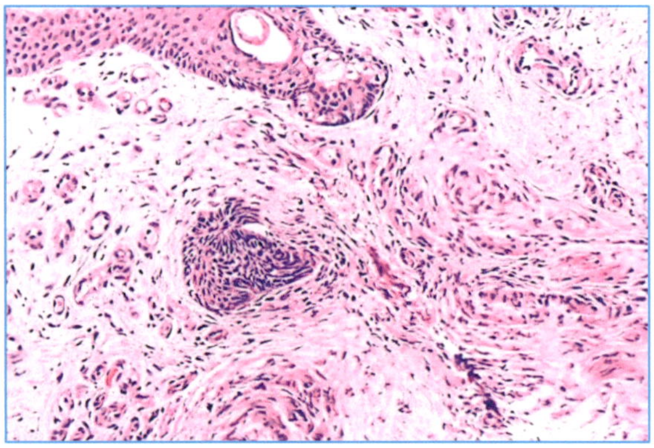

LDS with dermal vascular proliferation (stasis)

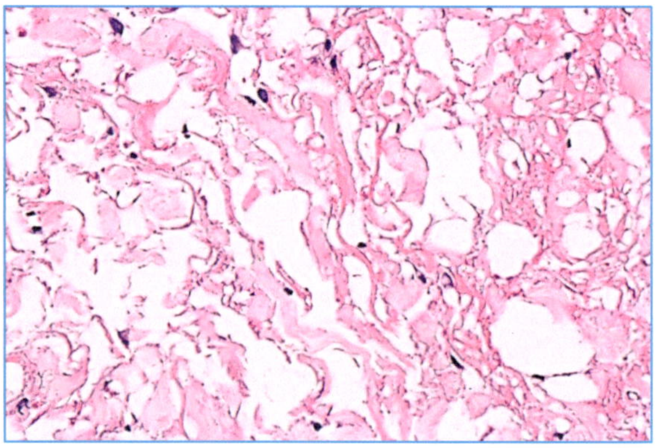

LDS with subcutaneous "feathery" changes

Chapter 12

SCLEREMA NEONATORUM

-widespread cutaneous induration
-affects sick, premature neonates
-within the first week of life
-starts on lower extremities and spreads upward
-prognosis is poor

Histopathology
-fine, **"needle-shaped feathery" cholesterol clefts**
-**very little or no inflammation**
-end up with subcutaneous septa widened by edema that eventually become sclerotic

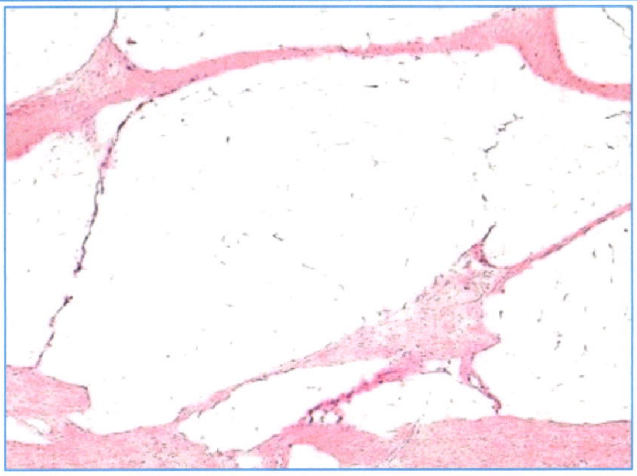

Late sclerema neonatum with sclerotic septa

SUBCUTANEOUS FAT NECROSIS OF THE NEWBORN/ POST-STEROIDAL PANNICULITIS

Subcutaneous fat necrosis of the newborn
-self-limited disease that presents at birth or in the first few days of life
-red to violaceous indurated nodules
-predilection for cheeks, shoulders, buttock, thighs
-obstetric trauma and cold are possible causes
-requires monitoring for hypercalcemia

Post-steroidal panniculitis
-occurs in children within 1 month after the withdrawal of steroid therapy
-multiple subcutaneous nodules that spontaneously regress
-cheeks are favored site

Histopathology
-**both entities** show **identical** features
-unremarkable epidermis and dermis
-lobular panniculitis with focal patchy fat necrosis
-characteristic crystallization of fat with **needle-shaped "feathery" cholesterol clefts ("maple leaf-like")**
-**mixed granulomatous inflammatory response**

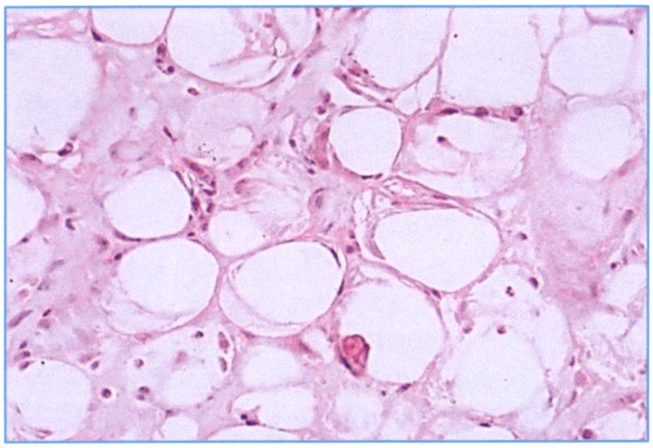

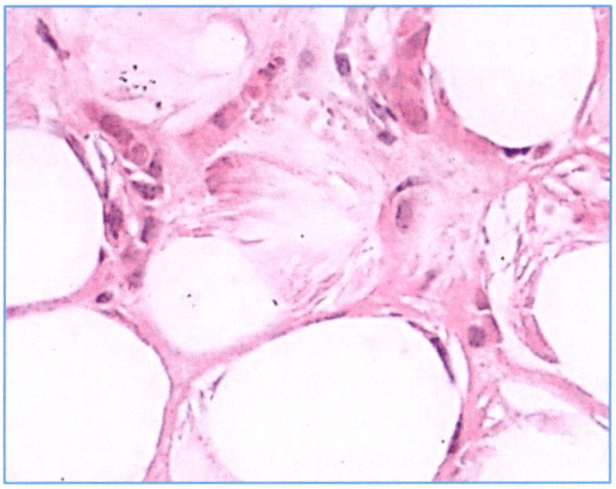

Early sclerema neonatorum with "feathery" cholesterol cleft and no inflammation

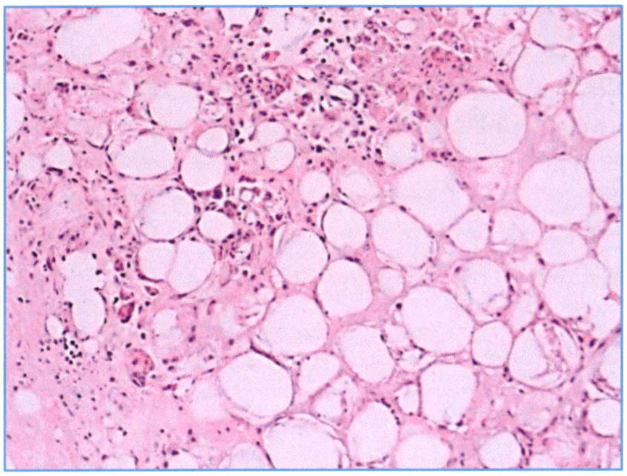

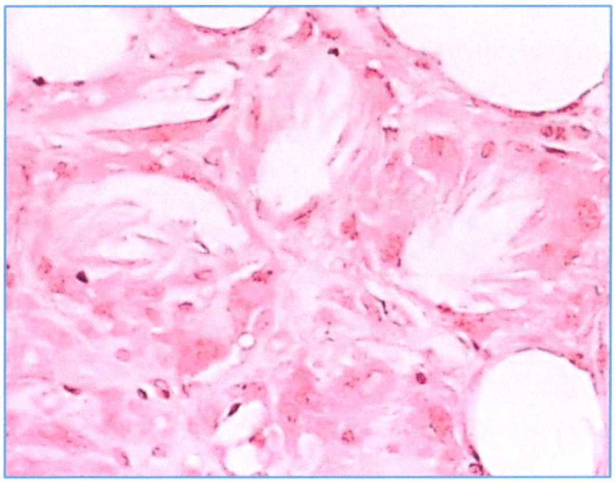

Subcutaneous fat necrosis of the newborn with "feathery" cholesterol cleft and mixed inflammation

Panniculitis

HOW TO APPROACH PANNICULITIS

DETERMINE THE PATIENT'S AGE

CHILD

-sclerema neonatorum	premature baby	"feathery crystals" + no inflammation + fibrosis
-subcutaneous fat necrosis of the newborn	term baby	"feathery crystals" + inflammation + no fibrosis
-post-steroid panniculitis	steroid withdrawal	"feathery crystals" + inflammation + no fibrosis

ADULT

SEPTAL PANNICULITIS

-erythema nodosum	septal fibrosis, histiocytes, lymphocytes, giant cells forming Miescher's granulomas

LOBULAR PANNICULITIS WITH SEPTAL SPILLOVER

WITH EOSINOPHILS

-eosinophilic panniculitis	no fibrosis	involves subcutis
-eosinophilic fasciitis	fibrosis	involves subcutis and fascia, can extend into dermis

WITH LYMPHOCYTES

-lupus panniculitis	patchy paraseptal lymphocytic aggregates + septal fibrosis
-subcutaneous panniculitis-like T cell lymphoma	diffuse lobular lymphocytic infiltrate

WITH NEUTROPHILS

-subacute Sweet's syndrome	normal adipocytes
-pancreatic panniculitis	saponified fat tissue necrosis
-α-1 antitrypsin panniculitis	septal hemorrhage + focal necrosis

WITH MIXED INFLAMMATION

-cytophagic histiocytic panniculitis	diffuse RBCs + emperipolesis
-traumatic fat necrosis	focal RBCs + variable adipocytes + foamy macrophages
-erythema induratum	neutrophilic vasculitis + vague granulomas

WITH MINIMAL INFLAMMATION

-lipodermatosclerosis	dermal stasis + septal fibrosis + lipomembranous fat necrosis

LOBULAR PANNICULITIS ONLY

-lobular panniculitis of unknown etiology (Weber Christian)	fat necrosis with mixed inflammation

Chapter 12

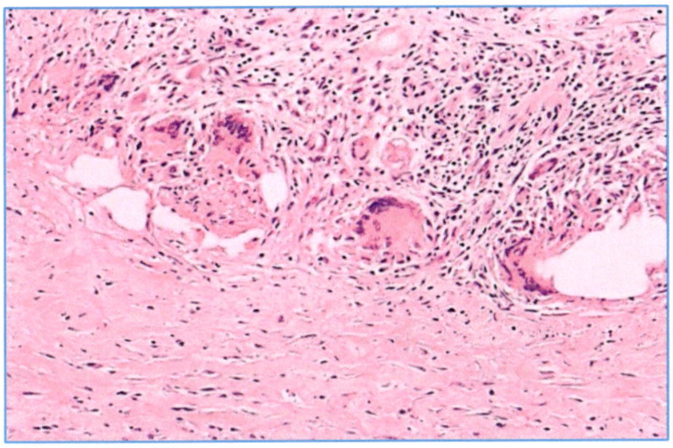

Erythema nodosum with Mischer's granuloma and fibrosis

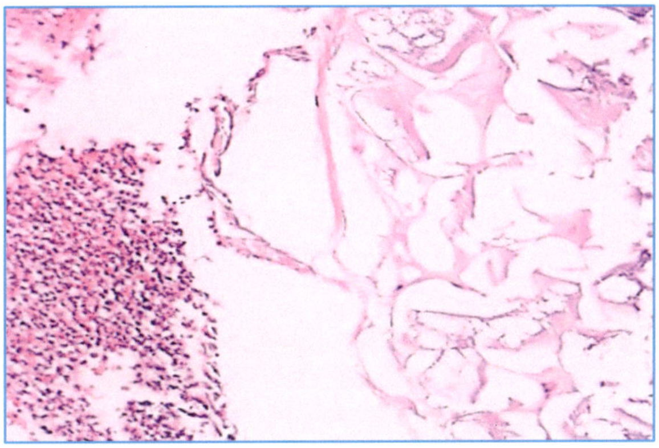

Pancreatic panniculitis with "saponification" of fat

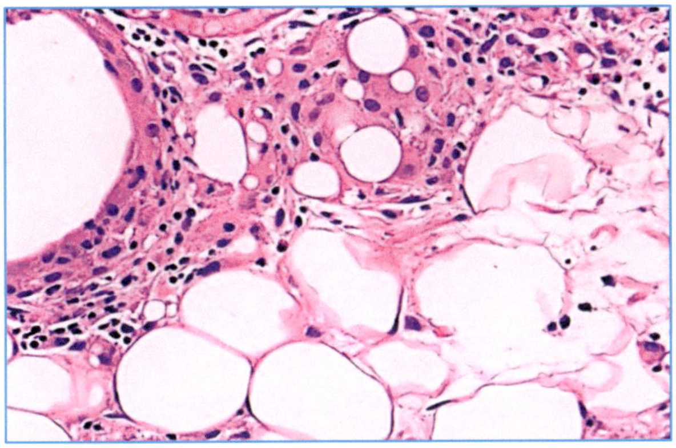

Traumatic fat necrosis with adipocytes of various size surrounded by inflammation with foamy histiocytes

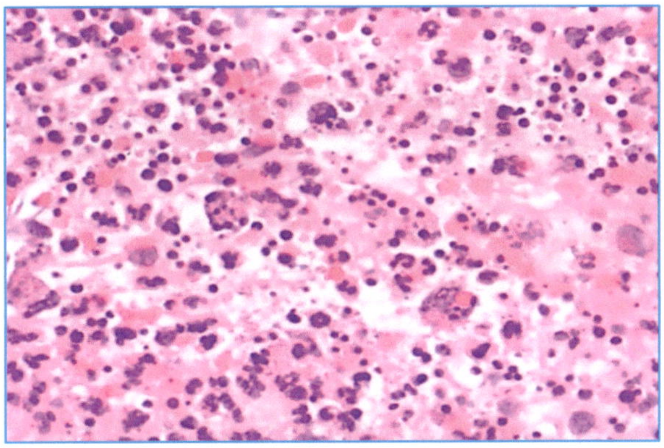

Cytophagic histiocytic panniculitis with histiocytes engulfing white and red blood cells

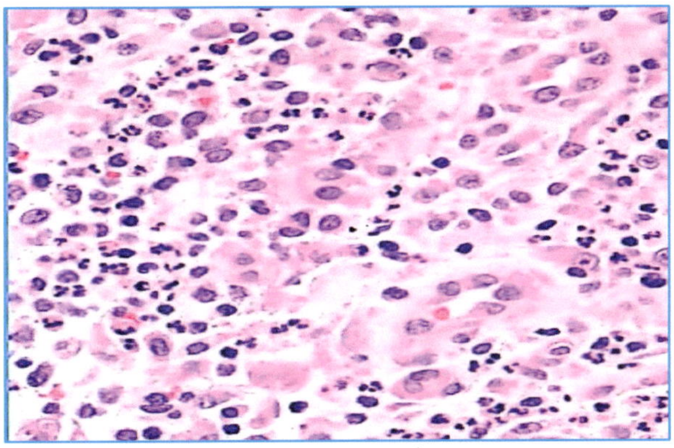

Alpha-1-antitrypsin panniculitis with neutrophils and RBCs

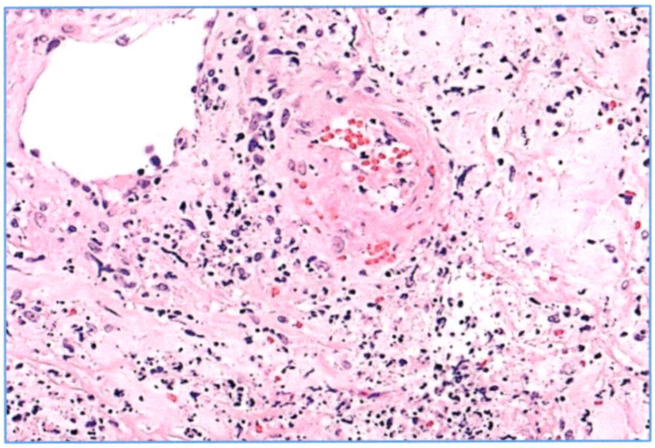

Nodular vasculitis with vascular fibrinoid deposition

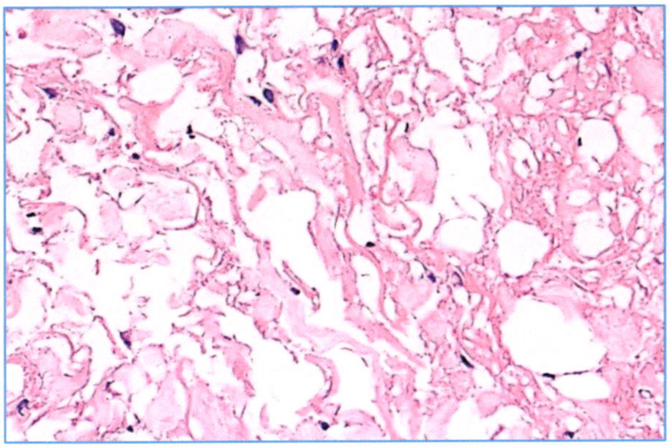

Lipodermatosclerosis with "feathery" degeneration of fat

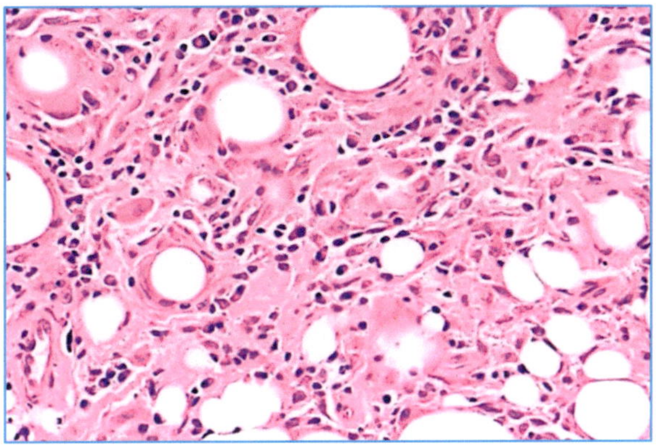

Weber Christian disease with mixed lobular panniculitis

Panniculitis

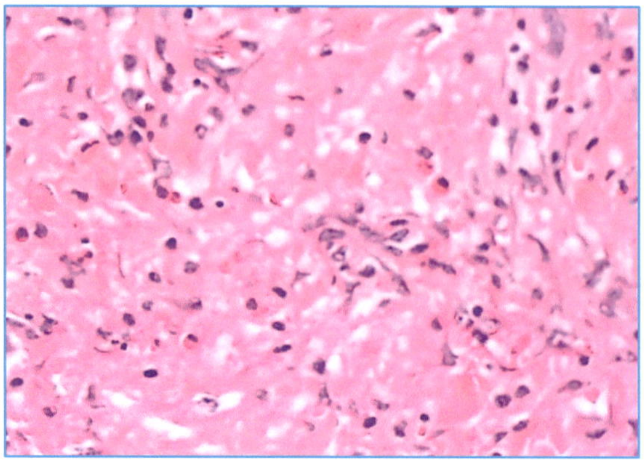

Eosinophilic fasciitis with sclerotic subcutis and fascia with eosinophils

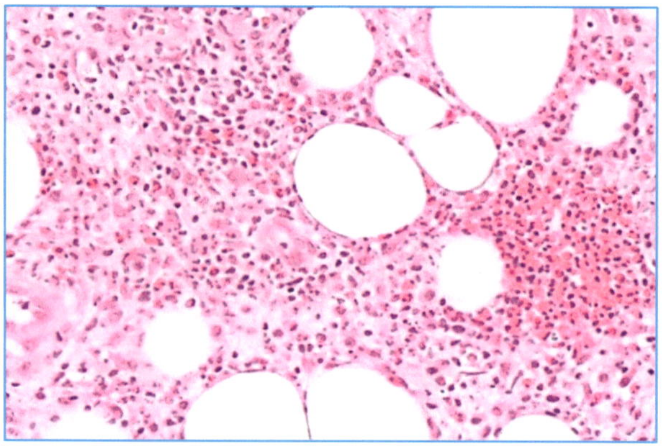

Eosinophilic panniculitis with numerous eosinophils and no fibrosis

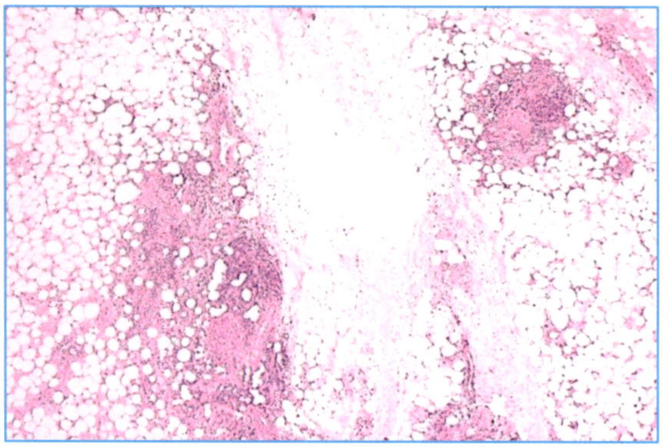

Lupus panniculitis with patchy lymphocytic inflammation and septal fibrosis

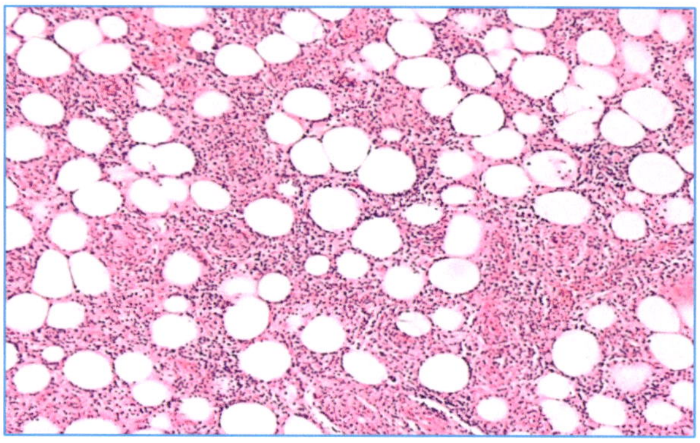

Subcutaneous panniculitis-like T cell lymphoma with diffuse lymphocytic inflammation

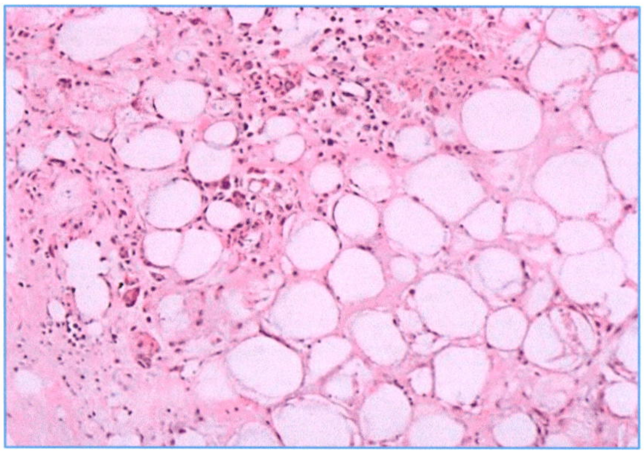

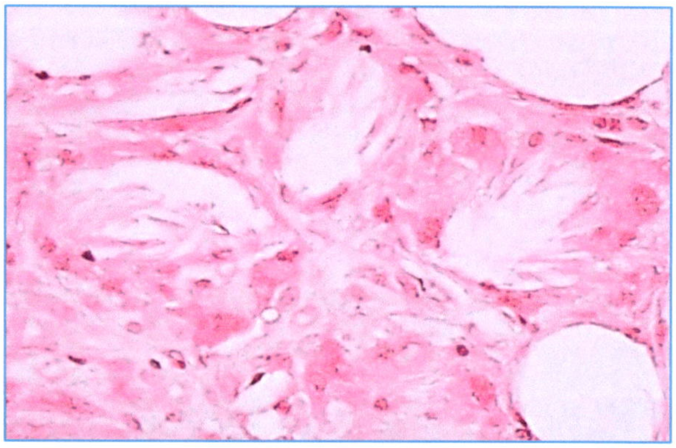

Subcutaneous fat necrosis of newborn with inflammation and “feathery” fat crystals

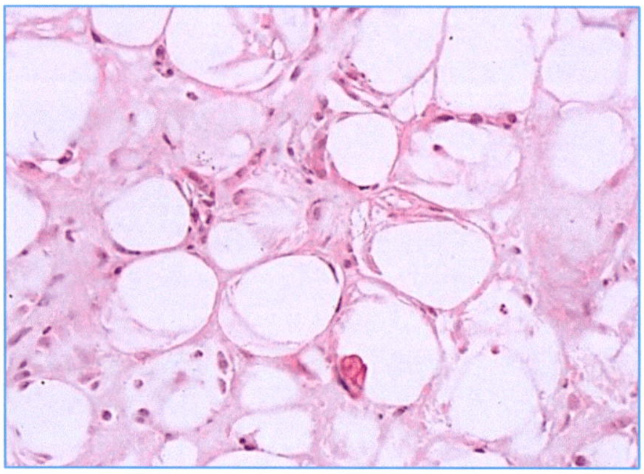

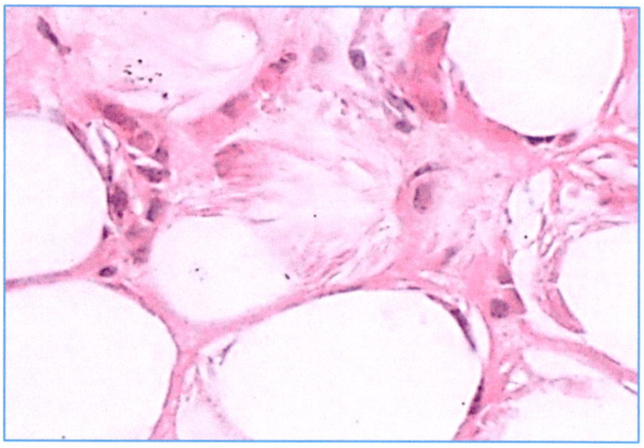

Sclerema neonatorum with minimal inflammation and “feathery” fat crystals

Chapter 13

ALTERATIONS OF COLLAGEN AND ELASTIN

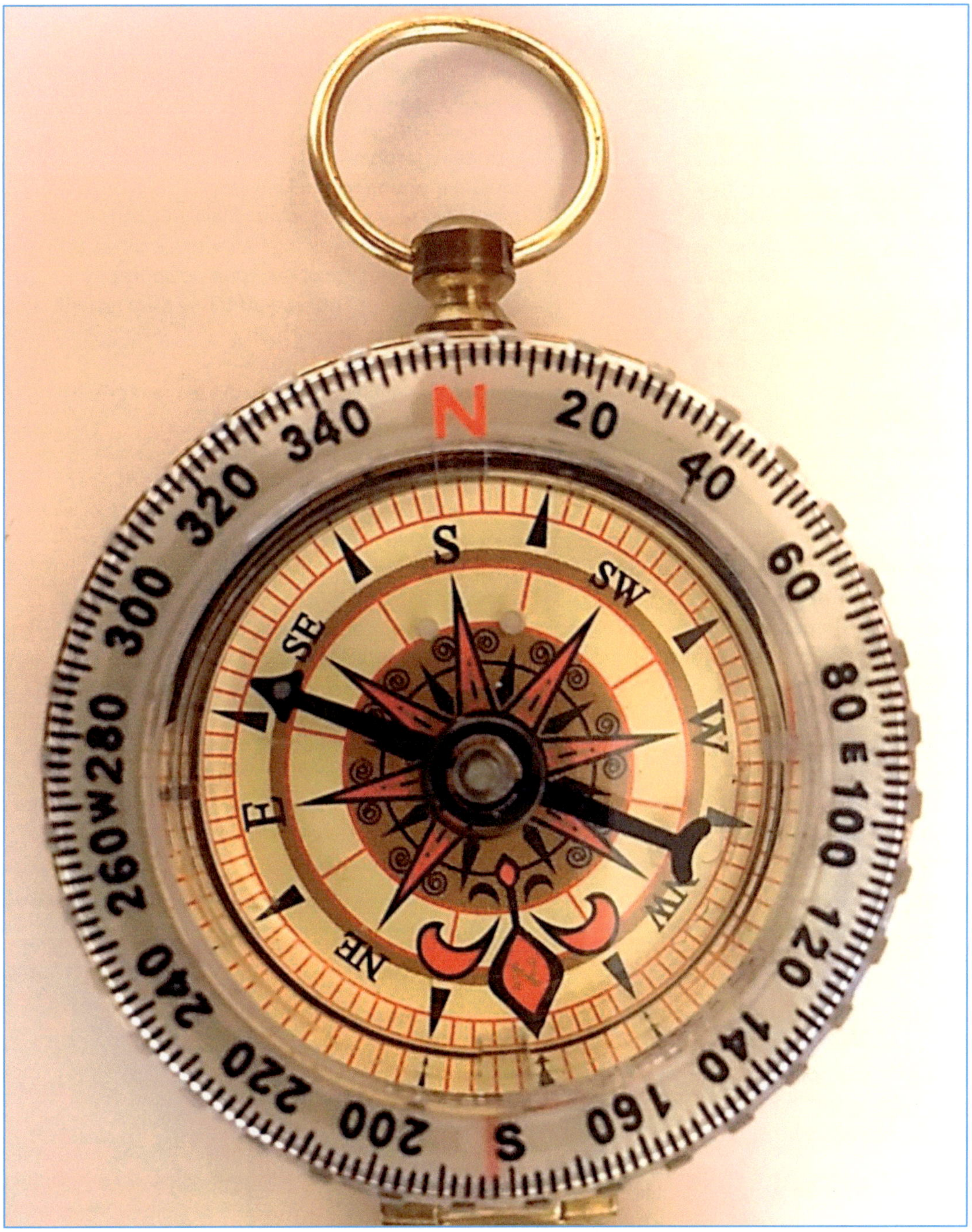

Alterations of collagen and elastin

SCLERODERMA (SYSTEMIC SCLEROSIS)

-systemic autoimmune condition characterized by vascular dysfunction and excess collagen deposition in skin and other organs
-more common in middle-aged women
-visceral sclerosis is present in addition to cutaneous lesions
-presents with symmetrical skin thickening, digital ulceration, salt and pepper hypopigmentation

Two subtypes:

Limited systemic sclerosis (CREST)
-thickening of skin on extremities and face
-**c**alcinosis cutis, **R**aynaud phenomenon, **e**sophageal dysmotility, **s**clerodactyly, and **t**elangiectasias
-less severe visceral involvement (lung/renal)
-classically positive anticentromere antibodies

Diffuse systemic sclerosis
-more generalized skin thickening
-severe pulmonary and renal disease
-classically positive anti scl-70 antibodies

Histopathology

-morphea and scleroderma have almost identical histomorphology
-square/rectangle-shaped biopsy
-thickened dermis and subcutis with **sclerotic collagen bundles**
-**atrophic or absent adnexal structures**
-remaining **eccrine glands are trapped** in fibrotic stroma
-perivascular lymphocytic infiltrate is present early on, but disappears in older lesions
-**loss of CD34+ fibroblasts**

MORPHEA

-variant of scleroderma localized to skin only (no systemic involvement)
-several clinical subtypes:

Plaque morphea
-the most common form
-single/multiple oval to round indurated plaques with a smooth, shiny surface and loss of hair
-margin has pale, lilac color when active
-trunk and proximal extremities are favored sites

Linear morphea
-most common form in children
-morphology like plaque morphea but with linear distribution and favoring lower extremities (#1), upper extremities, and head (*en coup de sabre*)
-can involve deeper tissue affecting limb growth and causing significant morbidity

Guttate morphea
-numerous small, pale, depressed macules with minimal induration, typically on trunk

Morphea profunda
-very rare variant that primarily affects deeper subcutaneous tissues (panniculum, fascia or even muscle)
-overlying skin can be normal or presents as hyperpigmented atrophic plaque
-paraspinal area is a favored site
-can cause deformity and joint restriction

Atrophoderma of Pasini and Pierini
-one or more large well-demarcated, depressed pigmented plaques with sharp, "cliff-drop" borders
-favors the trunk and upper arms of young females

Generalized morphea
-rare subtype with widespread involvement of indurated pigmented plaques of morphea
-spares the hands and face

EOSINOPHILIC FASCIITIS (SCHULMAN SYNDROME)

-most common in middle aged women with recent history of strenuous physical activity
-associated with eosinophilia, hypergammaglobulinemia, and arthralgia
-rapidly developing symmetrical edema and induration of forearms and legs ending with "woody" fibrosis
-sparing of hands/feet
-Raynaud's phenomenon is absent (unlike scleroderma)
-responds well to corticosteroid (unlike morphea profunda)

Histopathology

-thickening and **sclerosis of the subcutis and fascia (deeper sclerosis than seen in scleroderma)**
-variable number of lymphocytes and plasma cells with **scattered eosinophils**
-in more extensive cases, fibrosis extends into dermis

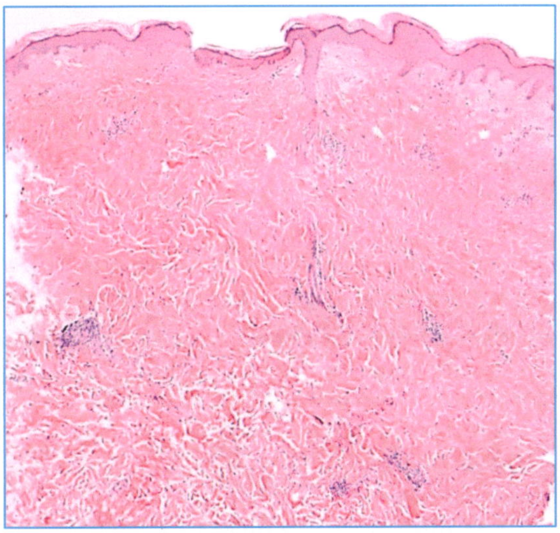

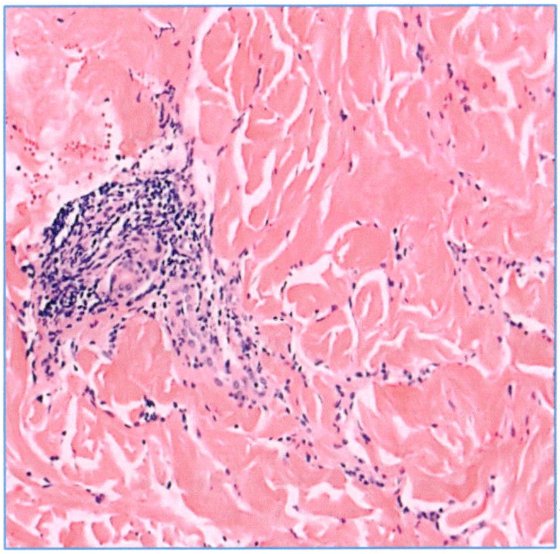

Morphea with thick sclerotic dermis and subcutis and absence of adnexal elements

Morphea with focal lymphocytic aggregate

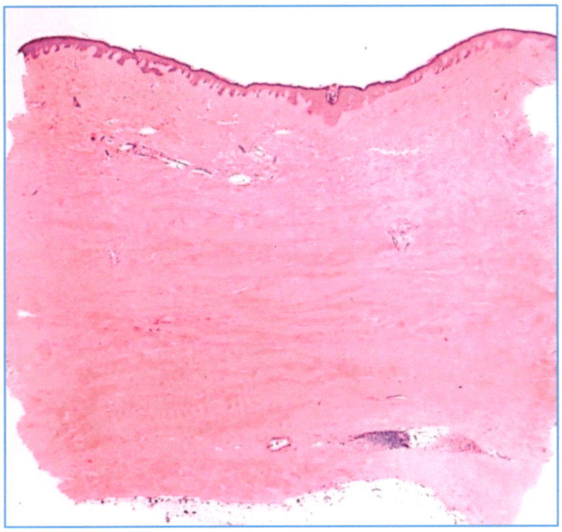

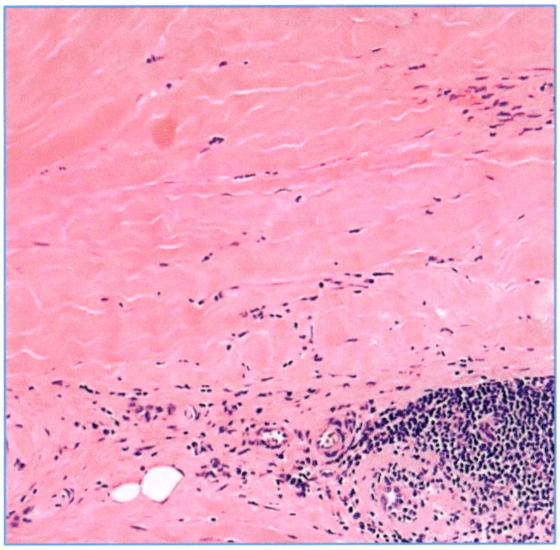

Scleroderma has similar histological appearance as morphea

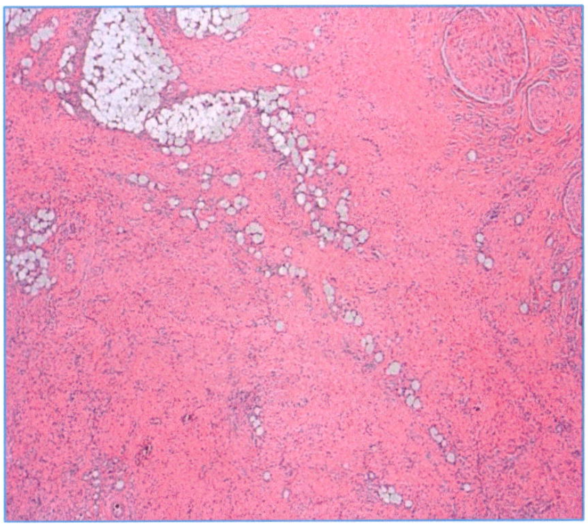

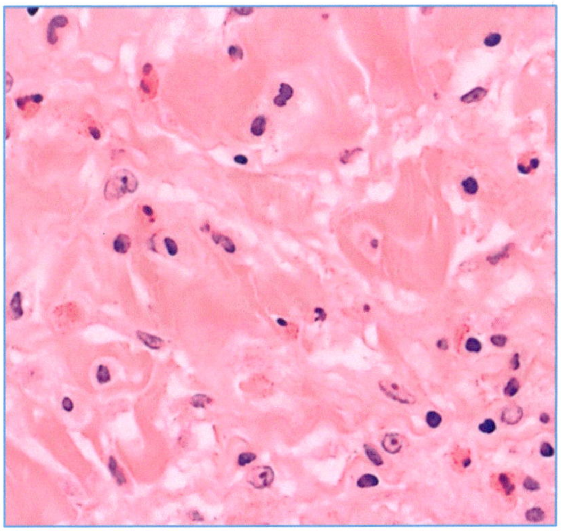

Eosinophilic fasciitis with sclerosis of subcutis and scattered eosinophils

Alterations of collagen and elastin

CONNECTIVE TISSUE NEVUS

-term describing hamartomatous lesions at any skin side, either **collagenomas** or **elastomas**
-skin-colored patches, plaques, or nodules
-associated with several syndromes:
Tuberous sclerosis
-Shagreen patch collagenoma on the lower back
MEN-1
-multiple pedunculated collagenomas
Proteus syndrome
-corrugated plantar collagenoma
Buscke-Ollendorf syndrome
-widespread small skin-colored papules (elastomas) and osteopoikilosis

Histopathology

-overgrowth of one connective tissue component
Collagenoma
-markedly **increased density** of haphazardly arranged **collagen fibers** in superficial and deep dermis as well as subcutaneous tissue
Elastoma
-appearance of normal skin with subtle increase of spaces between collagen fibers
-VVG stain for elastic fibers reveals **increased number of elastic fibers** with morphological alterations (fragmentation and irregular shapes)

SCLEREDEMA

-symmetrical hardening of skin causing indurated shiny skin with "wooden" appearance and loss of skin markings
-associated with infection (*Strep.*), monoclonal gammopathy, and diabetes
-predilection for upper trunk and extremities
-distal extremities are spared but face can be affected with difficulty opening mouth
-in diabetic patients lesions persist/progress
-in patients in which disease follows an infection, lesions resolve in months/years

Histopathology

-sclerotic dermis and subcutis
-**thick, sclerotic collagen bundles** with **normal number of fibroblasts**
-**collagen bundles separated by clear spaces**
-spaces filled with **mucin** (early on)
-**mucins disappear in older lesions**

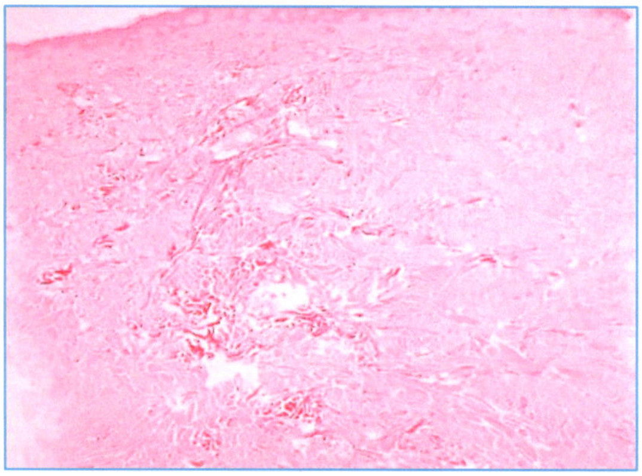

Scleredema with sclerotic dermis

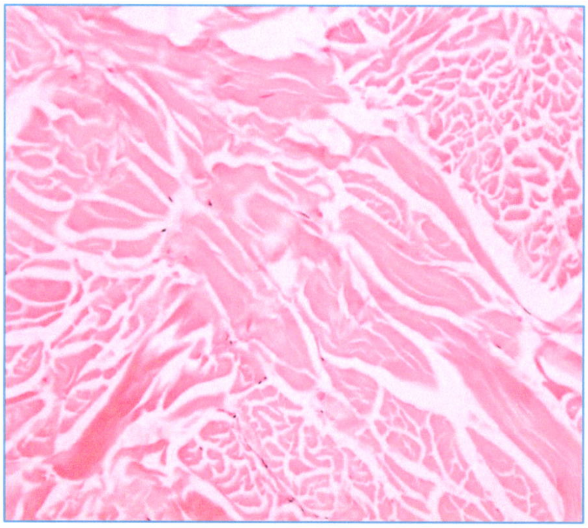

Scleredema with clear spaces between collagen fibers

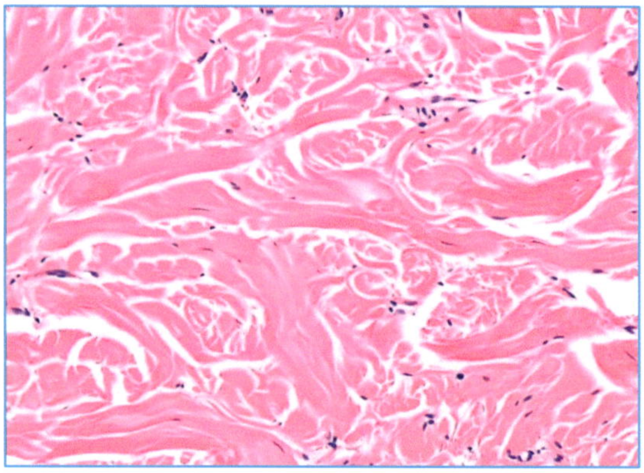

Collagenoma with increased density of collagen bundles

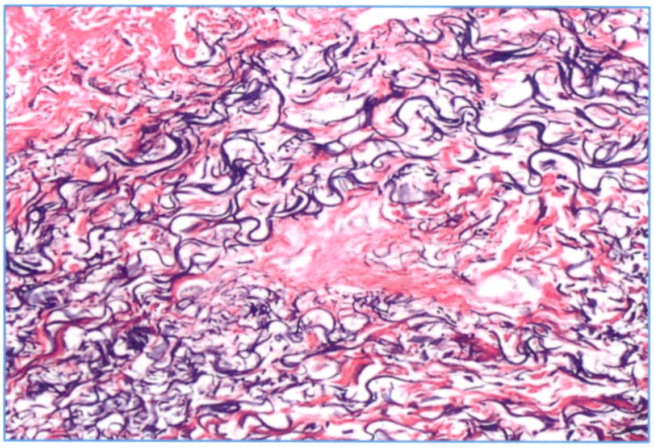

Elastoma with increased number of elastic fibers (VVG stain)

SCLEROMYXEDEMA (GENERALIZED LICHEN MYXEDEMATOSUS)

-chronic, progressive disease usually in middle-aged adults
-associated with IgG-λ monoclonal gammopathy
-characterized by multiple waxy papules that coalesce in plaques or are arranged in linear arrays
-predilection for dorsal hands, face, extensor extremities
-eventually develop diffuse infiltration with "woody" skin appearance
-may have systemic organ involvement (particularly GI and lung)

Histopathology

-**dermal fibroblastic proliferation** with **fibrosis** and **mucin deposition**
-**fibroblasts are CD34 positive** (unlike scleroderma)
-in **older lesions, mucin is less evident**
-mild perivascular lymphocytic inflammation

NEPHROGENIC SYSTEMIC FIBROSIS

-thickening and scarring of the skin and internal organs in patients with renal disease and a history of gadolinium-containing contrast exposure
-gradual onset of hyperpigmented, "woody" indurated plaques
-may have orange-peel or "pseudo-cellulite" appearance
-distribution is symmetric favoring extremities and trunk
-classically also have white-yellow scleral plaques

Histopathology

-requires deep biopsy to evaluate subcutaneous fat and fascia
-histology is **similar to scleromyxedema** but with more mucin
-**in addition**, it also **affects subcutaneous septa**

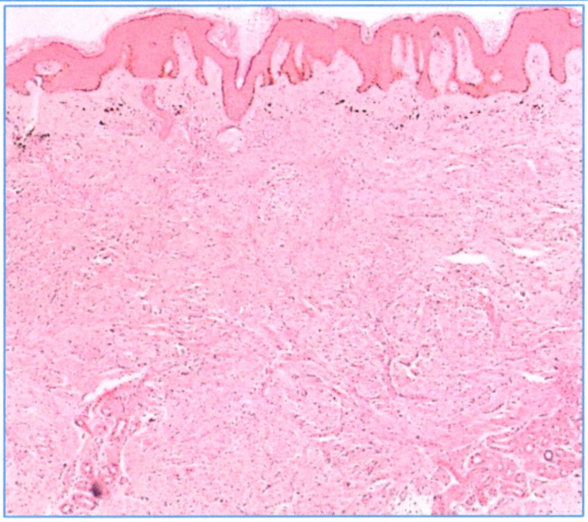
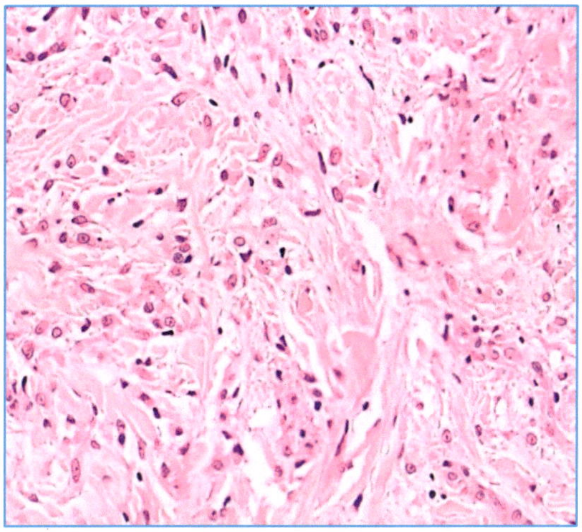

Scleromyxedema with fibrotic dermis with mucin and proliferation of dermal fibroblasts

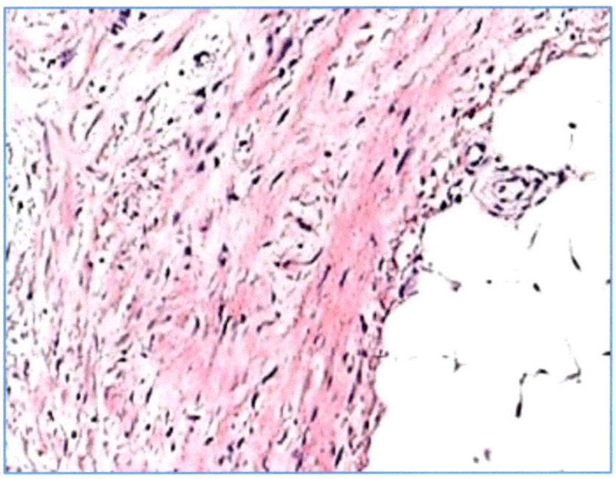
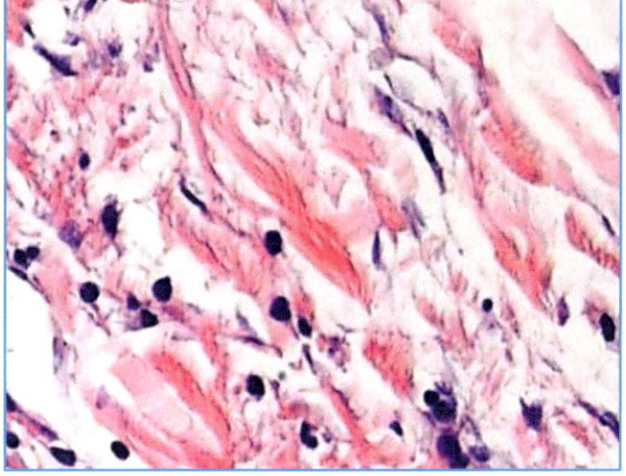

Nephrogenic systemic fibrosis with fibrosis and fibroblast proliferation in subcutis

Alterations of collagen and elastin

SCAR (CICATRIX)

-result of wound repair or final stage of scarring inflammatory disorders

Histopathology

-correlates with the time since injury

-within 24 hours- neutrophils appear at the edge of blood clot

-by day 3- macrophages replace neutrophils

-by day 5- granulation tissue forms

-by week 2- inflammation decreases, fibroblasts proliferate, and collagen forms

-by 4-5 weeks- **horizontally arrayed collagen ("East-West")** with **vertically oriented blood vessels** and **absence of adnexal structures**

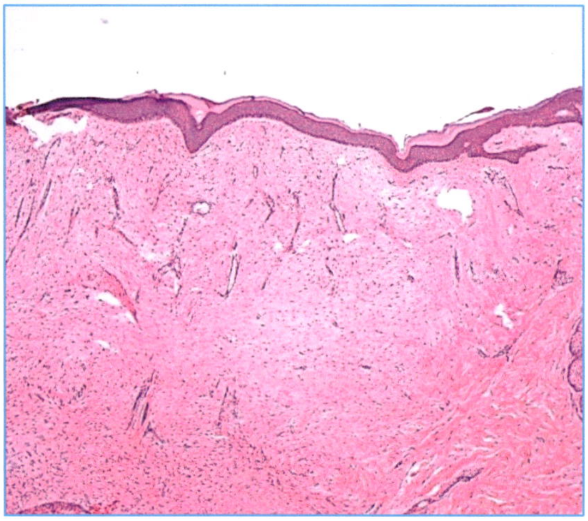

Scar with horizontally arranged collagen and vertically oriented blood vessels

HYPERTROPHIC SCAR

-nodular scar confined to the injury site

Histopathology

-atrophic epidermis

-dermal **adnexal structures are absent**

-scar has a **nodular shape**

-fibroblasts are increased in number

-fibroblasts, collagen bundles, and vessels have **swirling pattern,** but some vessels are still oriented perpendicular to epidermis

-mild chronic inflammation usually present

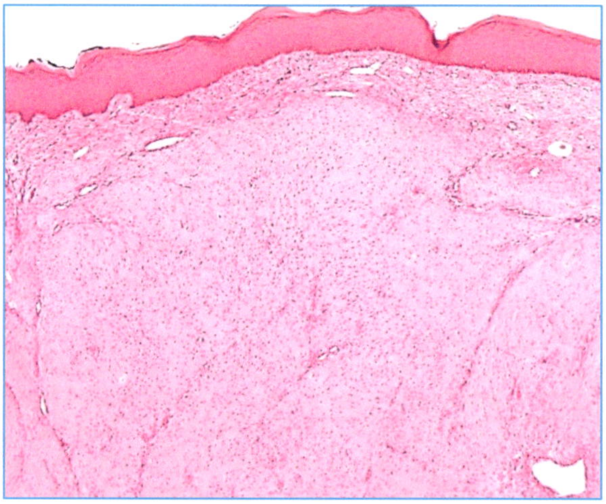

Hypertrophic scar has nodular shape and absent adnexal structures

KELOID

-raised, firm, frequently pedunculated hyperpigmented red-pink nodule of scar tissue that extends beyond the borders of initial injury

-early growth is red, tender and rubbery

-surface is usually smooth and shiny

-may occur at any site of previous injury with earlobe and chest being common sites

Histopathology

-epidermis is usually mildly atrophic

-dermal adnexal structures are absent

-normal dermal collagen is replaced with **thick, hyalinized collagen** bundles

-collagen is haphazardly organized and is **"bubble gum" dark pink** with some bluish collagen in between

-chronic lymphocytic inflammation can be present at the periphery

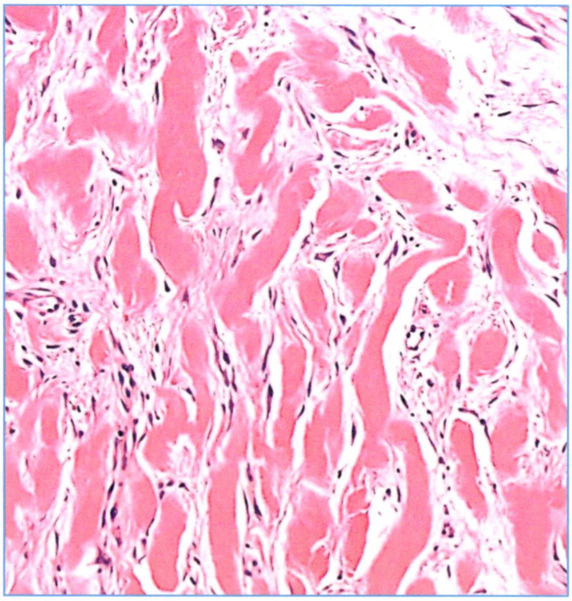

Keloid with "bubble gum" thick collagen

Chapter 13

APLASIA CUTIS CONGENITA

-congenital ulcer due to the absence of skin, with or without the absence of underlying structures
-most commonly affects the scalp, but any location of the body can be affected
-most children with aplasia cutis congenita have no other abnormalities
-can be seen in some syndromes such as trisomy 13, 4p deletion syndrome, epidermolysis bullosa (EB), ectodermal dysplasia, Adams-Oliver syndrome (AOS), and amniotic band sequence
-area heals with a scar and permanent alopecia

Histopathology
-rarely biopsied as it is a clinical diagnosis
-**cutaneous ulcer** with loss of epidermis and dermis
-later lesion shows **scar with absent appendages**
-subcutis is usually thin

FOCAL DERMAL HYPOPLASIA (GOLTZ SYNDROME)

-type of ectodermal dysplasia due to mutations or duplications/deletions in the *PORCN* gene on the X chromosome
-about 90% of patients are females
-multisystem disorder that affects the development of the skin, hands, feet, eyes, and teeth
-characterized by atrophic, linear streaks with soft yellowish nodules (fat herniation)
-sparse hair, absent or dystrophic nails, syndactyly/ectrodactyly ("lobster claw" deformity)

Histopathology
-**reduction in dermal thickness** with attenuation of dermal collagen
-**extension of adipose tissue into the dermis**

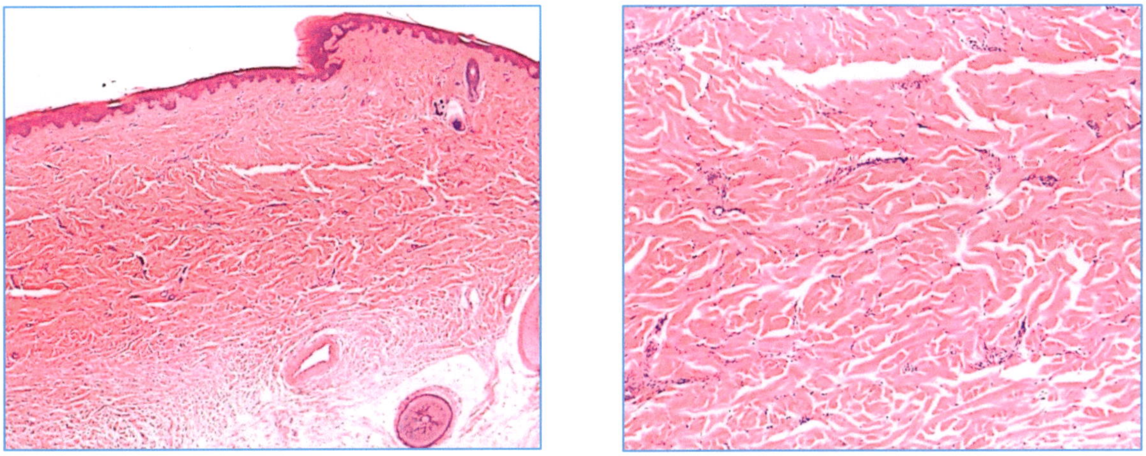

Older lesion of aplasia cutis appears as a scar with absent adnexal structures

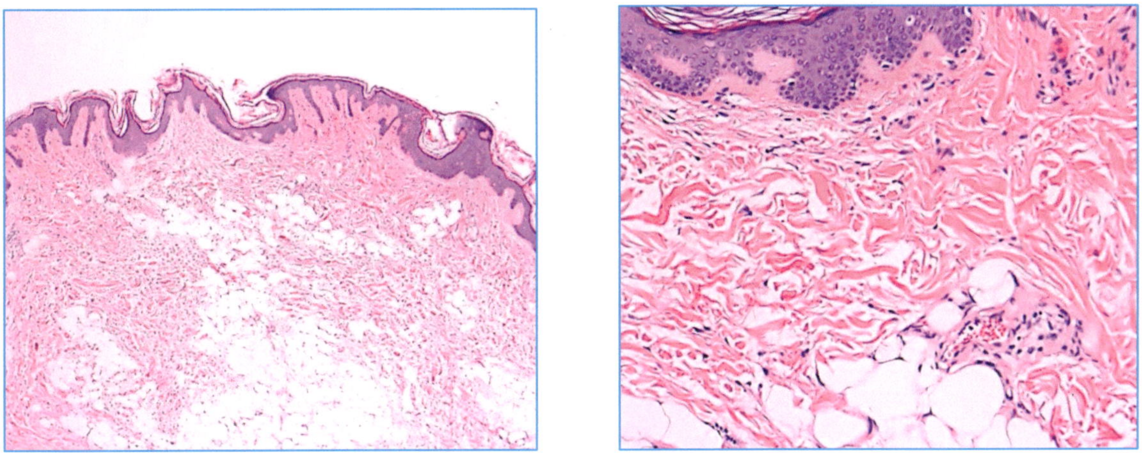

Focal dermal hypoplasia with thin dermis and adipose tissue high in the dermis approaching the epidermis

Alterations of collagen and elastin

ERYTHEMA AB IGNE

-skin change caused by long-term exposure to heat (e.g. heating blankets, fireplace)
-characteristic "net-like" reticulated red-brown patches on the affected area (resembles livedo reticularis)
-scaling and telangiectasia may be seen
-pigmentation gradually becomes permanent
-commonly seen on the lower legs (space heater, heating blanket), back or abdomen (heating pad)

Histopathology
-slightly atrophic epidermis, but otherwise unremarkable skin on H&E slides
-usually **"smudgy" dermal collagen**
-VVG elastic fiber stain demonstrates **fragmented elastic fibers in the midreticular dermis**

ANETODERMA (MACULAR ATROPHY)

-focal loss of elastin in the skin
-more common in young women (15-25 years of age)
-multiple, round, atrophic, skin-colored papules
-skin bulges outward or is slightly depressed
-most frequent sites are upper trunk and arms
-may be primary (idiopathic) or secondary (due to infections, autoimmune conditions, tumors, or inflammatory skin conditions)

Histopathology
-normal appearing skin on H&E slides
-no or minimal perivascular inflammation
-VVG elastin stain demonstrates significantly **decreased or completely absent elastic fibers**

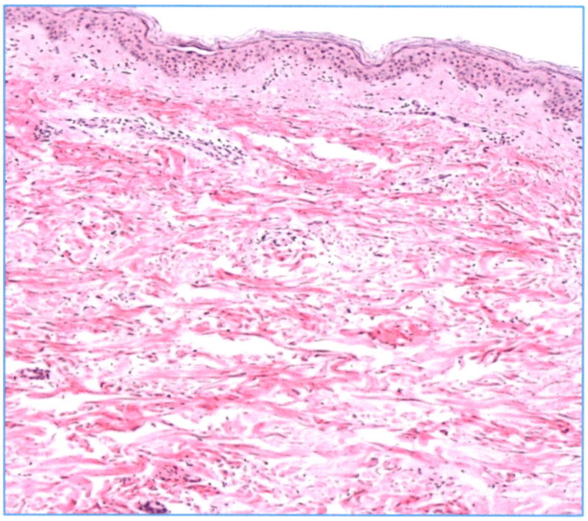

Erythema ab igne with smudgy dermal collage (H&E stain)

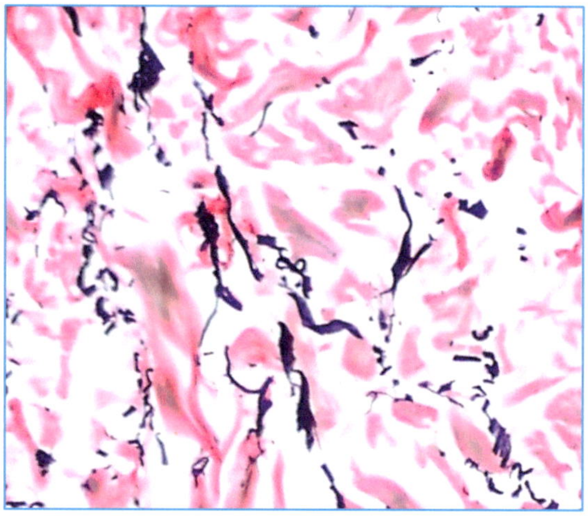

Erythema ab igne with fragmented elastic fibers (VVG stain)

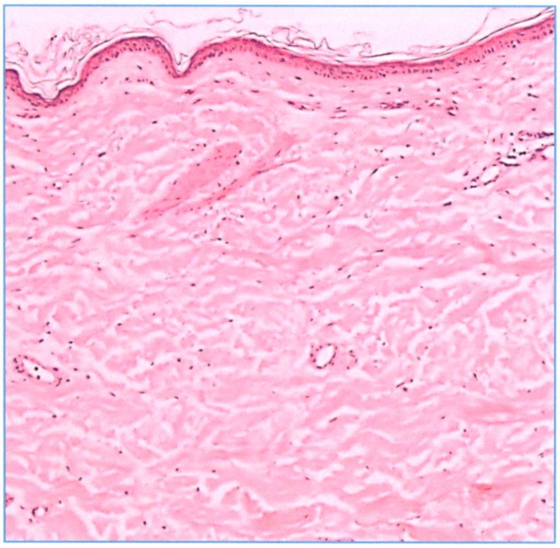

Anetoderma appears as normal skin on H&E stain

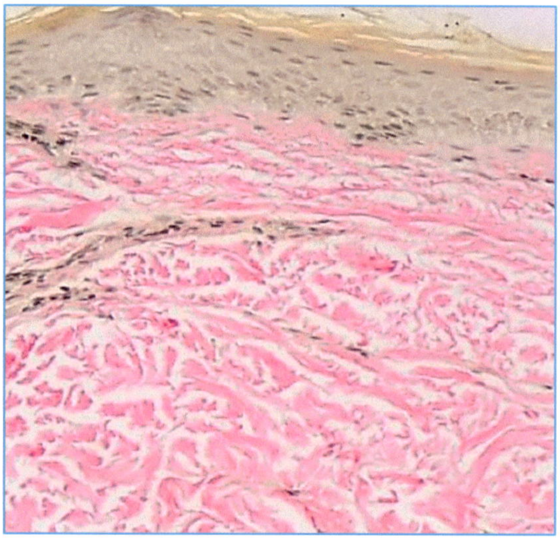

Anetoderma with absent elastic fibers on VVG stain

SOLAR ELASTOSIS (ACTINIC ELASTOSIS)

-skin atrophy and wrinkling due to chronic solar damage to the elastic fibers
-sign of aging and solar damage
-excessive solar elastosis is part of several clinical entities including
cutis rhomboidalis nuchae
-yellow "leather-like" skin on the neck with deep creases in a geometric pattern

Histopathology
-prominent **dermal elastic fibers with gray-blue appearance**
-**elastic fibers appear fragmented** and haphazardly oriented

COLLAGENOUS AND ELASTOTIC MARGINAL PLAQUES OF THE HAND (DEGENERATIVE COLLAGENOUS PLAQUES OF THE HAND)

-condition seen in elderly patients with extensive chronic sun exposure
-hyperkeratotic translucent papules/plaques arranged linearly on the lateral aspect of the hands

Histopathology
-epidermal acanthosis and hyperkeratosis
-**degenerated haphazardly arranged collagen and elastic fibers**
-**collagen and elastic fibers** appeared **entangled**
-elastic fibers have characteristic gray-blue color
-common focal calcifications

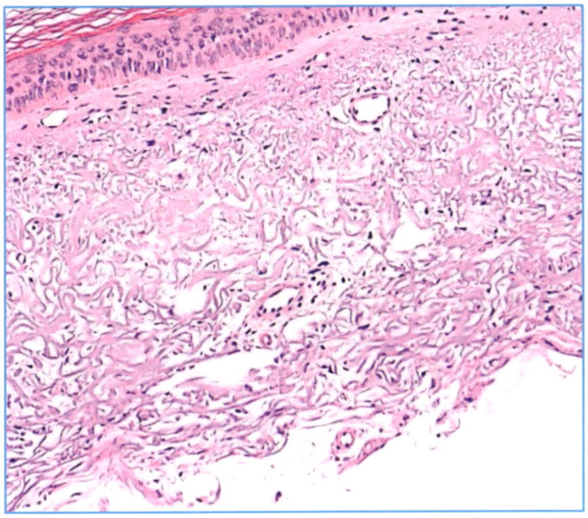
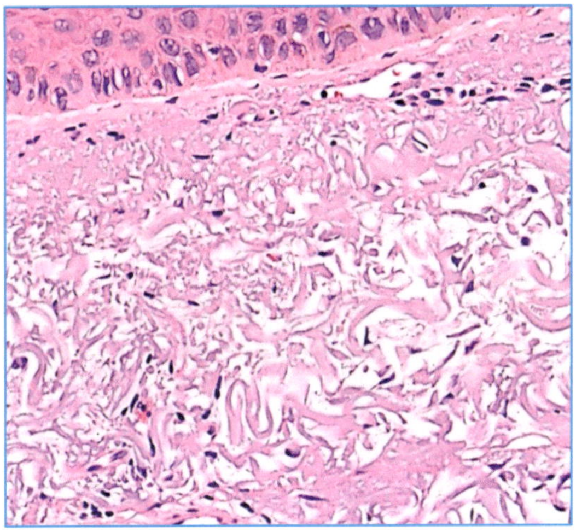

Solar elastosis with prominent fragmented elastic fibers

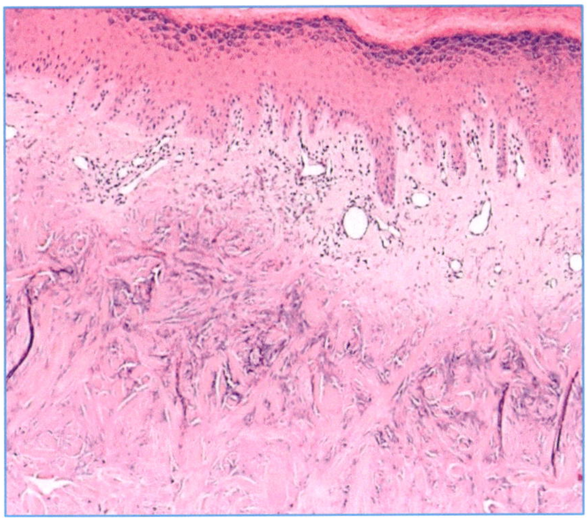
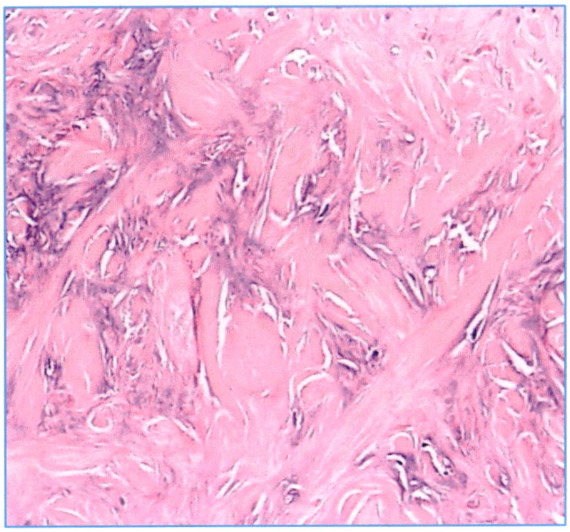

Collagenous and elastotic marginal plaques of the hand with entangled degenerated collagen and elastic fibers

Alterations of collagen and elastin

PERFORATING DERMATOSES

-group of conditions characterized by transepidermal elimination of collagen/elastin
-several clinical entities showing significant clinical and histological overlap

Elastosis perforans serpiginosa

-rare disease appearing in early adulthood
-more common in males
-annular or serpiginous arrangement of hyperkeratotic plaques
-keratotic papules along rim
-predilection for the lateral neck (#1), arms and face
-most cases are idiopathic but may be associated with **M**arfan's syndrome, **A**crogeria, **D**own's syndrome, d-**P**enicillamine therapy, **O**steogenesis imperfecta, **R**othmund-Thomson syndrome, **E**hlers-Danlos syndrome, and **S**cleroderma (**MAD PORES**)

Histopathology
-epidermal hyperplasia with **serpiginous epidermal channel** through which **elastic fibers are eliminated**
-**a keratinous plug** usually blocks the superficial part of channel
-lower portion of channel is filled with **pink-red, degenerated elastic fibers** and inflammatory cells

Perforating folliculitis

-associated with numerous diseases including psoriasis, juvenile acanthosis nigricans, primary sclerosing cholangitis, HIV infection, renal failure, and hemodialysis
-discrete, keratotic, follicular papules
-predilection for the extensor surfaces of the extremities and the buttocks
-may persist for months or years, although periods of remission often occur

Histopathology
-dilated and **distorted hair follicle**
-filled with **basophilic debris made of keratin and inflammatory cells**
-follicle is usually surrounded by chronic inflammation

Perforating calcific elastosis (periumbilical perforating pseudoxanthoma elasticum)

-rare disease most common in obese, multiparous, African Americans, middle-aged women
-presents as lax, well-circumscribed, reticulated, or cobble-stoned plaques with keratotic surface papules
-occurring in the periumbilical region

Histopathology
-acanthotic epidermis with pseudoepitheliomatous hyperplasia
-altered short, curled, and calcified elastic fibers throughout the dermis
-elastic fibers extruded through the skin by transepidermal elimination

Reactive perforating collagenosis

Familial variant
-extremely rare
-childhood onset of painless keratotic papules on the upper extremities and site of trauma
-lesions spontaneously regress in 6-8 weeks, leaving minor scarring
-lesions may recur throughout life

Acquired variant, Kyrle disease
-adult onset, commonly associated with diabetes and renal failure
-pruritic keratotic papules on the trunk and extremities with central "cone-shaped" plug
-when associated with renal failure, the term Kyrle disease is used
-predilection for legs (#1)
-occurs in 10% of patients on hemodialysis
-lesions heal spontaneously but new ones continue to develop

Histopathology
Familial variant
-irregular epidermal proliferation with hyperkeratosis
-central **"volcano-like"** indentation filled with **blue basophilic degenerated collagen** and acute inflammation

Kyrle disease
-wider lesion with hyperkeratotic epidermis
-more shallow central indentation filled with keratin
-**parakeratosis is present within the plug**
-mild dermal inflammation

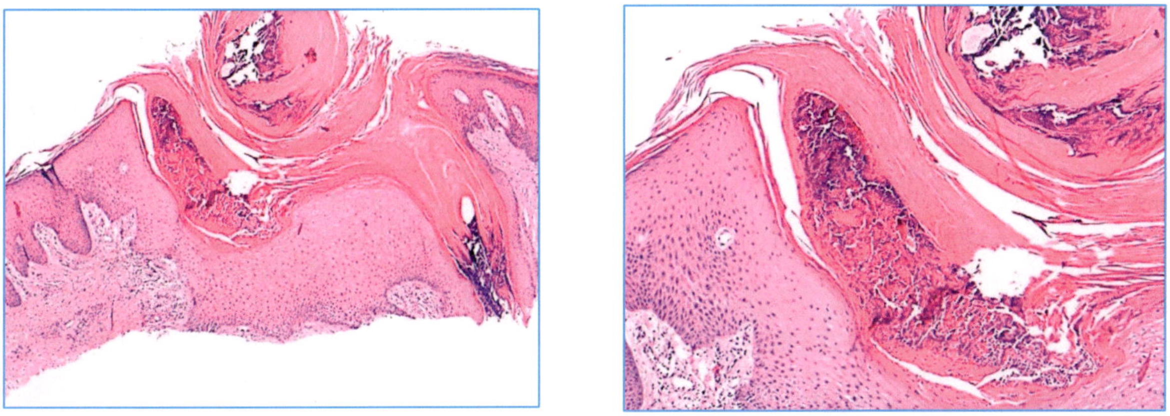

Perforating folliculitis with dilated and distorted hair follicle filled with debris made of keratin and inflammatory cells

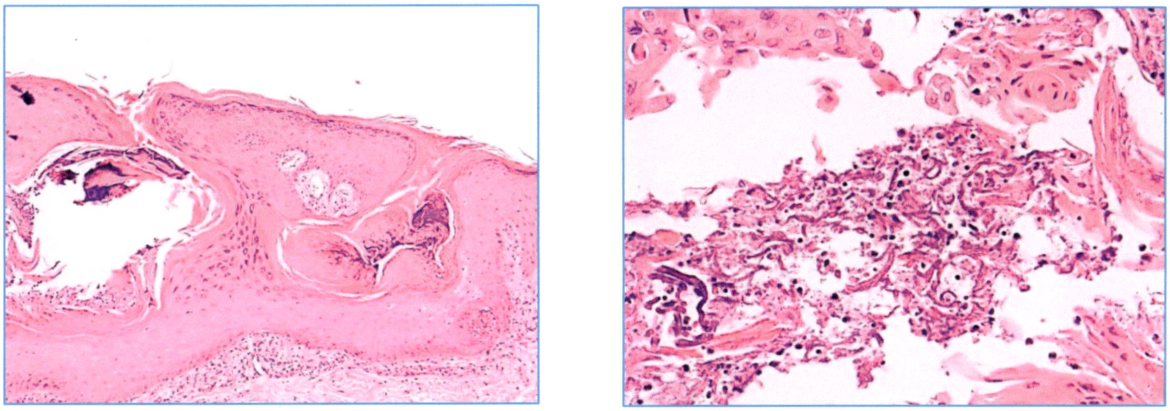

Elastosis perforans serpiginosa with irregular epidermis forming channel filled with degenerated pink elastic fibers and inflammation

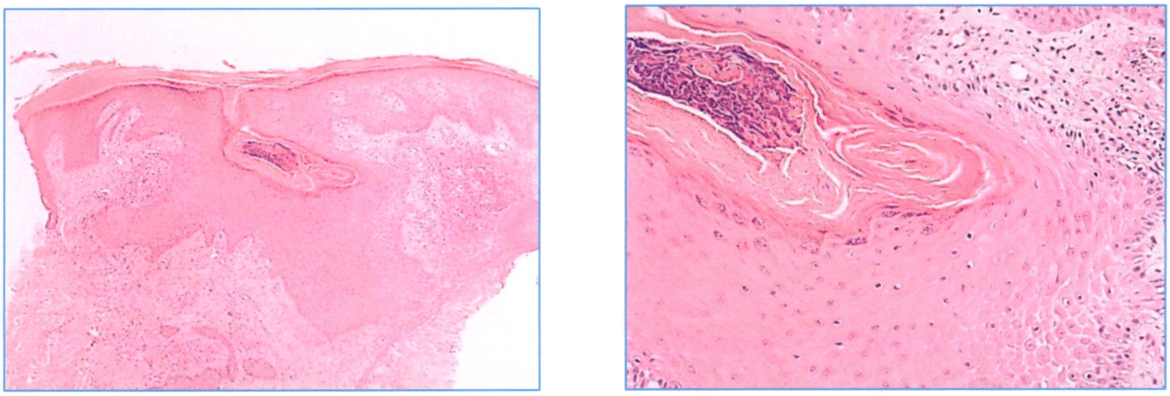

Reactive perforating collagenosis with deeper, "volcano shaped" epidermal indentation filled with basophilic collagen and inflammation

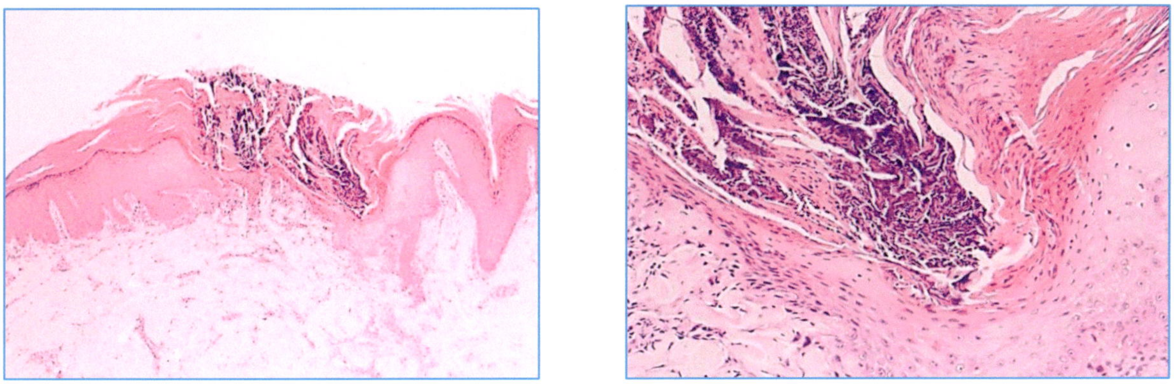

Kyrle disease with shallow epidermal indentation filled with basophilic collagen and keratin with parakeratosis

Alterations of collagen and elastin

CHONDRODERMATITIS NODULARIS HELICIS

-inflammatory skin condition of the ear, likely due to chronic pressure
-most commonly affects middle-aged or elderly men
-painful crusted nodule on the helix or antihelix of the ear
-surface is frequently ulcerated

Histopathology
-centrally **ulcerated hyperkeratotic, acanthotic epidermis**
-underlying ulcerated epidermis is prominent degenerated fibrin with **blue-gray chondroid appearance**
-surrounding **granulation tissue** is present

RELAPSING POLYCHONDRITIS

-uncommon chronic recurrent disease of cartilage
-most commonly affects ear (#1), nose, joint, respiratory tract
-frequently bilateral
-favors middle-aged individuals
-erythema, edema, and tenderness of the ear and/or nose
-recurrent episodes of disease results in flabby "cauliflower" ears and "saddle" nose
-25% fatality rate due to respiratory and cardiovascular complications

Histopathology
-focal vacuolization and **pyknosis of chondrocytes**
-perichondrial tissue with **mixed inflammation**

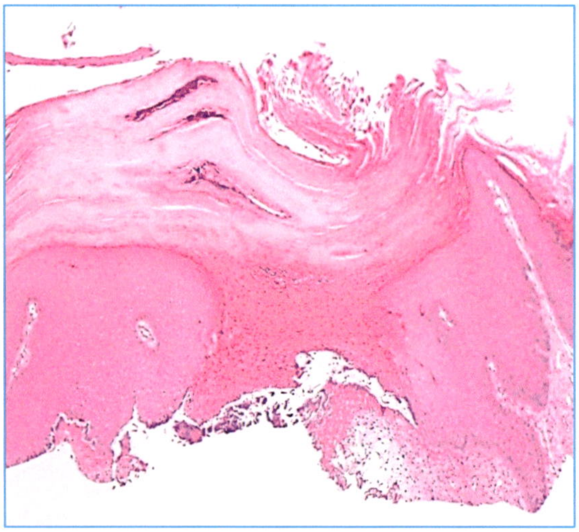

CNH with ulcerated hyperkeratotic, acanthotic epidermis

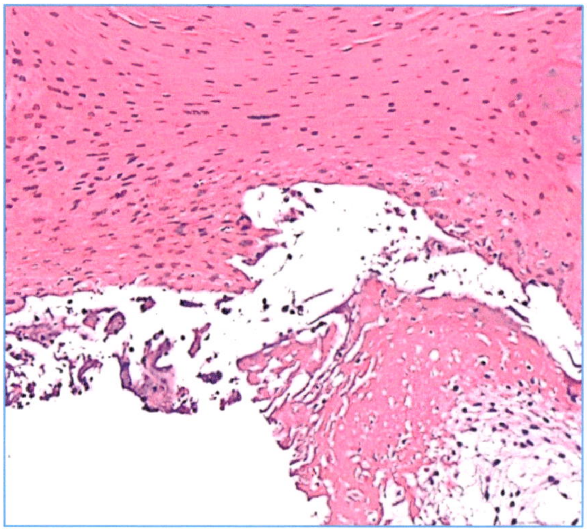

CNH with degenerated pink fibrin and bluish chondroid material

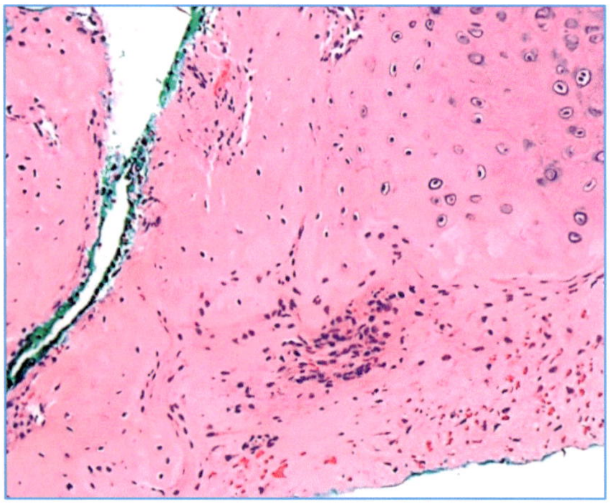

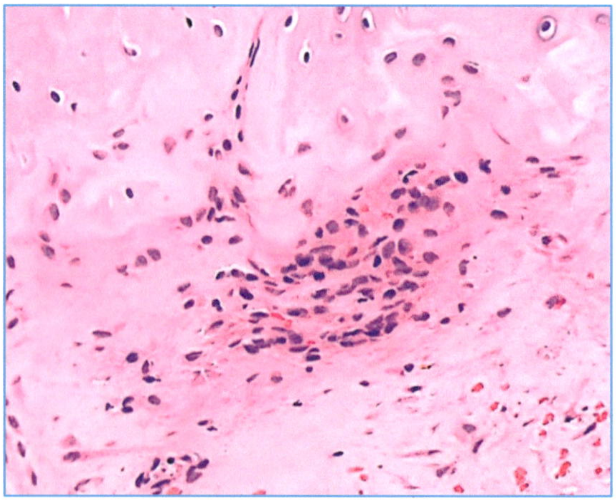

Relapsing polychondritis with pyknotic chondrocytes and mixed inflammation

PSEUDOXANTHOMA ELASTICUM

-autosomal recessive inherited disorder of connective tissue due to *ABCC6* gene mutation
-presents in childhood or early adulthood
-disturbance of elastic tissues in the skin, large blood vessels, and eyes
-characterized by yellowish papules that coalesce into plaques creating the appearance of "plucked chicken skin"
-skin is generally soft and lax and may gradually become loose and hang in folds
-popliteal and antecubital fossa, axilla, groin, and periumbilical areas are favored sites
-papules can also be present on the soft palate, labia, and vagina
-gastrointestinal hemorrhage, cardiovascular disease, claudication, and blindness are potential complications

Histopathology

-numerous scattered, fragmented, small elastic fibers in the dermis
-**elastic fibers are short, curled, and irregular**
-**calcium is deposited** on elastic fibers giving **crimson, dark purple-red color**
-VVG stain for elastics and Von Kossa stain for calcium can be used but are not necessary

CUTIS LAXA

-group of rare disorders characterized by loose, hanging skin that may occur in several inherited forms (AR, AD, XLR)
-can also be acquired
-when stretched, inelastic skin returns to place abnormally slowly
-easy bruising is not associated
-affects skin on the face, arms, legs, and trunk
-affected individuals and children have prematurely aged appearance and "bloodhound facies"
-the joints are often abnormally loose
-cardiovascular, pulmonary complications are common

Histopathology

-on H&E slides skin looks normal
-VVG special stain for elastic fibers shows diminished number of dermal elastic fibers
-residual elastic fibers are short, fragmented, and clumped

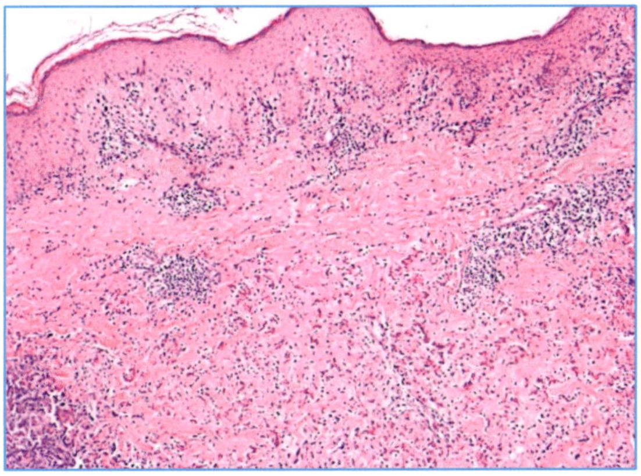

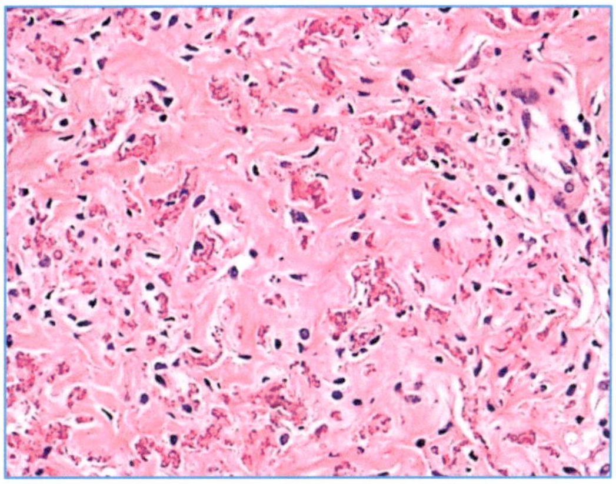

PXE with crimson colored, prominent, small and fragmented elastic fibers scattered in the dermis

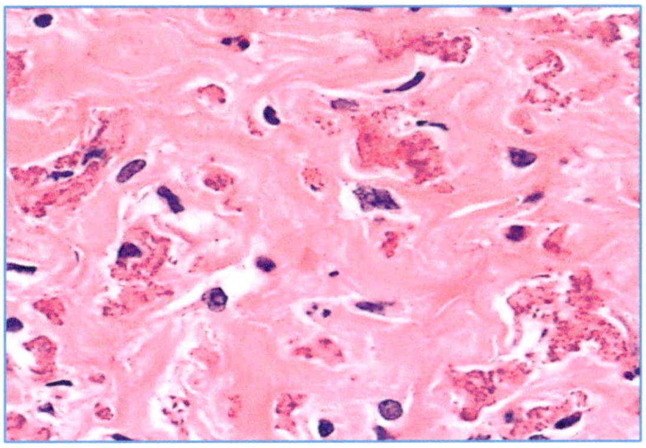

PXE with purple calcium deposits on broken elastic fibers

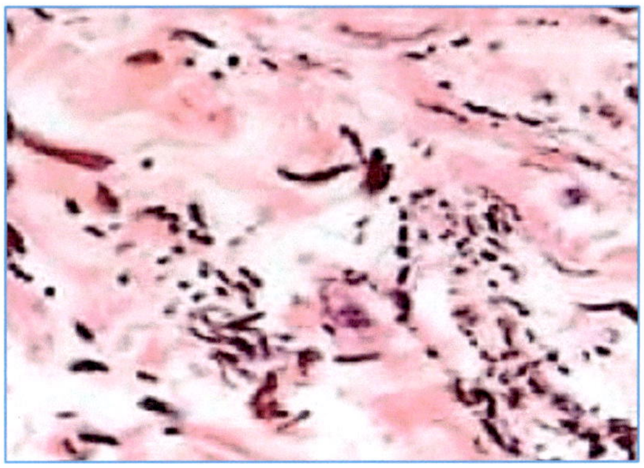

Cutis laxa with decreased number of short, fragmented elastic fibers (VVG stain)

Alterations of collagen and elastin

HOW TO APPROACH ALTERATIONS OF DERMAL COLLAGEN AND ELASTIN

IF SKIN APPEARS HISTOLOGICALLY NORMAL

-cutis laxa	loose hanging skin	short, fragmented elastic fibers (VVG)
-anetoderma	atrophic patches	decreased or absent elastic fibers (VVG)
-erythema ab igne	"net-like" patches	fragmented elastic fibers in mid dermis (VVG)

IF SCAR IS PRESENT

-scar	horizontal fibrosis with vertical vessels
-hypertrophic scar	nodular fibrosis with swirling vessels
-keloid	dark pink thick collagen
-aplasia cutis	newborn with an ulcer that scars

IF ADIPOSE TISSUE ABUT THE EPIDERMIS

-focal dermal hypoplasia

IF SKIN IS SCLEROTIC

-morphea/scleroderma	sclerotic dermis and subcutis	focal lymphocytic aggregates
-connective tissue nevus	thickened dermis and subcutis	no inflammation
-scleredema	thick collagen with empty spaces	variable mucin
-scleromyxedema	fibrosis with fibroblast proliferation	mucin
-nephrogenic systemic sclerosis	similar to scleromyxedema but with more mucin and involves subcutis	

IF ELASTIC FIBERS ARE DAMAGED

-solar elastosis	gray blue damaged elastic fibers
-collagenous and elastotic marginal plaques of the hand	gray blue damaged elastic fibers entangled with damaged collagen
-pseudoxanthoma elasticum	crimson colored Ca deposits on top of broken elastics

IF EPIDERMIS IS ULCERATED OR PERFORATED AND THERE IS CLINICAL CONCERN FOR SCC

-chondrodermatitis nodularis helicis	ear	excoriated epidermis with chondroid dermal material
-elastosis perforans serpiginosa	epidermal channel with elastin (pink)	
-reactive perforating collagenosis	epidermal channel with degenerated collagen (blue)	
-Kyrle disease	shallow epidermal lesion filled with keratin and parakeratosis	
-perforated folliculitis	distorted follicle with degenerated collagen (blue)	

Chapter 13

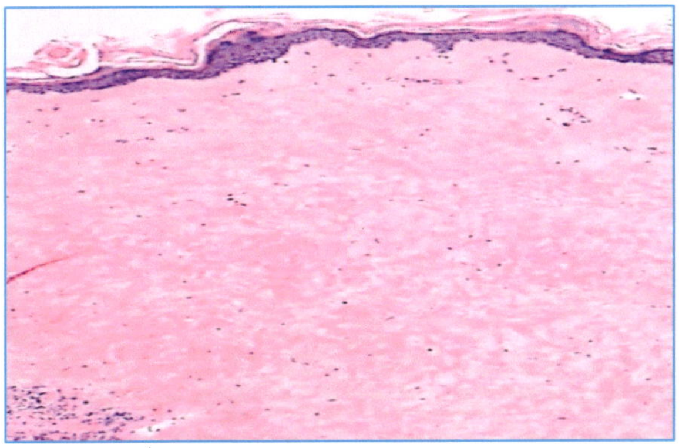

Morphea with fibrotic, square biopsy with no adnexae

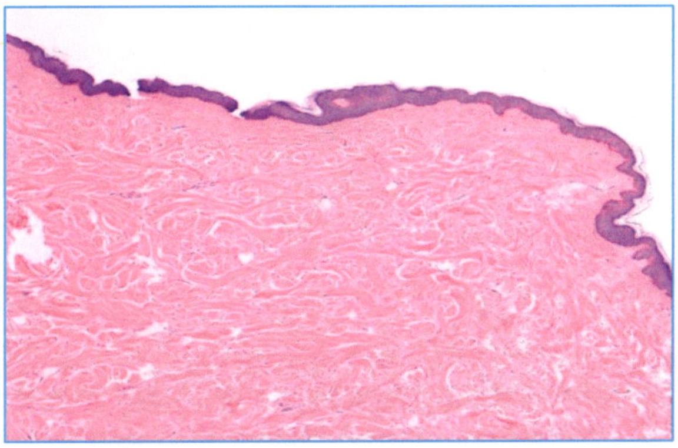

Collagenoma with histology similar to morphea; clinical correlation is necessary to separate them

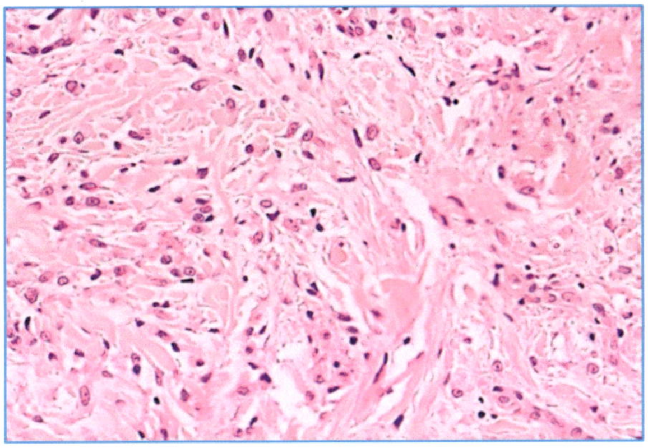

Scleromyxedema with sclerosis and numerous fibroblasts

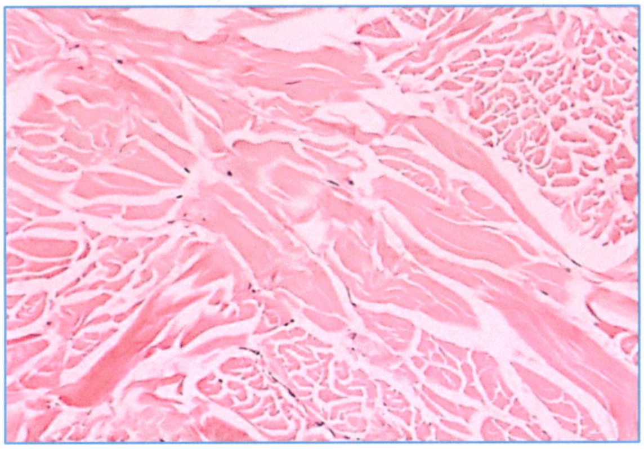

Scleredema with empty spaces in between collagen fibers

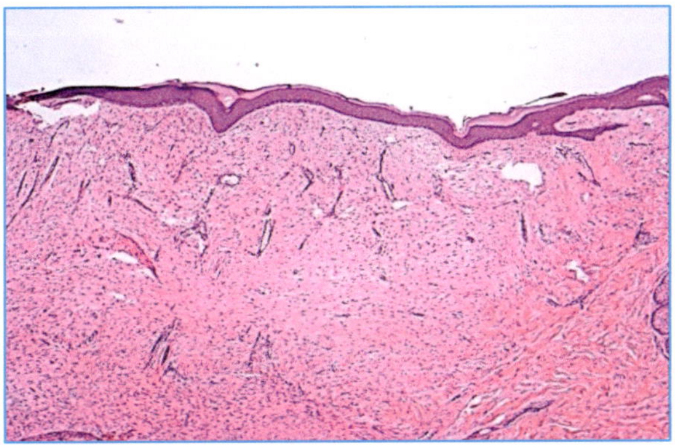

Scar with horizontal fibrosis and vertical vessels

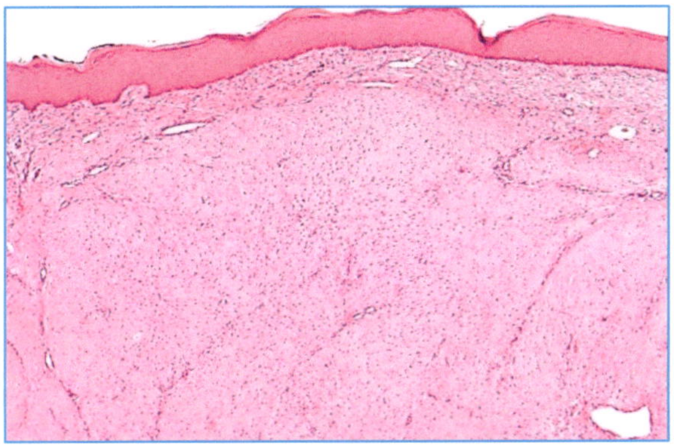

Hypertrophic scar with nodular fibrosis and irregularly oriented vessels

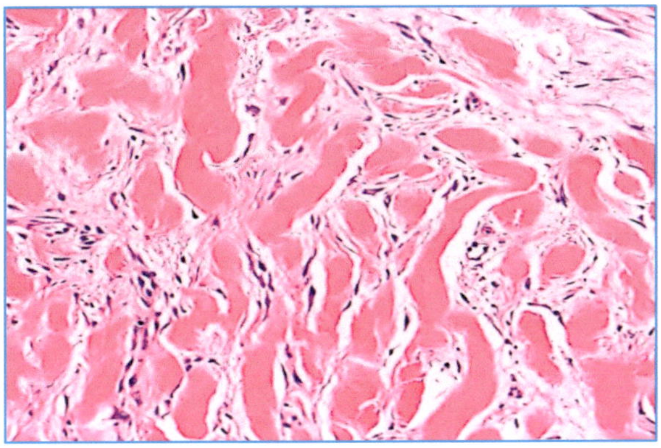

Keloid with thick, red-pink collagen

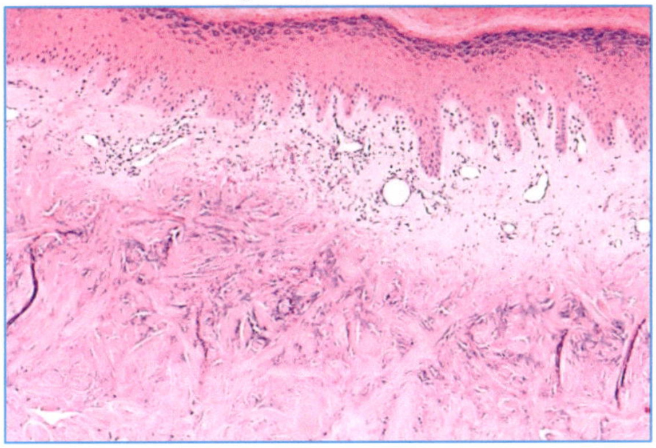

Collagenous and elastotic marginal plaques of the hand with entangled gray-blue collagen and elastic fibers

Alterations of collagen and elastin

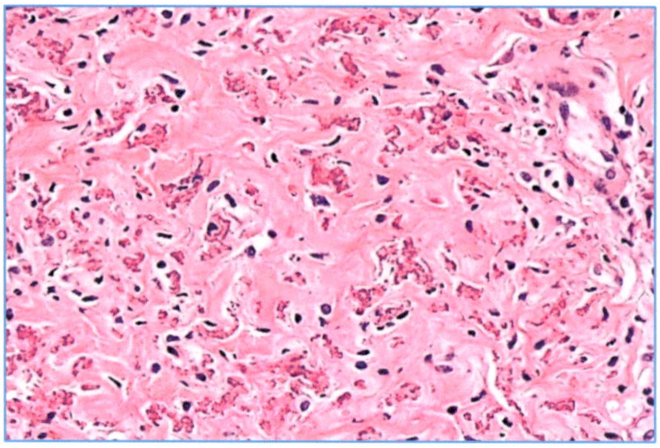

PXE with calcified, short, broken, purple-red elastic fibers

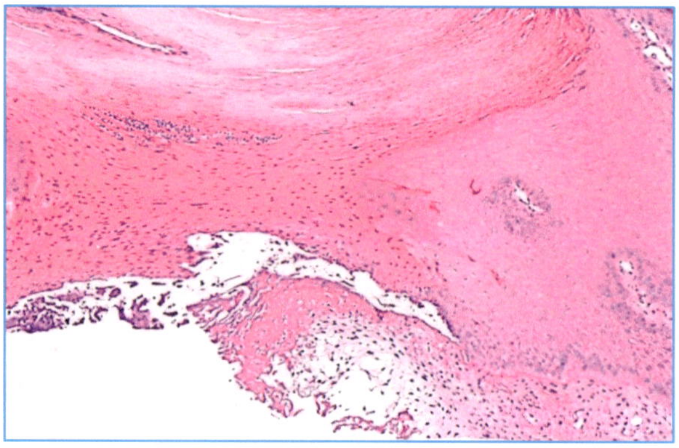

CDNH with dermal "cartilage-like" reaction

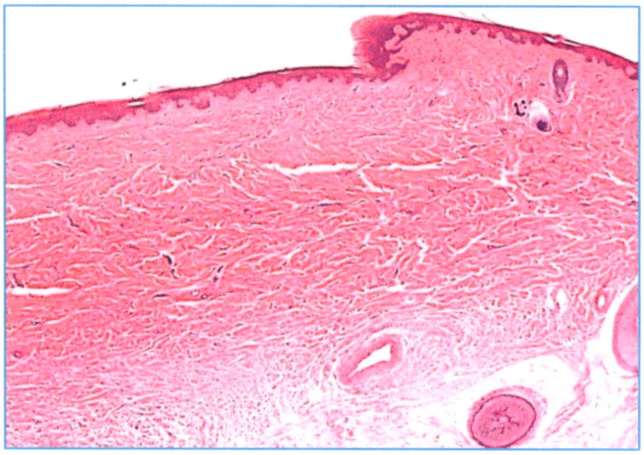

Aplasia cutis with sharply demarcated dermal scar

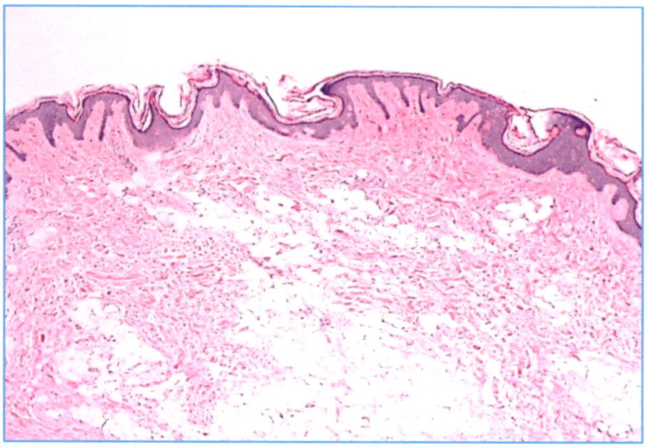

Focal dermal hypoplasia with adipose tissue abutting epidermis

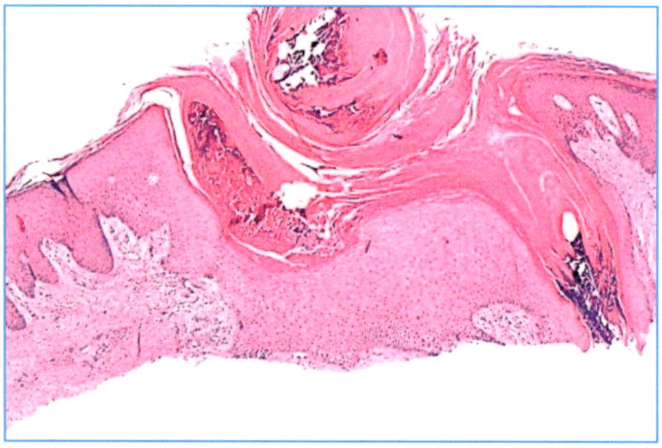

Perforating folliculitis with dilated, distorted follicle and basophilic debris

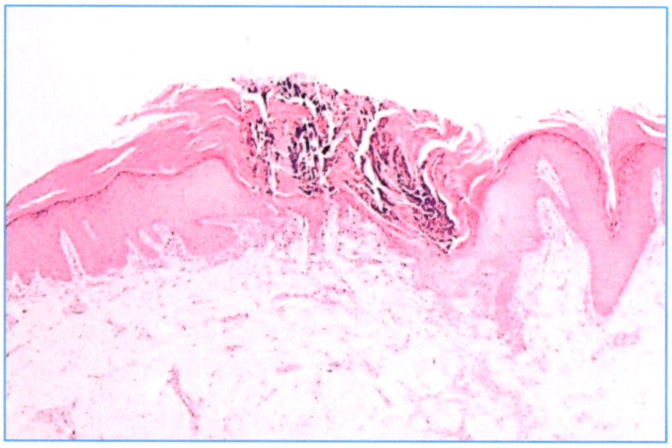

Kyrle disease with shallow indentation filled with keratin

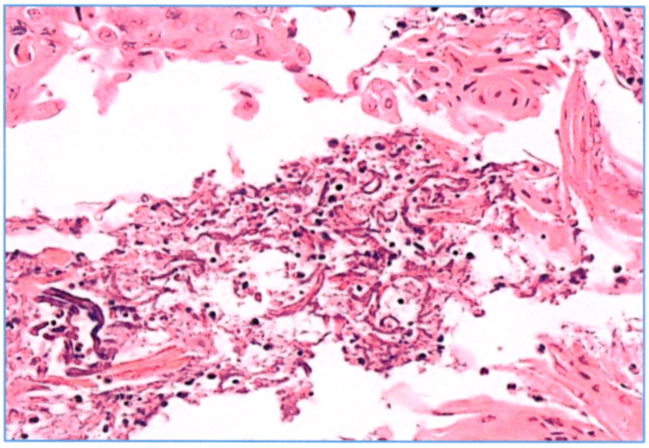

Elastosis perforans serpiginosa with eosinophilic, degenerated elastic fibers

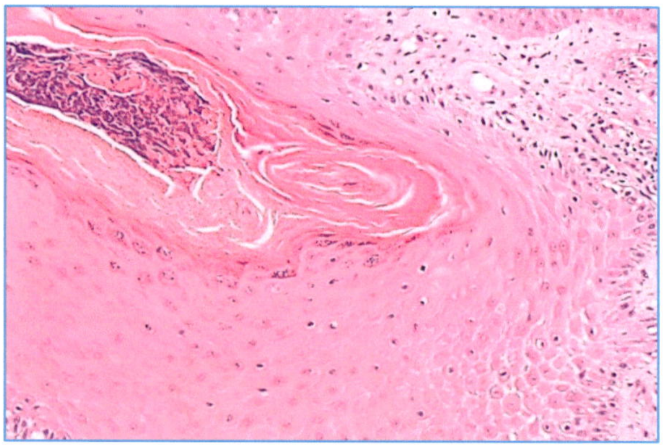

Reactive perforating collagenosis with basophilic, degenerated collagen

Chapter 14

DERMAL DEPOSITION DISORDERS

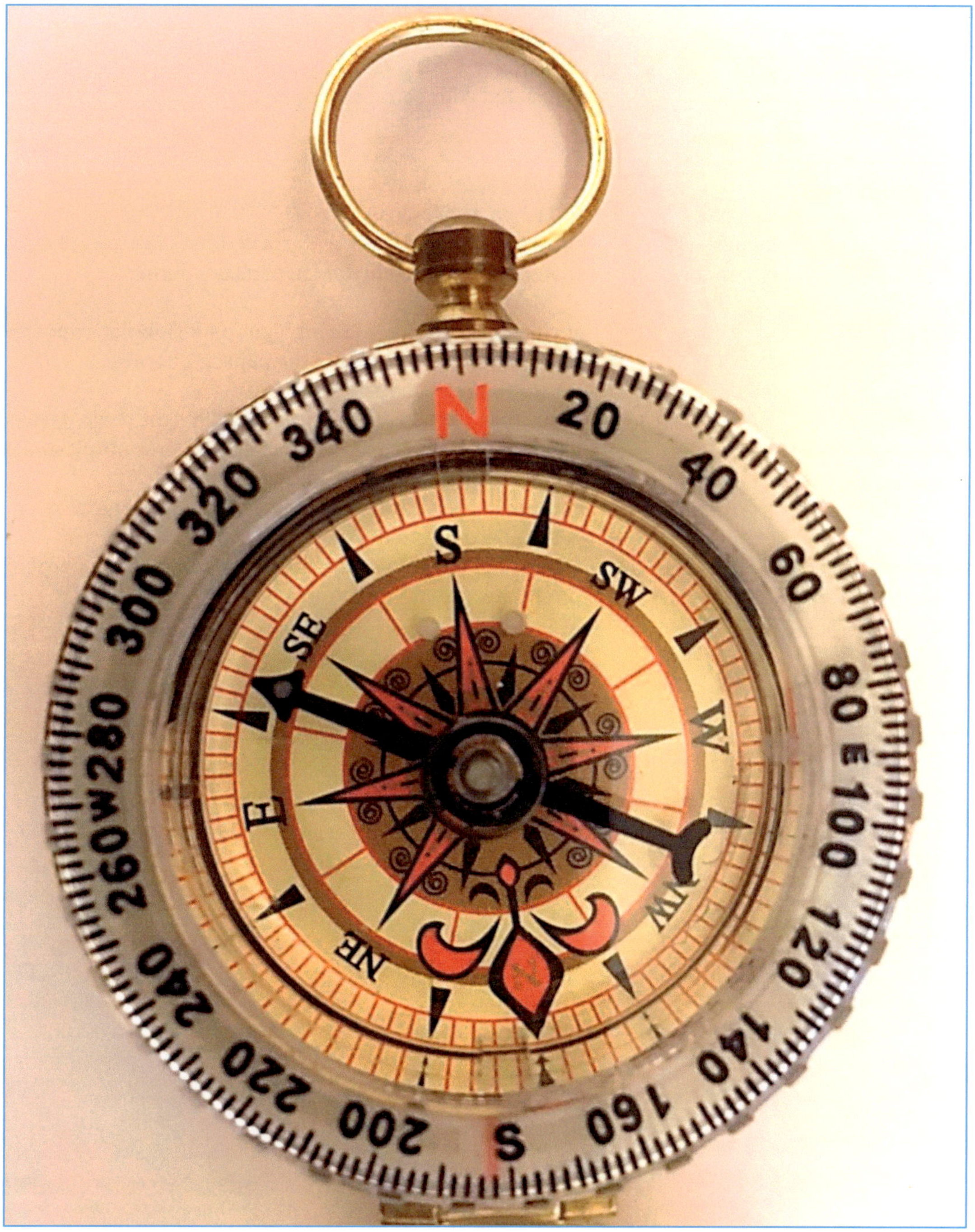

Dermal deposition disorders

AMYLOIDOSIS

-group of disorders characterized by extracellular amyloid distributions
-various clinical presentations divided into localized and systemic
- systemic is divided in primary systemic (deposits in the skin) and *secondary* systemic (skin rarely involved)

Localized amyloidosis

Lichen amyloidosis
-chronic, **itchy** condition
-numerous small waxy papules that coalesce into lichenified plaques
-extensor surface of lower extremities (particularly shins)

Macular amyloidosis
-**pruritic**, vague macules that coalesce and form a **"rippled" pattern**
-back is favored site

Nodular amyloidosis
-uncommon disorder
-single and rarely multiple brown-pink nodules or plaques
-extremities and face are favored sites
-can progress to systemic disease

Systemic amyloidosis

Primary systemic
-**non-pruritic** waxy papules on scalp, face, neck
-characteristic ecchymosis **"pinch purpura",** classically on eyelids
-carpal tunnel syndrome and macroglossia common
-idiopathic or associated with multiple myeloma (15%)
-kidney, heart, liver, GI tract are involved

Secondary systemic
-skin involvement is rare
-associated with chronic inflammatory disorders
-kidney, heart, liver, GI tract usually involved

Histopathology

Lichen amyloidosis
-**hypertrophic epidermis** with **small, light pink, round deposits** of **keratin derived amyloid** in papillary dermis

Macular amyloidosis
-**normal epidermis** with **scant, light pink globular deposits** of **keratin derived amyloid** in the papillary dermis

Nodular or plaque amyloidosis
-large mass of **cracked, immunoglobulin light chain derived pink amyloid** in the dermis and subcutis with present **plasma cells**

Primary systemic amyloidosis
-pink amyloid deposition around vessels and adnexal structures
-eventually amyloid fills the dermis
-**all types of amyloid** stains with **Congo Red** and has green birefringence with polarized light

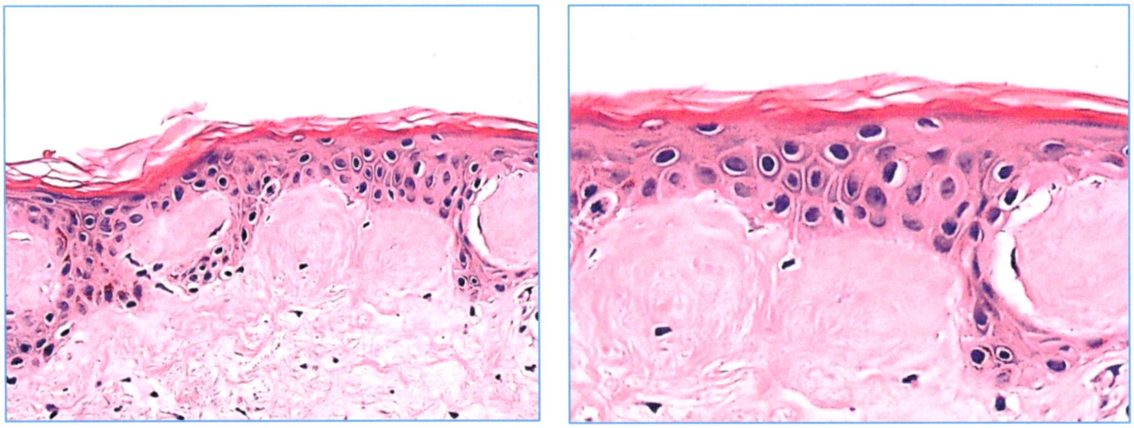

Macular amyloidosis with normal epidermis and pink deposits in papillary dermis

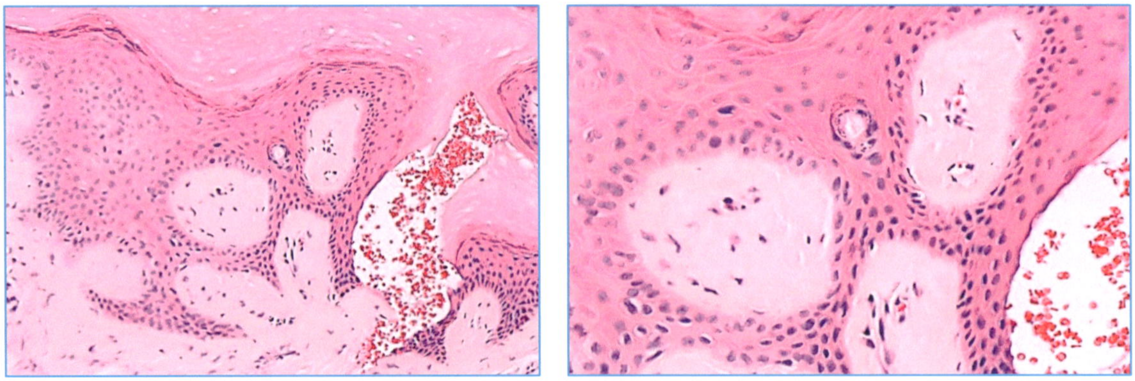

Lichen amyloidosis with hypertrophic epidermis and pink dermal deposits

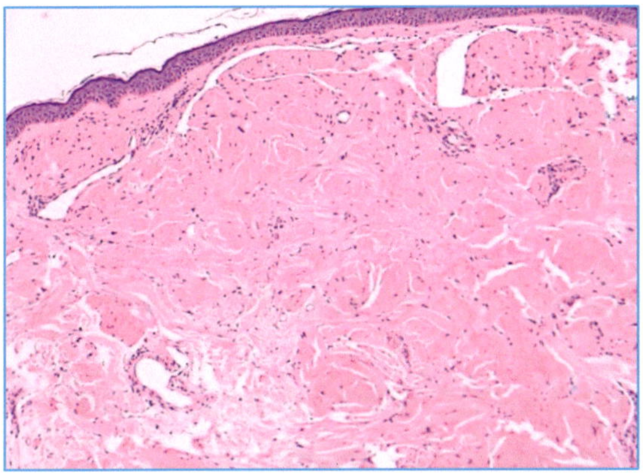

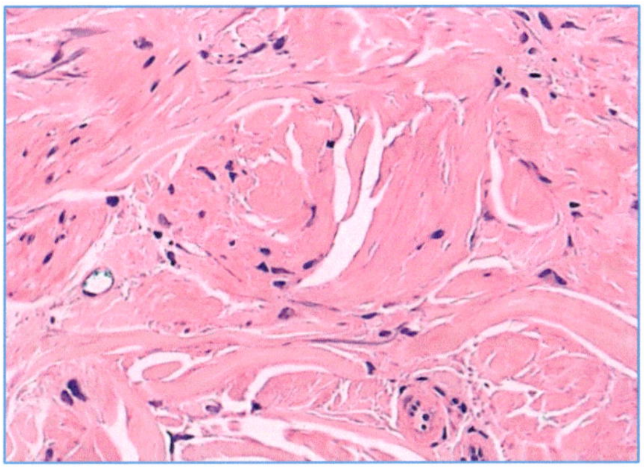

Nodular amyloidosis with large dermal deposits of pink, cracked amyloid

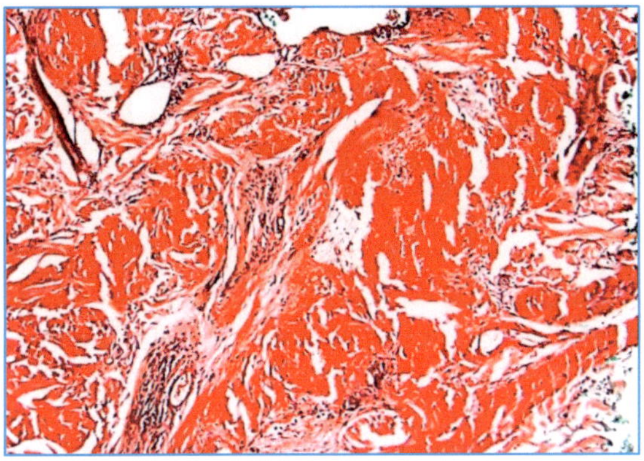

Nodular amyloid staining with nonpolarized Congo red stain

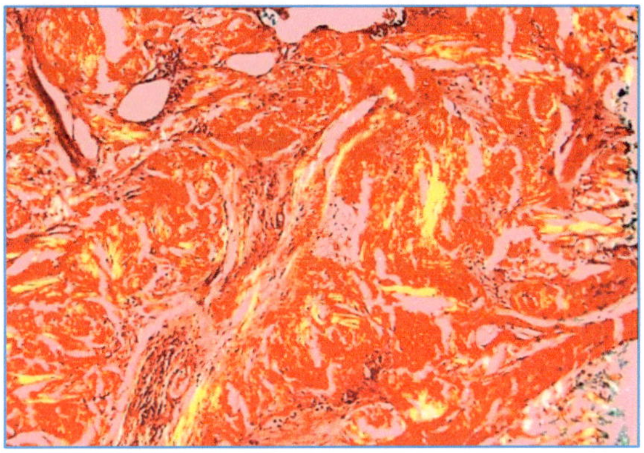

Nodular amyloid staining with polarized Congo red stain

COLLOID MILIUM

-degenerative, cutaneous deposition disorder

Adult type

-multiple translucent yellow or skin-colored papules that can form plaques
-minimal trauma leads to skin purpura
-induced by chronic UV exposure
-predilection for sun-exposed areas, face, hands, neck

Juvenile type

-very rare
-presents with papules/plaques on the face
-lesions are similar to lesions of adult type
-some present as part of erythropoietic protoporphyria

Histopathology of both types is very similar

Adult type

-**amorphous bluish pink** material with **irregular clefts** and **fissures** in the papillary dermis
-deposits **derived from degenerated elastic fibers**

Juvenile type

-**eosinophilic homogenous material** in the papillary dermis
-deposits are **derived from epidermal keratin**
-colloid **clefts are less prominent**

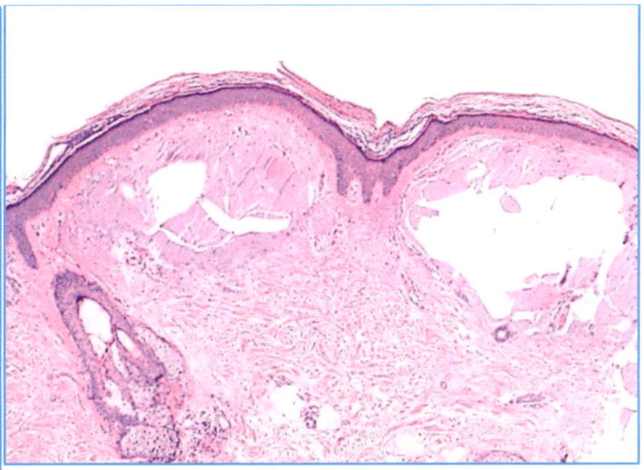

Adult type colloid milium with dermal bluish pink deposits with clefts and fissures

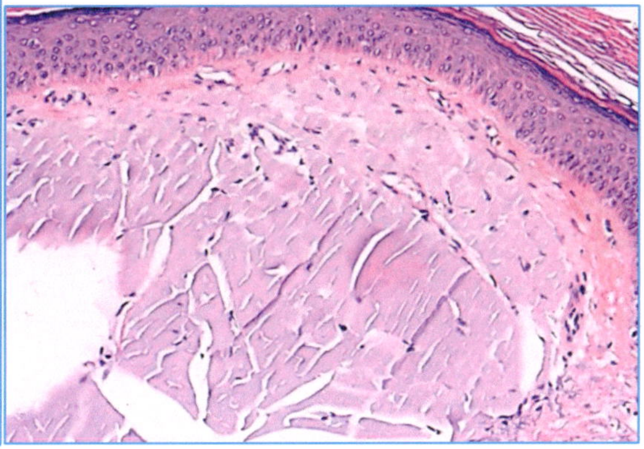

Dermal deposition disorders

MUCINOSIS

Group of cutaneous disorders that demonstrate presence of mucin

Digital mucous cyst

-benign cysts on the fingers/toes, typically at the distal interphalangeal (DIP) joints or in the proximal nail fold
-usually a solitary, 5-7 mm in size, skin-colored cystic nodule

Histopathology

-**acral skin** with attenuated epidermis and dermal mucin accumulation abutting the epidermis
-despite the name, it is **not a true cyst** but rather **pseudocyst** (epithelial lining is absent)

Focal dermal mucinosis

-adults with solitary flesh-colored papules or nodules
-predilection for face, trunk, proximal extremities

Histopathology

-atrophic epidermis with **poorly circumscribed dermal mucin**

Follicular mucinosis (alopecia mucinosa)

-erythematous firm plaque with alopecia, mostly on face, neck, or scalp
-if lesions are solitary or few in numbers, it usually follows benign course
-if there are multiple lesions, disease might be precursor or initial presentation of cutaneous T-cell lymphoma

Histopathology

-**intrafollicular mucin** with lymphocytic inflammation and **variable number of eosinophils**

Mucocele

-mucous pseudocyst in oral cavity
-most commonly occur on the inner surface of the lower lip (75% of cases)
-translucent to blue, mucous-filled, dome-shaped lesion
-single or multiple lesions may occur ranging from 1-15 mm in diameter.

Histopathology

-**submucosal mucin** surrounded by lymphocytes, histiocytes (muciphages) and some giant cells
-adjacent **salivary glands** are present

Myxedema

Generalized myxedema

-associated with **severe hypothyroidism**
-swollen face with puffiness around eyes
-swelling of arms and legs with non-pitting edema of hands

Pretibial myxedema

-associated with **hyperthyroidism**
-orange-colored, non-pitting, diffuse dermal infiltration on the lower legs

Histopathology

-prominent dermal and subcutaneous **mucin** with **normal number of fibroblasts**

Reticulated erythematous mucinosis (REM)

-chronic, indolent disease of women in 3-4th decade of life
-commonly start after intensive sun exposure
-erythematous reticulated plaques and patches favoring midline chest and back

Histopathology

-**perivascular lymphocytic infiltrate** with mildly separated collagen and **variable amount of dermal mucin**

Chapter 14

LICHEN MYXEDEMATOSUS

Scleromyxedema (**generalized lichen myxedematosus**)
-chronic, progressive disease usually in middle-aged adults
-multiple waxy papules that coalesce in plaques or are arranged in **linear** arrays
-predilection for dorsal hands, face (**"leonine facies"**), extensor extremities
-eventually develop diffuse infiltration with **"woody" skin** appearance
-usually **accompanied by monoclonal gammopathy** (IgGλ light chains) and may have systemic organ involvement, particularly GI and lung
-about 10% progress to multiple myeloma

Histopathology
-starts with disorganized collagen, fibroblast proliferation and **mucin separating collagen**
-established lesions show **CD34+ fibroblast proliferation** with significant **fibrosis and minimal mucin**

Papular mucinosis (localized lichen myxedematosus)
-**five localized forms** with **no gammapathy or systemic involvement**

Discrete papular lichen myxedematosus
-waxy, discrete firm papules on limbs and trunk
-may coalesce into nodules

Acral persistent papular mucinosis
-from few to over one hundred acral skin colored papules
-face and trunk are spared
-more common in women

Self-healing papular mucinosis
-sudden onset with ivory-colored papules on hands, neck, trunk
-in juveniles and young adults and commonly associated with acute arthritis
-spontaneously disappear over several months

Papular mucinosis of infancy
-yellow pink individual papules or localized grouping on the trunk and upper extremities
-at birth or soon after
-lesions persist and become static

Nodular lichen myxedematosus
-multiple yellowish nodules (6-10 mm) on the trunk or extremities

Histopathology
-focal or diffuse **mucin deposits** with variable fibroblast proliferation and **no fibrosis**

SCLEREDEMA (OF BUSCHKE)

-symmetrical hardening of subcutaneous tissue causing indurated shiny skin with "wood-like" consistency and loss of skin marking
-**type 1 scleredema** is an acute form that favor women and children
-typically starts with an infection, most often *Streptococcus pyogenes*
-hardening of face and neck skin quickly develops and spreads to the upper trunk and arms
-it usually improves spontaneously over six months to two years
-**type 2 scleredema** is not associated with infection and it starts more slowly and persists
-associated with abnormal paraproteins and multiple myeloma
-**type 3**, also called **scleredema diabeticorum**, occurs in diabetics, particularly adult men
-the skin of the neck and upper back slowly thickens over months or years and is persistent

Histopathology
-thick, **sclerotic collagen** separated by **"empty" spaces**
-the "empty" spaces contain **mucin that decreases and disappears with maturation** of the lesion

Dermal deposition disorders

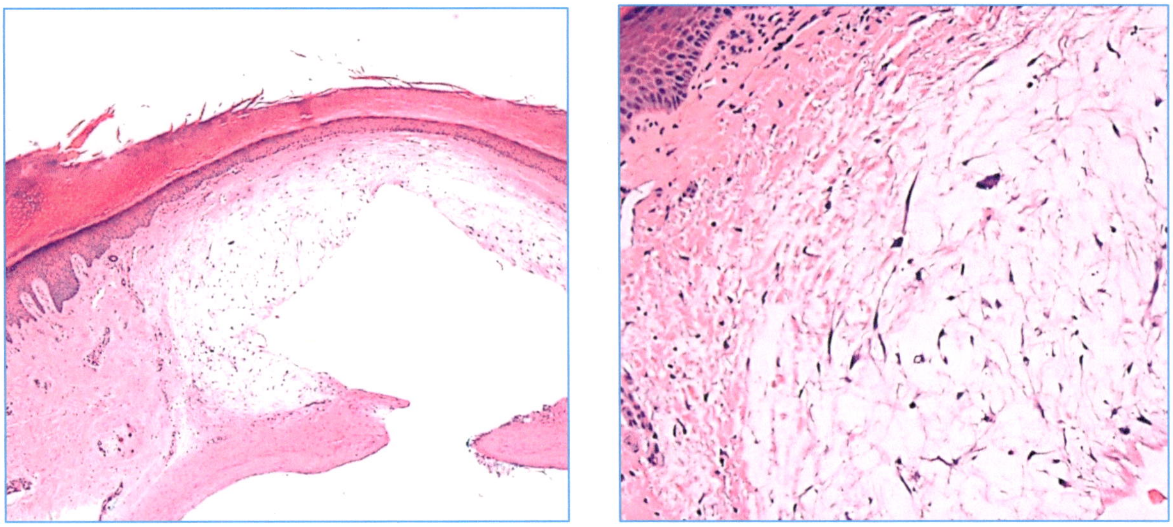

Digital mucous cyst with flattened acral epidermis and dermal accumulation of pale, bluish mucin

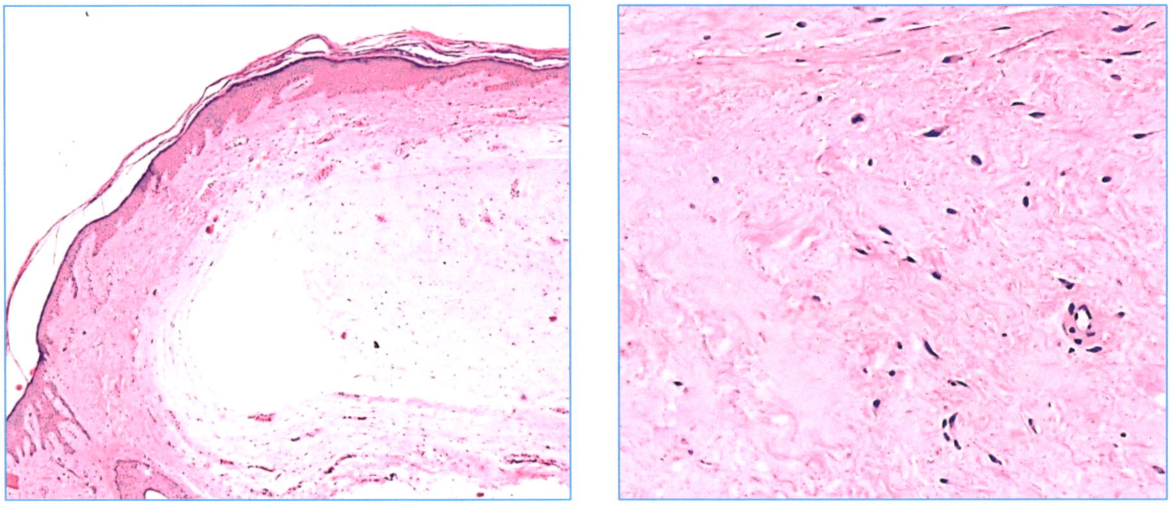

Focal dermal mucinosis forming dermal nodule filled with poorly circumscribed bluish mucin

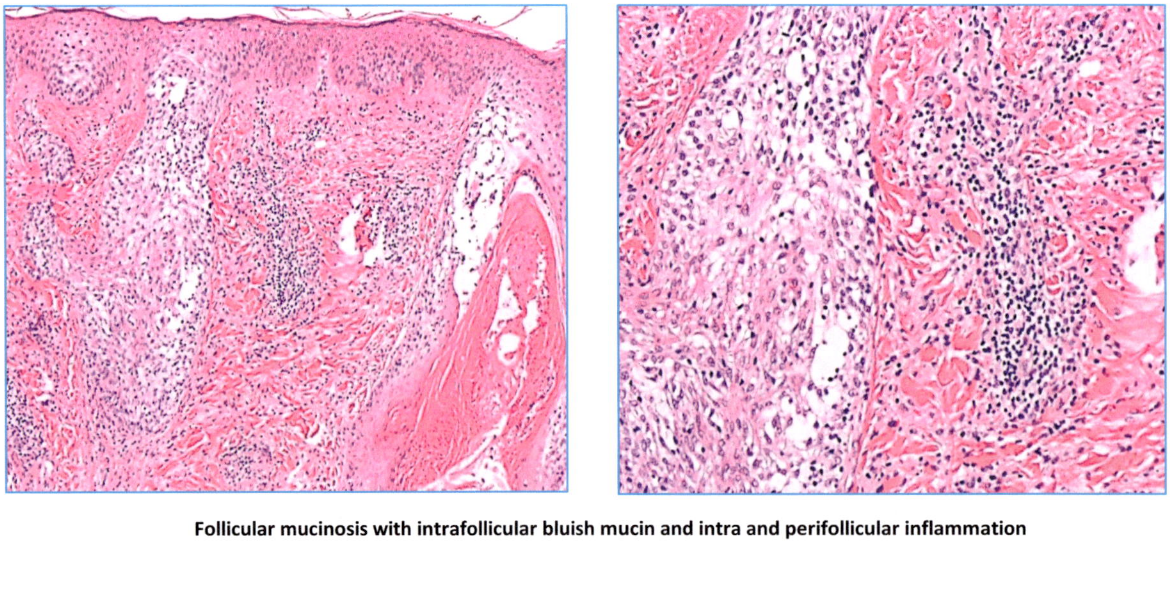

Follicular mucinosis with intrafollicular bluish mucin and intra and perifollicular inflammation

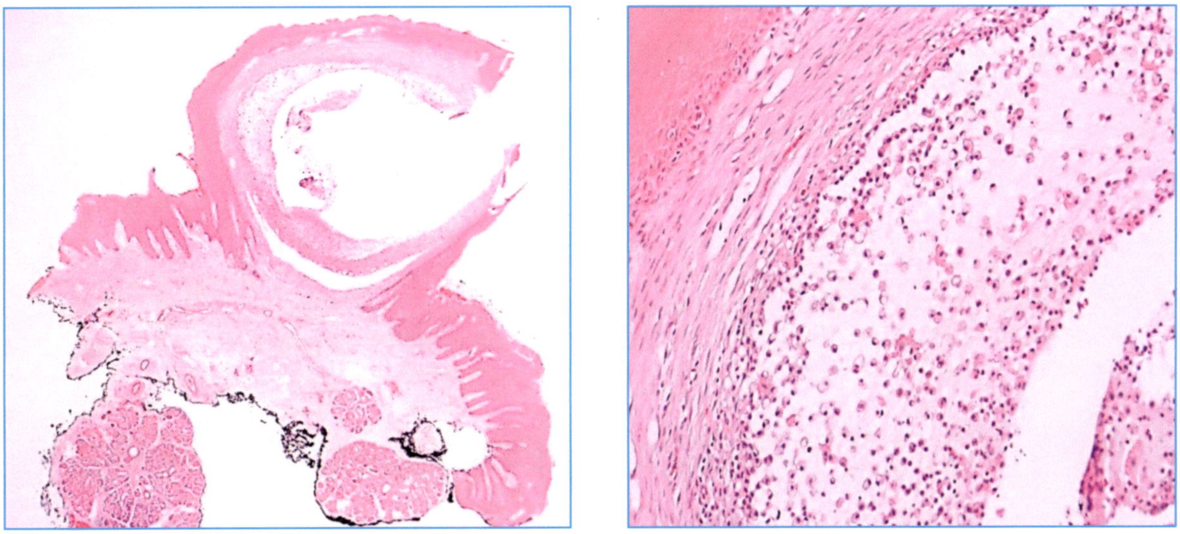

Mucocele next to salivary glands with mucin deposits surrounded by inflammation

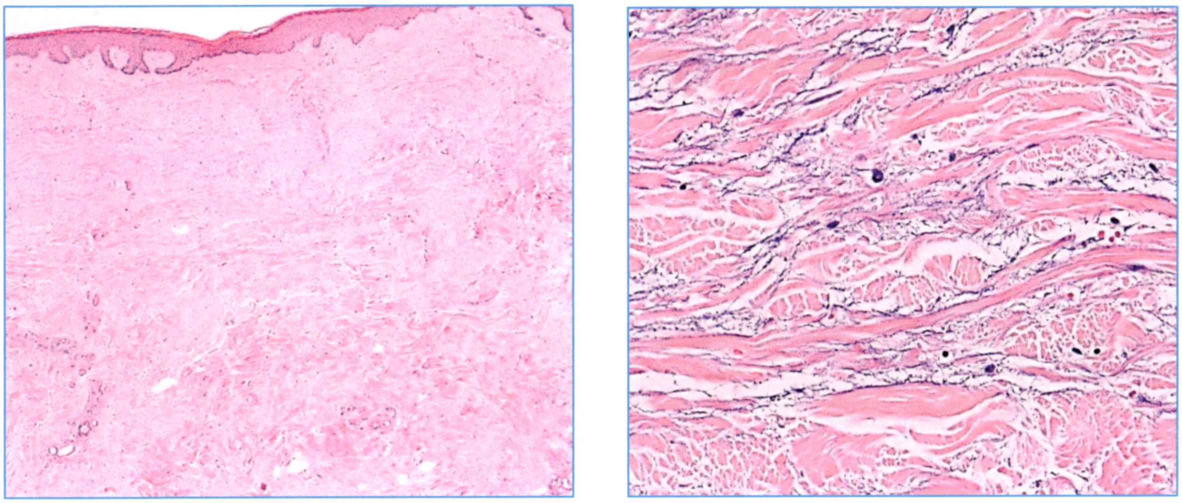

Myxedema with prominent dermal blue mucin in otherwise normal dermis

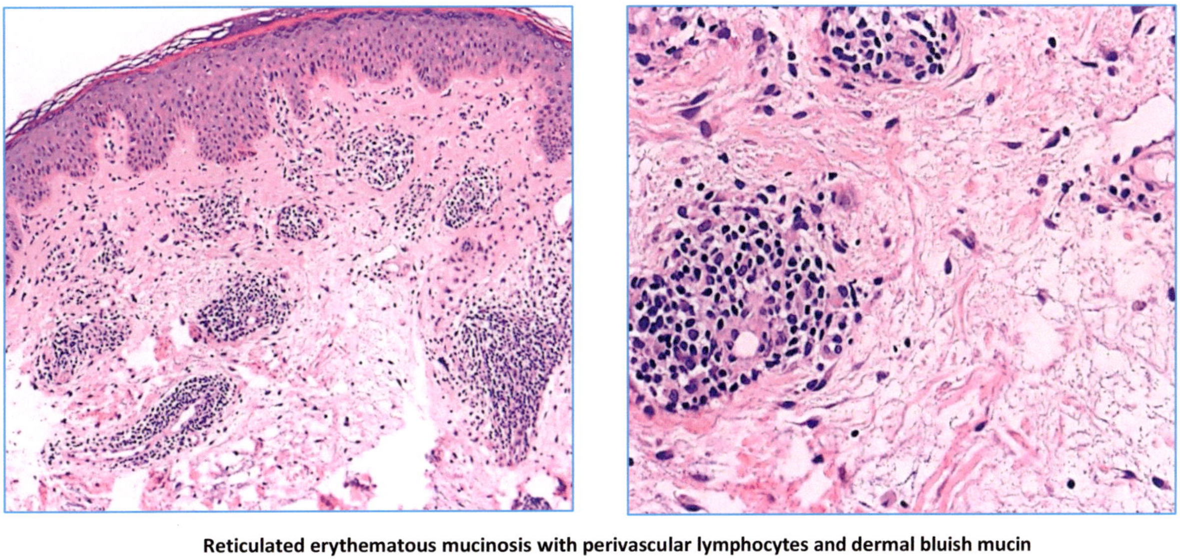

Reticulated erythematous mucinosis with perivascular lymphocytes and dermal bluish mucin

Dermal deposition disorders

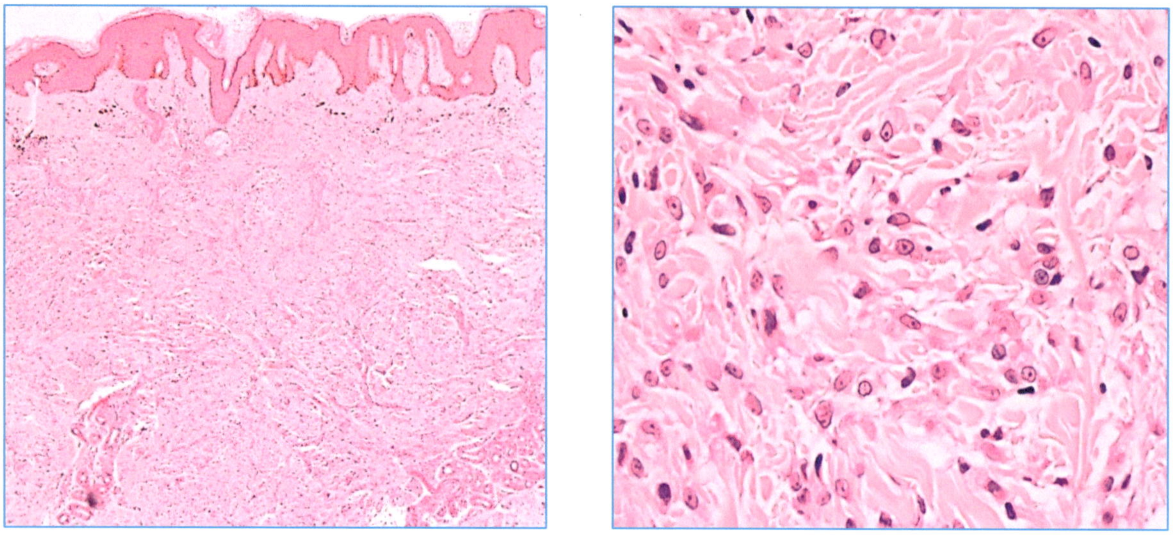

Scleromyxedema with fibroblast proliferation, fibrosis, and mucin

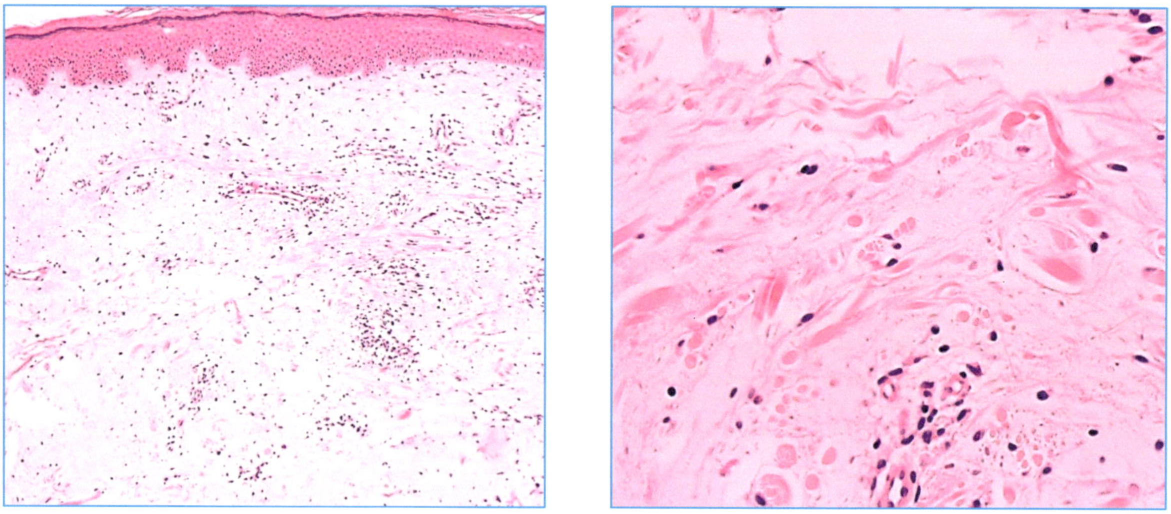

Papular mucinosis with diffuse deposit of bluish mucin with no significant dermal fibrosis

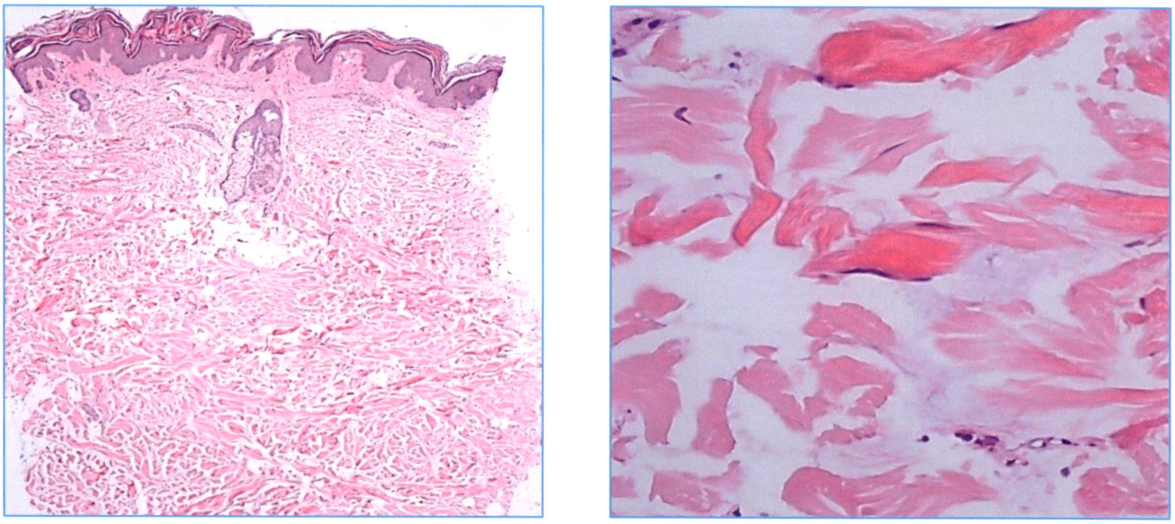

Scleredema with thick collagen separated by empty spaces, some filled with bluish mucin

Chapter 14

CALCINOSIS CUTIS

-dystrophic or idiopathic calcium deposition in the dermis with many clinical presentations

Subepidermal calcified nodule

-firm dermal nodule in young children of idiopathic etiology or associated with dermatomyositis

-head, ear, extremities are most common sites

Scrotal calcinosis

-calcified nodule(s) in the scrotum, probably the result of calcification of a ruptured epidermal inclusion cyst

Auricular calcinosis

-nodule(s) on one or both ears in older individuals

-associated with trauma, frost bite, and Addison disease

Tumoral calcinosis

-large nodule overlying the large joint

-more common in African Americans

Dystrophic calcification

-calcifications at a prior site of trauma or inflammation

-associated with dermatomyositis/collagen vascular diseases

Metastatic calcifications

-occurs in the setting of hypercalcemia

-associated with hyperparathyroidism, hypervitaminosis D

Histopathology

-**large, purple, amorphous calcium deposits** (Van Kossa stain positive) in deep dermis and subcutis

CALCIPHYLAXIS

-middle-aged and older patients

-more common in women

-classically seen in end stage renal disease

-**painful,** retiform, purpuric plaques arising from ischemia due to calcium depositions in blood vessels

-skin eventually becomes necrotic and ulcerates

-predisposition for fatty areas such as abdomen, buttocks

Histopathology

-dark purple calcium deposits in **subcutis** or deep dermis

-mostly **within the wall of small and medium sized vessels**

-focal fat necrosis and calcification of soft tissue

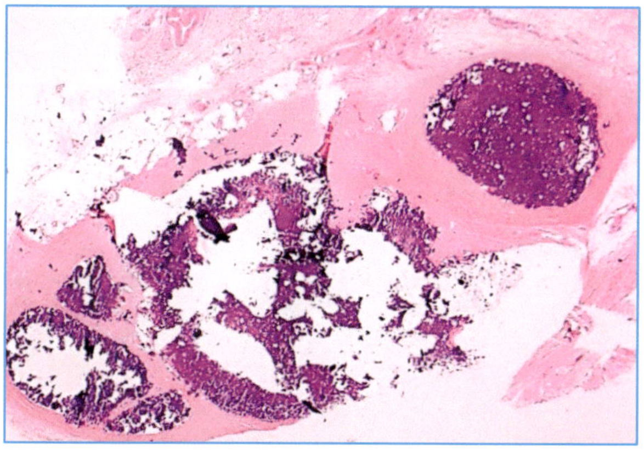
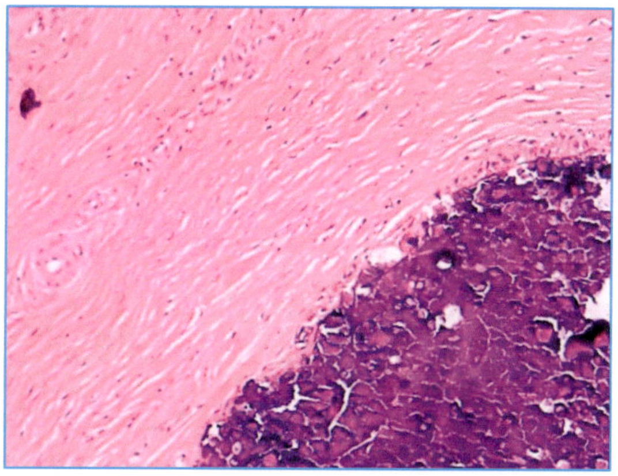

Calcinosis cutis with large dermal and subcutaneous deposits of calcium

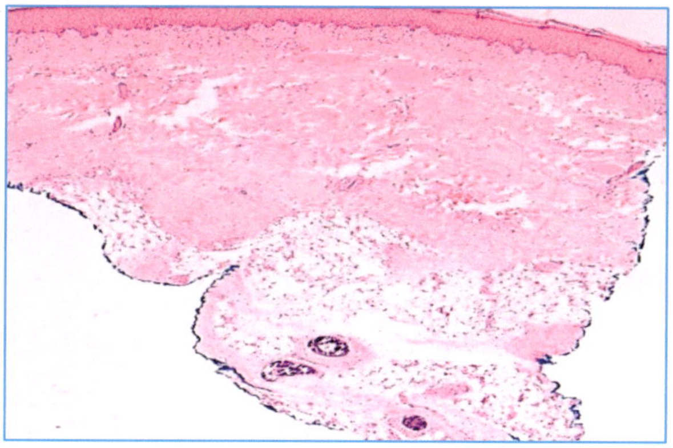
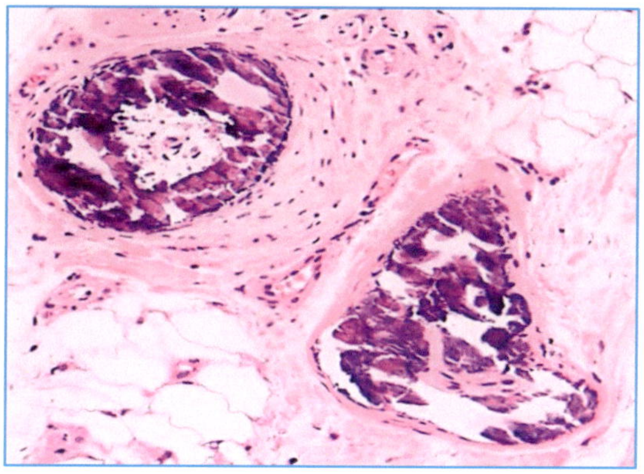

Calciphylaxis with intravascular calcium deposits in subcutis

Dermal deposition disorders

TATTOOS

-tattoos elicit initial inflammatory response that subsides leaving permanent tissue reaction
-occasional complications are well documented:
-allergic reaction -photosensitivity reaction
-keloid formation -granulomatous foreign body reaction
-infection (typically mycobacterial) introduced at time of tattooing
-**amalgam tattoo**: grey-blue or black area of discoloration on the mucous membranes of the mouth due to deposition of dental **a**malgam
-**Monsel's reaction**: reaction to 20% ferric subsulfate used for hemostasis in procedures (e.g. biopsy)
-presents as reddish-brown discoloration with a sharp demarcation from untreated skin

Histopathology
-**randomly distributed dermal black pigment with no inflammatory reaction**
-regardless of tattoo color on skin surface, on histological slides all tattoo dyes deposits were always black
-however, in more recent tattoos surface red dye also appears red on histological slide
-in **older** tattoos pigment becomes more **concentrated around dermal capillaries**
In the case of **hypersensitivity reaction:**
-lymphohistiocytic infiltrate with eosinophils with scattered tattoo pigment
-inflammation can be exuberant producing pseudolymphoma picture
In the case of **granulomatous foreign body reaction**:
-non-caseating granulomas with scattered tattoo pigment
In **amalgam tattoo:**
-black granular foreign body is present in submucosa
-surrounding fibrosis, **salivary glands**, and mild chronic inflammation
In **Monsel's reaction:**
-scar and large multinucleated histiocytes with granules and clumps of **dark brown pigment**

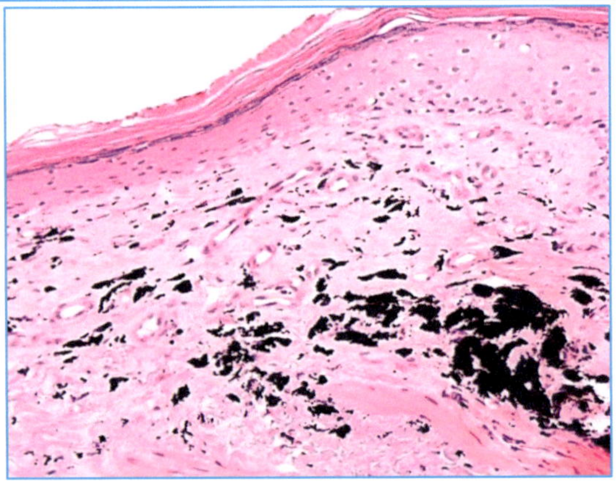
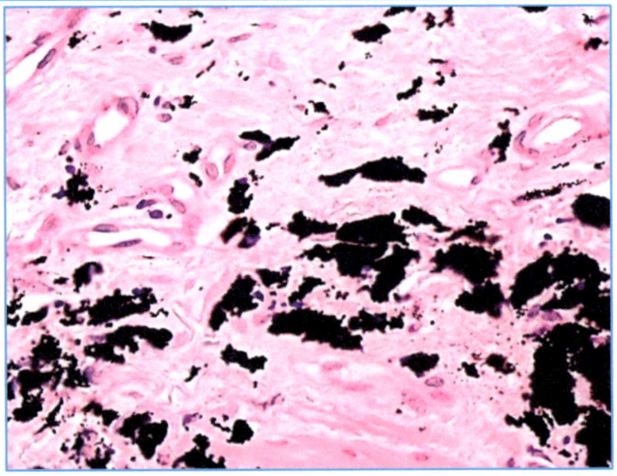

Tattoo with randomly distributed dermal black deposits

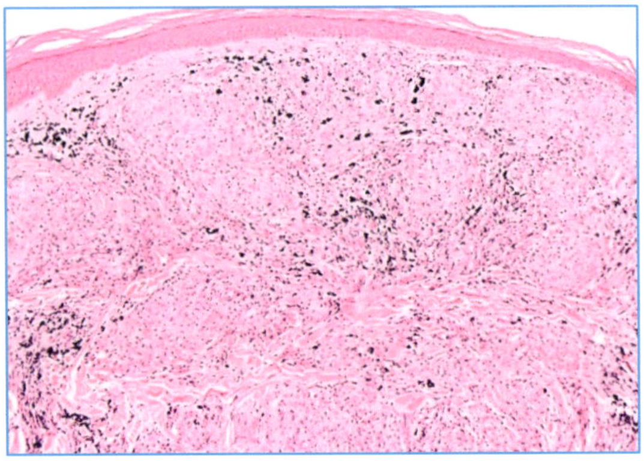
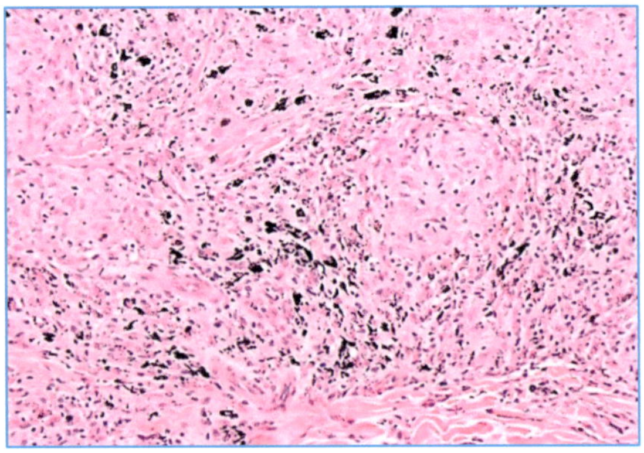

Histiocytes forming non-caseating granulomas with tattoo pigment

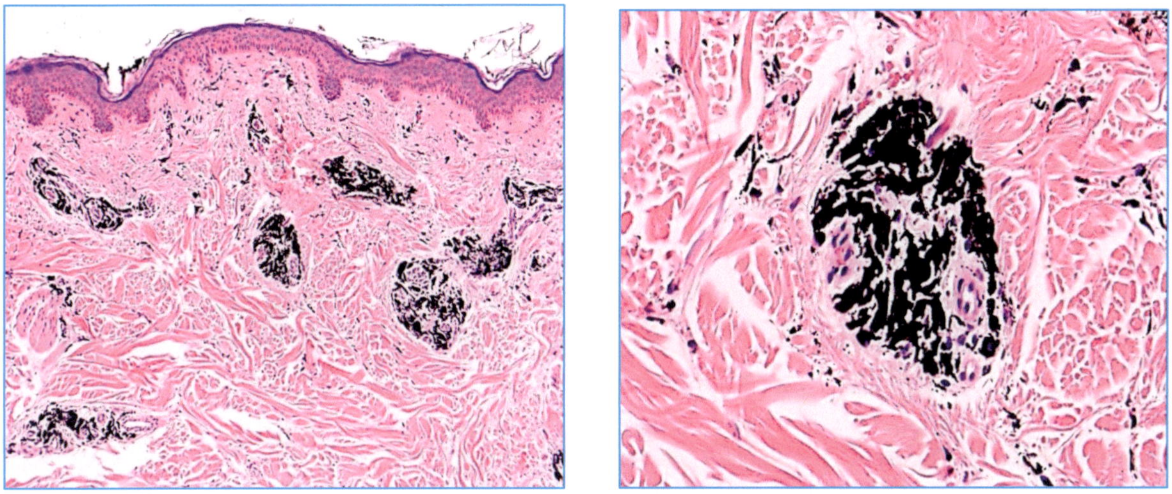

Old tattoo with perivascular deposits

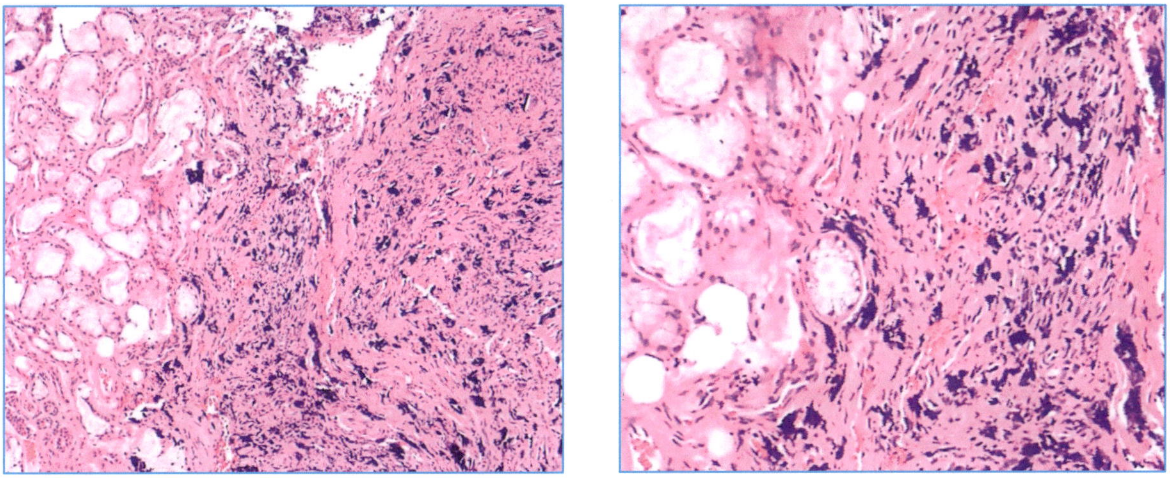

Amalgam tattoo adjacent to salivary glands

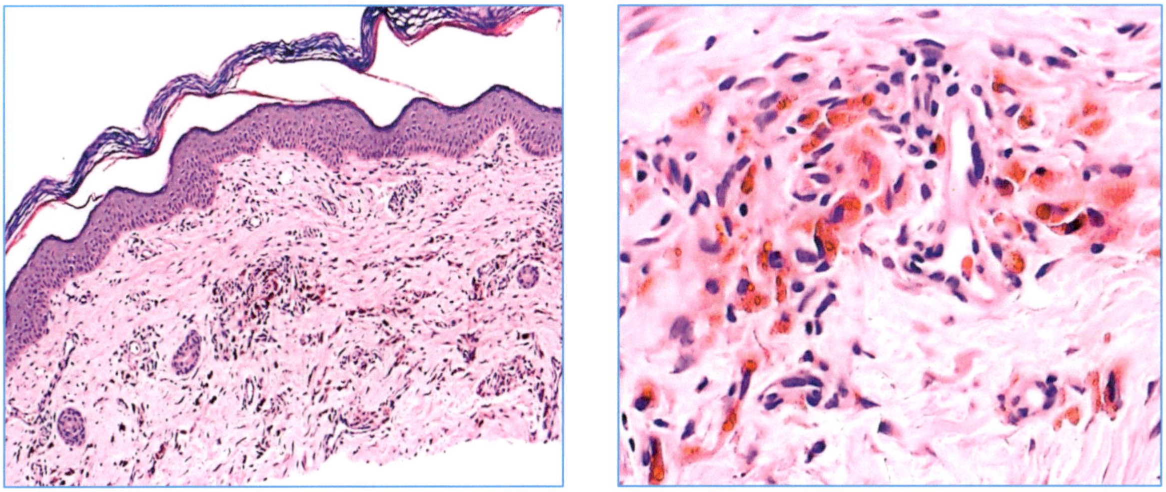

Monsel's reaction with brown pigment in dermal scar

Dermal deposition disorders

OCHRONOSIS

-caused by the accumulation of homogentisic acid in connective tissues
-skin appears bluish-grey because of a light-scattering phenomenon known as the Tyndall effect

Two types:

Endogenous ochronosis (alkaptonuria)

-inborn error of homogentisic acid metabolism with dark urine as the only indication of the disease for many years
-by third decade patients develop renal calculi, arthropathy, and cutaneous blue grey pigmentation
-skin changes have predisposition for pinna of the ear, tip of the nose, skin overlying cartilage or tendon

Exogenous ochronosis

-patients using high concentration of hydroquinone (#1), phenol, picric acid, or resorcinol for prolonged time
-blue grey hyperpigmentation occurs usually about 6 months after use on prominent parts of the face

Histopathology

-large irregular yellow brown **"ochre" colored** dermal deposits
-deposits have curved **"banana-shaped"** contour, so called **banana bodies**

GOUT

-condition caused by deposition of urates in the cartilage and skin
-due to abnormal uric acid metabolism
-primary complaint is acute inflammatory arthritis
-skin lesions present as intradermal or subcutaneous hard, erythematous papules or nodules **(gouty tophi)**
-metatarsal-phalangeal joint at the base of the big toe is affected most often
-beside finger joints, elbows and pinna of the ear are favored sites

Histopathology

-**brown-gray** amorphous deposits in the dermis and subcutis when tissue was fixed in **alcohol**
-deposits are **pink-gray** color if tissue was fixed in **formalin**
-deposits are surrounded by lymphocytes, histiocytes, and occasional giant cells

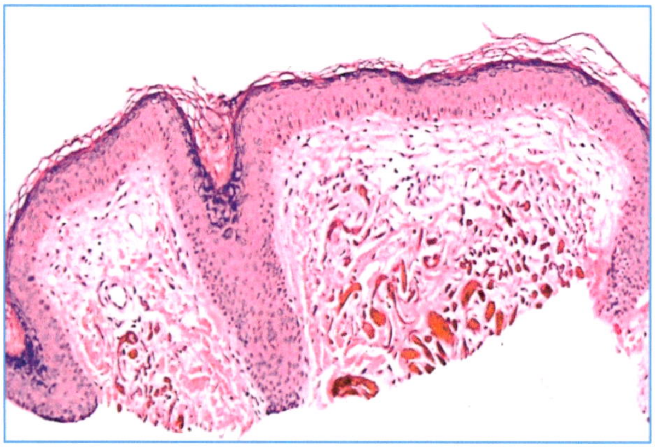

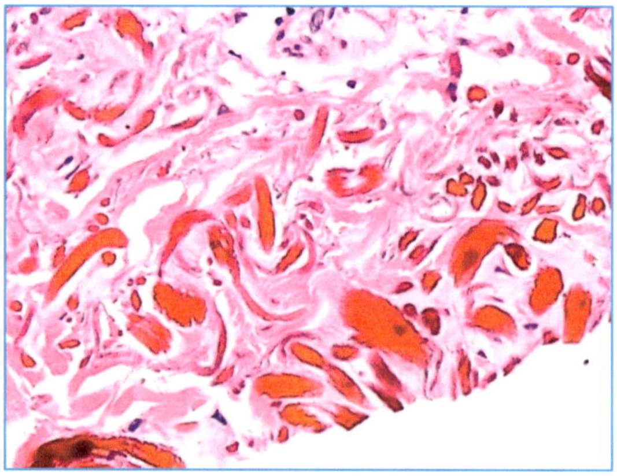

Ochronosis with ochre colored, "banana-shaped" deposits

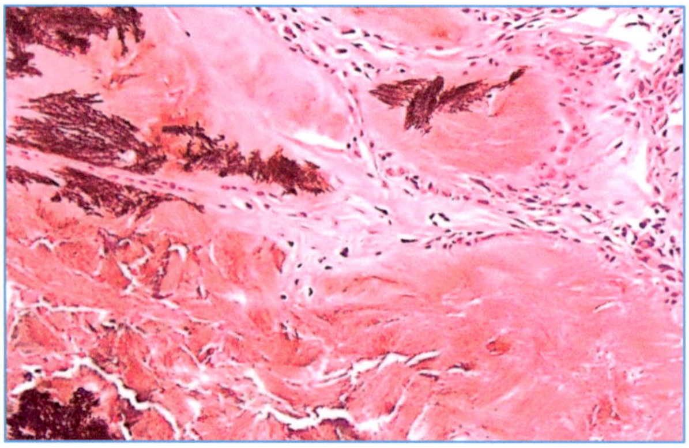

Brown-gray gout deposits fixed in alcohol

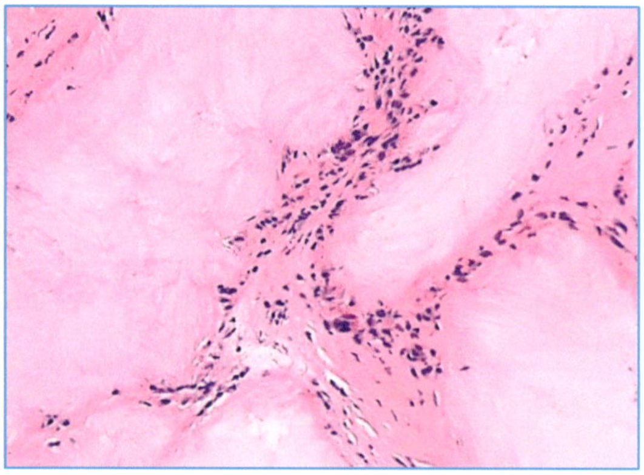

Pink-gray gout deposits fixed in formalin

CRYOGLOBULINEMIA

-precipitation of immunoglobulins that deposit in vessels resulting in vasculopathy or vasculitis

Type I

-deposition of monoclonal cryoglobulin antibodies that cause depositions but as they **do not have rheumatoid factor activity** there is no resulting vasculitis

-purpura, livedo reticularis, ulceration

-Raynaud's phenomenon with cold induced acrocyanosis (ears) common

-underlying leukemia, lymphoma, or multiple myeloma

Type II and Type III

-antibodies **with rheumatoid factor activity** (monoclonal in type II and polyclonal in type III) precipitate at cold temperature, activate complement, and cause vasculitis

-account for 80% of cases

-associated with connective tissue diseases, hepatitis B/C

-present as palpable purpura and urticarial lesions after cold exposure

-common system findings (arthralgia, myalgia, glomerulonephritis)

Histopathology

Type I: vasculopathy with dermal capillaries filled with **homogeneous, "baby pink" material** (PAS+)

Type II and **III**: **leukocytoclastic vasculitis** indistinguishable from other forms of LCV

LIPOID PROTEINOSIS (HYALINOSIS CUTIS ET MUCOSAE)

-sporadic or autosomal recessive disease due to mutation in *ECM1* gene

-the classic manifestation has **onset in infancy** with a **hoarse cry** due to laryngeal infiltration

-oral, pharyngolaryngeal mucosa is involved

-cutaneous lesions are small papules and/or pale yellow or large plaques

-favors face, particularly eyelid margins (**"string of pearls"**) and nostril edges

Histopathology

-**hyaline (glassy pink) depositions** that start around dermal vessels and sweat coils

-eventually the entire dermis is filled with pink cracked deposits similar to amyloid

-deposits are PAS positive and Congo Red negative or only weakly positive

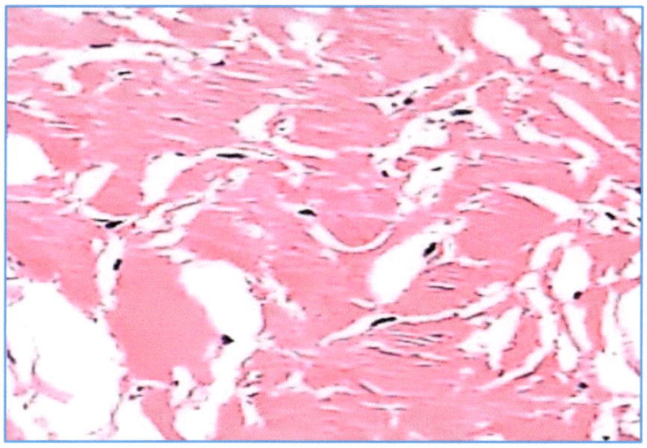

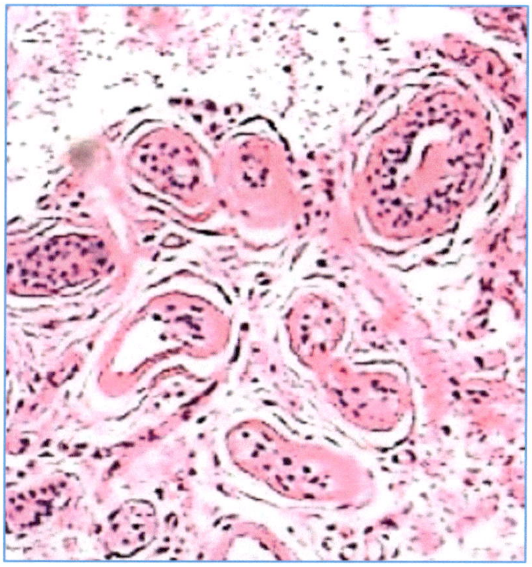

Lipoid proteinosis with diffuse or perieccrine hyaline deposits

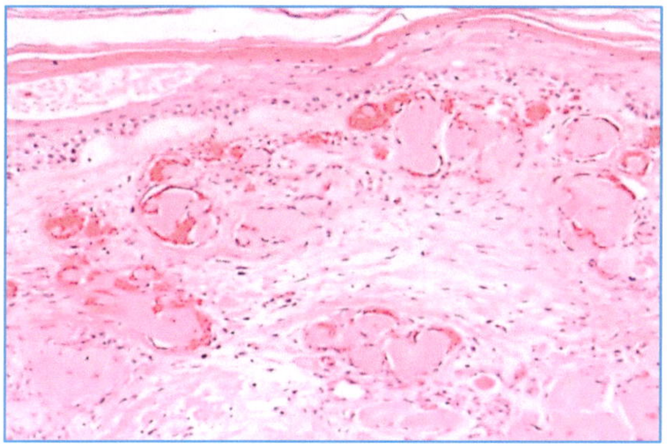

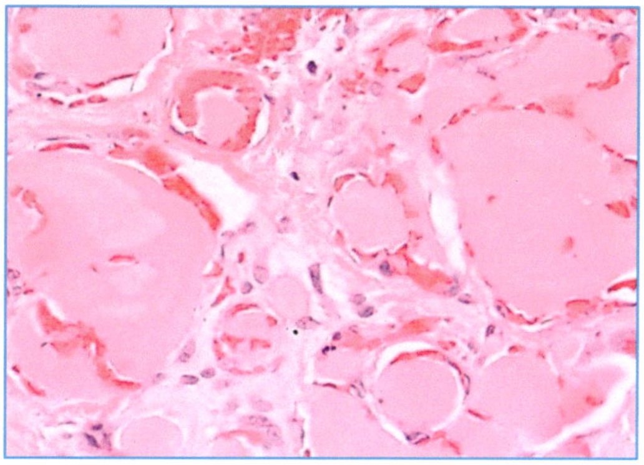

Cryoglobulinemia, type I, with vessels filled with baby pink smooth deposits

Dermal deposition disorders

ARGYRIA

-gradual accumulation of silver in the skin
-caused by excessive exposure to silver compounds or silver dust
-source of silver can be dietary supplements, medications (eye drops, silver sulfadiazine), or occupational
-skin color permanently purple or purple-gray
-can be generalized or localized
-mucous membranes and conjunctivae commonly affected

Histopathology
-dermis with brown/yellow granules and broken strands dispersed between collagen bundles
-**color is similar to ochronosis**
-**perifollicular** and **perieccrine** distribution is commonly seen
-inflammation is absent

CHRYSIASIS

-gradual accumulation of gold in the skin
-caused by excessive exposure to gold
-historically from prolonged use of intravenous, intramuscular or oral gold therapy for the treatment of rheumatoid arthritis
-rarely seen today
-blue-gray or purple pigmentation limited to light-exposed areas of the body and sclerae

Histopathology
-in early lesions, a deep granulomatous reaction within the deep subcutis is present
-in older lesions, there are subcutaneous sclerotic **nodules within the deep subcutis and subcutaneous fat**
-finely **refractile, yellow-brown gold granules** are present between thick collagen bundles

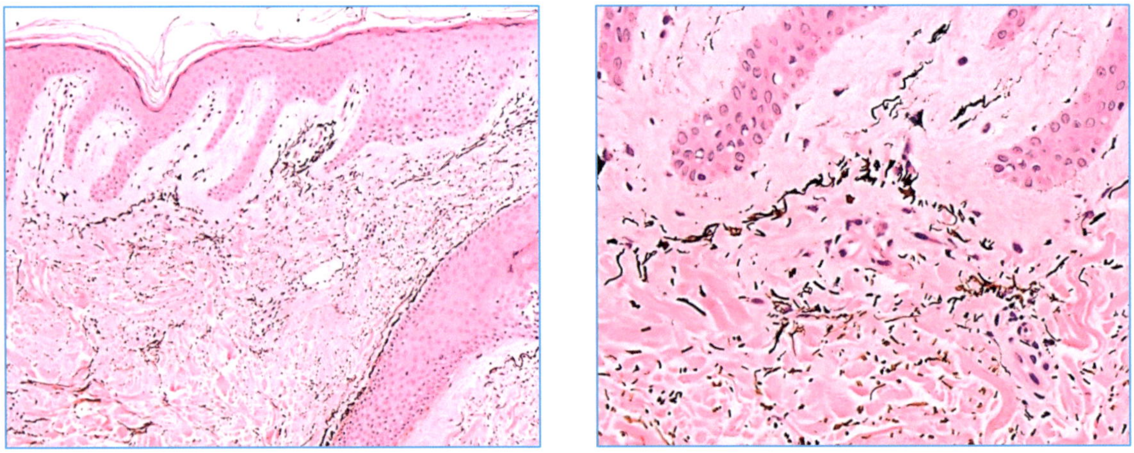

Argyria with yellow-brown deposits in between collagen and around hair follicles and sweat gland ducts

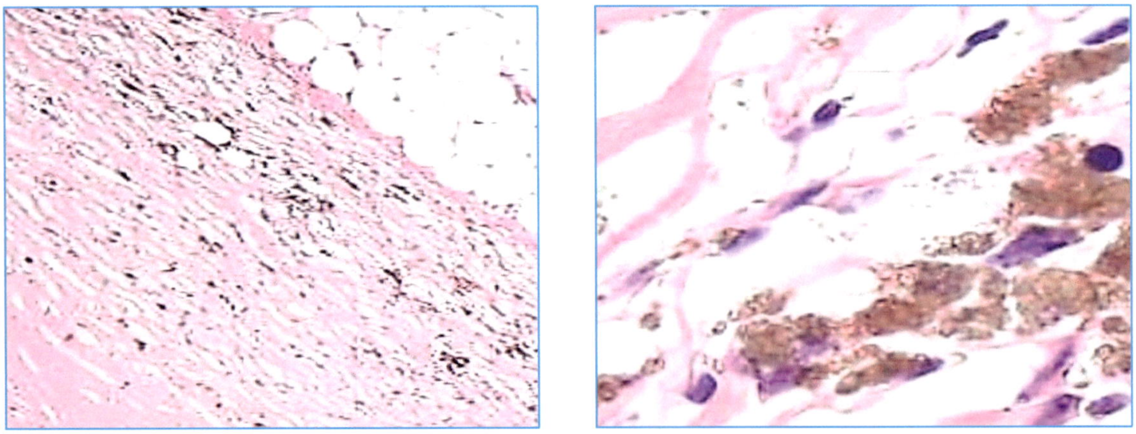

Chrysiasis with subcutaneous sclerotic nodule with yellow-brown granular deposits

MINOCYCLINE-INDUCED PIGMENTATION

-minocycline is a tetracycline antibiotic commonly prescribed for acne, rosacea, and other inflammatory skin disorders
-minocycline turns black when oxidized, leading to blue-black or blue-gray discoloration of the skin, nails, bulbar conjunctiva, oral mucosa, and/or teeth
-hyperpigmentation can occur after long-term minocycline therapy (at least 100 mg/day)

Type I *(most common)*
-blue-black pigmentation in areas of previous inflammation and scarring

Type II
-blue-gray pigmentation on the shins and forearms

Type III
-diffuse "muddy" brown pigmentation in sun exposed skin areas, typically face

Histopathology
-dark, **black to brown, subtle** dermal pigment
-pigment is present in macrophages and extracellularly
-**Types I and II** stain for iron and melanin
-**Type III** stains for melanin only

SILICONE (PARAFFINOMA, SCLEROSING LIPOGRANULOMA)

-inert material used for cosmetic purposes that mostly does not induce a reaction
-appears as empty rounded space in dermis and subcutis (**"Swiss cheese"** appearance)
-when it induces a reaction, it presents with larger irregular empty spaces embedded among histiocytes and lymphocytes with occasional giant cells (**sclerosing lipogranuloma**)

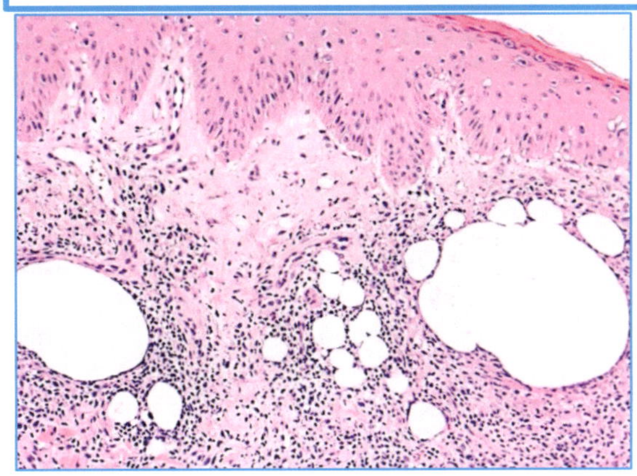

Sclerosing lipogranuloma with large empty spaces surrounded by lymphocytes, histiocytes and giant cells

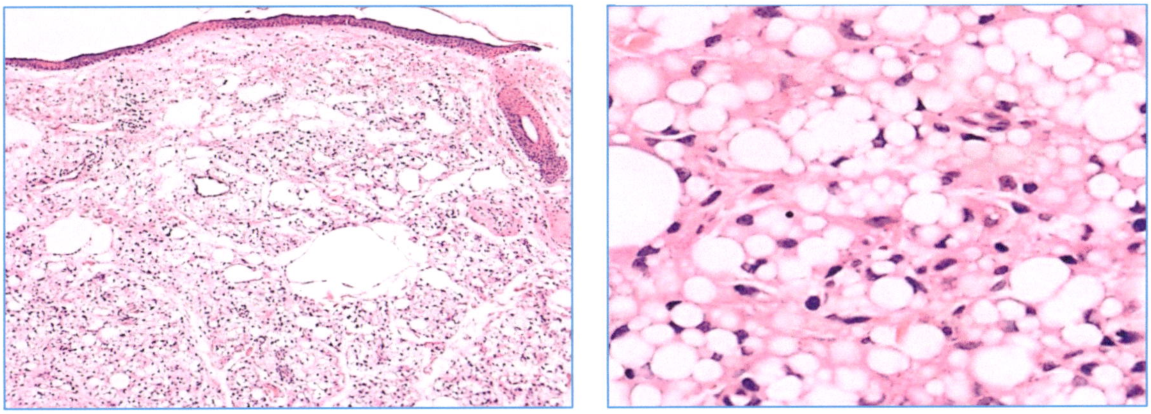

Silicone deposit in "Swiss cheese" pattern with no inflammation

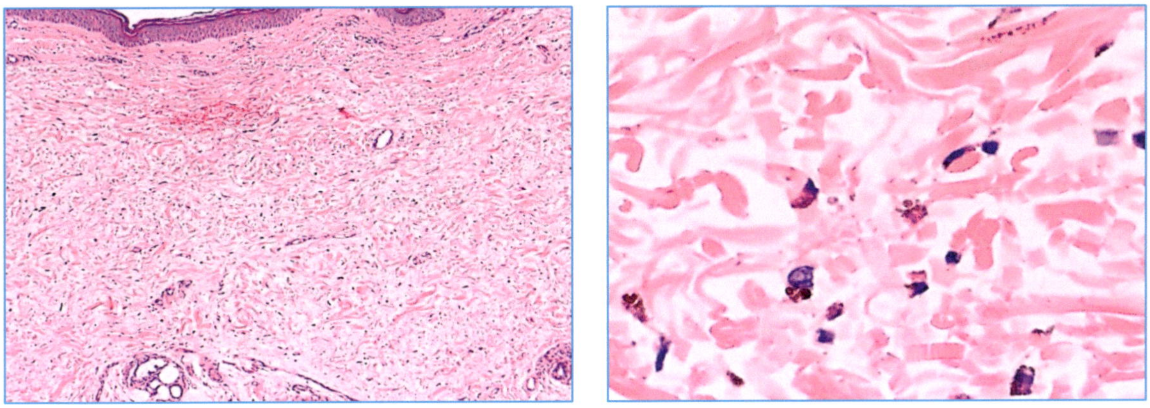

Minocycline black-brown deposit between collagen bundles

Dermal deposition disorders

HOW TO APPROACH DERMAL DEPOSITS

FIRST EXCLUDE MELANOCYTIC LESION

WHAT IS THE COLOR?

BROWN	**-Monsel's reaction**	in scar
RED-PURPLE (CRIMSON)	**-calcinosis cutis**	large lumps
	-calciphylaxis	in small and medium size vessels
YELLOW-BROWN (OCHRE)	**-ochronosis**	large banana-shaped deposits
	-argyria	small dusty periadnexal deposits
	-chrysiasis	small dusty deposits in subcutis
BLACK OR RED	**-tattoo**	superficial, easy to detect
BLACK-BROWN	**-minocycline**	superficial and deep, hard to detect
WHITE (EMPTY SPACES)	**-silicone**	Swiss cheese
LIGHT PINK	**-amyloid**	
	-lichen amyloidosis	hypertrophic epidermis
	-macular amyloidosis	normal epidermis
	-nodular amyloidosis	dermal nodules
	-cryoglobulins	in dermal vessels
	-hyalinosis	perieccrine early on
BLUE-PINK	**-colloid milium**	cracked deposits
GRAY-PINK	**-gout**	in formalin fixative
DARK BROWN-GRAY	**-gout**	in alcohol fixative
LIGHT BLUE	**-mucin**	
LOCATION	**-digital mucous cyst**	fingers
	-mucocele	mouth
	-pretibial myxedema	shin
	-follicular mucinosis	hair follicle
	-focal dermal mucinosis	face, trunk, extremities
FIBROSIS/FIBROBLASTS/ LYMPHOCYTES	**-REM**	mucin + perivascular lymphocytes
	-papular mucinosis	mucin, ↑fibroblasts, no fibrosis
	-scleromyxedema	↓mucin, ↑fibroblasts, fibrosis, does not involve subcutis
	-nephrogenic systemic sclerosis	mucin, ↑fibroblasts, fibrosis also involves subcutis
	-scleredema	fibrosis with empty space and variable mucin

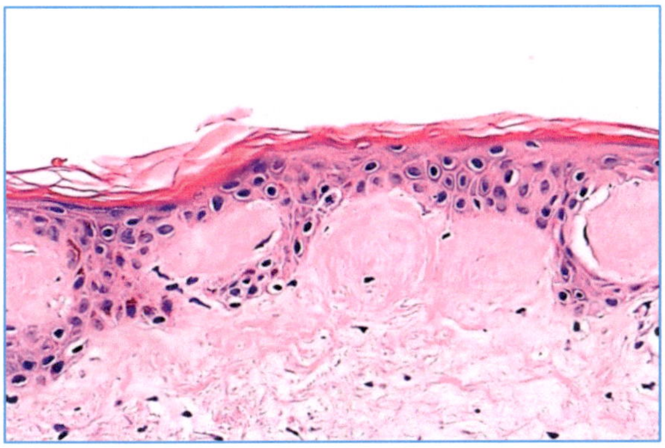

Macular amyloidosis

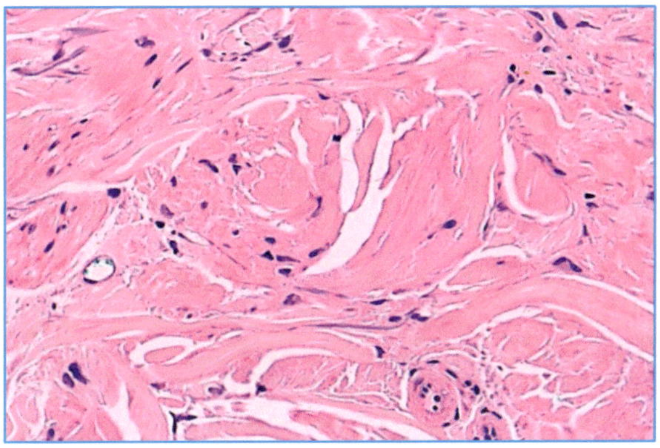

Nodular amyloidosis

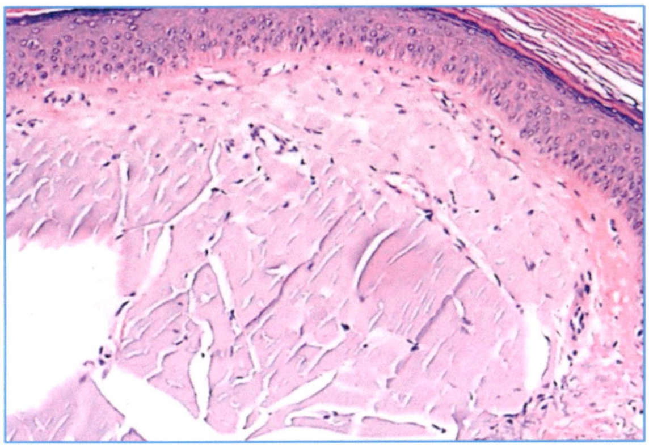

Colloid milium

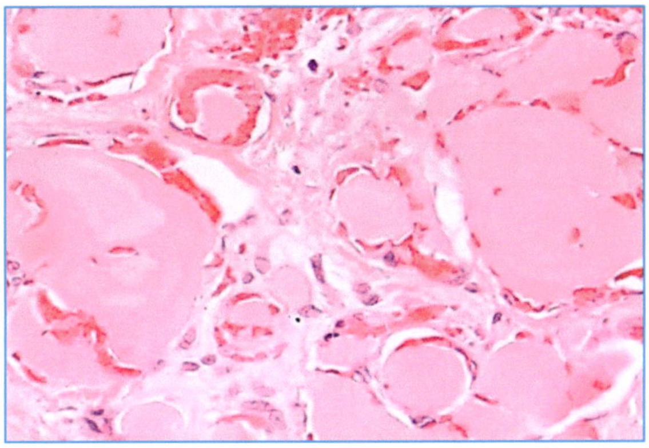

Cryoglobulinemia, type I

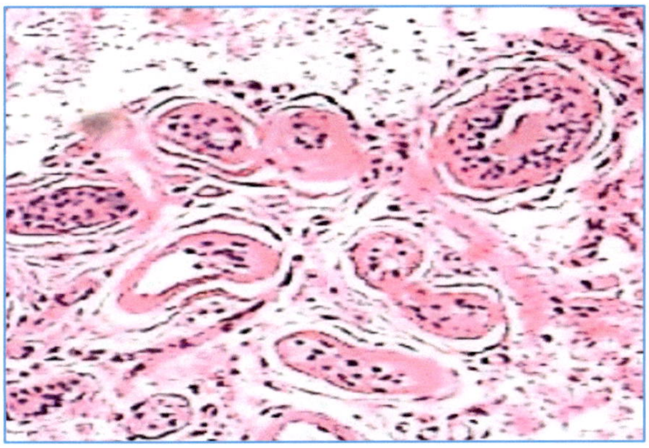

Hyalinosis

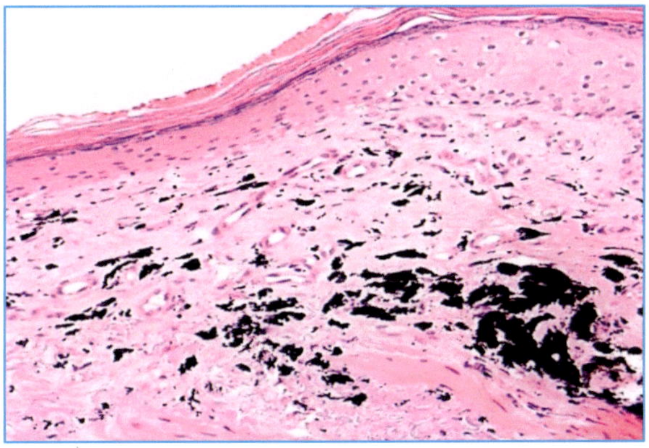

Tattoo

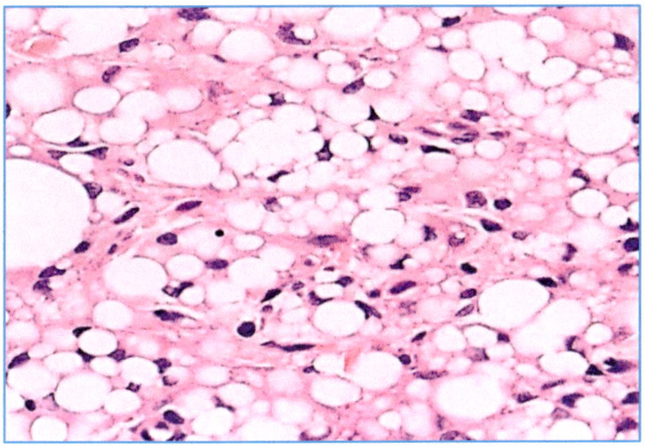

Silicone

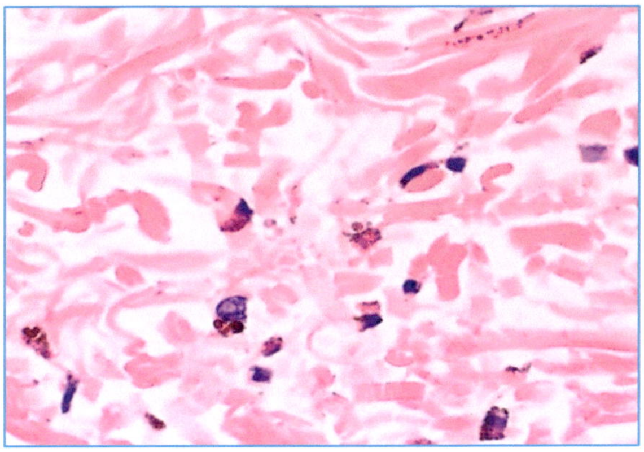

Minocycline

Dermal deposition disorders

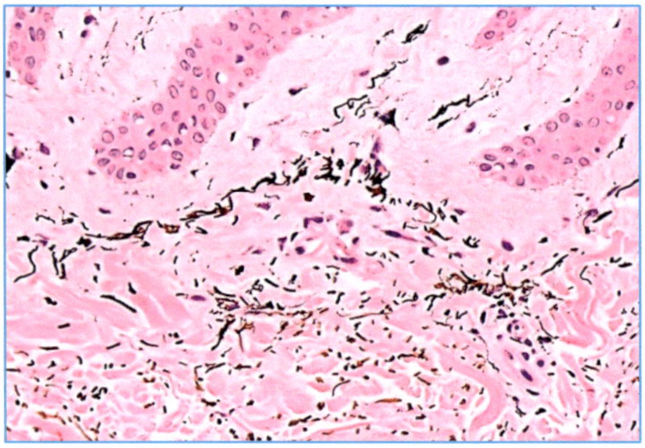

Argyria

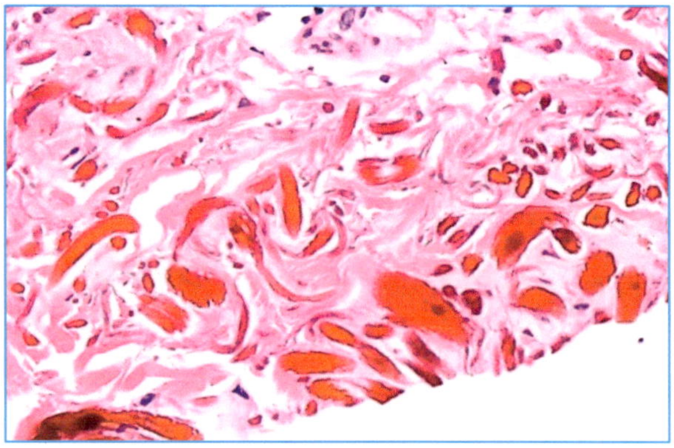

Ochronosis

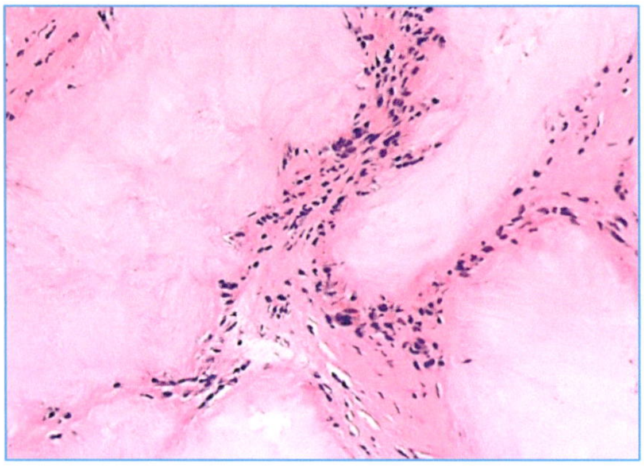

Gout fixed in formalin

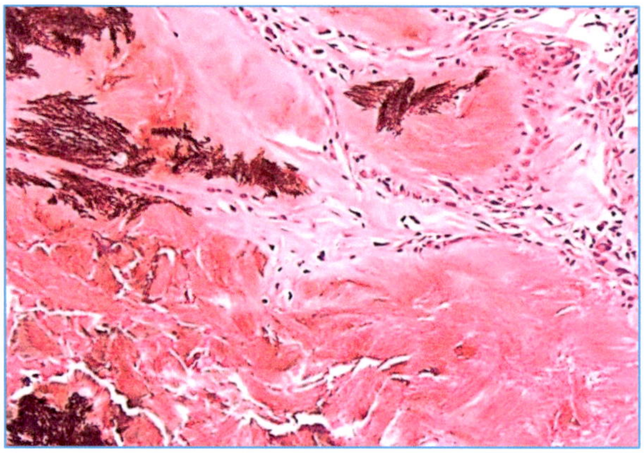

Gout fixed in alcohol

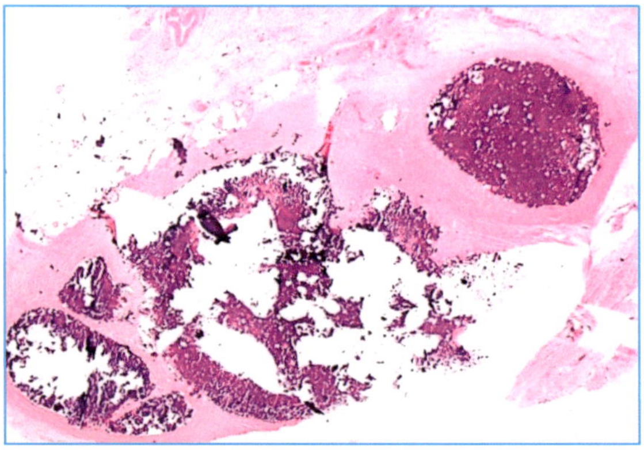

Calcinosis cutis

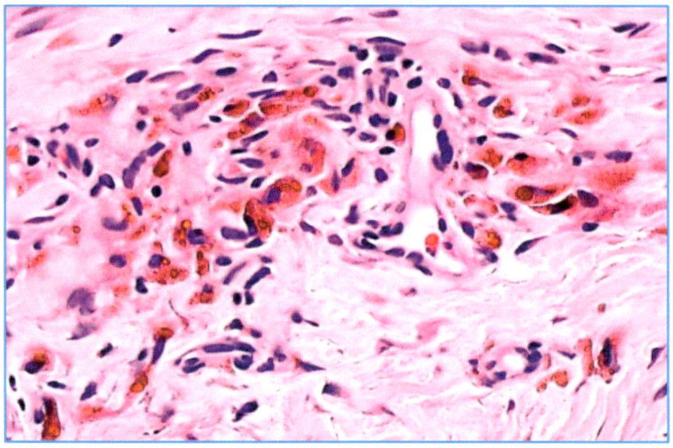

Monsel's reaction

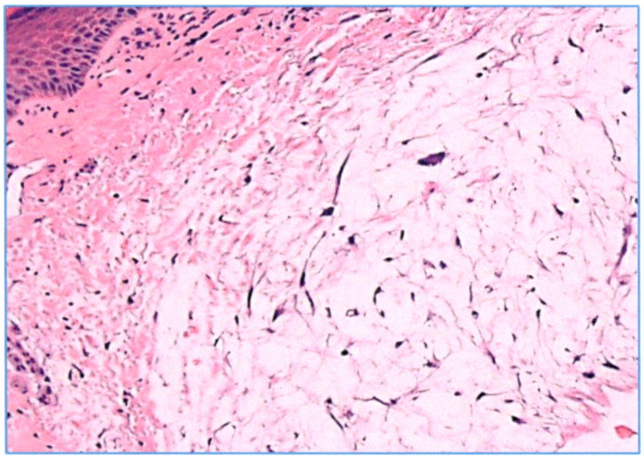

Digital mucous cyst

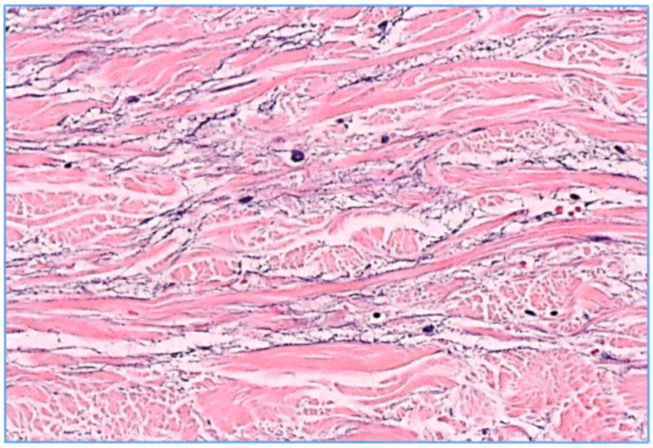

Myxedema

Chapter 15

FOLLICULITIS AND RELATED DISORDERS

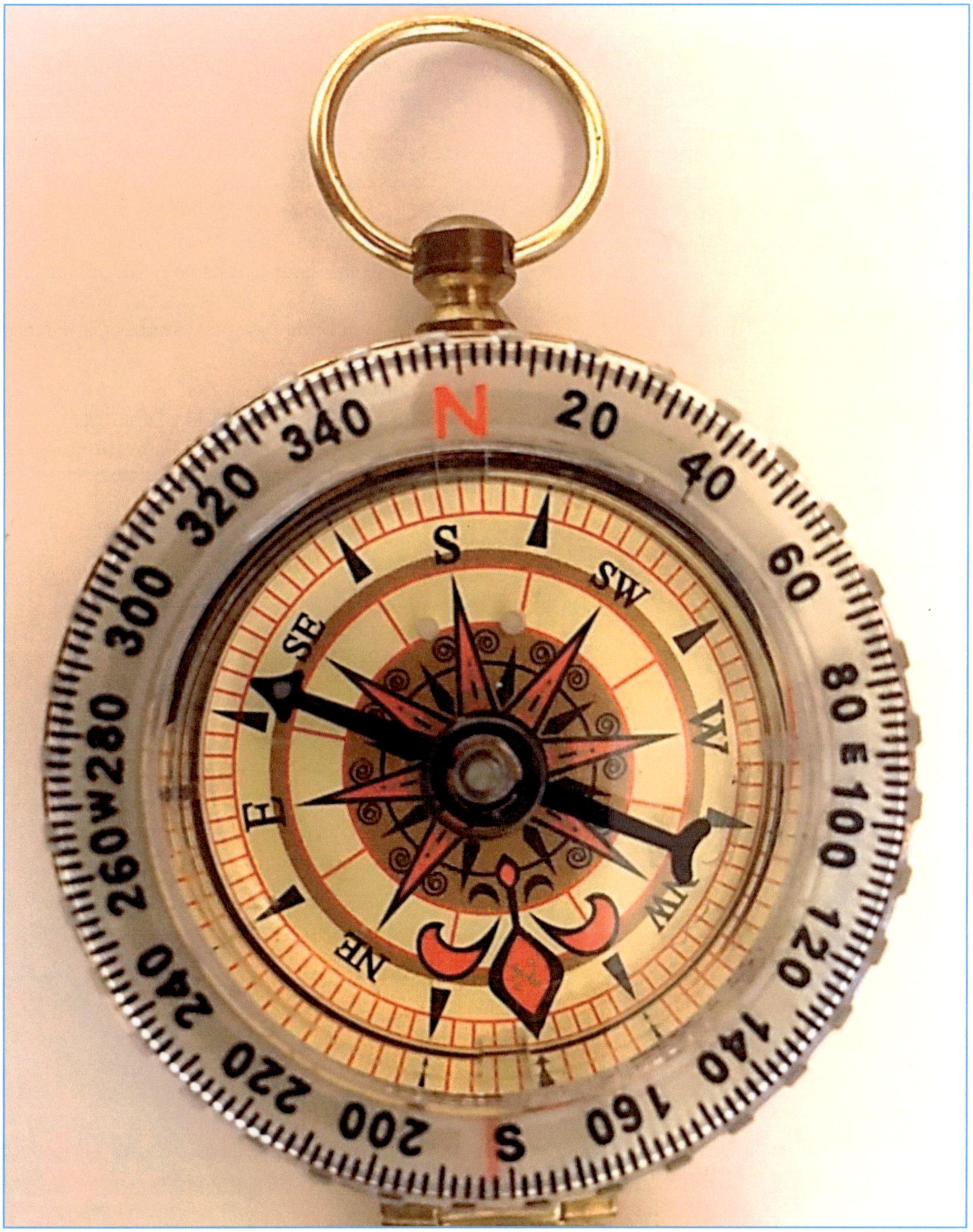

Folliculitis and related disorders

ACNE VULGARIS

-in adolescent individuals, more severe in men
-most frequent sites are face, back, and chest
-lesions start as comedones (closed pore = whitehead and open pore = blackhead)
-develop into erythematous papules, pustules, cysts, and nodules

Histopathology

-comedones are **dilated follicles** plugged with keratin and usually prominent **sebaceous glands**
-**no or minimally perifollicular inflammation**
-papules, pustules, nodules are **inflamed** form
-partially or completely ruptured follicle
-intra and perifollicular acute inflammation

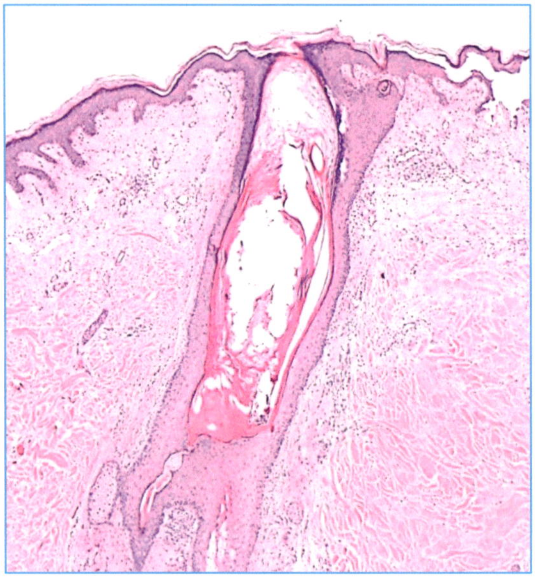

Comedo with dilated, keratin filled follicle and minimal inflammation

ACNE CONGLOBATA/ACNE FULMINANS

Acne conglobata

-form of cystic acne **without systemic symptoms**
-favors back, chest, and only rarely face
-nodules and cysts with sinus formation
-often heals with scarring

Acne fulminans

-most severe form of cystic acne with **systemic manifestations** (fever, arthralgia, sterile bone lesions)
-chest, shoulders, back of young men
-multiple suppurative nodules that ulcerate with black eschar and result in scarring

Histopathology

Acne conglobata

-ruptured follicles with extensive neutrophilic inflammation
-**keratin foreign body reaction, abscess,** and sinus tract formation

Acne fulminans

-exuberant "acne conglobata-like" changes
-**ulcer formation** (uncommon in acne conglobata)

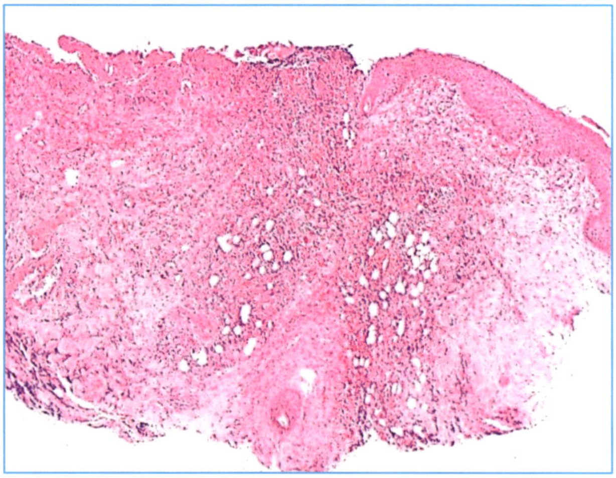

Acne fulminans with ulcer next to ruptured follicle and exuberant deep dermal acute inflammation

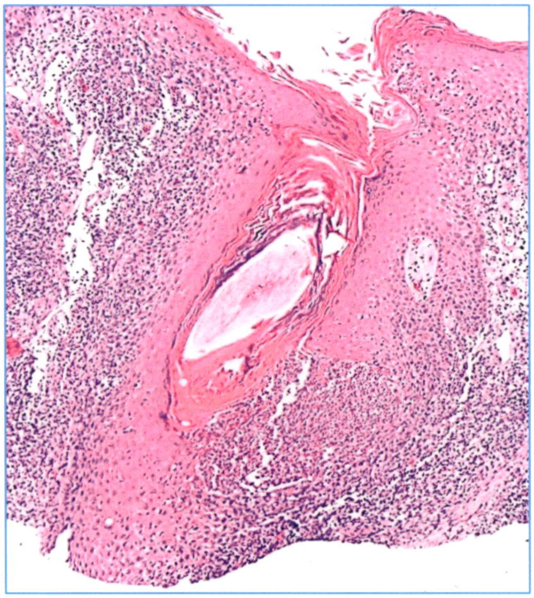

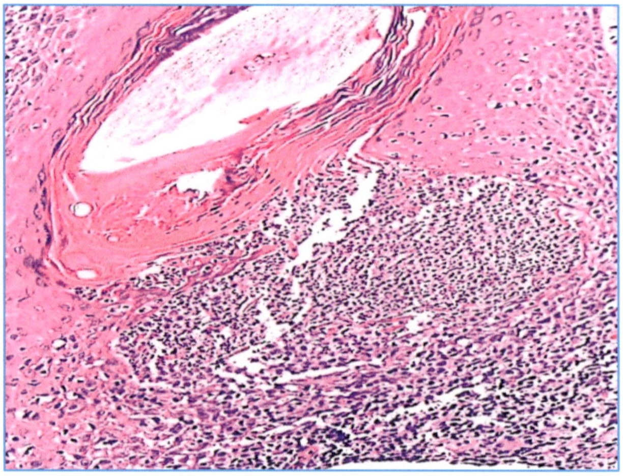

Pustular acne vulgaris with dilated, partially ruptured follicle surrounded by acute inflammation

Chapter 15

ACNE KELOIDALIS NUCHAE

-almost exclusively in young African American men
-occurs on the occipital scalp and posterior neck
-starts as mildly pruritic, follicular-based papules and pustules
-over time, raised plaques and firm scars develop and enlarge to resemble keloid
-scared area is largely hairless with a few tufted hairs

Histopathology

-early lesion resembles suppurative folliculitis with distorted follicles and numerous neutrophils
-in established lesions, hair follicles are destroyed
-**extensive fibrosis** with embedded **scattered naked hair shafts**
-mostly lymphoplasmocytic inflammation present
-**collagen bundles are prominent and dark pink in color like a keloid, but are thinner than true keloid bundles**

DISSECTING CELLULITIS

-rare inflammatory scalp condition
-more common in young African American men
-predilection for vertex and occipital scalp
-part of follicular occlusion tetrad (acne conglobata, hidradenitis suppurativa, dissecting cellulitis, pilonidal cyst)
-boggy plaques with scattered pustules and nodules
-subsequent scarring and permanent hair loss

Histopathology

-exuberant neutrophilic folliculitis
-**deep dermal abscess and sinus formation**
-destroyed hair follicles and **free broken hair shafts**
-in older lesions, more lymphocytes, macrophages, giant cells in addition to neutrophils
-**increased fibrosis and scar** formation

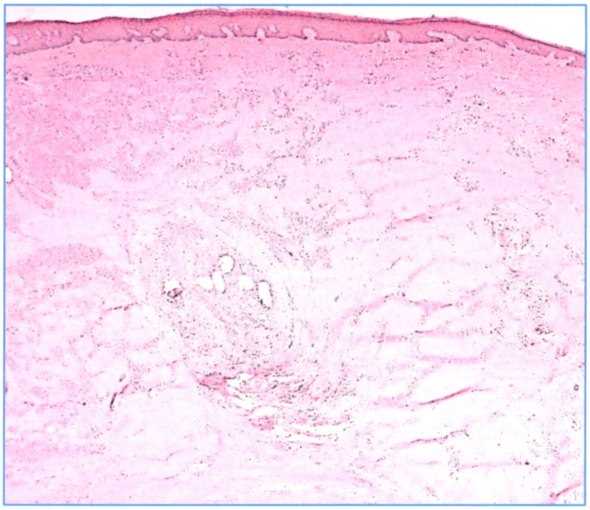
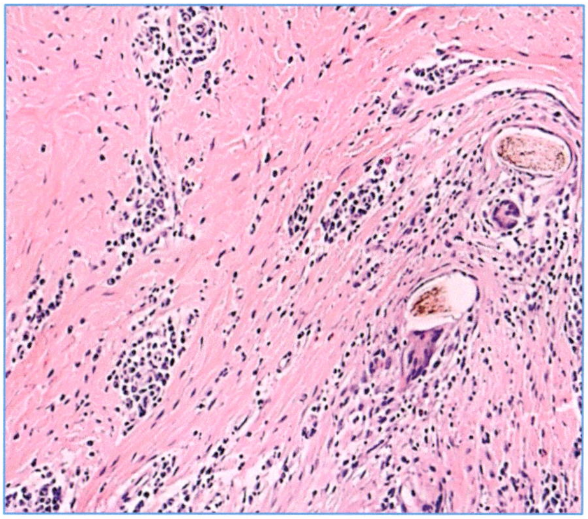

Acne keloidales nuchae with hair shaft remnants in thick "keloid-like" scar

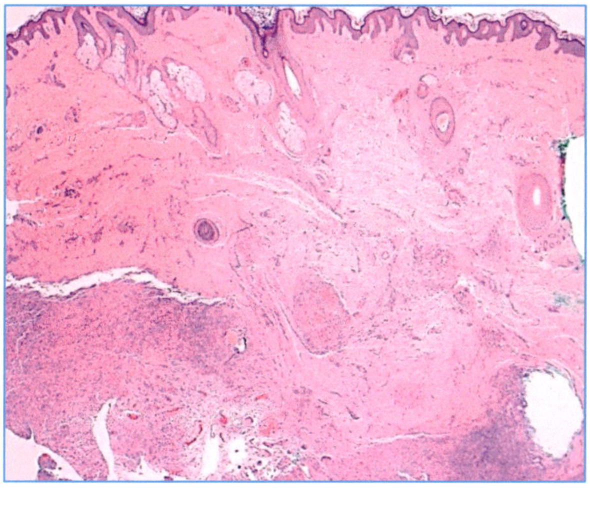
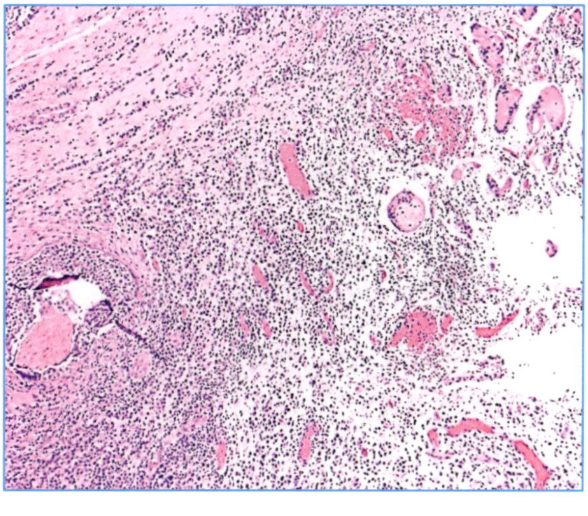

Dissecting cellulitis with exuberant deep subcutaneous neutrophilic inflammation and free broken hair shafts

Folliculitis and related disorders

FOLLICULITIS DECALVANS

-rare, chronic cicatricial (scarring) alopecia
-most common in African American males
-starts with redness, swelling, and pustules around the hair follicles
-develops into expanding patch of alopecia with peripheral pustules
-several hairs can be seen coming out of a single follicle
-scalp looks "tufted" like a toothbrush
-at the end the hairs are shed as the follicles are completely destroyed leaving a scar

Histopathology

-follicles are distorted and/or ruptured
-**abscess replaces follicle** (clinically pustule)

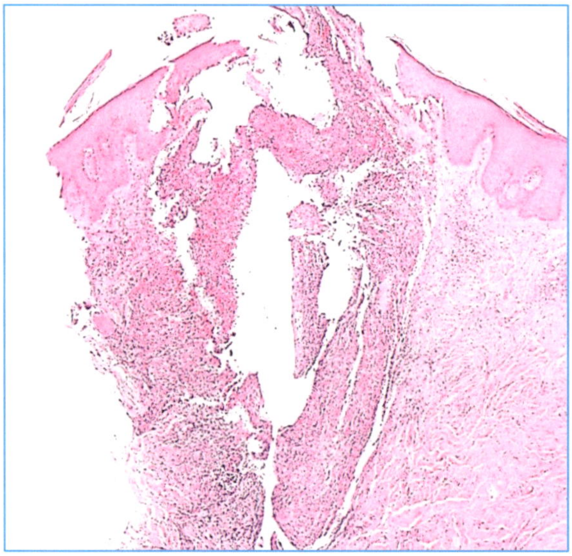

Folliculitis decalvans with ruptured follicle and abscess

HIDRADENITIS SUPPURATIVA

-chronic suppurative cicatricial disease of apocrine glands
-usually starts after puberty
-more common in African Americans
-develops in areas rich in apocrine glands
-in females, it is more common in axillary area and in males, in anogenital area
-inflamed painful nodules and sinus tracts
-heals with scarring

Histopathology

-starts with **suppurative folliculitis** and **neutrophilic hidradenitis**
-in older lesions, follicles are destroyed with **abscess formation and scarring**
-**foreign body keratin granulomas** are present around destroyed follicles

PILONIDAL SINUS

-red, painful, swollen mass in the sacrococcygeal region
-more common in men and associated with curly hair, obesity, sweating, and prolonged sitting
-hair shaft embedded in skin, causing foreign body reaction
-forms sinus with purulent draining

Histopathology

-**irregular sinus tract** lined by acanthotic squamous epithelium and granulation tissue
-dense acute inflammatory reaction
-**naked hair shafts** are easily detected
-often the **free hair shafts are seen in clusters**
-surrounding chronic inflammation with scarring

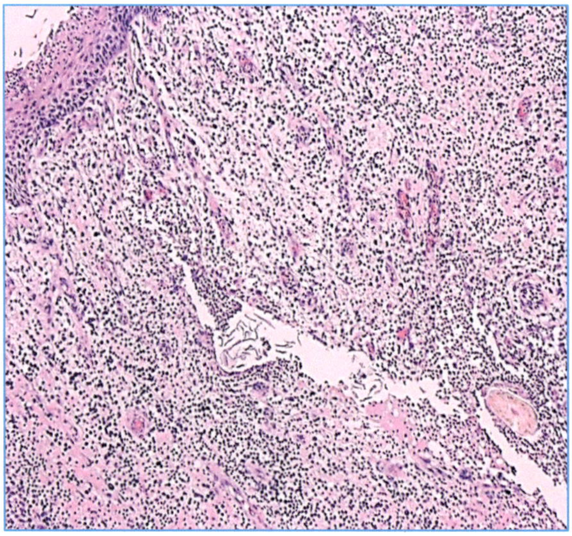

Hidradenitis suppurativa with numerous neutrophils

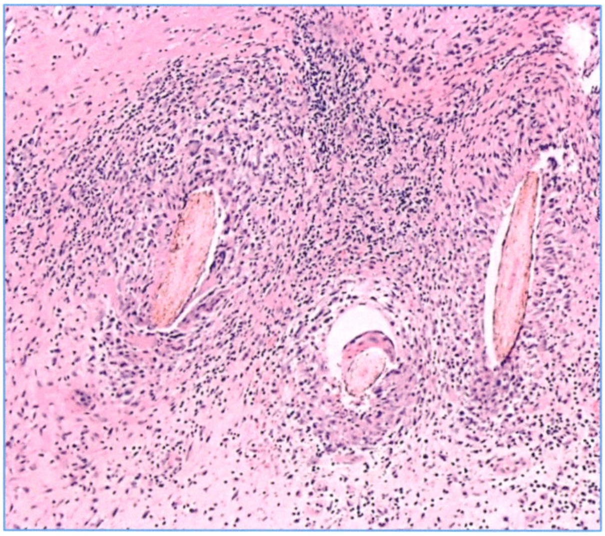

Pilonidal sinus with numerous naked hair shafts

Chapter 15

FOLLICULAR MUCINOSIS (ALOPECIA MUCINOSA)

-uncommon follicular inflammatory disorder
-predilection for face, neck, and scalp
-third and fourth decade of life
-present as erythematous follicular papules and firm plaques with alopecia
-may heal spontaneously or may be associated with mycosis fungoides (15-30% of cases)
-solitary or few plaques are usually associated with benign course
-multiple plaques may be presentation of cutaneous T-cell lymphoma

Histopathology
-**mucin is present within the hair follicle**
-variable presence of **intrafollicular lymphocytes and eosinophils**
-perifollicular lymphocytic infiltrate with **variable number of eosinophils**

EOSINOPHILIC FOLLICULITIS

-several clinical variants

Ofuji disease
-classically in young, middle-aged Japanese men
-multiple, very pruritic grouped follicular papules mainly on the face or back

AIDS associated eosinophilic folliculitis
-pruritic follicular papules common in advanced AIDS patients
-favoring scalp, face, neck, and upper chest

Eosinophilic pustular folliculitis of infancy
-pruritic dermatosis of young male infants
-characterized by scalp pustules that self-resolve

Histopathology
-follicular spongiosis
-**perifollicular and intrafollicular eosinophilic infiltrate**
-mild to moderate perivascular lymphocytic infiltrate

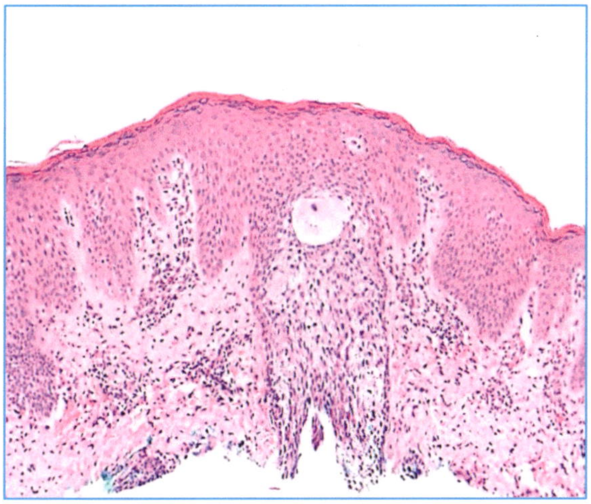
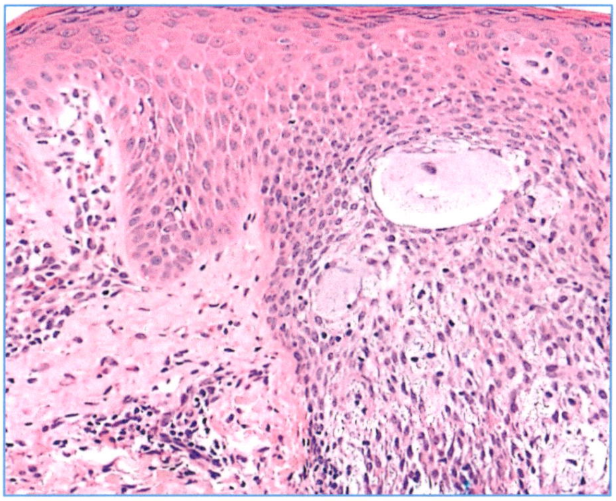

Follicular mucinosis with mucin within hair follicle and perifollicular mixed inflammation

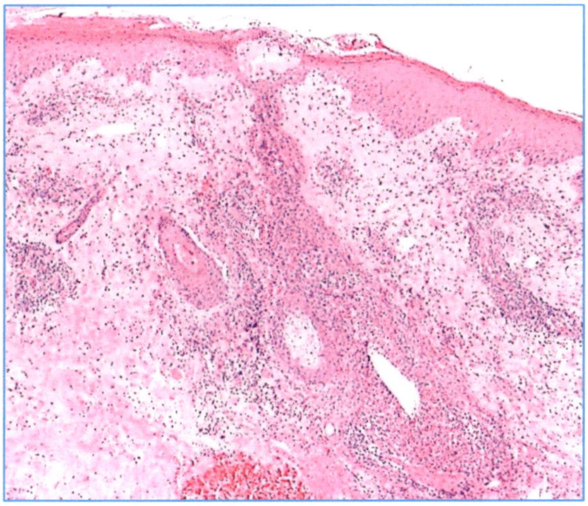
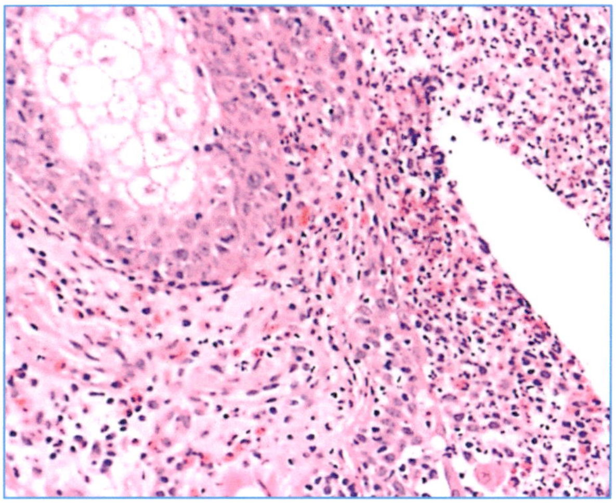

Eosinophilic folliculitis with follicular spongiosis and numerous intra and perifollicular eosinophils

Folliculitis and related disorders

KERATOSIS PILARIS (LICHEN PILARIS)

-common disorder starting in childhood with **"goosebumps" appearance**
-small hyperkeratotic follicular papules, typically on the upper arms

Lichen spinulosum (keratosis spinulosa)
-variant of keratosis pilaris usually seen in teenage boys
-usually symmetrical papules on elbows, knees, buttocks, and trunk

Histopathology
-**dilated hair follicle plugged with keratin**
-no or minimal perifollicular lymphocytic infiltrate

TRICHOSTASIS SPINULOSA

-usually in older adults but can occur at any age
-condition results from retention of numerous hairs surrounded by keratin in a dilated follicle
-appears dark and therefore can be confused with comedone
-common on face (particularly nose)

Histopathology
-keratin-plugged dilated hair follicle with **multiple pigmented hair shafts**

SCURVY

-clinical manifestation of severe vitamin C deficiency
-skin bruising and perifollicular hemorrhagic papules
-hairs curl and break off close to the follicular orifice (**"corkscrew" hairs**)

Histopathology
-dilated follicle with **follicular plugging**
-**multiple intrafollicular hair shaft fragments** (result of cross-sectioning of an individual curled hair shaft)
-**perifollicular red blood cell extravasation**

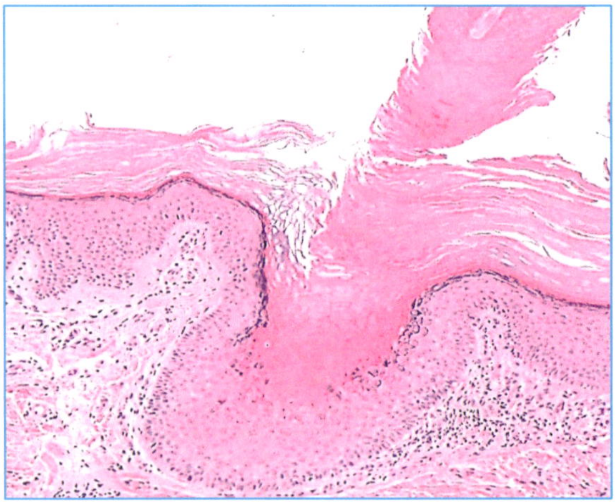

Keratosis pilaris with keratin plugged follicle

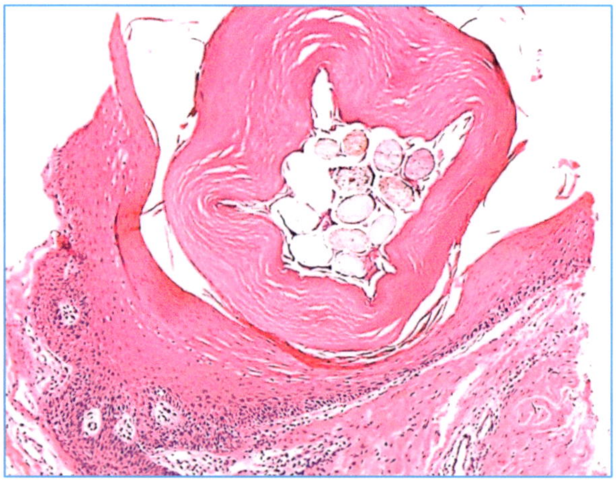

Trichostasis spinulosa with multiple pigmented hair shaft fragments

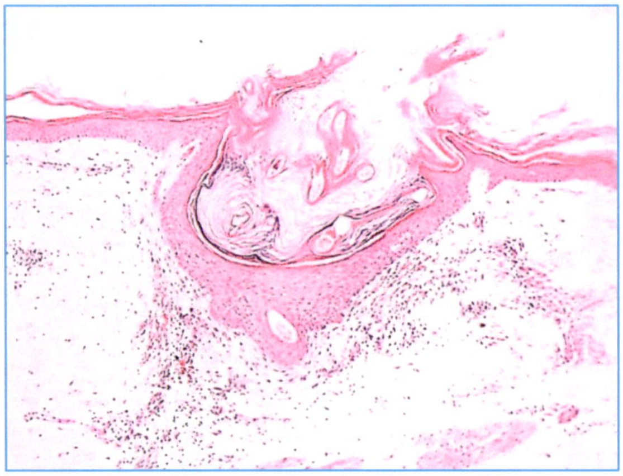

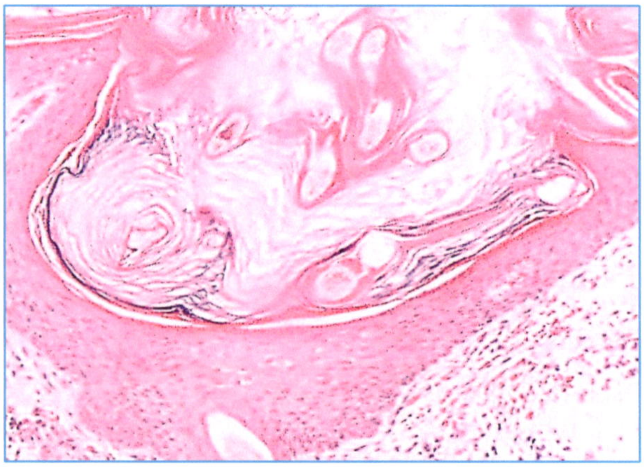

Dilated follicle of scurvy with multiple hair shaft fragments and perifollicular hemorrhage

Chapter 15

FOLLICULAR ECZEMA

-form of atopic dermatitis predominantly centered around the hair follicle
-red or skin-colored follicular papules or **"goosebumps" that don't go away**
-more common in African Americans and Asians

Histopathology
-mildly dilated **follicular infundibulum with spongiosis**
-lymphocytes are present in the infundibulum
-no or mild perifollicular lymphocytic inflammation

FOX-FORDYCE DISEASE (APOCRINE MILIARIA)

-results from plugging of apocrine glands
-usually in adolescents and young adults
-more common in females
-skin-colored, **very pruritic follicular papules**
-axilla is favored site

Histopathology
-usually very subtle
-follicular hyperkeratosis
-spongiosis of the follicular infundibulum adjacent to the entrance of the apocrine duct
-sparse perifollicular and perivascular lymphocytic infiltrate
-**focal foamy histiocytes adjacent to follicle next to apocrine duct**

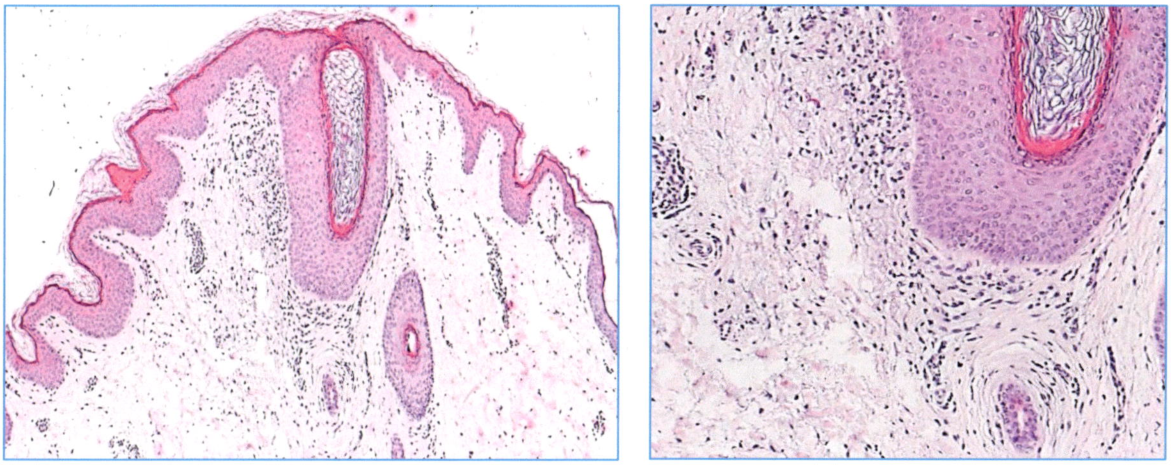

Fox-Fordyce disease with focal perifollicular foamy histiocytes in the vicinity of apocrine duct

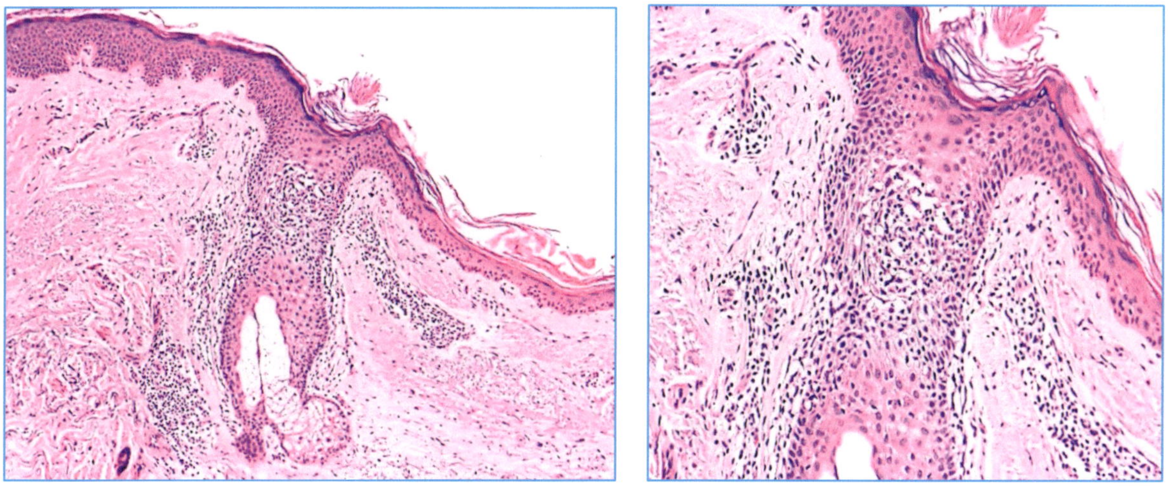

Follicular eczema with follicular spongiosis and perifollicular lymphocytes

Folliculitis and related disorders

BACTERIAL FOLLICULITIS

-superficial bacterial infection of hair follicles predominantly due to *Staphylococcus aureus*
-"hot tub" bacterial folliculitis is caused by *Pseudomonas*
-favors adolescents and young adult males
-predisposing factors are
  -maceration and occlusion
  -frequent shaving, waxing
  -history of atopic dermatitis and acne
  -use of topical corticosteroids
  -bathing in an inadequately cleaned hot tub/pool
-presents with one or more folliculocentric pustules
-may be itchy or mildly sore and heal without scarring
-hot tub folliculitis presents with papules and pustules on the trunk 12-48 hours after soaking
-a furuncles (boil) is a deeper painful abscess centered around a follicle
-a carbuncle is a cluster of furuncles with draining sinuses involving several follicles that heal with scarring

Histopathology

-distorted, dilated, and **usually ruptured follicle(s)**
-intra and perifollicular **neutrophilic inflammation**
-**bacterial elements** are found **within the ruptured follicle**

PITYROSPORUM FOLLICULITIS (MALASSEZIA FOLLICULITIS)

-superficial infection of hair follicle caused by *Malassezia* yeast (normal inhabitant of human skin that only causes disease under specific conditions)
-associated with excessive sweating, occlusions, and antibiotic and steroid use
-small uniform itchy papules and pustules
-favors forehead, chin, neck, trunk, and extensor aspect of the upper limbs

Histopathology

-**dilated keratin plugged hair follicles with fungal spores**
-mild perifollicular mixed inflammation
-hair follicle may rupture and then inflammation is more neutrophilic

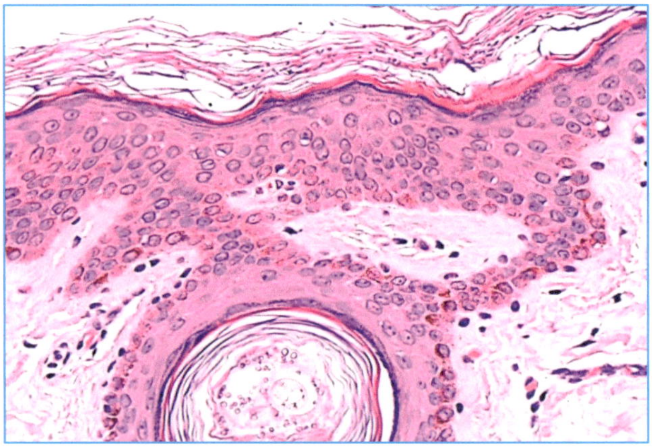

Pityrosporum folliculitis with fungal spores present in dilated follicle and in the stratum corneum

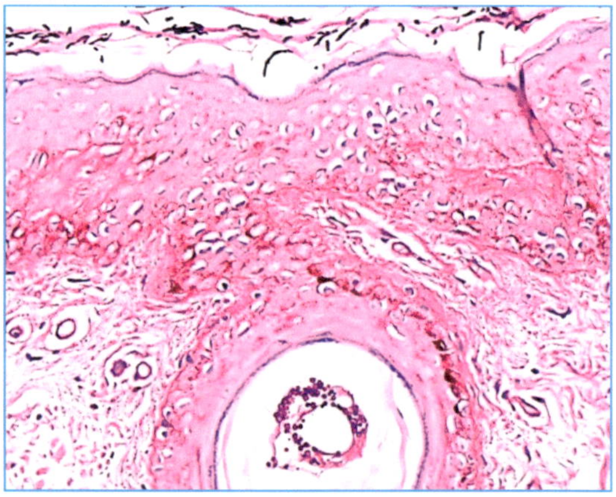

PAS stain outlines fungal spores

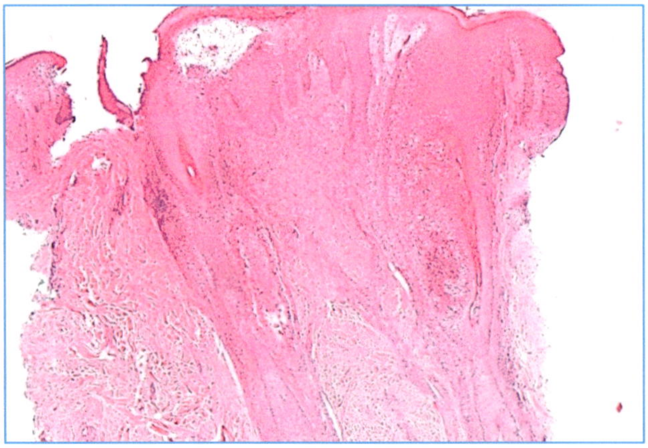

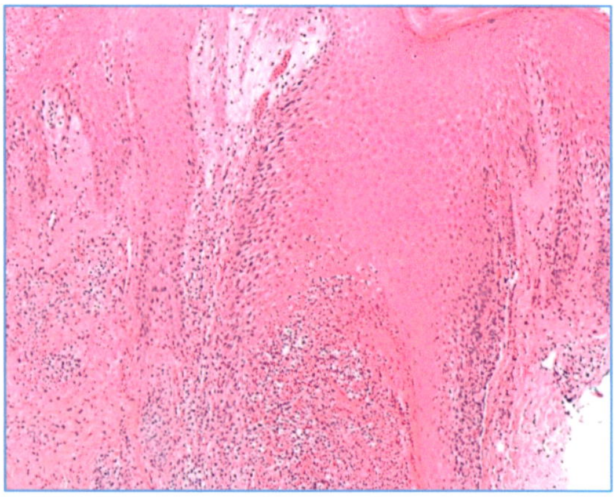

Bacterial (acute) folliculitis with neutrophilic inflammation

DEMODEX FOLLICULITIS

-superficial infection of hair follicle by *Demodex folliculorum,* saprophytic parasitic mite
-more frequent in **HIV patients and diabetics**
-very common in patients with **rosacea** and can cause itchy pustules with follicular scaling
-the role of *Demodex* mites in inflammatory skin conditions remains controversial as mites are commonly found in normal appearing facial skin of the elderly

Histopathology

-**dilated hair follicle with *Demodex* mite** within the follicle
-no or mild perifollicular lymphocytic inflammation
-occasional perifollicular granulomatous reaction

HERPETIC FOLLICULITIS

-rare infection of hair follicle by *herpes virus*
-more commonly due to *varicella zoster* than *herpes simplex*
-classically red follicular papules with vesicle and pustule formation, however over half of the cases lack vesicles or pustules

Histopathology

-ruptured follicle with intrafollicular vesicles filled with necrotic keratinocytes
-keratinocytes with **steel gray/purple nuclei** and **multinucleated keratinocytes** with **nuclear molding**
-intra and perifollicular acute inflammation

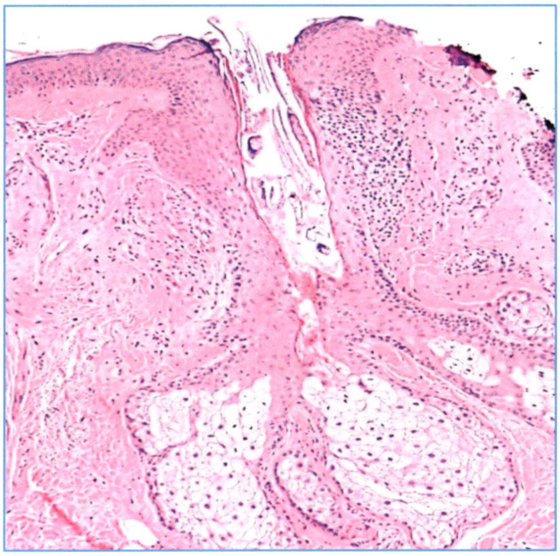
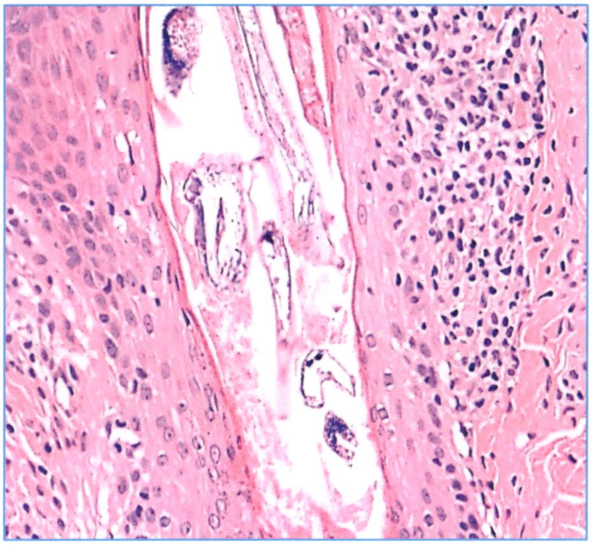

Demodex folliculitis with demodex mites within dilated follicle

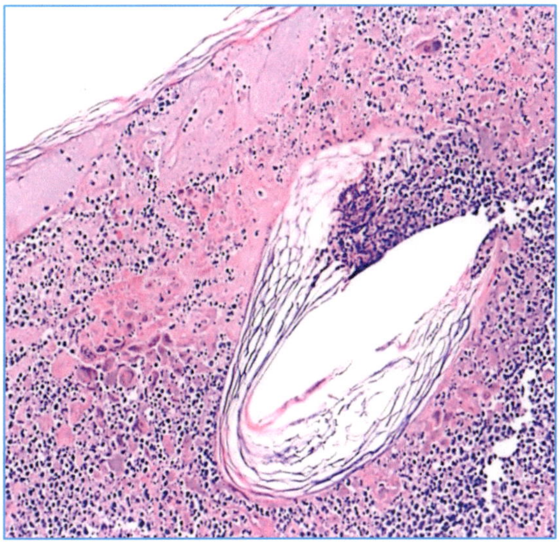
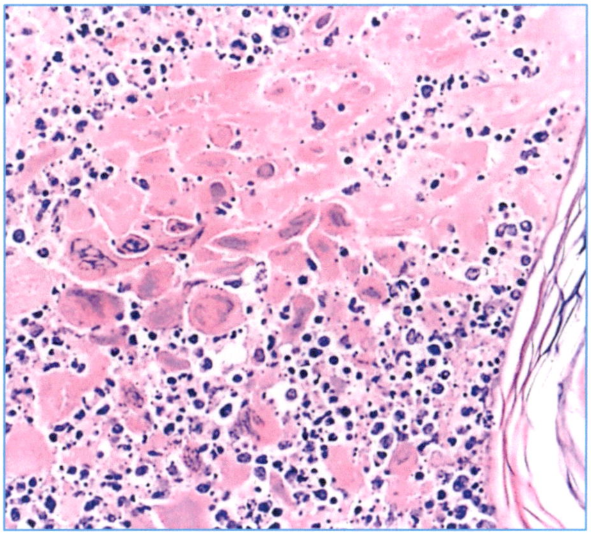

Herpes folliculitis with intranuclear viral inclusions

Folliculitis and related disorders

MAJOCCHI'S GRANULOMA

-fungal folliculitis mainly caused by dermatophytes (see more in the fungal chapter)
-patients usually have long-standing superficial fungal infection at another site (e.g. tinea corporis, onychomycosis)
-*Trichophyton rubrum* is # 1 cause
-classified into two forms:

Inflammatory form

-mainly observed in healthy individuals
-presents with red follicular papules, plaques, or less frequently nodules
-induced by trauma (e.g. shaving)
-mostly observed on the lower extremities

Granulomatous form

-related to immunosuppression
-usually presents as a red plaque or nodule
-favors upper and lower extremities and face

Histopathology

-**ruptured follicle** with exuberant intra- and perifollicular neutrophilic inflammation
-**abscess formation** is common
-in immunosuppressed patients, granulomatous infiltrate is also present
-**fungal spores and hyphae in and around hair shaft**

TINEA CAPITIS

-superficial fungal infection of the scalp (see more details in the fungal chapter)
-more common in children
-single/ multiple patches of non-scarring hair loss
-patches have **"black dot" pattern** due to broken **"comma-like" hairs** and scale

Histopathology

-epidermal hyperkeratosis with **no scarring** and **minimal perifollicular inflammation**
-in **endothrix** infections, caused by *Trichophyton tonsurans/violaceum,* the **hyphae extend within the hair shaft** and produce spores
-in **ectothrix** infections, caused by *Microsporum canis/audouinii*, **fungal forms coat the outside of the hair shaft without significant invasion of the shaft itself**

Kerion and **Favus** are more severe variants of tinea capitis causing scarring alopecia (see more details in the alopecia chapter)

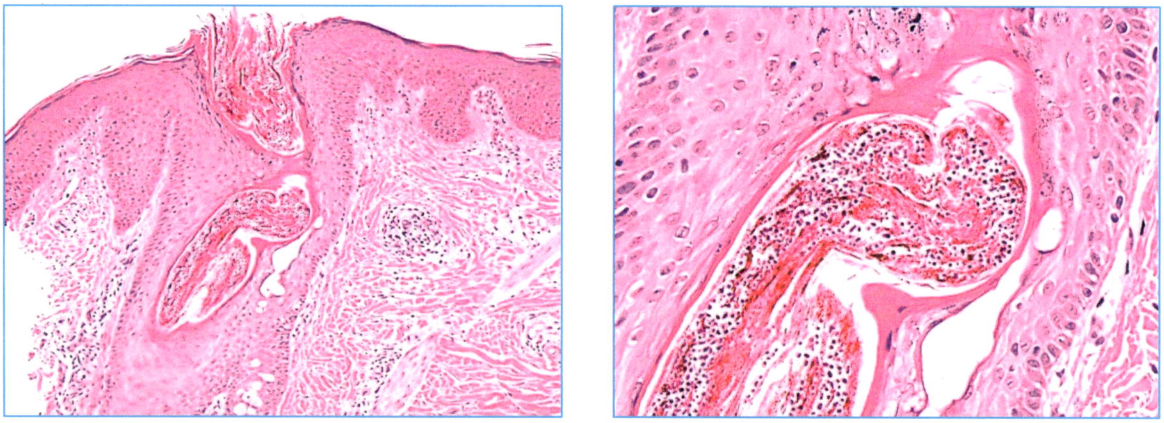

Tinea capitis with hyphae (endothrix) within the hair follicle

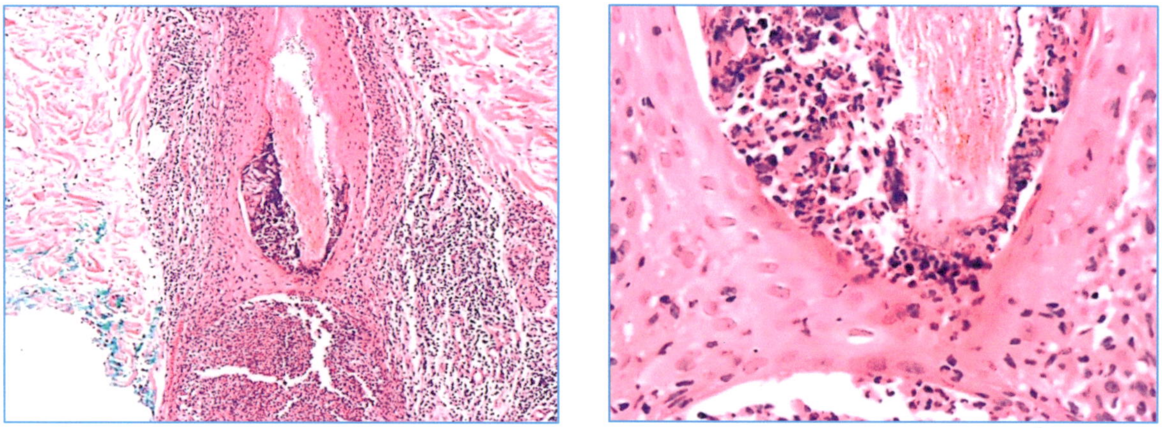

Majocchi's granuloma with ruptured follicle and fungal hyphae

Chapter 15

HOW TO APPROACH DISORDERS OF FOLLICLES

IF YOU SEE A FOLLICLE WITH EOSINOPHILS WITH OR WITHOUT MUCIN

-follicular mucinosis	variable eosinophils and **follicular mucin**
-eosinophilic folliculitis	numerous eosinophils and **no mucin**

IF YOU SEE A FOLLICLE THAT IS NOT ACUTELY INFLAMED AND

IS DILATED

-comedo	filled with keratin, no or minimal inflammation
-keratosis pilaris	filled with keratin plug forming horn, on upper arms
-trichostasis spinulosa	filled with multiple hair shaft fragments
-scurvy	filled with multiple hair shaft fragments and dermal hemorrhage
-pityrosporum folliculitis	normal follicular content with spores
-demodex folliculitis	normal follicular content with mites
-tinea capitis	hyphae in or outside hair shaft

IS NOT DILATED BUT IS SPONGIOTIC

-follicular eczema	follicular spongiosis in an atopic location
-Fox-Fordyce disease	focal spongiosis at the entrance of apocrine gland in axilla

IF YOU SEE A FOLLICLE THAT IS ACUTELY INFLAMED

Acute (early) lesions of the conditions listed below are similar	neutrophilic folliculitis with partial/full follicular destruction

Established lesions are similar but have some unique features

-acne vulgaris	face	
-acne conglobate	chest, back no systemic symptoms	abscess replaces follicle + extensive acute inflammation forming sinus
-acne fulminans	chest, black systemic symptoms	same as acne conglobate + ulcer
-folliculitis decalvans	Afr. Amer. vertex	abscess replacing follicle, forming pustules
-hidradenitis suppurativa	axilla, groin	hair shafts, abscess, scar
-pilonidal sinus	gluteal cleft	hair shafts, abscess, sinus tract
-dissecting cellulitis	Afr. Amer. vertex, scalp	hair shafts, deep abscesses
-acne keloidales nuchae	Afr. Amer. nape	hair shafts, extensive "keloid-like" fibrosis

WITH ORGANISMS

-bacterial folliculitis	*Staph. aureus*
-acne vulgaris	*Propionibacterium* can be seen
-herpes folliculitis	HSV, VZV viral nuclear inclusions
-Majocchi's granuloma	fungal spores and hyphae

Folliculitis and related disorders

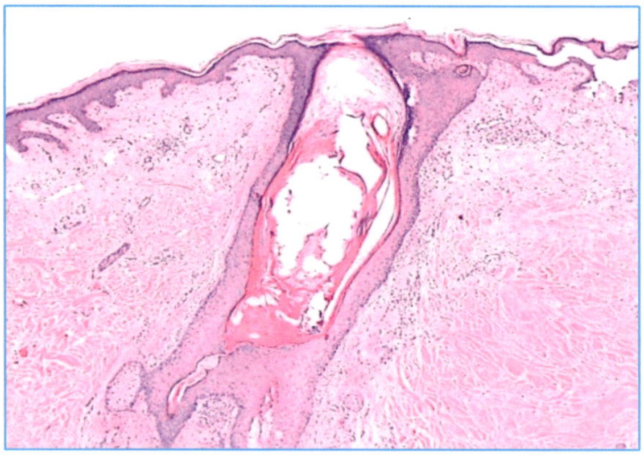

Comedo with dilated, keratin filled hair follicle

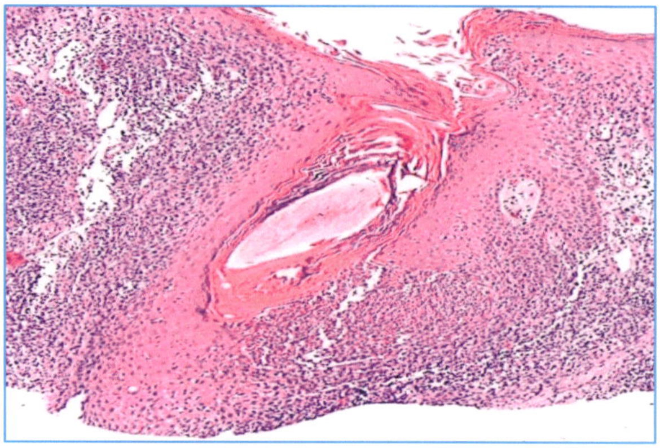

Acne vulgaris with acutely inflamed hair follicle

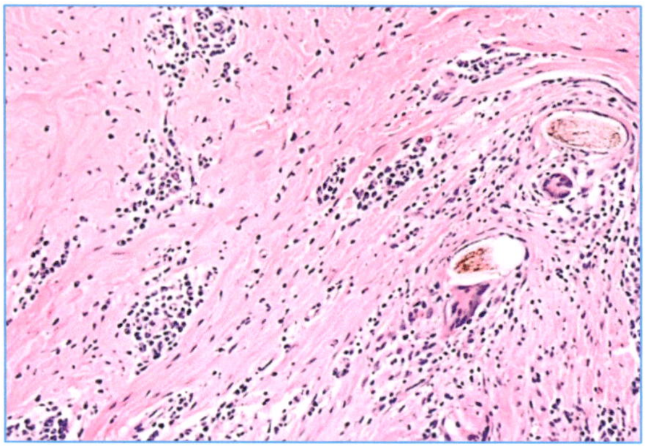

Acne keloidales with prominent "keloid-like" scarring

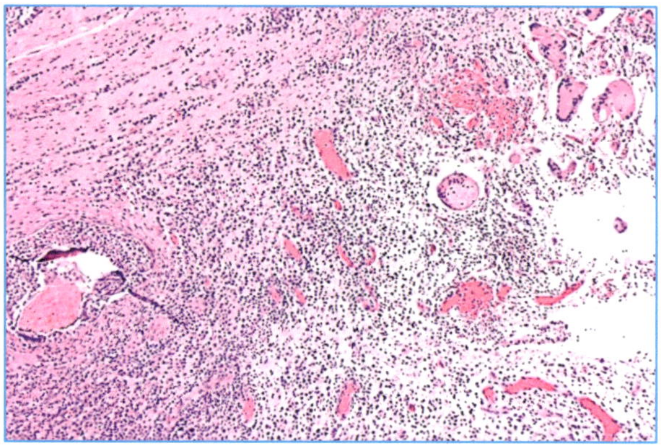

Dissecting cellulitis with exuberant deep acute inflammation

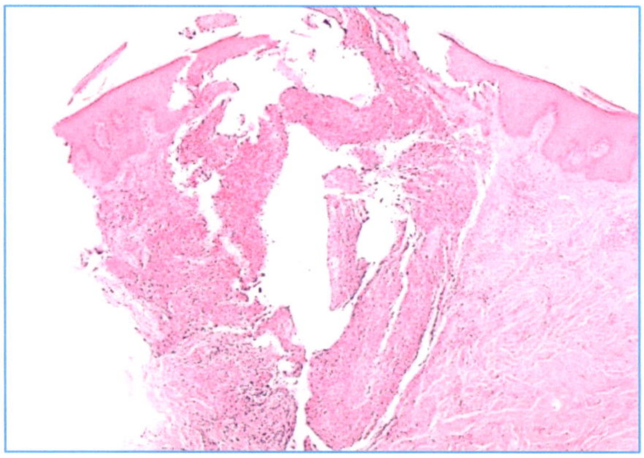

Folliculitis decalvans with destroyed follicle by acute inflammation

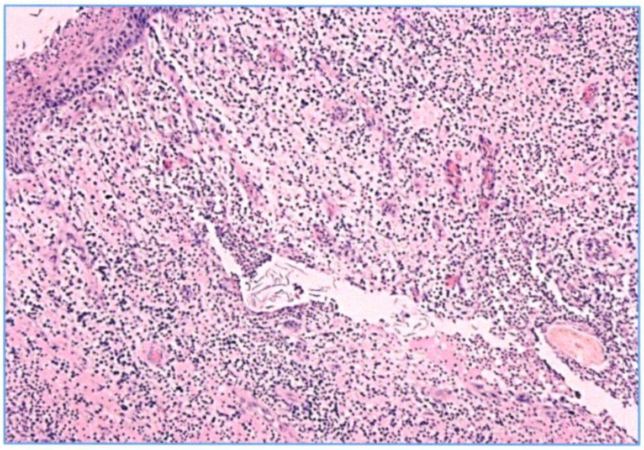

Hidradenitis suppurativa with dermal abscess

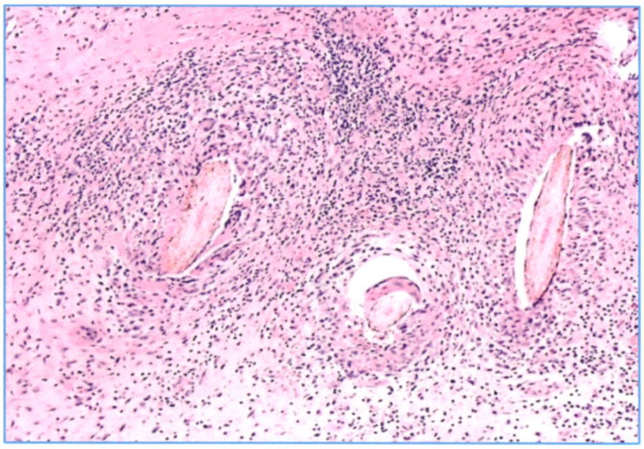

Pilonidal sinus with numerous naked hair shafts

All entities of follicular tetrad demonstrate remarkably similar histological features. Clinical correlation is of utmost importance.

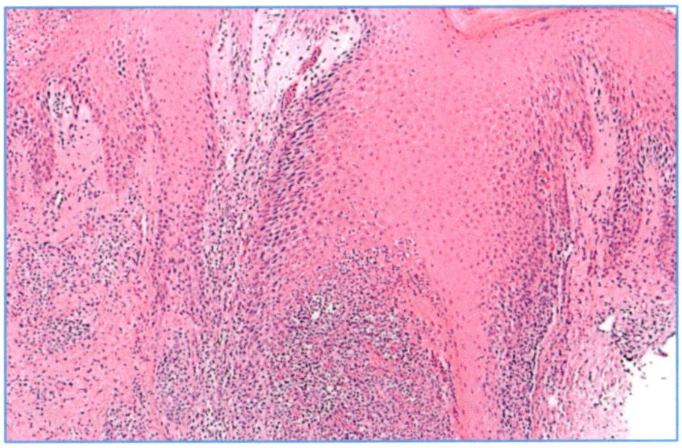

Bacterial folliculitis with neutrophilic inflammation in and around hair follicle

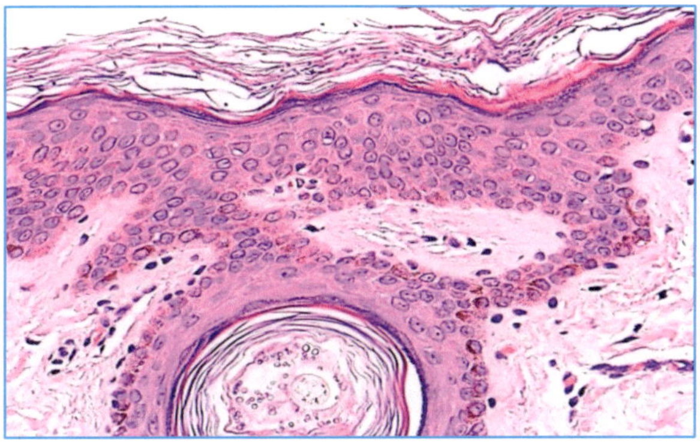

Pityrosporum folliculitis with spores within hair follicle and minimal inflammation

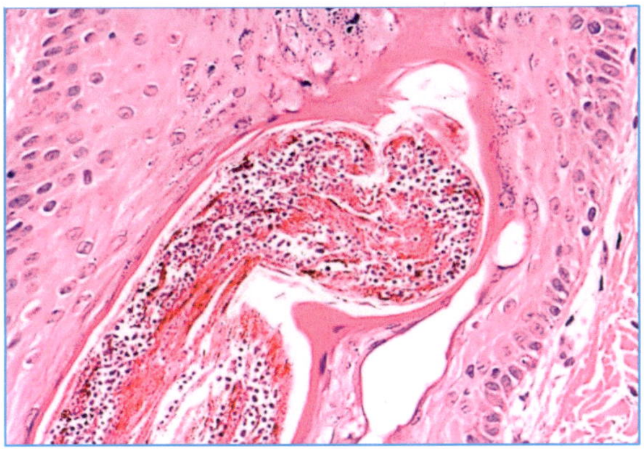

Tinea capitis with hyphae within the hair shaft (endotrix) and no inflammation

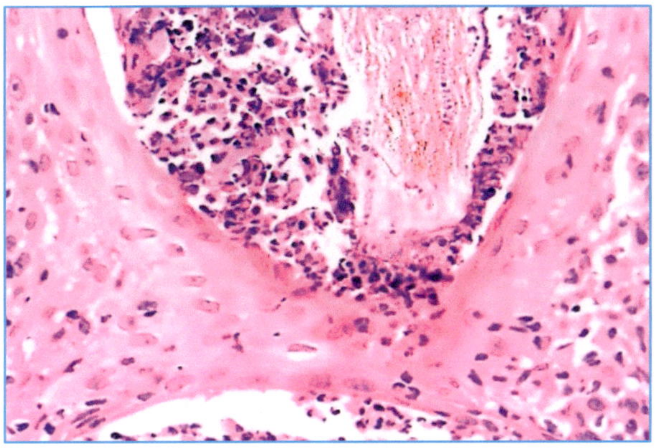

Majocchi's granuloma with hyphae within hair shaft and acute inflammation

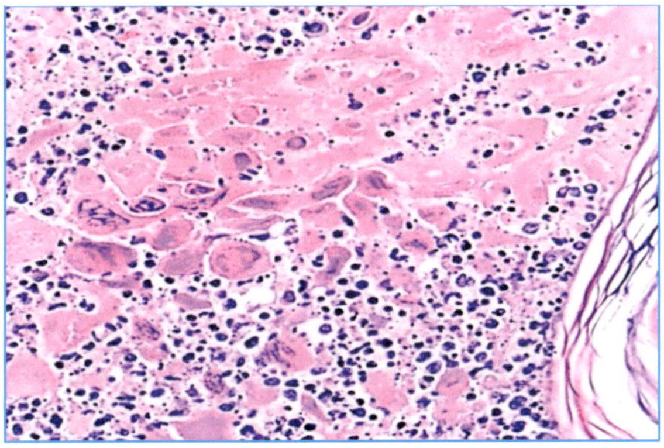

Herpes folliculitis with acute inflammation and viral inclusions

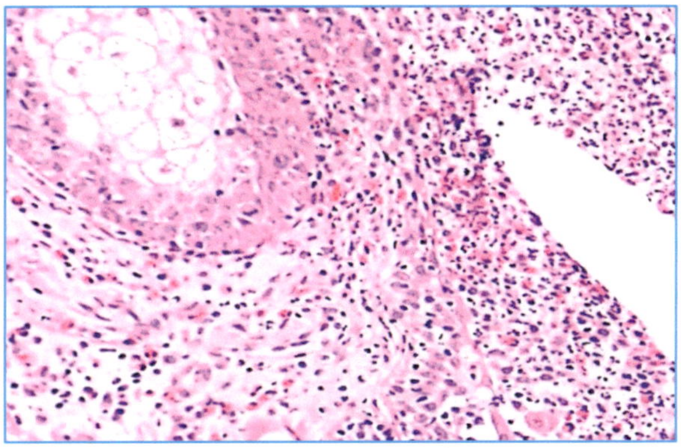

Eosinophilic folliculitis with eosinophils in and around hair follicle

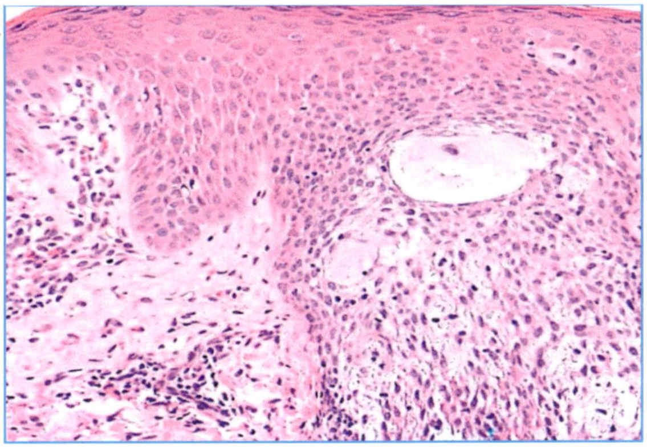

Follicular mucinosis with mucin within hair follicle

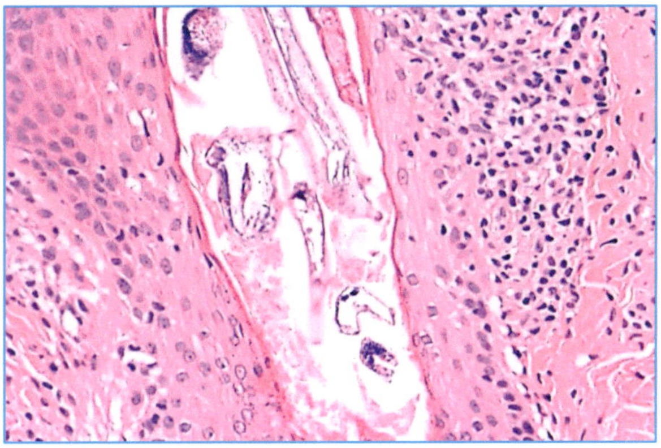

Demodex folliculitis with mites within hair follicle

Folliculitis and related disorders

Chapter 16

ALOPECIAS

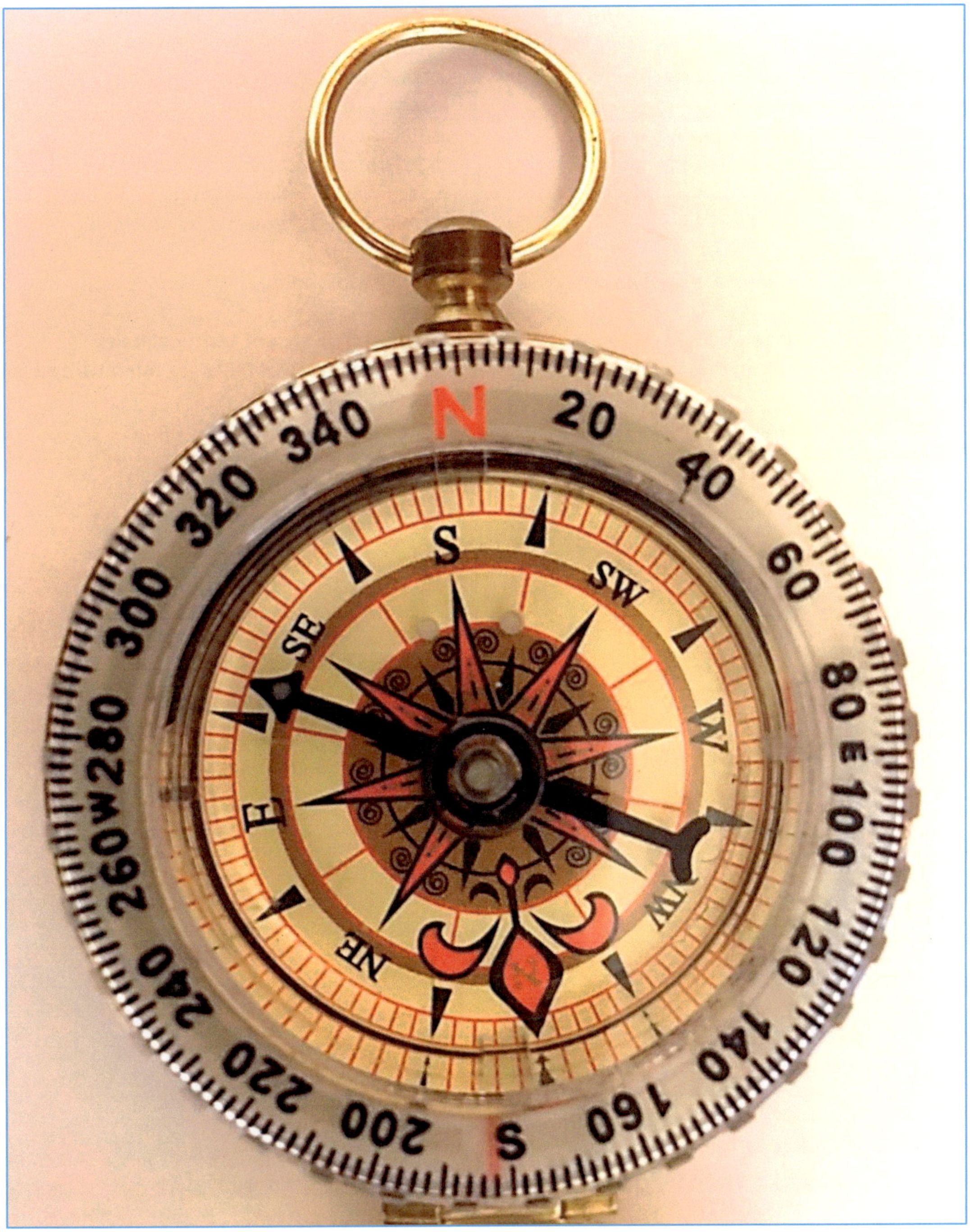

Alopecias

ALOPECIA AREATA

-**non-scarring alopecia** of autoimmune etiology due to CD8+ T cells targeting the hair follicles
-round areas of localized hair loss without scale or prominent erythema
-on dermoscopy perifollicular yellow dots and "exclamation mark" hairs can be seen
-over half occurs in patients before the age of 20

Variants:
-**alopecia totalis** with complete scalp hair loss
-**alopecia universalis** with whole body hair loss

Histopathology
-no scarring
-peribulbar lymphocytic infiltrate described as **"swarm of bees"**
-**decreased number of anagen hairs**
-**increased number of catagen/telogen hairs** (can be over 50%)
-remnants of anagen hair follicles presenting as **fibrous tracts** (also called **stellae or streamers**)

ANDROGENIC ALOPECIA

-**non-scarring**, hormonally driven form of hair loss
-affects 80% of men and 50% of women by age 70
-genetic predisposition (dominant inheritance with variable penetrance)
-in men, presents as frontotemporal hairline recession and diffuse hair thinning over frontal and vertex scalp
-in women, frontal hairline is preserved and there is hair thinning over the frontal scalp creating "Christmas tree" pattern around central part-line
-no scarring or inflammation
-terminal hair is replaced by fine vellus hair

Histopathology
-no scarring
-**decreased or absent terminal hairs**
-remaining terminal hairs are **miniaturized** (size of vellus hairs)
-**increased number of vellus hairs**
-prominent **sebaceous glands**
-follicular **fibrous tracts** present

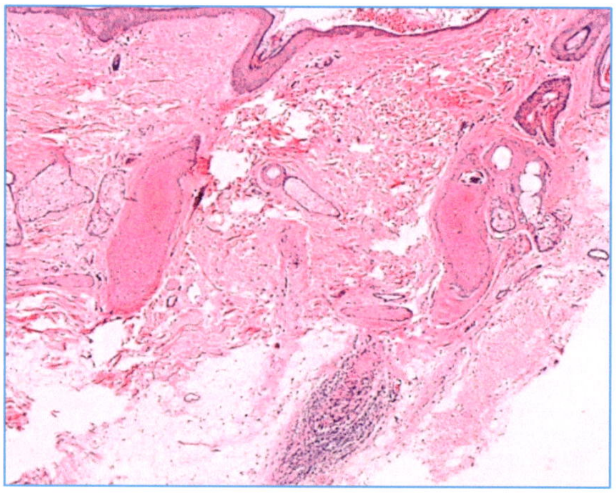

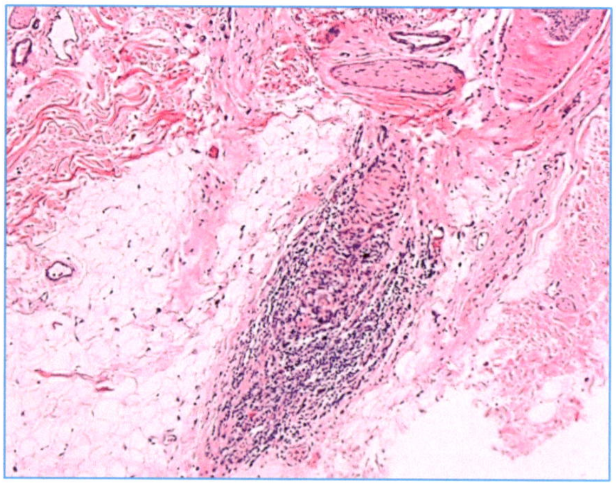

Alopecia areata with decreased number of anagen hairs and peribulbar lymphocytic inflammation

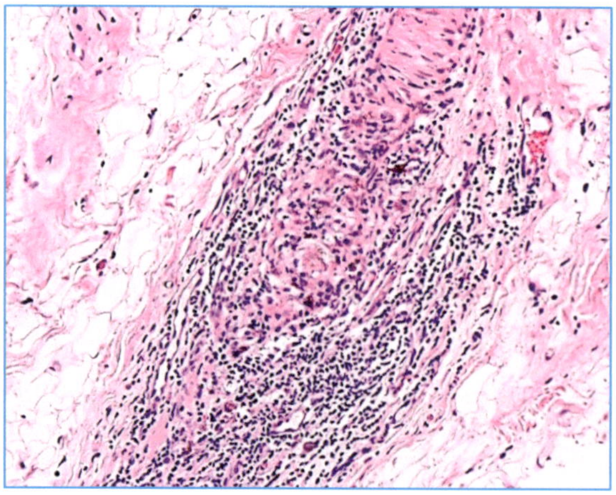

Alopecia areata with "swarm of bees"

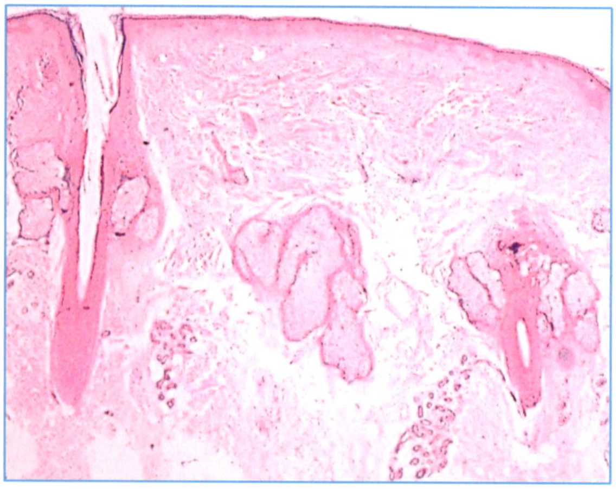

Androgenic alopecia with miniaturized hairs and prominent sebaceous glands

TELOGEN EFFLUVIUM

-**non-scarring alopecia** due to loss of telogen hairs in response to physiological or severe psychological stress (usually 3 months after event)
-precipitated by various stressful circumstances e.g. high fever, hemorrhage, crash diet, childbirth, chronic infection, systemic illnesses
-loss is diffuse and acute, but temporary, typically self-resolving within 6-12 months
-**positive hair pull test** (pull more than 5 hairs out of 50 grasped hairs)

Histopathology
-**no inflammation or scarring**
-normal terminal and vellus hair ratio and normal or slight decrease of hair density
-in **active** phase, **increased number of telogen hairs** (>20% but less than 50%; in normal hair it is <15%)
-in **chronic** phase, the biopsy appears like **normal scalp biopsy** (10-15% telogen hairs)

TRICHOTILLOMANIA

-self-induced, **non-scarring alopecia** resulting from patient pulling out his/her own hair
-classified under obsessive-compulsive and related disorders (along with skin-picking and body dysmorphic disorder)
-more common in children and young women
-can be associated with trichophagy (consumption of hair), which can result in formation of bezoars and intestinal obstruction
-large, irregular, and asymmetric patches of hair loss
-distribution often corresponds to the reach of dominant hand
-affected areas have broken hairs that are of uneven length

Histopathology
-increased number of catagen/telogen hairs (often >50%)
-**hair follicles are distorted**
-**no scarring and with minimal inflammation** only in superficial dermis
-presence of **empty hair follicles** and melanin **pigment cast** within the follicle
-follicular streamers can be present

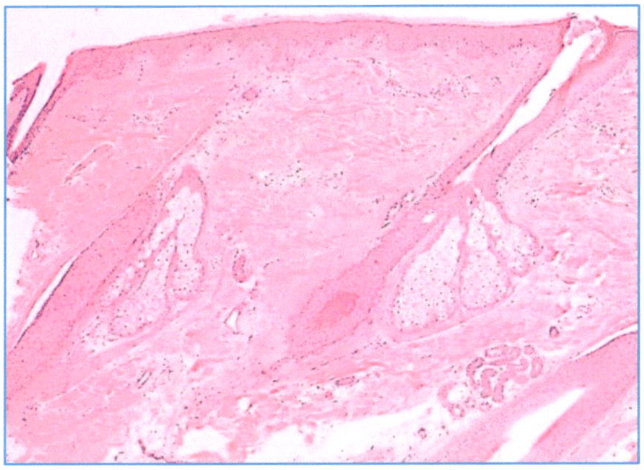

Telogen effluvium in active phase has increased number of telogen hairs

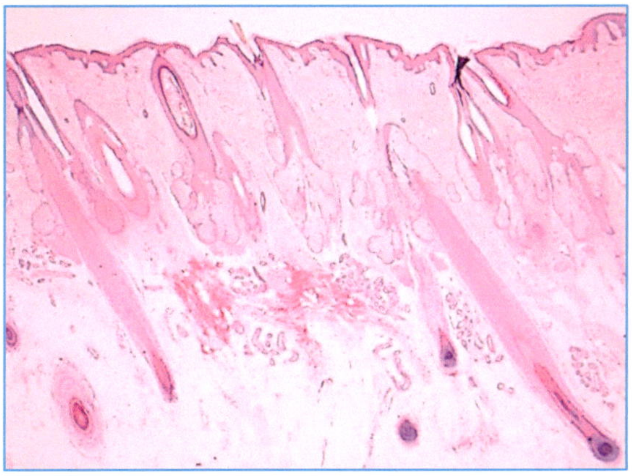

Telogen effluvium in chronic phase appears like normal scalp skin

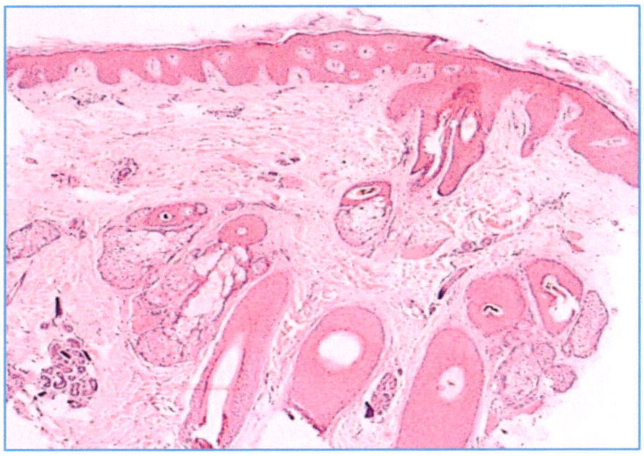

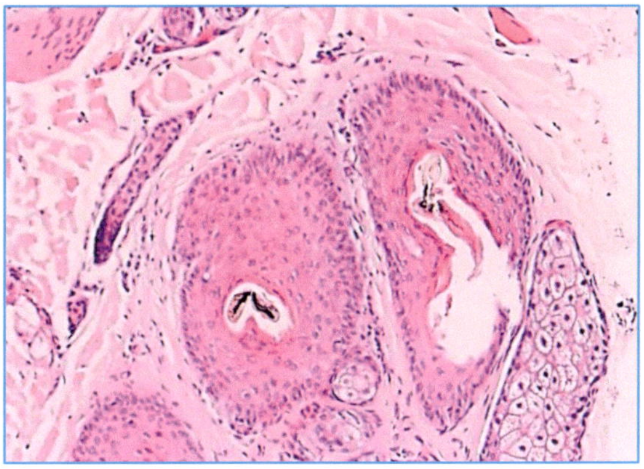

Trichotillomania with distorted hair follicles and pigment cast within the follicles

Alopecias

TINEA CAPITIS

-non-scarring alopecia
-superficial fungal infection of the scalp favoring children
-caused by dermatophytes that invade the hair shaft
-results in scaly, single/multiple patches of hair loss with short broken (**"black dot"**), and "**comma-shaped"** hairs

Histopathology
-epidermal hyperkeratosis with **no scarring** and minimal perifollicular inflammation
-in **endothrix** infections (e.g. *Trichophyton tonsurans/ violaceum*) **the hyphae extend within the hair shaft**
-in **ectothrix** infections (e.g. *Microsporum canis/ audouinii*) **fungal forms coat the outside of the hair shaft without significant invasion** of the shaft itself

KERION and **FAVUS** are variants of severe cases of **T. capitis** that **can cause scarring alopecia**

KERION
-result of the host's response to a fungal infection of the hair follicles
-presents as inflamed, boggy, purulent abscess on the scalp
-hairs within the kerion are loose and fall out, resulting in a bald area
-caused by *T. verrucosum*, *T. mentagrophytes*, and *Microsporum canis*
-frequently accompanied by secondary bacterial infection

Histopathology
-exuberant **suppurative folliculitis with abscess formation** and **fungal spores and hyphae**

FAVUS

-chronic fungal infection of the scalp, usually caused by *T. schoenleinii,* causing hair loss, atrophy, and scarring
-yellow crusting in "honeycomb" pattern on the scalp (scutula)
-each crust encircles a strand of hair which pierces the center
-uncommon in the US and confined to areas with malnutrition and poor living conditions
-occurs in both children and adults

Histopathology
-characteristic **scutula** (masses of keratinized as well as parakeratotic cells, exudate, and inflammatory cells intermingled with hyphae and spores)
-the **periphery of infected lesions has well-preserved hyphae**, while dead mycelium and granular debris (scutula) is present in the center

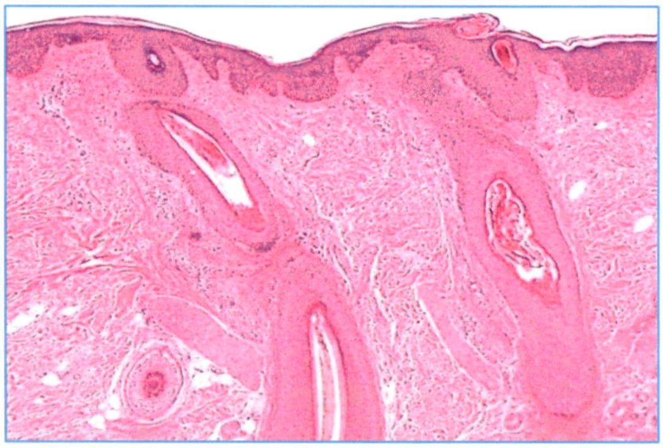
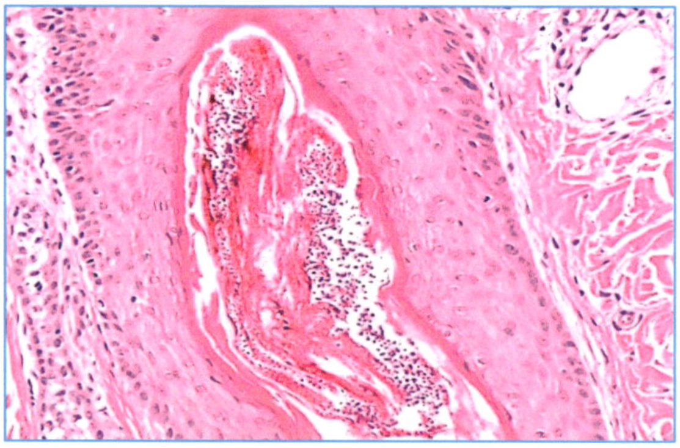

Tinea capitis with hyphae and spores within the hair follicle (endotrix)

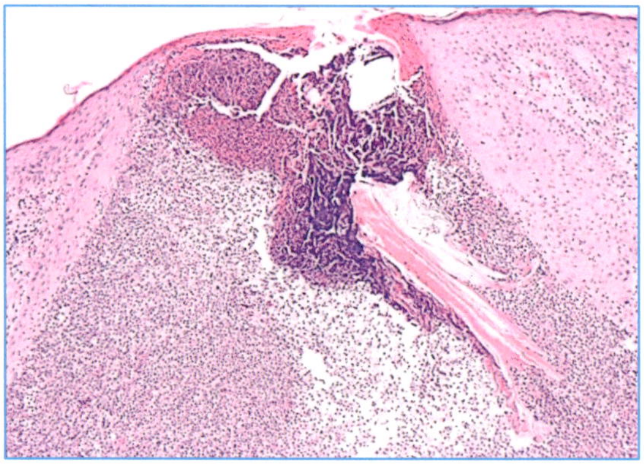

Kerion with suppurative folliculitis

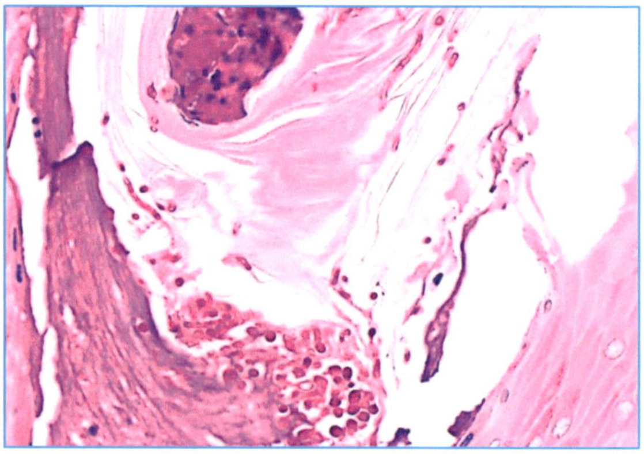

PAS stains fungal hyphae and spores in kerion

Chapter 16

DISCOID LUPUS ERYTHEMATOSUS

-most common variant of chronic cutaneous lupus erythematous
-sharply marginated, scaly, atrophic, red-white plaques on sun exposed area (scalp, nose, cheeks, ears, lower lip)
-follicular plugging is present
-on scalp results in **scarring alopecia** in affected area

Histopathology

-hyperkeratotic but atrophic epidermis with dilated **keratin-plugged follicles**
-interface **vacuolar changes** with focal necrotic keratinocytes
-thickened basement membrane and increased dermal mucin
-superficial and deep, **patchy, perivascular and periadnexal lymphocytic infiltrate** with tendency to accumulate around hair follicles
-**dermal scarring** is present

LICHEN PLANOPILARIS

-variant of lichen planus that involves hair follicles
-more common in middle-aged women
-hair loss is patchy and mostly on vertex
-perifollicular erythema, pruritus, and scaling are characteristic
-results in **scarring alopecia**
-half will have associated skin findings of lichen planus

Frontal fibrosing alopecia

-variant of LPP with frontal hairline recession and eyebrow loss

Lassueur Graham-Little Piccardi syndrome

-progressive "LPP-like" scarring alopecia of scalp, non-scarring hair loss of axilla and pubic area, and keratosis pilaris

Histopathology

-**upper part of the follicle** is surrounded by lichenoid infiltrate
-**inflammation abuts epidermal-dermal junction**
-no significant perivascular or perieccrine inflammation
-**dermal scarring** is present

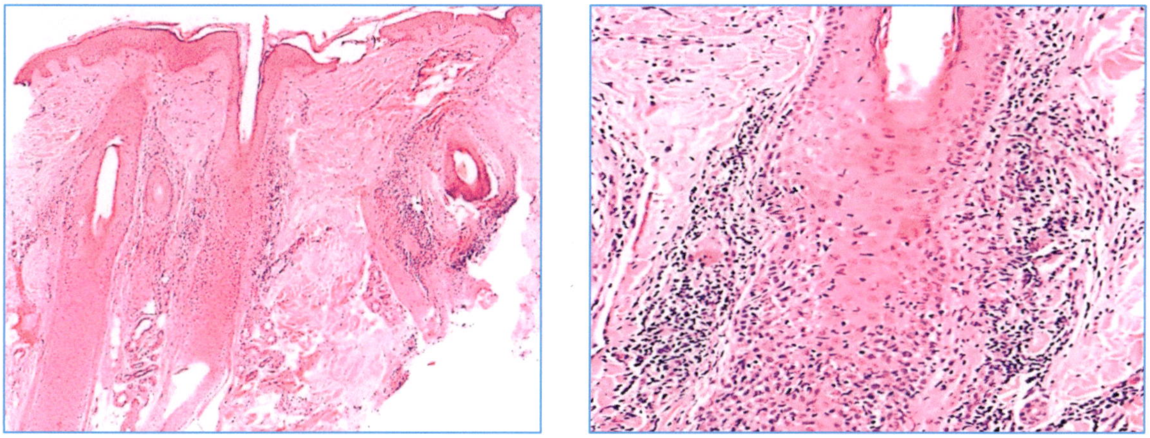

Lichen planopilaris with inflammation abutting upper half of the hair follicle

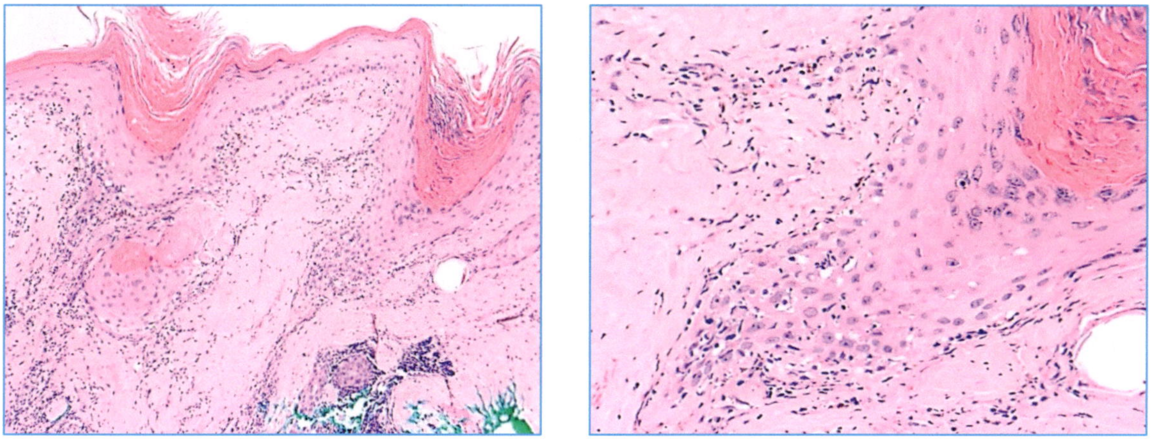

Discoid lupus erythematosus with dilated keratin-filled follicles, interface vacuolar changes, and patchy inflammation

Alopecias

ACNE KELOIDALIS NUCHAE

-**scarring hair loss** that occurs on the occipital scalp and posterior neck
-almost exclusively develops in young African American men
-starts as mildly pruritic, follicular-based papules and pustules on the nape
-with time, raised plaques and firm scars develop and enlarge to resemble a keloid
-resulting scarred area is hairless with a few tufted hairs

Histopathology

-early lesion resembles suppurative folliculitis with distorted follicles and numerous neutrophils
-in established lesions, **hair follicles are destroyed**
-extensive fibrosis with embedded scattered **"naked hair shafts"** (hair shafts without supporting structures)
-mostly lymphoplasmocytic inflammation present
-**collagen bundles are prominent** with dark pink color **like a keloid**, but are **thinne**r **than true keloidal collagens**

DISSECTING CELLULITIS

-rare inflammatory scalp condition
-more common in young African American men
-boggy plaques with pustules and fluctuant suppurative nodules with subsequent hair loss
-hair loss is permanent and **leaves scar** tissue
-predilection for vertex and occipital scalp
-it is a part of the follicular occlusion tetrad (acne conglobata, hidradenitis suppurativa, dissecting cellulitis, pilonidal cyst)

Histopathology

-exuberant neutrophilic folliculitis
-**deep dermal abscesses** and **sinus tract**
-destroyed hair follicles with free, broken "**naked hair shafts**"
-in older lesions, more lymphocytes, macrophages, and giant cells in addition to neutrophils
-increased fibrosis with scar formation

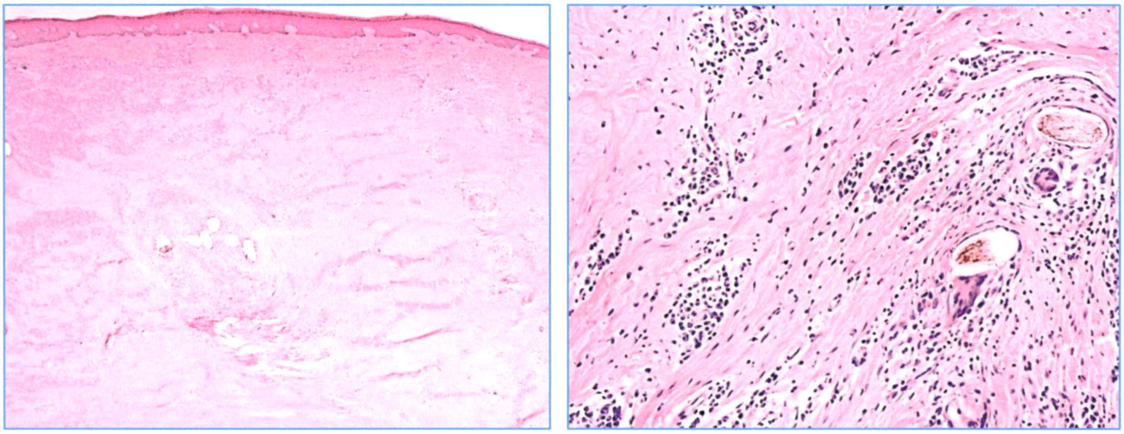

Acne keloidales nuchae with naked hair shaft embedded in "keloid-like" collagenous stroma

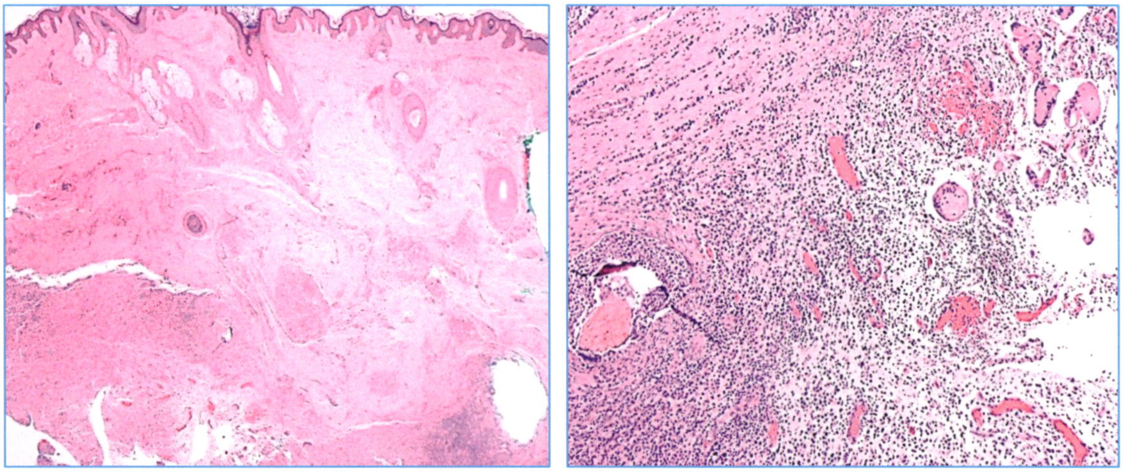

Dissecting cellulitis with deep dermal abscess and naked hair shafts embedded in inflammation

CENTRAL CENTRIFUGAL CICATRICIAL ALOPECIA (CCCA)

-chronic **scarring alopecia** in African American women
-associated with chemical or physical trauma (relaxers, hot comb use) or idiopathic
-usually starts at vertex and spreads outward
-initially may be boggy
-eventually results in scarring with loss of follicular openings
-scalp may appear shiny with multiple hairs emerging from a single follicular opening (**"doll hair"**)
-no clinical evidence of inflammation

Histopathology

-mild perifollicular lymphocytic inflammation around upper portion of the hair follicle
-**concentric fibrosis around upper hair follicle** segment (**"tree trunk fibrosis"**)
-**premature desquamation of inner root sheath** in non-inflamed follicle (found also in inflamed follicles in LPP, alopecia areata)
-absence of sebaceous glands
-in old lesions, histology is identical to pseudopelade

FOLLICULITIS DECALVANS

-**scarring alopecia** most common in African American males
-starts with redness, swelling, and perifollicular pustules
-expands to form patch of alopecia with peripheral pustules
-several hairs can be seen coming out of a single follicle (**"tufted"** appearance)
-in end stage, the hairs are shed as the follicles are completely destroyed, leaving a scar

Histopathology

-follicles are distorted and/or ruptured
-**suppurative neutrophilic folliculitis** and **abscess formation**
-follicles with multiple hair shafts can be seen
-prominent dermal scarring

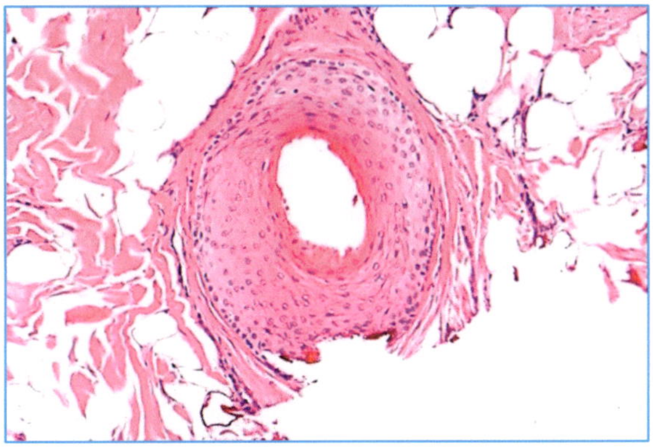

CCCA with premature desquamation of inner root sheath

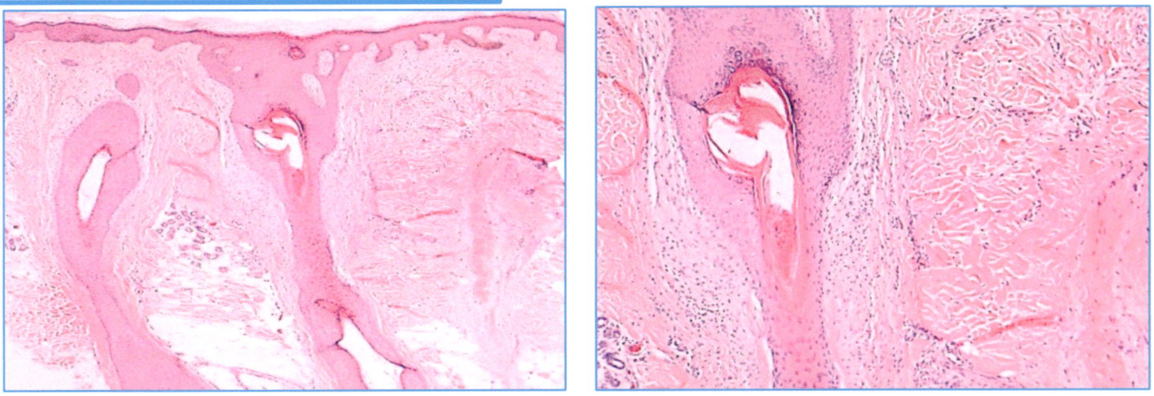

CCCA with concentric fibrosis around upper portion of the hair follicle

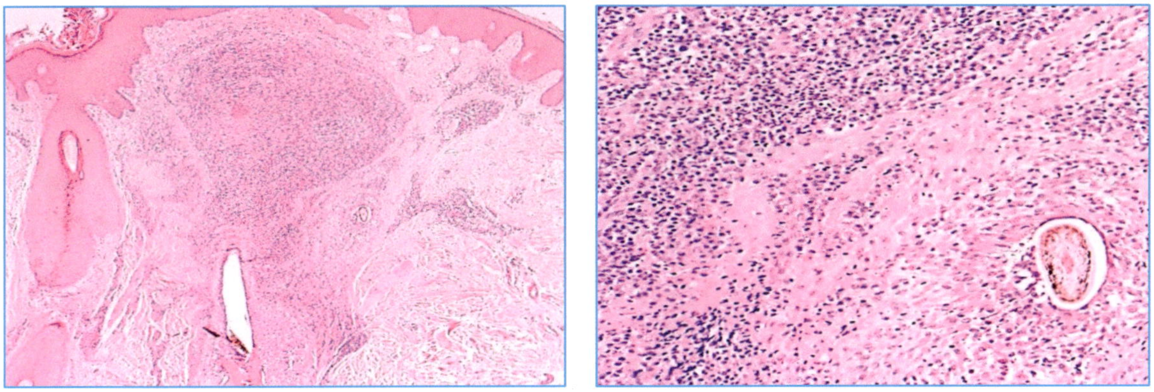

Folliculitis decalvans with suppurative folliculitis destroying hair follicle and forming abscess

Alopecias

EROSIVE PUSTULAR DERMATOSIS OF THE SCALP

-localized areas of pustules and eroded plaques with granulation tissue and lakes of pus
-typically affects the sun-damaged, bald scalp of older males
-frequently follows trauma or a surgical procedure (pathergy)
-complications are hair loss, secondary bacterial infection, and skin cancer
-often biopsied to exclude malignancy
-responds well to corticosteroid therapy

Histopathology

-**excoriated atrophic skin with serum crust with neutrophils**
-mixed dermal inflammatory infiltrate with **granulation tissue and scarring**
-findings are non-specific and clinical correlation is needed

TRACTION ALOPECIA

-loss of hair caused by repetitive or continuous and prolonged tension on hair follicles from styling patterns
-associated with occupational hair styles and behavioral patterns (e.g. ballerinas) or other hairstyles that cause tension
-more common in African Americans
-presents as localized hair loss typically on the frontal and temporal scalp with fractured hair
-hairs are retained along the temporal or frontal rims of hairline, **"fringe sign"**

Histopathology

-early stage is **similar to trichotillomania**
-**no inflammation or scarring**
-increased number of catagen/telogen hairs
-distortion of hair follicles
-occasional pigmented casts
-in late stages, number of terminal hairs is decreased and replaced by fibrous tracts
-resembles **"burned-out" scarring alopecia**

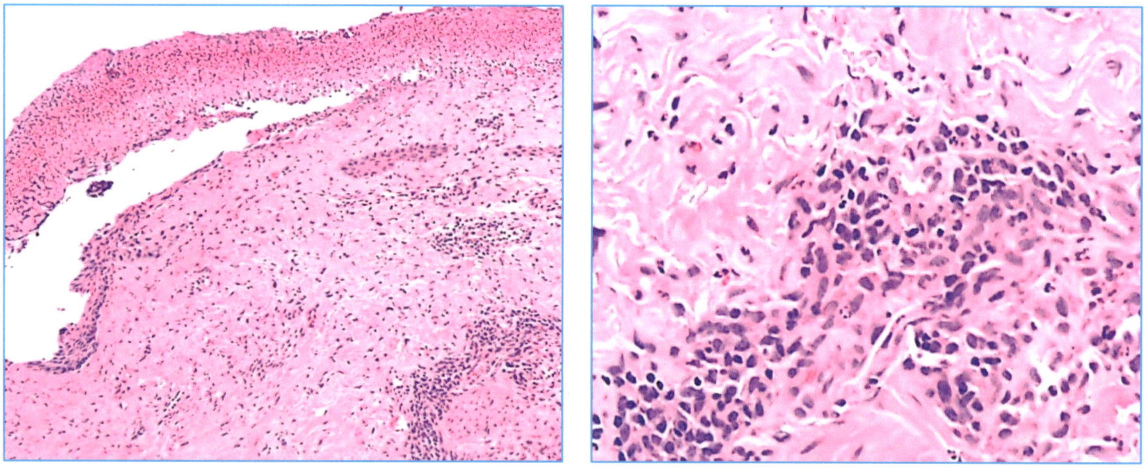

Erosive pustular dermatosis with excoriated epidermis covered with serum crust and dermal scarring and inflammation

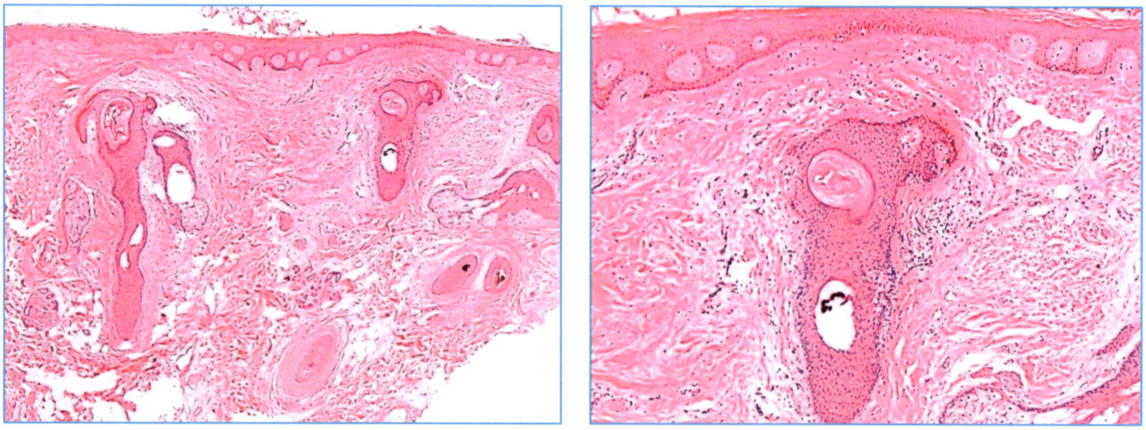

Non-scarring traction alopecia with distorted hair follicles, pigmented cast, and no inflammation

Chapter 16

PSEUDOPELADE OF BROCQ (IDIOPATHIC SCARRING ALOPECIA/IDIOPATHIC PSEUDOPELADE)

-term used to describe the end stage of any scarring alopecia when **etiology is unknown**
-any inflammatory skin disorder that affects the scalp (e.g. discoid lupus erythematosus, lichen planus, cicatricial pemphigoid) can lead to end stage scarring alopecia or pseudopelade
-typically, middle-aged women with patchy hair loss with no evidence of any inflammatory disease
-bald patches are slightly depressed and atrophic with completely absent hair follicles
-patches resemble "**footprints in the snow**" and can coalesce into larger areas

Histopathology
-**complete loss of hair follicles** and sebaceous glands
-replaced by bands of **fibrous scarring tissue** in the upper dermis
-**fibrous tracts** are usually present

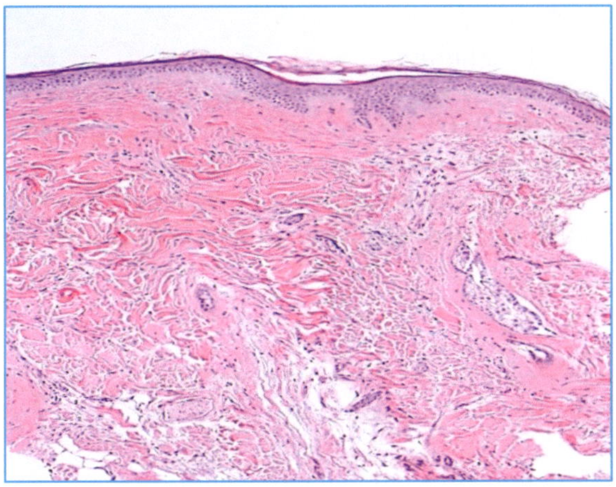

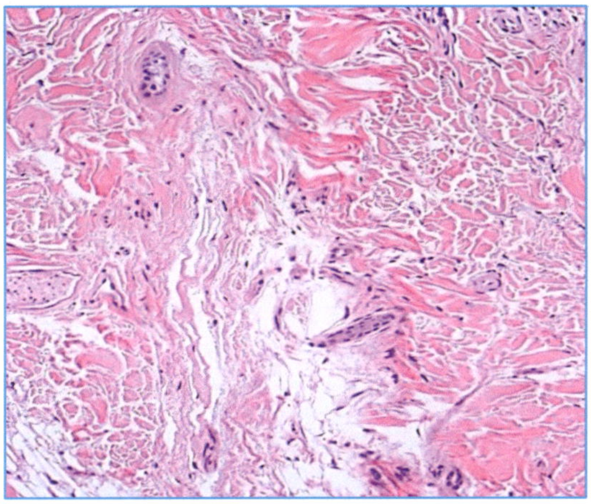

Pseudopelade of Brocq with complete absence of hair follicles and sebaceous glands. Fibrous tract is present.

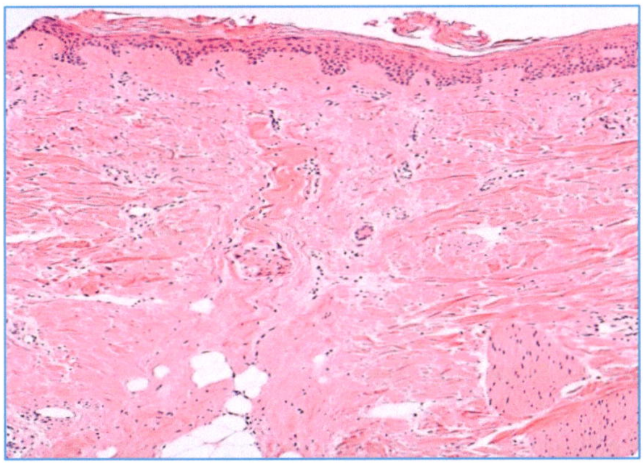

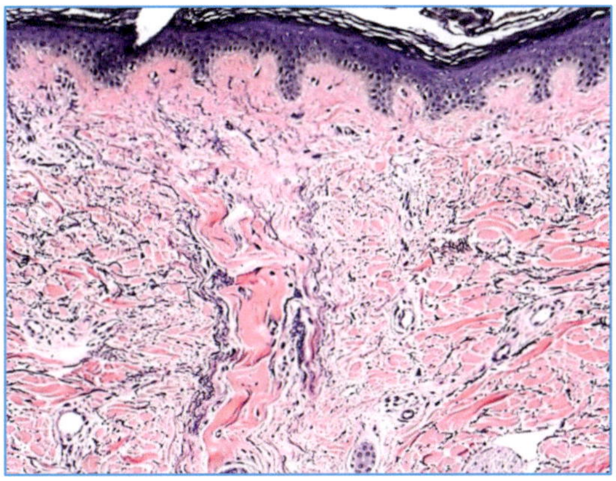

Pseudopelade of Brocq with scarring and fibrous tracts that are better visualized using elastin (VVG) stain on the right

Alopecias

HOW TO APPROACH ALOPECIA

IS THERE DERMAL SCARRING OR NO SCARRING?

SCARRING ALOPECIA WITH NEUTROPHILS

-folliculitis decalvans	suppurative folliculitis	crops of pustules	any area
-acne keloidales nuchae	suppurative folliculitis	"keloidal" scar	nape
-dissecting cellulitis	suppurative folliculitis	deep abscesses	vertex
-kerion, favus	suppurative folliculitis	hyphae/spores	
-erosive pustular dermatosis	epidermal erosions subcorneal non-follicular pustules	granulation tissue	bold scalp

SCARRING ALOPECIA WITH LYMPHOCYTES

-DLE	dilated plugged follicles	patchy infiltrate perivascular, perieccrine, perifollicular	mucin
-LPP/FFA	normal shaped follicles	"band-like" infiltrate around upper 1/3rd of follicle no perivascular/perieccrine lymphocytes	no mucin
-CCCA	distorted follicles	myxoid stroma/fibrosis/ lymphocytes around upper 1/3rd of follicle premature desquamation of inner root sheath	

SCARRING ALOPECIA WITH NO HAIR FOLLICLES

-pseudopelade — loss of all hairs and sebaceous glands replaced with scar and streamers

Note: Any scarring alopecia or end-stage traction alopecia can end as pseudopelade

NON-SCARRING ALOPECIA

-tinea capitis	fungal spores and hyphae in and around hair shaft
-alopecia areata	peribulbar inflammation ("swarm of bees")
-androgenic alopecia	↓terminal hairs + ↑sebaceous glands + miniaturized and vellus hairs
-telogen effluvium	in active phase ↑ telogen hair in chronic phase normal appearing biopsy
-trichotillomania	distorted follicles and melanin cast
-traction alopecia	early- distorted follicles and melanin cast (like trichotillomania) later- scarring (pseudopelade)

Note: Normal scalp has 85-90% anagen, 5-10% telogen, and 1-3% catagen hairs

In diagnosing non-scarring alopecia, counting ratio of different stages of hair development can be useful. Here is the summary:

-alopecia areata	↑ catagen/telogen hairs (over 50% and up to 70%)
-androgen alopecia	miniaturized terminal hairs
-telogen effluvium	↑ telogen hairs (over 20% but less than 50%)
-trichotillomania	↑ catagen/telogen hairs (over 50%)

Chapter 16

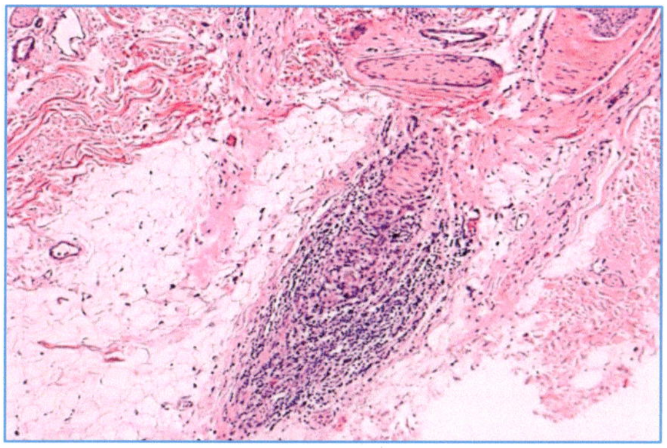

Alopecia areata with peribulbar lymphocytes

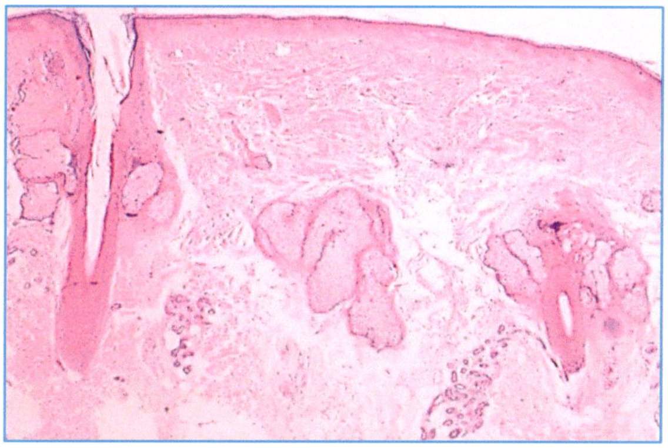

Androgenic alopecia with prominent sebaceous glands and miniaturized hairs

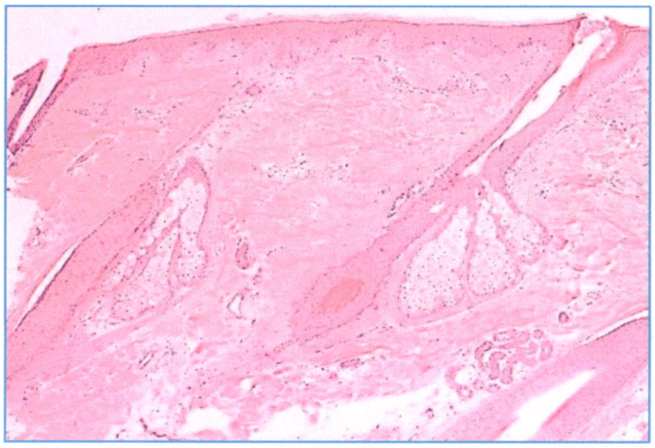

Telogen effluvium with telogen hair

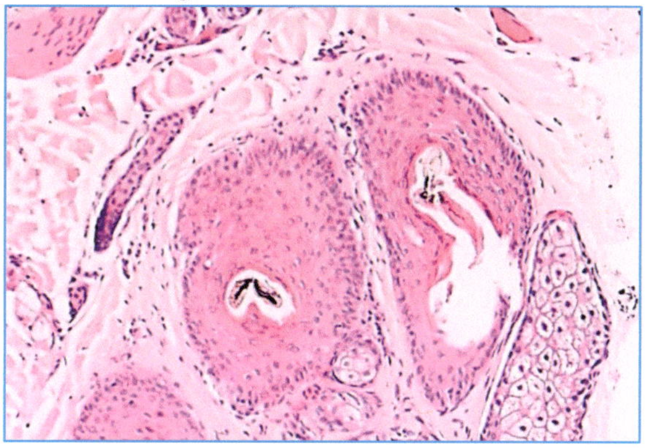

Trichotillomania with distorted hair follicles with pigment cast

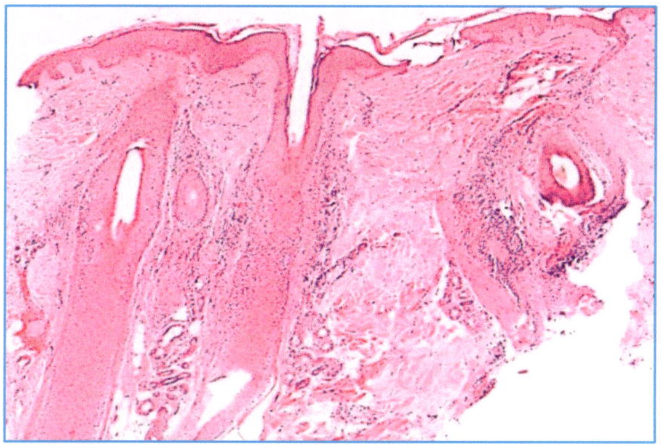

LPP with normal size follicles and perifollicular inflammation around upper portion of the follicle

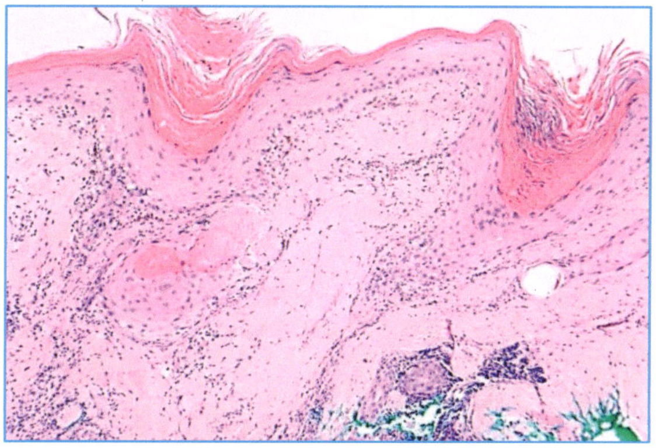

DLE with dilated plugged follicles with perifollicular and perivascular inflammation

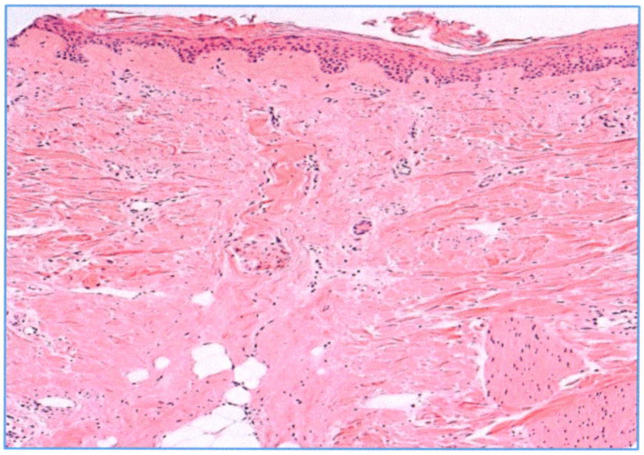

Pseudopelade scar with fibrous stella and no hair follicles

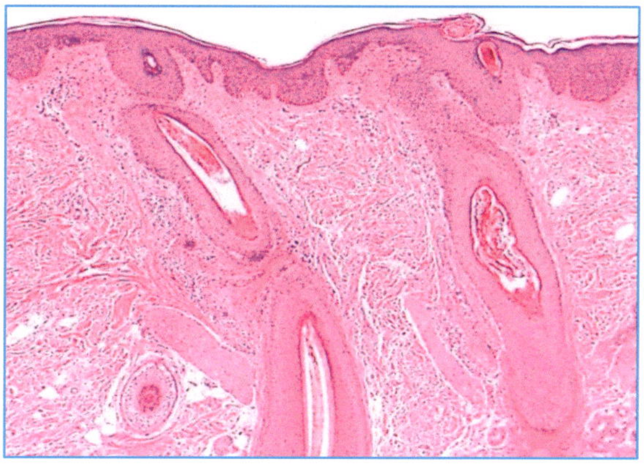

Tinea capitis with endothrix hyphae within hair shaft

Alopecias

Chapter 17

BACTERIAL INFECTIONS

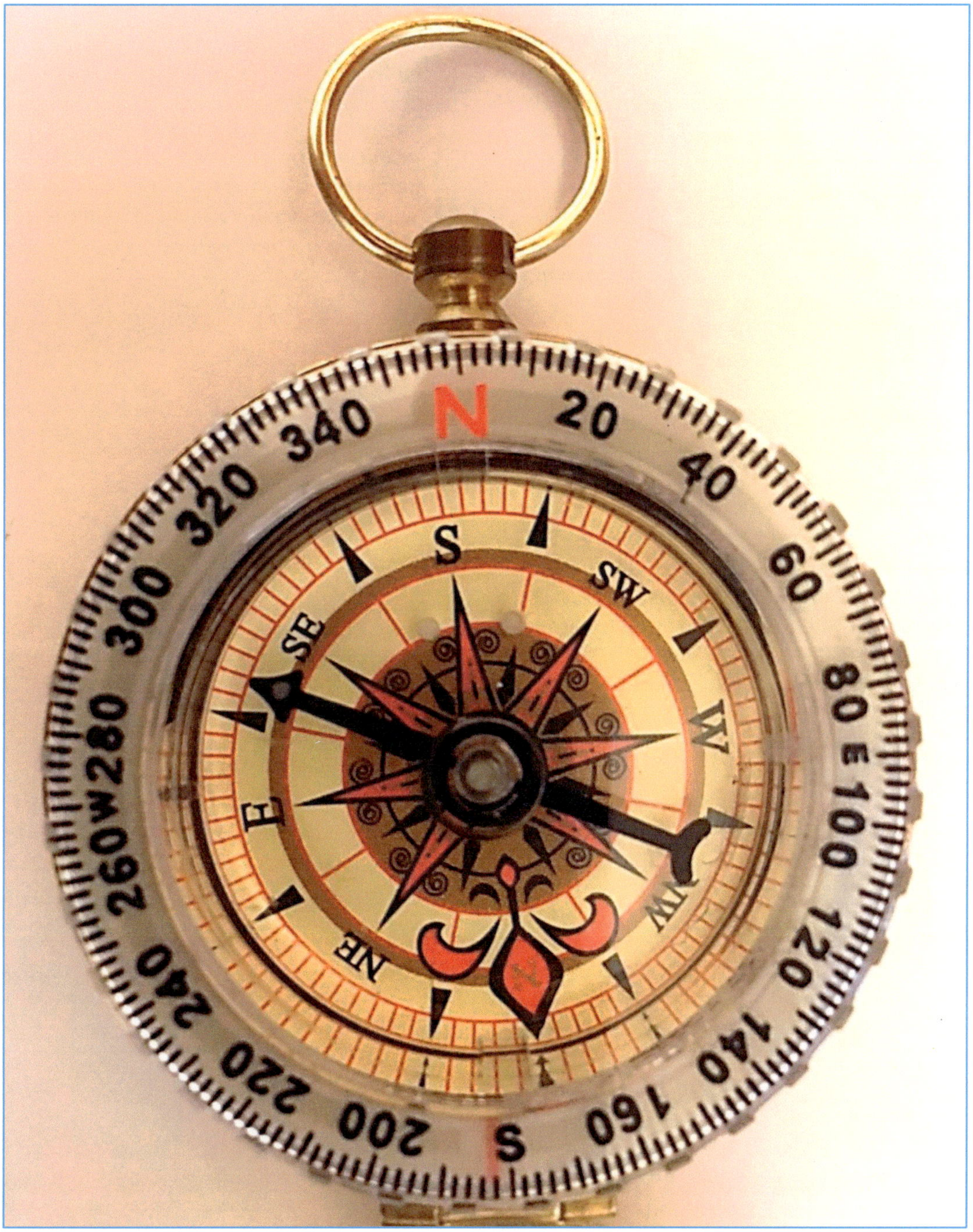

Bacterial infections

IMPETIGO/ ECTHYMA

Impetigo

-infection of the epidermis with *Staphylococcus aureus* (#1) and *Streptococcus pyogenes* (#2)
-it is the most common bacterial infection in children
-it presents more commonly as **non-bullous** and less commonly as **bullous form** (described in the chapter on intraepidermal blisters)
-non-bullous form presents with small vesicles/pustules that rupture forming erosions covered with golden yellow ("honey colored") crust
-predilection for face (perioral and perinasal), but also arms, legs, and buttock

Ecthyma

-deep variant of impetigo by *Streptococcus pyogenes* (#1)
-predisposing factors are warm, humid environment, atopic dermatitis, and prior antibiotic therapy
-ulceration with a thick, adherent, hemorrhagic crust
-predilection for ankles, feet, thighs, and buttock
-slowly resolves with scarring

Histopathology

Impetigo

-**subcorneal pustule filled with neutrophils**
-Gram positive bacteria present, but not always

Ecthyma

-ulceration of the skin with an inflammatory crust
-heavy **neutrophilic infiltrate in the reticular dermis**

ECTHYMA GANGRENOSUM

-epidermal and dermal bacterial infection caused by *Pseudomonas aeruginosa*
-typically in immunosuppressed patients
-usually indicates septicemia
-starts as erythematous macule that progress into a bulla
-ends with necrotic ulcer

Histopathology

-**epidermal, dermal, and subcutaneous necrosis**
-mixed inflammation with neutrophils
-**hemorrhage and vascular necrosis** sometimes with Gram-negative bacteria in the vessel wall

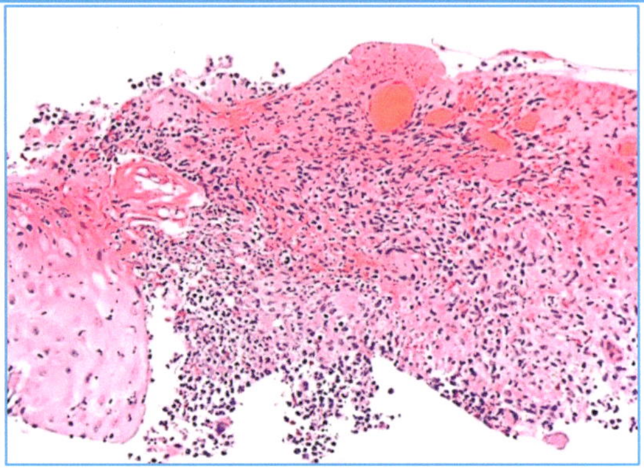

Ecthyma with ulcerated epidermis and epidermal and dermal neutrophils

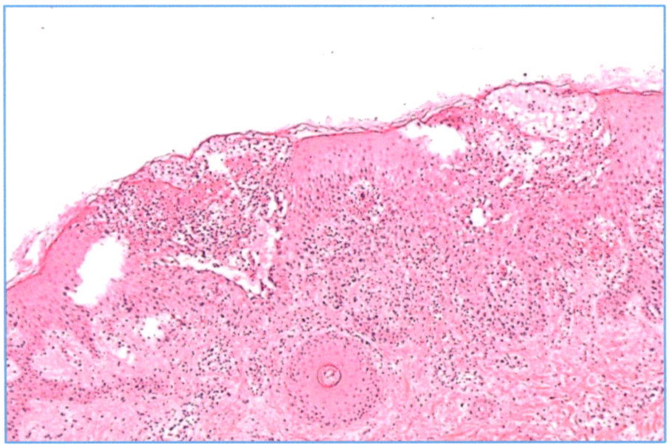

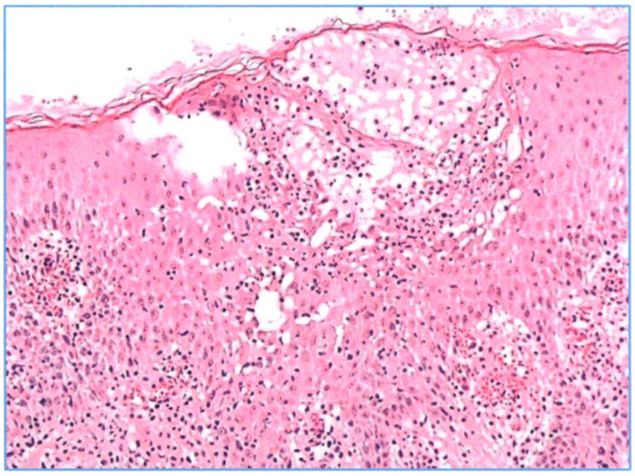

Impetigo with subcorneal neutrophilic pustule

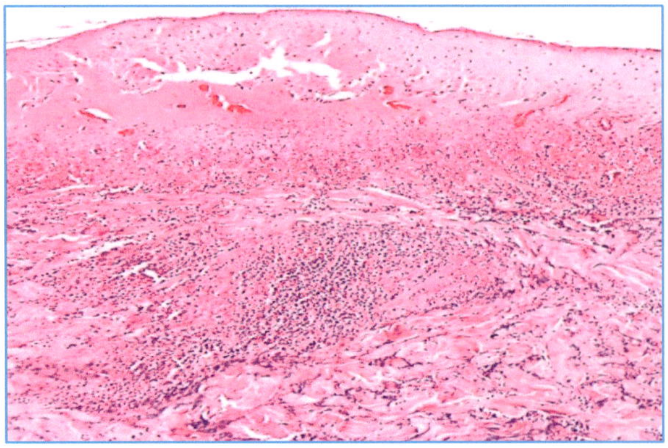

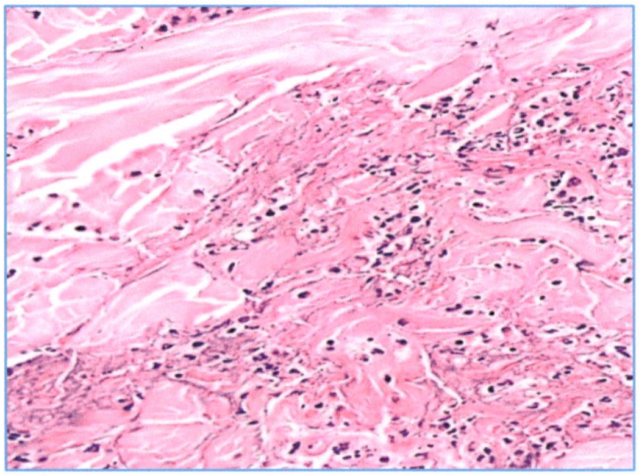

Ecthyma gangrenosum with extensive superficial and deep necrosis

Chapter 17

ERYSIPELAS/ CELLULITIS

-acutely spreading bacterial infections

Erysipelas

-due to group A *β–hemolytic Streptococcus*
-superficial variant of cellulitis
-red, hot, tender plaques with **sharp borders**
-predisposition for lower extremity and face

Cellulitis

-head/neck are favored sites in children (*S.aureous*)
-lower extremities are the most common site in adults (group A *β–hemolytic Strep)*
- red, tender, hot, **ill-defined** plaques
- sometimes with associated fever and lymphangitis

Histopathology

Erysipelas

-**dermal edema** that can form subepidermal blister
-dermal interstitial **neutrophilic infiltrate**
-bacterial stains are negative

Cellulitis

-superficial and deep dermal edema with dilated capillaries/ lymphatics
-superficial and deep dermal neutrophils with predominantly interstitial distribution, and therefore, easy to overlook

NECROTIZING FASCIITIS

-deep, life-threatening bacterial infection of fascia and soft tissue
-caused by group A *β–hemolytic Streptococcus* M types 1 and 3 in children
-typically caused by polymicrobial (*Streptococci, Staphylococci, E. coli, Clostridium, Bacteroides)* in adults
-diabetes, alcoholism, and immunosuppression are predisposing factors
-diffuse erythema, usually on the leg, that progresses to necrosis

Histopathology

-**necrosis of subcutis, fascia, and muscle**
-extensive neutrophilic inflammation
-**hemorrhage and vascular thrombosis**
-Gram stain positive for bacteria

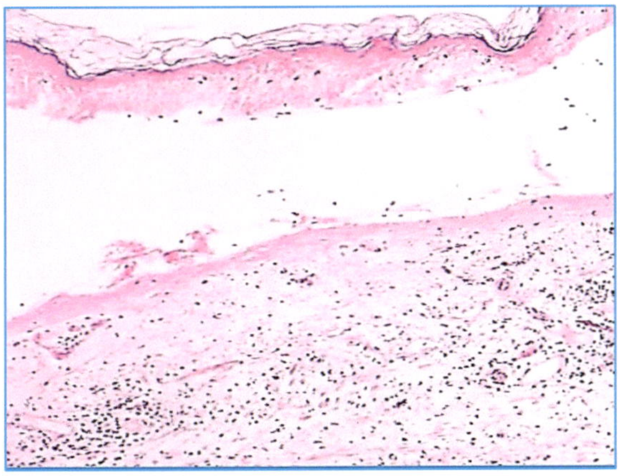

Erysipelas with subepidermal split, superficial dermal edema, and neutrophils

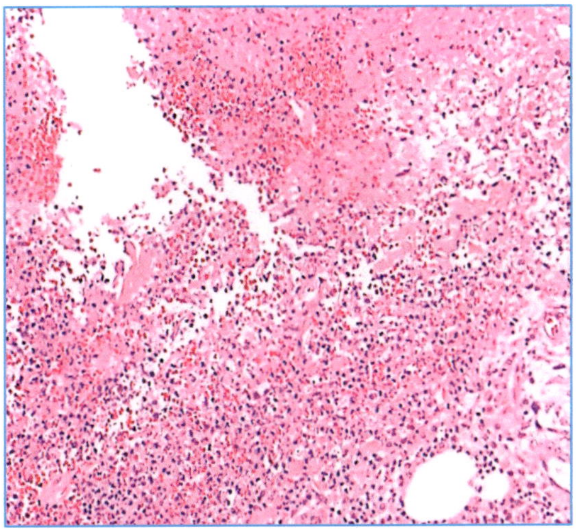

Necrotizing fasciitis with subcutaneous necrosis, neutrophils, and hemorrhage

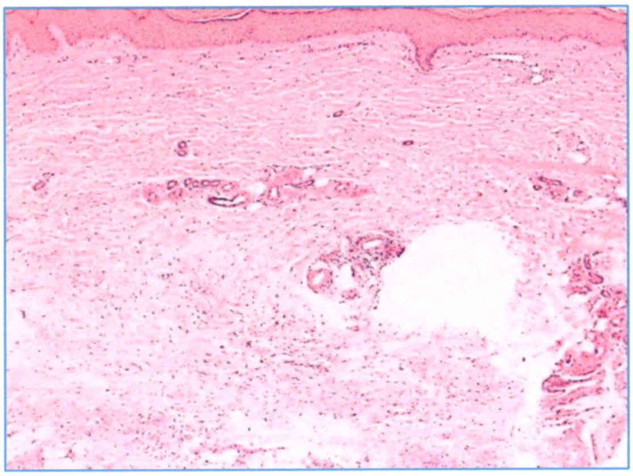

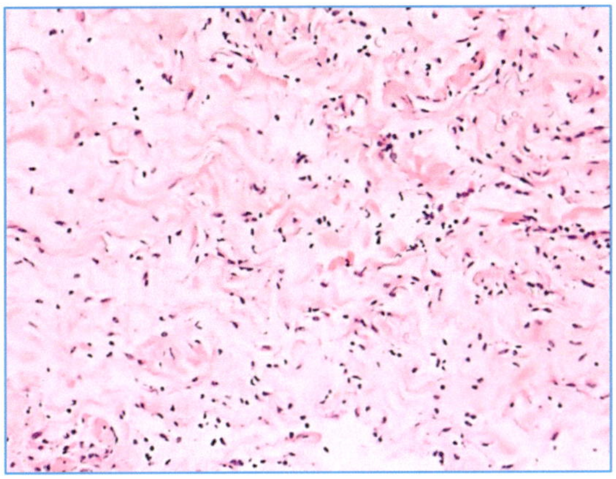

Cellulitis with diffuse dermal edema and deep interstitial neutrophils

Bacterial infections

ACTINOMYCOSIS/ BOTRYOMYCOSIS/ ACTINOMYCETOMA

-non-tender papules and nodules at site of inoculation
-lesion drains pus on pressure

Actinomycosis

-caused by filamentous *Actinomyces israelii*
-present in the normal flora of the mouth
-infection develops after oral trauma
-suppurative abscess draining yellow sulfur granules
-classic location is along mandible **("lumpy jaw")**

Botryomycosis

-associated with immunosuppression
-cutaneous and visceral form
-most caused by *Staphylococci*
-*Pseudomonas* and *Proteus* less frequently
-deep suppurative nodules that drain pus

Actinomycetoma (actinomycotic mycetoma)

-caused by *Nocardia* and more common in the tropics
-draining nodule favoring legs or neck

Histopathology

-dermal/ subcutaneous abscess and necrosis
-**"sulfur granules"** composed of filamentous bacteria (Actinomycosis, Actinomycetoma), Gram positive or Gram negative non-branching bacteria (Botryomycosis)
-"**starburst-like" eosinophilic material** composed of immunoglobulins and necrotic tissue surrounding granules (Splendore-Hoeppli phenomenon)

RHINOSCLEROMA

-chronic inflammatory disease of nose and upper respiratory tract
-common in tropical areas (Central and Latin America, Asia, Africa)
-caused by inhalation of *Klebsiella rhinoscleromatis*
-starts as non-specific rhinitis
-later presents as nasal swelling and ends up resolving with scarring and nose deformity

Histopathology

-biopsy of nasal skin or nasal mucosa
-dense histiocytic and lymphocytic infiltrate
-**numerous bacilli in foamy histiocytes (Mikulicz cells)**
-**plasma cells** with proteinaceous material (**Russell bodies**) are seen
-bacilli are best seen using Giemsa and Warthin Starry stains

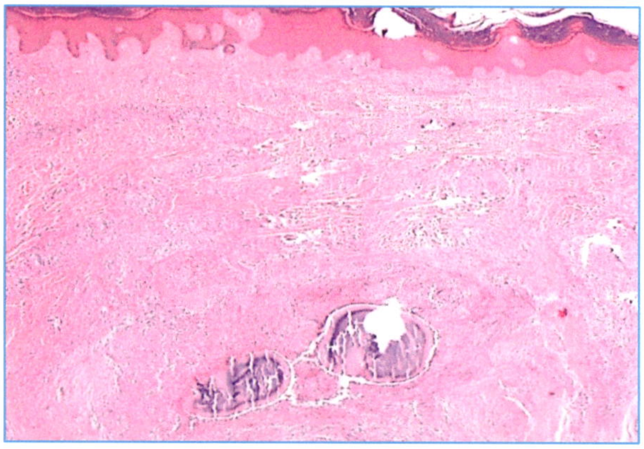
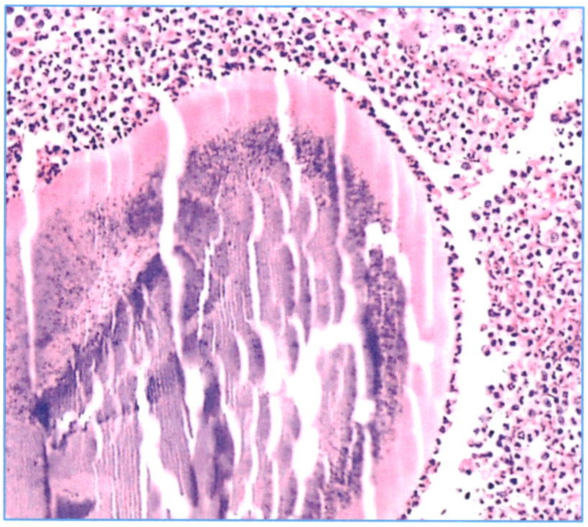

Botryomycosis with blue sulfur granules surrounded by "starburst-like" eosinophilic material

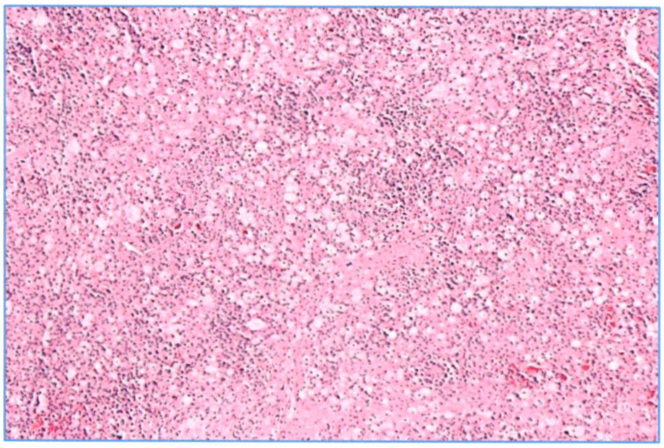
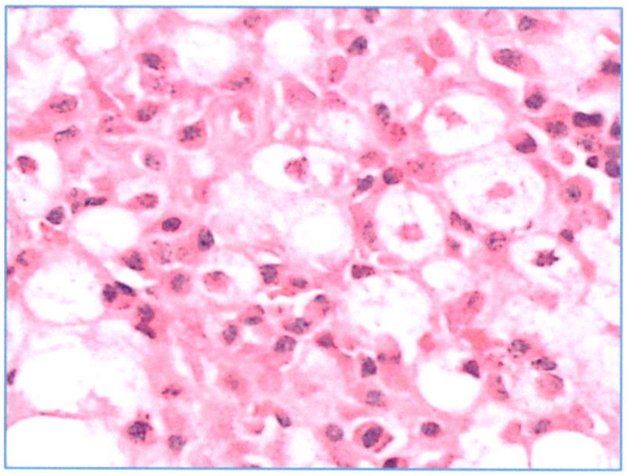

Rhinoscleroma with dense histiocytic infiltrate of foamy histiocytes and scattered plasma cells

Chapter 17

NOCARDIOSIS

-caused by *Nocardia brasiliensis*, a Gram-positive filamentous bacterium
-ubiquitous in soil
-cutaneous infection is usually seen in immunocompetent persons
-pulmonary and systemic infection is usually seen in immunocompromised persons
-three cutaneous clinical forms:

Primary superficial cutaneous form
-results from superficial skin inoculation
-presents with pus-filled blisters, ulcers, abscesses, or cellulitis
-can show sporotrichoid spread

Actinomycetoma (actinomycotic mycetoma)
-results from deep inoculation in subcutaneous tissue
-deep subcutaneous nodules with pus draining sinuses

Disseminated nocardiosis
-from the lung the infection is disseminated by blood to other organs including the skin

Histopathology
-**extensive neutrophilic infiltrate** in the dermis (superficial cutaneous form) and deep dermis and subcutis (actinomycotic form)
-abscess with necrosis is present
-**"sulfur granules"** are only seen in actinomycetoma variant
-Fite-Faraco and Gram stains detect fine filamentous bacteria

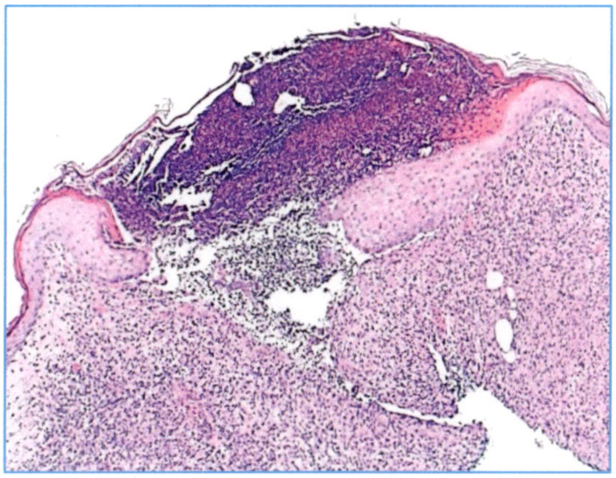

Superficial cutaneous nocardiosis ↑↓

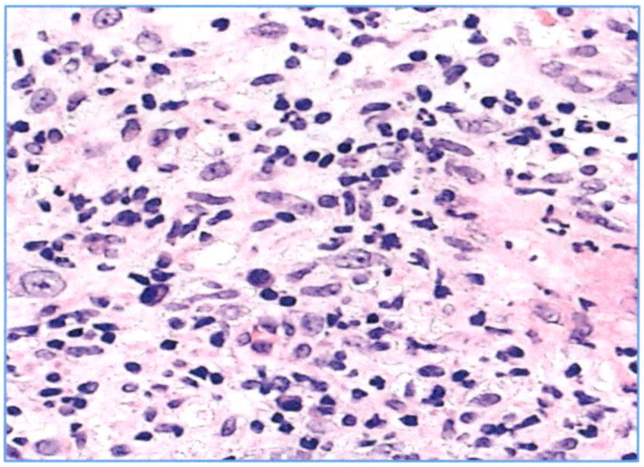

Neutrophilic inflammation

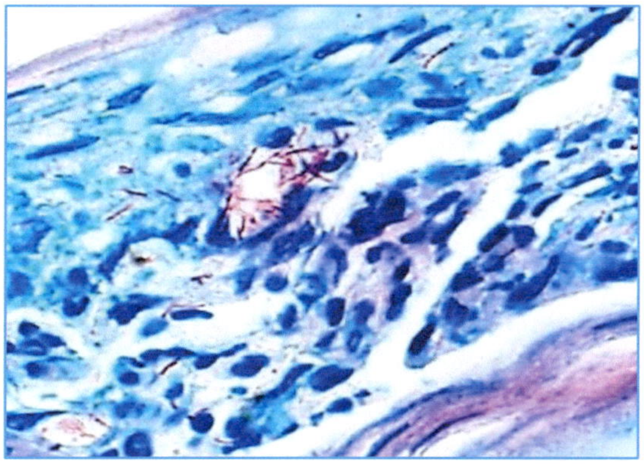

Fite-Faraco stain detects pink filamentous bacteria

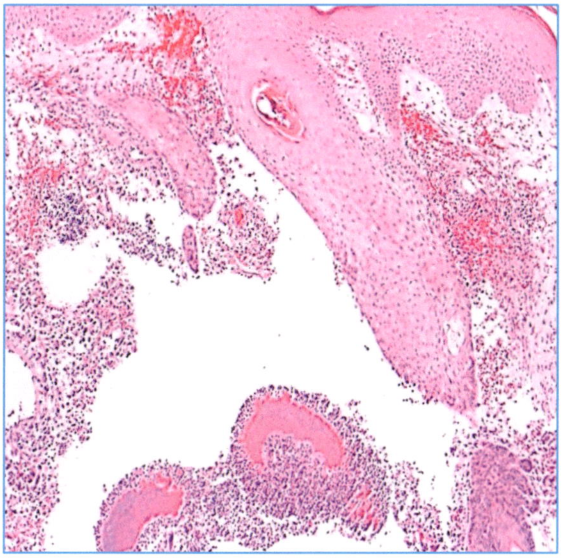

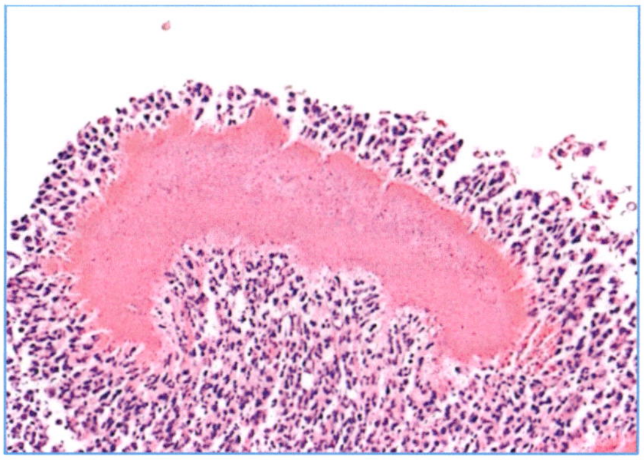

Actinomycetoma with sulfur granules within dermal neutrophilic abscess

TUBERCULOSIS

-infection caused by *Mycobacteria tuberculosis* with various cutaneous manifestations

Tuberculous chancre

-result of direct inoculation in patient without previous infection (no immunity)
-starts as a brown papule which ulcerates and becomes a sore with undermined edges

Tuberculosis verruca cutis

-result of direct inoculation in patients with high immunity (previous TB infection)
-solitary, hyperkeratotic, warty plaque

Scrofuloderma

-direct extension of infection from an underlying infected lymph node or bone
-in patients with low immunity
-presents as a nodule that ulcerates and has suppurative discharge
-favors neck, axilla, supraclavicular fossa

Lupus vulgaris

-most common form of cutaneous TB
-results from contiguous or hematogenous spread
-in patients with moderate to high immunity
-solitary, painful, red brown, "apple jelly" papules, plaques, or patches
-most often seen on the face around the nose, eyelids, lips, cheeks, ears, and neck

Orificial tuberculosis

-due to autoinoculation of skin or mucosa
-in patients with advanced TB and poor immunity
-clinically presents as an ulcer

Acute miliary tuberculosis

-hematogenous blood spread of TB in immunosuppressed patients
-multiple, small, crusted, blue-red papules

Lichen scrofulosorum

-tuberculoid reaction associated with tuberculous infections elsewhere in the body or in other parts of the skin
-more common in children and adolescents
-lichenoid eruption of minute, closely grouped papules
-papules are perifollicular and skin-colored to reddish brown
-mainly on abdomen, chest, back, and proximal part of limbs

Histopathology

-**caseous necrosis** is a distinctive form of coagulative necrosis in which the tissue maintains a **"cheese-like" appearance**
-if found it is highly suggestive of tuberculosis

Tuberculous chancre

-**necrotizing neutrophilic inflammation** and variable caseous necrosis

Tuberculosis verruca cutis

-**epidermal acanthosis and papillomatosis**
-granulomas with **variable necrosis**

Scrofuloderma

-prototypical TB granuloma with **extensive caseous necrosis** and abscess formation

Lupus vulgaris

-**well-formed granulomas with caseous necrosis**

Orificial tuberculosis

-**superficial ulcer** and underlying caseous necrosis

Acute miliary tuberculosis

-granuloma with variable caseous necrosis and **lymphoplasmocytic** inflammation

Lichen scrofulosorum

-**perifollicular granulomas** without caseous necrosis

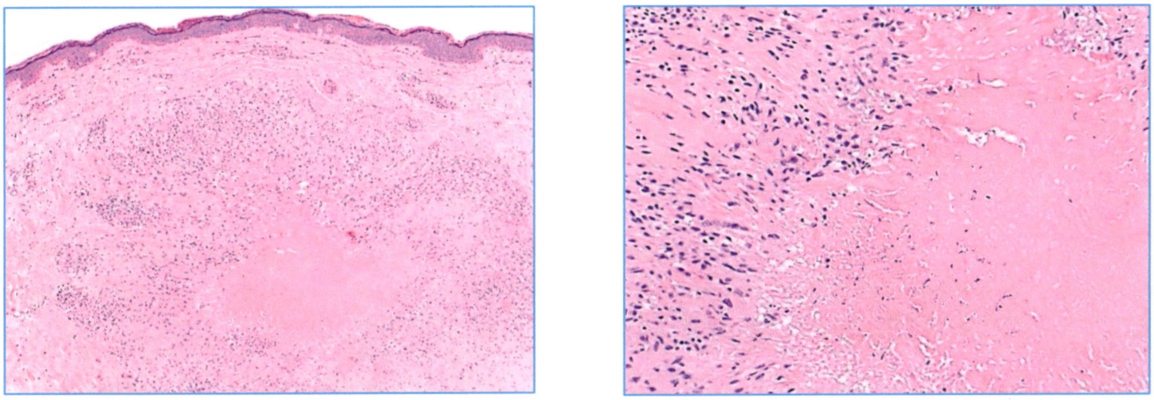

Scrofuloderma with extensive central caseating necrosis

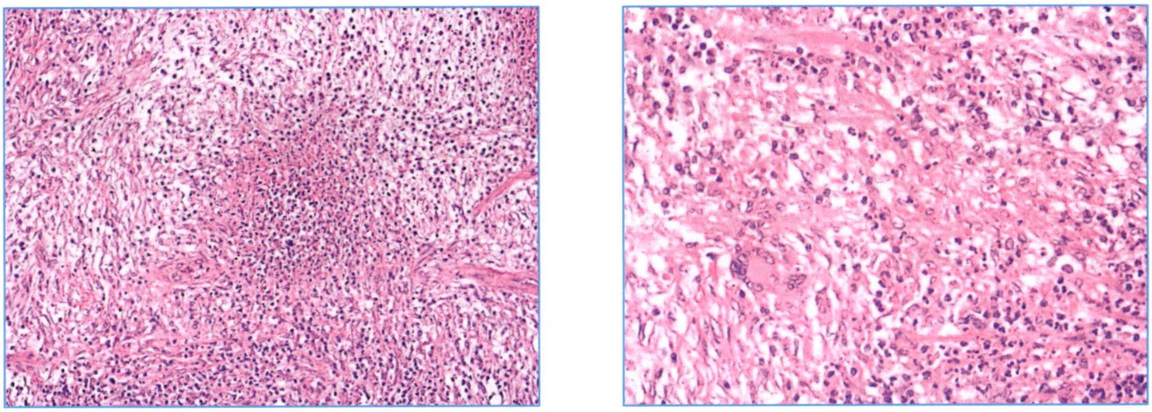

Tuberculous chancre with necrotizing neutrophilic inflammation

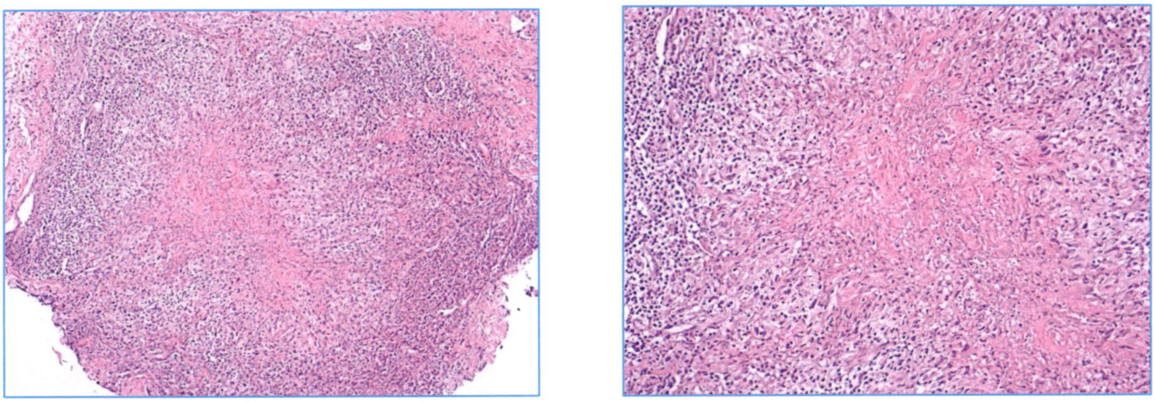

Lupus vulgaris granuloma with caseous necrosis

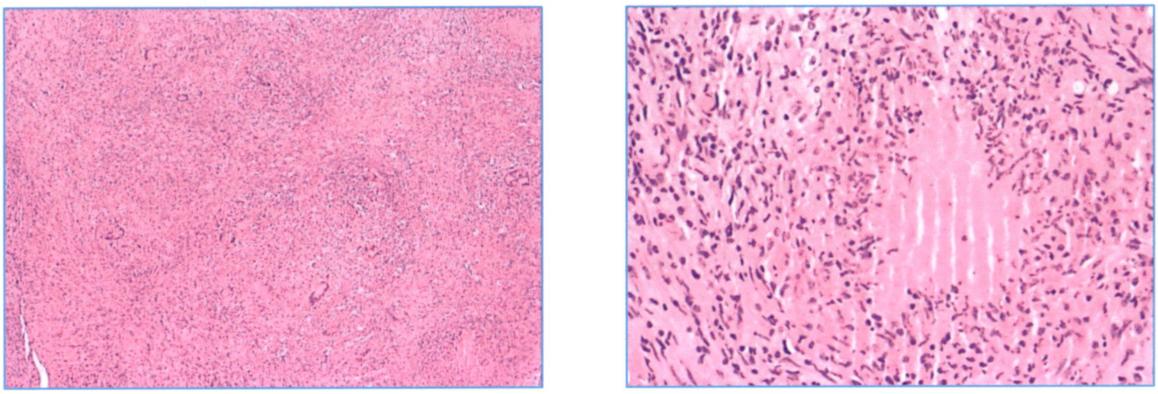

Orificial tuberculosis with caseous necrosis

Bacterial infections

ATYPICAL MYCOBACTERIAL INFECTIONS

M. avium-intracellulare (MAI)
-found in the environment
-opportunistic infection in the immunosuppressed
-primarily a pulmonary infection
-skin lesions are uncommon and non-specific

M. marinum
-contracted from infected fish, fish tanks, and swimming pools (**swimming pool or fish tank granuloma**)
-purple-red nodule at site of injury
-usually on hands and arms with sporotrichoid spread

M. ulcerans
-most common in central Africa
-causes **Buruli** nodules and large **ulcers** on extremities
-can extend to the bone

M. fortuitum, M. chelone, M, abscessus
(all rapid growers)
-present in water and soil and contaminated wounds
-abscess at the wound site and/or inflamed nodules with sporotrichoid spread

Histopathology

M. marinum
-vaguely necrotizing, but non-caseating granulomas

M. ulcerans
-epidermal ulceration with inflamed serum crust
-**extensive** dermal and deep subcutaneous **necrosis** and suppurative ulceration
-necrosis can extend to fascia and bone

M. fortuitum, M. chelone, M. abscessus
-suppurative dermal granulomas with necrosis and neutrophils in the center
-surrounding lymphocytes, histiocyte and giant cells

For all atypical mycobacterial infections diagnoses are best made via tissue culture, which should be time/temperature dependent, in addition to clinical correlation

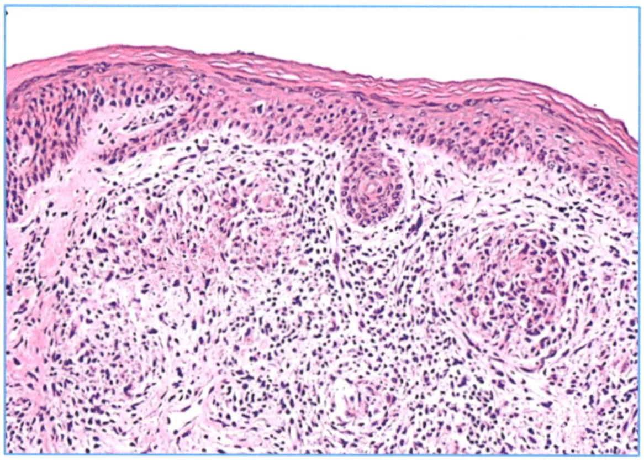
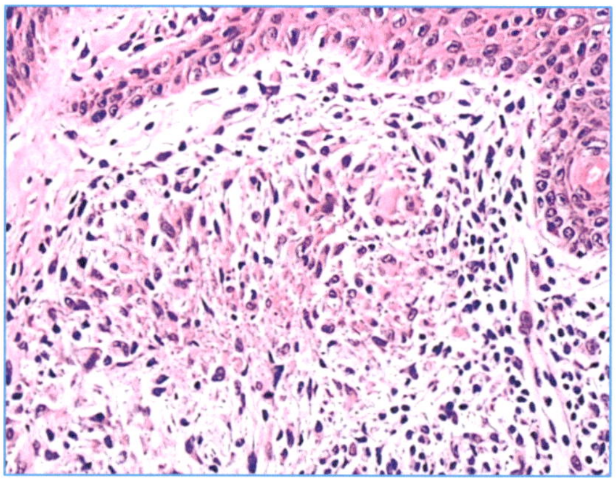

Swimming pool granuloma with focal necrosis that is non caseating

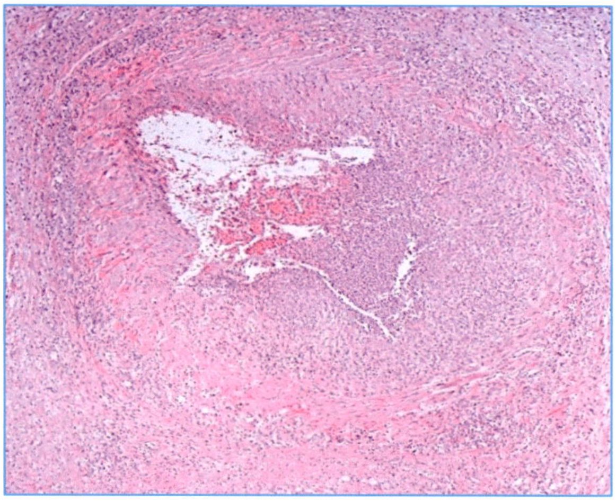
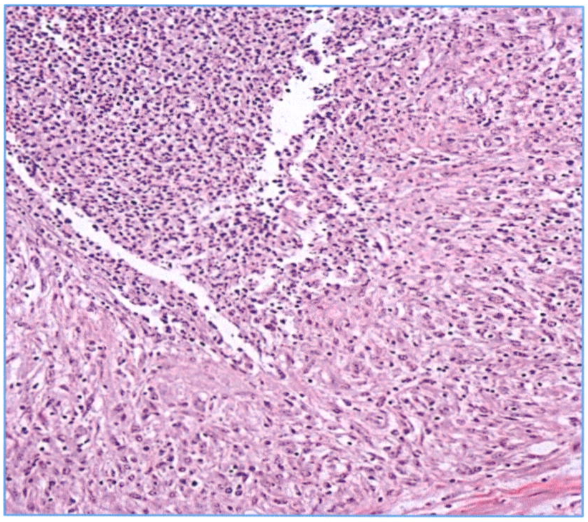

Buruli ulcer with neutrophilic aggregate and central necrosis

SYPHILIS (LUES)

-sexually transmitted disease caused by *Treponema pallidum*
-non-venereal endemic forms Bejel (*T. pallidum endemicum*), yaws (*T. pallidum pertinue*), pinta (*T. caratum*) are extremely rare in the US

Primary infection
-20-30 days after exposure
-painless, red, round/oval ulcer with indurated raised border (chancre) at site of inoculation
-chancre resolves within 1-5 weeks without scarring

Secondary infection
-6-8 weeks after primary infection
-lesions show great clinical variability **("the great mimicker")**
-usually starts as erythematous, **"ham colored"** macules on the head, face and neck
-progress to generalized, round to oval, copper-colored macules and papules
-classically involves the palms, soles, and oral cavity and can be localized to only these areas
-**condyloma lata** is manifestation of secondary syphilis presenting as soft, moist, flat-topped, pink papules in the genital area and mouth
-left untreated, secondary syphilis resolves within 2-10 weeks

Tertiary infection
-years or decades after primary infection
-presents as mucocutaneous gummae (hard nodules with ulceration), neurosyphilis (tabes dorsalis, meningoencephalitis), and/or cardiovascular syphilis (aortic aneurysm)

Histopathology

Primary infection
-epidermis is **ulcerated in the center** and ulcer **edge shows epidermal hyperplasia**
-ulcer bed is filled with dense infiltrate of lymphocytes and **numerous plasma cells**
-dermal capillaries are lined with plump endothelial cells
-Warthin Starry or Steiner stain demonstrates spirochetes

Secondary infection
-similar to clinical presentation, histology can be variable
-most common is the macular/spongiotic presentation with mildly spongiotic epidermis
-mild perivascular inflammation with **prominent plasma cells and vascular endothelial cells**

Condyloma lata
-psoriasiform epidermis or pseudoepitheliomatous hyperplasia
-focal small **intracorneal neutrophilic aggregates**
-dermal lymphohistiocytic infiltrate with numerous plasma cells
-capillary endothelial swelling is prominent

Tertiary infection
-**granulomatous dermatitis** with central necrosis

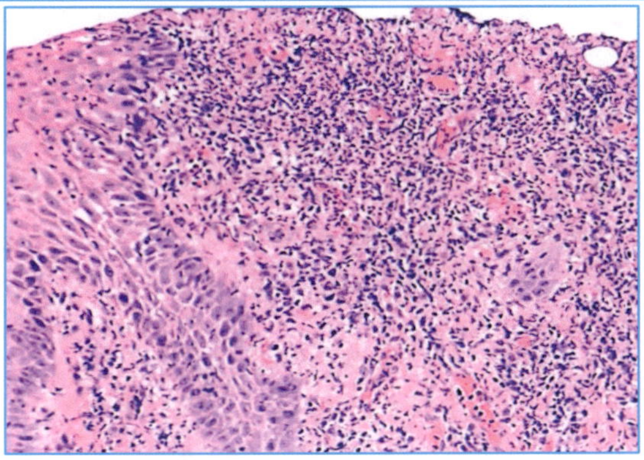

Primary chancre with central ulcer and epidermal hyperplasia at ulcer edge

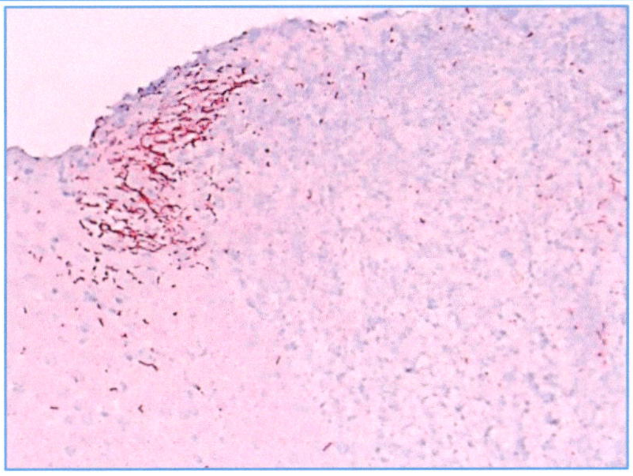

Warthin Starry stain detects spirochetes more prominent in abutting epidermis than in ulcer itself

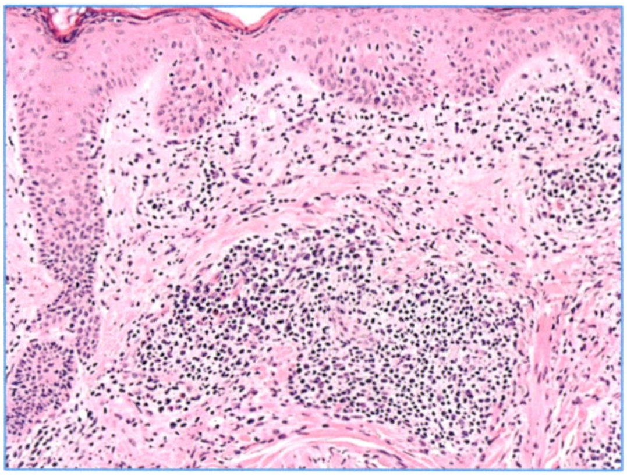
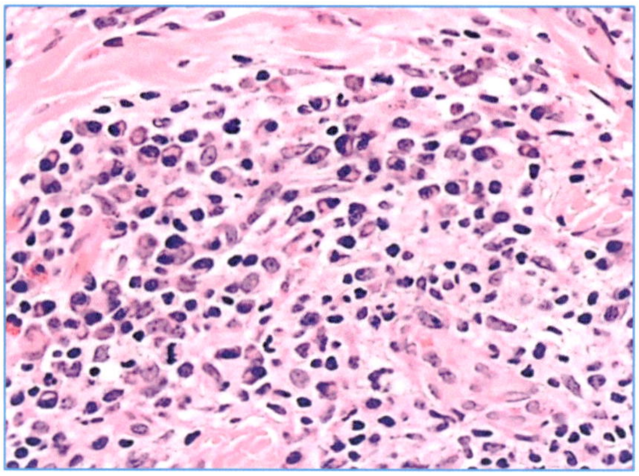

Morbilliform secondary syphilis with plasma cells

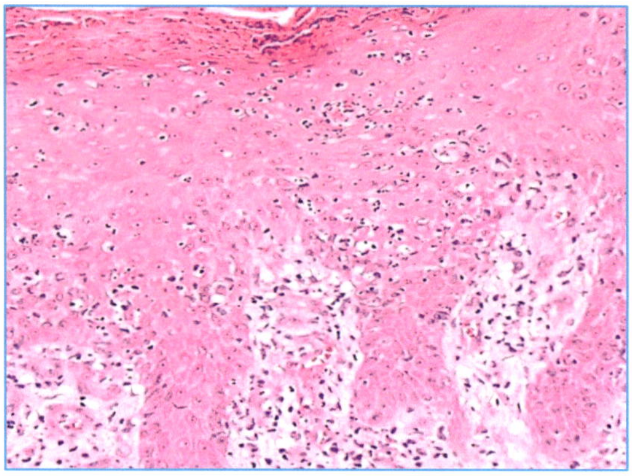
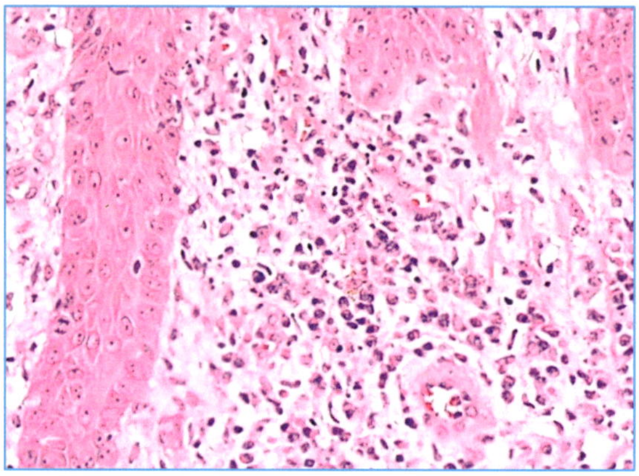

Psoriasiform secondary syphilis with epidermal neutrophils and dermal plasma cells

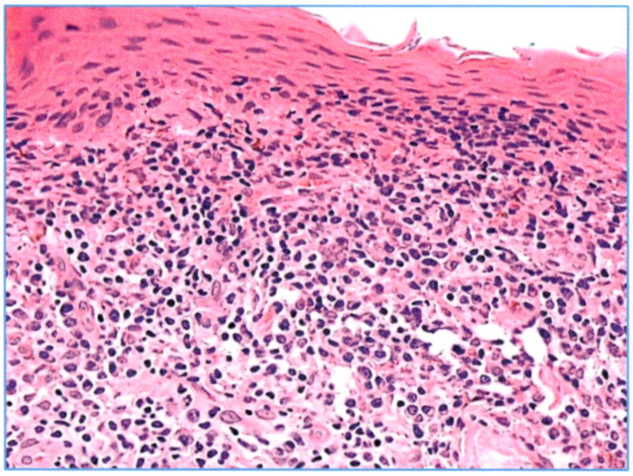

Lichenoid secondary syphilis

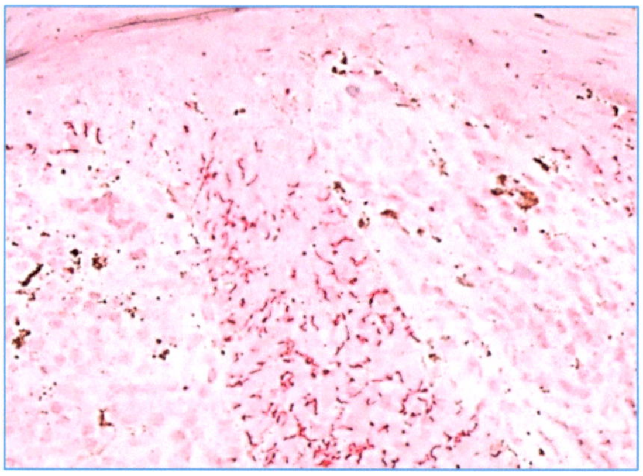

T. pallidum special stain (antibody stain)

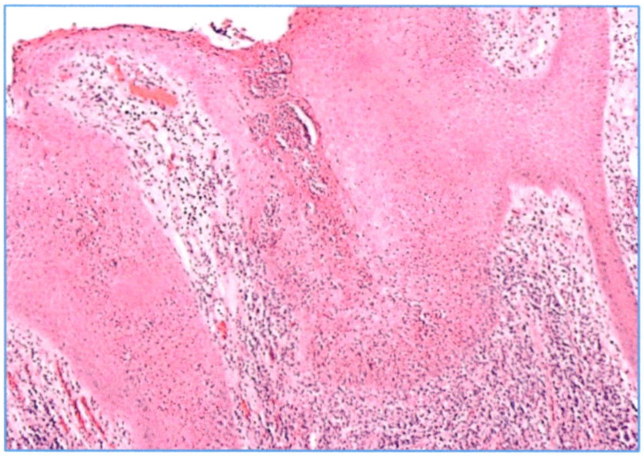
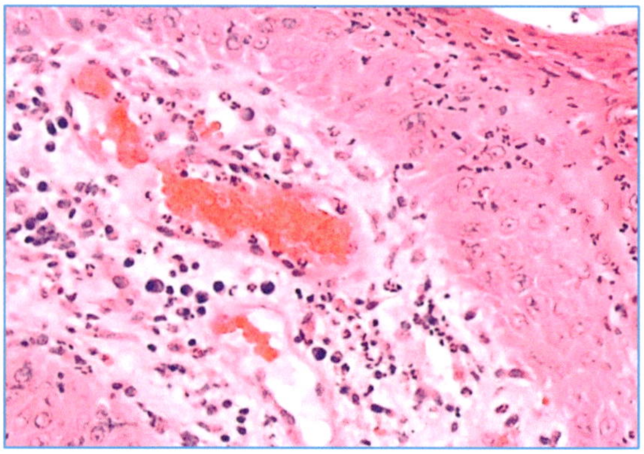

Condyloma lata with pseudoepitheliomatous hyperplasia, epidermal and dermal neutrophils, and dermal plasma cells

Chapter 17

GRANULOMA INGUINALE (DONOVANOSIS)

-sexually transmitted disease caused by *Klebsiella granulomatis* (formerly *Donovania*)
-begins as a firm papule or nodule in the genital area
-breaks down into **a painless ulcer** with an overhanging edge and exuberant **granulation tissue** (**"beefy red"** in color)
-unlike syphilitic chancre that self-heals, the ulcer becomes destructive to deeper tissue

Histopathology

-**ulcerated skin with exuberant granulation** tissue and mixed inflammation
-characteristic Donovan bodies (**"safety pin shaped"** organisms alone or in clusters within histiocytes) are **rarely seen**
-**diagnosis best made by taking smear** from the edge of the ulcer and staining with Giemsa or Warthin-Starry stain

CHANCROID

-sexually transmitted disease due to *Hemophilus ducreyi*
-**painful** purulent ulcer with undermined border
-can develop suppurative **inguinal adenopathy**

Histopathology

-epidermal ulcer with **three layers**
top- acutely inflamed serum crust
middle- granulation tissue
bottom- plasmolymphocytic infiltrate
-smear stained with Gram stain shows parallel strands of bacteria resembling **"school of fish"**

LYMPHOGRANULOMA VENEREUM

-transmitted by *Chlamydia trachomatis*
-common in tropics and rare in the US
-disease primarily involves lymphatic tissue with painful **adenopathy** of inguinal lymph nodes above and below inguinal ligament **("groove sign")**
-less prominent, commonly inconspicuous, small genital painless **ulcer** that heals rapidly

Histopathology

-ulceration with granulation tissue, mixed inflammation, and many plasma cells
-**Gamma-Favre bodies** in endothelial cells on Giemsa stain
-stellate microabscesses in a lymph node

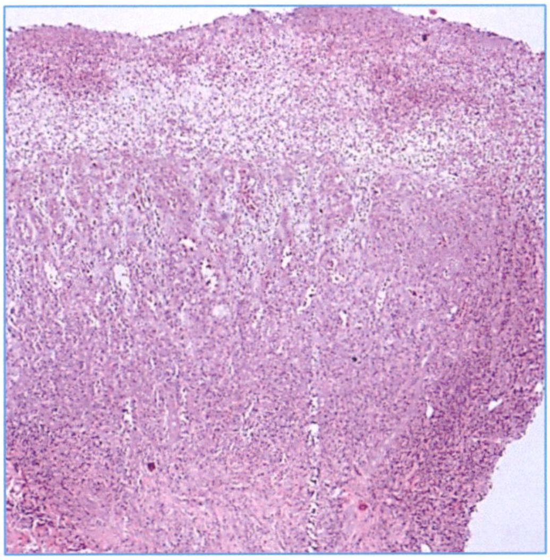

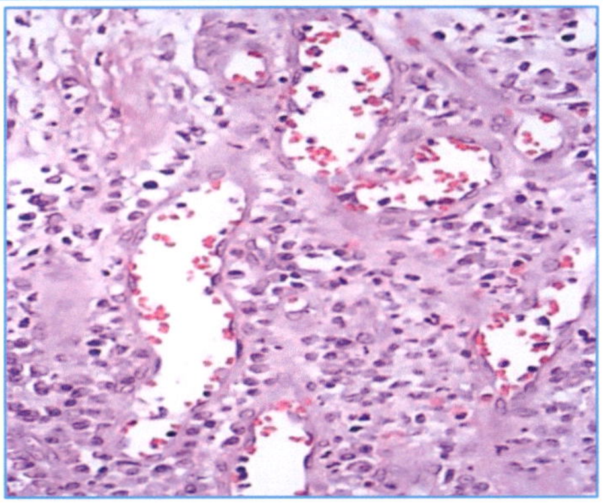

Chancroid with epidermal ulcer with three layers including the middle layer of granulation tissue

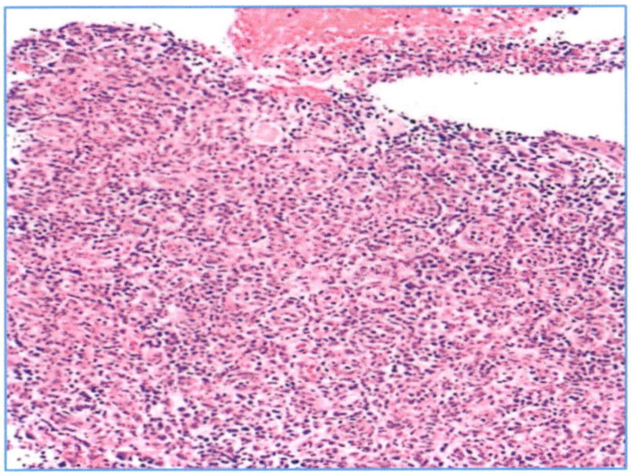

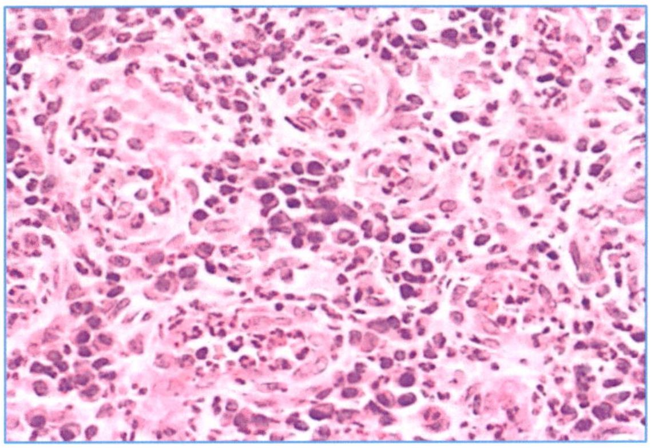

Lymphogranuloma venereum with granulation tissue with plasma cells

Bacterial infections

LYME DISEASE

-bacterial infection transmitted by the bite of an infected *Ixodes* tick
-caused by spirochete *Borrelia burdorferi* in the US and *B. garinii* and *B. afzelii* in Europe

Three clinical stages:

Stage 1

-**erythema migrans** is a macule at the site of the bite 7-14 days after tick attachment
-within days, macule obtains a distinct red border and partially cleared center **("bull's eye" appearance)**
-days to weeks after the primary lesion, up to half of patients develop disseminated erythema migrans lesions that are smaller than the original lesion
-systemic symptoms (fever, chills, headache)

Stage 2

-develops if stage 1 is untreated
-arthralgia (in 60% of patients), Bell's palsy (10%), cardiac complications (5%)
-in Europe (*B. garinii* and *B. afzelii*) 1% of patients develop **lymphocytoma cutis**
-presents as a red to purple nodule or plaque on earlobes, nipple/areola, and/or scrotum

Stage 3

-**acrodermatitis chronica atrophicans** seen only in Europe associated with *B. afzelii* infection
-initially ill-defined, violaceous discoloration on hands/distal extremities that may be tender
-ends with atrophic skin with "cigarette paper" appearance
-chronic arthritis, encephalomyelitis

Histopathology

Erythema migrans

-*Spirochetes* are identified only in a minority of cases
-superficial and deep perivascular and sometimes perieccrine lymphocytic infiltrate
-**loss of pilosebaceous elements**
-**plasma cells** seen in most but not all cases
-endothelial swelling and **dermal mucinosis can be seen**
-the histological findings are often non-specific and although they may be supportive, they are rarely diagnostic

Lymphocytoma cutis

-is a type of cutaneous pseudolymphoma
-diffuse dermal lymphocytic infiltrate with **numerous plasma cells**

Acrodermatitis chronica atrophicans

-in early lesions, the epidermis is normal with superficial and deep patchy perivascular inflammation with lymphocytes, **plasma cells, and focal mucin**
-in older lesions, the **epidermis is atrophic** with minimal dermal inflammation
-**dermal sclerosis** is present
-the histological findings are often non-specific and only supportive in the correct clinical setting

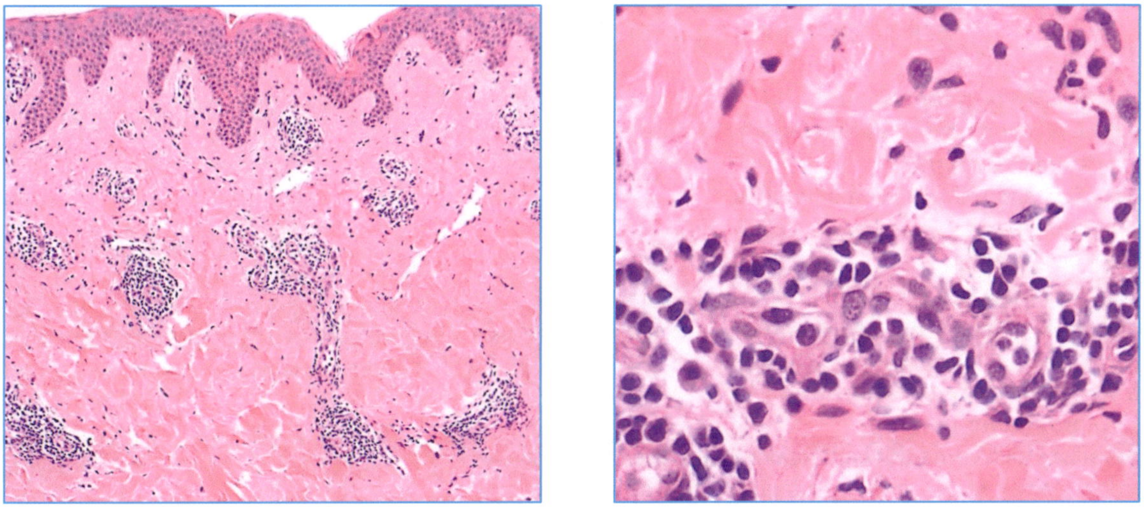

Erythema migrans with loss of pilosebaceous elements and perivascular plasma cells

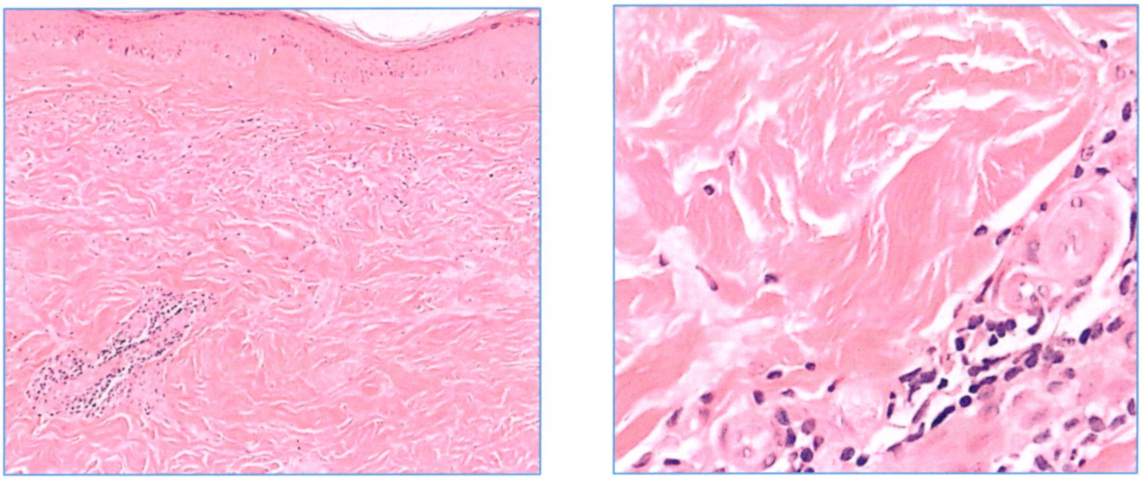

Acrodermatitis chronica atrophicans with atrophic epidermis, dermal sclerosis, and few plasma cells

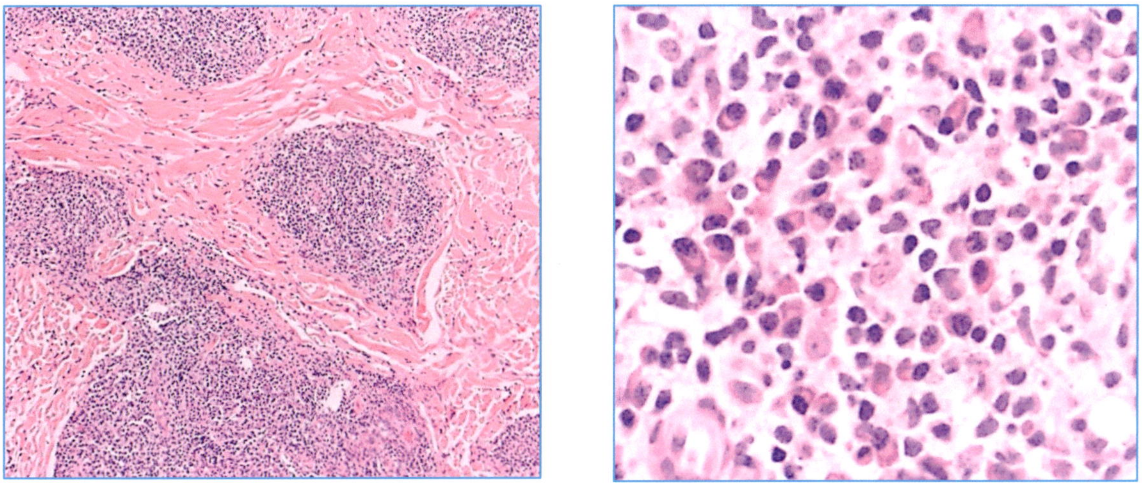

Lymphocytoma cutis with dense dermal inflammation with numerous plasma cells

LEPROSY (HANSEN'S DISEASE)

-caused by *Mycobacteria leprae*
-the clinical manifestations are related to the host response

Intermediate type

-the earliest and mildest form of leprosy
-few hypopigmented macules
-no loss of sensation

Tuberculoid type

-localized skin and/or nerve involvement
-few, well defined, hypopigmented, anesthetic, sharply defined macules
-any site of the body can be involved

Lepromatous type

-generalized involvement including skin, respiratory mucosa, adrenal glands, testes, and reticuloendothelial system
-small, hypopigmented, anesthetic macules that later become papules, plaques, and nodules with loss of hair
-lesions are symmetrical involving earlobes, face, arms, and buttocks
-facial involvement can cause "saddle" nose deformity or "leonine" facies

Borderline type

-has features in between tuberculoid and lepromatous leprosy

Immune response to *M. leprae* and reaction to therapy can produce various reactions causing a change in the clinical status:

Type 1 reaction (reversal reaction)

-inflammation with resulting redness/ulceration in preexisting lesions and neuritis

Type 2 reaction (erythema nodosum leprosum)

-vasculitis and "erythema nodosum-like" nodules appearing in previously not affected skin

Type 3 reaction (Lucio's phenomenon)

-vasculitis that results in shallow ulceration on the lower leg that heals poorly and recurs

Histopathology

Intermediate leprosy

-perivascular and perineural lymphohistiocytic infiltrate without granuloma formation

Tuberculoid leprosy

-perivascular and periadnexal histiocytes and lymphocytes
-histiocytic aggregates forming **"vague" non-caseating granulomas** often **adjacent to nerves**
-Fite-Farraco stain for **mycobacteria is usually negative**

Lepromatous leprosy

-**diffuse dermal and subcutaneous infiltrate of foamy macrophages** (**Virchow cells**)
-common **Grenz zone**
-absence of adnexal structures
-**numerous mycobacteria** detected by Fite-Farraco stain

Borderline leprosy

- histomorphology in between tuberculoid and lepromatous type

Type 1 reaction

-similar to borderline leprosy with increase in number of lymphocytes and few giant cells

Type 2 reaction

-similar to borderline leprosy with mixed infiltrate of neutrophils and lymphocytes
-vasculitis may be present

Type 3 reaction

-similar to lepromatous leprosy with a necrotizing vasculitis and resulting necrosis and ulceration

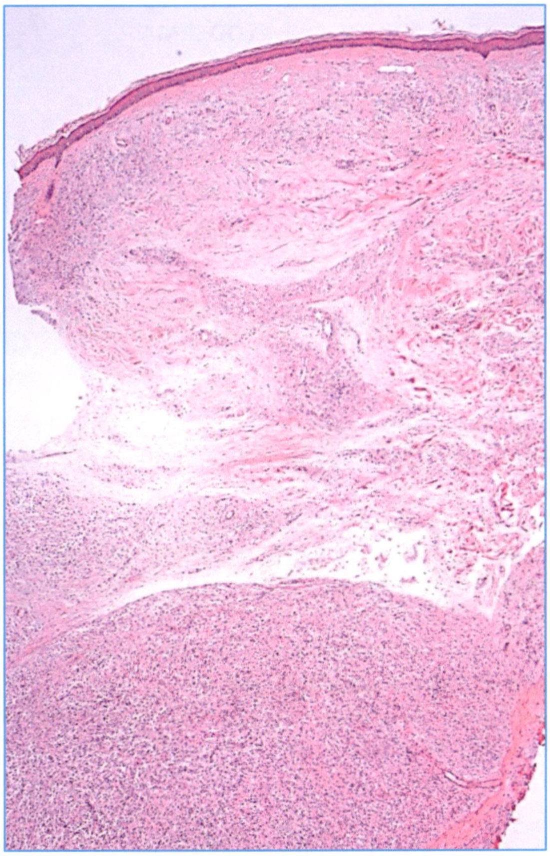

Lepromatous leprosy ↑↓

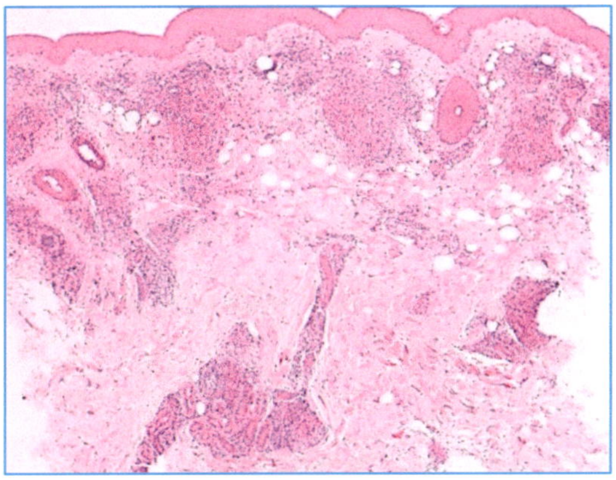

Tuberculoid leprosy ↑↓

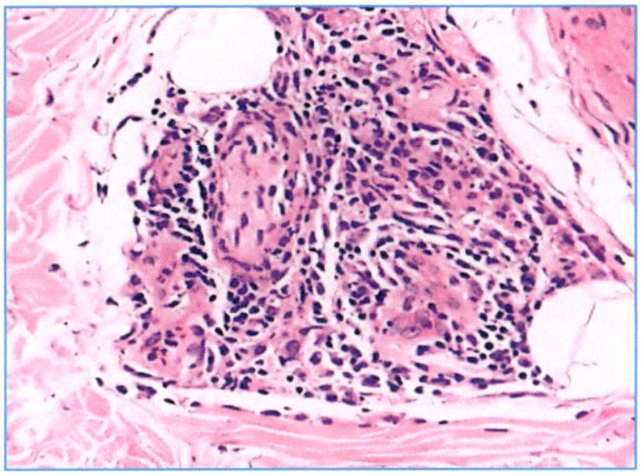

Perineural histiocytic inflammation

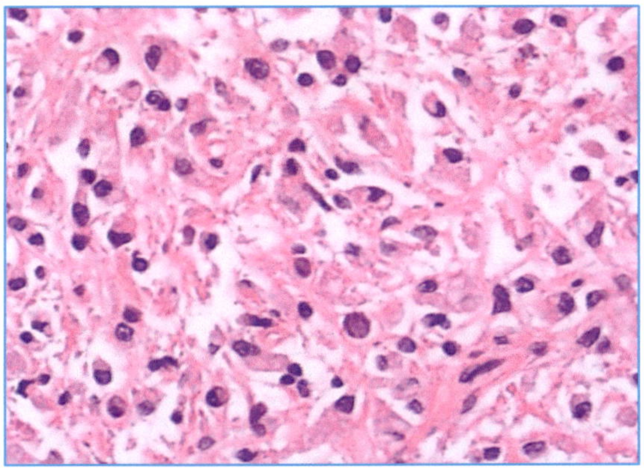

Diffuse foamy histiocytes

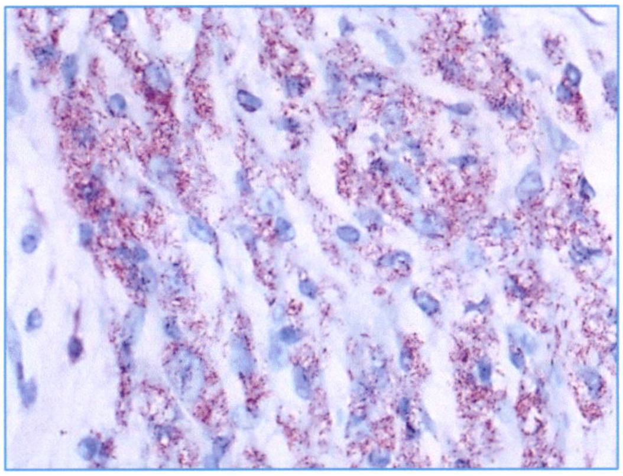

Fite-Farraco stains mycobacteria leprae

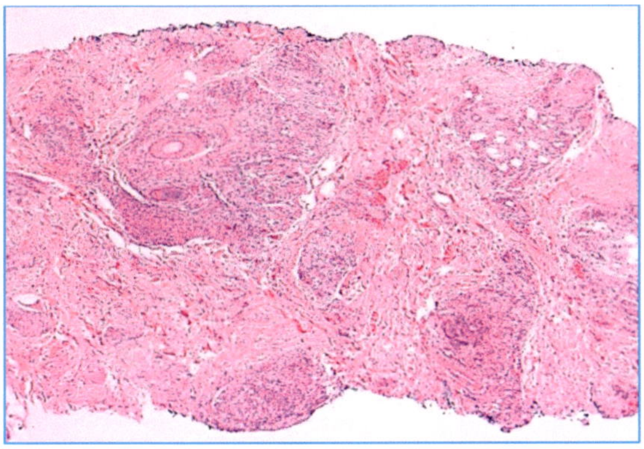

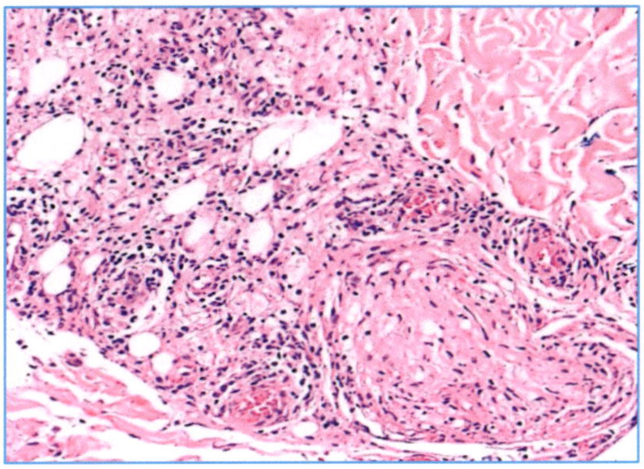

Erythema nodosum leprosum with patchy periadnexal and perineural mixed inflammation

Bacterial infections

BACILLARY ANGIOMATOSIS

-caused by *Bartonella henselae* or *B. quintana*
-mostly in HIV or other immunosuppressed patients
-solitary or multiple, "dome-shaped" red papules or nodules
-older lesions have friable surface resembling a pyogenic granuloma

Histopathology
-**proliferation of vessels** with plump endothelial cells and open lumina
-**neutrophils with nuclear dust** in between small vascular channels
-**hemorrhage is common**
-bacteria in areas rich with neutrophils
-best detected with Warthin-Starry silver stain

BLASTOMYCOSIS-LIKE PYODERMA

-rare, cutaneous bacterial infection of skin
-seen in malnourished individuals
-presents as thick verrucous surfaced plaques and papules with draining sinuses on trunk and extremities
-*Staph. aureus, Pseudomonas, and Proteus* are most common isolated organisms

PYODERMATITIS/PYOSTOMATITIS VEGETANS

-probably a reactive, rather than infectious process
-only normal bacteria (probable superinfection) present
-presents as erythematous, vesiculopustular, exudative, vegetating plaques
-usually localized in the inguinal and axillary folds (pyoderma) or lips (pyostomatitis)
-associated with ulcerative colitis and Crohn's disease

Histopathology of **these two diseases is identical**
-**pseudoepitheliomatous hyperplasia**
-intraepidermal and subepidermal neutrophilic or eosinophilic **microabscesses** with **bacteria**
-dermal acute inflammation

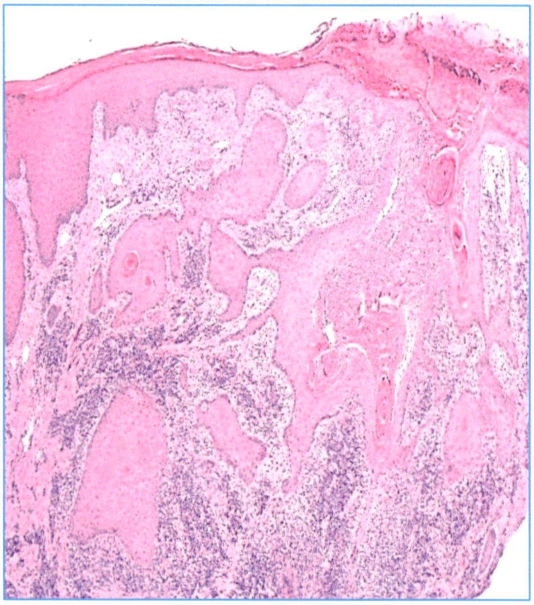

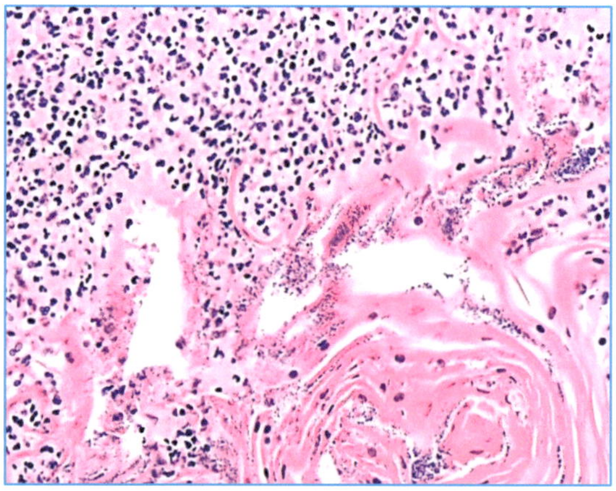

Pyoderma vegetans with extensive pseudoepitheliomatous hyperplasia, microabscesses, and bacteria

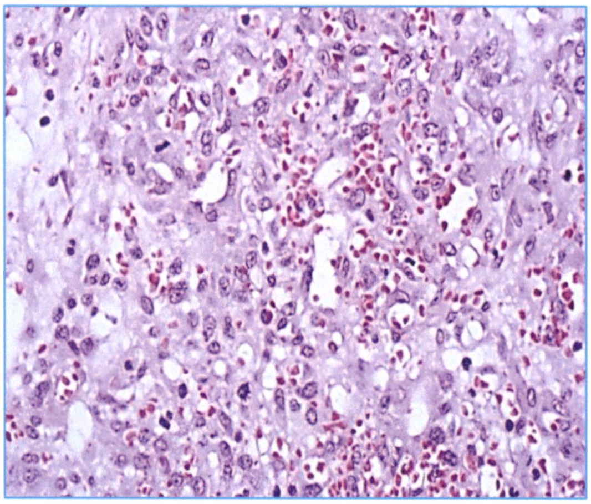

Bacillary angiomatosis with vascular proliferation

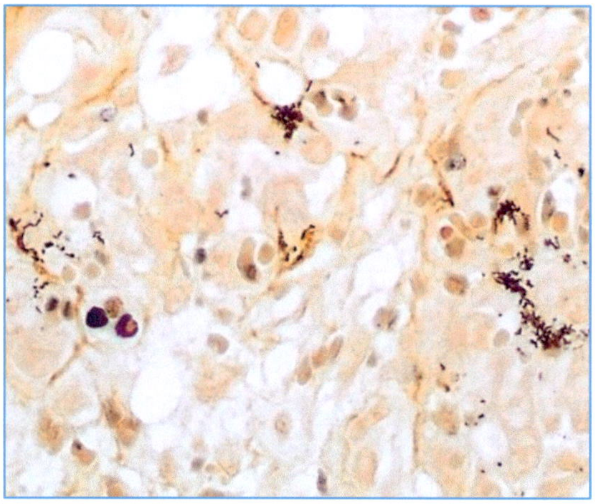

***Bartonella h.* detected with silver stain**

STAPHYLOCOCCAL SCALDED SKIN SYNDROME (SSSS)

-caused by epidermolytic exotoxin from *group 2 Staphylococcus aureous* at a distant site
-occurs in infants and children under the age of five and adults with renal failure
-rapidly evolves to desquamating disorder that involves the entire body
-starts with redness in the intertriginous areas (neck, groin, axilla) and perioral radial fissuring
-rapidly spreads involving the entire body but sparing the palms and soles
-the skin exfoliates in sheets

Histopathology
-**subcorneal separation** with split in the granular layer
-below the split, epidermis is normal
-**no or minimal inflammation**
-**no bacteria** seen as the disease is caused by hematogenous spread of exfoliatoxin

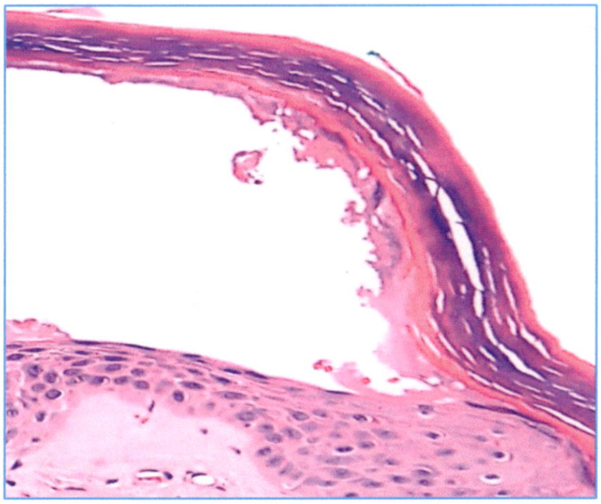

SSSS with subcorneal split and no inflammation

MENINGOCOCCEMIA

-usually young children and adolescents
-over half of the patients develop petechiae with purpura that may progress to ecchymosis, bullae, and necrosis
-predilection for trunk and lower extremities
-very ill patients with fever, chills, hypotension, and meningitis

GONOCOCCEMIA

-dissemination of gonorrhea infection
-characterized by cutaneous lesions, polyarthralgia, and tenosynovitis
-lesions typically appear acral, around joints, and are usually multiple
-evolves from petechiae or papules into vesicles or pustules on a necrotic or hemorrhagic base
-usually spares the face, scalp, and mouth

ROCKY MOUNTAIN SPOTTED FEVER

-caused by bacteria *Rickettsia rickettsii* and transmitted by *Dermacentor* tick bites to humans
-generalized skin eruption, initially with blanchable red macules which progress to petechiae/palpable purpura
-usually, initially involves the extremities
-then spreads centrally to the trunk
-mortality is up to 20% without therapy

Histopathology of **all 3 diseases is similar**
-**septic leukocytoclastic vasculitis and venulitis** with neutrophilic infiltrate, nuclear dust, focal fibrin thrombi, and capillary wall necrosis
-red blood extravasation can be prominent
-bacteria can be found within thrombi and in the wall of capillaries

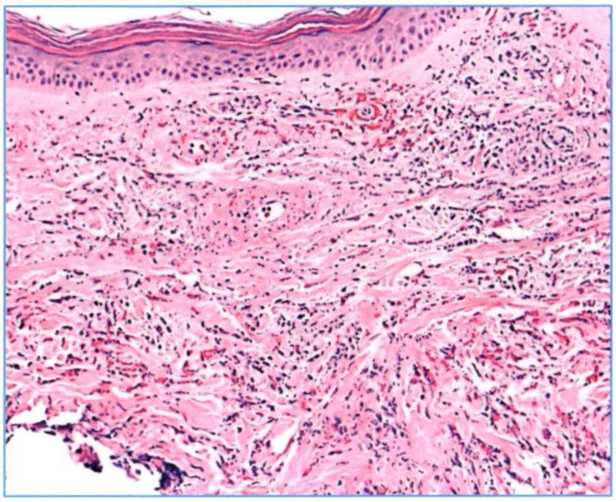

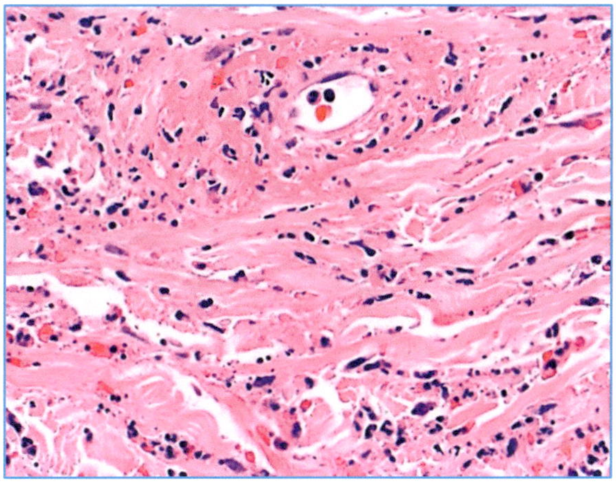

Meningococcemia with leukocytoclastic vasculitis

Bacterial infections

ERYTHRASMA

-superficial infection by *Corynebacterium Minutissimum* in moist intertriginous areas
-red-brown, slightly wrinkled patches
-bacteria produce porphyrins that show **coral red** fluorescence on Wood's lamp examination

Histopathology
-mild epidermal hyperkeratosis, **focal parakeratosis**, and spongiosis
-minimal to mild perivascular lymphocytic inflammation
-**bacteria in the stratum corneum**

PITTED KERATOLYSIS

-bacterial infection with *Kytococcus sedentarius*
-presents as small depressions or pits on acral sites with frequent malodor
-predilection for soles, particularly the weight-bearing areas
-palms can also be affected but less frequently

Histopathology
-rarely biopsied
-acral hyperkeratotic epidermis
-**shallow epidermal indentations filled with keratin**
-no dermal inflammation
-**bacteria are present in the pits**

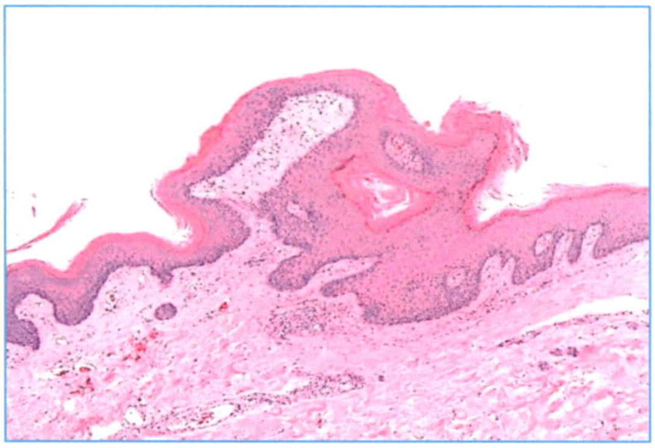

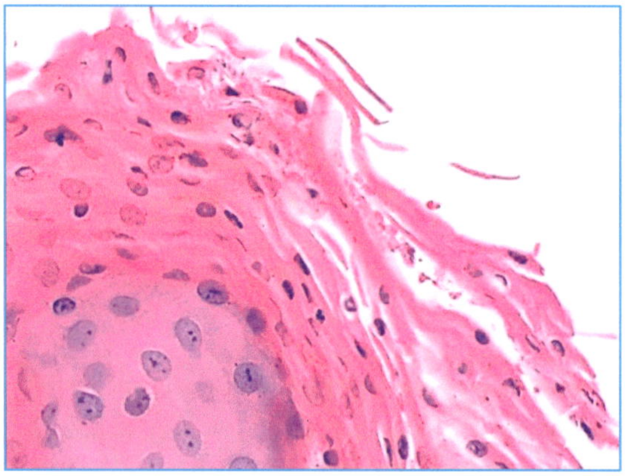

Erythrasma with focal parakeratosis

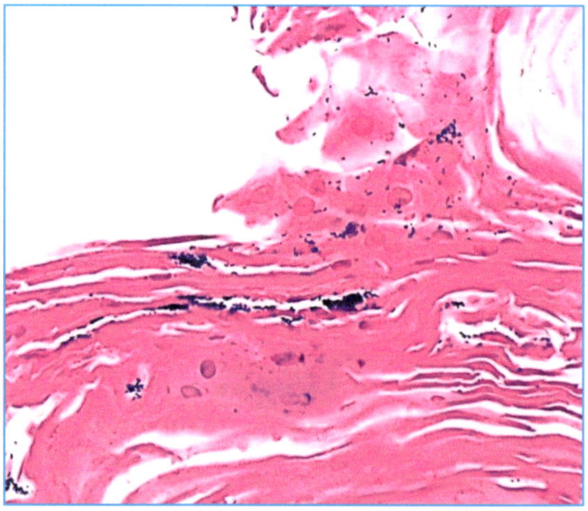

Corynebacterium in the stratum corneum (Gram stain)

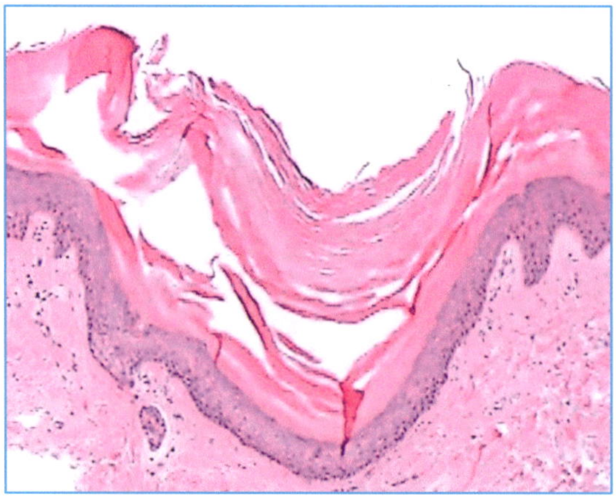

Pitted keratolysis with epidermal pit

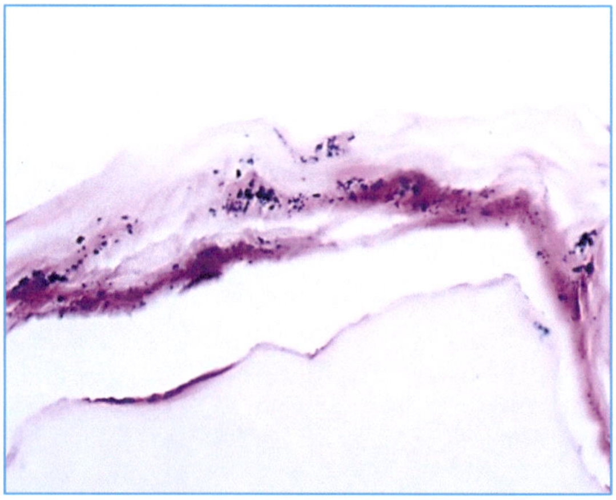

Kytococcus sed. stained with Gram stain

Chapter 17

HOW TO APPROACH BACTERIAL INFECTIONS

NORMAL APPEARING SKIN WITH NO OR MINIMAL INFLAMMATION

-SSSS	young children/dialysis patients	no bacteria
-erythrasma	intertriginous area	bacteria present
-pitted keratolysis	palms	bacteria present

SPONGIOTIC DERMATITIS WITH PLASMA CELLS

-secondary syphilis	numerous plasma cells
-erythema migrans	few plasma cells and focal mucin
-acrodermatitis chronica atrophicans	few plasma cells and sclerosis

PSORISIFORM DERMATITIS WITH PLASMA CELLS

-condyloma lata

PSEUDOEPITHELIOMATOUS HYPERPLASIA WITH MICRO ABSCESSES AND FUNGAL STAINS ARE NEGATIVE

-pyoderma vegetans

SUBCORNEAL NEUTROPHILIC PUSTULE

-impetigo

EDEMA WITH SCATTERED NEUTROPHILS

-erysipelas	dermal edema and neutrophils
-cellulitis	dermal and subcutaneous edema and neutrophils

EXTENSIVE TISSUE NECROSIS

-ecthyma gangrenosum	more superficial	epidermis, dermis, subcutis
-necrotizing fasciitis	deeper	subcutis, fascia, muscle

LEUKOCYTOCLASTIC VASCULITIS WITH MICROTHROMBI

-meningococcemia, gonococcemia, Rocky mountain spotted fever	septic LCV

VASCULAR PROLIFERATION RESEMBLING KAPOSI SARCOMA

-bacillary angiomatosis	neutrophilic nuclear dust + bacteria (unlike KS)

DERMAL HISTIOCYTIC INFLAMMATION

-lepromatous leprosy		diffuse infiltrate of foamy histiocytes
-tuberculoid leprosy		periadnexal and perineural foamy histiocytes
-rhinoscleroma	respiratory mucosa	diffuse infiltrate of foamy histiocytes +plasma cells

DERMAL GRANULOMA PRESENT AND FUNGAL STAINS ARE NEGATIVE

with caseating necrosis	favor	**-tuberculosis**
with neutrophils	favor	**-atypical mycobacterium**

"SULFUR GRANULES" PRESENT

-actinomycosis	oral	filamentous bacteria (*Actinomyces*)
-botryomycosis		cocci
-actinomycetoma	leg, neck	filamentous bacteria (*Nocardia*)

GENITAL LESIONS (CLINICAL INFORMATIAL IS CRUCIAL)

-primary syphilis	painless ulcer	granul. tissue + plasma cells	self-heals
-granuloma inguinale	painless ulcer	granul. tissue + plasma cells	destructive
-chancroid	painful ulcer	supur. lymphadenitis	3 tissue layers
-lymphogranuloma ven.	rarely ulcerates	suppur. lymphadenitis	granul. tissue +plasma cells

Bacterial infections

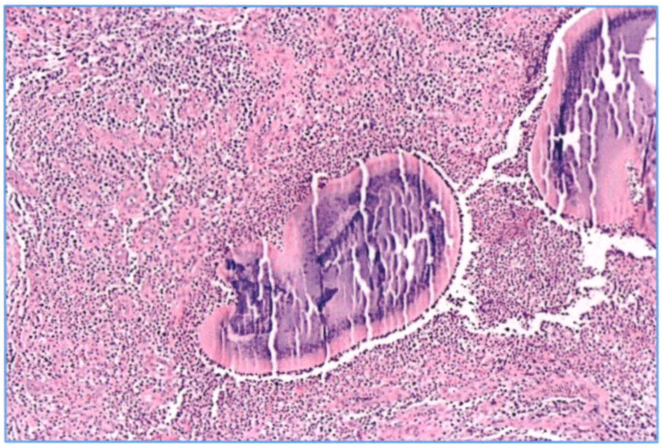

Actinomycosis with abscess and "sulfur granules"

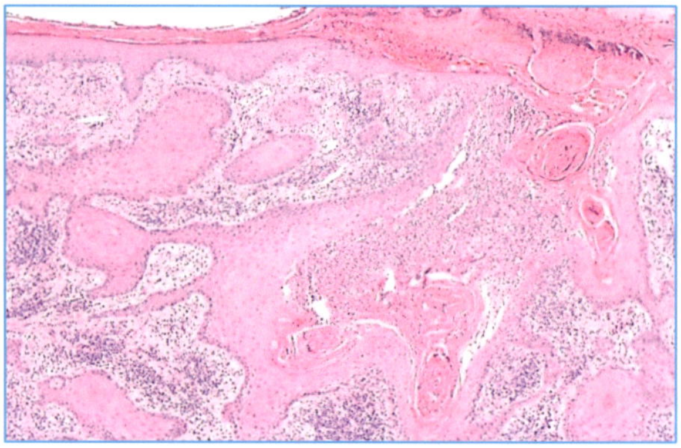

Pyoderma vegetans with pseudoepitheliomatous hyperplasia and microabscesses

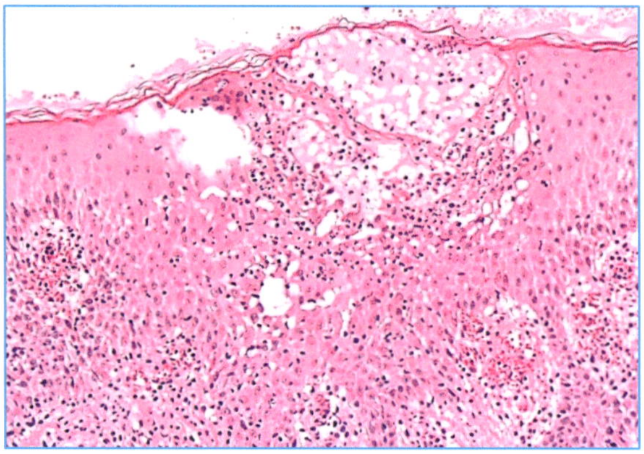

Impetigo with subcorneal neutrophilic pustule

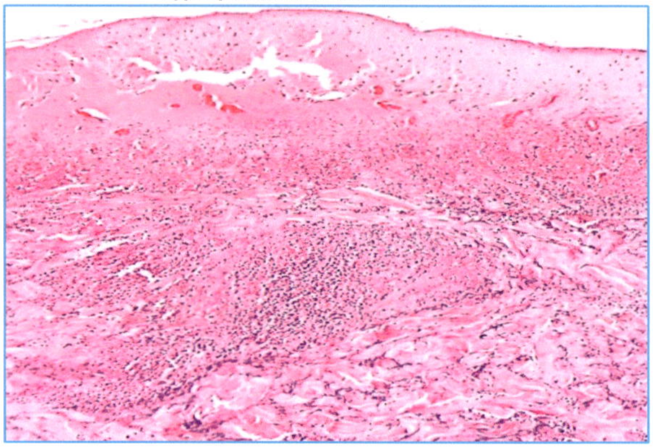

Ecthyma gangrenosum with epidermal, dermal, and subcutaneous necrosis

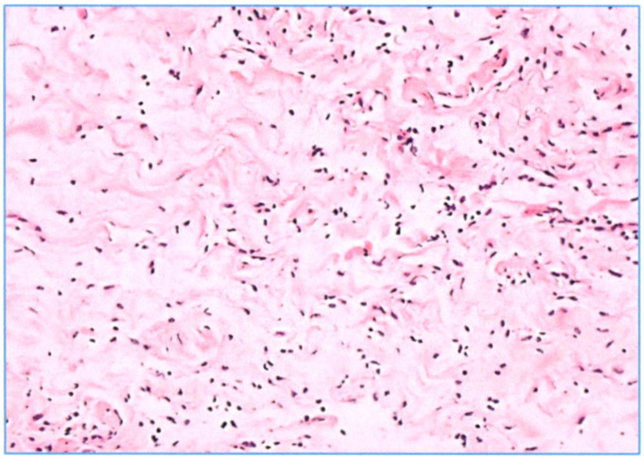

Cellulitis with dermal and subcutaneous edema and scattered neutrophils

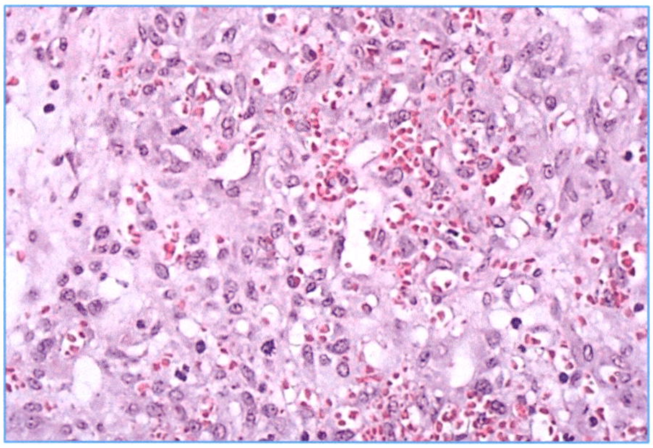

Bacillary angiomatosis with vascular proliferation and neutrophilic nuclear dust

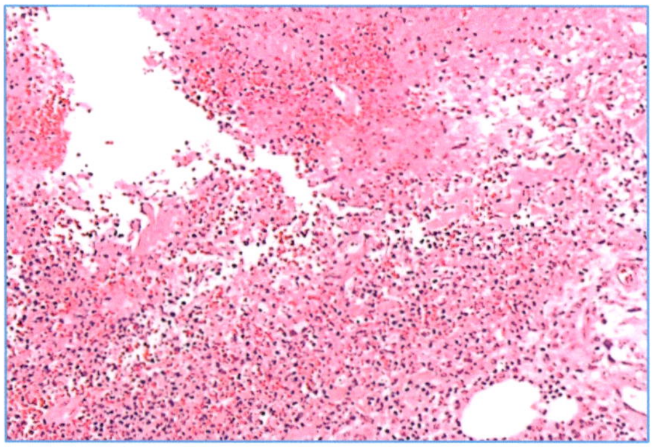

Necrotizing fasciitis with necrosis and acute inflammation of subcutis and fascia

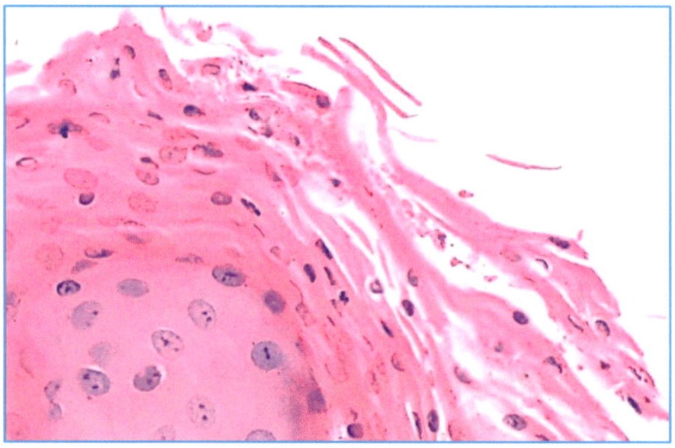

Erythrasma with bacteria hiding in normal appearing skin with focal parakeratosis

Chapter 17

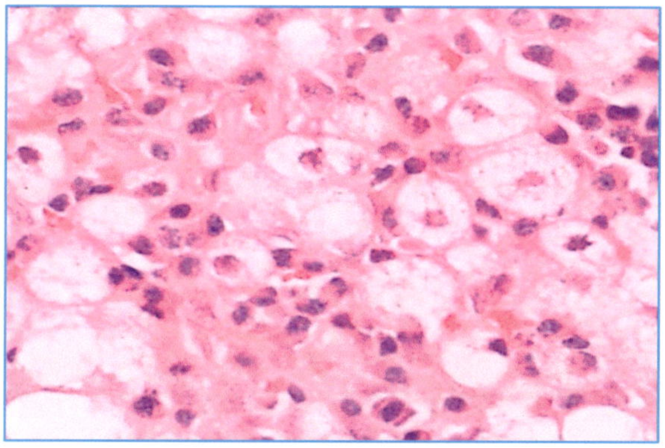

Rhinoscleroma with "dusty" histiocytes and plasma cells

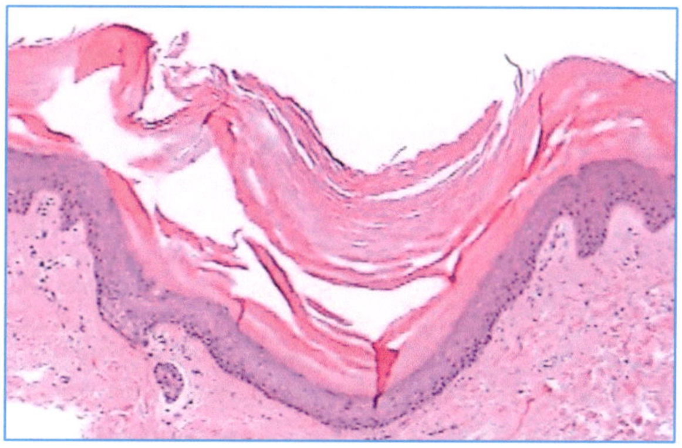

Pitted keratolysis with shallow epidermal indentation filled with keratin

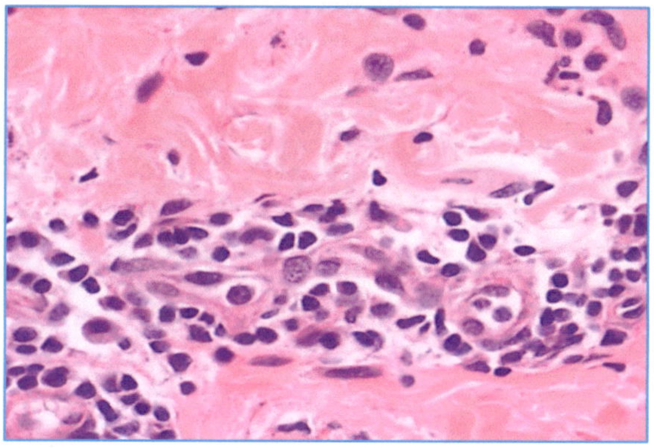

Erythema migrans with perivascular plasma cells and mucin

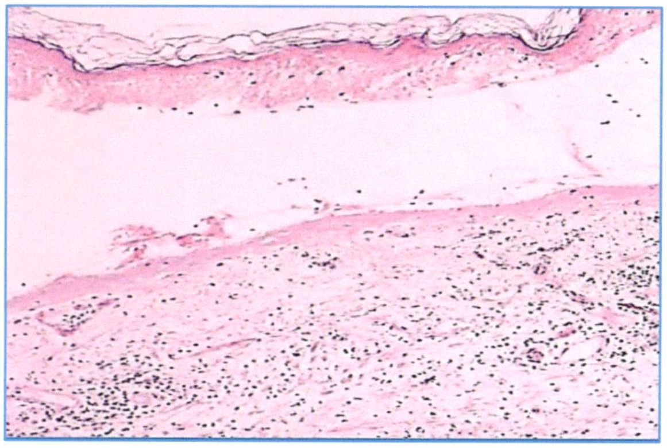

Erysipelas with dermal edema with scattered neutrophils; common subepidermal blister

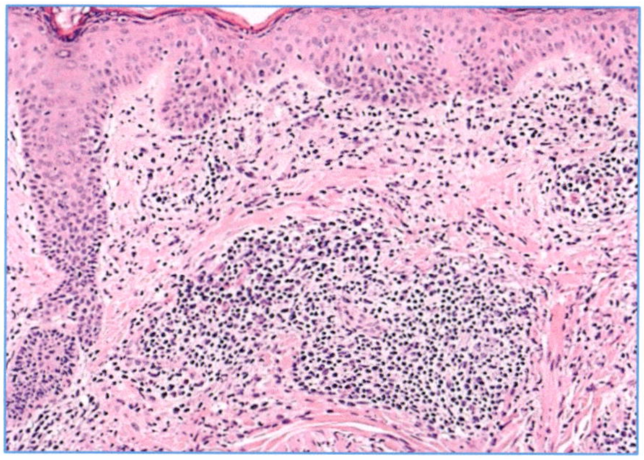

Secondary morbilliform syphilis with spongiotic epidermis and numerous dermal plasma cells

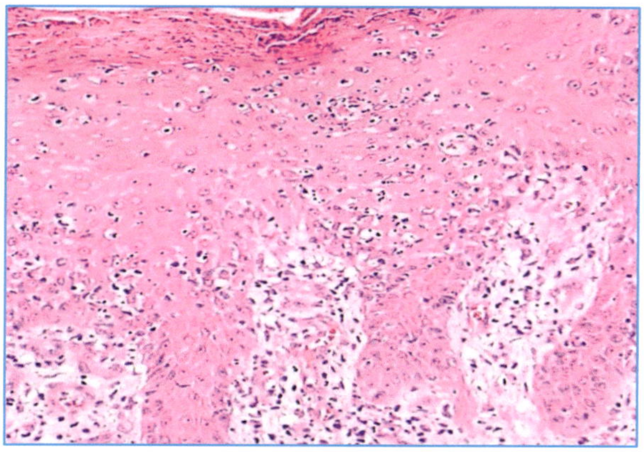

Codyloma lata with psoriasiform epidermis and epidermal neutrophils and dermal plasma cells

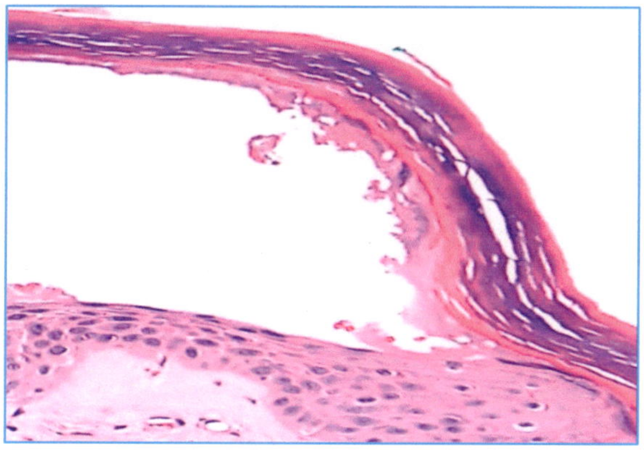

SSSS with "cell-poor" separation of stratum corneum

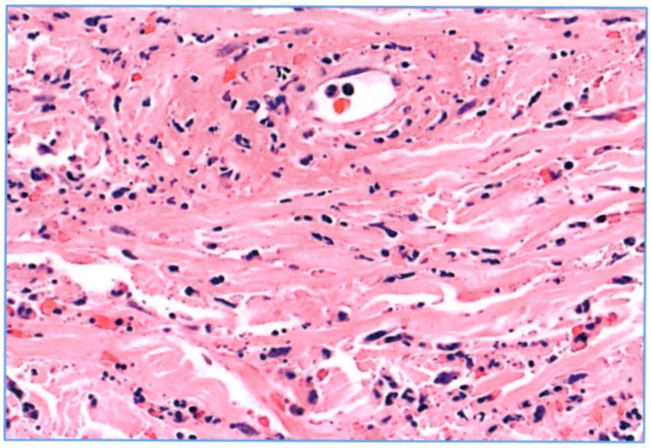

Septic LCV with vascular damage and nuclear dust

Bacterial infections

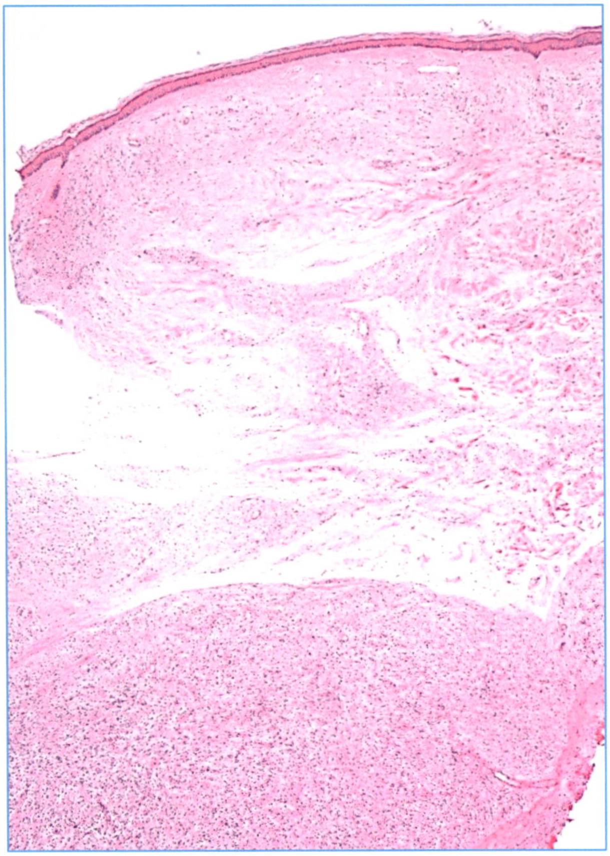

Lepromatous leprosy with diffuse histiocytic infiltrate

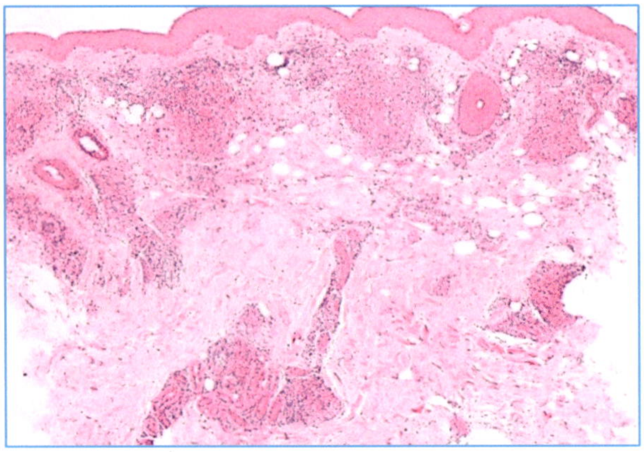

Tuberculoid leprosy with perivascular and periadnexal lymphohistiocytic inflammation

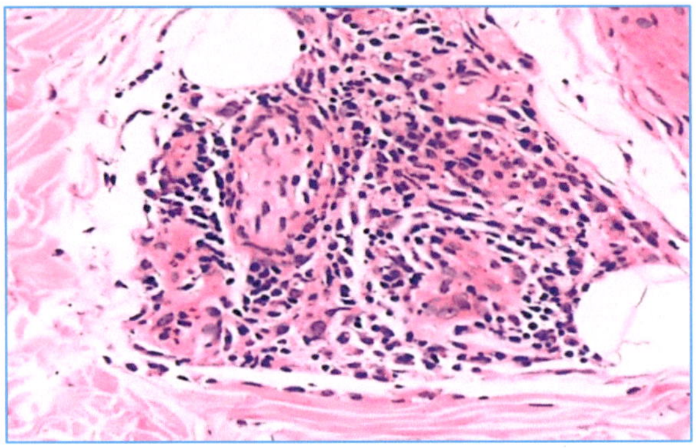

Tuberculoid leprosy with perineural histiocytic inflammation

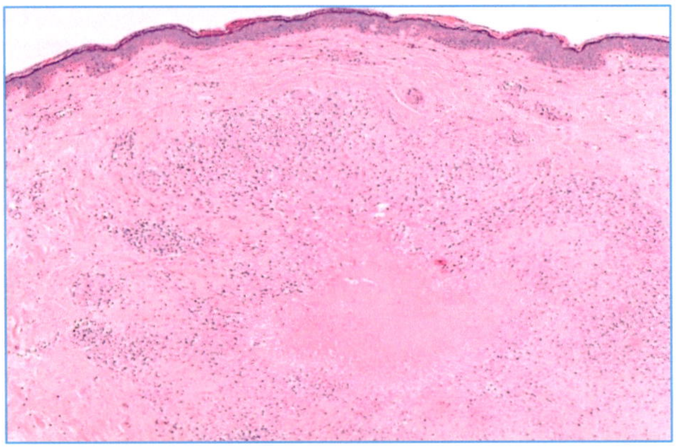

TB scrofuloderma with caseating granuloma

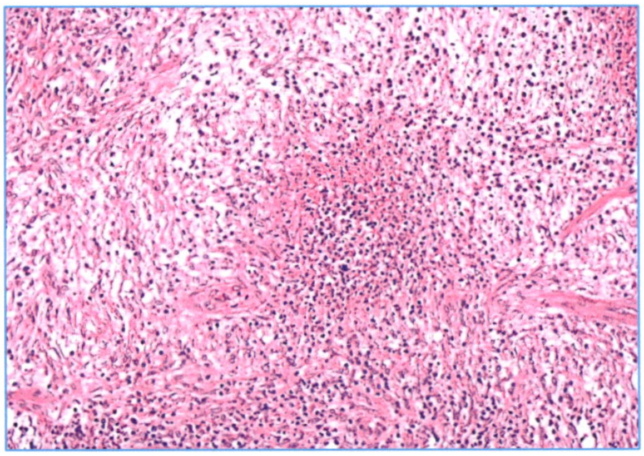

Tuberculous chancre with necrotizing granuloma

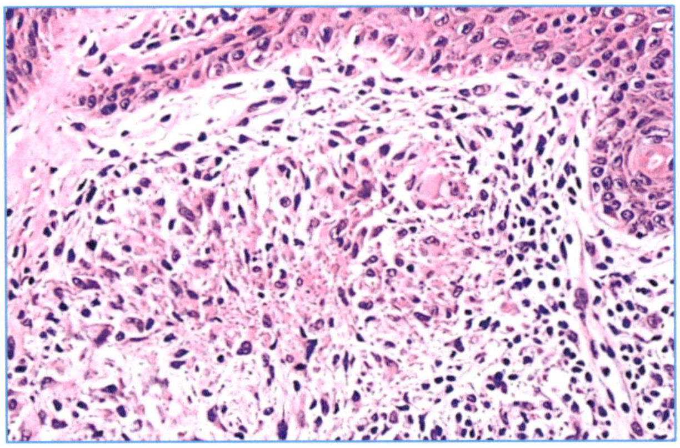

Swimming pool granuloma with focal non-caseating necrosis

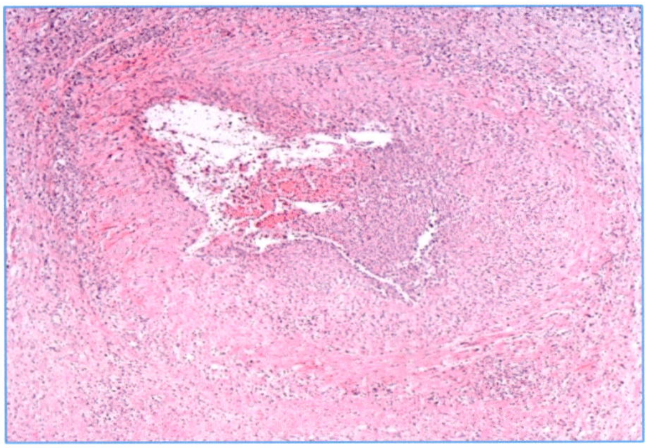

Buruli ulcer with abscess and central necrosis

Chapter 18

FUNGAL INFECTIONS

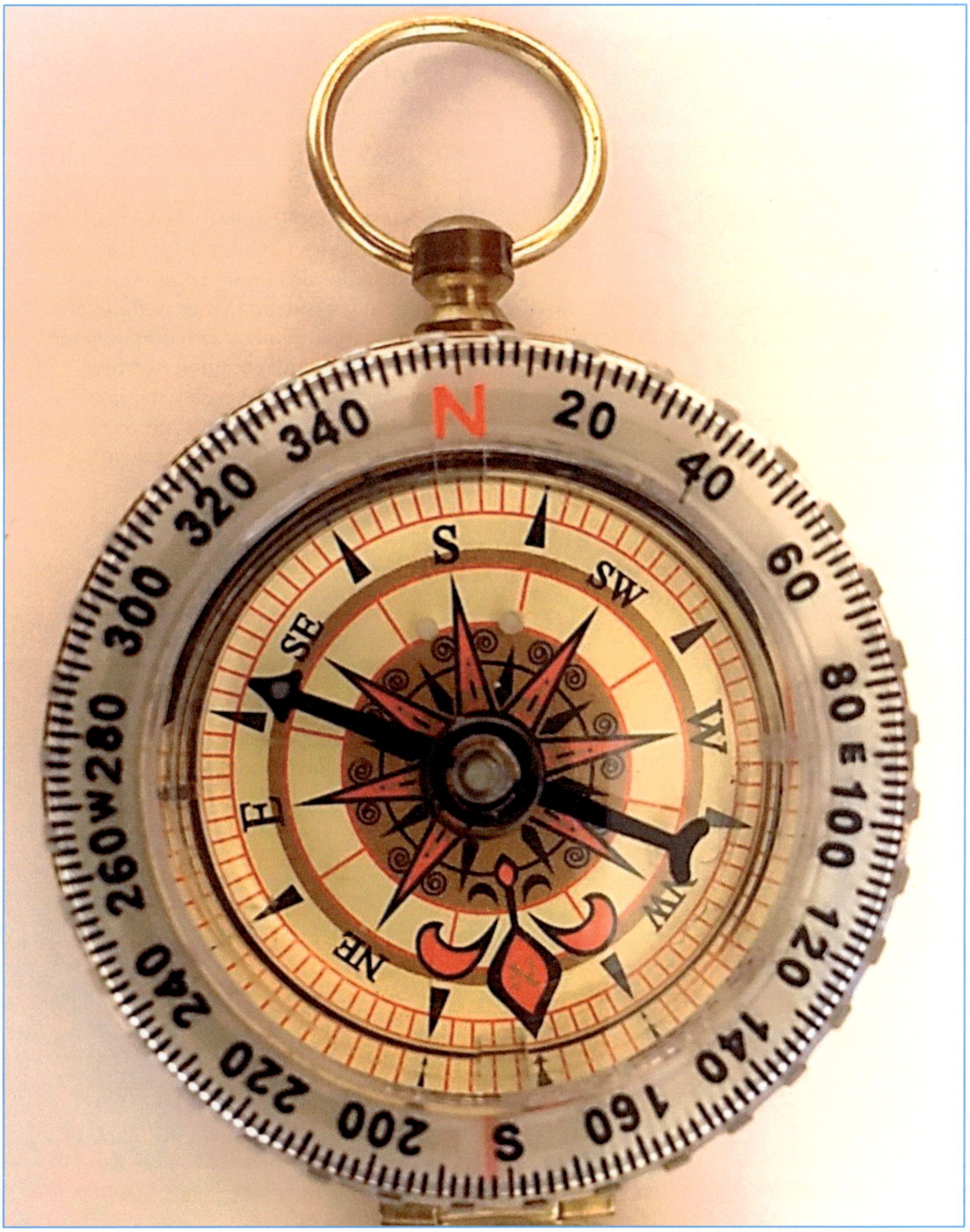

Fungal infections

CHROMOBLASTOMYCOSIS	PHAEOHYPHOMYCOSIS
-localized chronic fungal infection of skin and subcutaneous tissue -caused by *Fonsecaea pedrosoi* (most common), *Phialophora verrucosa, Fonsacea compacta, Cladosporium (Cladophialophora) carrionii* -found in the soil and decaying vegetation -more common in subtropical and tropical climates -usually introduced via traumatic cutaneous inoculation with a thorn or splinter -starts as a small papule, usually on the lower leg -slowly progresses into a verrucous hyperkeratotic plaque Histopathology -**epidermal pseudoepitheliomatous hyperplasia** -extensive dermal and subcutaneous neutrophilic inflammation with scattered giant cells -multiple epidermal/dermal micro abscesses -round brown spores **(Medlar bodies or "copper pennies"**) seen specially in micro abscesses and giant cells -**Medlar bodies** can be individual, in clusters, or chains -**hyphae** are **not seen**	-caused by heterogenous group of dematiaceous (pigmented) fungi *Exophiala jeanselmei* (most common), *Wangiella dermatitidis, Alternaria bipolaris, Rhinocladiella mackenziei* -usually introduced via traumatic cutaneous inoculation with a thorn or splinter -presents as a verrucous lesion or more commonly subcutaneous nodules -extremities, particularly fingers, are favored Histopathology -**pseudoepitheliomatous hyperplasia** (in verrucous lesions) **or normal epidermis** in nodular lesions (more common) -dermal and subcutaneous nodules of mixed inflammation with predominant **neutrophils and common necrosis** -**pigmented brown septate hyphae** and budding **yeast** that stain with Fontana-Masson melanin stain in addition to PAS and GMS stains

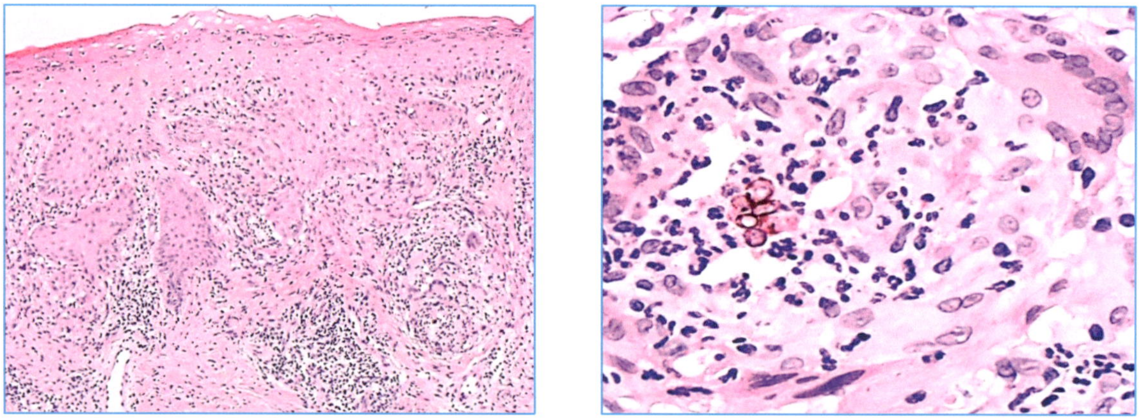

Chromoblastomycosis with pseudoepitheliomatous hyperplasia and pigmented "copper pennies" spores

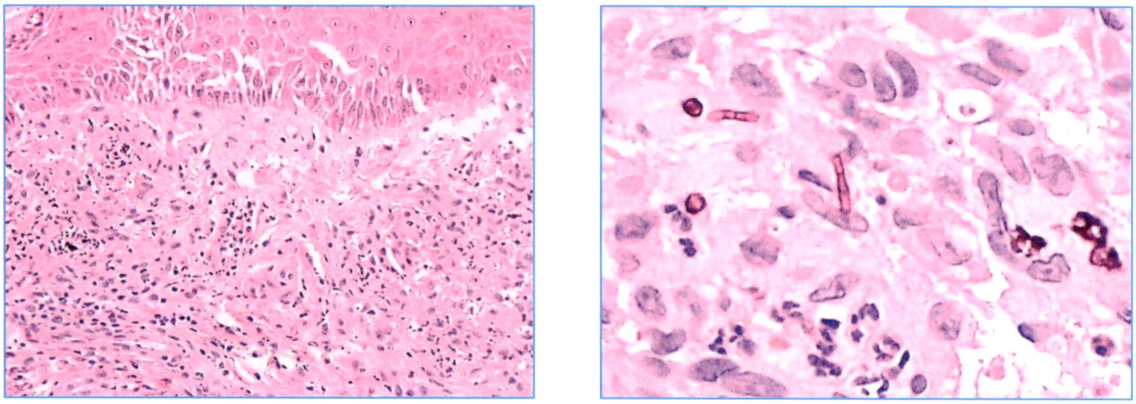

Phaeohyphomycosis forming dermal nodule with brown, pigmented spores and septate hyphae

ASPERGILLOSIS

-opportunistic, **angioinvasive** fungal infection with *Aspergillus fumigatus,* found ubiquitously in soil
-seen in immunosuppressed patients
-primary infection of lungs occurs by inhalation
-skin infection is less frequent and occurs by direct inoculation (catheter, wound site)
-presents as either papules, plaques, nodule with necrotic center, hemorrhagic bullae, or ulcers

Histopathology

-acute dermal and subcutaneous inflammation with neutrophils and abscess formation
-**vascular invasion** and **necrosis** are common
-**narrow, septate, bluish** hyphae branching at **45º**

MUCORMYCOSIS (ZYGOMYCOSIS)

-opportunistic infection caused by *Mucor, Rhizopus, Absidia*, and *Cunninghamella* genera
-seen in HIV, diabetes, burns, leukemia, and transplant patients
-classically presents as indurated necrotic plaque surrounded by cellulitis, most commonly on the face
-usually acquired via respiratory tract (rhinocerebral subtype involves nasal or oral mucosa in diabetic patients) or by direct skin inoculation through trauma

Histopathology

-extensive dermal and subcutaneous necrosis
-variable inflammation depending on status of patient's immunosuppression
-broad, **non-septate**, **irregularly shaped ("sausage" like), hollow, pink hyphae (resemble big straws cut in cross section)**
-hyphae branch at **90º angle**

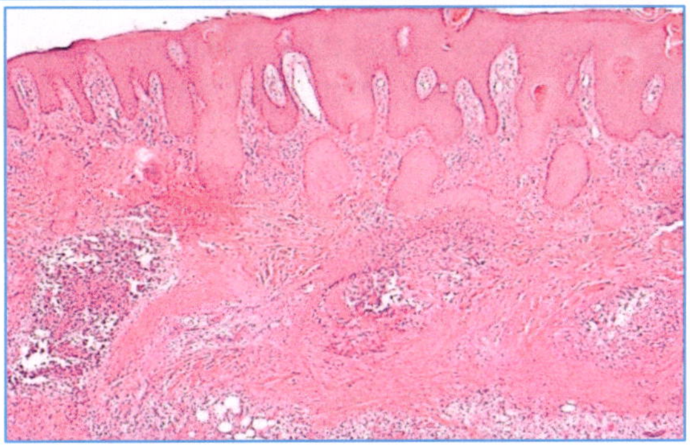

Aspergillosis with dermal abscess

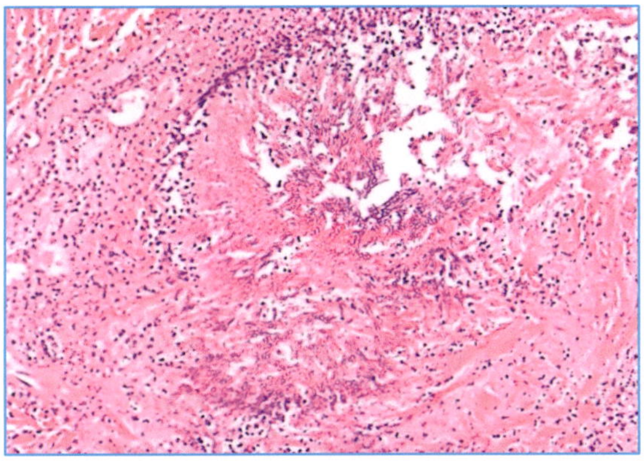

Aspergillosis with fungal vascular invasion

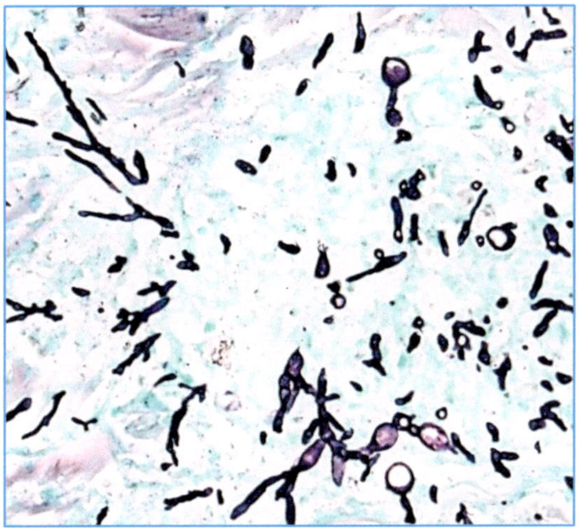

Aspergillosis with hyphae branching at 45º angle (GMS stain)

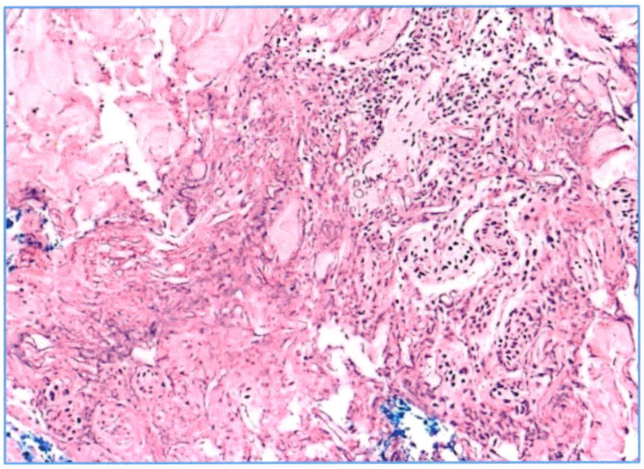

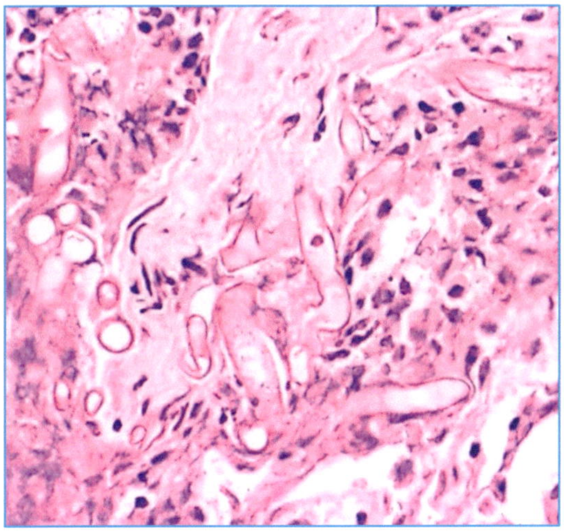

Mucormycosis with broad, hollow hyphae in necrotic tissue

Fungal infections

COCCIDIOIDOMYCOSIS (VALLEY FEVER)

-fungal infection caused by *Coccidioides immitis* or *C. posadasii*
-endemic in the southwest United States
-common cause of community-acquired pneumonia in the endemic areas
-occasionally hematogenous dissemination causing cutaneous verrucous papules/nodules with occasional ulceration
-infection can also occur via direct skin inoculation

Histopathology
-irregular epidermis with pseudoepitheliomatous hyperplasia or ulcer
-acute and chronic inflammation with giant cells
-**large spherules** (10-100 μm) with **prominent pink wall**
-**numerous endospores** within spherule

CRYPTOCOCCOSIS

-fungal infection caused by *Cryptococcus neoformans,* present in bird (pigeon) dropping
-endemic on the US Pacific coast
-mostly seen in immunocompromised patients
-respiratory tract is portal of entry and primary disease site
-cutaneous lesion results from hematogenous dissemination to the skin
-primary skin lesions are rare
-cutaneous lesions present as papules and nodules that can be molluscoid (central umbilication)
-favors the face (around mouth) and neck

Histopathology
-yeast (5-10 μm) has a unique **thick, mucinous capsule**
-stain with India ink, mucicarmine, GMS, PAS
-presents in two forms:
gelatinous form
-numerous yeasts and **mucin** with minimal inflammation
granulomatous form
-histiocytic/ lymphocytic inflammation with fewer yeasts

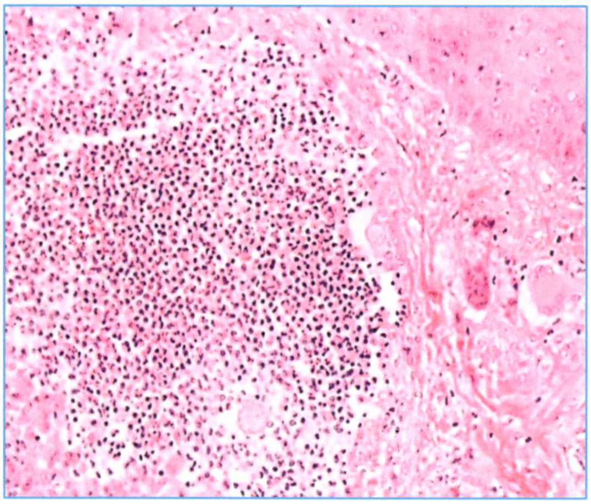

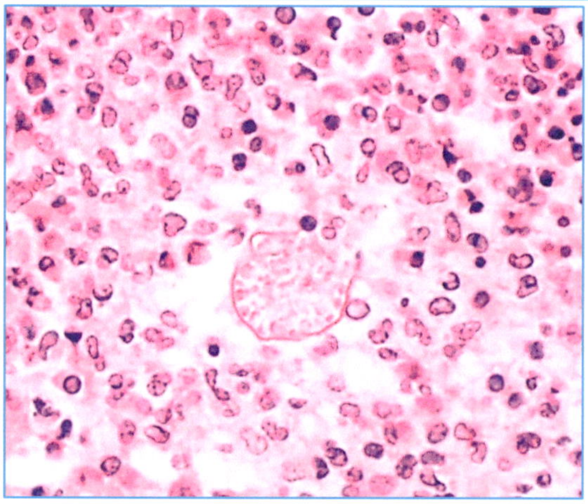

Coccidioidomycosis with large spherule filled with numerous endospores surrounded by acute inflammation

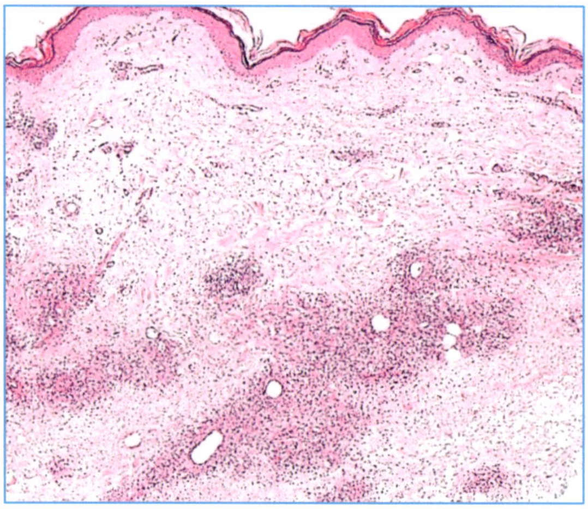

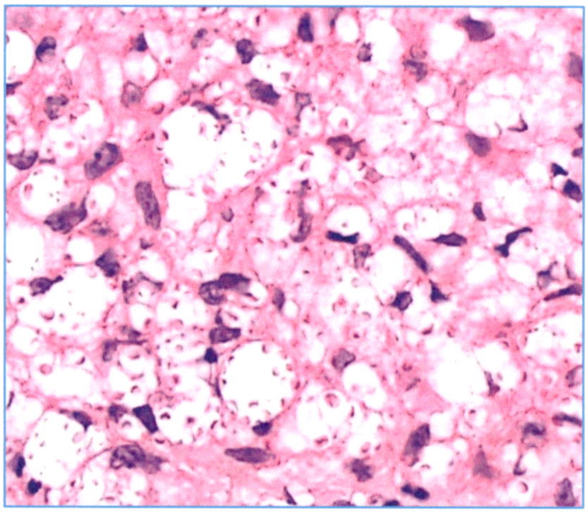

Gelatinous form of cryptococcosis with cryptococci in pale mucinous background

Chapter 18

BLASTOMYCOSIS (NORTH AMERICAN BLASTOMYCOSIS)

-endemic fungal disease caused by *Blastomyces dermatitidis*
-infects both healthy and immunosuppressed individuals
-endemic in Great Lakes and Ohio and Mississippi river valleys
-occurs through inhalation of spores which causes pneumonia (most common presentation)
-subsequent hematogenous dissemination to skin, CNS, and bones can then occur
-skin lesions present as crusted, verrucous plaques or nodules that may ulcerate with common facial involvement
-primary cutaneous inoculation is uncommon

Histopathology

-epidermis is either acanthotic with **pseudoepitheliomatous hyperplasia** or **ulceration**
-dermal mixed inflammation with **neutrophils predominating**
-scattered **giant cells and microabscess**
-**refractile, thick-walled spores** (8-18 μm) that can have single, **broad based buds**

HISTOPLASMOSIS

-primary pulmonary infection with *Histoplasma capsulatum*
-endemic in eastern and central parts of the US
-common in soil with bird and bat feces (caves)
-infection occurs through inhalation with subsequent hematogenous dissemination to the skin and mucosal surfaces
-healthy individual and immunosuppressed patients can develop systemic infection but cutaneous involvement is more common in immunosuppressed people
-secondary skin involvement presents as erythematous, necrotic, hyperkeratotic or molluscoid papules/nodules

Histopathology

-excoriated epidermis or epidermis with **pseudoepitheliomatous hyperplasia**
-diffuse dermal and subcutaneous **histiocytic infiltrate** with lymphocytes and granulomas can form
-**macrophages contain intracellular yeast (2-5 μm)** with basophilic crescent shaped nucleus
-yeast is surrounded by a **clear halo (pseudocapsule)** and can show **narrow-based budding**
-organisms are **evenly spaced** within histiocytes

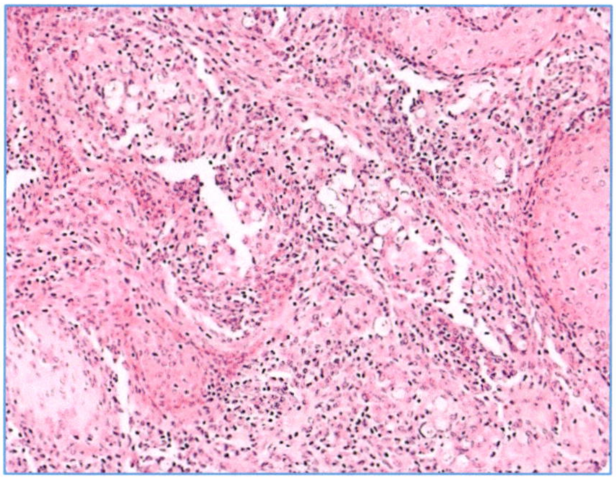

Blastomycosis induced pseudoepitheliomatous hyperplasia

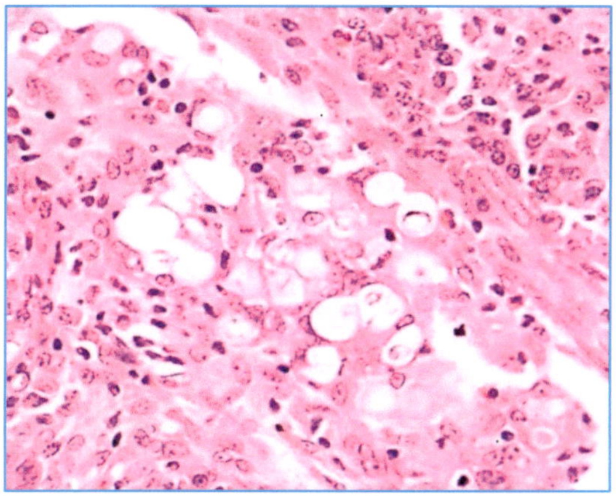

Blastomycosis with refractile, thick-walled spores

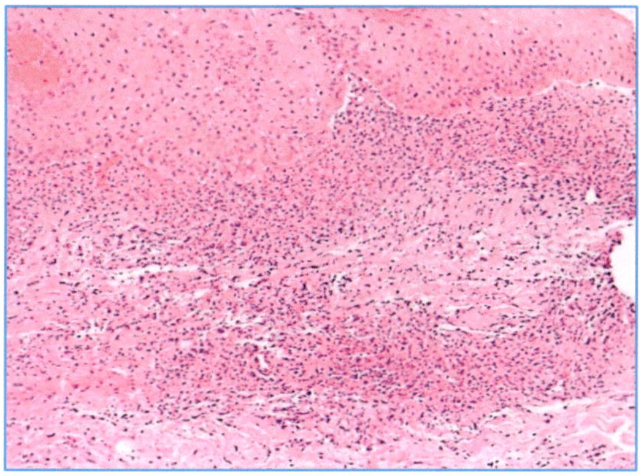

Histoplasmosis induced pseudoepitheliomatous hyperplasia

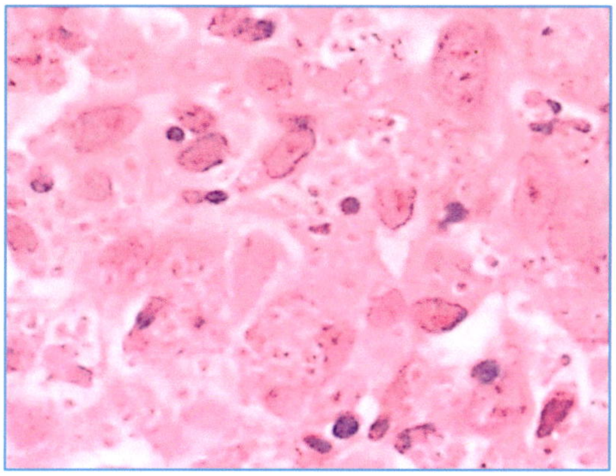

Histoplasmosis with intracellular yeasts with clear halo

Fungal infections

PARACOCCIDIOIDOMYCOSIS (SOUTH AMERICAN BLASTOMYCOSIS)

-fungal infection caused by *Paracoccidioides brasiliensis* and *Paracoccidioides lutzii*
-present in soil and endemic to southern US, Mexico, and Central and South America
-inoculation typically occurs by respiratory tract
-widely disseminates and affects the lymph nodes, liver and spleen
-skin lesions result from contiguous spread, hematogenous spread, or direct inoculation
-classic lesions are classically perioral pustules that turn into painful ulcers, with small spots of bleeding

Histopathology
-irregular epidermis with **psudoepitheliomatous hyperplasia or ulcer** and mixed inflammation **with giant cells and microabscesses**
-**round yeast that are variable in size (4-60 µm)**
-large round fungal form with circumferential narrow-based yeast buds, resembling a "**Mariner's wheels**"

RHINOSPORIDIOSIS

-chronic infectious disease caused by *Rhinosporidium seeberi*
-traditionally thought to be a fungus but is an aquatic protistan parasite
-endemic in India, Sri Lanka, and Brazil
-characterized by the formation of red-purple, polypoid, fleshy masses on the mucosa
-involves the upper respiratory tract and mucosa of the nose, conjunctiva, and urethra

Histopathology
-polypoid lesion of **nasal mucosa** with **gigantic sporangia** (10 to 350 µm)
-sporangia (capsular structures containing spores) contain innumerable endospores
-surrounding chronic inflammatory response consisting of lymphocytes, histiocytes, plasma cells, and eosinophils
-rupture of the sporangia causes microabscess formation

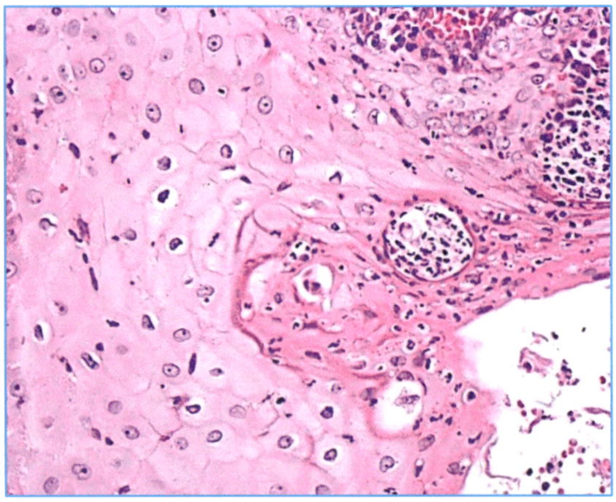
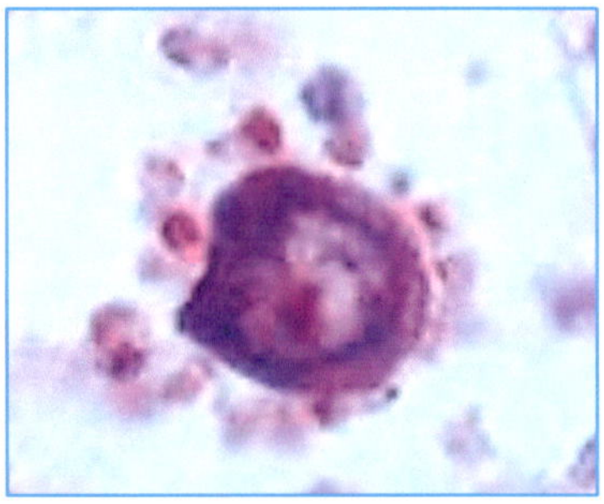

Paracoccidioidomycosis with pseudoepitheliomatous hyperplasia and microabscesses containing "Mariner's wheel" fungal elements

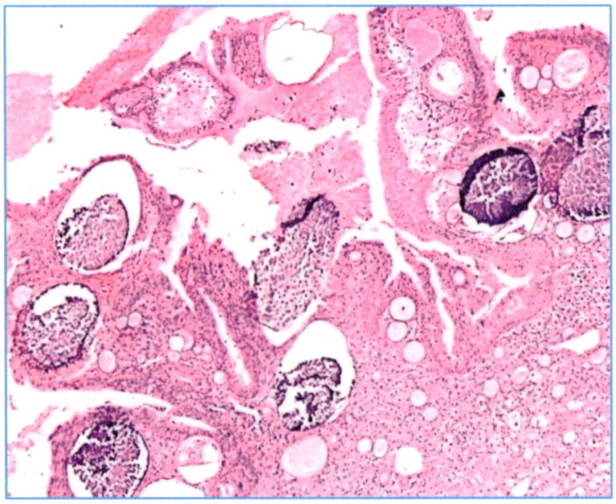
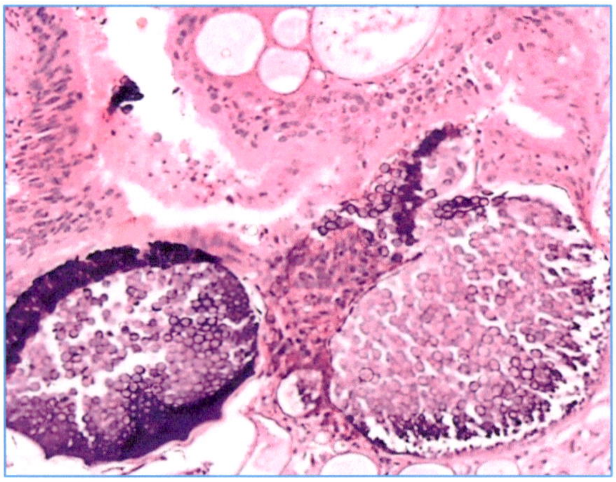

Rhinosporidiosis with gigantic sporangia containing numerous endospores

LOBOMYCOSIS

- fungal infection of the skin caused by *Lacazia loboi* (formerly named *Loboa loboi*)
- almost exclusively found in South America, particularly the Amazon basin
- can infect humans and dolphins
- humans are infected by traumatic implantation of the fungus with incubation period estimated to be between 1–2 years
- affects mainly exposed skin areas, such as the auricles and upper and lower limbs
- presents as a slow growing papule that becomes plaque or nodule (over periods of months or years)
- it ends up as "keloid-like" lesion

Histopathology

- dense dermal **histiocytic inflammation** with variable giant cells
- large round/oval **thick-walled** fungal elements (6-12 μm) in chains **"pop bead-like"**
- fibroblast proliferation with **keloidal collagen** present **only in the older lesions**

SPOROTRICHOSIS

- **"rose gardener's disease"**
- caused by traumatic implantation of *Sporotrix schenkii,* a dimorphic fungus found in soil
- presents as a papule or nodule at the site of injury
- hands are the most common site
- spreads via the lymphatics in an ascending manner to form a chain of subcutaneous nodules

Histopathology

- pseudoepitheliomatous hyperplasia
- **dermal suppurative inflammation** with neutrophils and necrosis
- round to oval, **"cigar shaped"** spores (2-6μm)
- *Sporotrix* asteroid body occasionally seen (yeast forms surrounded by eosinophilic material)
- **generally fungal elements are usually few and hard to find**
- if there is clinical suspicion for sporotrichosis and tissue stains are negative, tissue culture is highly recommended

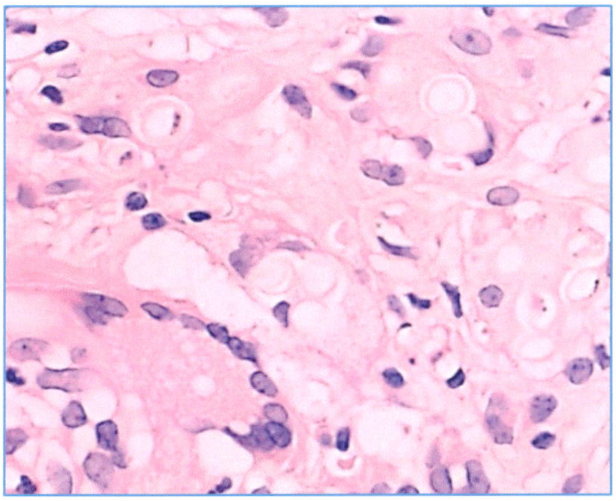

Lobomycosis with "pop bead-like" spores

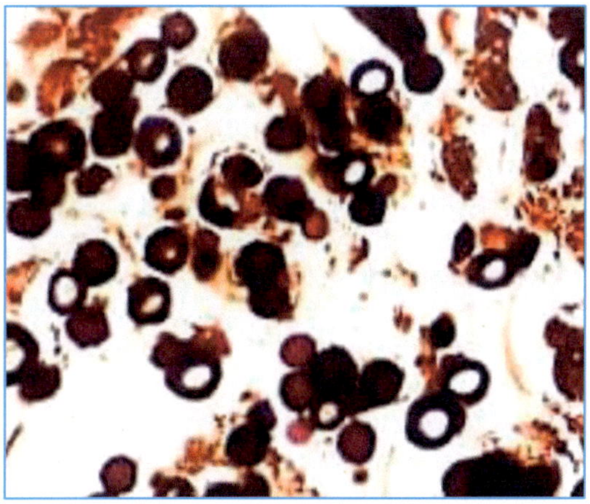

Lobomycosis with thick-walled spores (GMS stain)

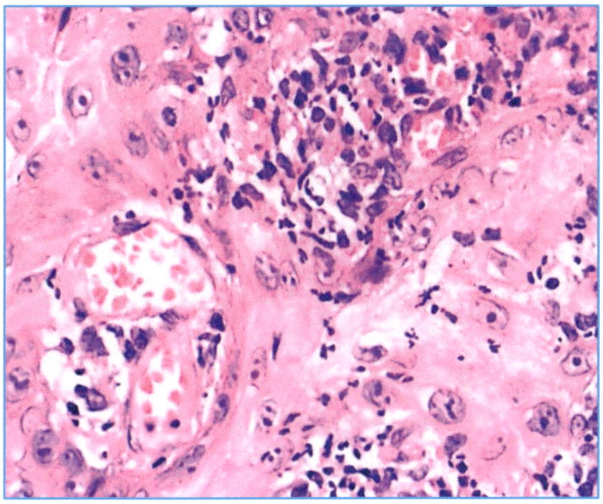

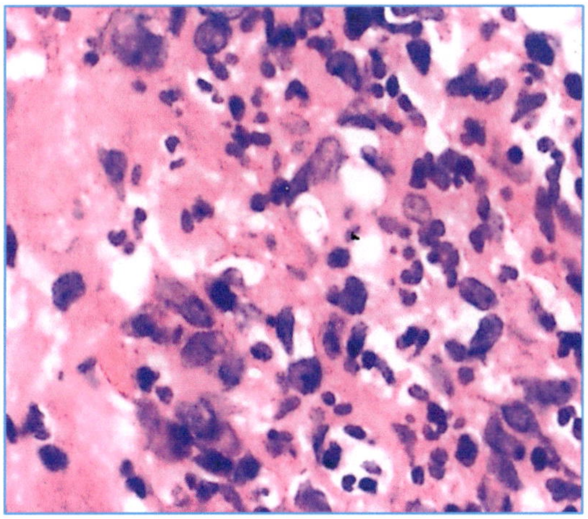

Sporotrichosis with pseudoepitheliomatous hyperplasia and extensive neutrophilic inflammation surrounding round spore

Fungal infections

DERMATOPHYTOSIS (TINEA)

-dermatophytes are related filamentous fungi capable of infecting non-viable keratinized tissue including stratum corneum, nails, and hair
-three genera: *Epidermophyton, Microsporum,* and *Trichophyton*
-tinea is a clinical term for dermatophyte infection modified according to the anatomical site

Tinea capitis
-dermatophyte infection of the scalp
-follicular inflammation manifesting as scaling plaques/patches or boggy nodules that drain pus
-can result in alopecia
-*Kerion* and *Favus* are variants of *T. capitis*
-described in more detail in the alopecia chapter

Tinea faciei
-dermatophyte infection of the face
-sharply marginated erythematous scaly annular plaque with elevated border and central regression

Tinea cruris ("jock itch")
-dermatophyte infection of the groin/inguinal folds
-more common in males
-well-demarcated, erythematous, scaly, annual plaque

Tinea manum
-dermatophyte infection of the hand
-scaling patches confined to hands
-well-demarcated borders with central clearing

Tinea barbae
-dermatophyte infection of the mustache or beard of men
-follicular pustules, exudation, and crusting, sometimes coalescing into boggy plaques on the lower face

Tinea pedis ("athlete's foot")
-dermatophyte infection of the feet
-pink scaly patches on the feet, often the soles ("moccasin scale")
-erosion and maceration between toes

Tinea corporis ("ringworm")
-dermatophyte infection on all other body sites
-small to large scaling, erythematous plaque with central clearing

Onychomycosis
-dermatophyte infection of the nails
-subungual hyperkeratosis and onycholysis with yellow discoloration

Majocchi's granuloma
-fungal folliculitis
-described in more detail in the folliculitis chapter

Histopathology depends on the anatomical site

In **moist** skin areas
-spongiotic epidermis with intraepidermal neutrophilic vesicles
-fungal hyphae **horizontally oriented** usually present above the granular layer with **"holes in thickened pink stratum corneum"**
-requires PAS or GMS stains to definitively identify hyphae

In **dry** skin areas
-normal-appearing skin, so called "invisible dermatosis"
-stratum corneum appears more compact, orthokeratotic
-focal mounds of parakeratosis above orthokeratosis, usually accompanied with few neutrophils
-careful examination will reveal **horizontally oriented hyphae** that are **"sandwiched"** in between parakeratosis and orthokeratosis
- PAS or GMS stains are required to definitively identify hyphae

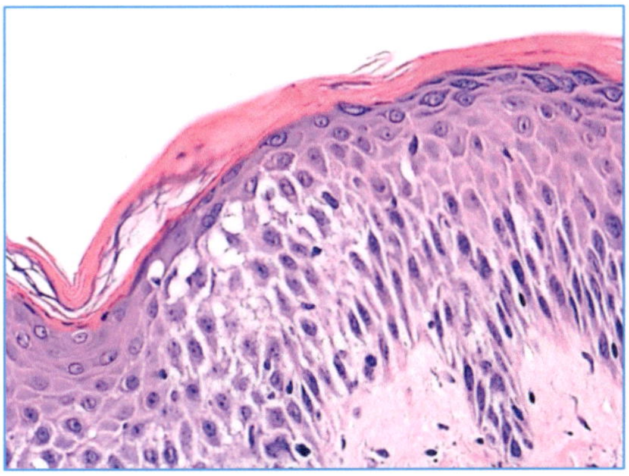

Tinea faciei with subtle epidermal spongiosis

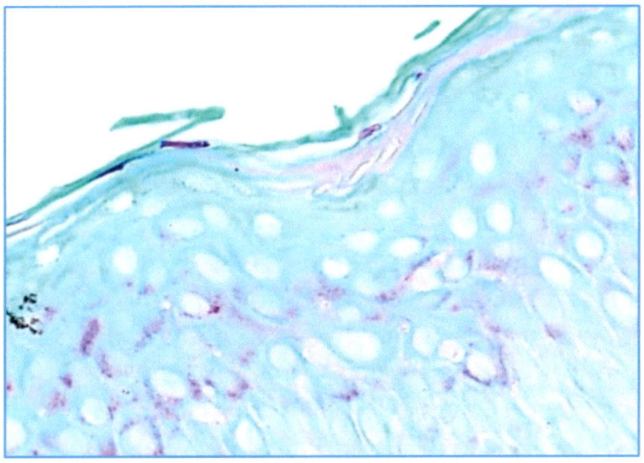

Tinea faciei with PAS stain with green counterstain that detects hyphae in the stratum corneum

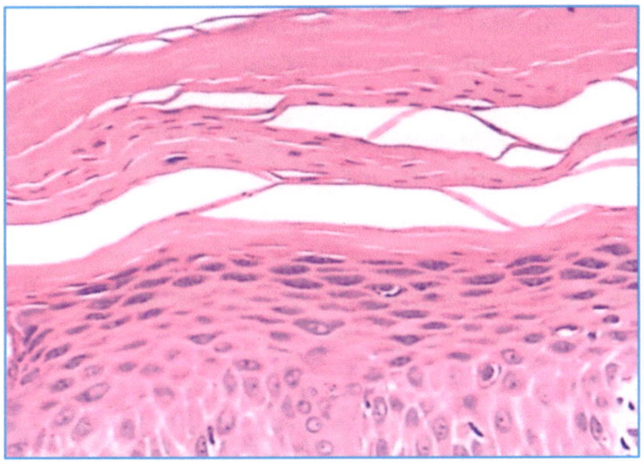

Tinea corporis with "sandwich" sign

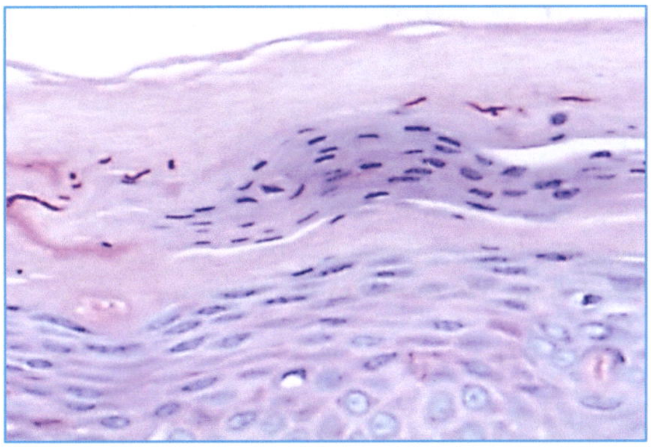

Horizontally oriented hyphae between parakeratosis and orthokeratosis (PAS stain with hematoxylin counterstain)

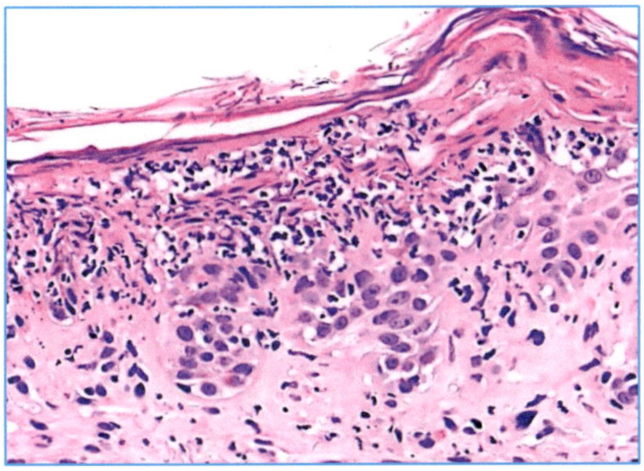

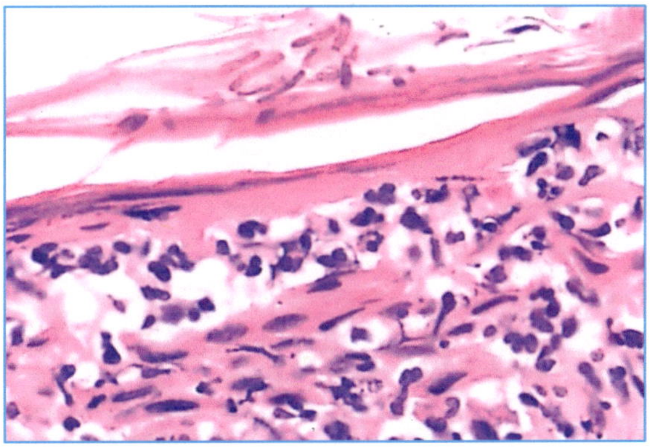

Tinea cruris with intraepidermal neutrophils and horizontally oriented hyphae above micropustule

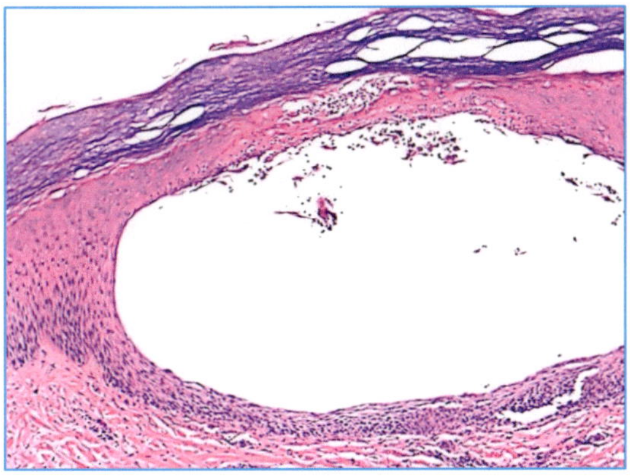

Tinea pedis with large intraepidermal vesicle with neutrophils

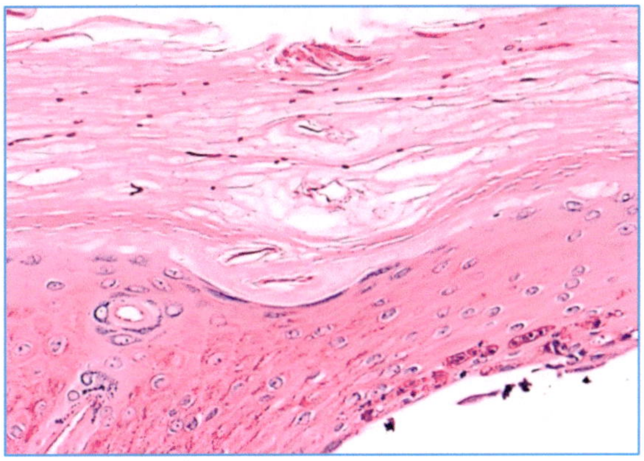

Tinea pedis with hyphae in the roof of the vesicle (PAS stain)

Fungal infections

TINEA VERSICOLOR (PITYRIASIS VERSICOLOR)

-superficial fungal infection caused by the overgrowth of yeasts *Malassezia globosa* and *M. furfur*
-yeast forms of *Malassezia* species are normal commensal organisms of the skin
-more common in warm humid climates and among adolescents with darker skin
-presents with hypo/hyperpigmented or pink macules (hence versicolor) with fine scaling
-asymptomatic or mildly pruritic
-upper back and chest (seborrheic areas) are preferred sites

Histopathology
-hyperkeratotic epidermis
-**no or very mild** superficial dermal perivascular **lymphocytic infiltrate** (less than in tinea corporis)
-elongated hyphae **("spaghetti/ziti")** and spores **("meatballs")** in the stratum corneum

ONYCHOMYCOSIS (TINEA UNGUIUM)

-fungal infection of the nails caused by dermatophytes (*Trichophyton rubrum* and *T. interdigitale*), but also yeast (*Candida* species) and molds
-typically starts as a white-yellow discoloration of the nail
-nail than develops ungual hyperkeratosis and onycholysis (separation/lifting from nail bed)

Clinically divided into:

Distal subungual onychomycosis (most common)
-involves hyponychium and distal nail bed

Proximal subungual onychomycosis
-white spot appears beneath proximal nail fold

Superficial white onychomycosis
-white, chalky plaque on dorsal nail plate

Candidal onychomycosis
-hyperkeratosis and nail bed destruction

Histopathology
-nail fragment with dermatophytes arranged parallel within keratin plates

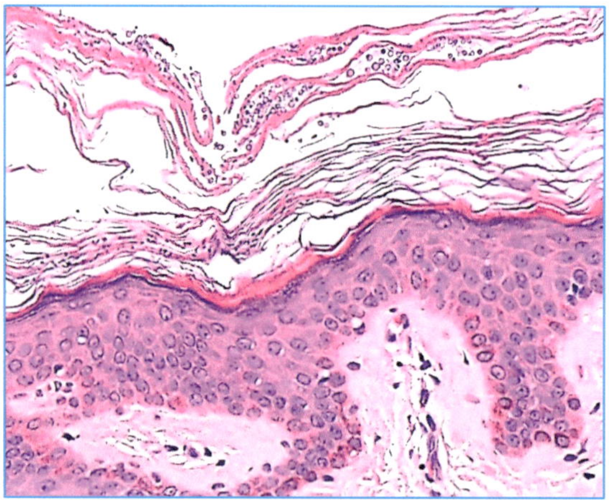
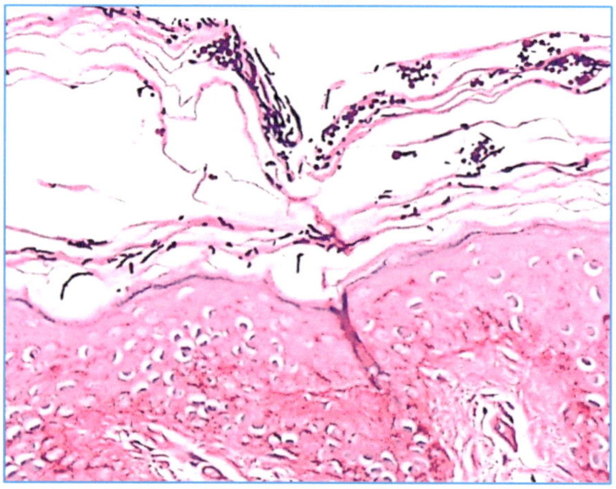

Tinea versicolor with "spaghetti meatballs" fungal elements in the superficial stratum corneum (H&E stain on the left and PAS stain on the right)

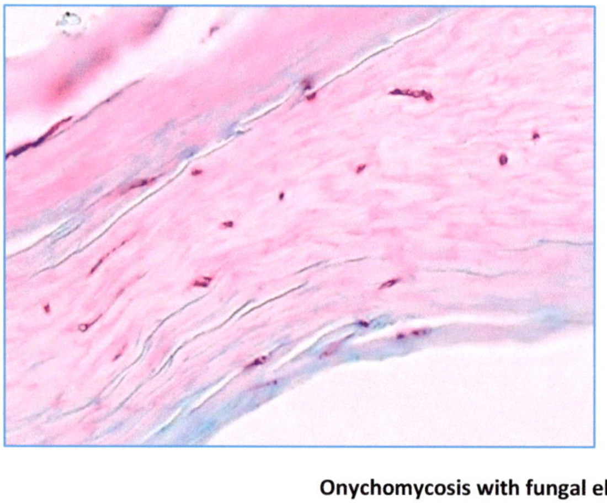
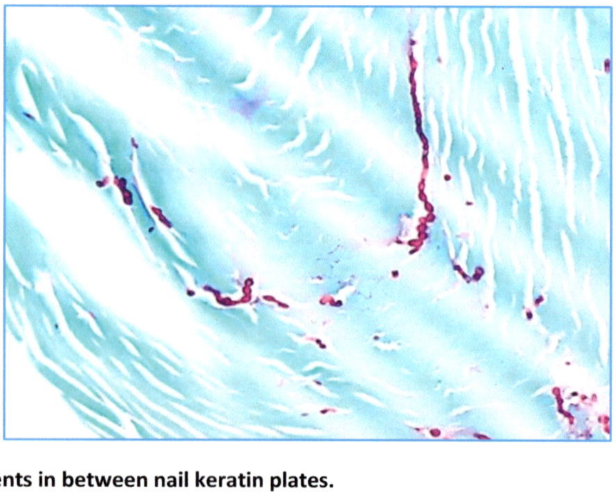

Onychomycosis with fungal elements in between nail keratin plates. PAS stain with hematoxylin (left) and methylene blue (right) counterstain.

CANDIDIASIS (MONILIASIS)

-superficial fungal infection due to **Candida** species, most commonly *Candida albicans*
-more common in young children, the elderly, and diabetic and immunosuppressed patients
-favors moist cutaneous sites (intertriginous areas)
-presents as erythema with papular and pustular lesions
-mucosal candidiasis presents with friable moist white plaques (e.g. thrush)

Histopathology
-epidermis with prominent stratum corneum
-epidermal parakeratosis with neutrophils
-neutrophils usually form small **subcorneal pustules** but sometimes can be quite large
-spores, branching pseudohyphae, and hyphae are present
-**hyphae grow in a vertical orientation** in addition to the typical horizontal orientation (unlike tinea)

TINEA NIGRA

-asymptomatic infection by *Hortaea werneckii*
-more common in the tropics
-slowly enlarging brown or black macule or patch, sometimes mistaken for a pigmented lesion
-favors palms and palmar side of fingers

Histopathology
-hyperkeratotic acral epidermis
-usually numerous **thick brown septate hyphae** limited to the stratum corneum
-no dermal inflammation

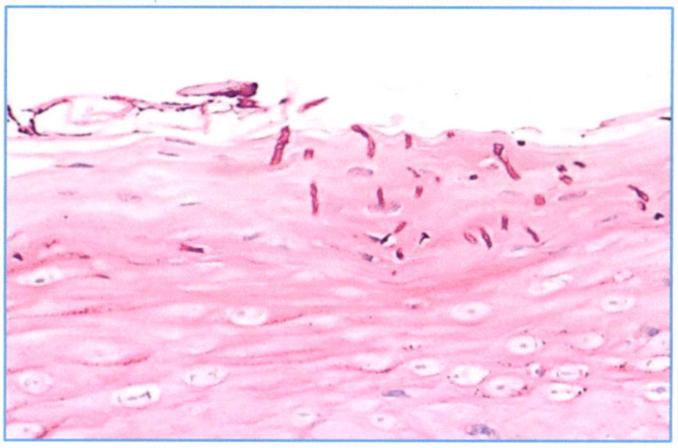

Candidiasis with vertically oriented hyphae (PAS stain)

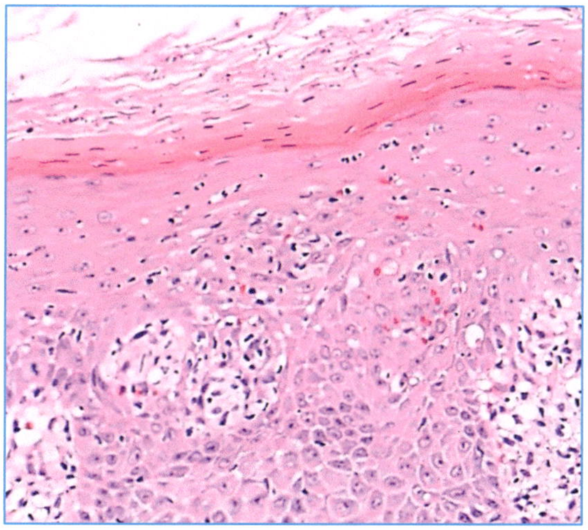

Candidiasis with subcorneal neutrophils

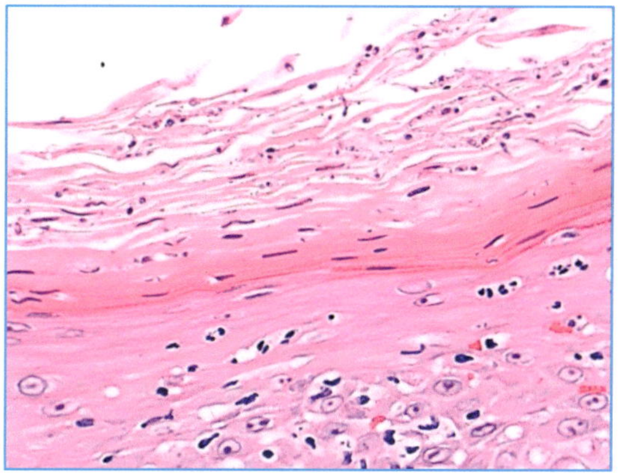

Candidiasis with spores and hyphae

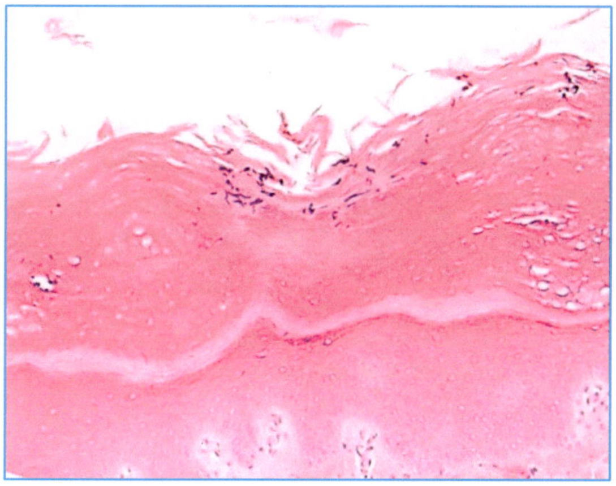

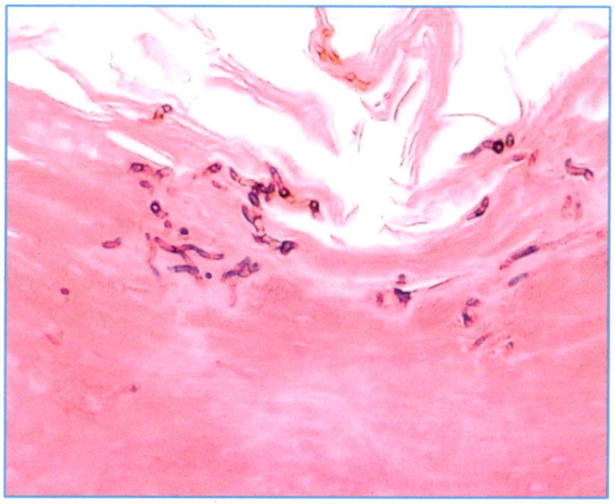

Tinea nigra with thick brown hyphae in superficial stratum corneum

Fungal infections

FUSARIOSIS

-fungal infection caused by fungus *Fusarium sp.* often found as mold in soil and on plants
-more common in the immunosuppressed and patients with severe burns
-infection occurs via skin inoculation typically at the wound/burn site with subsequent hematogenous spread (fungemia), sepsis, and a high mortality rate
-presents with erythematous plaques that may become purpuric and necrotic

Histopathology

-in immunosuppressed patients there is minimal cutaneous inflammation and extensive necrosis
-hyphae are numerous and **vascular invasion is extensive**
-**hyphae branch at 45º angle**, like *Aspergillosis,* and tissue culture is needed to separate them
-in immunocompetent patients, there is extensive acute inflammation with minimal necrosis and few hyphae

EUMYCETOMA

-chronic fungal infection by *Madurella* spp.
-slow growing papules and nodules at the site of inoculation that drain pus containing black grains
-favor lower leg, particularly feet (Madura foot)

Histopathology

-dermal/ subcutaneous abscess and necrosis
-**"sulfur granules"** composed of non-pigmented fungal elements surrounded by **"starburst-like" eosinophilic material** composed of immunoglobulins and necrotic tissue (**Splendore-Hoeppli phenomenon**)

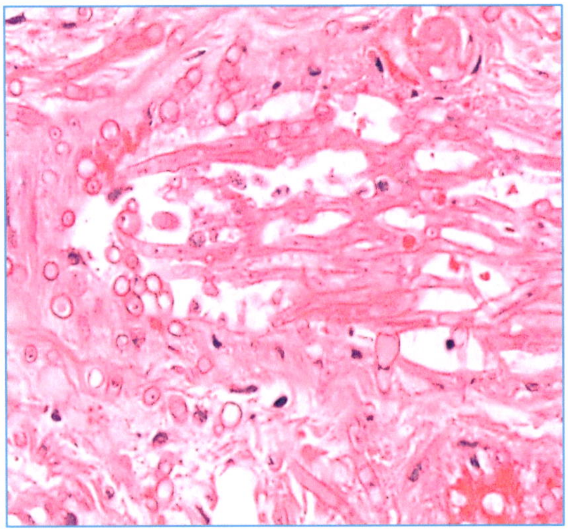

Fusariosis with branching hyphae invading vessel wall

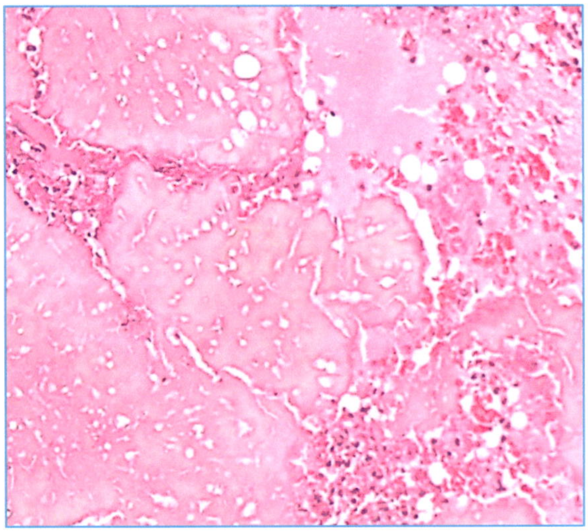

Eumycetoma with fungal hyphae within "sulfur granules"

PROTOTHECOSIS

-results from traumatic implantation of *Prototheca* spp. of unicellular algae
-ubiquitous in nature, especially in decaying organic matter
-presents as nodular or papular skin lesion with or without ulceration at the site of implantation

Histopathology

-variable inflammation from mild to granulomatous
-algae form **septate morulae** in **"daisy"** or **soccer ball"** appearance

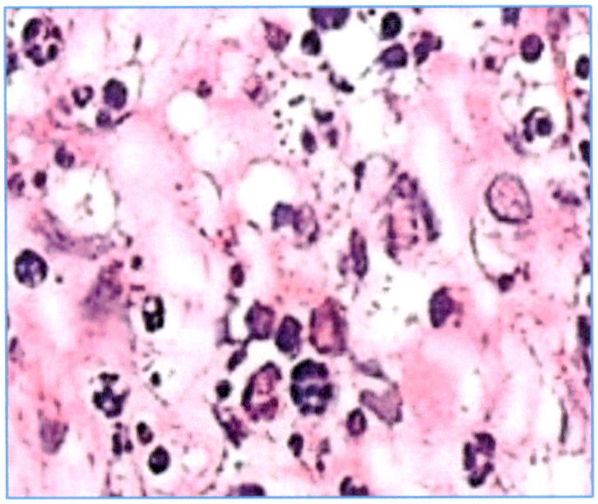

Protothecosis with morulae in "soccer ball" appearance

Chapter 18

HOW TO APPROACH FUNGAL INFECTIONS

DETERMINE LOCATION OF INFLAMMATION

SUPERFICIAL (EPIDERMAL)

-dermatophytes	minimal inflammation in dry skin area	horizontal hyphae in stratum corneum
	epidermal neutrophils in moist skin area	horizontal hyphae in stratum corneum
-candidiasis	epidermal neutrophils	horizontal + vertical hyphae
-tinea versicolor	minimal inflammation	"spaghetti meatballs" (hyphae + spores)
-tinea nigra	no inflammation acral site	brown black hyphae

DEEP (DERMAL)

WITH PIGMENTED FUNGAL ELEMENTS

-chromoblastomycosis	reactive epidermis	"copper pennies"	no hyphae
-phaeohyphomycosis	dermal nodular reaction	pigmented spores and septate hyphae	

WITH EASILY IDENTIFIED FUNGAL ELEMENTS

-mucormycosis		thick non septate hyphae	90º angle branching
-aspergillosis	vascular invasion	septate hyphae	45º angle branching
-fusariosis	vascular invasion	septate hyphae	45º angle branching

Tissue culture is required to distinguish aspergillosis from fusariosis

WITH DERMAL MUCIN

-cryptococcosis spores within focal or large mucin lakes

WITH LARGE SPHERULES

-rhinosporidiosis	larger	10-350 μm	dark purple wall	respiratory mucosa
-coccidioidomycosis	smaller	10-100 μm	pink wall	

WITH DERMAL SPORES BUT NO HYPHAE OR MUCIN

-paracoccidioidomycosis	South American blasto	4-60 μm	"Mariner's wheel"
-blastomycosis	North American blasto	8-18 μm	broad-based budding
-lobomycosis	Brazil	6-12 μm	"pop beads"
-sporotrichosis	gardeners	2-6 μm	"cigar-shaped"

WITH HISTIOCYTES WITH TINY CYTOPLASMIC DOTS

-histoplasmosis	tiny fungal spores	2-5 μm	+ GMS, PAS stains

Two diseases mentioned below have similar histology to histoplasmosis but are not fungal diseases

-leishmaniasis	parasite amastigote	2-4 μm	+ Giemsa stain
-rhinoscleroma	bacteria respiratory mucosa	2-3 μm	+ Giemsa stain

All fungi will stain with PAS and GMS stains.
Cryptococci also stain with Indian ink (capsule) and mucin stains e.g. mucicarmine, Alcian Blue.

Fungal infections

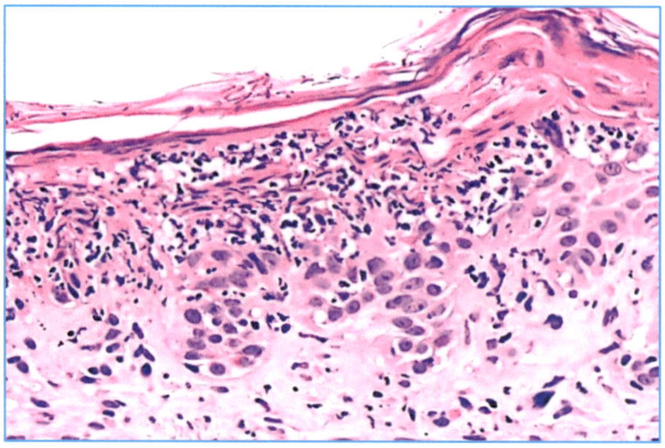

Tinea corporis with hyphae hiding in compact stratum corneum with neutrophils

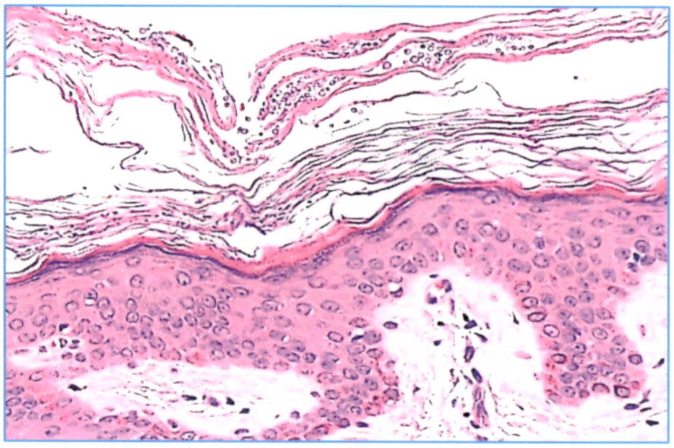

Pityriasis versicolor with hyphae and spores in "spaghetti and meatballs" pattern

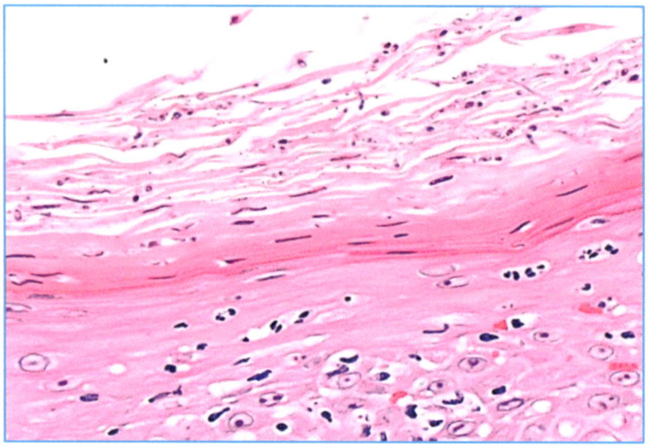

Candidiasis with hyphae growing in horizontal and vertical plane (unlike tinea)

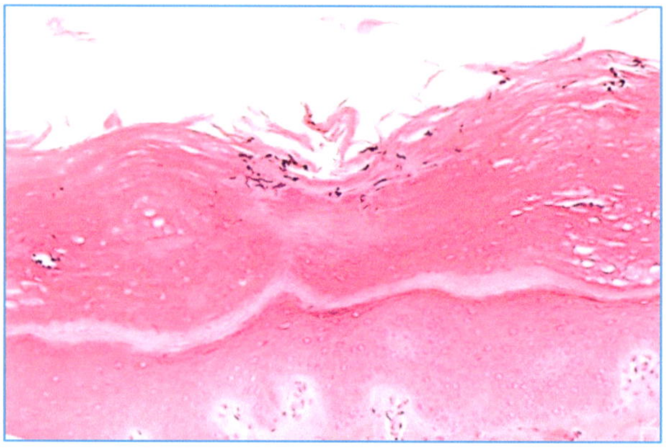

Tinea nigra with thick brown septate hyphae

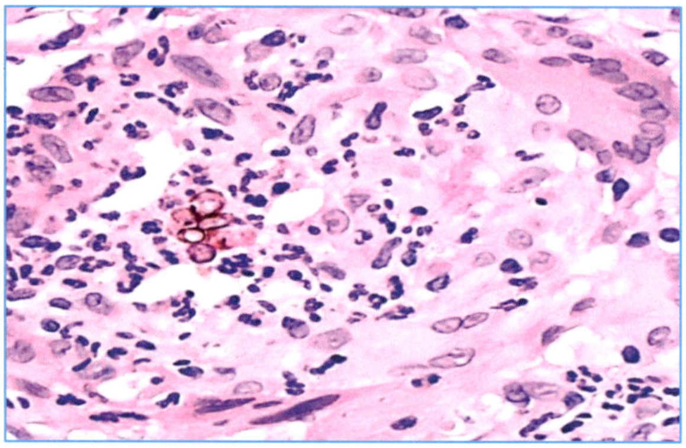

Chromoblastomycosis with round brown spores, "copper pennies"

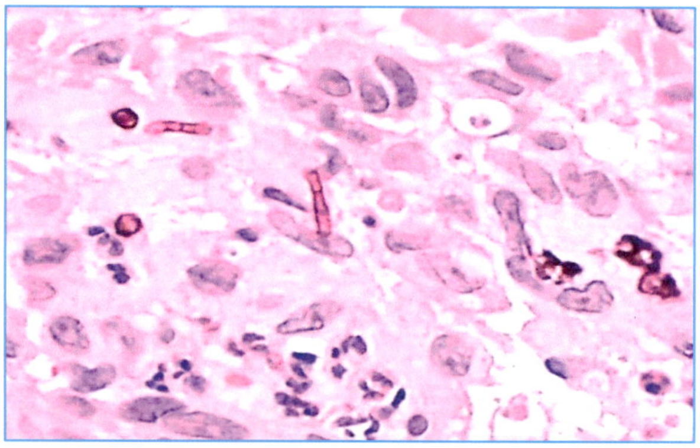

Phaeohyphomycosis with pigmented, septate hyphae and spores

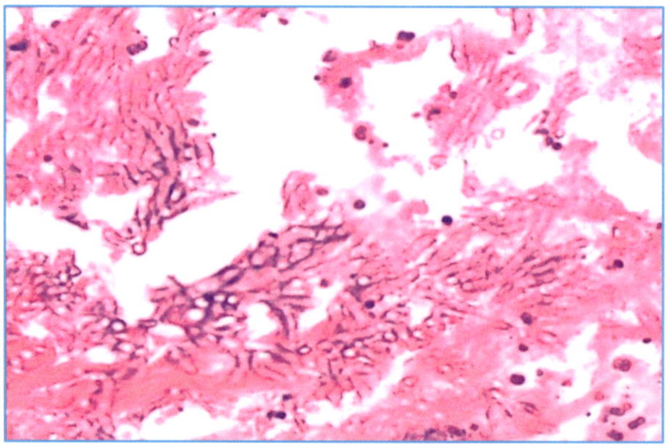

Aspergillosis with hyphae that are septate and branch at 45º angle

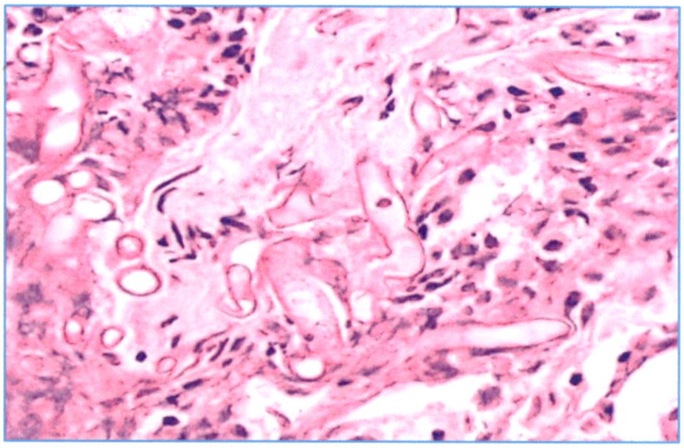

Mucormycosis with non-septate, irregularly shaped hyphae ("sausage like") that branch at 90º angle

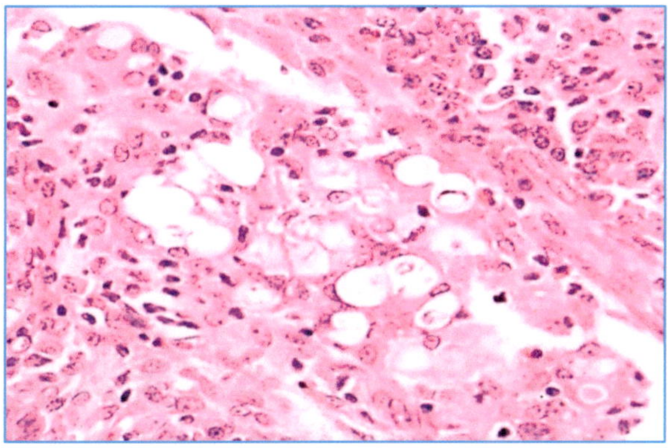

Blastomycosis with thick-walled large spores in mixed inflammation

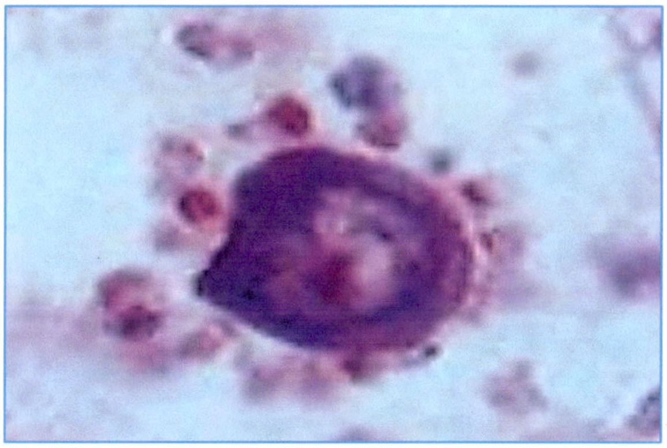

Paracoccidioidomycosis with “mariner’s wheel”

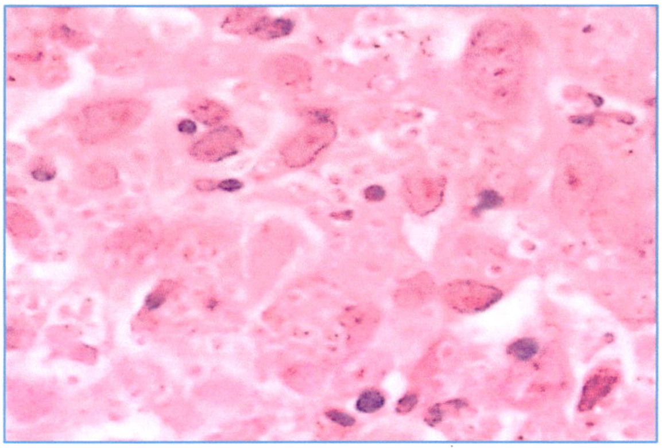

Histoplasmosis evenly spaced spores within histiocytes

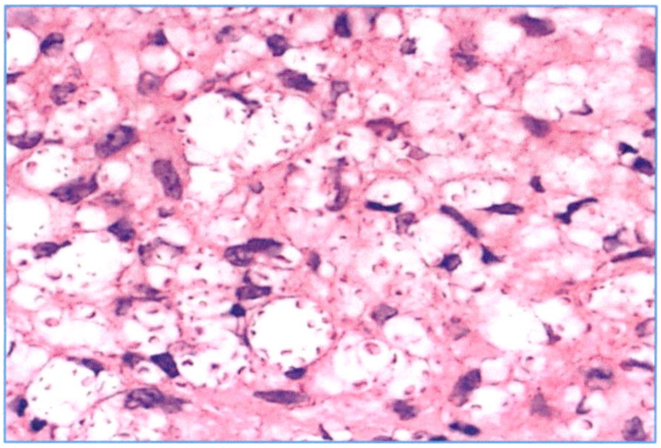

Cryptococcosis yeast in mucinous pale background

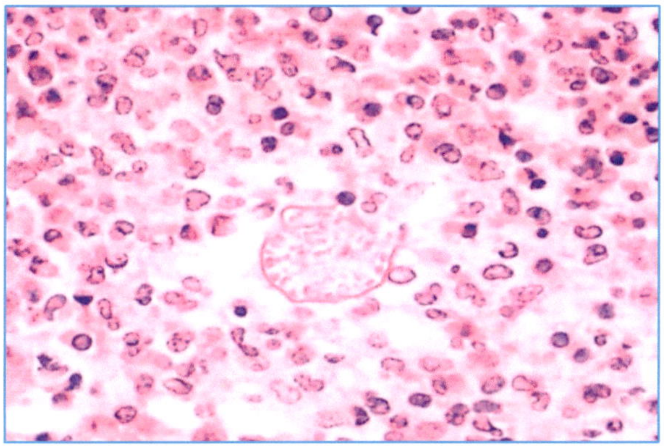

Coccidiodidomycosis with smaller sporangia with pink wall

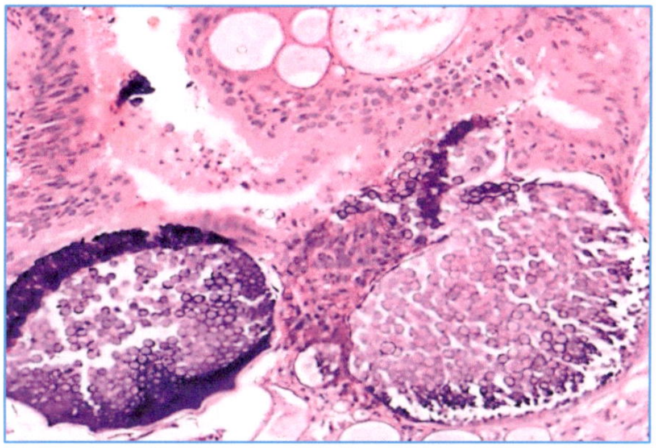

Rhinosporidiosis with large sporangia

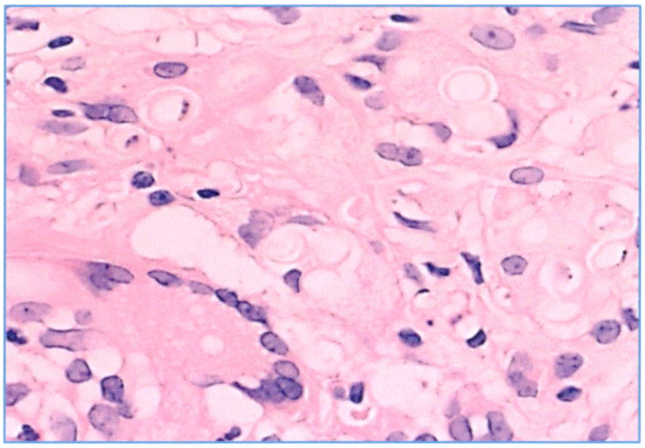

Lobomycosis with histiocytic infiltrate with spores “pop beads”

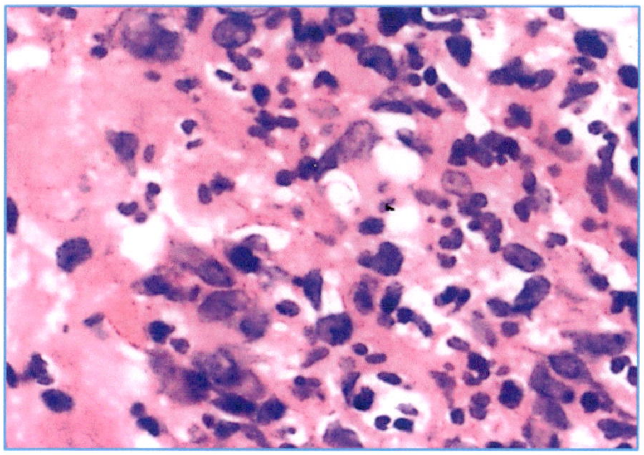

Sporotrichosis with round spore hidden in necrosis and neutrophilic inflammation

Fungal infections

Chapter 19

VIRAL INFECTIONS

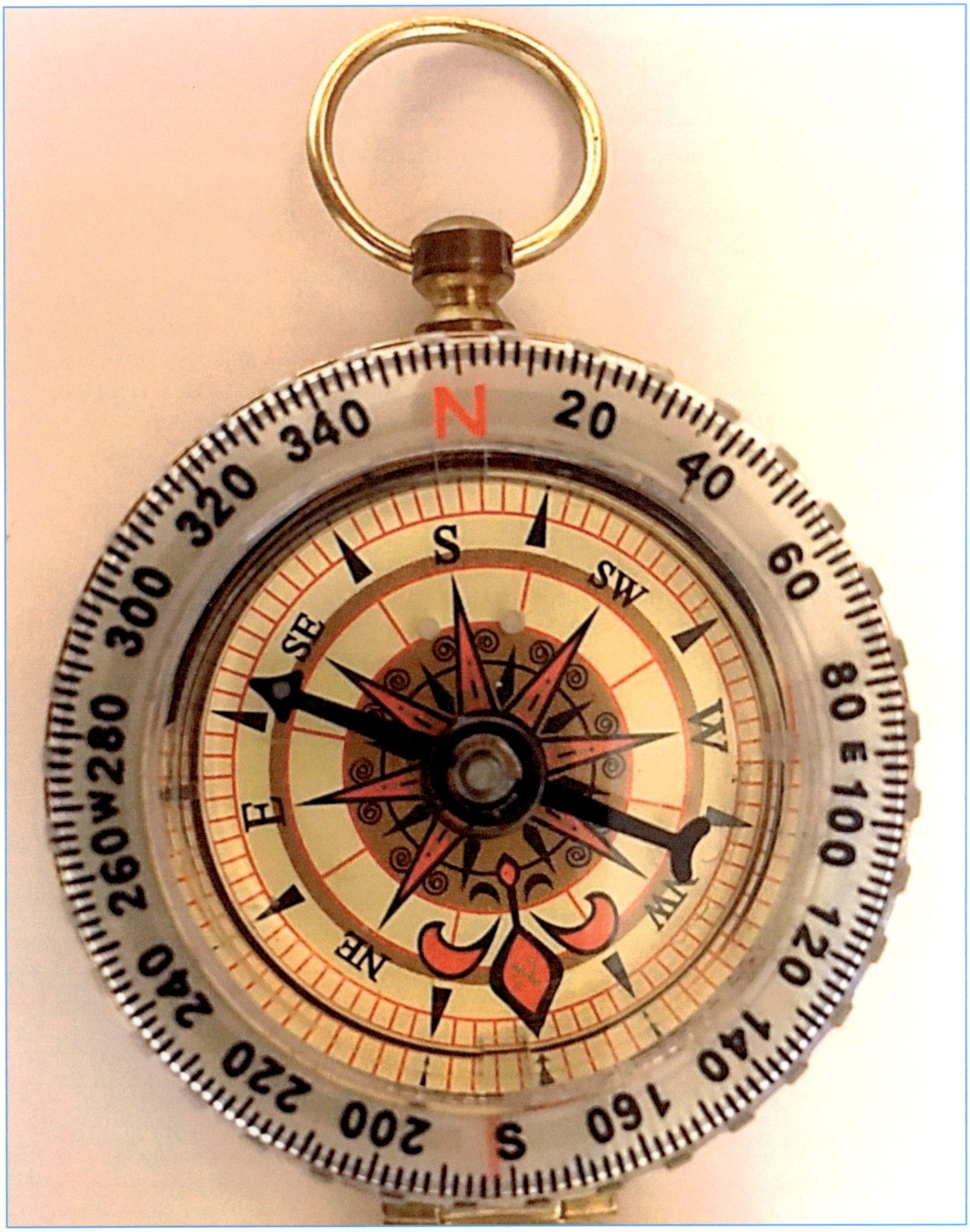

Viral infections

HUMAN PAPILLOMA VIRUS INFECTIONS (HPV)

Different types of HPV cause different clinical manifestations

Verruca vulgaris (common wart): HPV types 1, 2, 4

-flesh-colored, hyperkeratotic papules with hyperkeratotic, papillomatous surface

-hands are favorite site, but can occur anywhere

Verruca plana (flat wart): HPV types 3, 10

-flat-topped, skin-colored or light brown papules

Verruca plantaris (myrmecia), verruca palmaris: HPV types 1, 2, 4

-sometimes painful, deep-seated hyperkeratotic papule, plaque, or nodule on palms or soles

Epidermodysplasia verruciformis: HPV types 3, 5, 8, 9, 12

-rare autosomal recessive condition characterized by high susceptibility to HPV

-widespread warts on face, hands, feet

-highly susceptible to developing squamous cell carcinoma

Condyloma acuminatum (genital wart): HPV types 6, 11

-filiform to "cauliflower-like", skin-colored to pink lesions clustered in genital area

Histopathology

-all lesions caused by HPV have **koilocytes** (HPV infected keratinocytes) in the upper part of the epidermis

-**koilocytes** are large cells with **small, dark, "raisin-shaped" nucleus surrounded by clear cytoplasm**

-different HPV lesions differ by the epithelial shape and quality of keratohyaline granules

Verruca vulgaris

-exophytic **"church spire" shaped** lesion with epidermal kyperkeratosis, papillomatosis, and hypergranulosis

-columns of epidermal parakeratosis

Verruca plana

-hyperkeratotic, **flat to wavy epidermis** with hypergranulosis and no or minimal papillomatosis

Verruca plantaris (myrmecia)/palmar wart

-**exophytic and endophytic** hyperkeratotic epidermis with papillomatosis

-epidermis pushes into dermis

-prominent granulosis with **large, prominent, dark purple granules**

Epidermodysplasia verruciformis

-architecturally can resemble verruca vulgaris or verruca plana

-keratinocytes with **distinctive blue-gray-pink swollen cytoplasm** and **grouped koilocytes**

-individual cells can have **clear intranuclear space and perinuclear halo**

Condyloma acuminatum

-large **polypoid lesion** that is wider than exophytic

-epidermal hyperplasia with parakeratosis and hypergranulosis

-**koilocytes are less prominent** compared to other HPV lesions

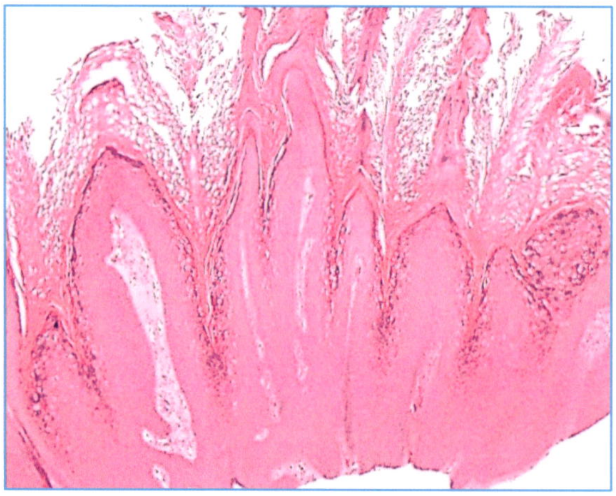

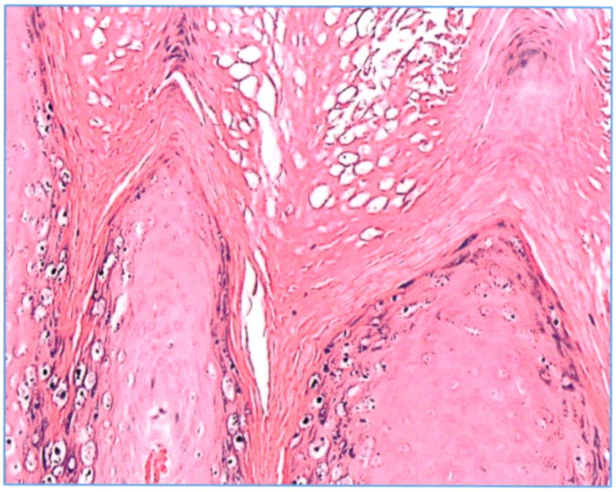

Verruca vulgaris with "church spire" shape and superficial epidermal koilocytes

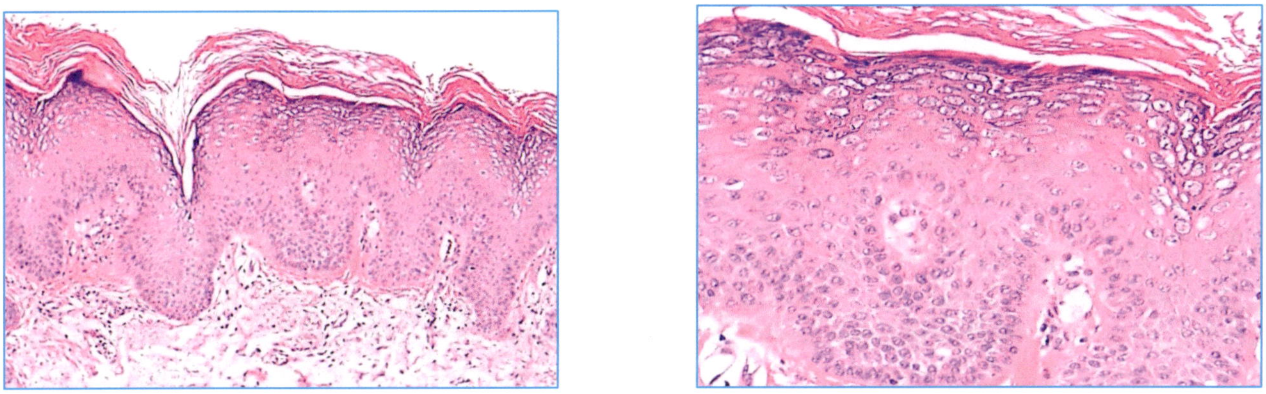

Verruca plana with wavy epidermis and koilocytes in superficial portion of the epidermis

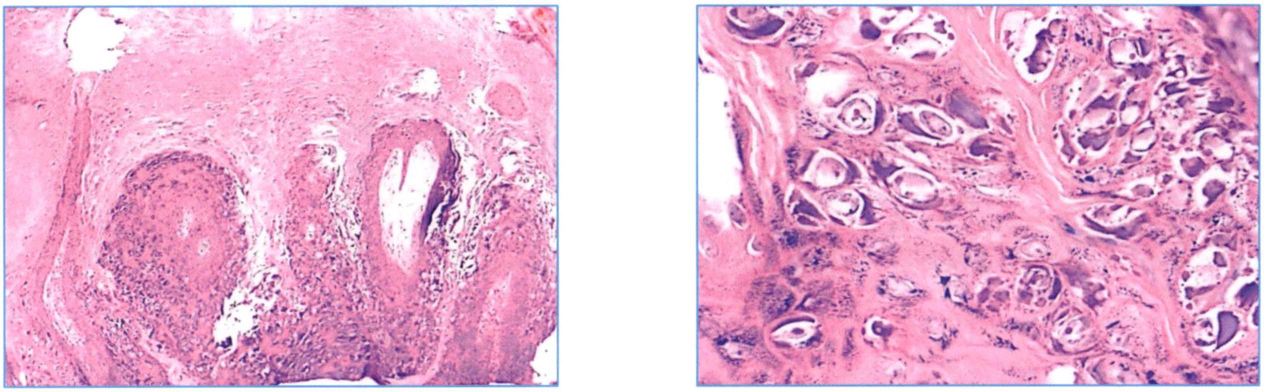

Plantar wart (myrmecia) with exophytic and endophytic epidermis containing coarse, dark purple granules

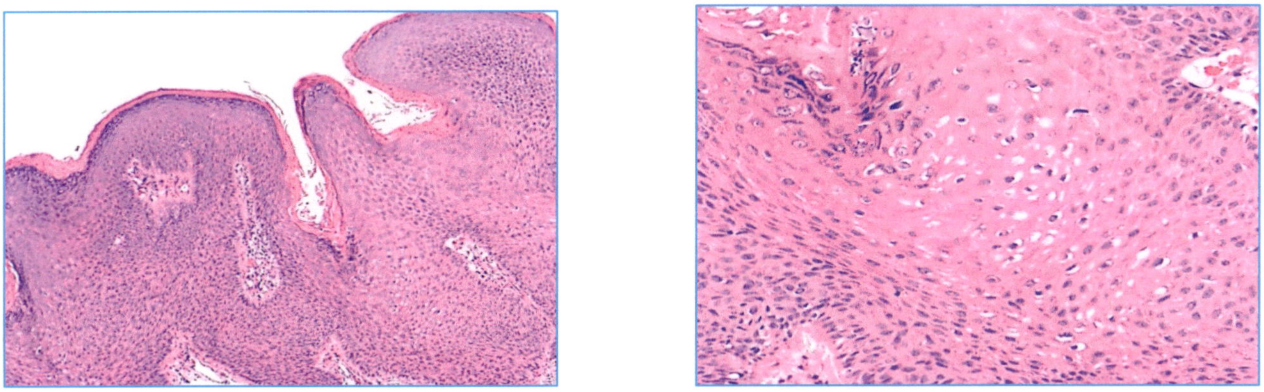

Polypoid lesion of condyloma acuminatum with subtle presence of koilocytes

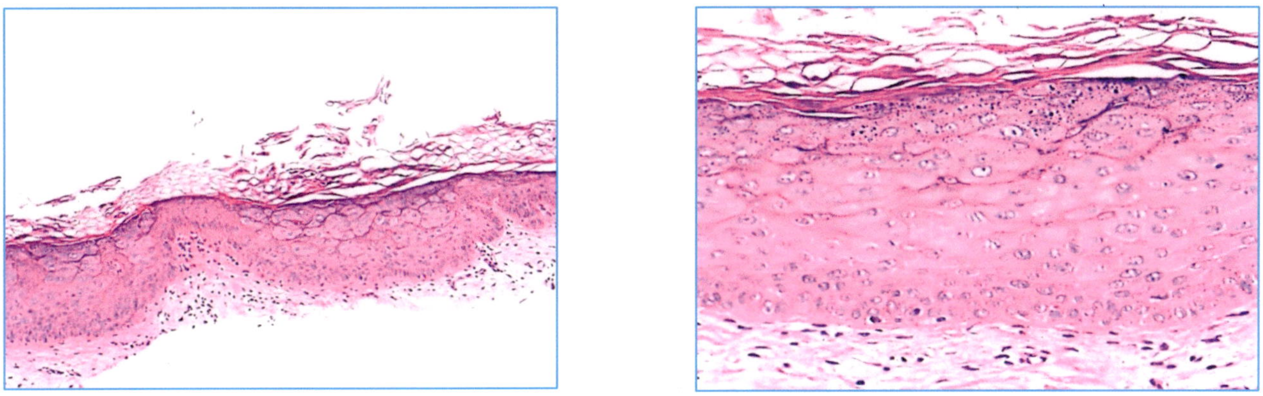

Epidermodysplasia verruciformis with clustered, swollen, pink-gray keratinocytes

Viral infections

HERPES VIRUS INFECTION

Herpes simplex

-acute, self-limited, viral infection
-HSV-1 (HHV-1) causes mostly an oral and facial infection while HSV-2 (HHV-2) causes mostly a genital infection
-grouped red macules that rapidly become painful vesicles ("dew drops on a rose petal") that erode and form crusts

Herpes zoster

-VZV virus (HHV-3) causes *chicken pox*, a common viral disorder in children
-crops of macules evolve to erythematous vesicles
-lesions are characteristically in various stages of healing, pruritic, and heal without scarring if not secondarily infected
-virus resides dormant in the dorsal root or cranial nerve ganglions
-*herpes zoster (shingles)* is reactivation of VZV in adults
-more common in immunosuppressed individuals
-patients typically experience a prodrome (itch, tingling, hyperesthesia) before the eruption
-red macules that rapidly become vesicles surrounded by erythema in a dermatomal distribution

Histopathology

-herpes simplex, herpes zoster, and chicken pox have the same histological features
-immunoperoxidase stains for HSV or VZV herpes virus are needed to distinguish them
-ulcerated epidermis with vesicle
-vesicles contains acantholytic keratinocytes with **"steel gray" nuclei**
-many keratinocytes have intranuclear eosinophilic inclusion bodies (**Cowdy A body**)
-**multinucleated keratinocytic giant cells** with nuclear **molding** are present
-exuberant acute and chronic inflammation

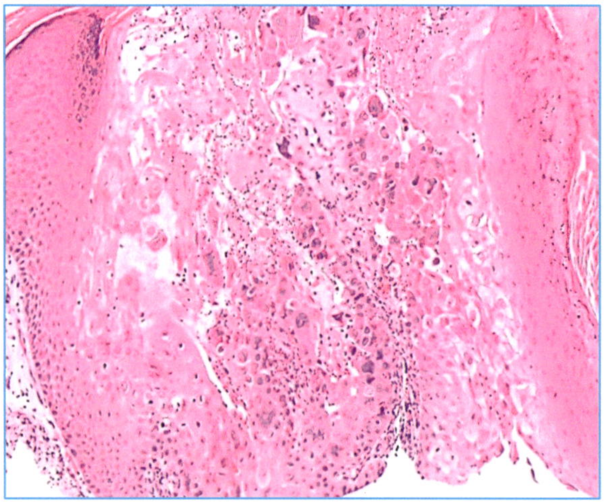

Epidermal vesicle with herpes virus infection

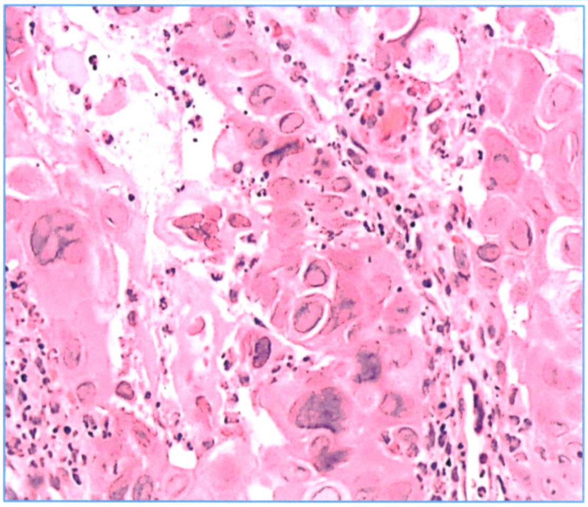

Herpetic intraepidermal eosinophilic inclusions

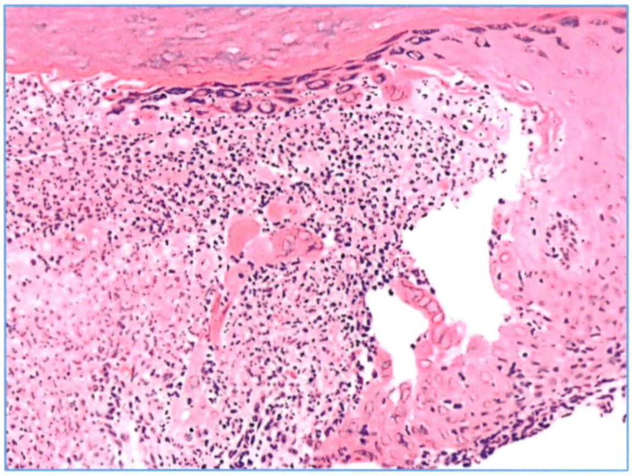

Acute inflammation surrounding viral inclusions

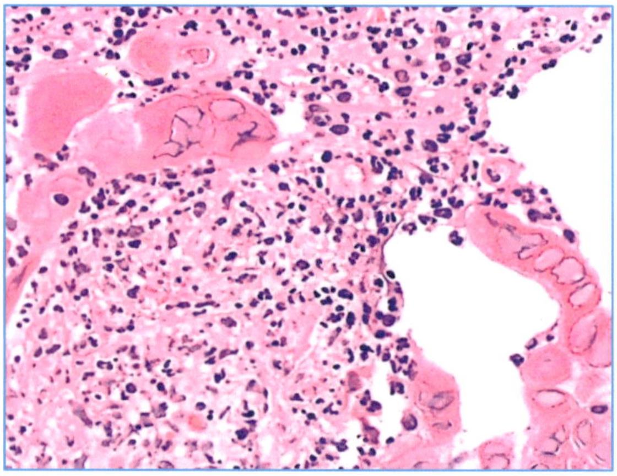

Nuclear molding of steel gray nuclei

VIRAL EXANTHEMA

-umbrella term describing transient cutaneous eruption found in conjunction with viral infections
-most common in children and sometimes immunosuppressed adults
-the most common childhood viral exanthems include measles (rubeola), rubella (German measles), varicella (chickenpox), erythema infectiosum (fifth disease), roseola (exanthema subitum), and infectious mononucleosis (EBV infection)
-patterns and onsets vary by clinical type, but classically present as a generalized eruption of erythematous macules, papules, and occasionally vesicles
-clinically mimic morbilliform drug eruption that more commonly affects adults

Histopathology

-usually histologically non-specific and clinical correlation is crucial
-mild epidermal spongiosis and a mild perivascular lymphocytic infiltrate
-in **measles**, **"Warthin-Finkeldy" cells** (giant cells with multiple overlapping nuclei) can be seen in the epidermis
-in **dengue fever**, there is **red blood cell** extravasation
-in **rubella**, there are atypical lymphocytes in the dermis (**Turk cells**)
-in **Zika** exanthema, scattered **dermal neutrophils** are present
-in **HIV** exanthema, few epidermal **necrotic keratinocytes** are present

MOLLUSCUM CONTAGIOSUM

-self-limited, viral infection caused by the poxvirus *Molluscum contagiosum*
-transferred by skin to skin contact
-most common in children, adolescents, and immunosuppressed adults
-skin-colored papules with a central umbilication
-predilection for face, eyelids, neck, axilla, and anogenital area

Histopathology

-**"cup-shaped"**, inverted, acanthotic squamous epithelium
-keratinocytes in the stratum corneum and stratum spinosum contain **large eosinophilic inclusions** molluscum bodies (**Henderson-Patterson bodies**)
-molluscum bodies occupy almost the entire infected cell

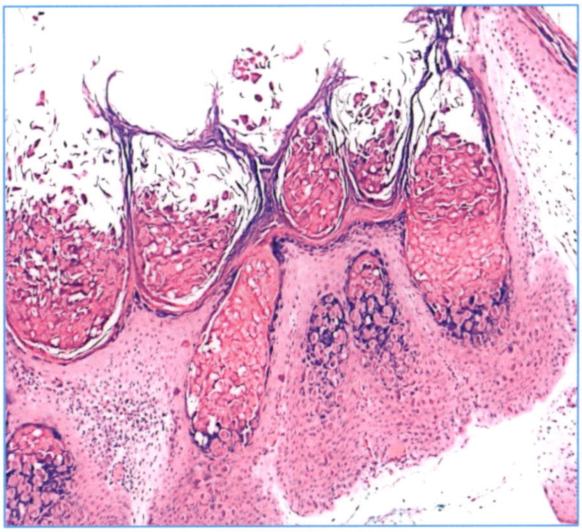

"Cup-shaped" molluscum contagiousum

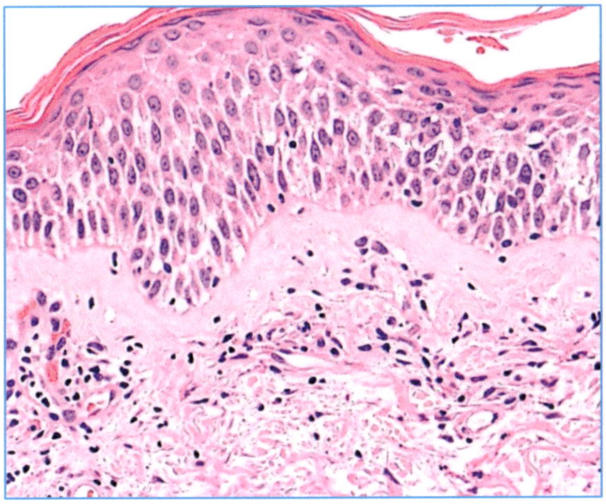

Viral exanthema with non-specific spongiotic dermatitis

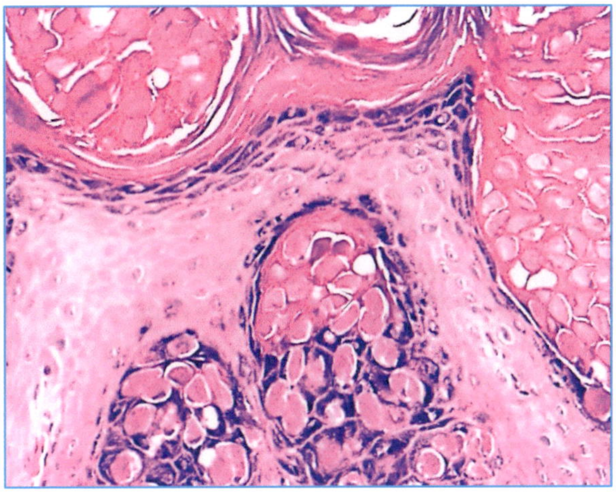

Molluscum contagiousum with large eosinophilic inclusions

Viral infections

HAND FOOT AND MOUTH DISEASE

-viral infection most commonly caused by *Coxsackie virus A16*
-more common in summer and fall
-favors children younger than 10 years of age
-can occur in adults with less typical lesions and distribution
-starts with prodrome of fever and malaise
-then develops few to numerous erythematous macules and oval, deep-seated, gray vesicles on the hands, feet, and buttock
-erosions are seen in the oral cavity

Histopathology
-epidermal spongiosis with intraepidermal vesicles
-focal epidermal necrosis with **"lace-like" epidermal reticular degeneration**
-no inclusion bodies or giant cells (unlike herpes)
-variable dermal lymphocytic and neutrophilic inflammation

ORF (ECTHYMA CONTAGIOSUM)/ MILKER'S NODULES

-zoonotic diseases of sheep, goats, and cows
-caused by a *parapox virus* (orf) or *paravaccinia virus* (milker's nodule)
-lesions primarily occur on the hands at site of inoculation
-transmitted to human by direct contact with infected sheep/goats (orf) or infected cow udders (milker's nodules)
-milker's nodules are generally multiple
-orf nodule is usually solitary
-presents with a targetoid, red-blue pustules/nodules that slowly enlarge and may become ulcerated

Histopathology
-orf and milker's nodules have the same histology
-irregular epidermal acanthosis with pale keratinocytes in the upper epidermis
-keratinocytes contain eosinophilic cytoplasmic inclusions **resembling small molluscum bodies**
-**dermal capillary proliferation** forming granulation tissue
-later, lesion becomes necrotic, ulcerated, with serum crust and neutrophils

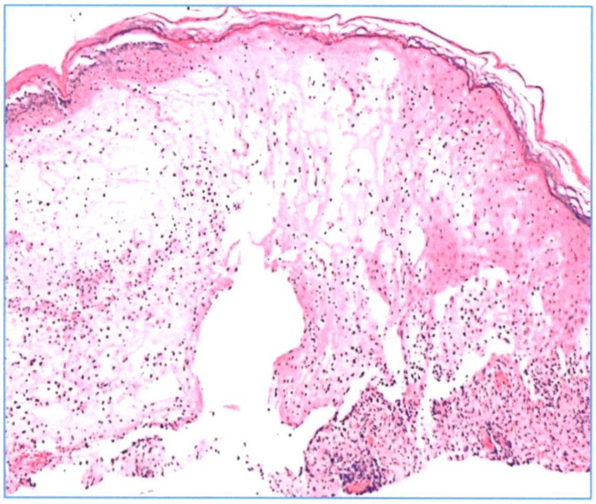

Hand foot mouth disease with epidermal necrosis

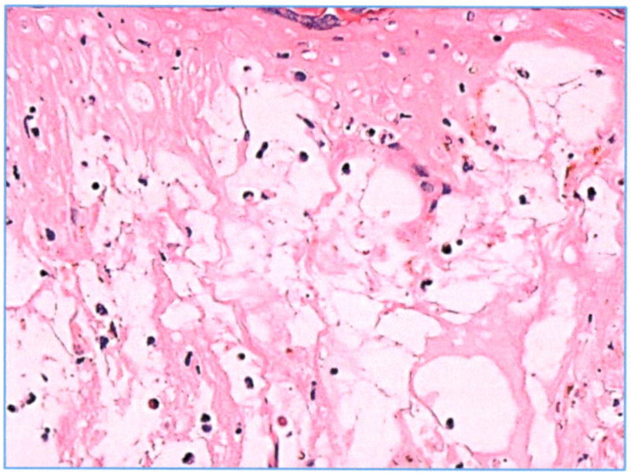

Hand foot mouth disease with "lace-like" appearance of necrotic, separated keratinocytes

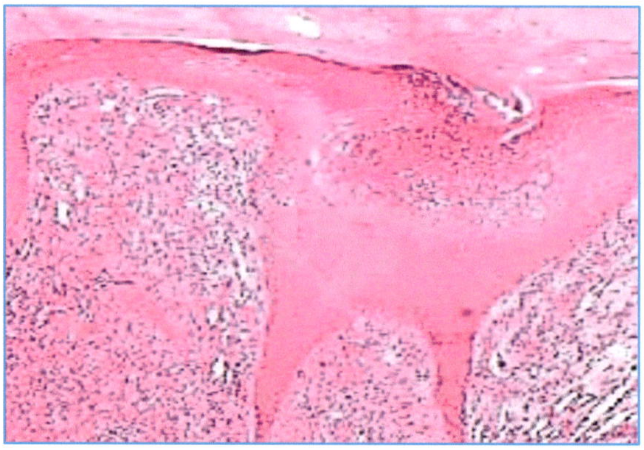

Orf with irregular epidermal acanthosis and dermal vascular proliferation

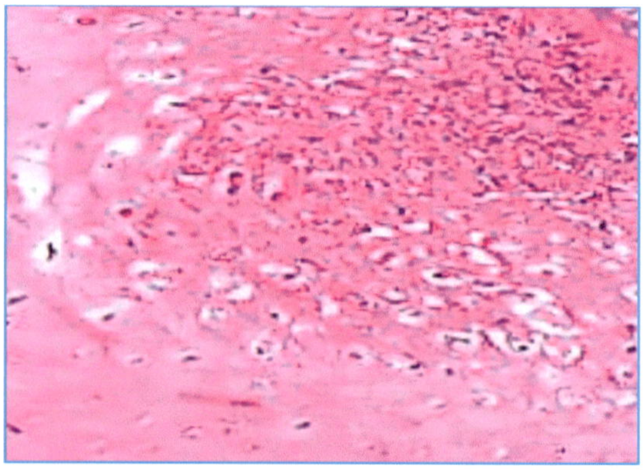

Orf with pink cytoplasmic inclusions within keratinocytes

Chapter 19

CYTOMEGALOVIRUS

-common viral infection transmitted via direct contact, bodily fluids, organ transplants, and blood transfusion
-about half of Americans are infected by age 40
-most of infections in healthy individuals are asymptomatic or sometimes develop "mononucleosis-like" syndrome
-typically, in that case the cutaneous manifestation is a non-specific, morbilliform exanthem
-congenital infection causes a "blueberry muffin" baby with generalized purple papules and nodules and hearing loss
-in immunocompromised adults (HIV) can cause ulcers, vesiculobullous hemorrhagic nodules, or verrucous lesions

Histopathology
-non-specific dermal infiltrate
-enlarged endothelial cells of dermal vessels
-large eosinophilic inclusion with a clear halo, so-called **"owl's eye"** seen in nuclei of few endothelial cells (**Cowdy A body**)

GIANOTTI-CROSTI DISEASE (PAPULAR ACRODERMATITIS OF CHILDHOOD)

-viral exanthem with specific clinical findings common in children
-most commonly caused by EBV in the US, and hepatitis B worldwide
-symmetric, monomorphic eruption of skin-colored to pink papules
-most commonly involves the limbs (elbows, knees) and face (cheeks) of children (1-6 years old)
-trunk is frequently spared
-self-limited and resolves in 1-2 months

Histopathology
-changes are **not specific** and clinical correlation is required
-mild acute/ subacute spongiotic dermatitis
-**dermal edema** is common

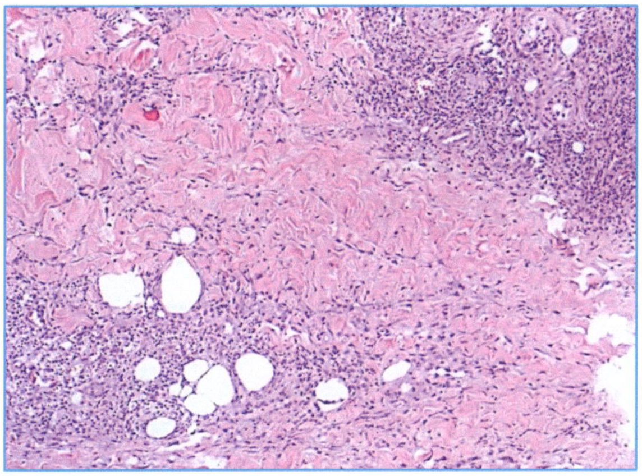

CMV with non-specific dermal inflammation

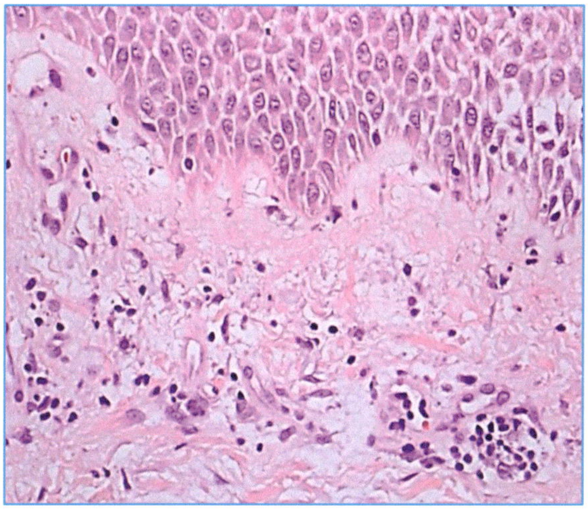

Non-specific spongiotic dermatitis of Gianotti-Crosti disease

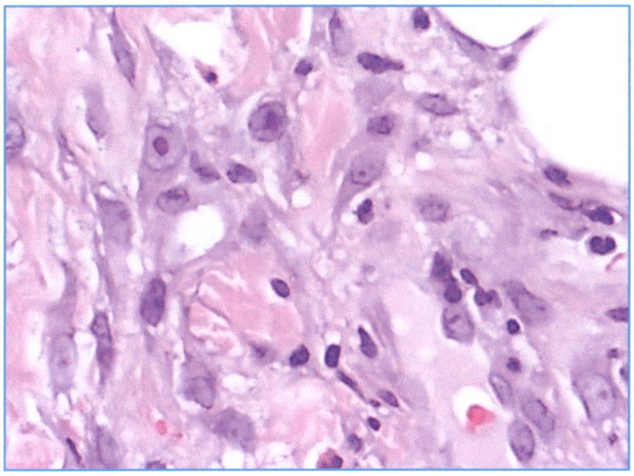

CMV with "owl's eye" inclusions in endothelial cells

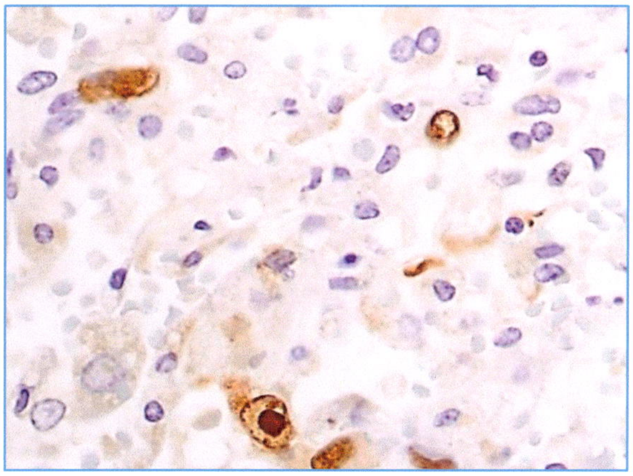

CMV inclusions highlighted with CMV IHC stain

Viral infections

HOW TO APPROACH VIRAL INFECTIONS

EPIDERMIS IS NECROTIC WITH VESICLES

-herpes	multi-nucleated keratinocytes, nuclear molding, steel gray nuclei
-hand foot and mouth disease	epidermal "lacy-like" reticular degeneration

KOILOCYTES ARE PRESENT
(keratinocytes with dark small nuclei and clear cytoplasm)

-verruca vulgaris	epidermis in shape of Gothic church spires
-verruca plana	epidermis in shape of undulated waves
-**condyloma acuminatum**	epidermis in umbonate (rounded knob) shape
-epidermodysplasia verruciformis	swollen pink-gray keratinocytes
-plantar/palmar wart	endophytic shape and dark purple coarse keratohyaline granules

LESION IS "CUP-SHAPED"

-plantar/palmar wart	koilocytes
-molluscum	keratinocytes with large pink inclusions

LESION IS ON THE HANDS

-hand foot and mouth disease	intraepidermal vesicles with reticular degeneration
-orf/milker's nodule	pink inclusions in keratinocytes (baby molluscum) with a dermal vascular proliferation
-verruca vulgaris	shape of Gothic church spires and koilocytes

CHILD WITH DIFFUSE RASH AND UNSPECIFIC SPONGIOTIC DERMATITIS

-viral exanthema	clinical correlation needed to determine the cause

ACUTELY INFLAMED SKIN IN AN IMMUNOSUPPRESSED PATIENT WITH NEGATIVE TISSUE CULTURE

-CMV	prominent eosinophilic inclusions in dermal endothelial cells

Chapter 19

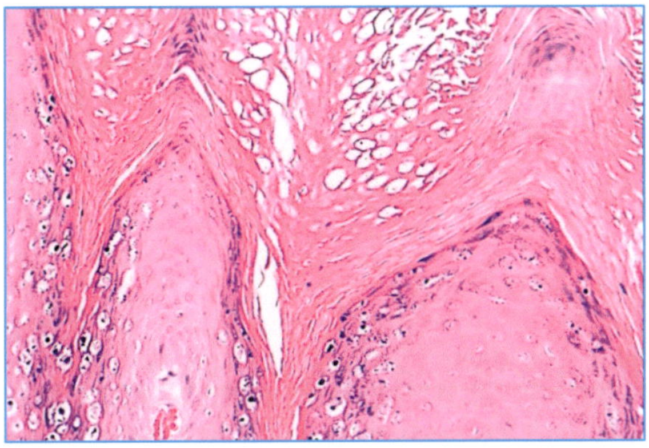

Verruca vulgaris with papillomatous epidermis and koilocytes

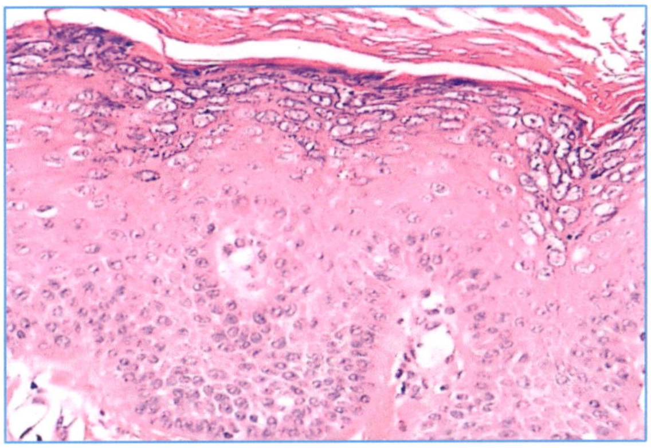

Verruca plana with wavy epidermis and koilocytes

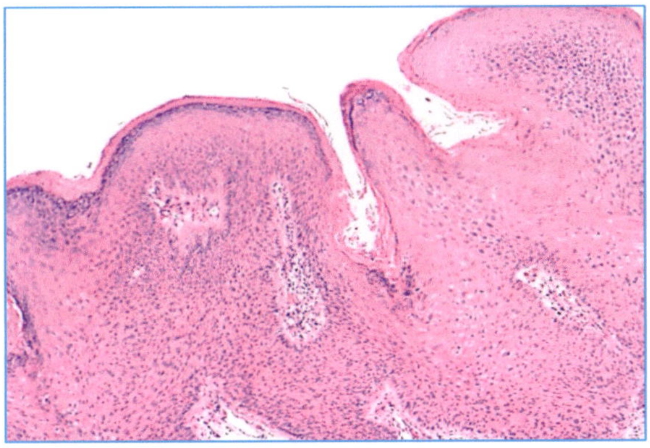

"Knob-like" shaped condyloma acuminatum with few koilocytes

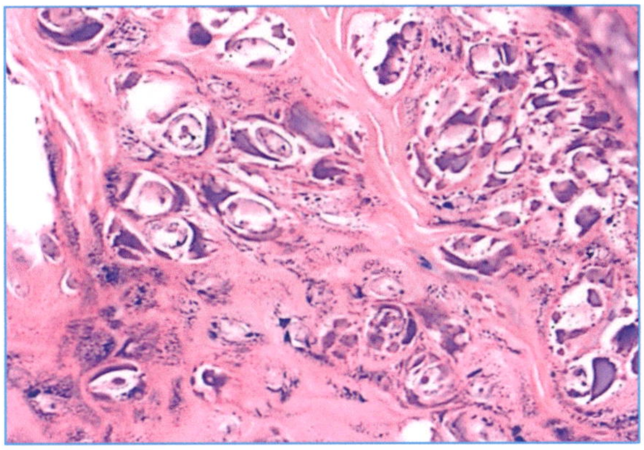

Myrmecia with lumpy, prominent, dark purple, irregular granules

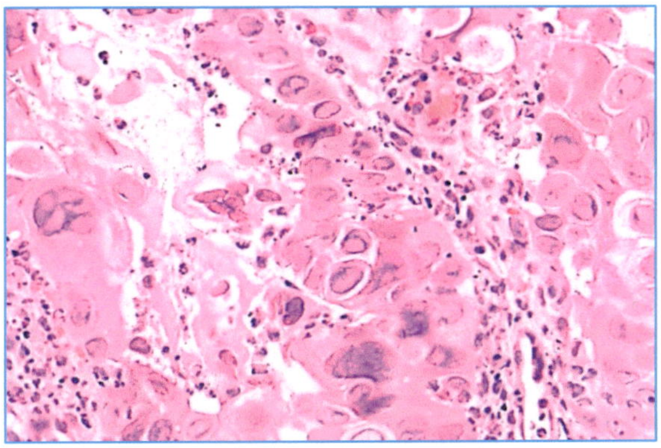

Herpes with multinucleated keratinocytes
with steel gray nuclei

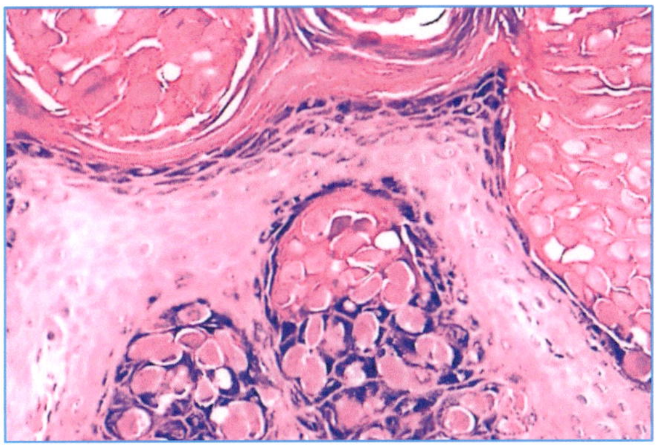

Molluscum with keratinocytes with large pink inclusions

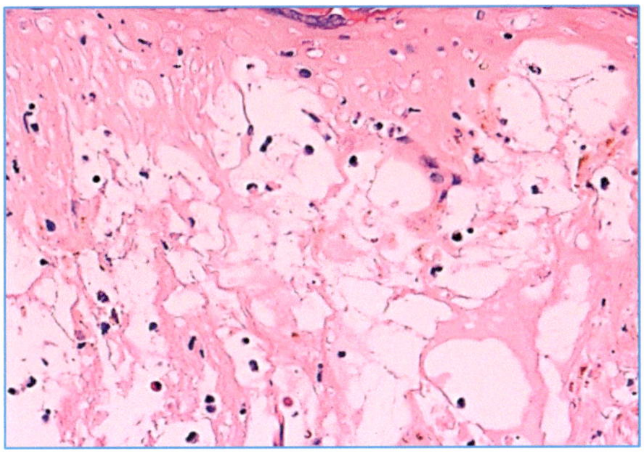

Hand foot mouth disease with epidermal necrosis and
reticular degeneration

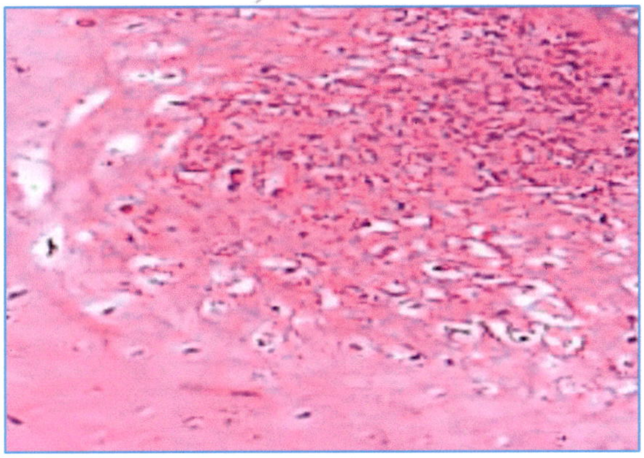

Orf with pink cytoplasmic inclusions
within keratinocytes

Viral infections

Chapter 20

PARASITIC INFECTIONS

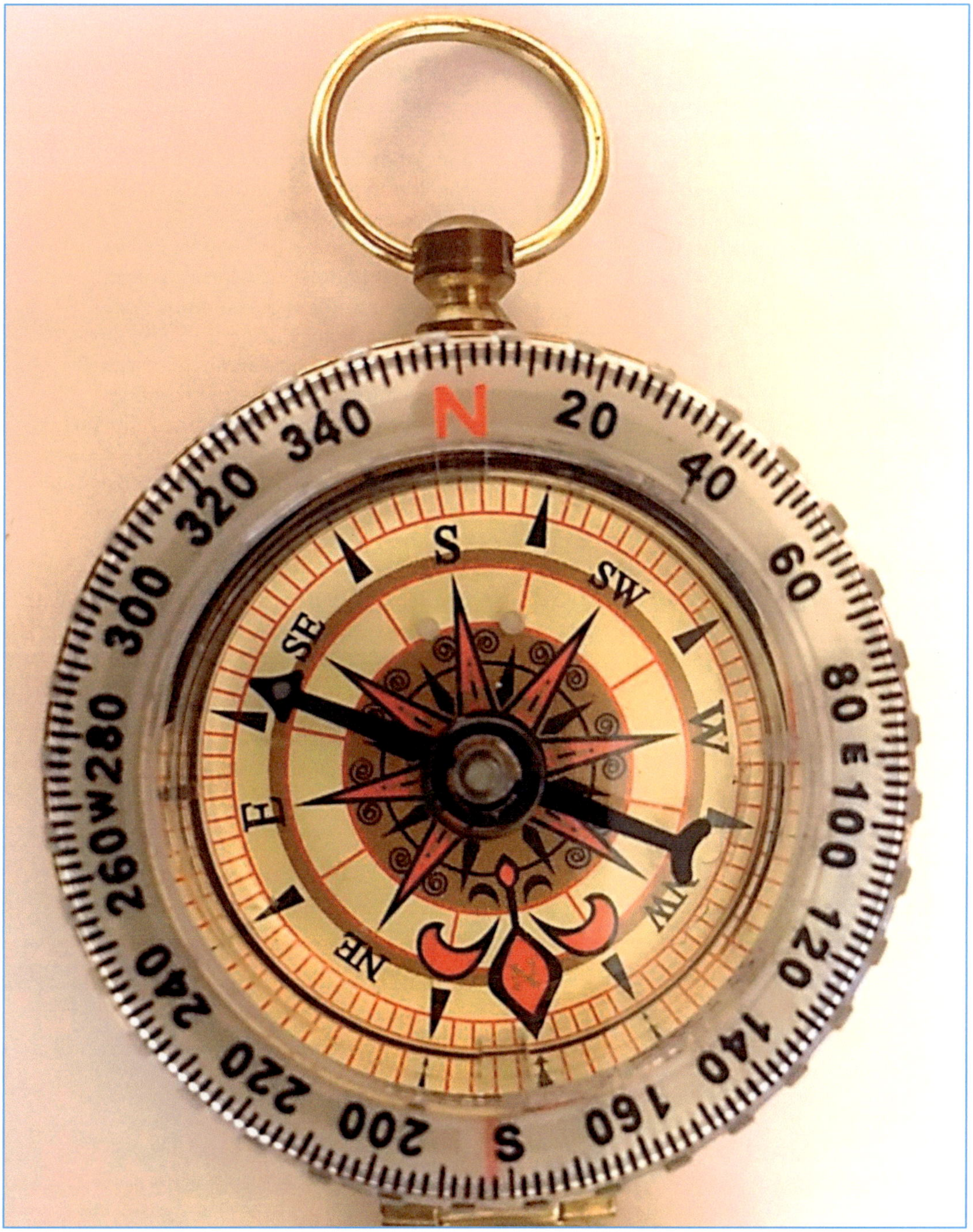

Parasitic infections

DEMODEX

-two species of commensal mites that live on the skin: *Demodex folliculorum* and *D. brevis*
-one-third of children and young adults, half of adults, and two-thirds of the elderly carry them
-the role of *Demodex* mites in rosacea and acne remains controversial
-D. *folliculorum,* saprophytic parasitic mite of the hair follicle, can cause itchy pustules with follicular scaling

Histopathology

-**dilated hair follicle with *Demodex* mite**
-very mild perifollicular lymphocytic infiltrate
-occasional perifollicular granulomatous reaction

SCABIES

-infestation with mite *Sarcoptes scabiei*
-finger webs, wrists, genitalia, feet, and buttocks are favored sites
-intraepidermal **burrows** (skin-colored ridges in linear pattern ending with a small vesicle/papule) are diagnostic
-**generalized pruritus** is typical

Variants:

Crusted or Norwegian scabies- severe infestation in immunocompromised or debilitated patients with marked hyperkeratosis, scaling, and crusting

Nodular scabies- red-pink or brown persistent nodules usually in children
-scrotal skin is the most common site

Histopathology

-epidermal acanthosis and hyperkeratosis
-**scabies mite** within stratum corneum
-frequently only **"pig tails"**, mite remnants, are present
-numerous epidermal and **dermal eosinophils**
-**Norwegian scabies**-mites are numerous and epidermis is markedly hyperkeratotic
-**nodular scabies**- mites are seen less frequently and dermal lymphoid follicles with admixed eosinophils are present

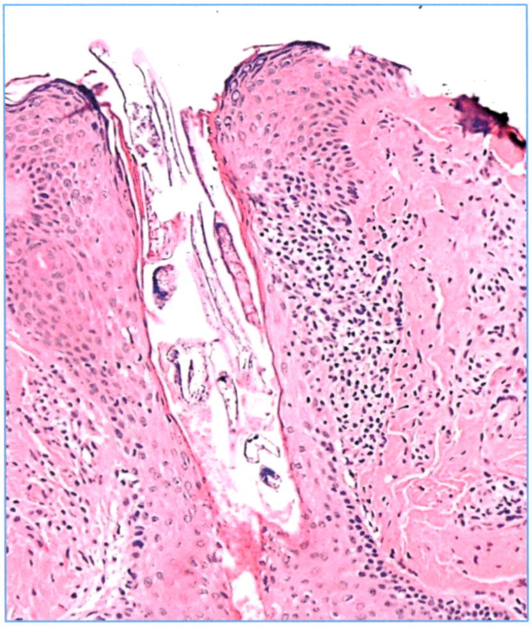

Demodex within hair follicle

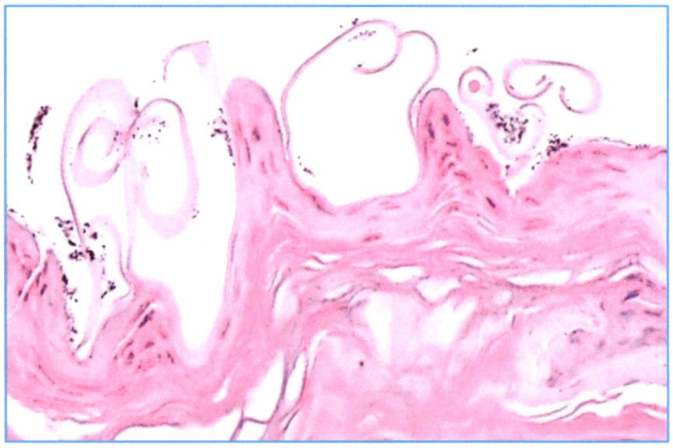

Scabies "pig tails"

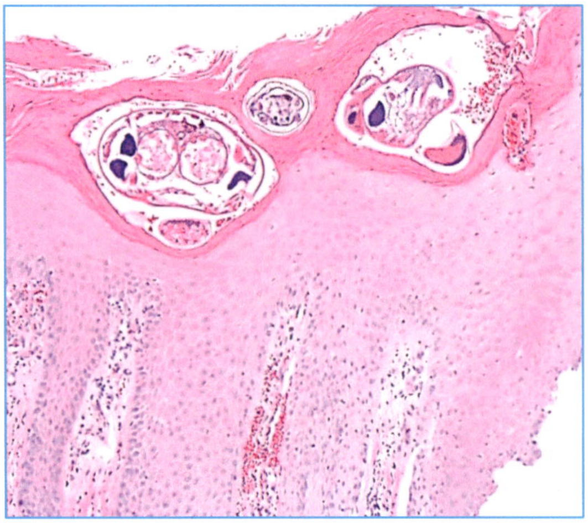

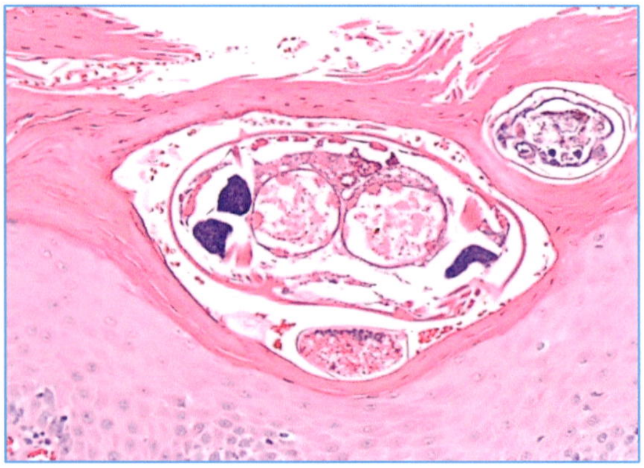

Scabies with mites in epidermal burrows

LEISHMANIASIS

-protozoan infection caused by various subspecies of *Leishmaniasis* transmitted by the sandfly
-symptomatology depends on the subspecies

Mucocutaneous leishmaniasis

-caused by *L. braziliensis* in New World
-destruct mucosa of lip, nose, and pharynx

Visceral leishmaniasis (Kala-azar)

-more common in Old World than New World
-caused by *L. donovani*
-systemic infection of liver, spleen, bone marrow, and skin ulceration at bite site

Cutaneous leishmaniasis

-caused by *L. major, L. tropica* in Old World and *L. mexicana, L. braziliensis* in New World
-solitary papule or nodule at the site of the bite
-ulcerate resembling volcano crater or becomes verrucous
-may have sporotrichoid spread
-in New World commonly presents as **"chiclero's ulcer"** on ear
-skin lesions heal spontaneously **leaving life-long scars**

Histopathology

-epidermis is often ulcerated or shows hyperkeratosis and acanthosis
-extensive dermal lymphohisticytic infiltrate with admixed neutrophils, eosinophils, and plasma cells
-**small oval amastigotes** (2 µm) with "bar-shaped" kinetoplasts are **present within histiocytes** (histoplasmosis is larger 2-5 µm)
-Giemsa stain identifies amastigotes in cells

PEDICULOSIS

-obligate ectoparasites that feed on blood

Head lice (*Pediculus humanus capitis*)

-most frequent in children aged 3–10 and their families and is spread by direct contact
-less common in African Americans due to differences in hair texture

Pubic lice (*Pthirus pubis*) or **"crabs"**

-found in pubic hair or eyelashes
-skin bluish macules (maculae ceruleae) at bite sites

Body lice (*Pediculus humanus corporis*)

-live and lay eggs on clothing
-more common in the homeless
-vector for epidemic typhus, trench fever, and relapsing fever
-cause rash/pruritus as an allergic reaction

Histopathology

-all three have 3 pairs of legs and 2 antennae
-pubic louse is shortest and widest and has front **"crab-like"** pincher claw
-body and head lice have slimmer, longer body with body louse being the longest

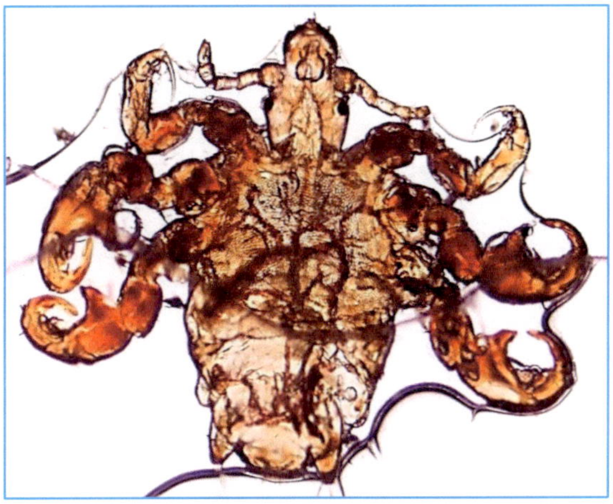

Pubic louse with "crab-like" pincher claws

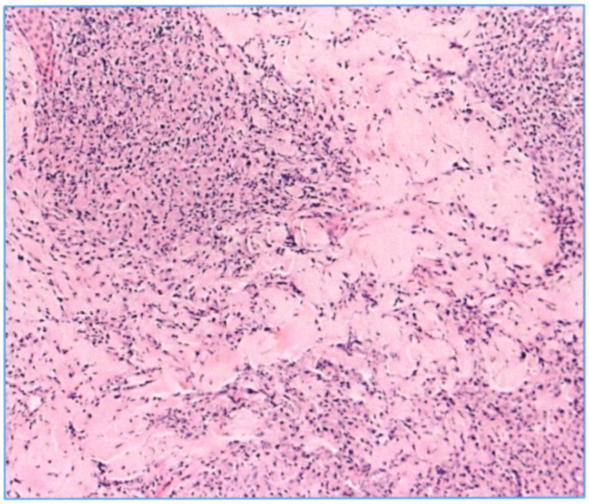

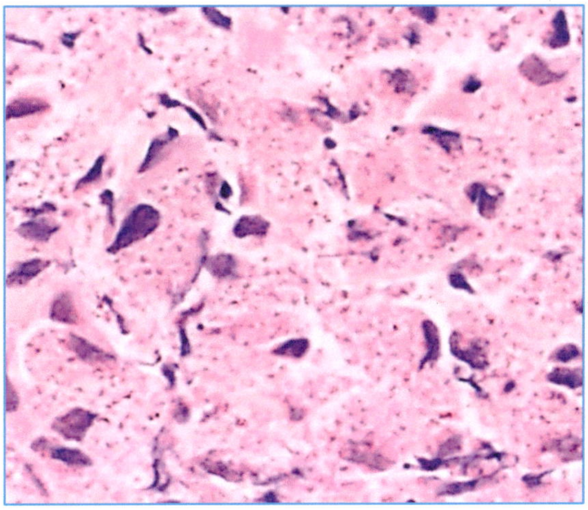

Leishmaniasis with histiocytes filled with small oval amastigotes

Parasitic infections

CUTANEOUS LARVA MIGRANS/LARVA CURRENS

-cutaneous **larva migrans** caused by *Ancylostoma braziliense*
-usually on the feet from ground contaminated by animal feces
-**larva currens** caused by *Strongyloides stercoralis*
-results from autoinfection by larva in feces
-both show itchy, erythematous, linear, or serpiginous tract
-appears days but sometimes even months after exposure to larvae
-eruption extends a few centimeters per day
Histopathology
-spongiotic epidermis with eosinophils
and **extensive dermal hypersensitivity reaction**
-dermal edema is common
-larva is **rarely** found in biopsy specimen

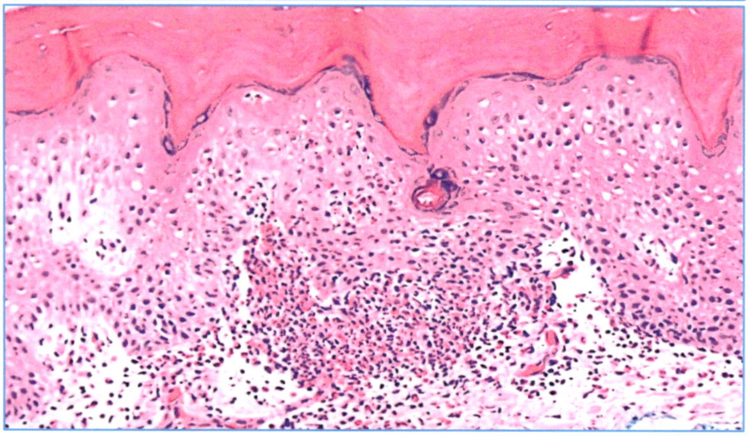

Larva migrans burrow with dermal edema and numerous epidermal and dermal eosinophils

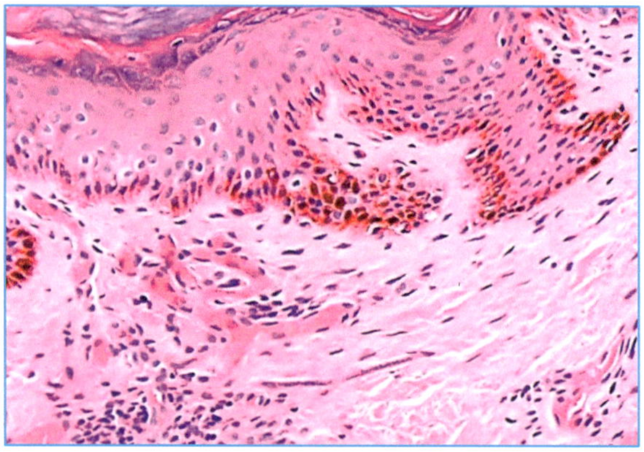

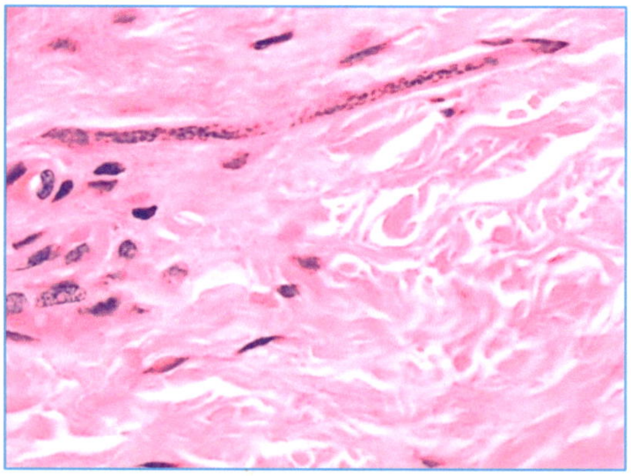

Larva in the dermis

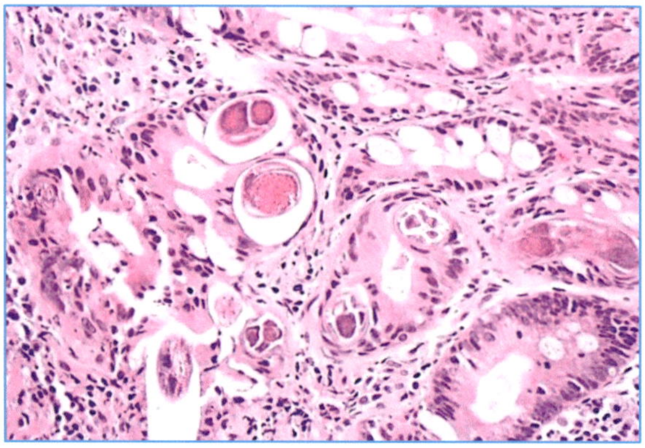

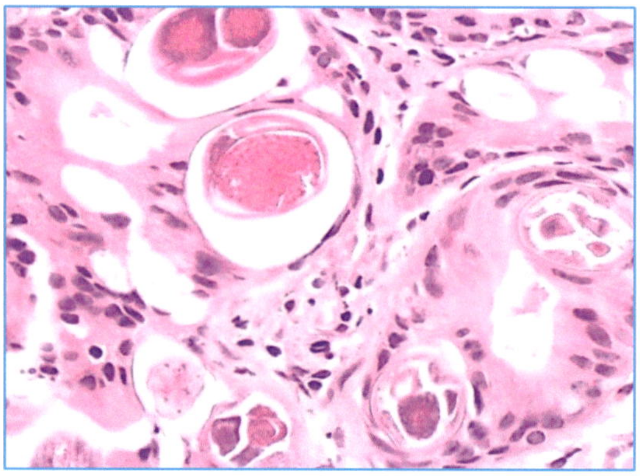

Strongyloides ova in rectal mucosa

ONCHOCERCIASIS

-caused by parasite *Onchocerca volvulus*
-transmitted to humans by the black fly
-occurs mainly in sub-Saharan Africa and a few isolated areas in the Americas (Brazil, Colombia, Guatemala, Mexico, and Venezuela)
-the death of microfilariae induces intense inflammatory reactions causing skin and eye symptoms
-presents with very pruritic macular rash and itchy papules/nodules
-skin loses elasticity, causing **"hanging groin"**
-sometimes the pigmentation of the skin is affected causing **"leopard skin"**

Histopathology
-**microfilaria** can be detected in skin and eye
-dermal inflammation varies from no inflammation to exuberant inflammation with eosinophils
-worms develop from larva in the subcutis
-**worm** is surrounded by **extensive fibrosis**

SCHISTOSOMIASIS

-caused by *Schistosoma* trematode worms
-*S. mansoni*, *S. japonicum*, *S. intercalatum*, and *S. mekongi* cause intestinal disease
-*S. haematobium* causes urinary disease
-mostly in Africa, Asia, and South America
-all subspecies can cause skin rash as an allergic reaction to the parasite
-presents as maculopapular eruption, comprising discrete erythematous raised lesions that vary in size from 1 to 3 cm
-nodules can also arise at the site of percutaneous penetration by *schistosome* cercariae

Histopathology
-mixed inflammation that varies from minimal inflammation to exuberant inflammation with eosinophils
-**calcified dead ova** are present in very fibrotic stroma

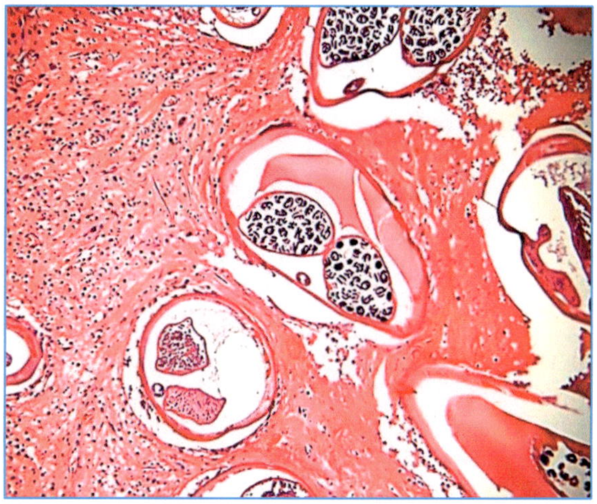

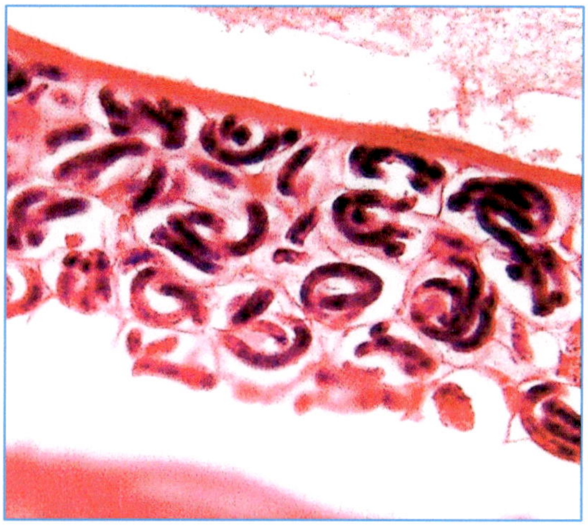

Onchocerciasis with numerous microfilarias within worm

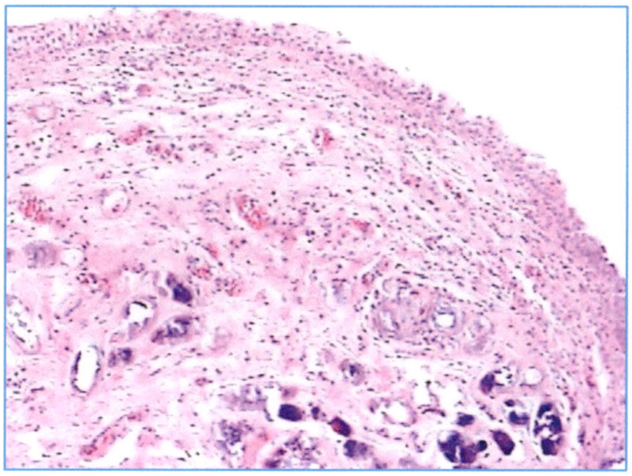

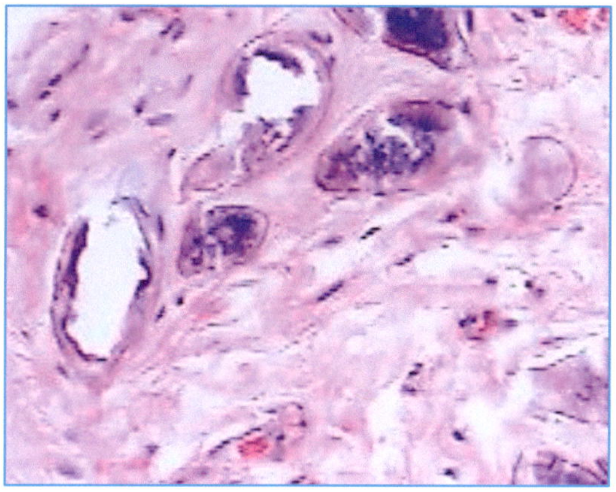

Schistosomiasis with calcified ova

Parasitic infections

PROTOTHECOSIS

-rare infection by alga-like organism *Prototheca wickerhamii* or *P. zopfii*
-at site of traumatic inoculation in immunocompromised people
-presents as vesiculobullous and ulcerative lesion with pustule and scab

Histopathology

-acute inflammatory or granulomatous inflammation
-organisms have thick-walled spherical bodies
-it shows internal septation resembling **morula or "daisy" form**

DIROFILARIA

-genus of nematodes
-round worms spread by mosquitoes
-human dirofilariasis is caused by *D. immitis* and *D. repens*
-present as a painful lump under the skin or infection of the eye

Histopathology

-**nematode** with **laminated cuticle** and **circumferential muscle** in the subcutis
-surrounding mixed or granulomatous inflammation

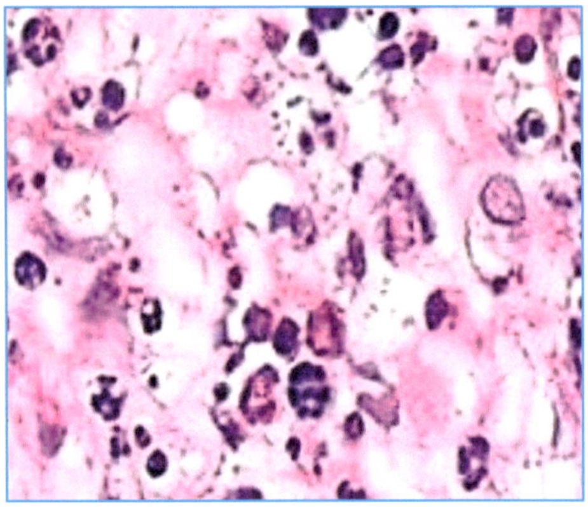

Protothecosis "daisy like" algae surrounded by inflammation

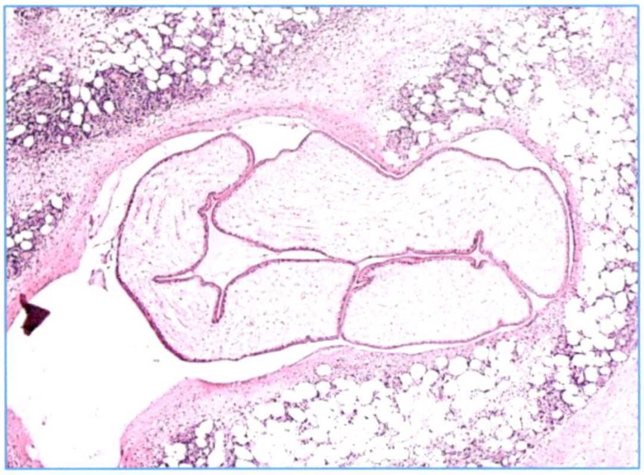

Dirofilaria nematode in the subcutis

ACANTHAMOEBIASIS

-caused by *Acanthamoeba* and *Naeglaria,* soil and water amebae
-primary manifestation of infection is keratitis and meningoencephalitis
-cutaneous lesions in immunosuppressed patients
-can present as papules, ulcers, or nodules

Histopathology

-granulomatous or diffuse neutrophilic inflammation and common vasculitis
-characteristic trophozoites with **"bull's eye"** appearance within giant cells
-**wrinkled ectocysts** are present

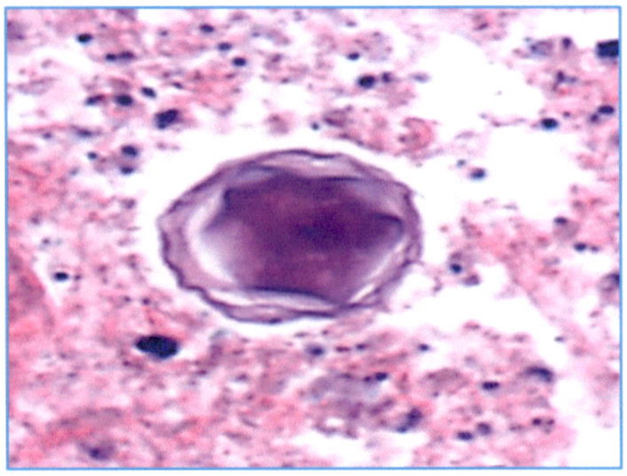

Wrinkled ectocyst of acanthamoeba

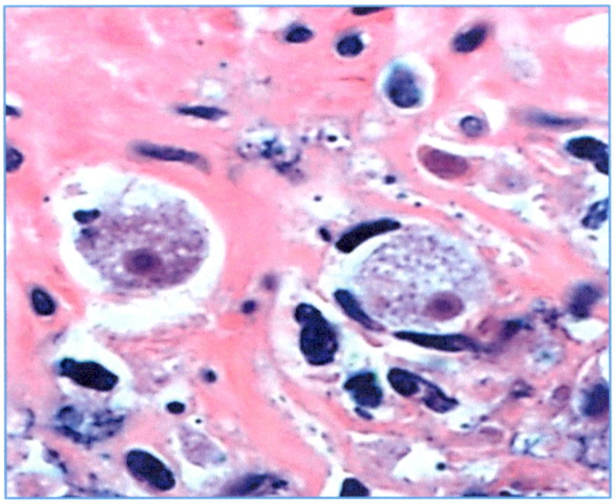

"Bull's eye" of acanthamoeba trophozoites

MYIASIS (BOTFLY)

-infestation of human skin by fly larvae (human botfly is most common)
-wound myiasis occurs when the fly lays eggs in an open wound
-furuncular myiasis (caused by the human botfly in tropical areas) involves a mosquito as the vector to carry fly eggs
-painful furuncle containing larva develops at the site of the bite

Histopathology
-dermal acute inflammation with larvae present
-full-grown larva is **13-15 mm** in length

TUNGIASIS

-skin infestation with the burrowing sand flea (*Tunga penetrans* or related species)
-the tunga flea is native to the West Indies and Caribbean region, but has spread to Africa, Latin America, and India
-lesions are characterized by a white patch with a black dot in the center
-because of limited jumping ability of the tunga flea, the most common sites of infection are the feet and ankles
-will heal spontaneously in 2 weeks as the flea dies and skin sheds

Histopathology
-in the early lesion, the bulk of the flea is intraepidermal
-the flea than penetrates the upper dermis to feed from blood vessels
-it forms dermal burrow with flea (**1-3 mm in size**) surrounded by acute inflammation and scarring
-burrow is open to the surface for the flea to breathe and lay eggs that fall out through the epidermal opening

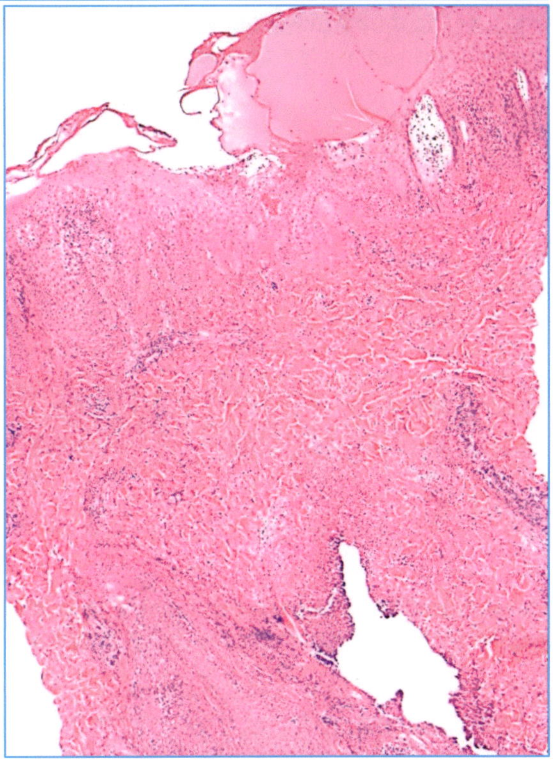

Botfly larva embedded in deep dermis inducing prominent inflammation

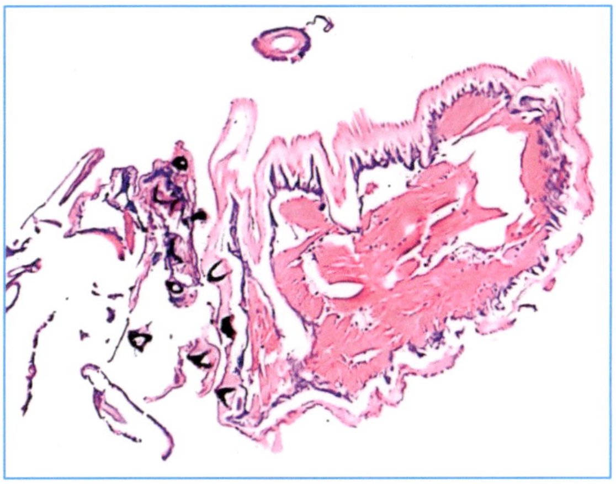

Myiasis larva

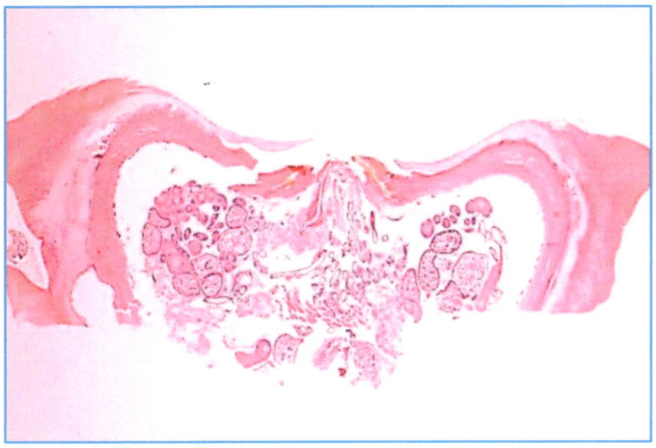

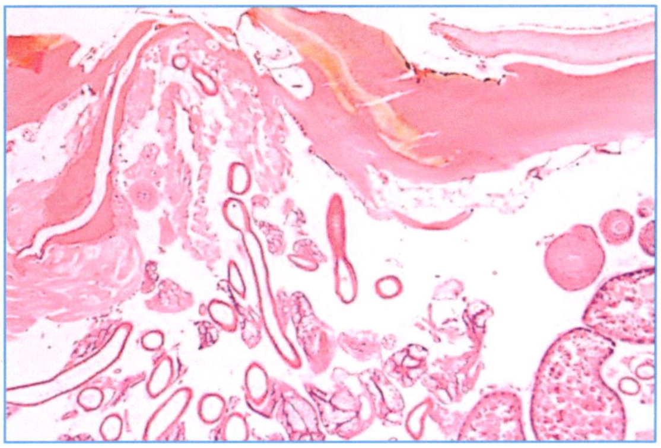

Tungiasis flea

Parasitic infections

HOW TO APPROACH PARASITIC INFECTIONS

IF YOU SEE EPIDERMAL MITES

-scabies	mite(s) in stratum corneum, **see note**	
-demodex	mite(s) in hair follicle	

AN INSECT IN NECROTIC SKIN

-myasis	fly larva	13-15 mm in size
-tungiasis	flea	1-3 mm in size

DIFFUSE HISTIOCYTES WITH SMALL DOTS

-leishmaniasis	parasite amastigote	(2-4 μm)	+ Giemsa stain
-rhinoscleroma	bacteria	(2-3 μm)	+ Giemsa stain, on respiratory mucosa
-histoplasmosis	tiny fungal spores	(2-5 μm)	+GMS, PAS stains

NUMEROUS DERMAL AND EPIDERMAL EOSINOPHILS

-larva migrans/larva currens	most of the time you will not find cutaneous larva
-scabies	many times you will not find intra epidermal mites

DERMAL CALCIFIED PARASITE OVA

-schistosomiasis

OVA IN SCLEROTIC DERMIS/SUBCUTIS

-onchocerciasis microfilarias

NEMATODE WITH LAMINATED CUTICLE

-dirofilaria

"DAISY FORM" SPHERICAL BODIES

-protothecosis

TROPHOZOITES WITH "BULL'S EYE"

-acanthamoebiasis

NOTE: In many cases of scabies, mites are not present in biopsy material and biopsy and scraping should be repeated. Sometimes if repeat biopsies are negative, empirical treatment should be considered based on strong clinical suspicion.

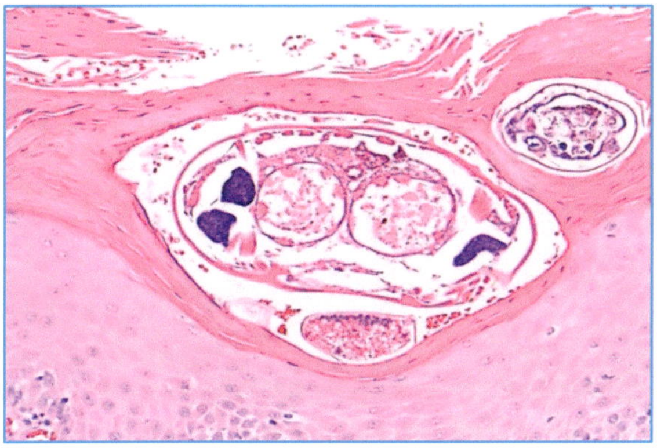
Scabies with intracorneal mite

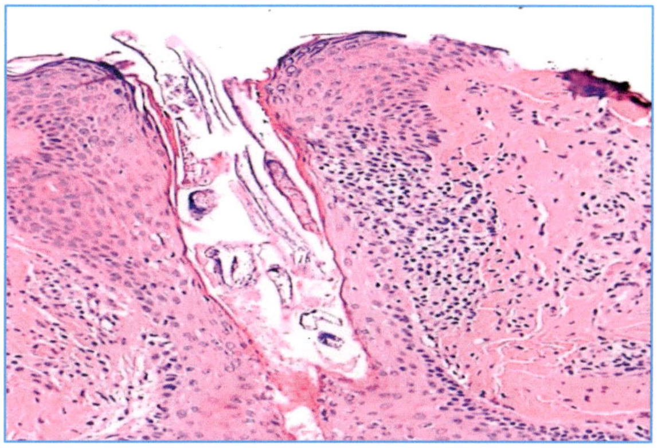
Demodex mite in hair follicle

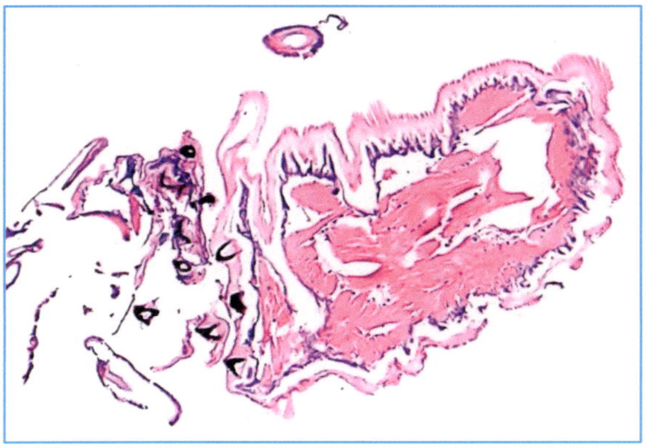
Myiasis 13-15 mm in length

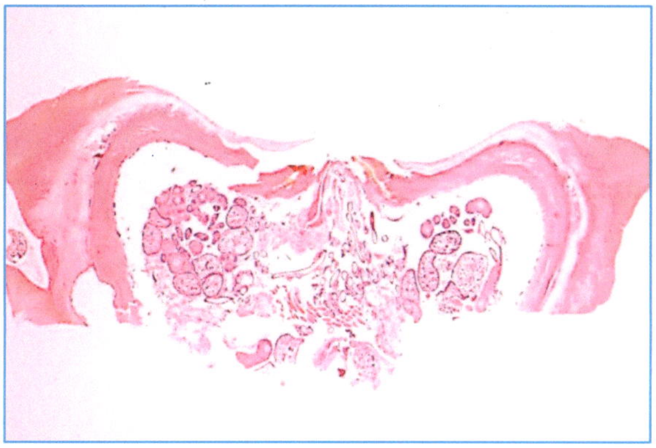
Tungiasis 1-3 mm in length

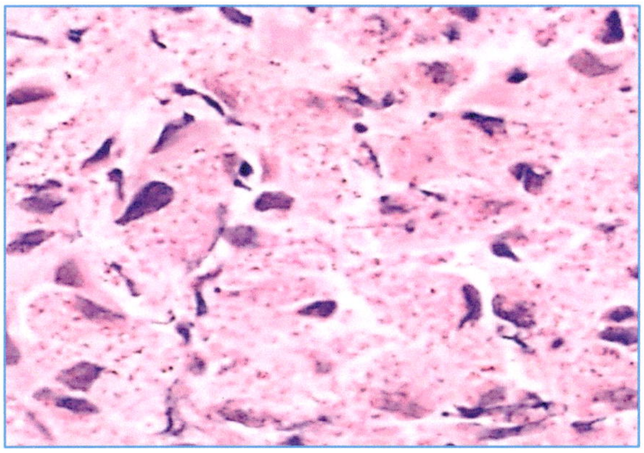
Leishmaniasis with histiocytes with dotted appearance

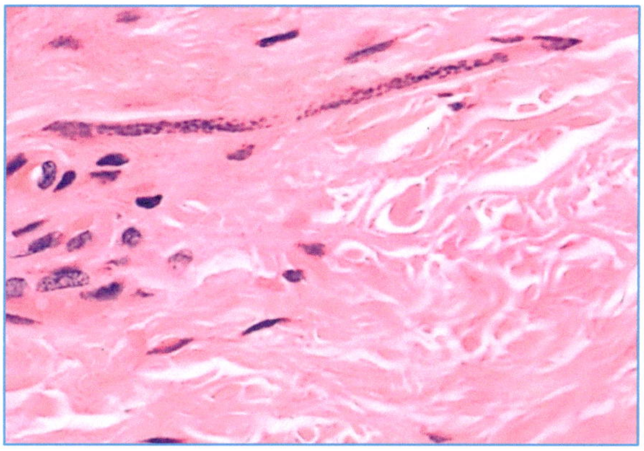
Larva migrans with "lancet-shaped" dermal larva

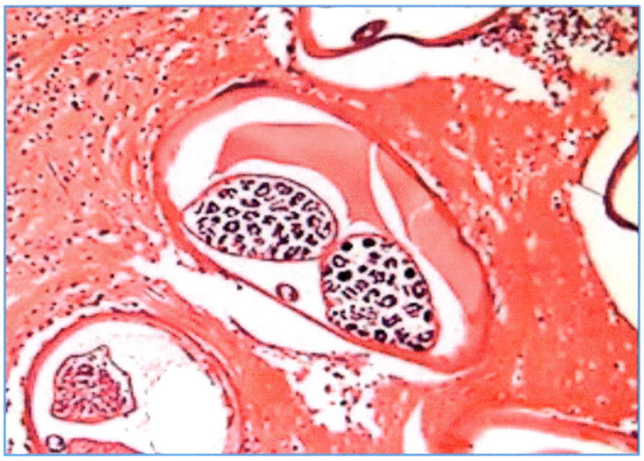
Onchocerciasis with microfilaria in subcutaneous worm

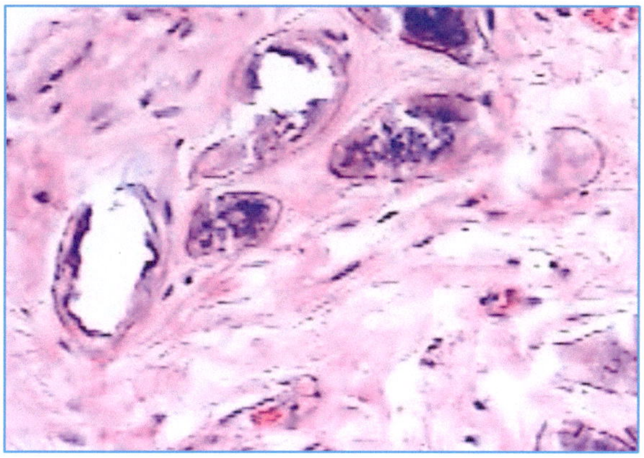
Schistosomiasis with calcified dead ova in fibrotic stroma

Parasitic infections

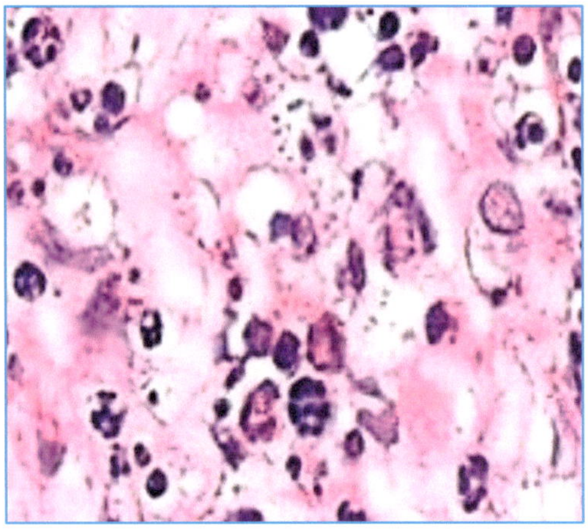

Prototheca with "daisy-like" algae

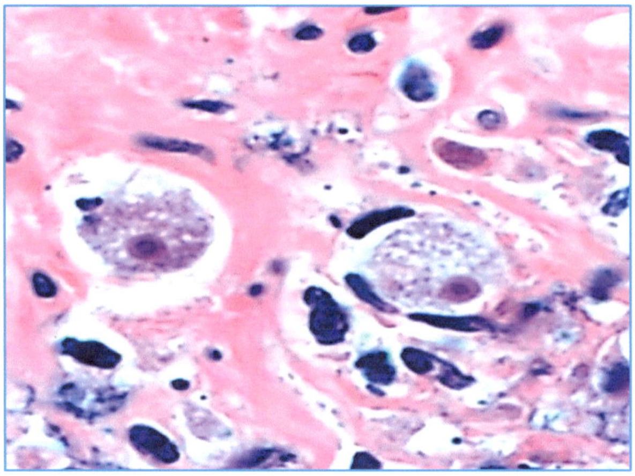

Acanthamoebiasis with trophozoites with "bull's eye"

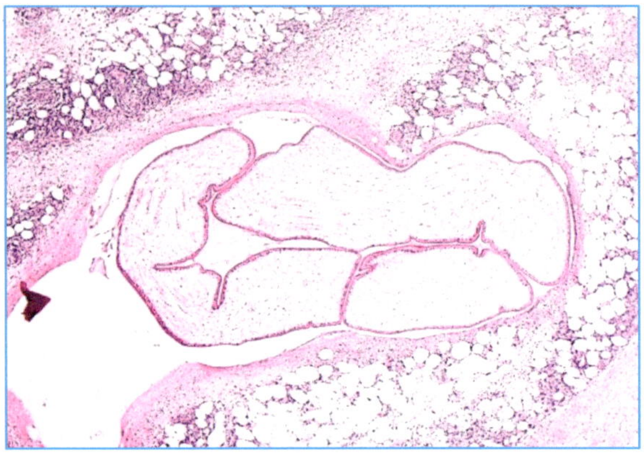

Dirofilaria with nematode with laminated cuticle

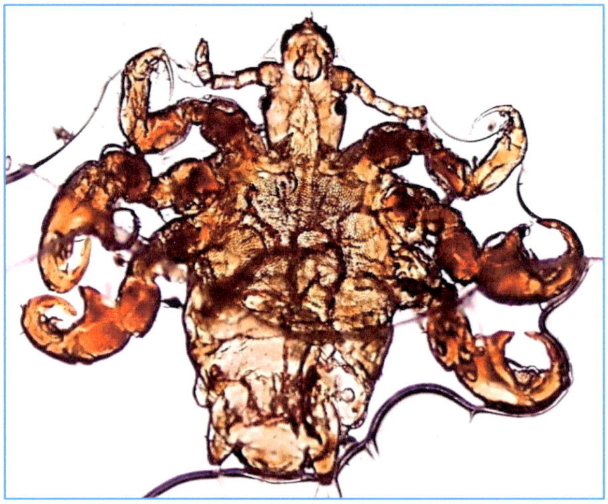

Pubic louse

Chapter 21

DRUG REACTIONS

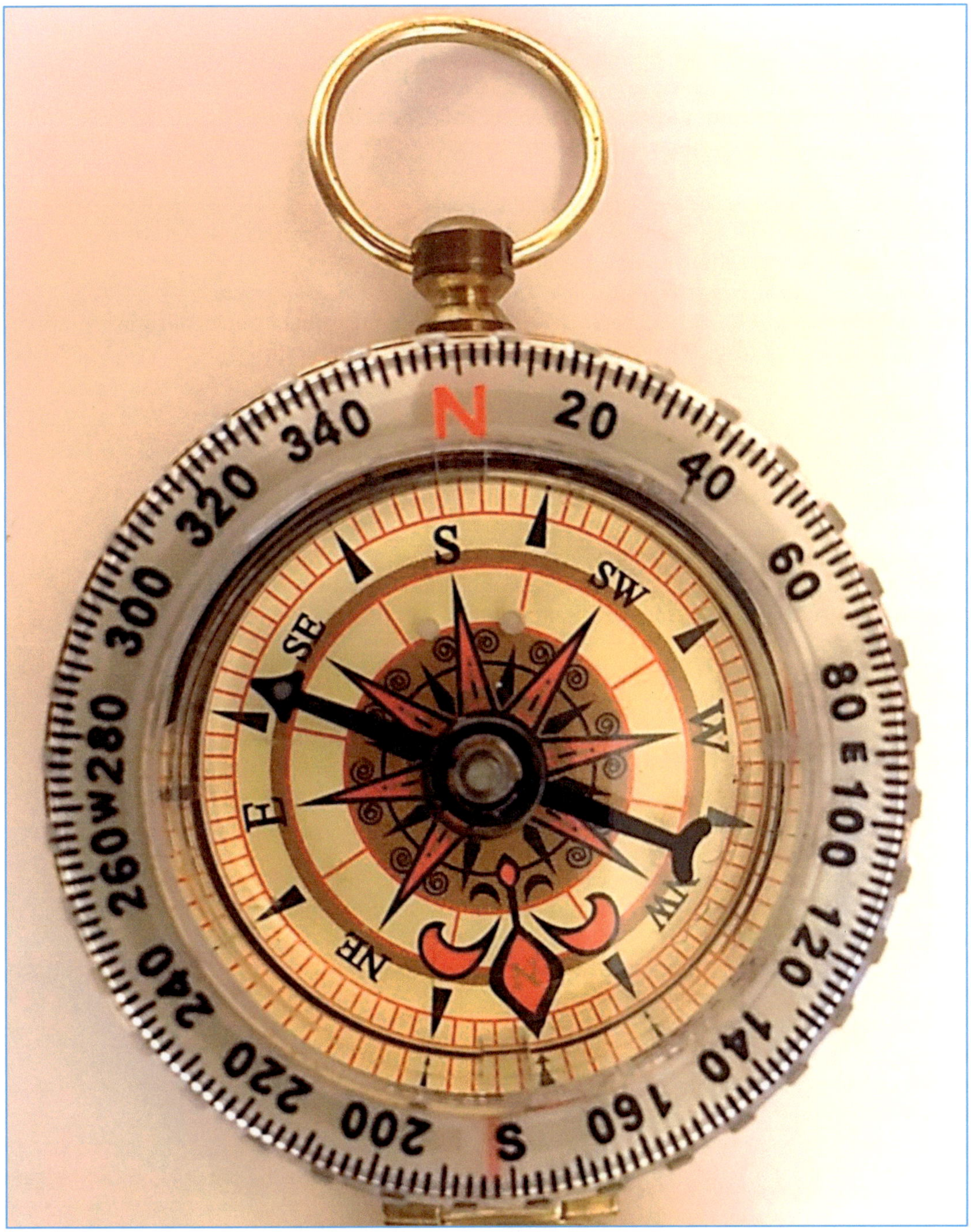

Drug reactions

HOW TO APPROACH DRUG REACTIONS

DRUG REACTIONS MIMIC VARIOUS SKIN DISEASES CLINICALLY AND HISTOLOGICALLY

Clinical presentations:

Acanthosis nigricans- nicotinic acid, glucocorticosteroids, oral contraceptives
Acneiform- corticosteroids
Acute generalized erythematous pustulosis- penicillin, aminopenicillins, macrolides, quinolones, sulfonamides, hydroxychloroquine, terbinafine, diltiazem
Bullous- barbiturates
Erythroderma- allopurinol, penicillamine, sulfonamide, gold
Exanthematous (most common type) -penicillin, carbamazepin, allopurinol, NSAID, sulfonamide
Neutrophilic eccrine hidradenitis- cytarabine, antracycline
EAC- finasteride, piroxicam, hydroxychloroquine, amitriptyline, and spironolactone
Erythema multiforme/toxic epidermal necrolysis- sulfa, allopurinol, carbamazepin, dilantin
Fixed drug reaction- tetracyclin, sulfonamides, salicilates, NSAID, barbiturate
Hyperpigmentation- estrogen, minocycline, chloroquine
Lichenoid- gold, arsenic, chlorthiazide, chloroquine
Lupus erythematosus- hydralazine, chlorpromazine
Necrosis- warfarin
Palmoplantar erythrodysaestesia- cytarabine, doxorubicin
Pemphigus- penicillamine
Photoallergic drug reaction- NSAIDs, sulfonamide, quinine
Phototoxic drug reaction- tetracycline, NSAIDs, fluoroquinolone, psoralen
Pseudolymphoma- ACE-inhibitors, anticonvulsants, beta and Ca-channel blockers
Psoriasiform- practolol
Urticaria- NSAID, ACE inhibitors, Ca-channel blockers
Vasculitis- sulfonamides, penicillin

Histopathology
-only a few drug reactions have unique histopathology

Acute generalized erythematous pustulosis
-subacute epidermal spongiosis
-**subcorneal or intraepidermal neutrophilic pustules**, varying from small to large
-mild dermal edema, with dermal mixed inflammation and rare eosinophils

Fixed drug reaction
-**interface vacuolar changes** with **focal necrotic keratinocytes**
-**dermal pigment incontinence** is characteristic
-variable perivascular lymphocytic infiltrate
-dermal eosinophils, neutrophils can be seen

Photoallergic and Phototoxic dermatitis
-discussed in detail in the spongiotic dermatitis chapter
-in short, they are akin to allergic or contact dermatitis with necrotic keratinocyte in the upper epidermis

-most drug reactions show histology of specific inflammatory disorder with the presence of eosinophils
-therefore, **whenever you see eosinophils in the biopsy, think of drug reaction**
e.g. **exanthematous drug eruption**- spongiotic dermatitis with eosinophils
lichenoid drug reaction- lichenoid dermatitis with eosinophils
psoriasiform drug reaction- psoriasiform dermatitis with eosinophils
"EAC-like" drug reaction- EAC with eosinophils
drug induced vasculitis- vasculitis with eosinophils

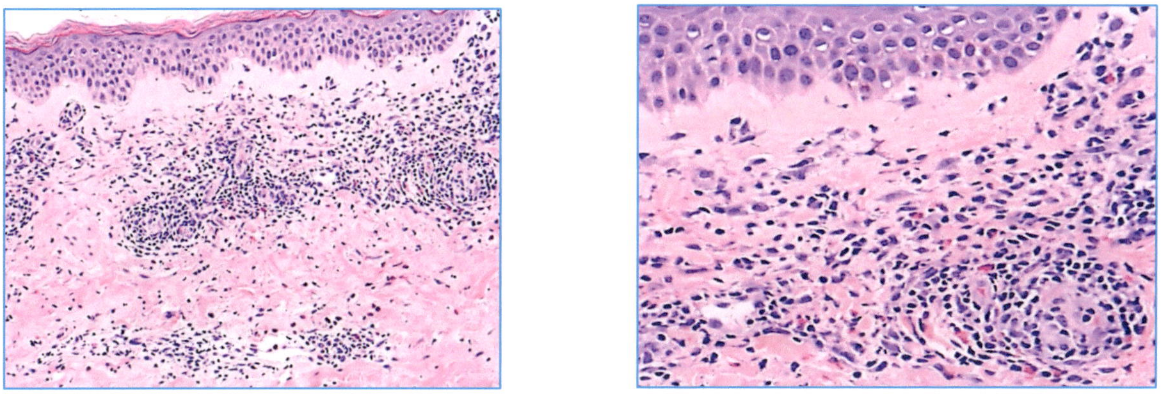

Exanthematous drug reaction with mild epidermal spongiosis, dermal lymphocytes, and numerous eosinophils

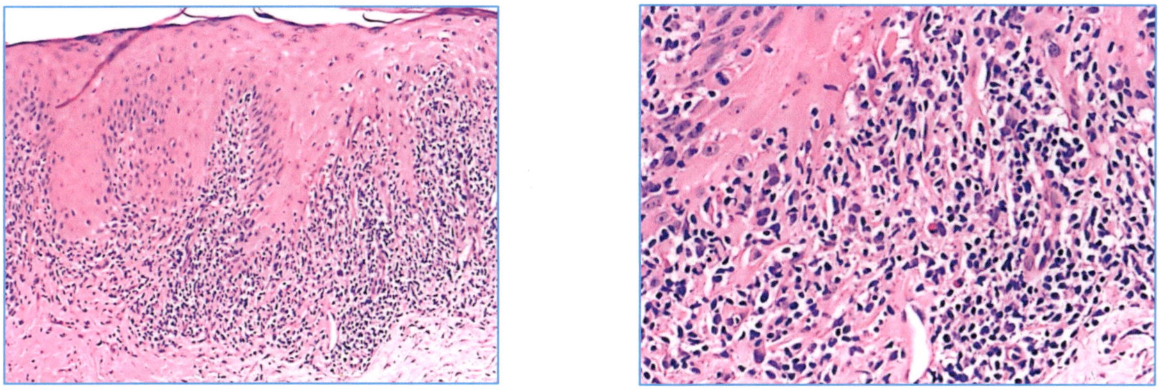

Lichenoid drug reaction with dermal, "band-like" lymphocytic infiltrate with scattered eosinophils

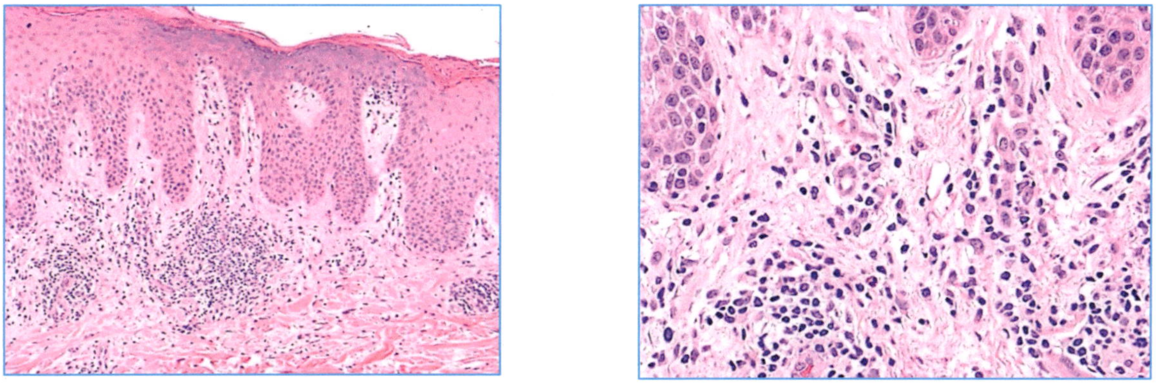

Psoriasiform drug reaction with psoriasiform epidermis with dermal lymphocytes and eosinophils

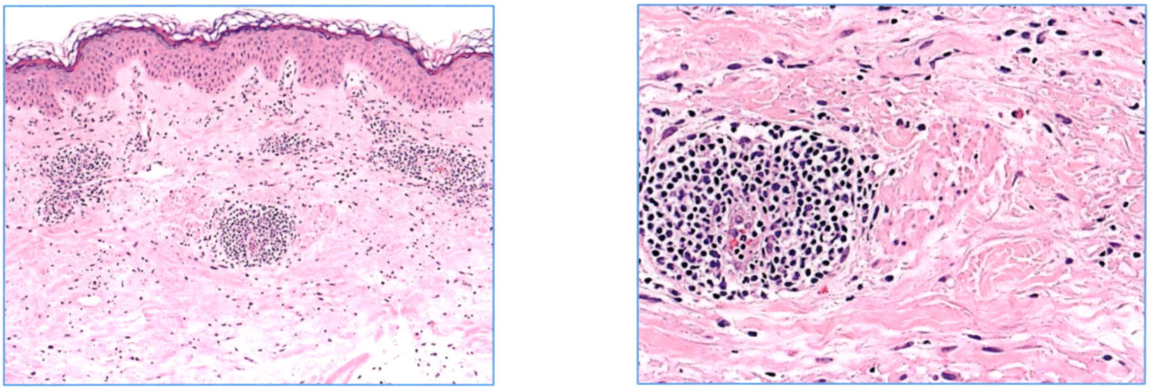

"EAC-like" drug reaction with tightly cuffed perivascular lymphocytes and scattered eosinophils

Drug reactions

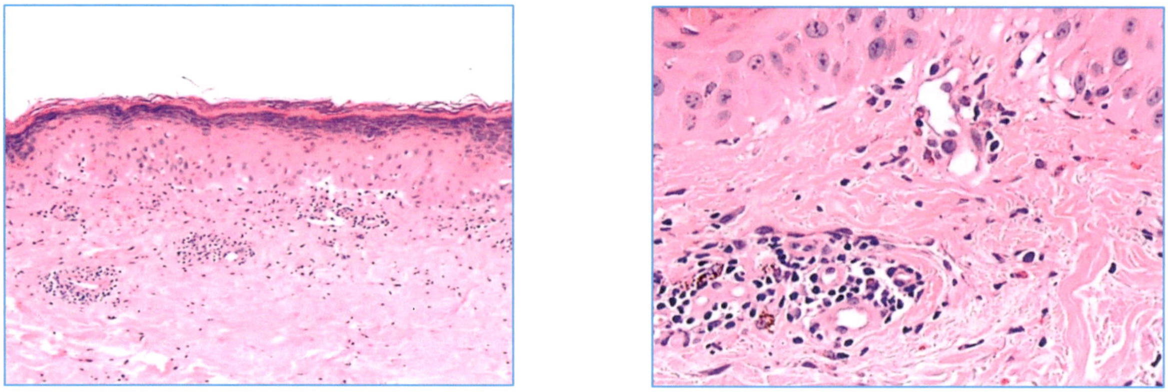

Fixed drug reaction with focal interface vacuoles, dermal pigment incontinence, and few eosinophils

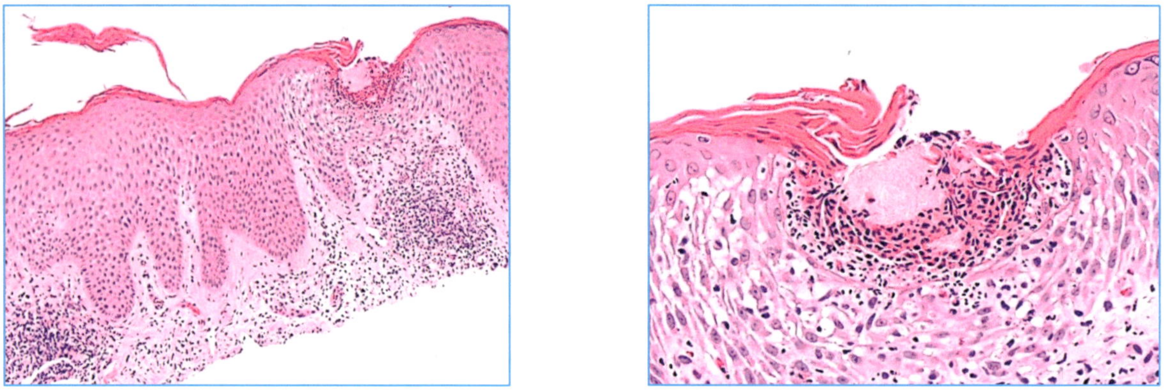

AGEP with epidermal spongiosis, subcorneal neutrophilic pustule, and few eosinophils

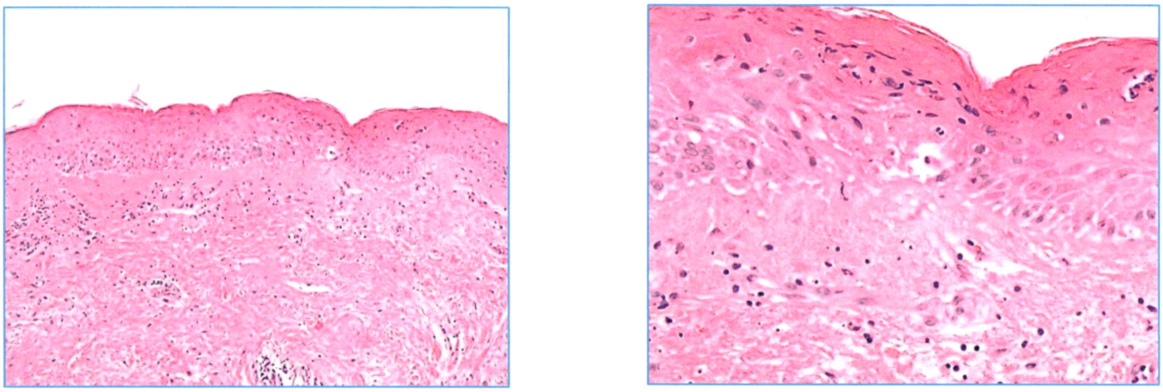

Phototoxic drug reaction with superficial necrotic keratinocytes and dermal neutrophils

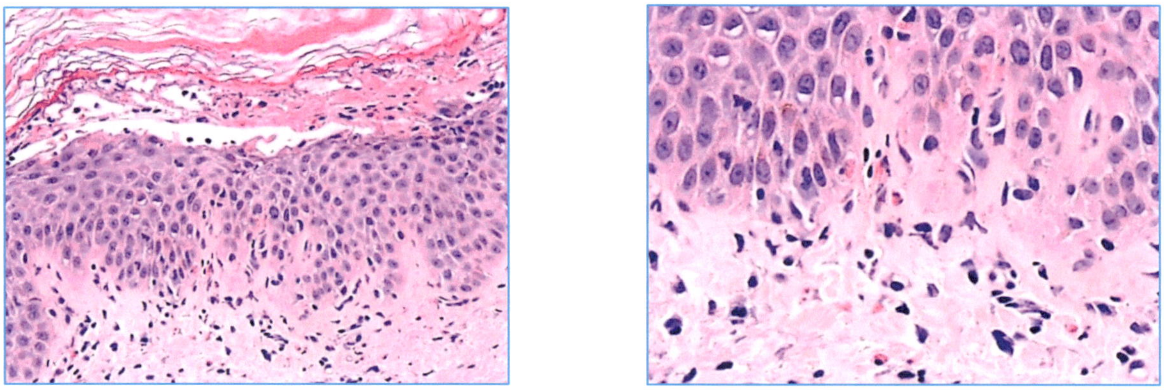

Photoallergic drug reaction with superficial necrotic keratinocytes and dermal eosinophils

Chapter 22

EXOGENOUS SKIN INSULTS

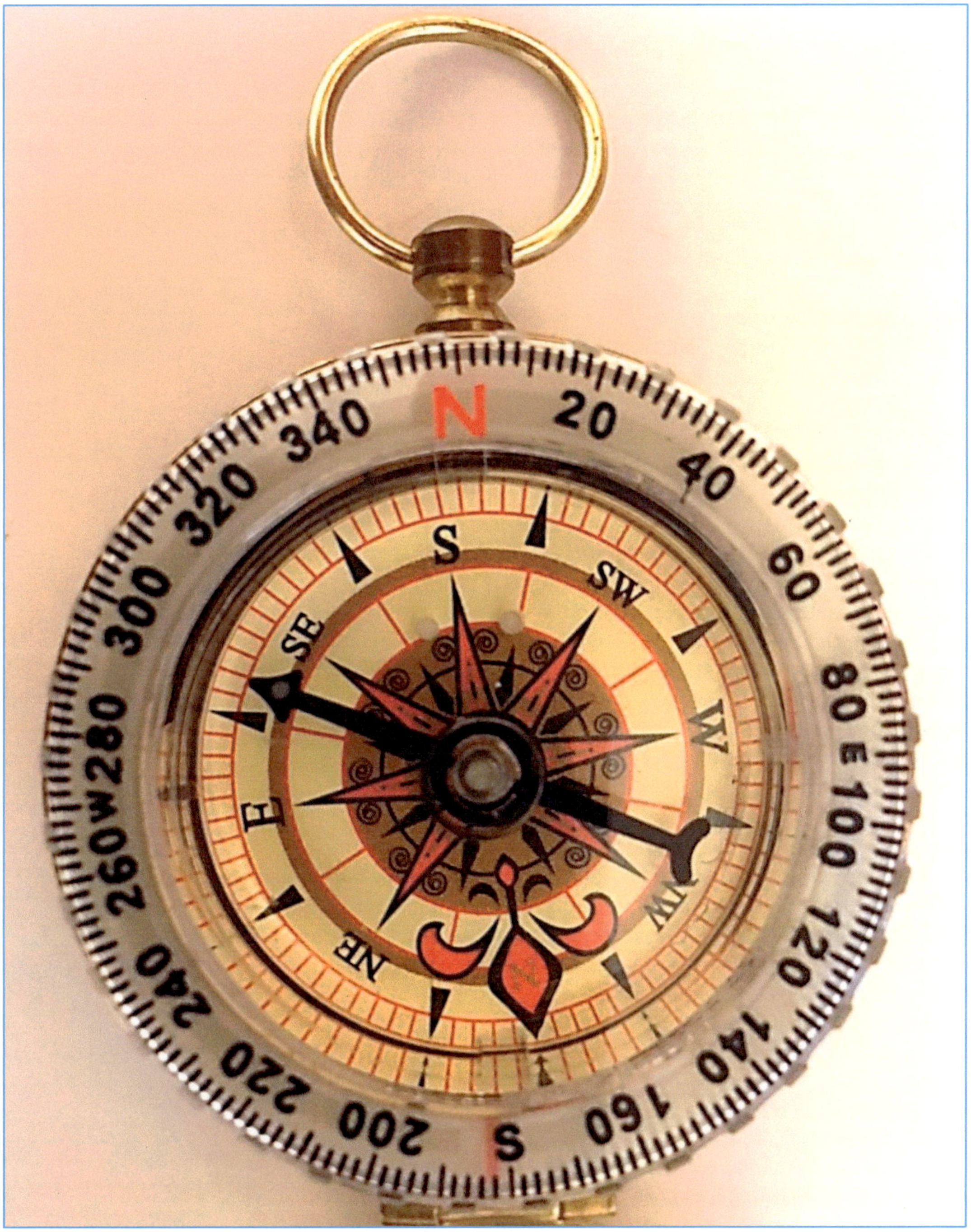

Exogenous skin insults

REACTION TO SUNLIGHT

ACUTE

Sunburn

-tender, bright erythema and mild edema of the skin several hours following sun exposure
-sharp demarcation from skin not exposed to sunlight
-never biopsied, but would show mild epidermal spongiosis and individual necrotic keratinocytes **("sun-burn cells")**

Photoallergic and Phototoxic dermatitis

-discussed in detail in the spongiotic dermatitis chapter
-in short, they are akin to allergic and irritant contact dermatitis with necrotic keratinocytes in the upper epidermis
-photoallergic dermatitis more commonly has scattered eosinophils
-phototoxic dermatitis more commonly has scattered neutrophils

Polymorphous light eruption (PMLE)

-discussed in detail in the dermal inflammation chapter
-in short, prominent dermal edema with dermal lymphocytic inflammation

CHRONIC

Actinic prurigo

-rare idiopathic photodermatosis
-classically affects the face, neck, and dorsal surface of the upper extremities
-usually manifests in the spring as a symmetric, intensely pruritic, eczematous, papulonodular dermatitis, and can persist into the winter months
-typically present in childhood, before puberty
-has a strong genetic component and is more commonly seen in Native Americans of North, Central, and South America

Histopathology non-specific

-acute and subacute forms resemble PMLE
-chronic form resembles prurigo nodularis

Hydroa vacciniforme

-very rare photodermatosis that appears in spring, with recurrences throughout the summer months
-mostly affects children and is more commonly diagnosed in females
-sun-exposed areas are affected most, and include the face, ears, hands, and lower limbs
-symptoms usually start about 30 minutes to 2 hours after sun exposure, with mild burning, itching, or stinging
-patients then develop tense vesicles and papules
-facial swelling is also common
-lesions heal with pale, depressed scars

Histopathology

-epidermal necrosis with intraepidermal vesicle
-focal dermal hemorrhage and lymphocytic infiltrate

Chronic actinic dermatitis (actinic reticuloid)

-itchy, red, lichenified, eczematous patches and plaques sharply demarcated at areas of sun exposure
-patients frequently have a history of allergic contact dermatitis (particularly to plants) preceding onset
-usually in elderly men, on chronically-sun damaged skin

Histopathology

-irregular psoriasiform epidermis with a preserved granular layer
-focal spongiosis with **lymphocytic epidermal exocytosis** (resembling mycosis fungoides)
-dermal lymphocytic infiltrate with dermal fibrosis

Chapter 22

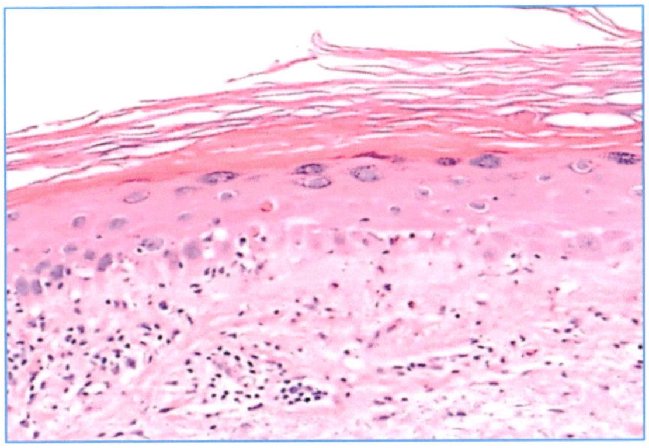

Sunburn with epidermal necrotic "sun-burn" cells

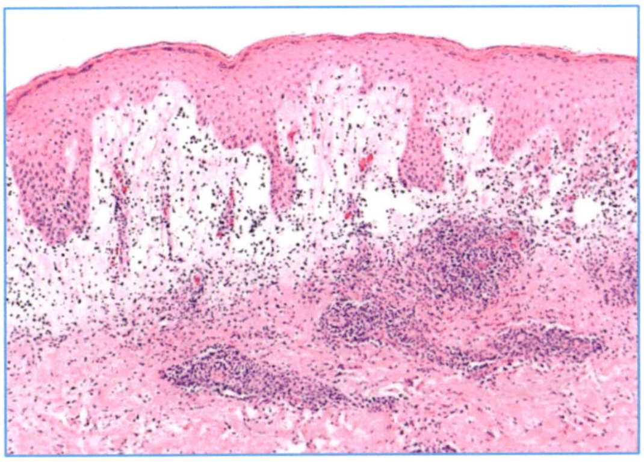

PMLE with linear papillary edema and lymphocytes

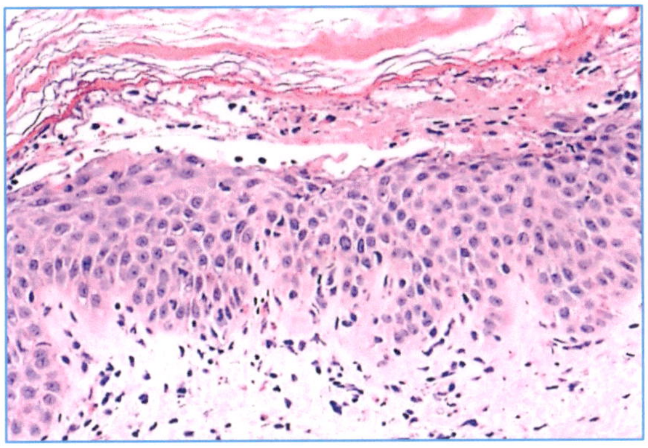

Photoallergic dermatitis with necrotic keratinocytes and eosinophils

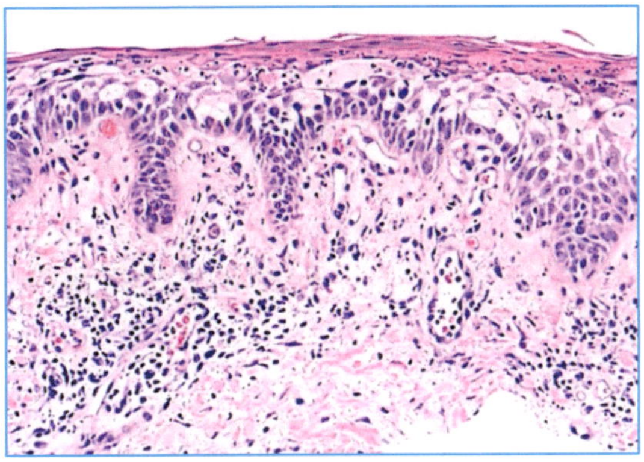

Phototoxic dermatitis with necrotic keratinocytes and neutrophils

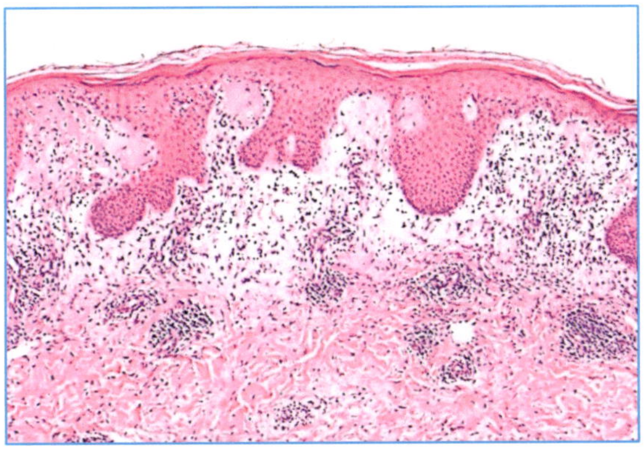

Subacute actinic prurigo resembles mild PMLE

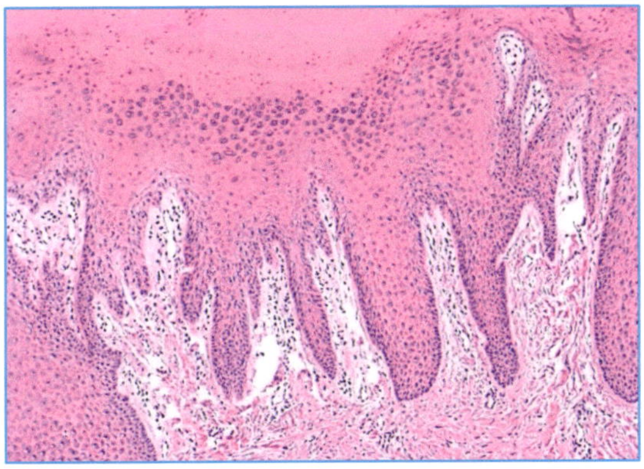

Chronic actinic prurigo resembles prurigo nodularis

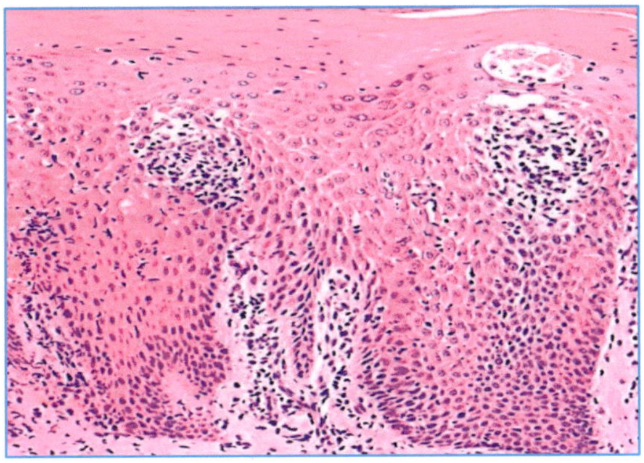

Chronic actinic dermatitis with epidermal lymphocytes resembling mycosis fungoides

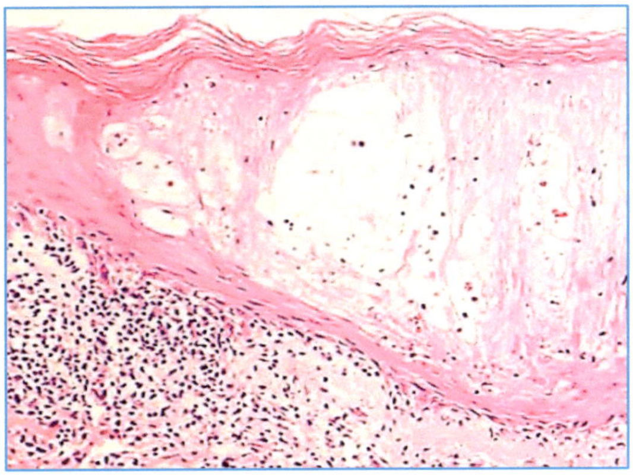

Hydroa vacciniforme with epidermal necrosis and intraepidermal vesicle

Exogenous skin insults

HEAT INJURY

ACUTE

First degree burns

-congestion of superficial vessels causing erythema, commonly followed by peeling (e.g. sun burn)
-partial or full epidermal necrosis with **no dermal damage**

Second degree burn is divided into

superficial- vesicles and blisters that recover without scarring
deep- skin is pale and anesthetic, recovers with scarring

-**full-thickness epidermal necrosis** with serum crust
-**dermal damage** is mild/moderate, and at least **some appendages** (hair follicles, etc.) are **preserved**

Third degree burn

-presents as an ulcerated wound that heals with necrotic eschar and scarring (e.g. electrical burn)
-**necrosis of dermis and portion of subcutis**
-**appendages are destroyed** and necrotic eschar covers the burn

Fourth degree burn

-full thickness destruction and **necrosis of skin, underlying fat, and even tendons** if present

CHRONIC

-present as **erythema ab igne**
-caused by long-term exposure to heat (e.g. heating blankets, fireplace)
-"net-like" reticulated red-brown patches at site of heat exposure (typically lower legs, lower back)
-clinically resembles livedo reticularis
-pigmentation occurs gradually and is permanent in later stages

Histopathology

-at first glance appears as unremarkable skin on routine H&E slides
-slightly **atrophic epidermis** and **"smudgy" dermal collagen**
-demonstrates **fragmented elastic fibers** in the mid reticular dermis (Verhoeff-Van Gieson stain for elastin)

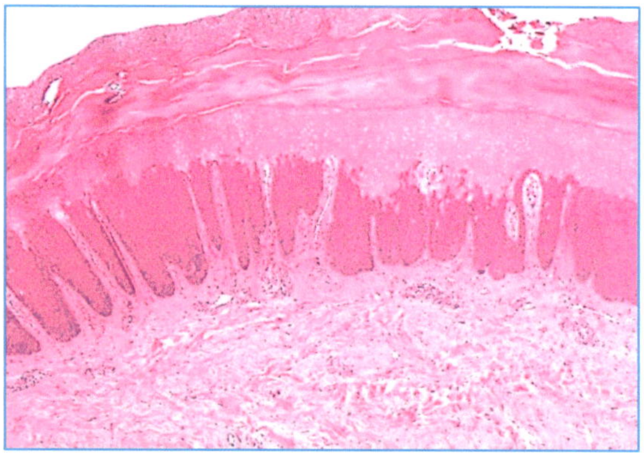

1st degree acute burn with partial epidermal necrosis

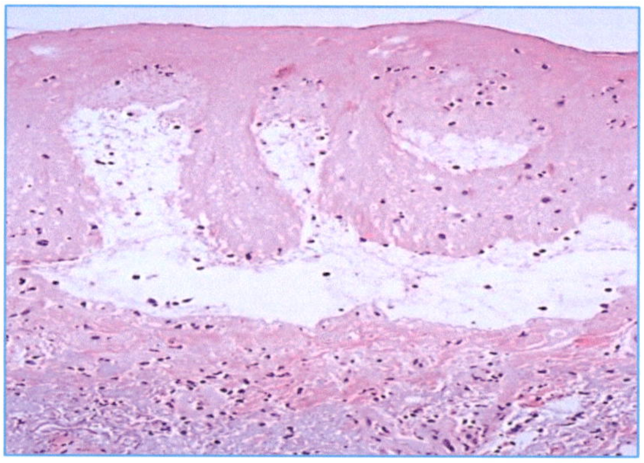

2nd degree acute burn with epidermal and partial dermal necrosis

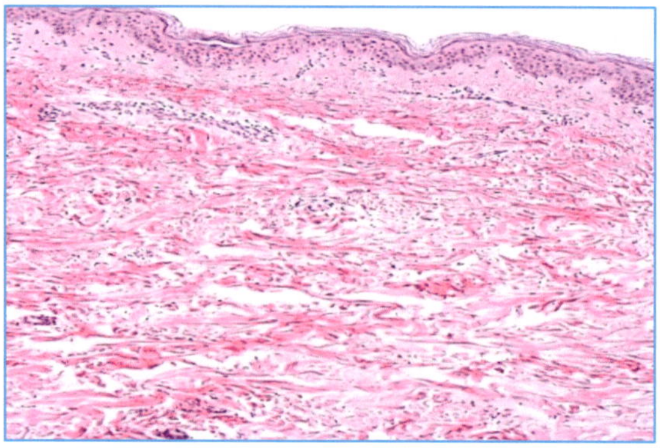

Erythema ab igne with "smudgy" dermal collagen

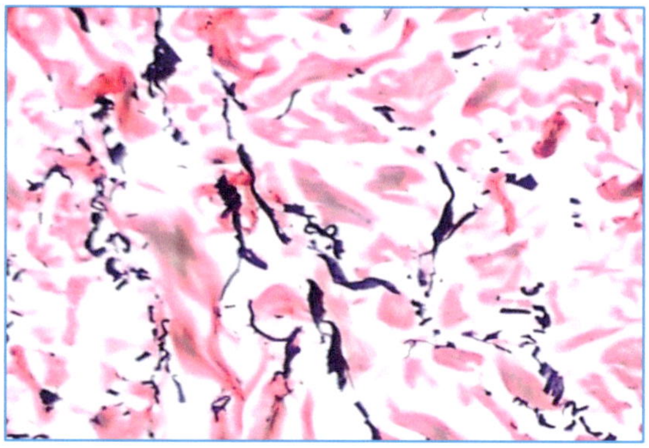

Erythema ab igne with fragmented elastic fibers (VVG stain)

Chapter 22

ELECTROCAUTERY ARTIFACT

-electrocautery instruments reduce bleeding and the risk of hematoma
-direct or alternating current is passed through a resistant metal wire electrode, generating heat
-the heated electrode is then applied to living tissue to achieve hemostasis

Histopathology
-thermal injury to tissue causes tissue necrosis and associated histological artifact
-**nuclei** of cells are **elongated and hyperchromatic**
-**cytoplasm** appears **"smudgy" purple**
-**cell outlines are blurred**
-keratinocytes have an elongated **"hair-like"** appearance

FREEZE ARTIFACT

-a tissue processing artifact
-occurs if tissue fixed in formalin is transported (or stored) at temperature close or below 0 °C
-can also occur if tissue is frozen with liquid nitrogen prior to the biopsy

Histopathology
-**intracytoplasmic empty vacuoles**
-most prominent in epidermis
-evenly distributed in epidermal keratinocytes
-vacuoles represent ice crystals and resemble glycogen

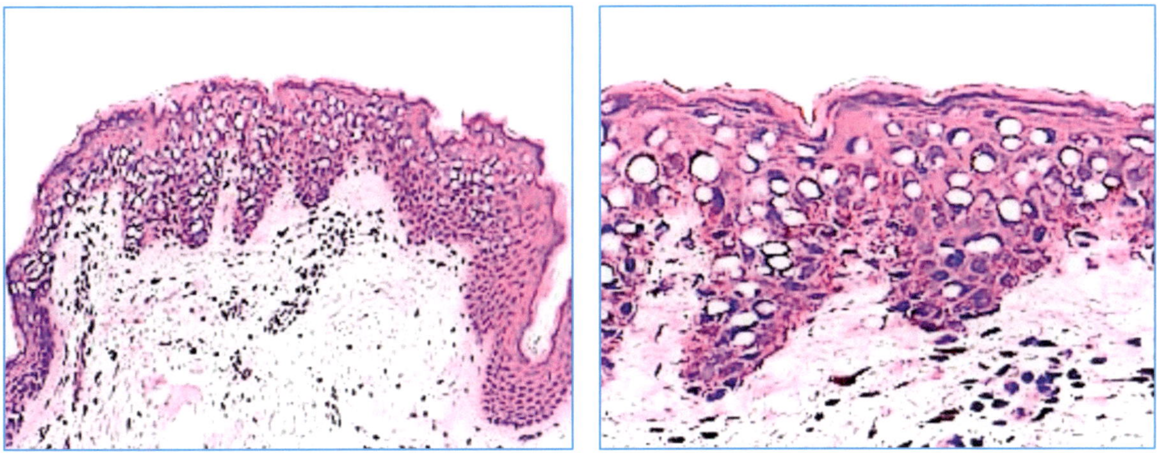

Freeze artifact creates keratinocytes with white intracytoplasmic vacuoles

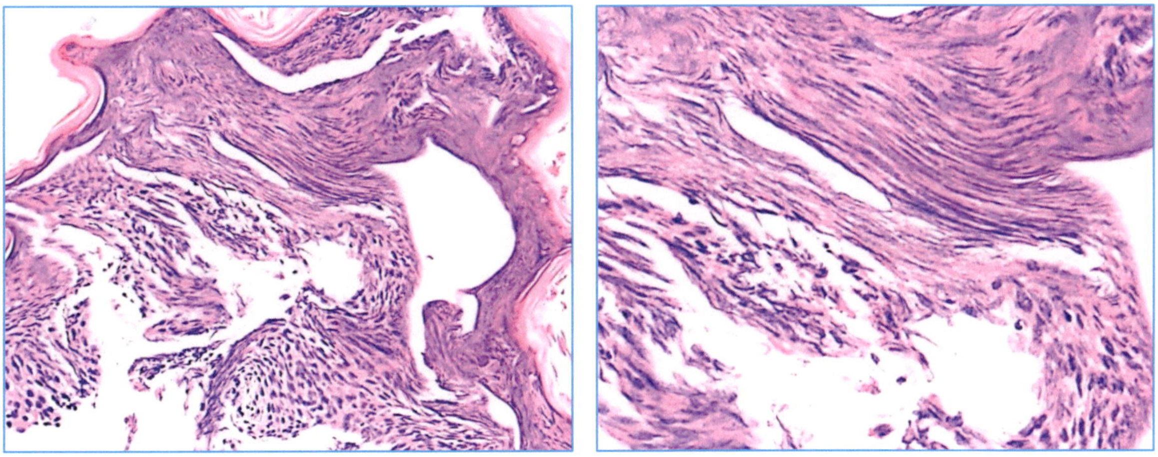

Electrocautery artifact with elongated, purple, "hair-like" keratinocytes

Exogenous skin insults

COLD INJURY

Frostnip

-a mild cold injury caused by freezing of the top layers of the skin, managed by gentle rewarming
-reversible and manifests with numbness and a white, hard skin surface, but soft deep tissue
-favors cheeks, earlobes, fingers, and toes

Frostbite (chilblains, pernio, perniosis)

-more severe injury that includes all layers of skin
-the skin appears white with a "wooden" indurated feel
-numbness and possibly anesthesia present
-**First-degree frostbite** presents with hyperemia, mild itching, and edema; no blistering or peeling of the skin
-**Second-degree frostbite** shows blistering and desquamation
-**Third-degree frostbite** is associated with necrosis of the skin and the subcutaneous tissue with ulceration

Note: misleading dermatological terms

Chilblain pernio- form of chronic lupus erythematosus
Lupus pernio- form of cutaneous sarcoidosis

Histopathology

-normal (1st degree) to necrotic epidermis (3rd degree)
-linear **papillary dermal edema** with blisters
-superficial and deep lymphocytic infiltrate with common red blood cell extravasation
-common **perieccrine lymphocytes and dermal microthrombi**

RADIATION DERMATITIS (RADIODERMATITIS)

Acute radiodermatitis

-24-hour latency period before skin erythema appears
-erythema lasts 2-3 days, but can reappear after 3-6 days, and last for several weeks if dose was high

Chronic radiodermatitis

-results from chronic "sub-erythematous" doses of radiation
-skin atrophy, hypopigmentation, and telangiectasias
-skin appears dry, thin, and shiny

Histopathology

Acute radiodermatitis

-not biopsied as it is a clinical diagnosis

Chronic radiation dermatitis

-shows **"sick dermis"**
-epidermal atrophy with **dermal fibrosis**
-**large telangiectasias** and reactive endothelial cells
-**absence of adnexal structures** with **atypical stellate fibroblasts**

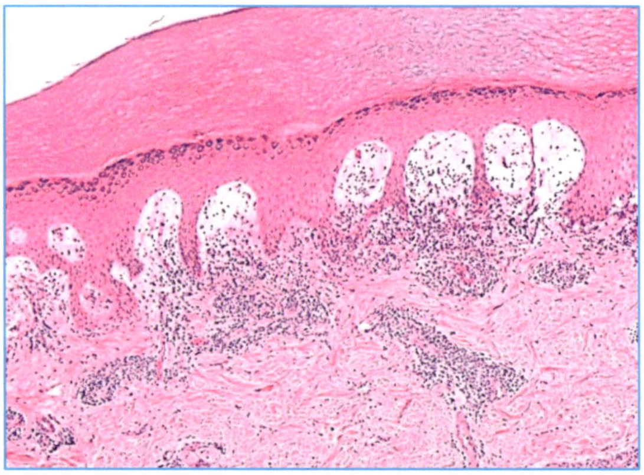
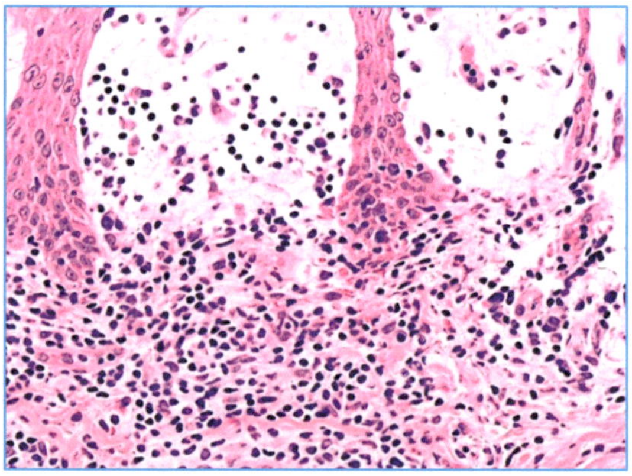

First degree frostbite with papillary dermal edema and lymphocytic inflammation

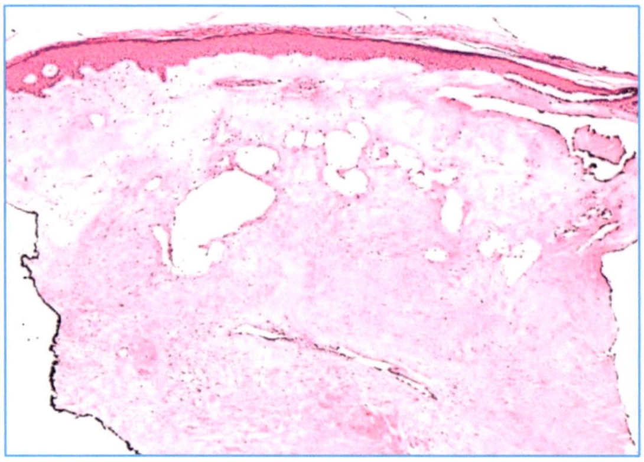
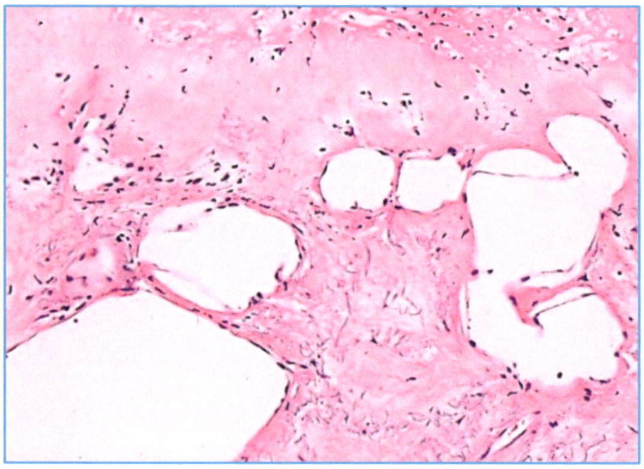

Chronic radiation dermatitis with sclerotic dermis, absent adnexal structures, and dilated capillaries

Chapter 22

ARTHROPOD BITES

Skin reaction depends on the kind of insect

Bedbugs- red, itchy papules, commonly in linear pattern **"breakfast, lunch, and dinner"** sign
Bee/wasp- painful red papule with surrounding blanching
Flea- itchy urticarial papules, often on the ankles and legs
Fire ants- grouped, itchy, tender, sterile papules and vesicles with erythema
Mosquitoes- raised, itchy, pink papules
Spider- erythema with localized swelling and pain, possible ulceration, and necrosis
Ticks- leaves targetoid lesion

There are varieties of tick families. Those relevant to dermatologists are:

Ixodes family
-transmit Lyme disease and babesiosis

Dermacentor family
-transmit Rocky Mountain spotted fever, tularemia, Colorado tick fever

Ornithodors family
-transmit relapsing fever

Histopathology

-varies depending on the age of the lesion

Ant, bee, wasp, or spider bites are similar

New lesions

-spongiotic epidermis with **central ulceration** and serum crust
-superficial and deep, **"V-shaped"** lymphohistiocytic infiltrate
-perivascular and interstitial **eosinophils and neutrophils**
-dermal edema with focal dermal necrosis and abscess formation can be seen

Older lesions

-epidermis is intact, but mildly spongiotic
-dermal edema can be prominent with blister formation
-inflammation is more diffuse (not so "V-shaped"), and more mixed with less eosinophils and neutrophils

Flea and **bedbugs**

-more **lymphocytic inflammation** with less neutrophils and eosinophils

Tick bite

-skin is excoriated at the site of the bite
-dermal necrosis and mixed inflammation with **neutrophils more prominent** than eosinophils
-**mouthpiece** of a tick is commonly attached

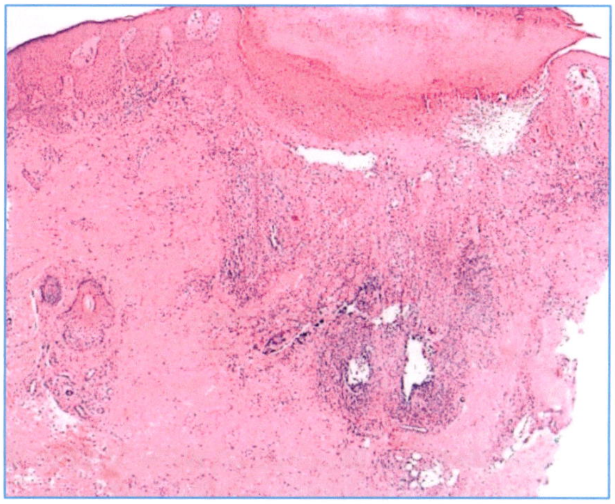

Arthropod bite with epidermal ulceration and "wedge shaped" acute inflammation with eosinophils

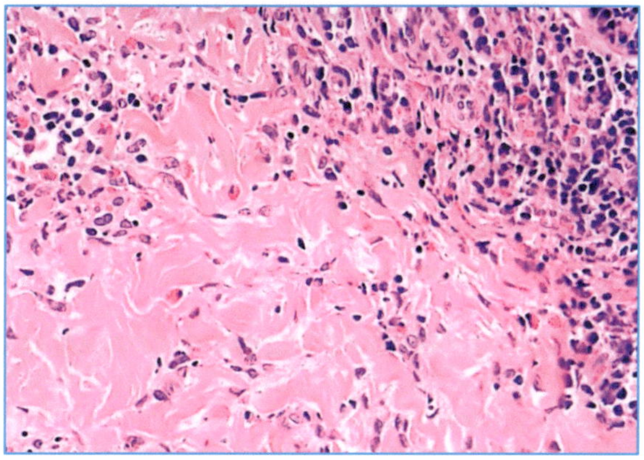

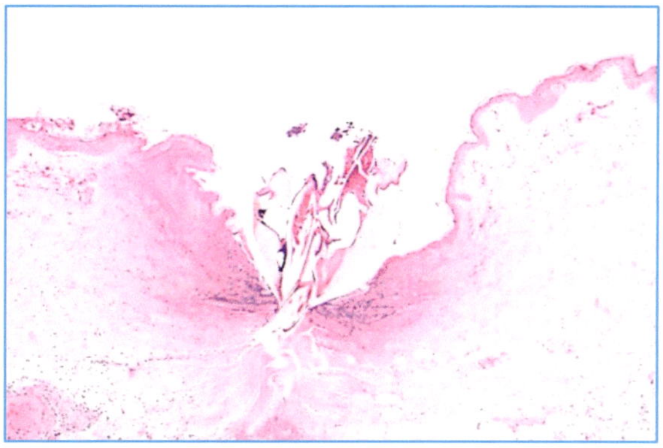

Tick mouthpiece attached to ulcerated, inflamed skin

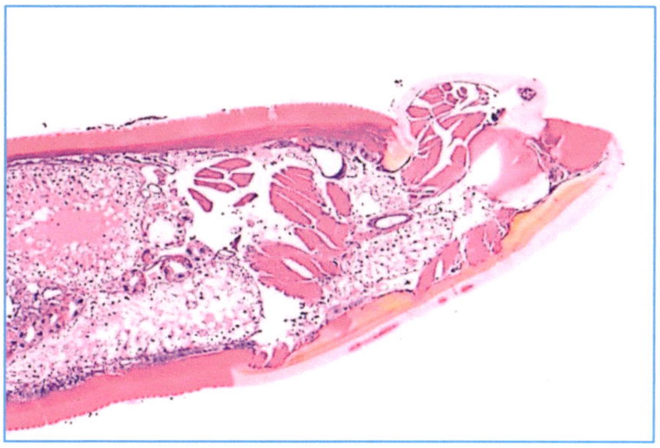

Intact tick

Exogenous skin insults

HOW TO APPROACH EXOGENOUS SKIN INSULTS

SKIN LOOKS NORMAL

-erythema ab igne	VVG stain highlights fragmented elastic fibers

EPIDERMIS IS NECROTIC

-hydroa vacciniforme	with intraepidermal vesicle
-burn	no intraepidermal vesicle
-frost bite	no intraepidermal vesicle

EPIDERMIS IS EXCORIATED WITH "WEDGE SHAPED" DERMAL INFLAMMATION

-arthropod bite

PSORISIFORM EPIDERMIS WITH EPIDERMAL LYMPHOCYTES

-chronic actinic dermatitis

SPONGIOTIC EPIDERMIS WITH NECROTIC KERATINOCYTES

-phototoxic dermatitis	with dermal neutrophils
-photoallergic dermatitis	with dermal eosinophils

EMPTY VACUOLES PRESENT IN EPIDERMAL KERATINOCYTES

-freeze artifact

SMUDGY TISSUE WITH "HAIR-LIKE" KERATINOCYTES AND ELONGATED NUCLEA

-electrocautery artifact

SCLEROTIC DERMIS AND DILATED VESSELS

-chronic radiation dermatitis

PROMINENT SUPERFICIAL DERMAL EDEMA

-PMLE	with dermal lymphocytes
-pernio	with dermal and perieccrine lymphocytes

Chapter 22

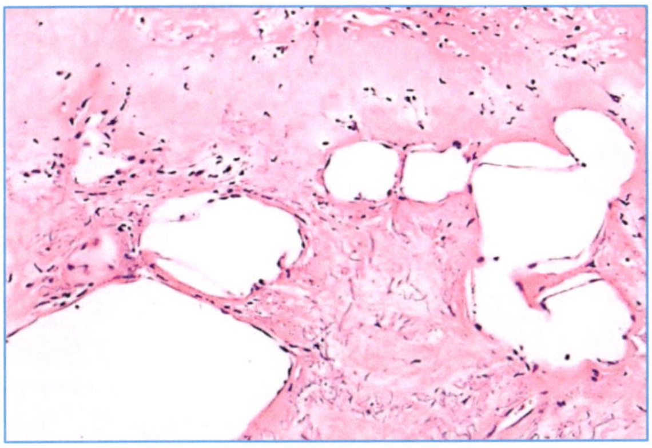

Radiation dermatitis with dilated vessels in hyalinized stroma

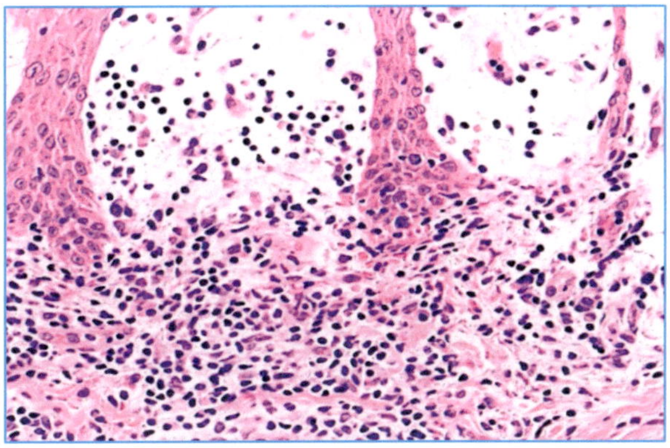

Frostbite with dermal edema and perivascular and perieccrine lymphocytes

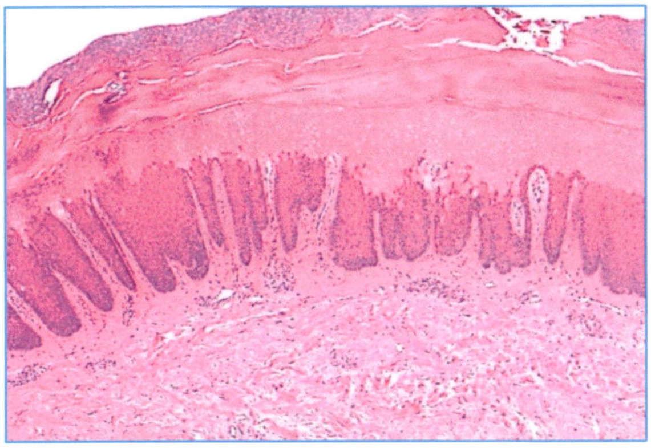

First degree burn with necrotic epidermis

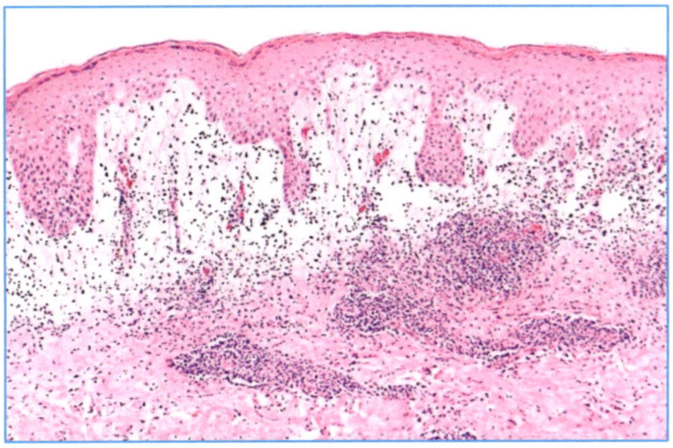

PMLE with dermal edema and lymphocytic inflammation

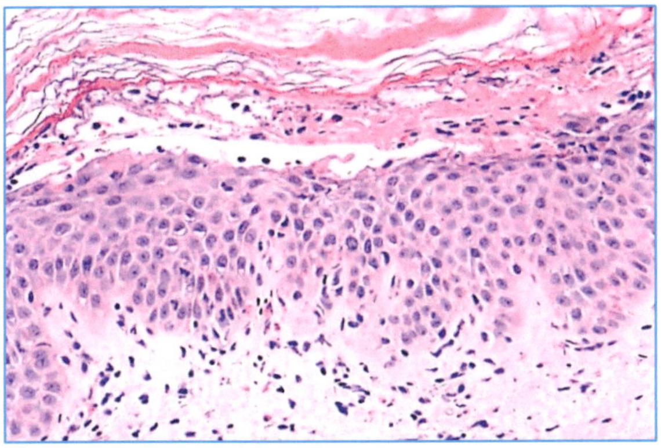

Photoallergic contact dermatitis with superficial necrotic keratinocytes with eosinophils

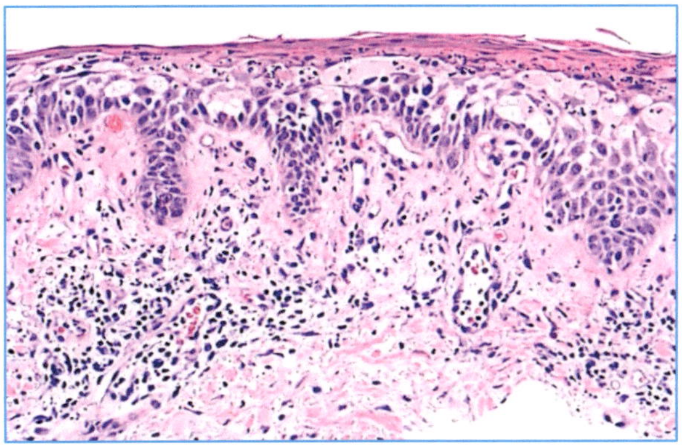

Phototoxic contact dermatitis with superficial necrotic keratinocytes and neutrophils

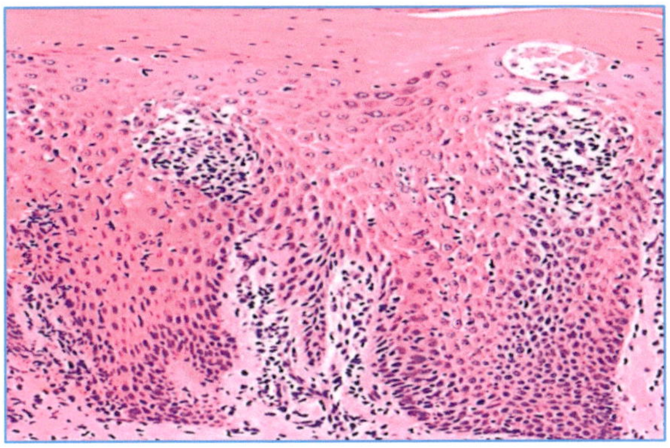

Actinic reticuloid with psoriasiform epidermis with spongiosis and epidermal lymphocytes

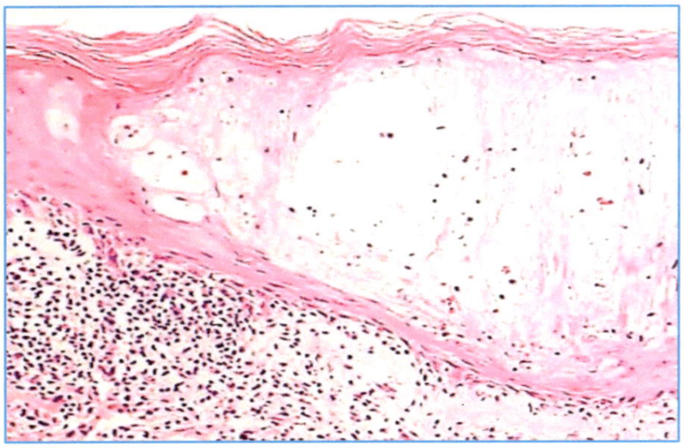

Hydroa vacciniforme with epidermal necrosis and intraepidermal vesicle

Exogenous skin insults

Chapter 23

DISORDERS OF PIGMENTATION

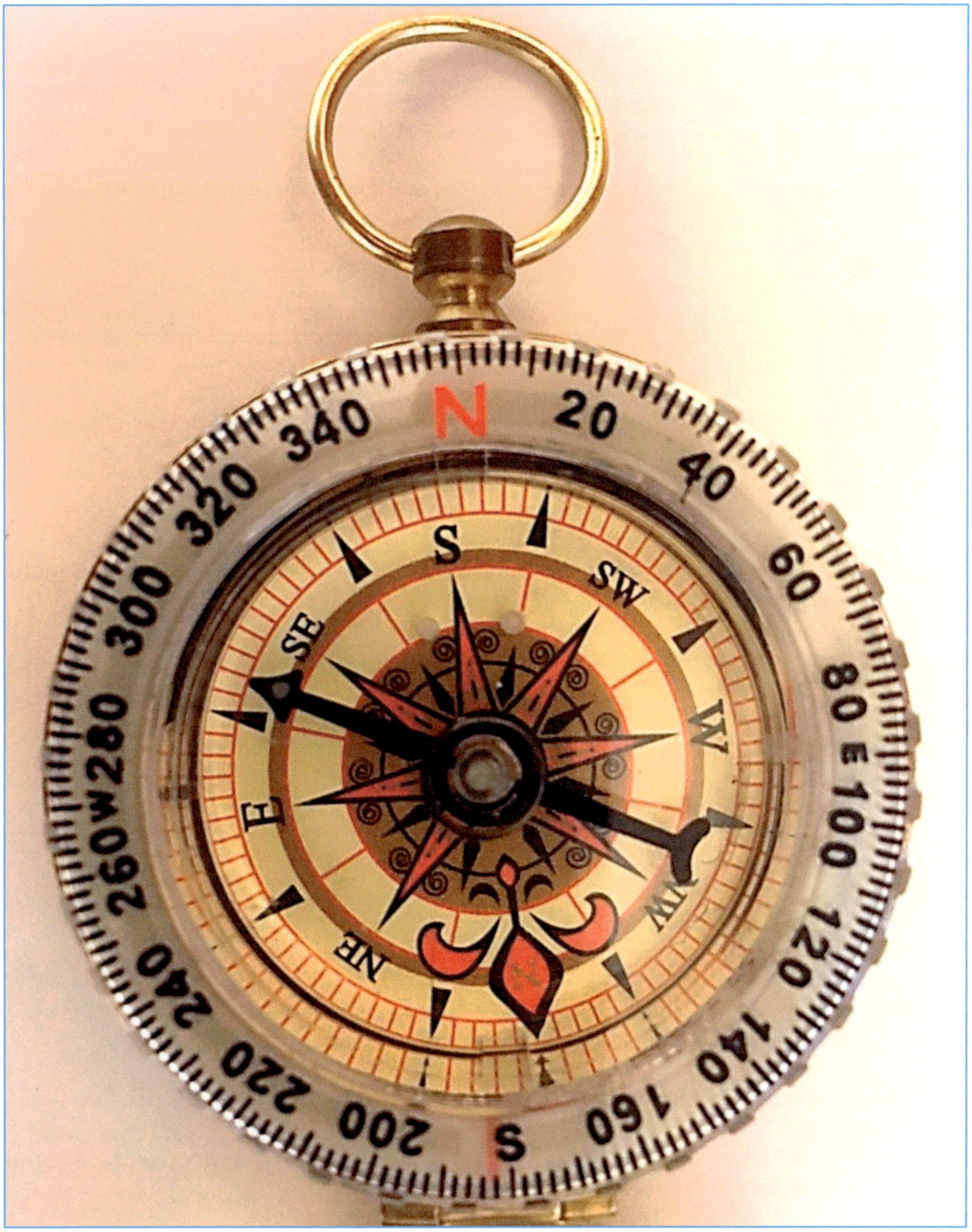

Disorders of pigmentation

HYPERPIGMENTATION

Generalized (diffuse) hyperpigmentation

-has numerous causes:
- -hormonal (Addison's disease, Nelson's syndrome, POEMS syndrome, thyrotoxicosis, estrogen)
- -liver diseases (primary biliary cirrhosis, hemochromatosis)
- -cancer (lung carcinoma, neurofibroma, lymphoma)
- -metal ingestion (silver, gold, arsenic, lead, iron)
- -drugs (e.g. chlorpromazine, busulphan, amiodaron)
- -malabsorption and infection (e.g. tuberculosis)

-diffuse hyperpigmentation is more obvious in the skin creases of the palms, soles, flexures, scars, along the nails

Histopathology

-normal epidermal architecture with **hyperpigmentation (increased melanin) of basal layer keratinocytes**

Localized hyperpigmentation

Café au lait macules (CALM)

-present in childhood
-irregular light brown macules or patches with smooth borders, typically on covered areas of the body
-multiple CALMs (>6) with **smooth borders ("coast of California")**, typically on covered areas of the body, are associated with **NF type1**
-large CALMs with ragged "coast of Maine" borders are associated with **McCune-Albright syndrome,** favoring head, neck, shoulder, lower back, and buttock

Histopathology

-wavy epidermis with **increased melanin at the epidermal basal layer**
-slightly increased number of melanocytes
-the epidermal melanocytes of an isolated café-au-lait macule will have **excessive numbers of melanosomes (epidermal melanotic hypermelanosis)**
-the café-au-lait macules associated with NF type 1 and McCune-Albright syndrome have **increased proliferation of epidermal melanocytes (epidermal melanocytic hyperplasia)**

Ephelides (freckles)

-light to dark brown flat macules prominent during summer that fade during winter

Histopathology

-wavy epidermis with **increased melanin pigment** and normal number of melanocytes

Lentigines can be divided into

Solar lentigo

-sun induced, well-circumscribed, pigmented spot that is round, oval, or irregular in shape
-typically found as groups of similar lesions on sun-exposed sites

Lentigo simplex

-single or multiple lesions, not induced by sun exposure, that present at birth or more commonly in early childhood
-majority are not associated with any medical diseases but a small number are associated with:

Peutz-Jeghers syndrome

-lentigines on the lips and oral mucosa with GI polyposis

Leopard syndrome

-**L**entigines and café au lait spots, **E**KG abnormalities, **O**cular hypertelorism, **P**ulmonary stenosis, **A**bnormal genitalia, **R**etardation of growth, **D**eafness

Carney complex (and its subsets **LAMB syndrome** and **NAME syndrome**)

-lentigines, myxomas, endocrine overactivity

Histopathology **of lentigines**

-**both** solar lentigo and lentigo simplex have **elongated epidermal rete ridges** with **prominent intraepidermal melanin**
-number of melanocytes is mildly increased and focal dermal pigment incontinence can be present
-**difference between them** is that **solar lentigo has dermal solar elastosis** whereas **lentigo simplex has no solar elastosis**

Chapter 23

Melasma (chloasma)

-brown patches on the cheeks, nose, and forehead that worsen in the summer
-mostly observed in women and darker skin types and associated with pregnancy, oral contraception

Histopathology

-**increased epidermal melanin**
-**absent interface changes** (unlike erythema dyschromicum perstans or fixed drug reaction)
-dermal solar elastosis and dermal melanophages, but only in 1/3rd of cases

Post inflammatory hyperpigmentation (PIH)/ post inflammatory pigment alteration (PIPA)

-mostly observed in darker skin types and may follow any inflammatory skin disease
-in can also be caused by a drug reaction (e.g. antimalarial drugs, clofazimine, tetracycline, bleomycine)
-manifests as hyperpigmented macules/patches in the distribution of the prior skin condition

Histopathology

-**normal epidermis** (unlike erythema dyschromicum perstans or fixed drug reaction)
-**dermal pigment incontinence** and **mild perivascular lymphocytic infiltrate**

Erythema dyschromicum perstans (ashy dermatosis)

-well-circumscribed round to oval or irregular patches on the face, neck and trunk that are grey in color
-symmetric distribution and involve the trunk, but commonly spread to the face and extremities
-most often affects darker-skinned patients and young adults
-cause is idiopathic although medications, pesticides, infections with parasites, and HIV has been implicated

Histopathology

-**minor vacuolar degeneration** of the basal layer in early lesions
-pigmentary incontinence with **dermal melanophages** in more established patches.

Becker's nevus

-hyperpigmented plaque sometimes with hypertrichosis on the chest/shoulder of younger men
-onset around puberty, may be androgen mediated

Histopathology

-**epidermal acanthosis** and elongated rete ridges with basal layer hyperpigmentation
-increased number of haphazardly arranged **smooth muscles in the dermis**
-number of **hair follicles** sometimes increased

Dowling Degos disease

-rare autosomal dominant disease due to *keratin 5* mutation that usually starts in early adulthood
-reticulate macular hyperpigmentation in the axilla and groin
-associated with "comedone-like" lesions on the back and neck and perioral scars
-**Galli-Galli disease is a variant of Dowling-Degos** (also due to *keratin 5* mutation)
-presents as 1-2 mm, slightly keratotic, red brown papules in a reticulated pattern

Histopathology

-**"finger-like" downgrowth** of the epidermis
-hyperpigmentation at the tips of the rete ridges and small horn cysts can be seen
-Galli-Galli has the same histology with additional focal suprabasal acantholysis

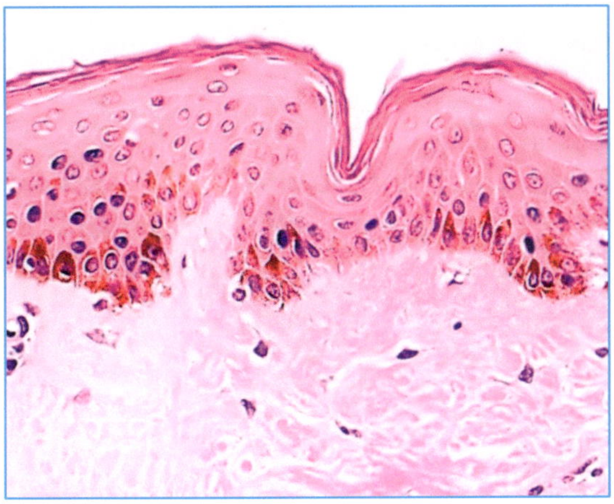

Café au lait spot with increased melanin in wavy epidermis

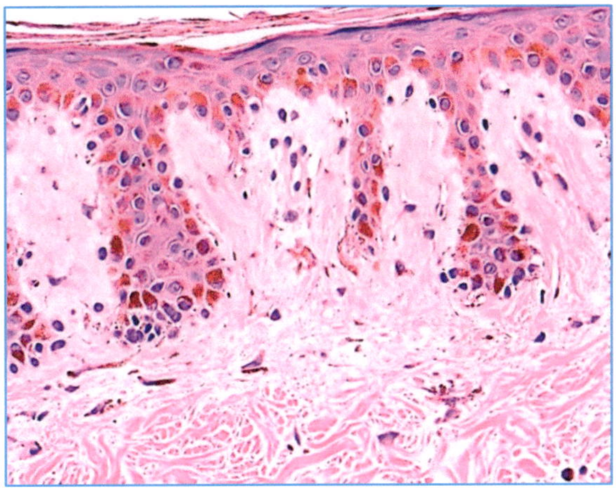

Lentigo simplex with elongated, hyperpigmented rete ridges

Disorders of pigmentation

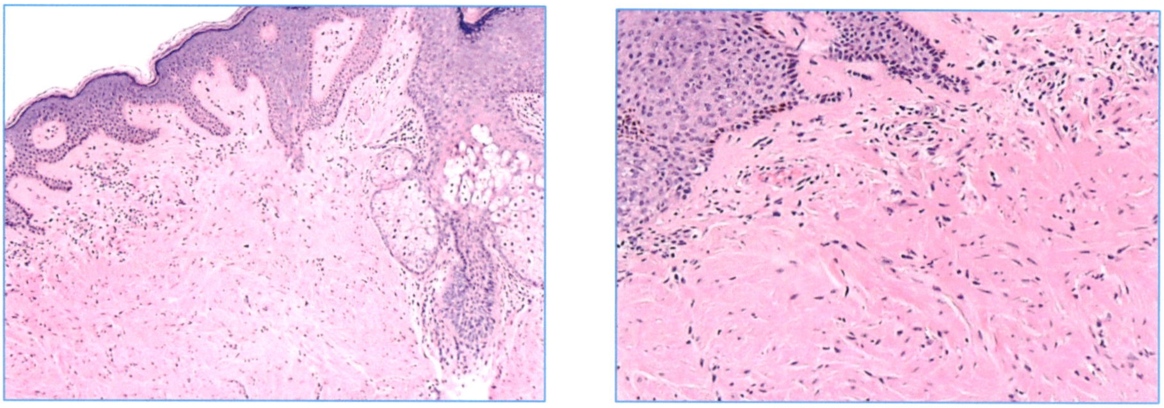

Becker's nevus with acanthotic, pigmented epidermis and numerous dermal smooth muscle bundles

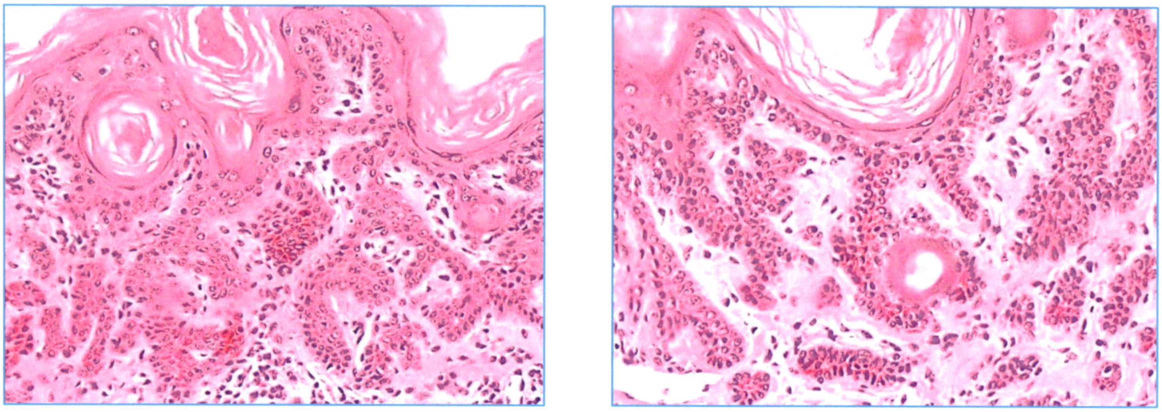

Dowling-Degos disease with "finger-like" downgrowth of the epidermis

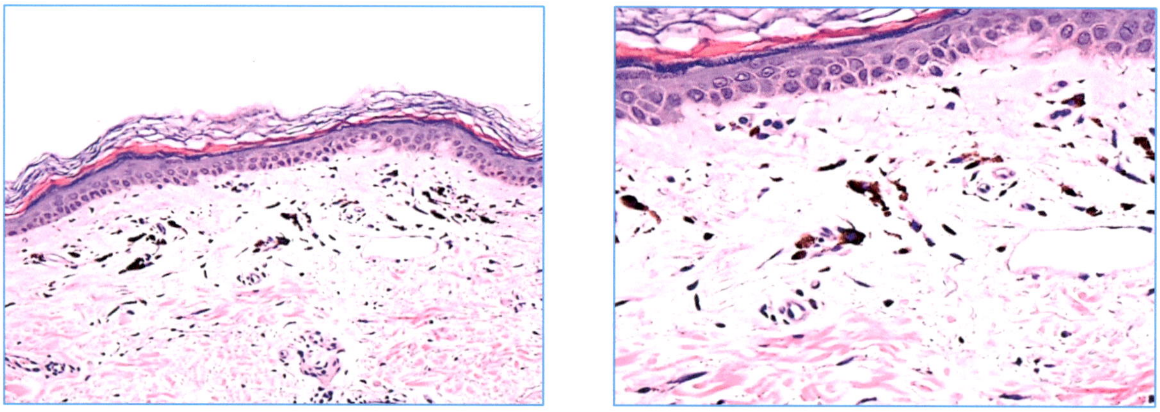

PIPA with prominent dermal pigment incontinence

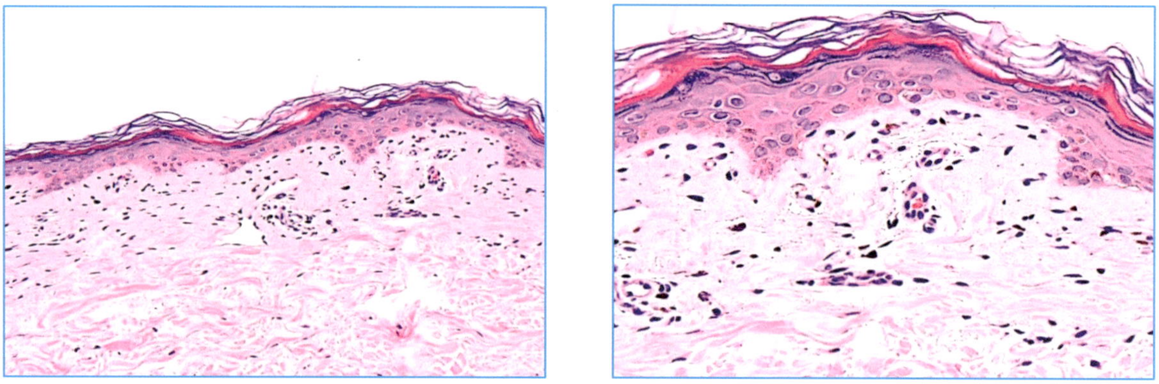

Melasma with normal epidermis with increased epidermal melanin and minimal dermal pigment

Chapter 23

HYPOPIGMENTATION

Multiple diseases show hypopigmentation but histopathology is remarkably similar

Albinism

-genetically heterogenous group of disorders due to defects in melanin and melanosome production or transport
-variable absence of pigment of the skin, hair, and eyes

Histopathology

-skin appearance is unremarkable on H&E slides
-epidermal **melanocytes are present** in normal number
-**absent or decreased** amount of **melanin**

Chediak-Higashi syndrome

-progressive fatal disease due to mutation in the *LYST* or *CHS1* gene
-decreased NK and T cell cytotoxicity
-oculocutaneous albinism, immunodeficiency, and neurological defects

Histopathology

-**same as albinism** and has additional presence of **giant melanosomes** detected by electron microscopy (EM)

Hermansky-Pudlak syndrome

-autosomal recessive disease due to a variety of mutations in *HPS* gene family
-oculocutaneous albinism with bleeding diathesis

Histopathology

-**same as albinism** but EM demonstrates **dysfunctional melanosomes**

Griscelli syndrome

-autosomal recessive disease due to mutations in *MYO5A, RAB27A*, or *MLPH* gene
-silvery-gray sheen of the hair and the light-colored skin with immunodeficiency and neurological defects

Histopathology

-same as in albinism

"Ashleaf" macules of tuberous sclerosis

-ashleaf shaped hypopigmented spots on the trunk and extremities
-present from birth or early childhood
-usually the first cutaneous presentation of tuberous sclerosis

Histopathology

-normal or decreased number of melanocytes and **melanin amount is reduced but not completely absent**
-findings **similar but not identical to albinism**
-EM demonstrates reduction in number, size, and melanization of **melanosomes** which **form aggregates** within keratinocytes

Nevus depigmentosus

-probably due to a sporadic defect in embryonic development
-solitary partially hypopigmented macule with ragged border present at birth
-typically remains stable and only increases in size as the body grows

Histopathology

-normal or decreased number of melanocytes
-melanin amount is reduced but not completely absent (**same as in ash-leaf macule**)
-EM demonstrates **decrease in transfer** of **melanosomes to keratinocytes**

Hypomelanosis of Ito

-hypopigmented streaks following Blaschko's lines
-present at birth or shortly after
-multiple chromosomal abnormalities associated

Histopathology

-**similar** findings **as albinism**
-normal number of melanocytes and reduction but not complete absence of melanin
-EM demonstrates poorly formed melanocytic organelles and reduced number of melanosomes

Progressive macular hypomelanosis

-multiple, circular, poorly defined pale and non-scaly spots that coalesce
-mainly affects the trunk and rarely extends to the arms, legs, or neck
-the course of the disease is variable; some resolve in 3–5 years and others remain stable or even progress

Histopathology

-**same as albinism**

Pityriasis alba

-typically patches of hypopigmentation with no surface changes
-favors face (particularly cheeks) of children and adolescents with atopic dermatitis
-thought to represent low grade atopic dermatitis
-resolves spontaneously after a number of years

Histopathology is **non-specific**

-mild spongiosis and perivascular lymphocytic infiltrate
-normal number of melanocytes with decreased melanization

Disorders of pigmentation

Vitiligo

-autoimmune disease where the immune system attacks melanocytes leading to depigmentation
-can affect all ages and skin types
-chalk white depigmented macules that may progressively enlarge, easily identified on Wood's lamp examination
-six clinical types based on extent and distribution
-generalized (#1), localized, segmental, universal, acrofacial, and mucosal

Histopathology

-skin appears unremarkable on H&E slides
-total **absence** of functioning **melanocytes** with **no melanin**
-at the advancing border of the lesion, melanocytes are decreased in number and may be increased in size

Chemical leukoderma (occupational vitiligo)

-acquired depigmentation caused by repeated exposure to chemicals (classically phenol #1)

Histopathology

-same as vitiligo

Piebaldism

-autosomal dominant condition due to mutation in c*KIT* or *SNAI2*
-discrete patches of depigmentation with characteristic hyperpigmented macules within hypopigmented areas
-characteristic white forelock (triangular or rhombus-shaped white patch on the frontal scalp with white hair)

Histopathology

-same as vitiligo

Waardenburg syndrome

-rare autosomal dominant disease due to mutation in *PAX3, MITF, SNAI2*, or *SOX10* gene
-a white forelock or patches of light skin (similar to piebaldism), bright blue eyes, and hearing loss
-usually the first cutaneous presentation of tuberous sclerosis

Histopathology

-same as vitiligo

Idiopathic guttate melanosis

-numerous (10-30) small hypopigmented macules primarily on shins and forearms
-usually occurs after age 40

Histopathology

-atrophic epidermis with redaction (more common) or absence of melanocytes and melanin

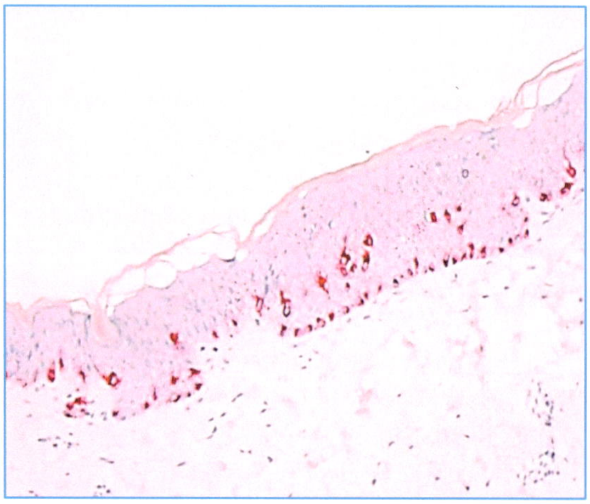

Melan-A stain demonstrates normal number of melanocytes (red dots) in albinism

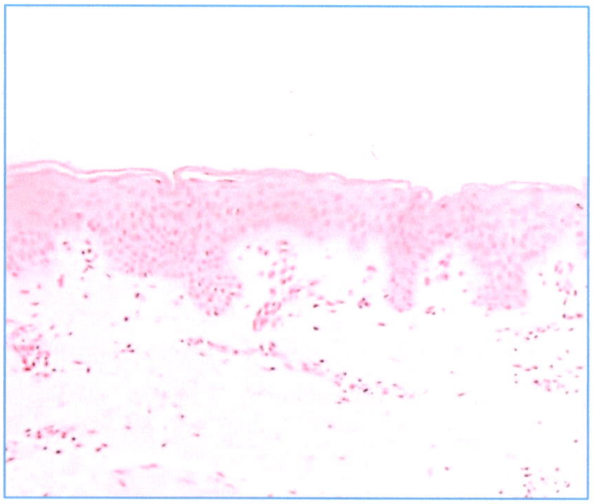

Fontana Masson stain for melanin demonstrates complete absence of melanin in albinism

Chapter 23

HOW TO APPROACH HYPERPIGMENTED LESIONS

FIRST, EXCLUDE THE POSSIBILITY OF A MELANOCYTIC LESION

DETERMINE IF HYPERPIGMENTATION IS

GENERALIZED

-generalized hyperpigmentation		associated with endocrine diseases, malignancy, infectious diseases, drugs, metal ingestions

LOCALIZED

ELONGATED PIGMENTED RETE RIDGES ("DIRTY SOCKS")

-solar lentigo	middle aged or older	solar elastosis
-lentigo simplex	childhood	no solar elastosis

WAVY HYPERPIGMENTED EPIDERMIS

-ephelides	smaller	disappear or lighter in winter
-café au lait	larger	sporadic or associated with NF-1 and McCune-Albright syndrome

DERMAL PIGMENT INCONTINENCE

-melasma	increased epidermal melanin
-post inflammatory hyperpigmentation	normal epidermal melanin
-erythema dyschromicum perstans	focal interface vacuolar changes

RESEMBLE SEBORRHEIC KERATOSIS

-Dowling Degos disease	axilla, groin (unlike SK)
-Galli Galli disease	axilla, groin + focal epidermal acantholysis

INCREASED DERMAL SMOOTH MUSCLE

-Becker's nevus

HOW TO APPROACH HYPOPIGMENTED LESIONS

NORMAL NUMBER OF MELANOCYTES AND DECREASED OR NO MELANIN

Multiple disorders with same histology and clinical presentation, history, and electron microscopy help to separate them

-albinism	at birth	variable generalized pigment dilution
- Hermansky-Pudlak syndrome	at birth	bleeding + oculocutaneous albinism
-Chediak-Higashi syndrome	at birth	infections + oculocutaneous albinism
-Griscelli syndrome	at birth	albinism + immunodeficiency + neuro impairment
-"ashleaf" of tuberous sclerosis	at infancy	usually first sign of tuberous sclerosis
-nevus depigmentosus	birth/childhood	single stable patch
-hypomelanosis of Ito	at birth	follows Blaschko's lines+ neurological findings
-pityriasis alba	children+ adolescents	associated with eczema

DECREASED NUMBER OR NO MELANOCYTES AND DECREASED OR NO MELANIN

- vitiligo		depigmented milky white patches
-piebaldism		congenital white forelock
-Waardenburg syndrome		congenital white forelock + deafness
-idiopathic guttate hypomelanosis	shin	small (guttate) hypopigmented macules

NOTE: DON'T FORGET TINEA VERSICOLOR AS A POSSIBLE CAUSE OF HYPOPIGMENTATION

Disorders of pigmentation

Chapter 24

CUTANEOUS HETEROTOPIC LESIONS

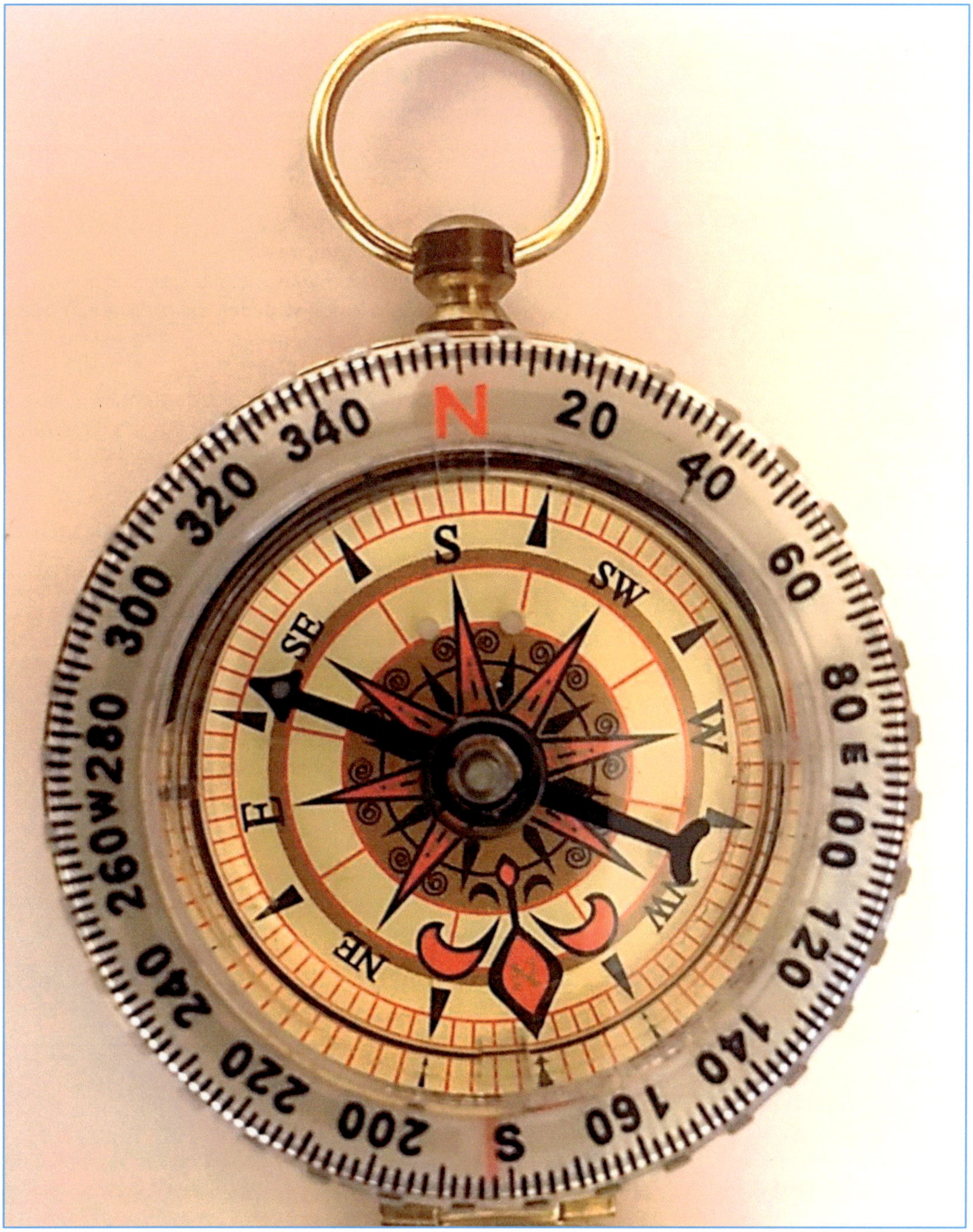

Cutaneous heterotopic lesions

ACROCHORDON
(SKIN TAG, FIBROEPITHELIAL POLYP)

-is not ectopic tissue but a benign growth
-predilection for areas of friction (axilla, neck, groin)
-more common in obese people and pregnant women
-polypoid, soft, skin-colored papules attached by a thin, pedunculated stalk

Histopathology
-**polypoid** lesion with **hyperkeratotic, acanthotic epidermis** and **absent adnexal structures**
-variably sclerotic collagenous stroma

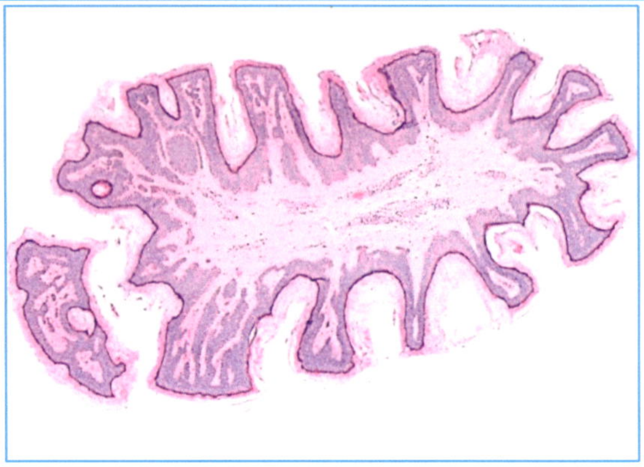

Polypoid skin tag with absent adnexal structures

SUPERNUMERARY/ RUDIMENTARY DIGIT

-congenital extra digit on hand or feet
-can be classified into 3 distinct categories based on location: postaxial (ulnar), preaxial (radial), and central polydactyly
-ulnar polydactyly is the most common type
-presents as a smooth or verrucous papule, most frequently on lateral aspect of a newborn's fifth finger
-represents amputation (traumatic) neuroma from in utero amputation

Histopathology
Supernumerary digit
-presents as miniaturized finger
-polypoid lesion with **central cartilage or bone**
-nail can be present
Rudimentary digit
-present histologically as traumatic neuroma
-polypoid lesion with numerous large neural structures haphazardly organized
-no bone or cartilage

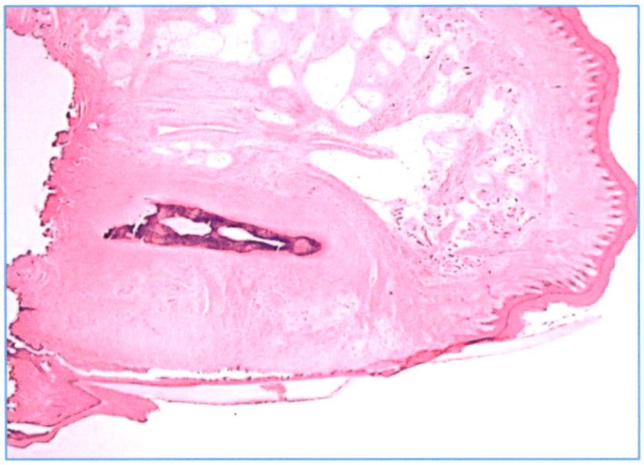

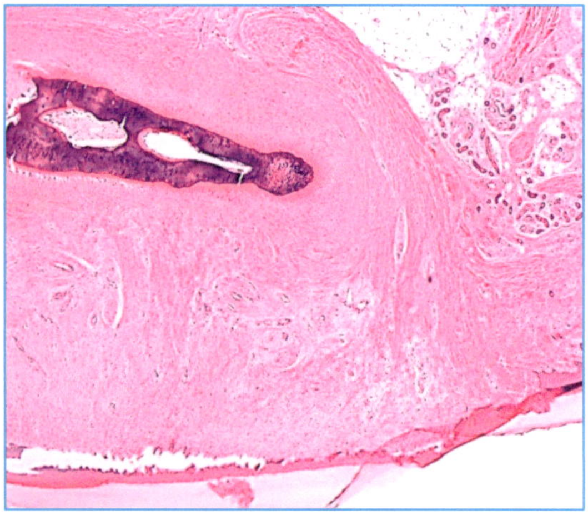

Supernumerary digit with central bone and attached nail

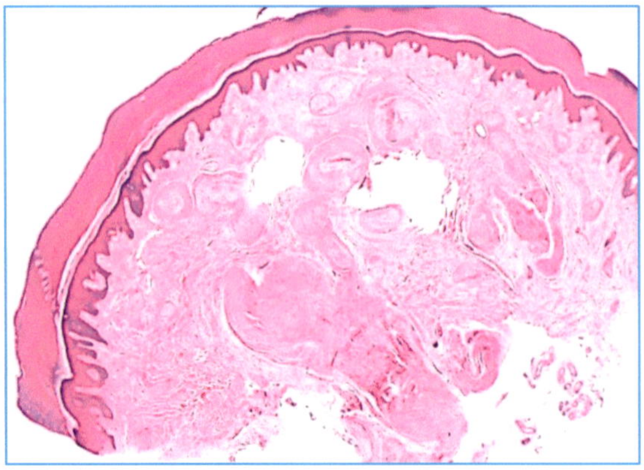

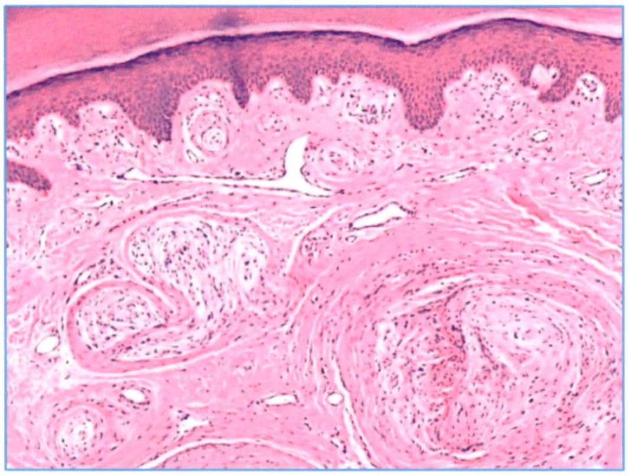

Rudimentary digit with numerous large, haphazardly organized dermal neural structures

Chapter 24

ACCESSORY BREAST TISSUE (SUPERNUMERARY BREAST)

-usually not evident until puberty
-typically appears as swelling/nodule in axillary area
-can occur anywhere along the milk line
-occasionally can include accessory nipple

Histopathology
-normal **mammary glands** surrounded by mature fat

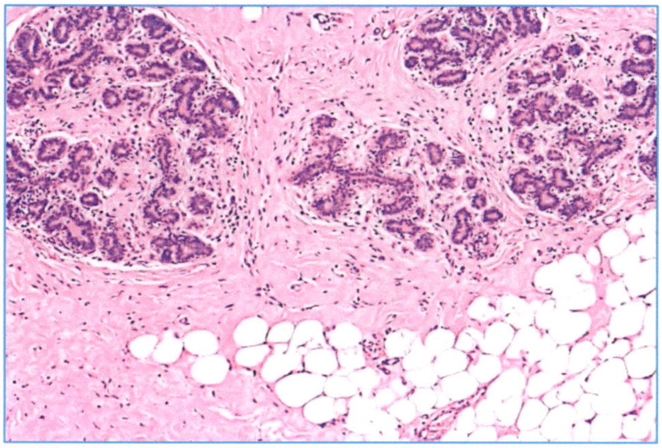

Accessory breast with mammary glands surrounded by fibroadipose tissue

SUPERNUMERARY NIPPLE

-solitary, slightly pigmented nodule present at birth
-may occur anywhere along the pathway of the embryonic milk line

Histopathology
-bares resemblance to normal nipple
-mild epidermal papillomatosis and hyperpigmentation
-**prominent dermal smooth muscles**
-**mammary ducts** and **glands** are present

ACCESSORY TRAGUS

-classically solitary **preauricular** nodule or papule
-can occur anywhere along the 1st branchial arch
-present at birth
-incidental or part of several genetic syndromes (Goldenhar, Treacher-Collins syndrome)

Histopathology
-polypoid lesion with **prominent vellus hairs**
-central fibroadipose tissue and **cartilage**

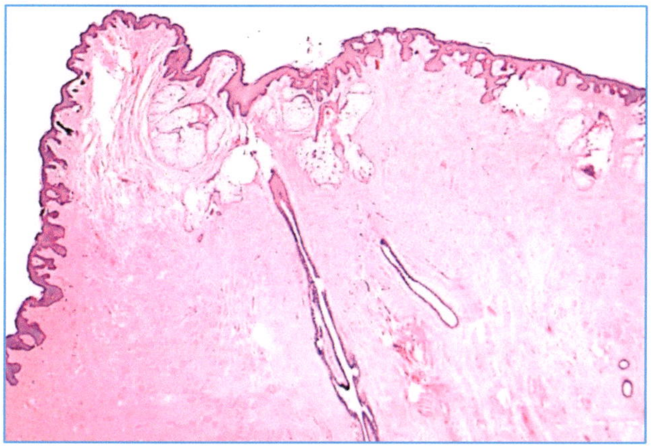

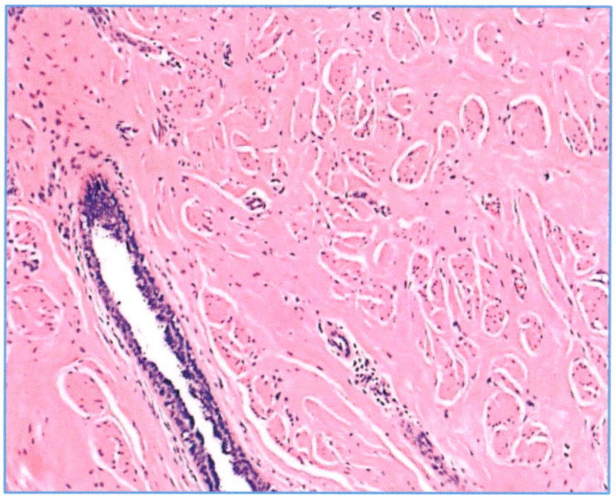

Supernumerary nipple with epidermal papillomatosis, mammary ducts, and prominent muscle bundles

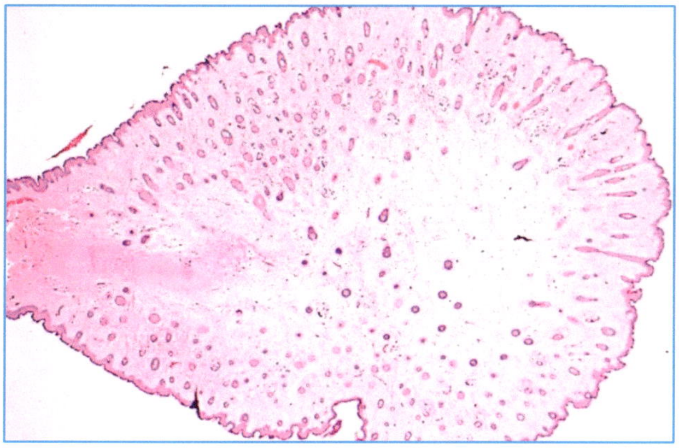

"Tag-like" accessory tragus

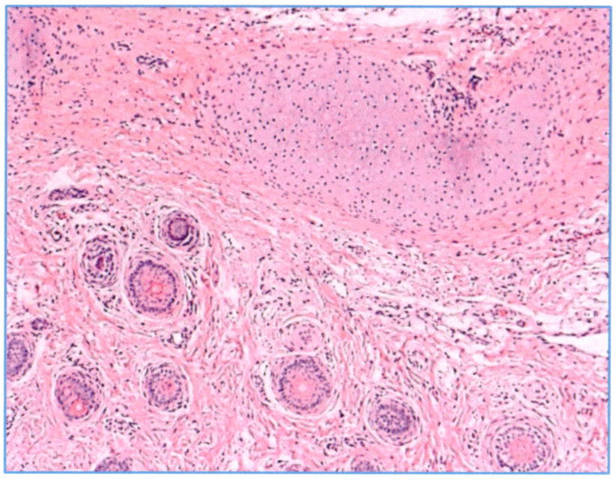

Accessory tragus with vellus hair and central cartilage

Cutaneous heterotopic lesions

ENDOMETRIOSIS

-endometrium-like tissue, consisting of glands and/or stroma, found outside the uterine cavity including skin
-most commonly near or around the umbilicus
-has a tendency to occur in scars (70%) but also in normal tissue
-presents as a single, firm nodule with color depending on the amount of hemorrhage and depth of the glands
-changes in size and color in correlation with menstrual cycle

Histopathology
-**uterine glands and stroma embedded in scar tissue**
-glands lining is CK7+, ER+, PR+ and varies in thickness depending on menstrual phase
-blood is common within the glands

HETEROTOPIC NEURAL TISSUE (NASAL GLIOMA)

-congenital malformation that presents at birth or early in life
-presents as a subcutaneous nodule (60%) at the bridge of the nose, polypoid mass within the nasal cavity (30%), or mixed (10%)

Histopathology
-normal epidermis with dermal and subcutaneous neural tissue
-**made mostly of normal glial tissue** that resembles a hypercellular scar and special stains are required to confirm diagnosis
-**occasionally neurons are present**, making diagnosis very easy

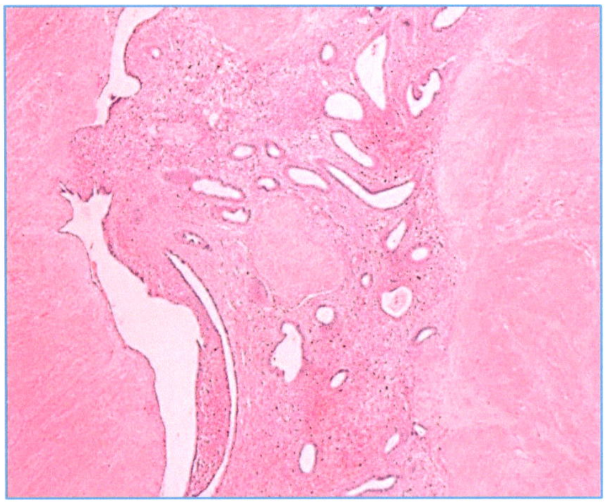

Endometriosis with uterine glands and stroma in scar

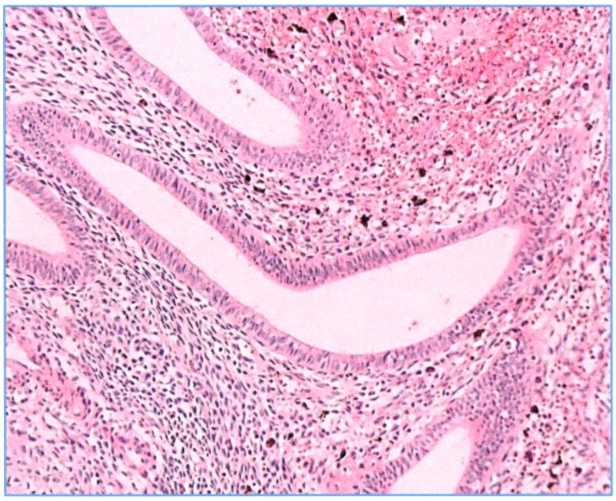

Hemorrhage and hemosiderin are present in the stroma

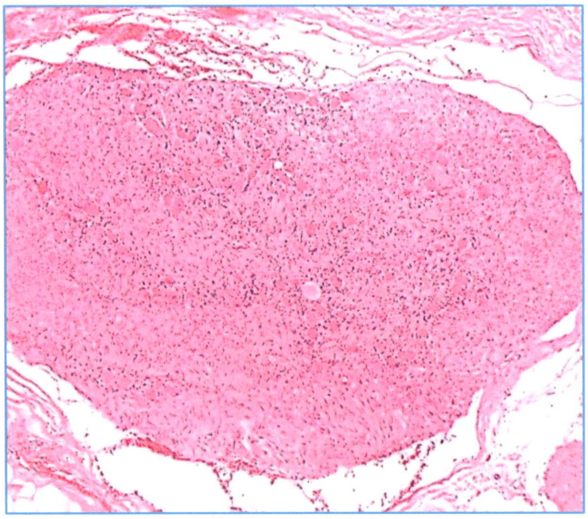

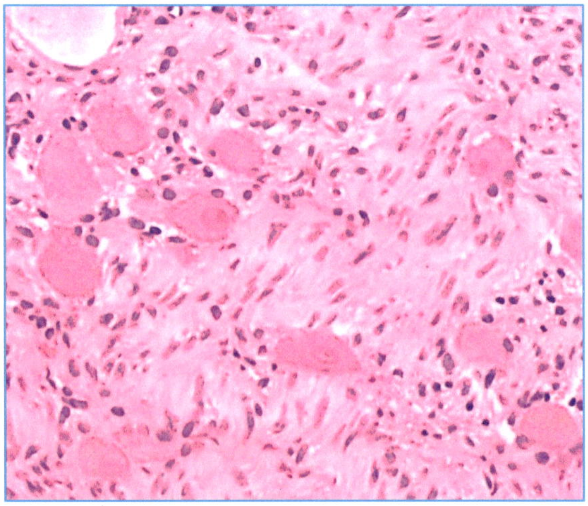

Heterotopic neural tissue with neurons surrounded by glial tissue

Chapter 24

HOW TO APPROCH HETEROTOPIC LESIONS

POLYPOID LESIONS

ANSWER IS IN THE CORE

-acrochordon	central core of fibroconnective tissue without hair follicles
-supernumerary digit	core contains bone/cartilage, nail can be present
-rudimentary digit	core contains large neural structures
-accessory tragus	core contains cartilage and vellus hairs
-supernumerary nipple	core contains mammary glands and smooth muscle

HETEROTOPIC TISSUE

RECALL NORMAL HISTOLOGY FROM THE FIRST YEAR OF MEDICAL SCHOOL

-heterotopic neural tissue	brain tissue from bridge of the nose
-endometriosis	uterine glands and stroma around umbilicus
-accessory breast	mammary glands and stroma in axilla

Cutaneous heterotopic lesions

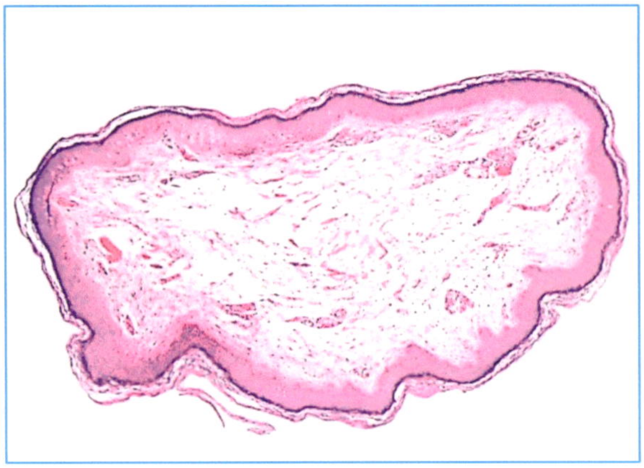

Acrochordon with fibrotic stroma

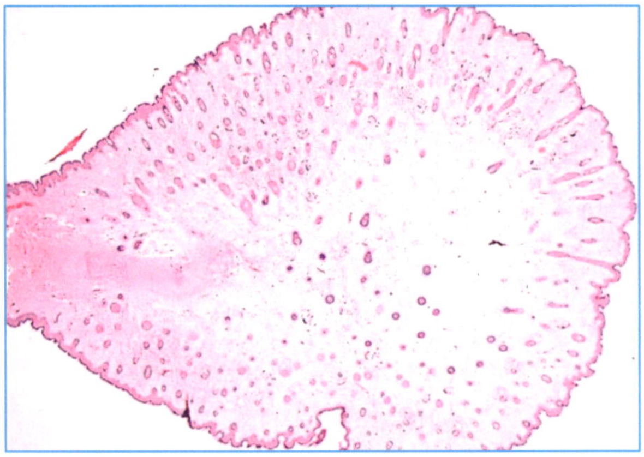

Accessory tragus with central cartilage and vellus hairs

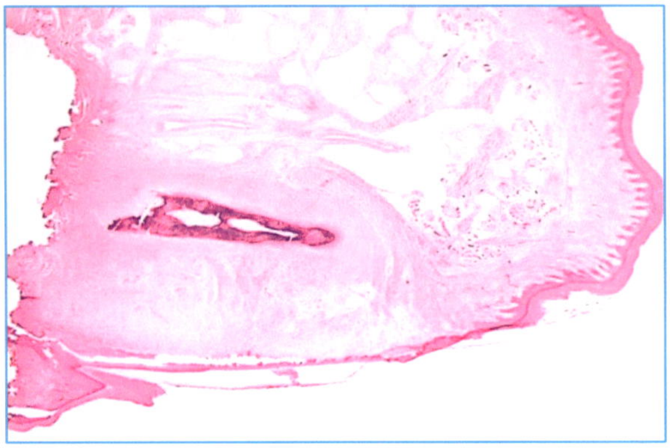

Supernumerary digit with central bone and nail

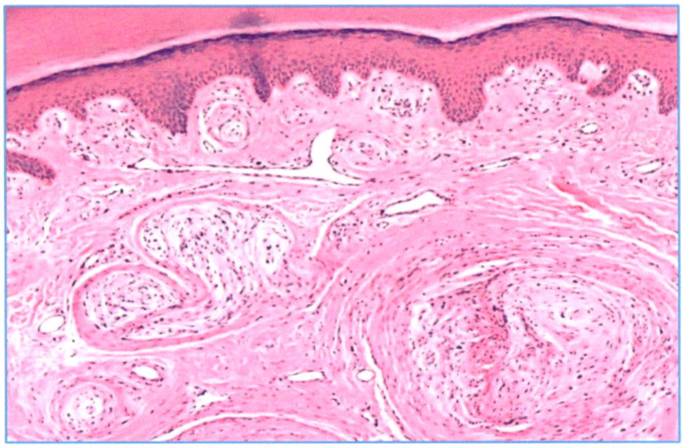

Rudimentary digit with numerous nerves

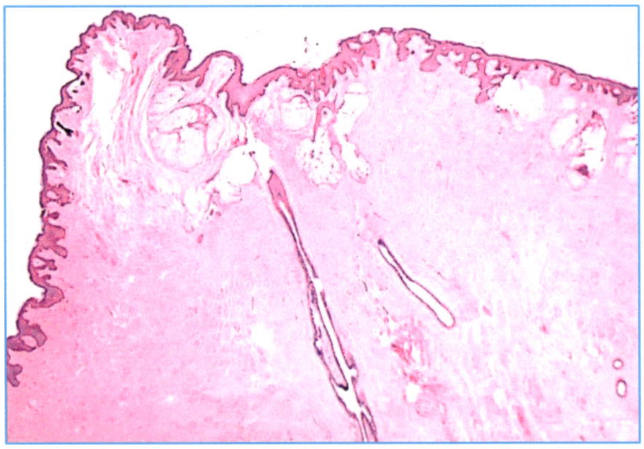

Supernumerary nipple with mammary glands
and numerous dermal muscles

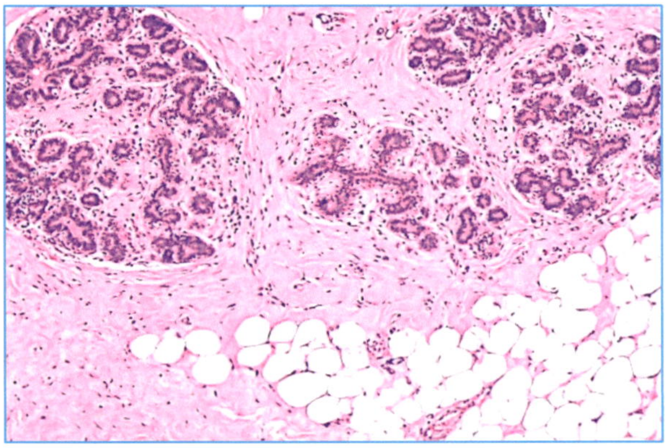

Accessory breast with mammary glands and no ducts

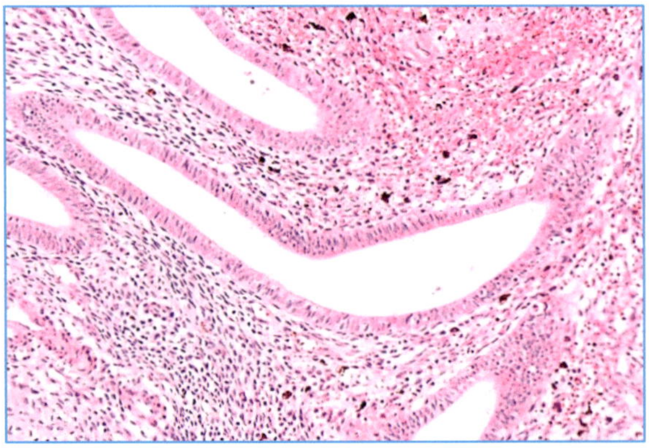

Endometriosis with uterine glands and hemorrhagic stroma

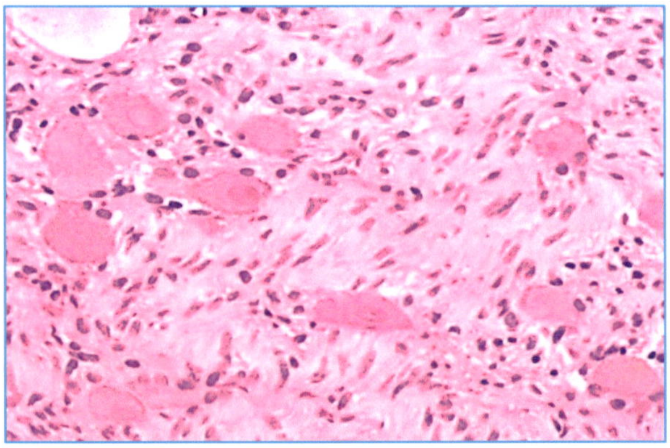

Heterotopic neural tissue with neurons and glial tissue

Chapter 25

CUTANEOUS CYSTIC LESIONS

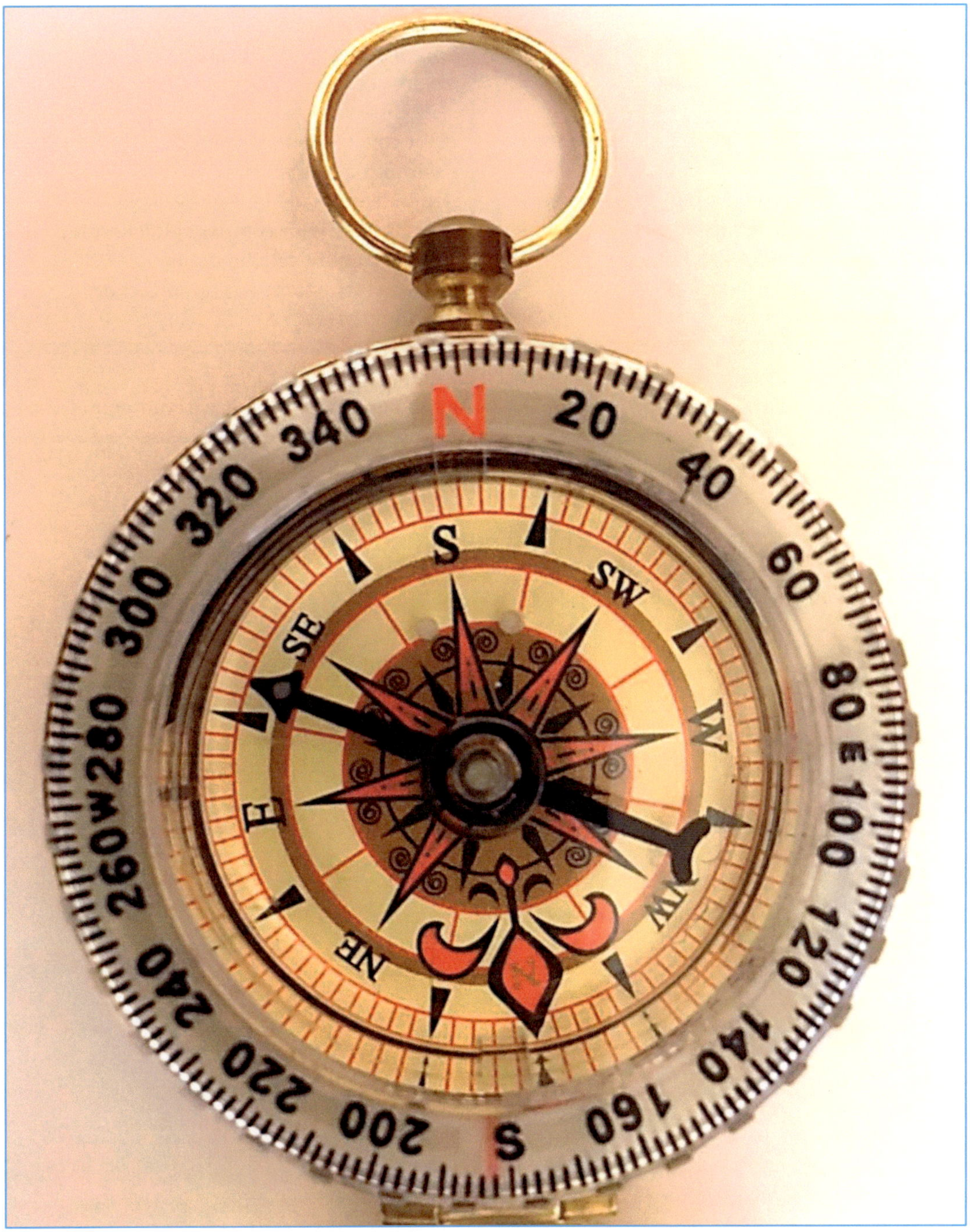

Cutaneous cystic lesions

EPIDERMAL INCLUSION CYST

-most common cutaneous cyst, presents as a skin-colored, firm, mobile subcutaneous nodule, often with punctum
-slow growing and painless (unless ruptured)
-associated with acne, injury, and Gardner's syndrome
-favored sites are face, neck, and trunk

Histopathology

-cyst lined with flat, stratified, keratinized **squamous epithelium with granular layer**
-cyst is **filled with laminated (layered, flaky) keratin**
-adnexal structures are **not attached** to the cyst wall
-if rupture occurs, a keratin foreign body reaction with giant cells develops

PILAR CYST (TRICHILEMMAL CYST)

-second most common cutaneous cyst
-originates from the outer hair root sheath
-presents as round bumps with a smooth surface texture
-painless unless ruptured
-predilection for the scalp (90%)
-more common in women

Histopathology

-cyst covered with stratified epithelium **without granular layer**
-epithelium made of 3-4 cells layer
-cyst is filled with **compact pink keratin** with **frequent calcifications**
-adnexal structures are not attached to the cyst wall

HYBRID CYST- represents hybrid between epidermal inclusion cyst and pilar cyst
-portion of the cyst lining has granular layer and another portion is without granular layer

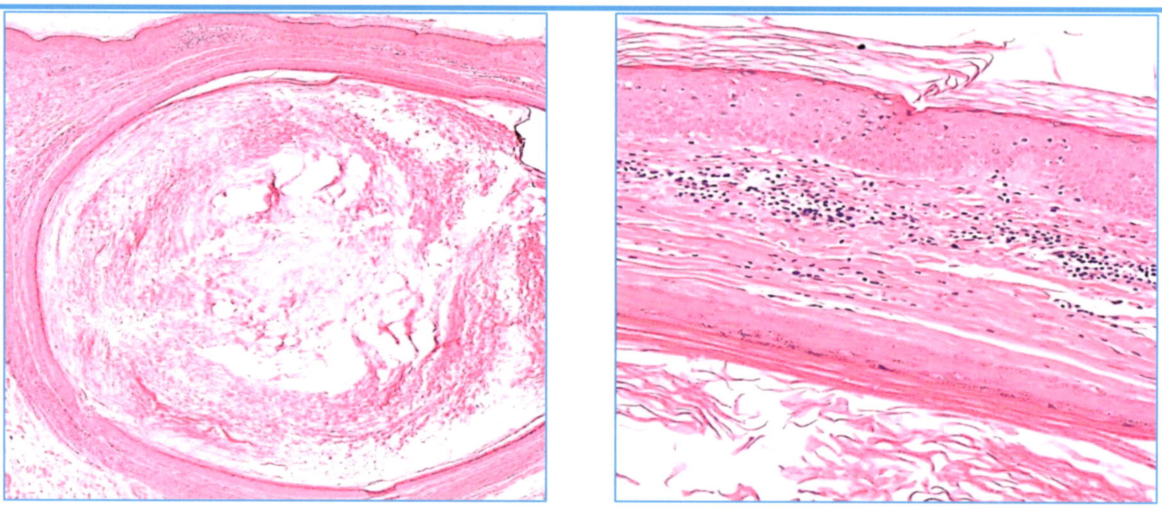

Epidermal inclusion cyst has lining with granular layer and is filled with flaky keratin

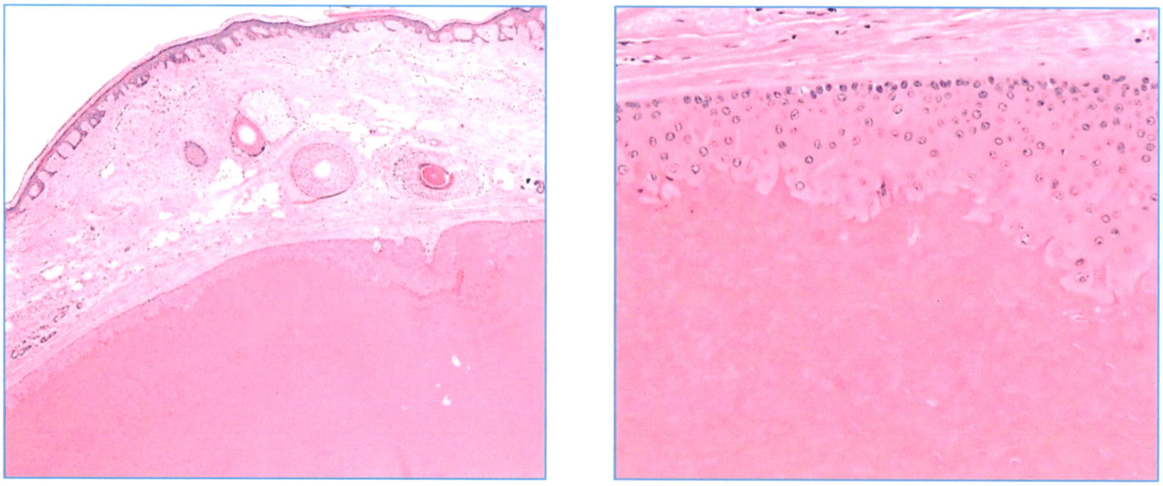

Pilar cyst has lining without granular layer and is filled with compact keratin

PROLIFERATING EPIDERMAL INCLUSION CYST

-epidermal inclusion cyst with proliferating epithelial lining
-presents as an enlarging subcutaneous nodule
-more common in men
-most common in anogenital area and scalp

Histopathology

-**a portion of normal epidermal inclusion cyst** usually present
-**squamous epithelium proliferates into the cyst lumen**
-proliferative areas are made up of bland squamous epithelium
-sometimes squamous eddies can be present (resembling seborrheic keratosis)
-squamous **proliferation can also extend outward** from the cyst
-no significant cytological atypia present
-important to carefully examine because in 10-20% of cases, squamous cell carcinoma arises in the outward proliferating epithelium

PROLIFERATING PILAR CYST (PROLIFERATING TRICHILEMMAL CYST)

-pilar cyst with proliferating epithelial lining
-more common in older women
-as in typical pilar cyst, scalp is favored site
-presents as an enlarging subcutaneous nodule

Histopathology

-**a portion of a normal pilar cyst** usually seen
-tumor has nodular cystic appearance and is relatively well circumscribed
-lobules of squamous epithelium are seen **extending into the cyst cavity**
-lobules also extend into the adjacent connective tissue **"rolls and scrolls"**
-tumor demonstrates **trichilemmal keratinization** without a granular layer
-no significant atypia or mitosis
-non-infiltrating borders

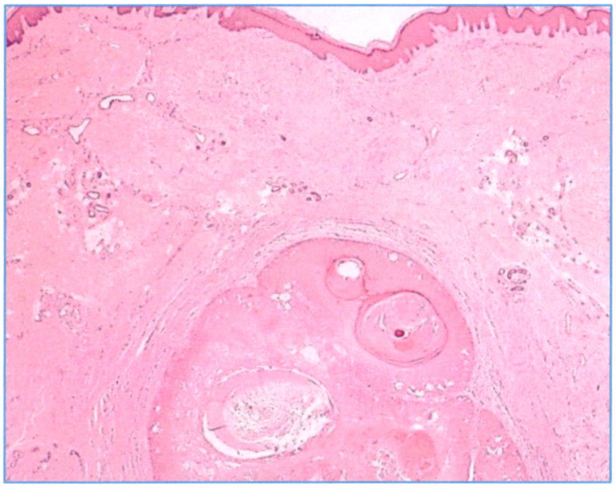

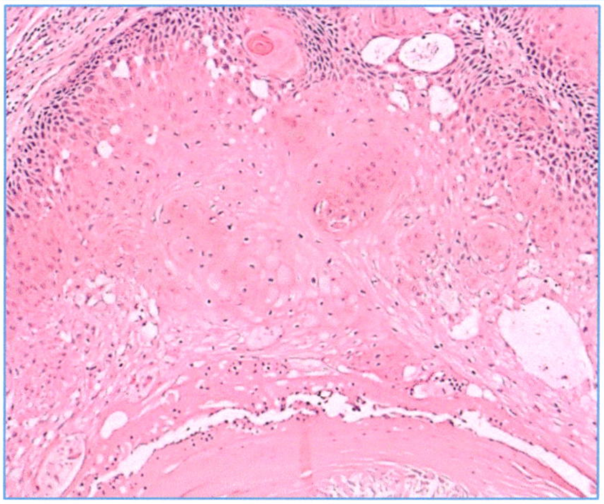

Proliferating epidermal inclusion cyst with proliferating squamous epithelium filling lumen of the cyst

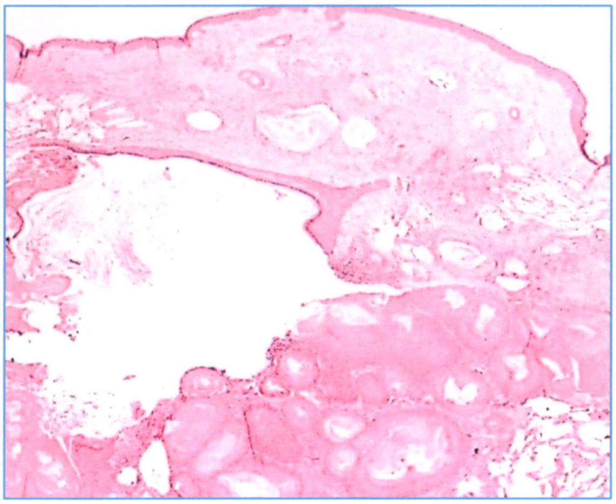

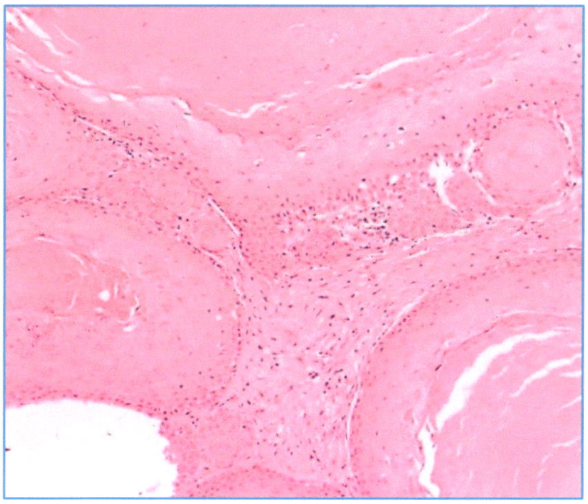

Proliferating pilar cyst with proliferating trichilemmal epithelium

Cutaneous cystic lesions

MILIA

-small, white-yellow papule
-primary location is on the eyelids, cheeks
-occurs at any age, even in infants
-can develop secondary to trauma or blistering diseases (porphyria cutanea tarda, bullous lichen planus, epidermolysis bullosa)
-there is also a rare eruptive form

Histopathology

-small superficial dermal cyst
-wall made of flat atrophic stratified squamous epithelium with central keratinous material
-**resembles miniature epidermal inclusion cyst**

VERRUCOUS CYST

-rare benign cyst clinically resembling epidermal inclusion cyst
-predominantly on the face, neck, and trunk
-often have overlying punctum

Histopathology

-cyst lined with acanthotic squamous epithelium
-**prominent irregular keratohyalin granules and koilocytes**
-squamous eddies reminiscent of inverted follicular keratosis can be present

DERMOID CYST

-present at birth or soon after
-results from inclusion of embryonic epithelium at the lines of fusion
-lateral eyebrow/canthus, midline forehead, and neck are common locations

Histopathology

-lined by **keratinizing squamous epithelium**
-**hair follicles and sebaceous glands are attached to the cyst wall**
-common **hair shaft fragments within the lumen**

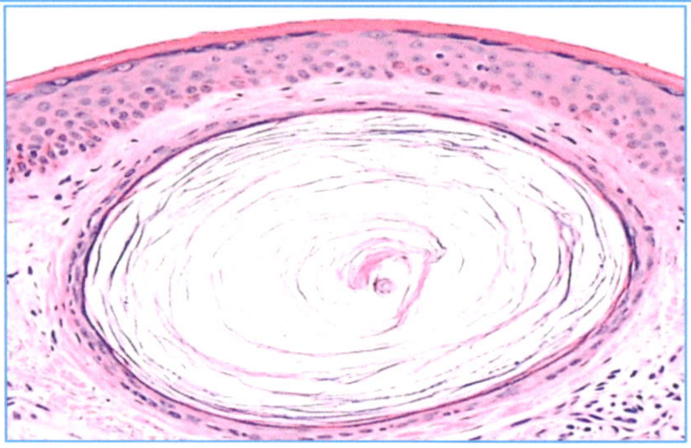

Milia lined with atrophic squamous epithelium

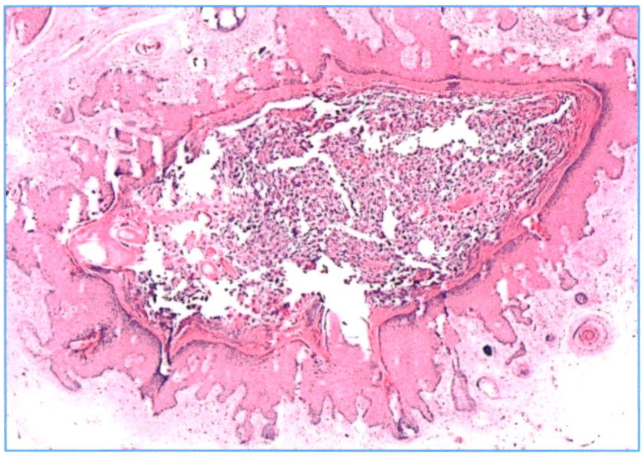

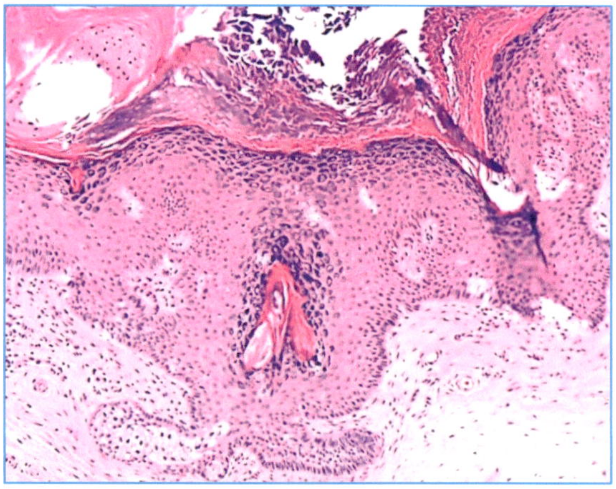

Dermoid cyst lined with squamous epithelium with attached hairs and sebaceous glands

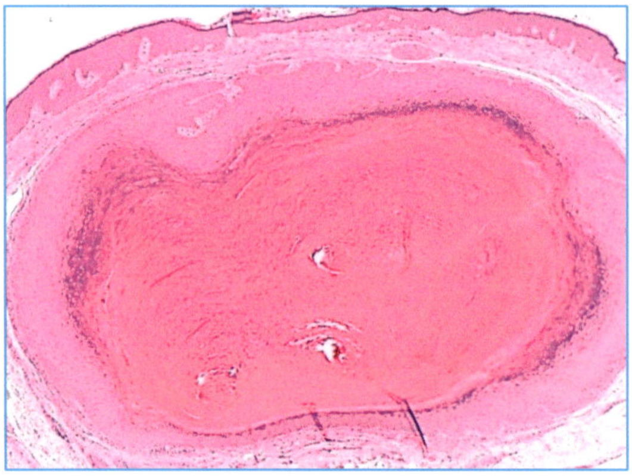

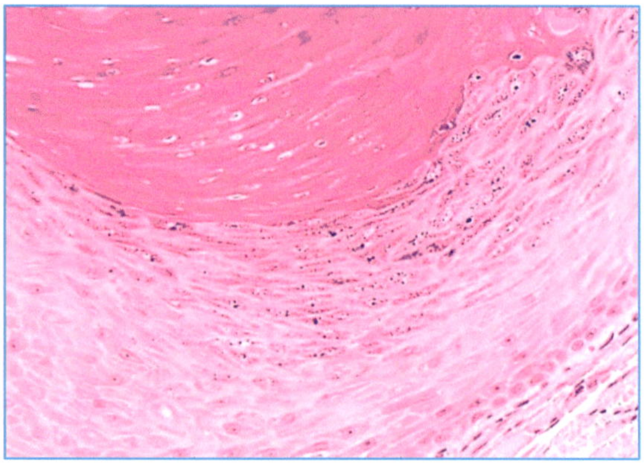

Verrucous cyst lined with squamous epithelium with changes resembling wart

PIGMENTED FOLLICULAR CYST

-solitary pigmented subcutaneous nodule
-often clinically mistaken for nevus
-predilection for the face
-more common in men

Histopathology

-dermal cyst with a flat, thin, stratified squamous epithelium
-lumen is filled with keratin
-pathognomonic finding is **multiple pigmented hair shafts in the lumen**

VELLUS HAIR CYST

-single or multiple small, red or brown papules, classically on the central chest
-eruptive vellus hair cysts occur in childhood/adolescence and can be inherited in autosomal dominant manner
-if it presents as a solitary lesion, it is not inherited

Histopathology

-dermal cyst lined with stratified squamous epithelium with granular layer
-**epithelium is flattened** and made of only few (3-4) layers of keratinocytes
-**multiple not pigmented vellus hairs** and **loose keratin** present in the lumen

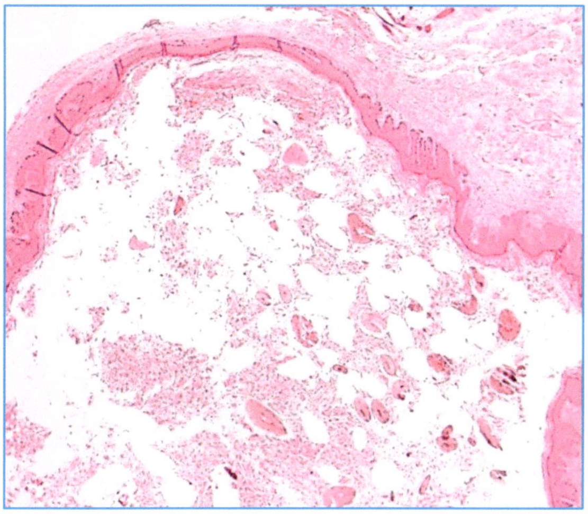

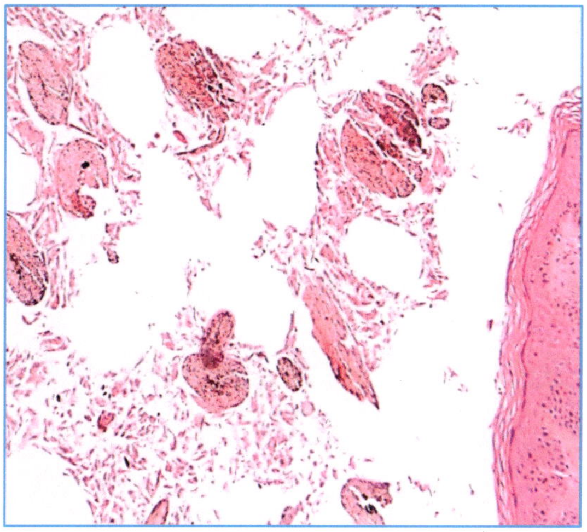

Pigmented follicular cyst with multiple pigmented hair shafts

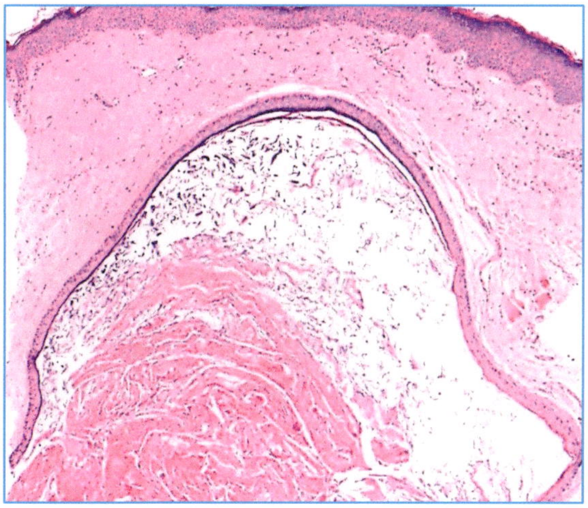

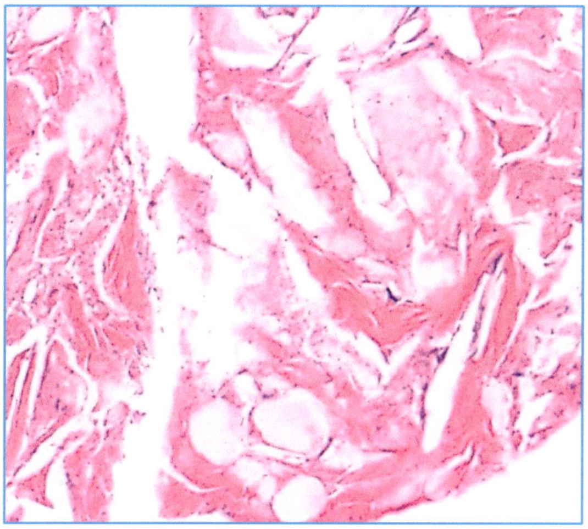

Vellus hair cyst with multiple not pigmented hair shafts

Cutaneous cystic lesions

HIDROCYSTOMA (ECCRINE and APOCRINE HIDROCYSTOMA)

-arises from eccrine or apocrine glands
-slow growing, painless, translucent, blue papules
-favors head and neck area with periorbital area being the most common site

Histopathology
-cyst has wavy outline and usually empty lumen
-**lined with two layers of cells**, an outer flat myoepithelial cells and inner cuboidal cells
-if of eccrine origin, cuboidal cells do not have snouts (decapitation secretion)
-if of apocrine origin, **apocrine snouts** present

STEATOCYSTOMA

-skin-colored to yellow papules, most often on the chest but can occur on the upper arms, axilla, or face
-may be solitary (steatocystoma simplex), usually appearing in adults, or multiple (steatocystoma multiplex), presenting during adolescence
-steatocystoma multiplex is inherited in an autosomal dominant fashion due to mutations in the *keratin* 17 gene

Histopathology
-cyst with folded, **corrugated** lining made of thin stratified squamous epithelium
-granular layer is absent
-characteristic **"saw teeth" shaped compact pink cuticle** forming cyst wall
-**sebaceous glands arise from the wall**

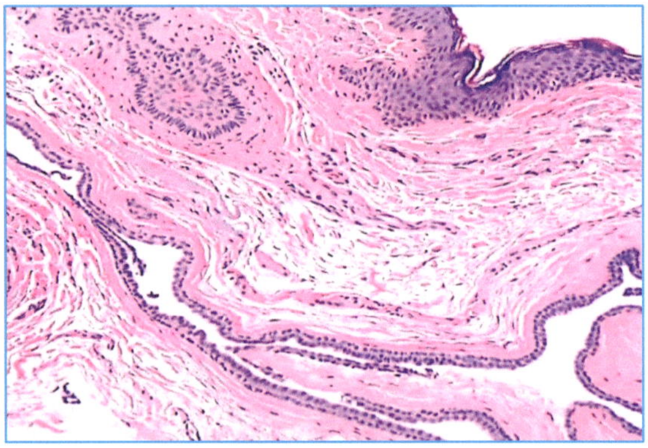

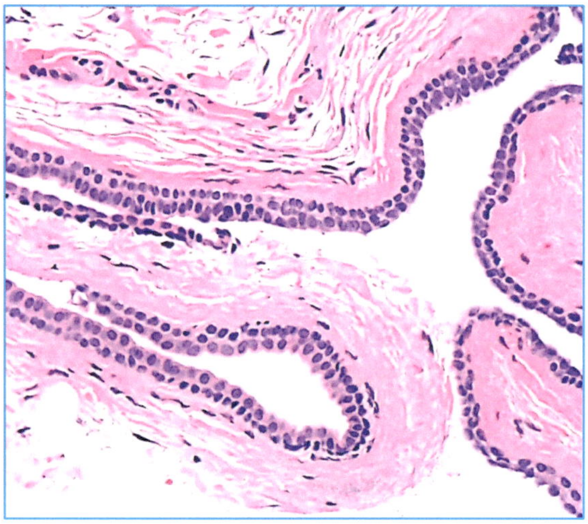

Hidrocystoma lined with uniform two cells layer

KERATOCYST

-rare cutaneous cysts that favor head/neck
-associated with nevoid basal cell carcinoma syndrome (Gorlin syndrome), resulting from mutation in *PTCH1* gene
-cutaneous keratocysts are much less frequent than odontogenic keratocysts

Histopathology
-characteristic **"saw teeth" shaped** compact **pink cuticle** on the surface
-**sebaceous glands** are **NOT attached**

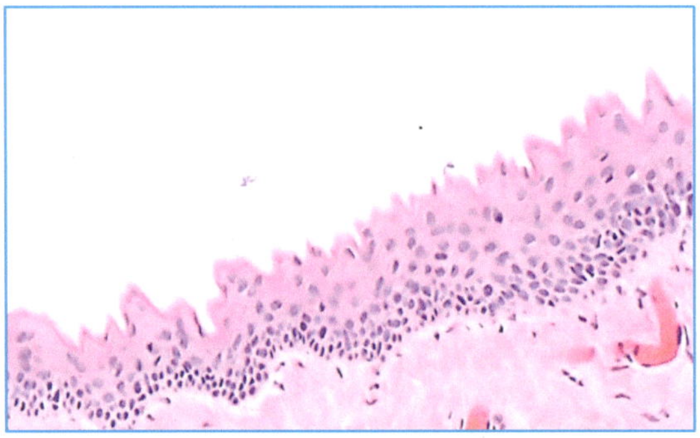

Keratocyst with "saw teeth" shaped pink cuticle

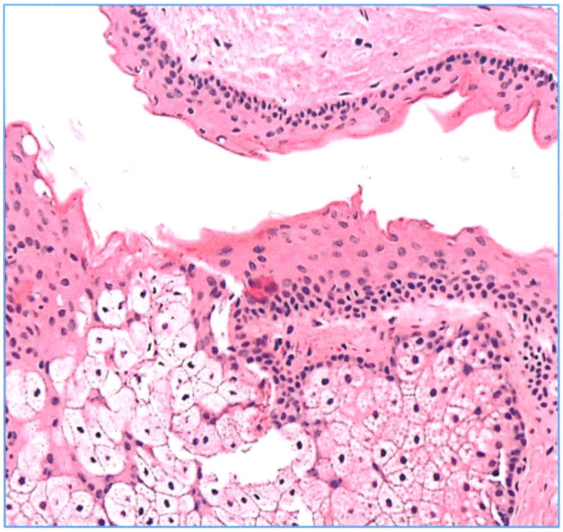

Steatocystoma with "saw teeth" shaped pink cuticle and attached sebaceous glands

BRANCHIAL CLEFT CYST

-developmental abnormality arising from embryogenic remnant of the branchial arches
-subcutaneous solitary mass typically presenting in 2nd-3rd decade of life
-accounts for almost 20% of neck masses in children (2nd after thyroglossal cyst)
-favors anterior border of the sternocleidomastoid muscle (lateral neck)
-secondary infection can cause rapid swelling

Histopathology
-cyst lined with mostly stratified squamous epithelium and focally ciliated columnar cells
-**heavy lymphoid infiltrate** in the cyst wall
-**germinal centers** are seen

BRONCHOGENIC CYST

-developmental abnormality arising from an abnormal budding of the tracheal diverticulum
-typically discovered in childhood
-predisposition for anterior neck or chest (presternal or suprasternal)
-symptoms may arise because of airway compression

Histopathology
-cyst with respiratory lining
-characteristic **ciliated pseudostratified columnar epithelium** with scattered **goblet** (mucin producing) **cells**
-**smooth muscle and cartilage** can be occasionally found in the wall

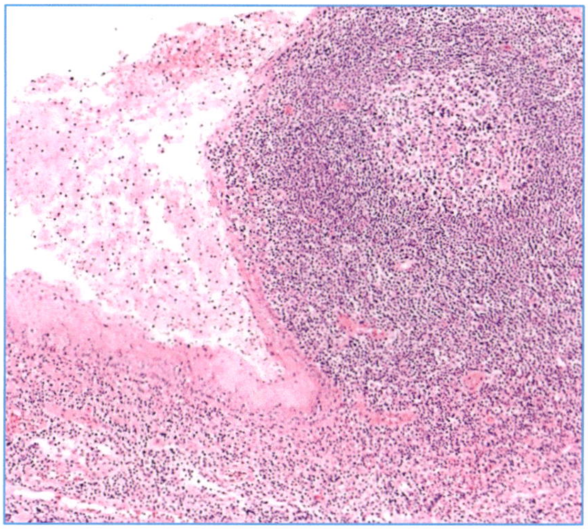

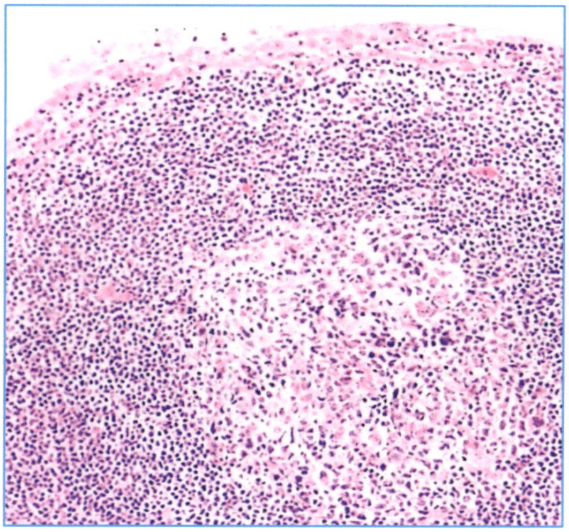

Bronchial cleft cyst with prominent lymphoid tissue and pale germinal center

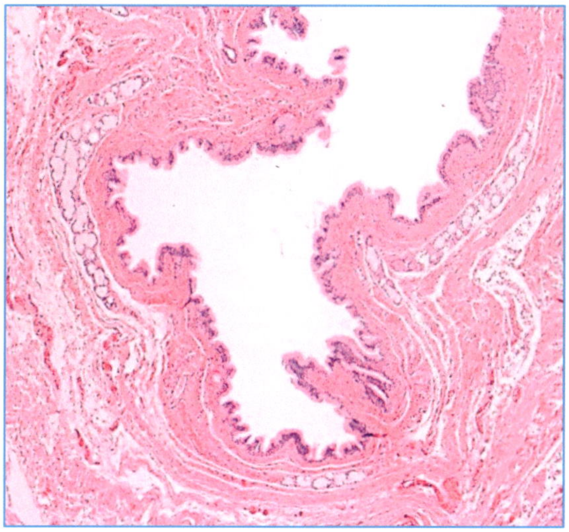

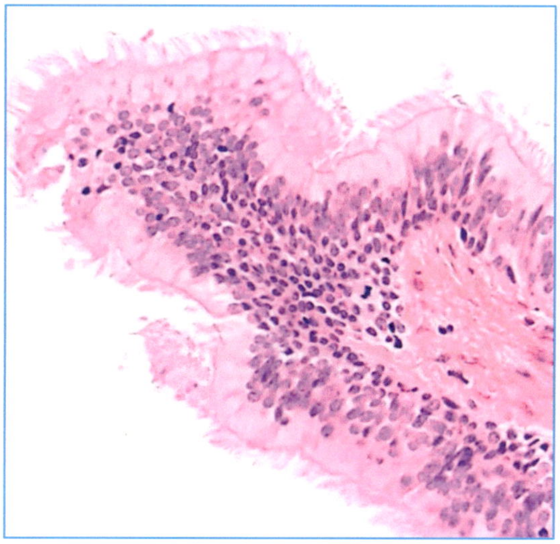

Bronchogenic cyst with ciliated pseudostratified columnar lining

Cutaneous cystic lesions

CERVICAL THYMIC CYST

-rare cyst that occurs when the thymopharyngeal duct, an embryonic structure connecting the nascent thymus with the embryonic pharynx, fails to close and disappear
-more often affecting the left side of the neck
-usually found near the carotid sheath
-manifests during the first decade of life
-slow, painless mass in the region between the angle of mandible and sternum

Histopathology

-flattened cuboidal epithelium or stratified squamous epithelium line the cyst wall
-**Hassall's corpuscles** (concentric pink structures made of epithelial reticular cells) and **lymphoid tissue** found adjacent to the cyst lining

THYROGLOSSAL CYST

-developmental abnormality seen in children and adolescents
-forms from a persistent thyroglossal duct
-presents as palpable, asymptomatic, deep midline neck mass
-the mass moves with swallowing
-**most frequent nodular neck lesion in children**

Histopathology

-cyst wall made of ciliated columnar/cuboidal cells
-**thyroid follicles** (small glands filled with pink content) are present near the cyst wall

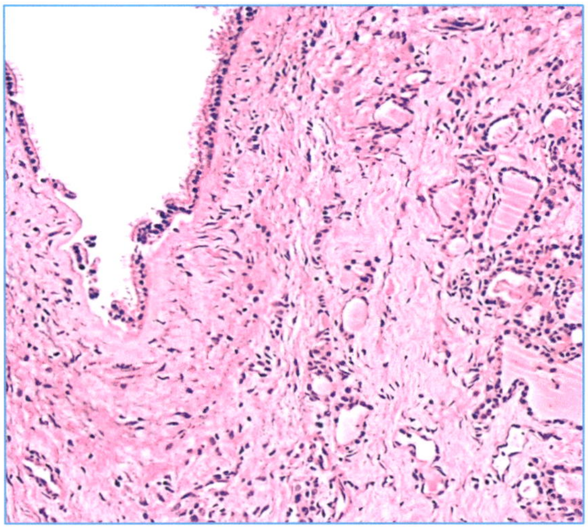

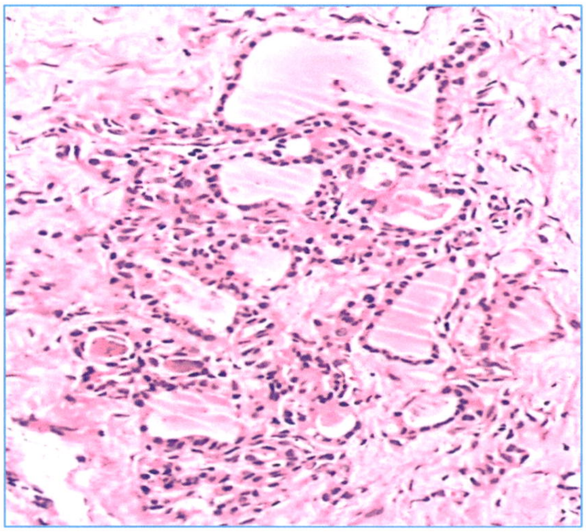

Thyroglossal cyst with columnar lining and adjacent thyroid follicles

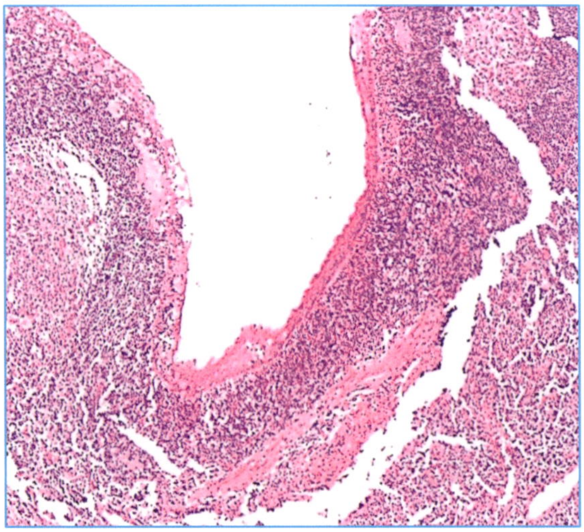

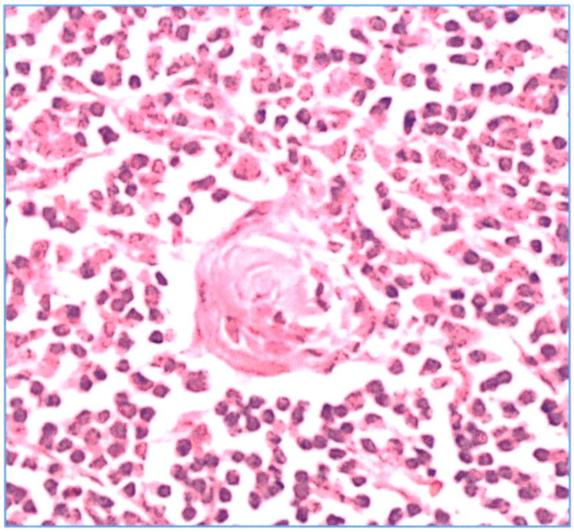

Cervical thymic cyst with prominent lymphoid tissue and pink concentric Hassall's corpuscle

CUTANEOUS CILIATED CYST/ CILIATED CYST OF THE VULVA

-rare benign cysts thought to be remnants of Müllerian duct
-most common on the lower extremities of young women
-comes to the attention of the patient with growth after puberty
-may be tender, but many are asymptomatic
-the ciliated cyst of the vulva is a variant which occurs at the vulvar vestibule
-usually small and non-tender, but larger cysts may cause discomfort

Histopathology
-**ciliated** cuboidal or columnar **lining**
-focal squamous or mucinous metaplasia can be seen

MEDIAN RAPHE CYST

-cyst resulting from abnormal separation of the urethral epithelium during development
-presents as a papule on the **midline, ventral aspect of the penis**
-may be first noted due to pain during intercourse

Histopathology
-the lining is usually **pseudostratified columnar epithelium**
-less frequently, may have mucinous glandular epithelium or a mixture of mucinous, transitional, and squamous epithelia

URACHAL CYST

-rare cyst from remnants of urachus that connect umbilicus and bladder during embryogenesis
-periumbilical deep subcutaneous nodule
-usually clinically silent but becomes painful when infected

Histopathology
-**lined by transitional urothelium** with underlying connective tissue
-lining can also be cuboidal or flat

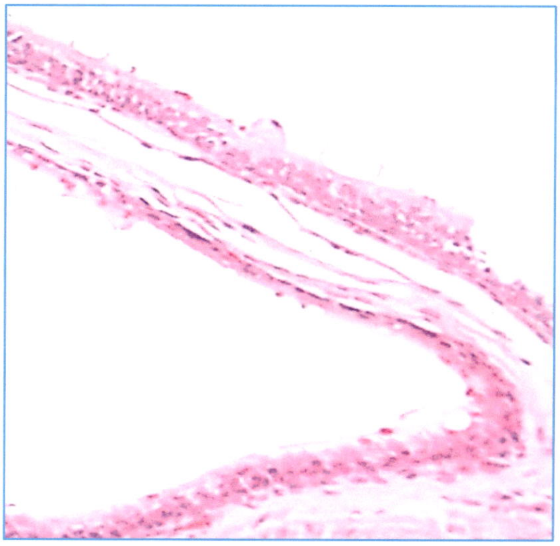

Urachal cyst with transitional urothelial epithelium

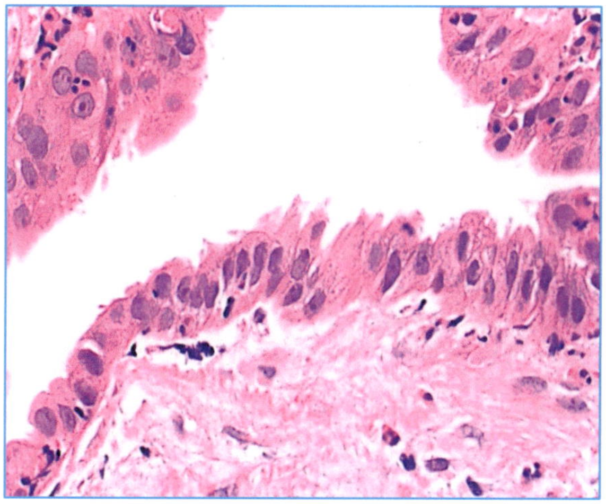

Cutaneous ciliated cyst with ciliated columnar lining

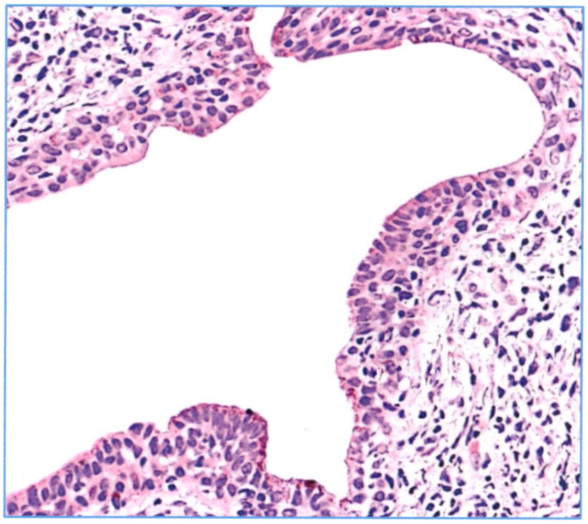

Median raphe cyst with pseudostratified columnal lining

Cutaneous cystic lesions

DIGITAL MUCOUS CYST

-benign, solitary, translucent, bluish pseudocysts of the digits
-occurs over the distal interphalangeal joints and at the base of the nail
-predilection for fingers over toes
-if drained, exudes clear gelatinous material

Histopathology
-it is a **pseudocyst,** meaning there is **no epithelial lining**
-**acral skin** with dense fibrous tissue encircling a **mucinous dermal nodule**

GANGLION CYST/SYNOVIAL CYST

-fluid-filled subcutaneous nodule associated with a joint or tendon sheath
-most often occurs on the dorsal wrist along the joint line
-occasional pain or numbness may occur

Histopathology
-large **irregularly shaped pseudocyst**
-no epithelial lining
-in a synovial cyst, **lining is fibrotic** with **synovial cells** on the surface
-in ganglion cyst, **lining is fibrotic without synovial cells**

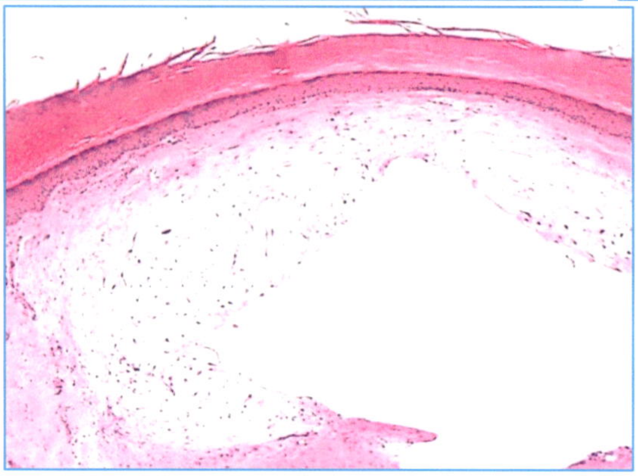

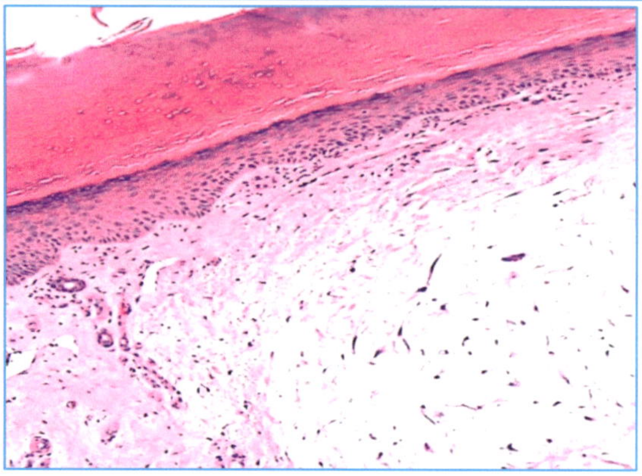

Digital mucous cyst of acral skin with accumulation of bluish dermal mucin

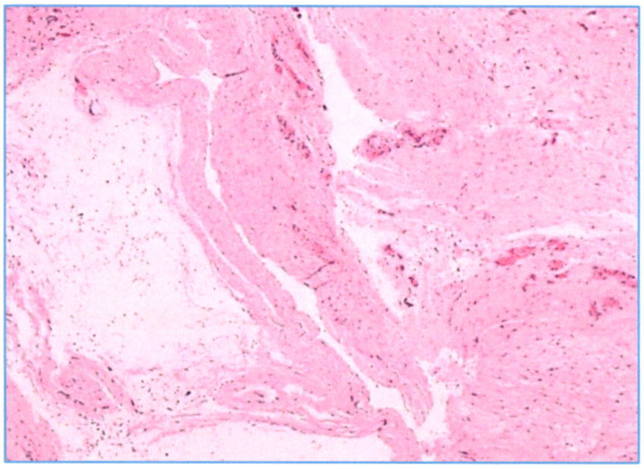

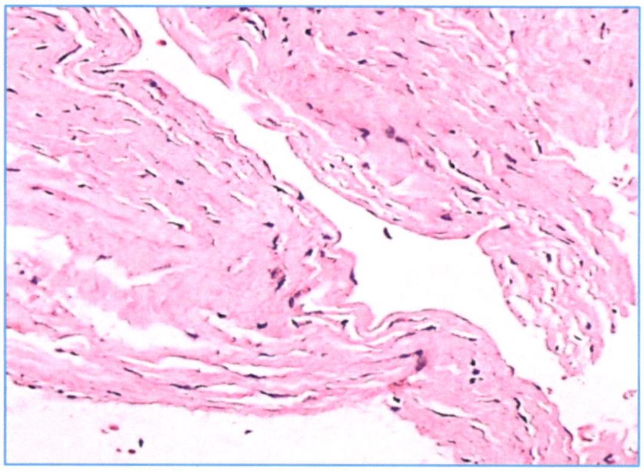

Ganglion cyst with fibrotic tissue surrounding irregular open spaces

PSEUDOCYST OF THE AURICLE

-cystic swelling of the upper anterior part of the ear
-arises over the period of a few weeks
-most common in men, associated with chronic trauma (wrestling, cell phone use)

Histopathology
-pseudocyst within the cartilage
-appears as **cracked cartilage**
-chondrocytes appear focally degenerated
-inflammation is not present

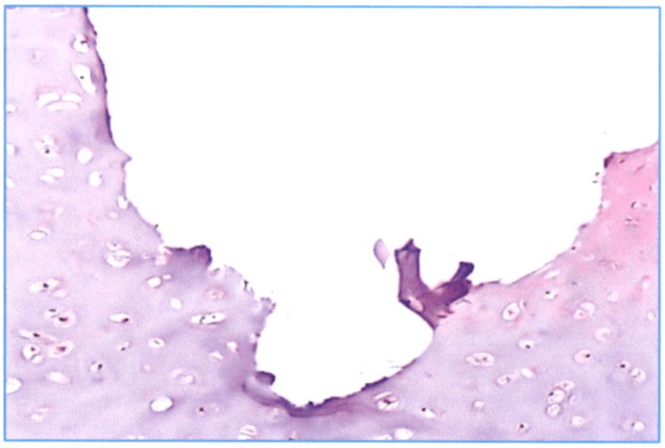

Pseudocyst of the auricle with degenerated chondrocytes

Chapter 25

HOW TO APPROACH CYSTIC LESIONS

DETERMINE IF WALL IS MADE OF EPITHELIUM (TRUE CYST) OR FIBROUS TISSUE (PSEUDOCYST)

CYSTS

LINED WITH SQUAMOUS EPITHELIUM WITHOUT A GRANULAR LAYER

-pilar (trichilemmal) cyst	typically on scalp

LINED WITH SQUAMOUS EPITHELIUM WITH A GRANULAR LAYER:

-epidermal inclusion cyst	large cyst filled with keratin
-milia	small cyst with thin wall (2-4 layers) filled with keratin
-verrucous cyst	keratohyaline granules + focal koilocytes
-pigmented follicular cyst	like EIC + pigmented hair shafts within cyst
-vellus hair cyst	like EIC + multiple vellus hairs within cyst
-dermoid cyst	like EIC + attached hair follicles and sebaceous glands
-statocystoma	"saw teeth" shaped cuticle + attached sebaceous glands
-keratocyst	"saw teeth" shaped cuticle + no sebaceous glands

LINED WITH SQUAMOUS EPITHELIUM WITH AND WITHOUT GRANULAR LAYER

-hybrid cyst	part EIC + part pilar cyst

LINED WITH CILIATED/CUBOIDAL CELLS AND/OR VARIABLE SQUAMOUS EPITHELIUM

-bronchogenic cyst	mostly ciliated epithelium
-branchial cleft cyst	mostly squamous epithelium and only focal ciliated + heavy lymphoid infiltrate abuts wall + vague germinal centers
-cervical thymic cyst	mostly cuboidal and focal squamous epithelium + heavy lymphoid infiltrate abuts wall + Hassall's corpuscle
-thyroglossal cyst	ciliated and cuboidal epithelium + adjacent thyroid follicles
-cutaneous ciliated cyst	small cyst with ciliated lining, on lower extremities or vulva
-median raphe cyst	small cyst with columnar lining, on penis
-urachal cyst	columnar/transitional epithelium, periumbilical
-hidrocystoma	two layers of cuboidal cells, on face

LINED WITH EPIDERMIS THAT PROLIFERATES INWARD AND OUTWARD

-proliferating pilar cyst	trichilemmal epidermis without a granular layer
-proliferating epidermal cyst	epidermis with a granular layer

PSEUDOCYSTS (NO EPITHELIAL LINING)

-digital mucous cyst	dermal mucin surrounded by fibrous tissue	digits
-synovial cyst	irregular spaces lined with synovial cells	wrist
-ganglion cyst	irregular spaces lined with fibroblasts	wrist
-pseudocyst of auricle	crack in degenerated cartilage	ear
-pilonidal sinus (cyst)	ruptured follicle + hair shafts + gran. tissue	intergluteal

Cutaneous cystic lesions

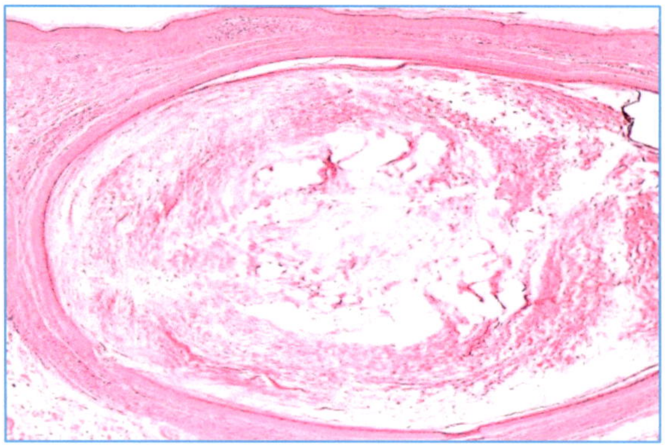

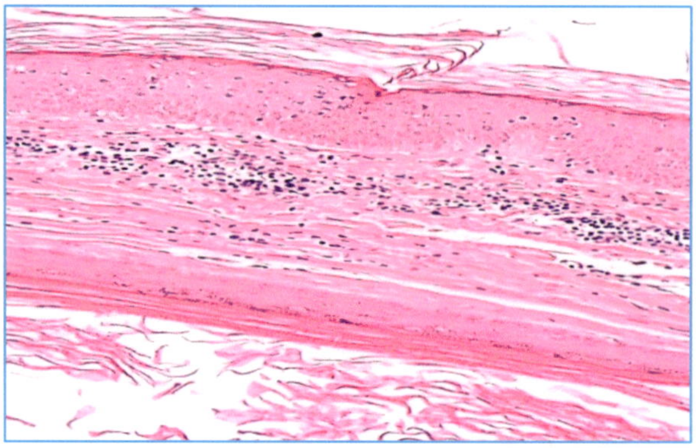

EIC with epidermal lining containing granular layer

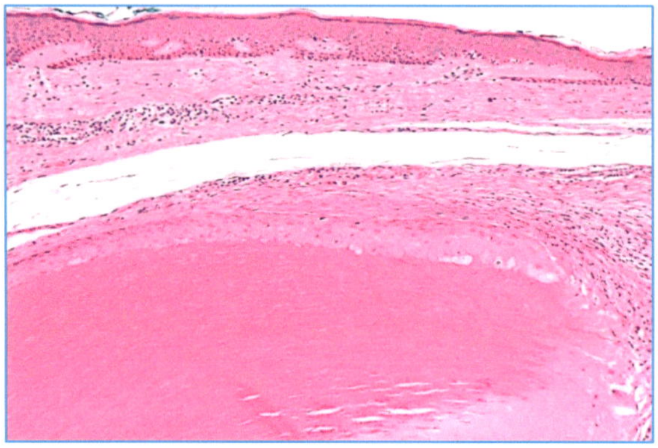

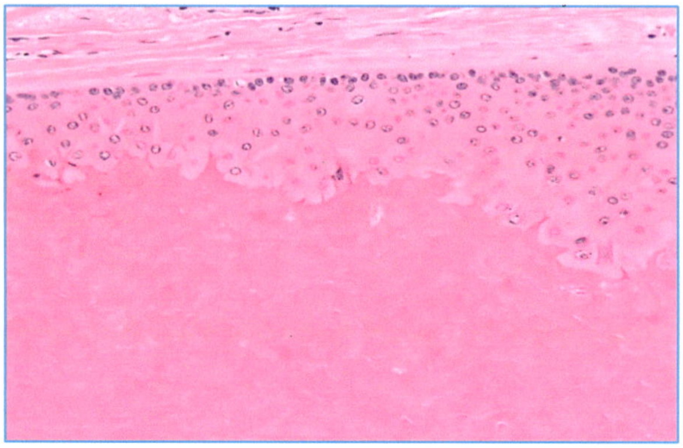

Pilar cyst with epidermal lining without granular layer

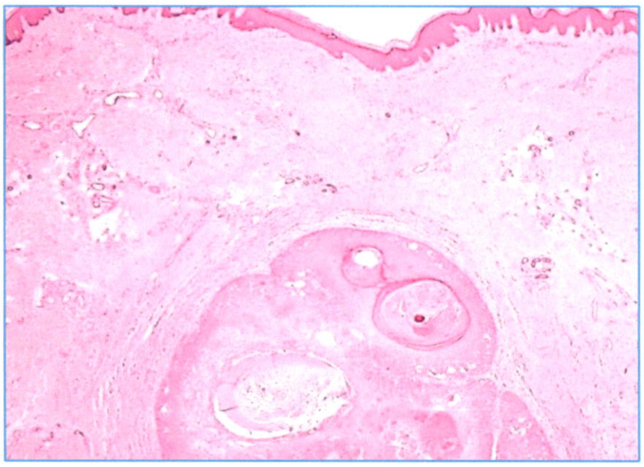

Proliferating EIC with growth within or outside of cyst

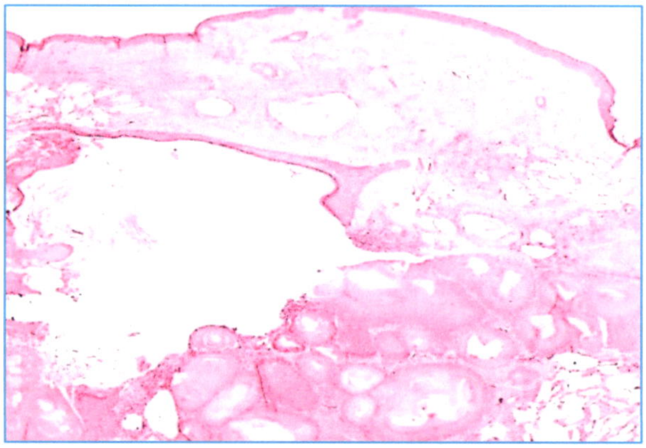

Proliferating pilar cyst with growth inside and outside of cyst

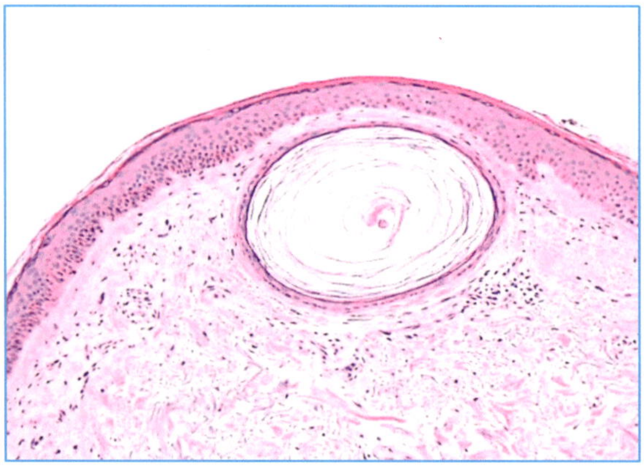

Milia looks like miniaturized EIC

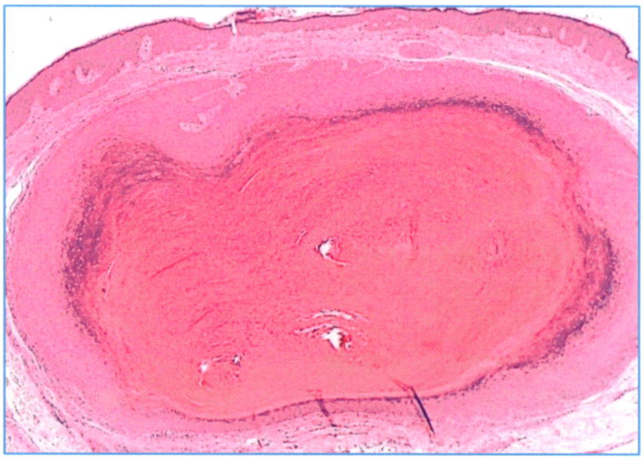

Verrucous cyst looks like EIC with koilocytes

Chapter 25

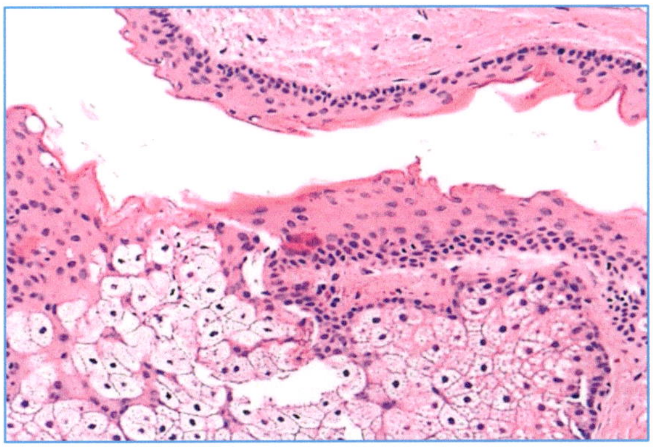

Steatocystoma with "saw-tooth" cuticle and sebaceous gland

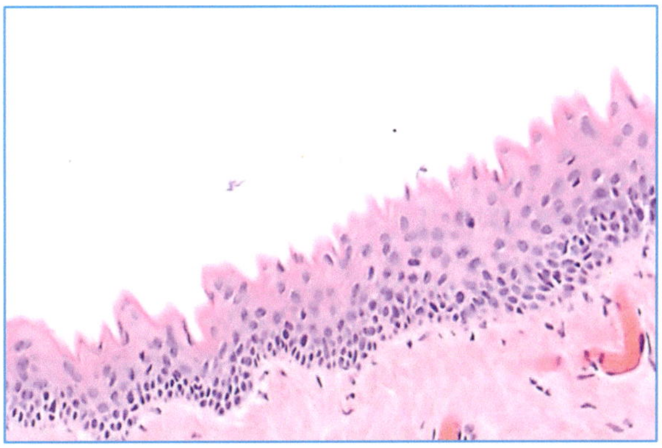

Keratocyst with "saw-tooth" cuticle and no sebaceous glands

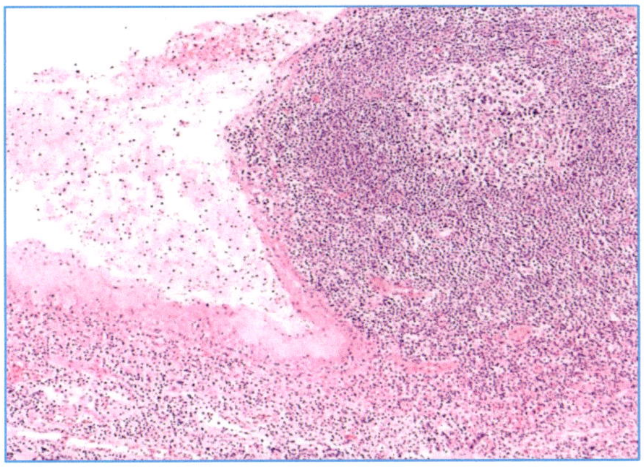

Bronchial cleft cyst with lymphocytic infiltrate and germinal center

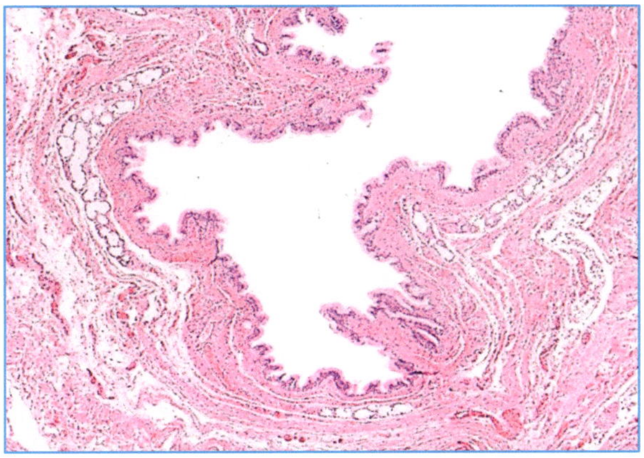

Bronchogenic cyst with ciliated lining

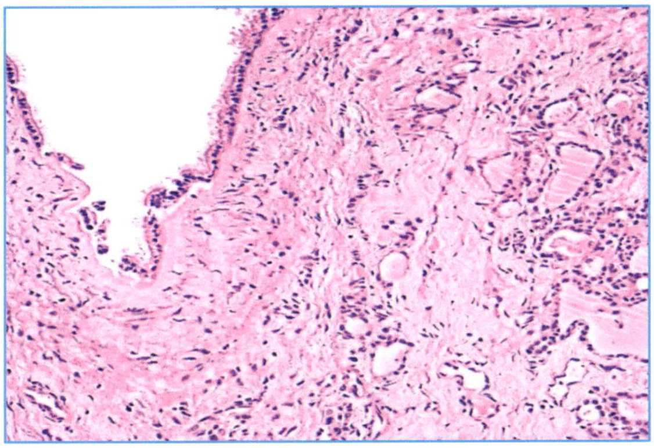

Thyroglossal cyst with adjacent thyroid follicles

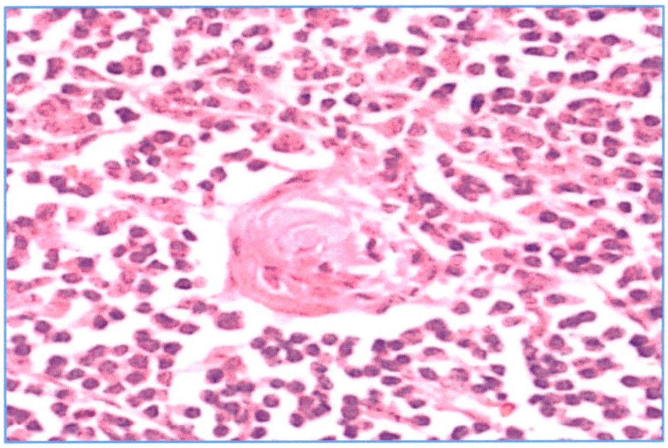

Cervical thymic cyst with Hassall's corpuscle

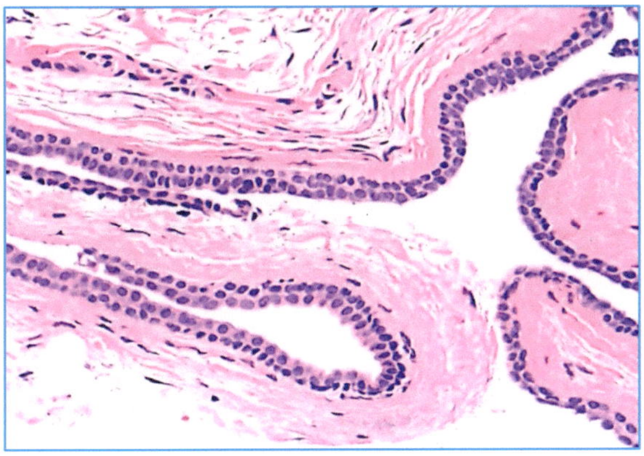

Hidrocystoma with cuboidal lining two cell layers thick

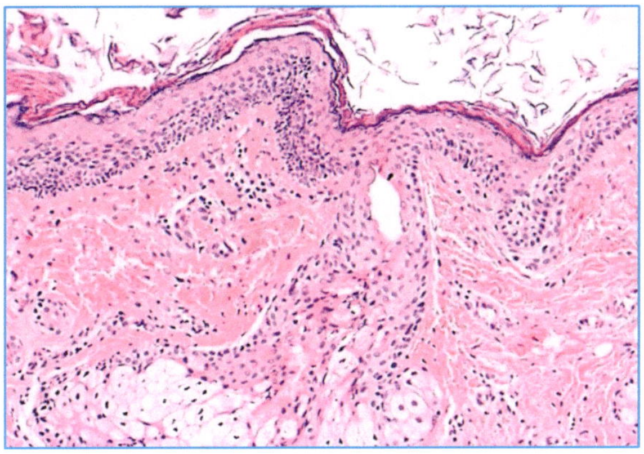

Dermoid cyst with attached pilosebaceous units

Cutaneous cystic lesions

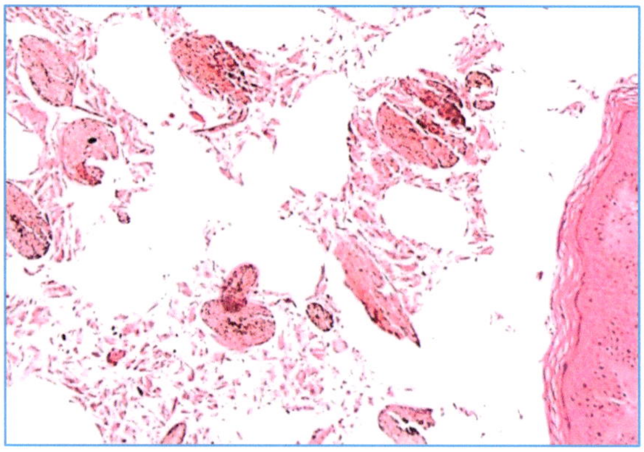

Pigmented follicular cyst is "EIC-like" with pigmented hairs

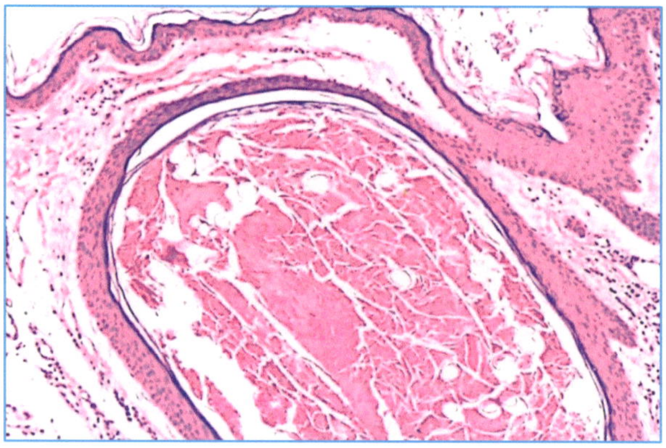

Vellus hair cyst is "EIC-like" with non-pigmented vellus hairs

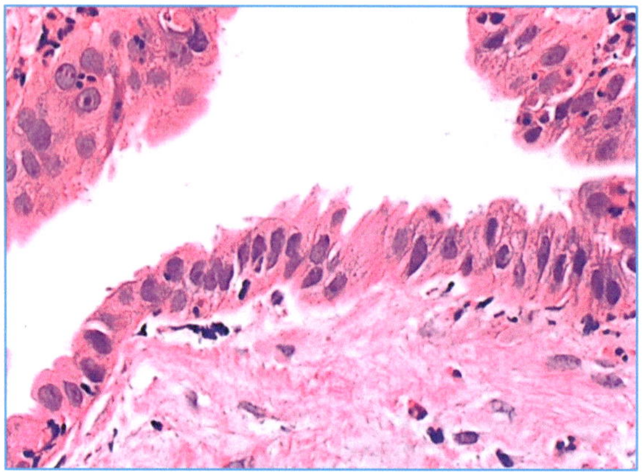

Cutaneous ciliated cyst with ciliated lining

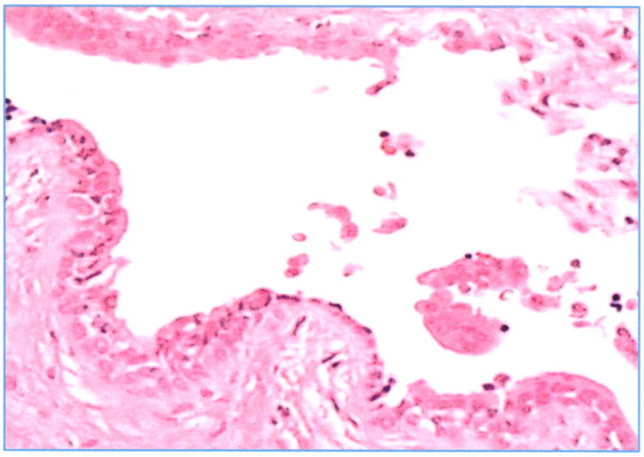

Median raphe cyst is penile cyst with cuboidal lining

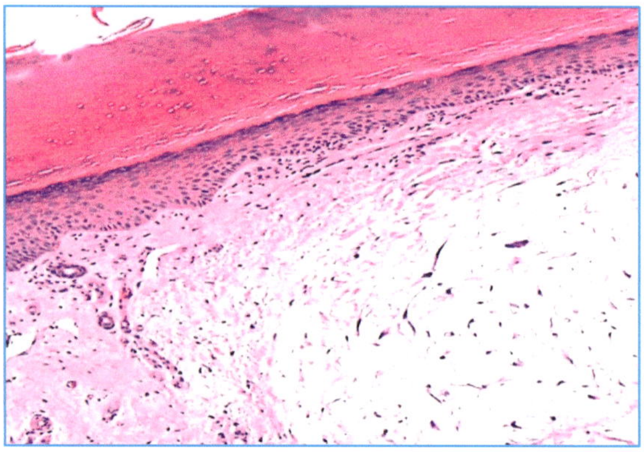

Digital mucous cyst with dermal mucinous aggregate

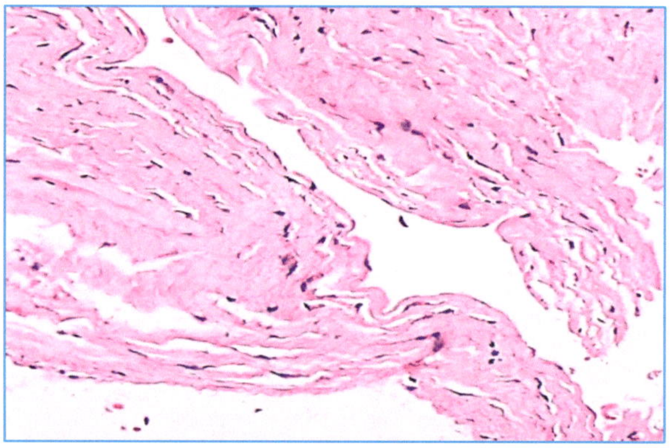

Ganglion cyst is pseudocyst with fibroconnective tissue lining

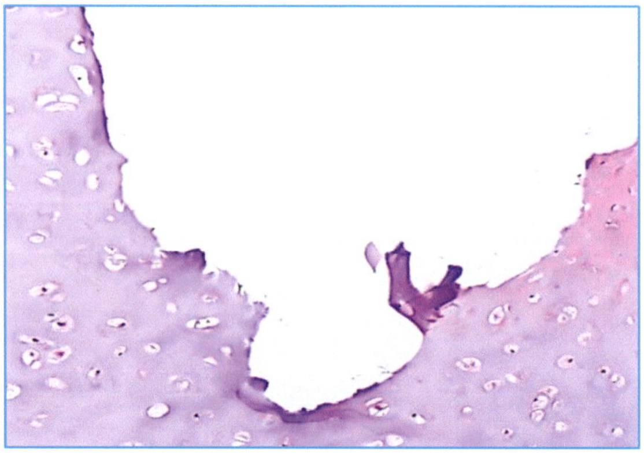

Pseudocyst of the auricle with fissure in cartilage

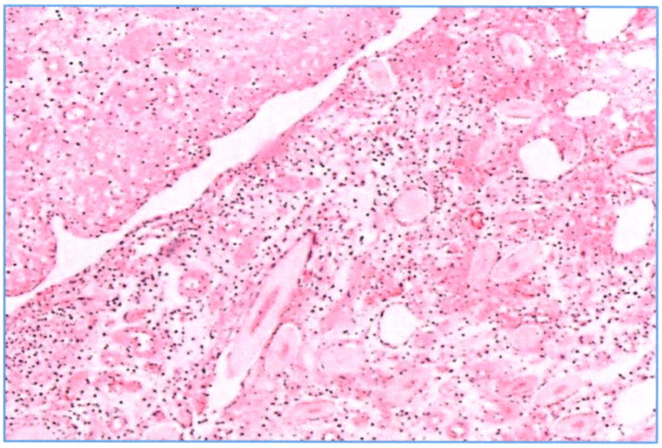

Pilonidal cyst (sinus) with
naked hair shafts in granulation tissue

Chapter 26

EPIDERMAL TUMORS

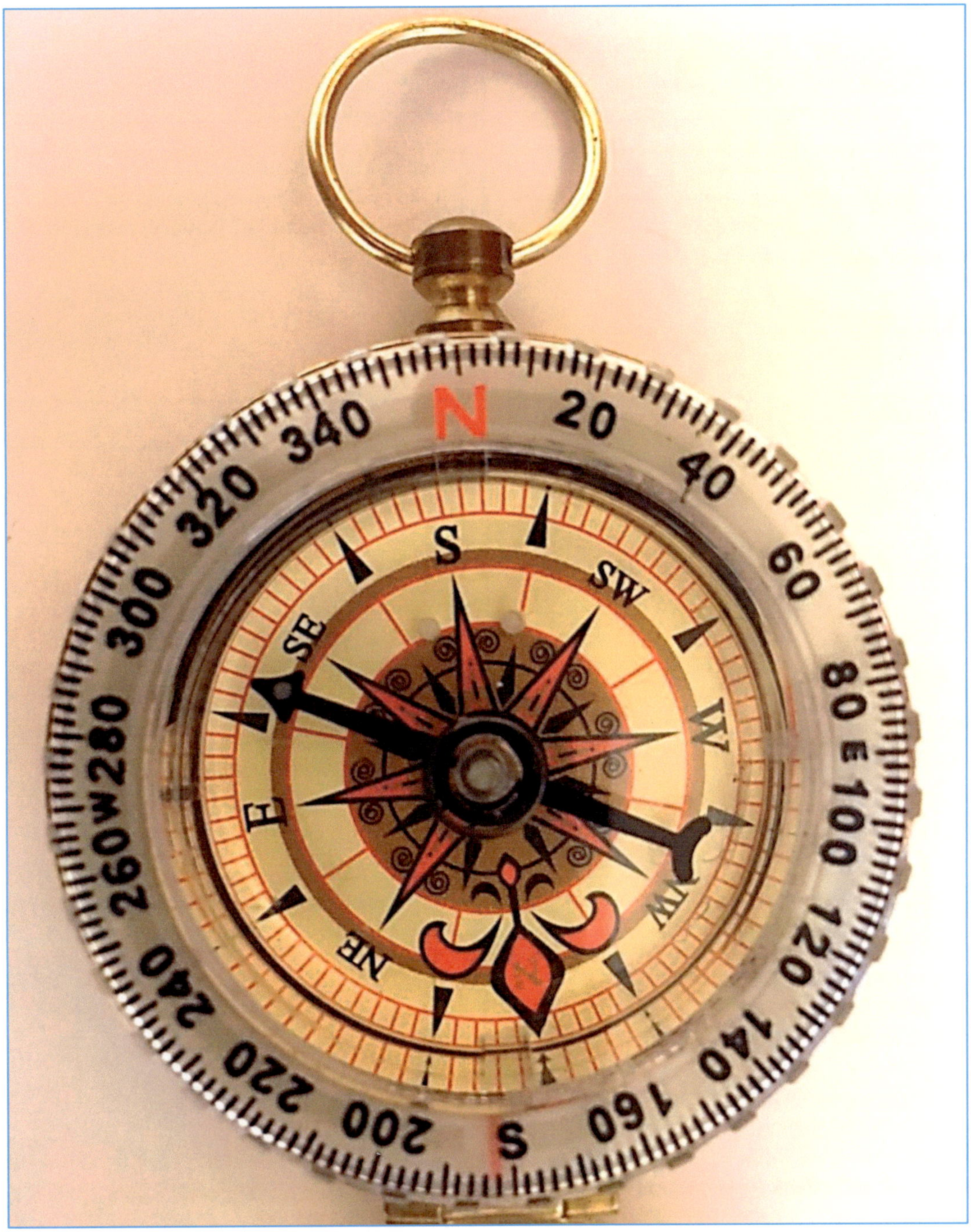

Epidermal tumors

EPIDERMAL NEVUS

-benign hamartoma of the epidermis
-presents at birth or in early childhood
-associated with multiple syndromes: Proteus, Child, McCune-Albright, Klippel-Trenaunay, and epidermal nevus syndrome
-verrucous, dark brown patches, papules, nodules
-typically, in linear or whirled pattern (Blaschoid)

Histopathology
-various histological presentations
-typically shows **irregular papillomatosis** and variable hyperkeratosis and hypergranulosis
-**minimal hyperpigmentation** of epidermal basal layer

ACANTHOSIS NIGRICANS

-velvety thickening and hyperpigmentation of the skin
-favors axillae, neck, and groin
-related to heredity, endocrine disorders (diabetes), obesity, and rarely malignancy (GI cancer)

Histopathology
-wavy epidermis with hyperkeratosis and mildly thinned epidermis (despite name)
-mild epidermal hyperpigmentation
-epidermal **"box-like" (square) rete ridges**

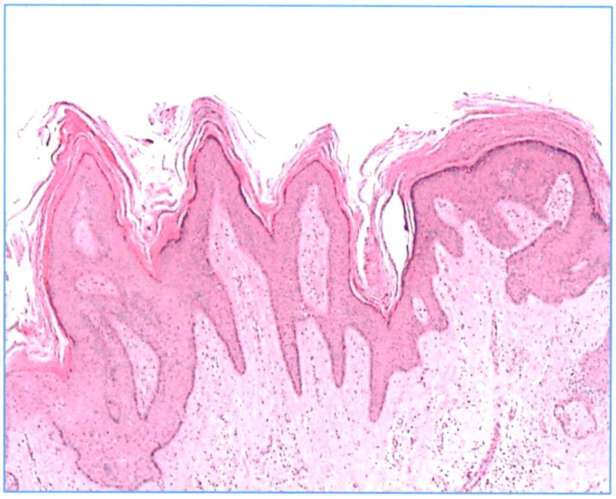

Epidermal nevus with irregular papillomatosis

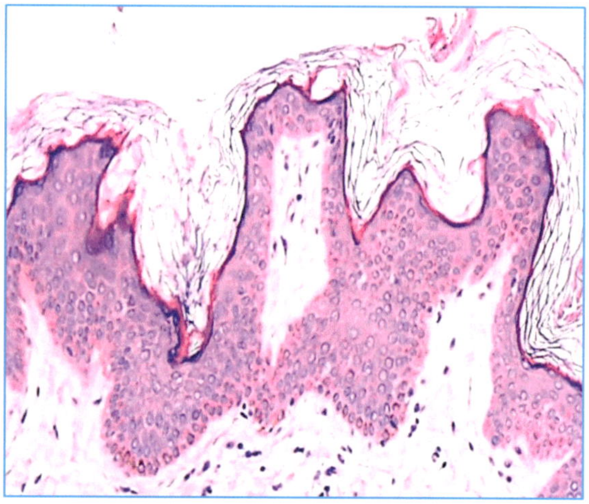

Acanthosis nigricans with squared rete ridges

CONFLUENT AND RETICULATED PAPILLOMATOSIS OF GOUGEROT AND CARTEAUD (CARP)

-more common in women and African Americans
-asymptomatic, small, hyperpigmented velvety macules and papules in "net-like" pattern
-favors the chest and interscapular region

Histopathology
-hyperkeratosis with papillomatosis
-mild hyperpigmentation of basal layer
-"finger-like" epidermal rete

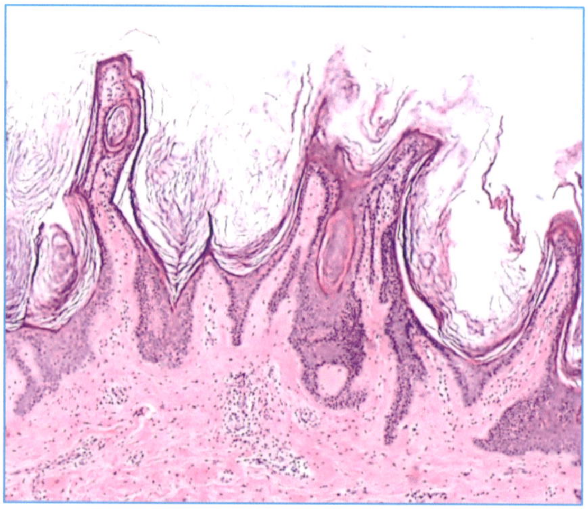

CARP with "finger-like" epidermal rete

ACANTHOLYTIC ACANTHOMA/ ACANTHOLYTIC DYSKERATOTIC ACANTHOMA

-solitary benign papule or nodule
-predilection for the trunk of the elderly

Histopathology
-well circumscribed lesion
-**flat or mildly indented** epidermis
-hyperkeratosis, papillomatosis, and acanthosis
-**keratinocytic acantholysis (discohesion) through upper 2/3rd of the epidermis** (hence the name **acantholytic acanthoma**)
-**can have dyskeratosis (corp ronds and grains)** in the upper half of the epidermis (**acantholytic dyskeratotic acanthoma**)
-in both types **lower third** of the epidermis appears **normal**

WARTY DYSKERATOMA

-solitary benign umbilicated papule
-favors sun exposed skin (head, neck)
-middle-aged and elderly

Histopathology
-**"cup-shaped"** invaginated lesion
-can be associated with a follicle
-**suprabasal clefting** with **acantholytic and dyskeratotic** cells
-resembles split seen in pemphigus vulgaris
-villi are formed at the base
-**lumen filled with keratinous material**

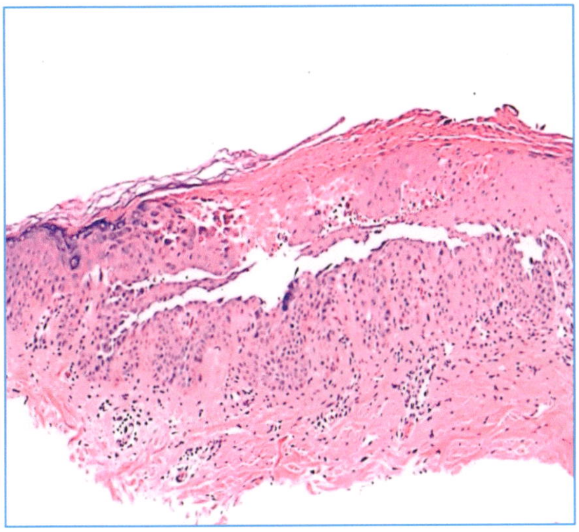
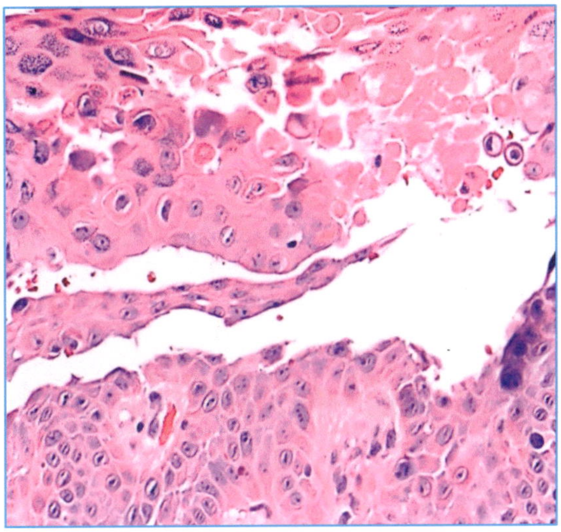

Mildly indented acantholytic dyskeratotic acanthoma with acantholysis and discohesive keratinocytes in the upper portion of the epidermis

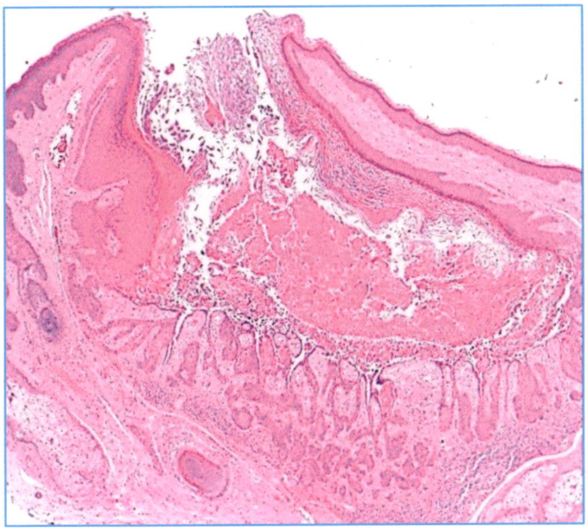
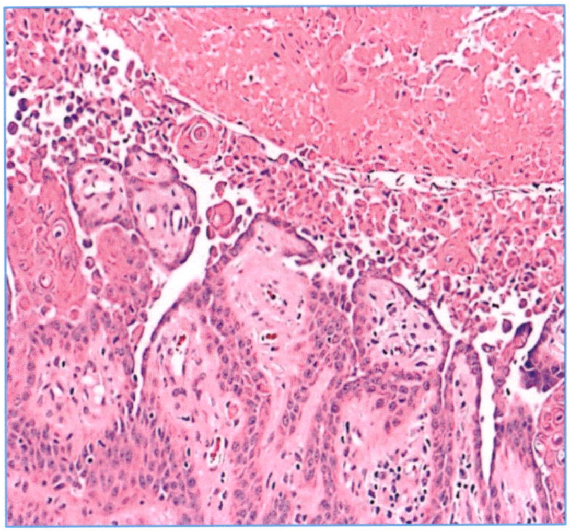

"Cup-shaped" warty dyskeratoma with suprabasal cleft and epidermal acantholysis and dyskeratosis

Epidermal tumors

EPIDERMOLYTIC ACANTHOMA

-discrete, keratotic, "wart-like" papule
-more common on extremities of adults
-can appear in the genital area raising concern for genital warts

Histopathology

-hyperkeratotic acanthotic epidermis
-granular layer **keratinocytes** have **pale vacuolated cytoplasm**
-**coarse basophilic granules** present in the granular layer and **eosinophilic granules** in granular and spinous layer

LARGE CELL ACANTHOMA

-small, skin-colored, or mildly hyperpigmented papules or plaques
-lesions are well demarcated and scaly
-favor sun exposed skin of middle-aged or elderly individuals

Histopathology

-mildly thickened epidermis with hyperkeratosis
-keratinocytes are uniformly enlarged (roughly twice the size of cells of normal neighboring uninvolved epidermis)
-no evidence of cellular atypia
-sharply demarcated from normal epidermis
-mild hyperpigmentation of the basal layer

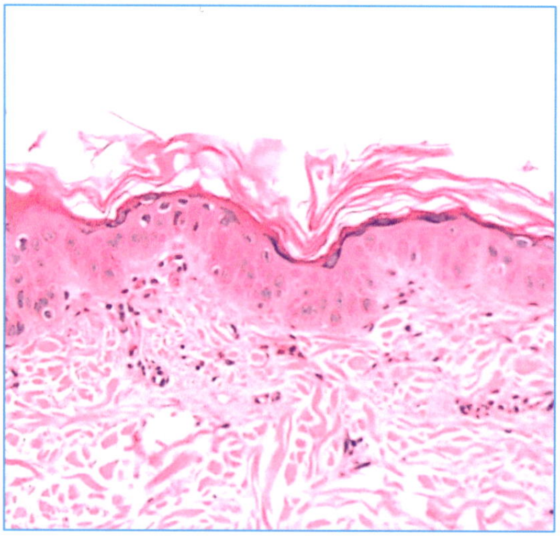

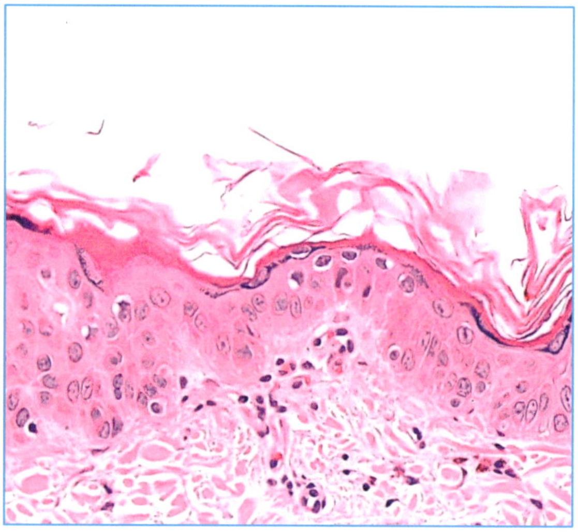

Large cell acanthoma with large keratinocytes without atypia

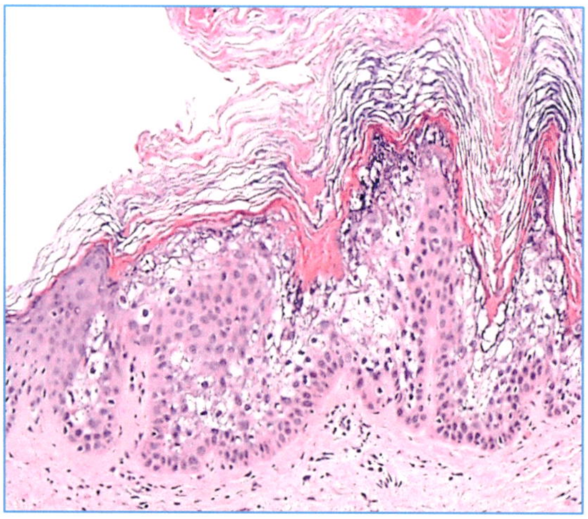

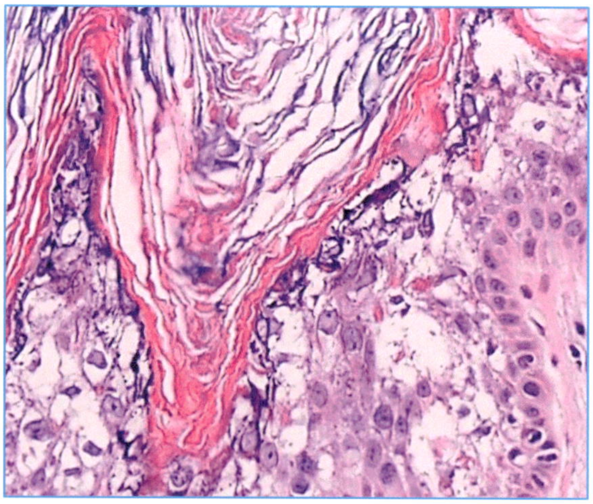

Epidermolytic acanthoma with pale keratinocytes and blue and pink coarse granules

Chapter 26

PRURIGO NODULARIS (PICKER'S NODULE)

-nodular counterpart of lichen simple chronicus
-"dome-shaped", itchy papules and nodules, commonly grouped
-appears at any area of body that is easily accessible to scratching
-classically spares mid upper back, **"butterfly sign"**

Histopathology
-**"dome-shaped"** lesion
-acanthotic, psoriasiform epidermis with **hyperkeratosis, hypergranulosis**
-no epidermal atypia
-**papillomatosis** varies from regular to very irregular
-papillary dermis is fibrotic with dermal scarring and lymphocytic inflammation

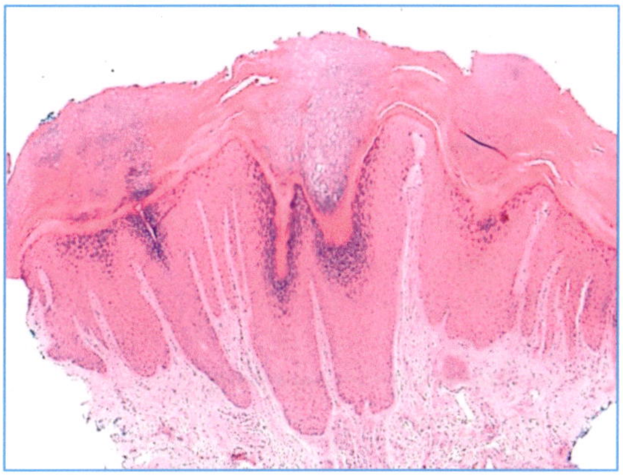

"Dome-shaped" lesion of prurigo nodularis

PSEUDOEPITHELIOMATOUS HYPERPLASIA

-benign reactive pattern of the epidermis
-can closely simulate squamous cell carcinoma
-result of chronic irritation and probably represents a variant of prurigo nodule
-it can also be induced by surgery, infection, halogens, or a granular cell tumor

Histopathology
-**florid hyperplasia** of squamous epithelium with invagination into dermis
-epithelial proliferation with irregular downgrowth of epidermis
-rete are bulbous and irregular forming irregular growth patterns with common keratin cysts entrapped in proliferating epidermis
-squamous eddies can be present
-**minimal keratinocytic atypia** and mild to moderate dermal inflammation

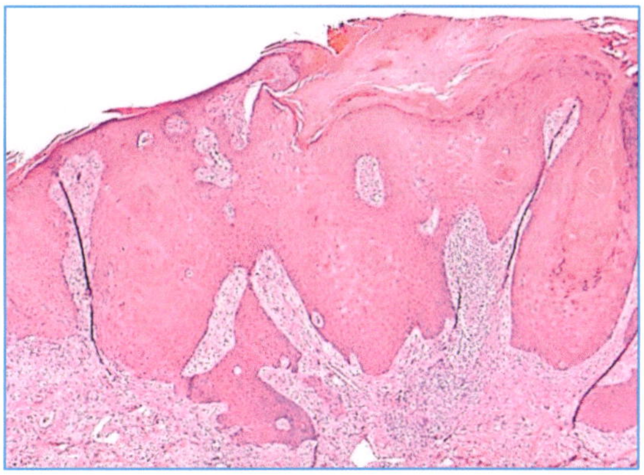

Pseudoepitheliomatous hyperplasia

HALOGENODERMA

-results from ingestion of iodides, bromides, or fluorides
-takes months of continued exposure to develop
-can sometimes be acute (e.g. iodine containing radiocontrast)
-commonly presents as papules/nodules that progress to a vegetating verrucous lesion that can ulcerate
-can also present as acneiform rash

Histopathology
-exuberant **pseudoepitheliomatous hyperplasia** with **intraepidermal micropustules**
-dermal acute and chronic inflammation
-occasional dermal giant cells

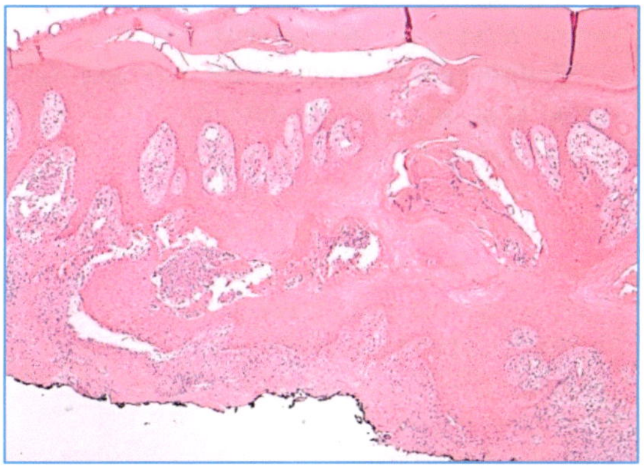

Halogenoderma with epidermal micropustules

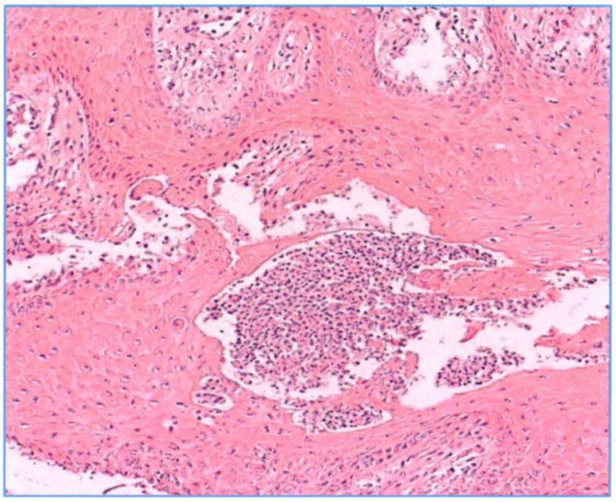

Epidermal tumors

SEBORRHEIC KERATOSIS

-very common benign epidermal tumor of adults
-**waxy or verrucous,** pink or brown papules with **"stuck on" appearance**
-well defined border with rough surface and uniform color
-the rapid onset of multiple seborrheic keratoses can be paraneoplastic sign (Leser–Trélat sign)

Dermatosis papulosa nigra

-variant of seborrheic keratosis in African Americans
-autosomal dominant with variable penetrance
-multiple, small, pigmented papules on the face

Histopathology

-proliferation **of small, uniform keratinocytes** in a variety of patterns
-all variants have acanthosis and hyperkeratosis
-**horn pseudocysts** are present in most variants except macular, digitated, and clonal

Acanthotic type

-most common type
-broad lesion with smooth borders
-**horn pseudocysts** can be very large

Macular type

-**early SK** with mild papillomatosis and acanthosis
-has a flat surface and mimics lentigo or dysplastic nevus
-**no horn cysts** and are usually pigmented

Pigmented (melanoacanthoma) type

-same as acanthotic type but with lots of **melanin in keratinocytes**

Papillomatous hyperkeratotic type

-"Gothic church spire"-like papillomatosis
-hyperkeratosis and acanthosis with only occasional horn pseudocysts

Reticulated (adenoid) type

-elongated epidermis with reticulated **"net-like" pattern**
-usually pigmented

Clonal type

-acanthotic epidermis with uniform keratinocytes in "**nesting" pattern**

Irritated type

-"pseudoepitheliomatous-like" hyperplasia
-characteristic **squamous eddies**
-dermal lymphocytic infiltrate
-mild to moderate cytological atypia

Digitated type

-hyperkeratosis and uniform papillomatosis thinner than in hyperkeratotic type
-no increase in number of basaloid cells or horn pseudocysts
-"lentigo-like" digitated proliferation

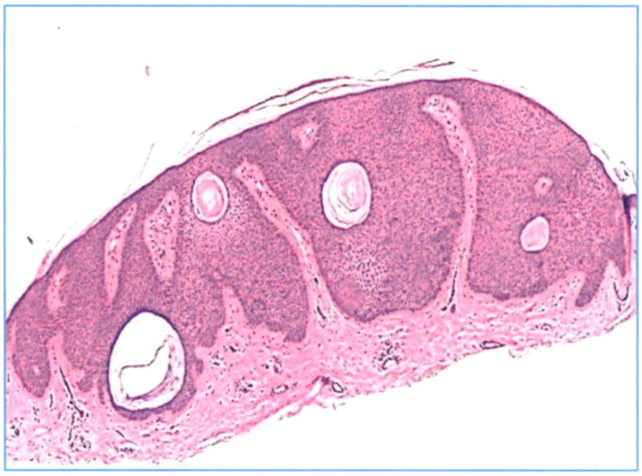

Acanthotic SK with uniform keratinocytes and pseudocysts

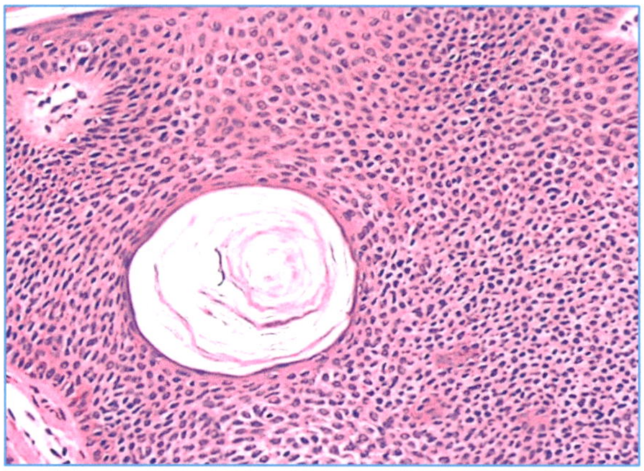

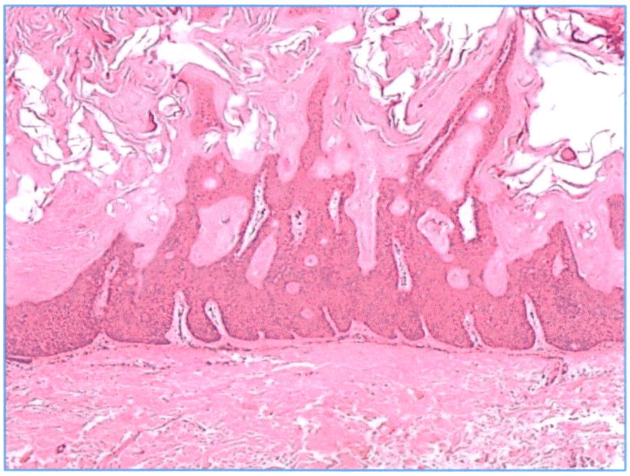

Papillomatous hyperkeratotic SK with "Gothic church spires"

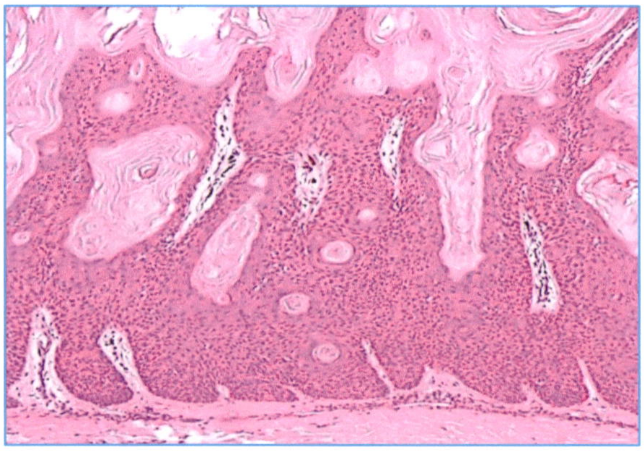

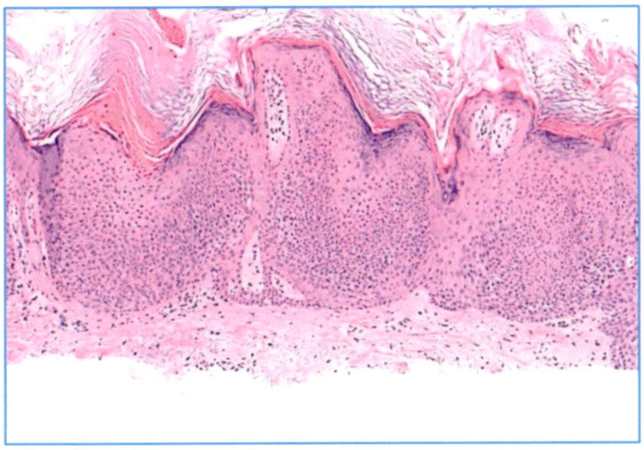
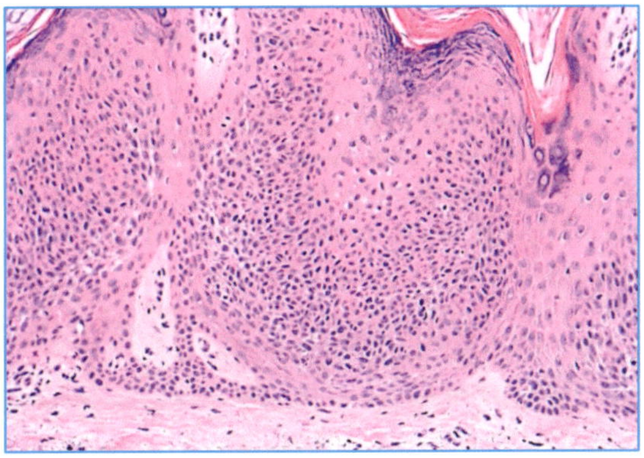

Clonal SK with uniform proliferation of keratinocytes in "nest-like" pattern

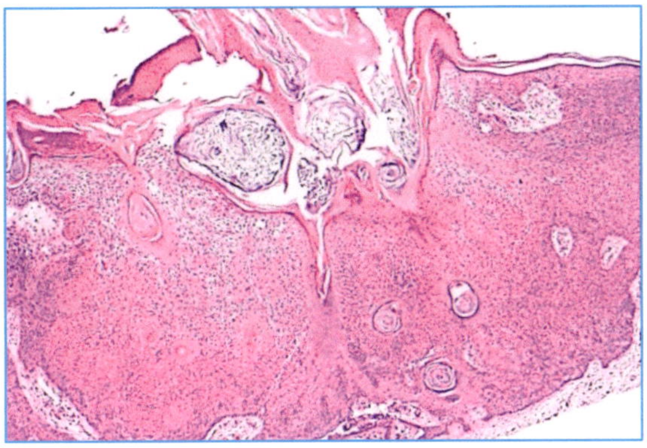
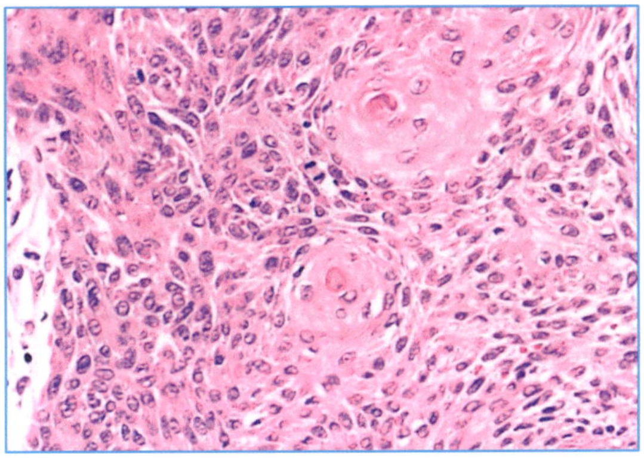

Irritated SK with squamous eddies

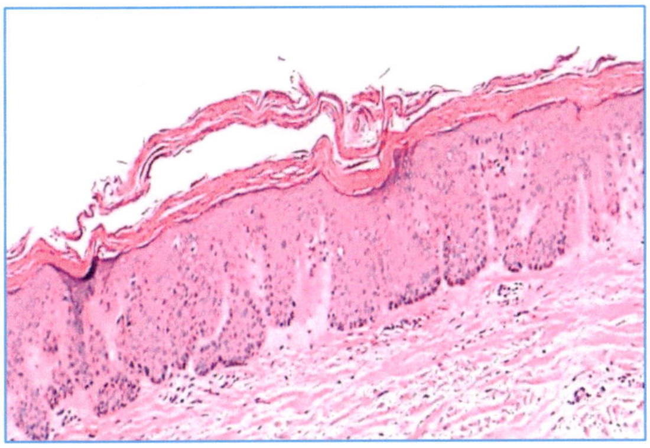
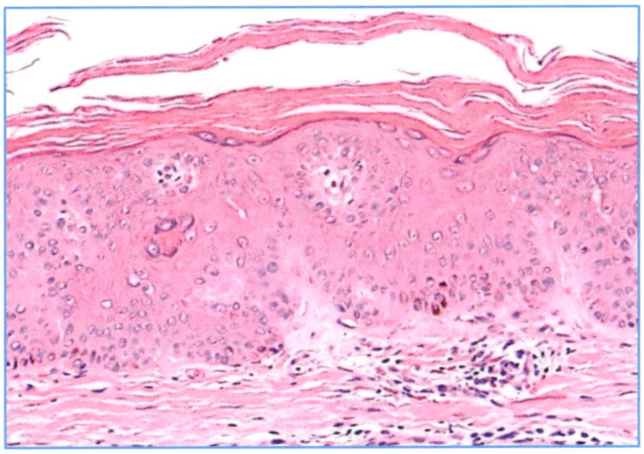

Macular SK that mimic lentigo and does not have pseudocysts

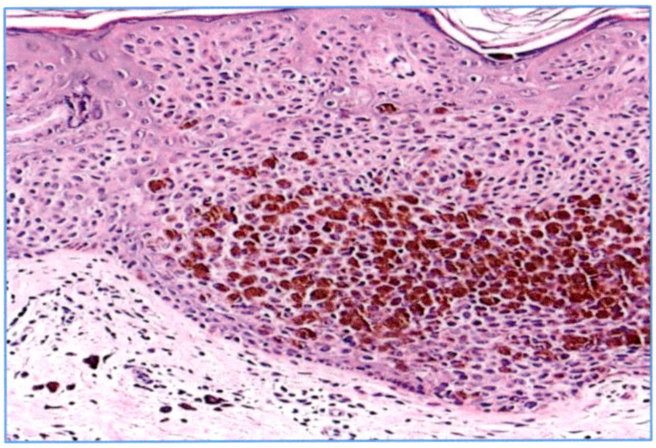

Pigmented SK with abundant melanin

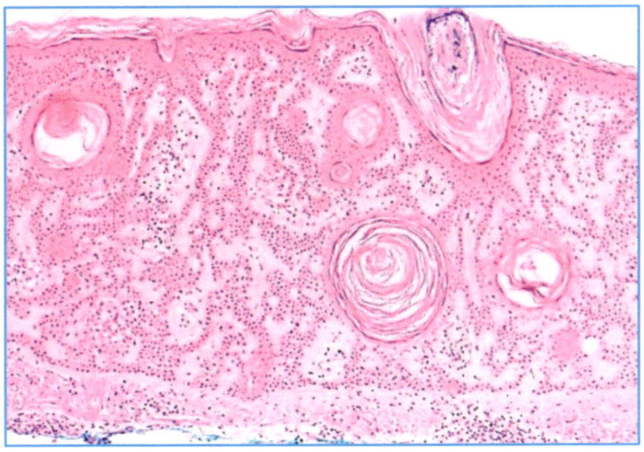

Reticulated SK in "net-like" pattern

ACROKERATOSIS VERRUCIFORMIS OF HOPF

-rare autosomal dominant disease
-appears at birth or in early childhood
-small, verrucous, flat papules resembling flat warts on the hands and fingers
-like Darier's disease, it is associated with defects in the *ATP2A2* gene
-however, the specific mutations found in the *ATP2A2* gene in acrokeratosis verruciformis have never been found in Darier's disease

Histopathology

-hyperkeratosis, regular acanthosis and papillomatosis
-**"church spire-like" appearance**
-**no horn cysts**
-resembles papillomatous/digitated seborrheic keratosis

STUCCO KERATOSIS

-probably a variant of seborrheic keratosis (digitated SK)
-multiple, small, pale, white-yellow keratotic papules, resembling stucco splattered on the skin
-commonly found on lower legs and feet

Histopathology

-hyperkeratosis and regular papillomatosis ("church spire" pattern)
-no increase in number of basaloid cells or horn pseudocysts

These two entities have almost identical histopathology. Therefore, clinical correlation is paramount to separate them.

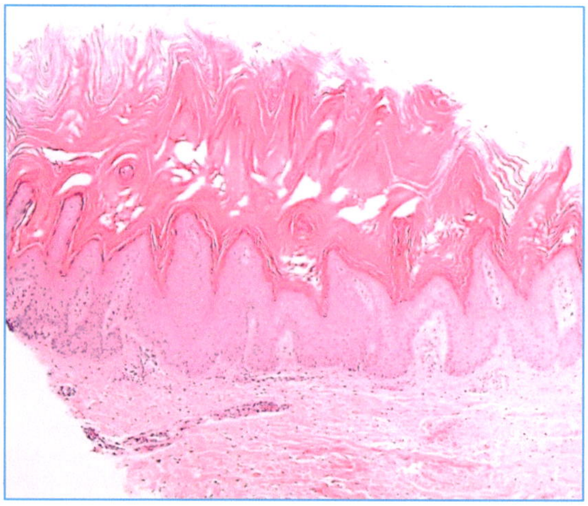

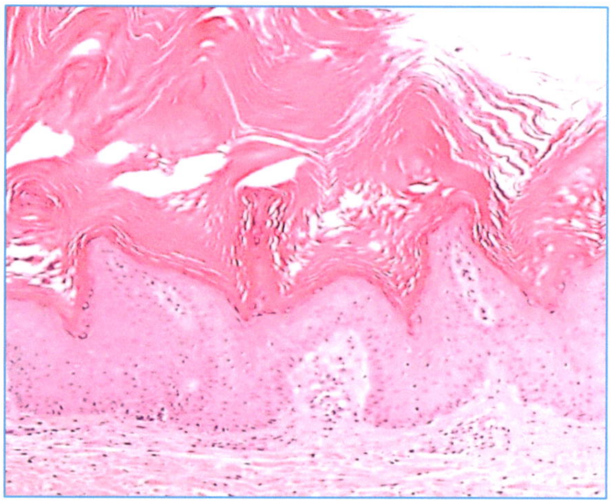

Acrokeratosis verruciformis with "church spire-like' appearance

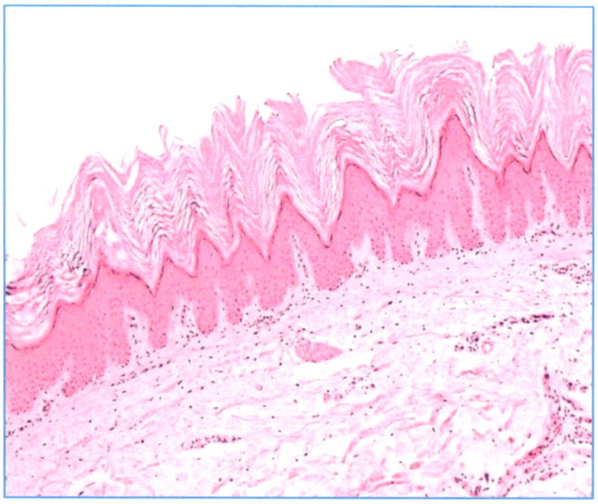

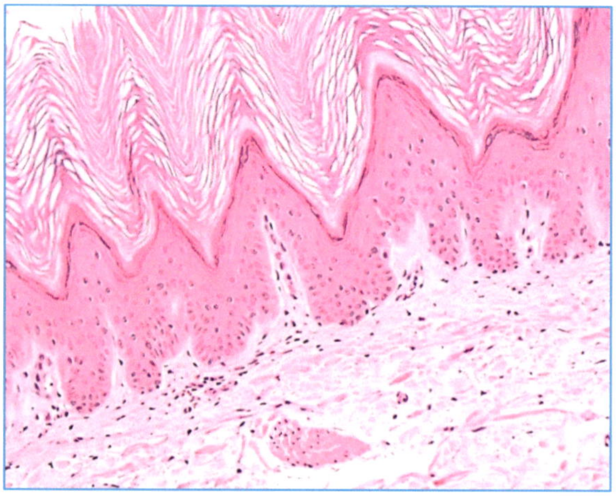

Stucco keratosis with hyperkeratosis and regular papillomatosis

Chapter 26

CLEAR CELL ACANTHOMA

-benign, solitary, firm, red-brown, well-circumscribed plaque or nodule
-favors lower legs of elderly individuals
-typically has a crusted, scaly peripheral collarette and vascular puncta on the surface
-characterized by slow growth

Histopathology

-**well-demarcated** epidermal proliferation
-**psoriasiform** epidermal hyperplasia
-uniform keratinocytes that have **pale-staining cytoplasm** due to excess glycogen (PAS positive)
-cells are uniform with no atypia
-basal layer may not be as pale
-variable number of **neutrophils scattered** over epidermis

INVERTED FOLLICULAR KERATOSIS

-regarded as a variant of seborrheic keratosis
-solitary, flesh-colored nodule
-favors head (particularly cheeks, upper lip), neck

Histopathology

-**endophytic** and sometimes **endo-exophytic** proliferation of benign keratinocytes
-nodule made of basaloid cells at the periphery and squamoid cells in the center
-**squamous eddies** are characteristic features
-no significant cellular atypia although occasional mitosis can be seen

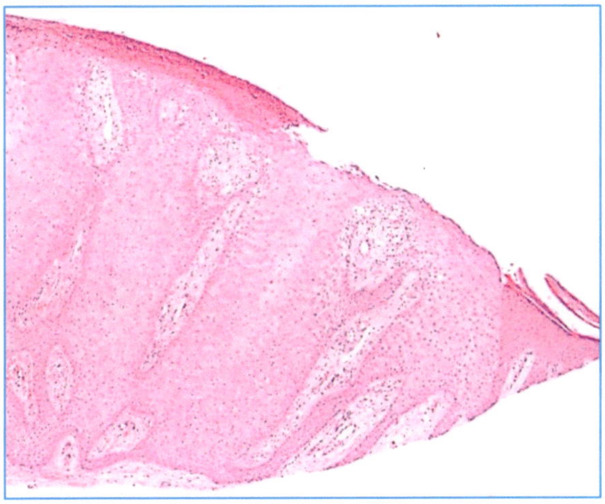

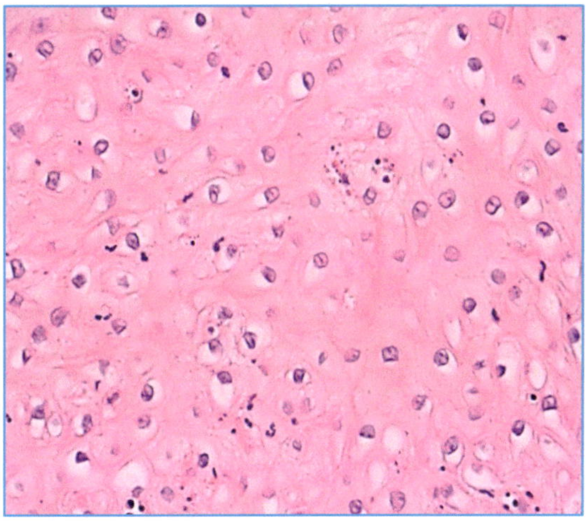

Clear cell acanthoma with clear cells and scattered neutrophils

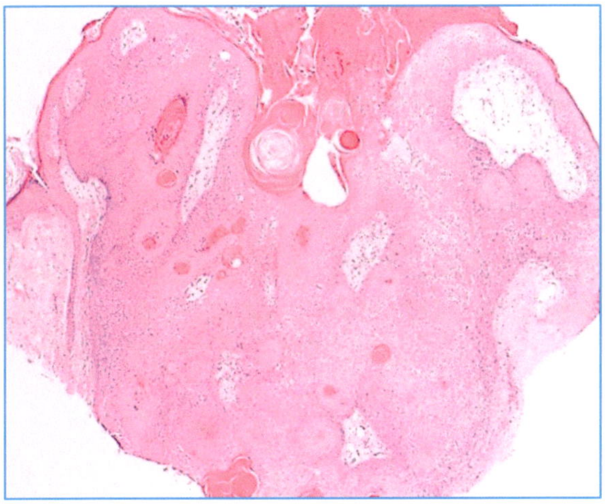

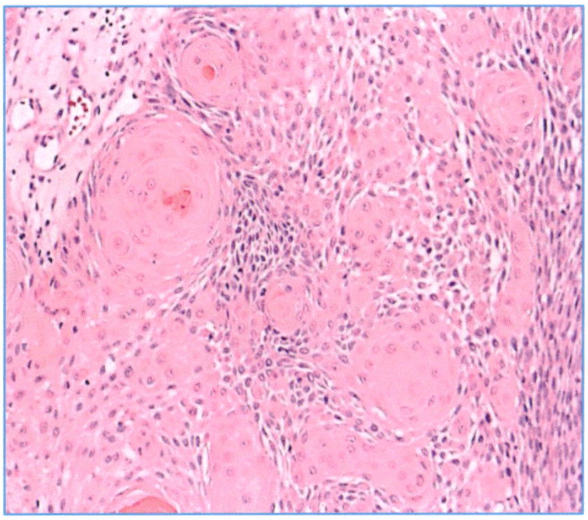

Endo-exophytic silhouette of inverted follicular keratosis with squamous eddies

BASAL CELL CARCINOMA

-most common skin cancer due to prolonged, intermittent UV exposure
-common on sun exposed areas of light-skinned middle-aged and elderly people
-pearly pink papule or nodule with **arborizing telangiectasias**
-can show pigmentation and ulceration
-can also present as white, waxy, "scar-like" lesion (morpheaform BCC)
-can occur in children in Gorlin syndrome (nevoid basal cell carcinoma syndrome) where it **clinically resembles nevus**, and is due to mutation in *PTCH1* gene
-fibroepithelioma of Pincus BCC variant presents as a nodule on the **lower back**

Histopathology
-multiple variants with variable architecture
-common to most of them are **small basaloid tumor cells**, **peripheral palisading** of tumor cells, tumor **stromal retraction,** and **mucinous blue stroma**

Superficial type- multiple foci of basaloid cell islands along epidermo-dermal junction
Nodular type- large islands (nodules) of basaloid cells with frequent epidermal ulceration
Micronodular type- proliferation of multiple smaller basaloid dermal nests
Morpheaform type- narrow strands of basaloid cells in fibrotic stroma, minimal stromal retraction, and poor palisading
Infundibulocystic type- basaloid folliculocystic spaces
Fibroepithelioma of Pincus- polypoid lesion with thin cords of basaloid cells forming "net-like" appearance
Pigmented type- usually nodular type with numerous melanophages
Clear cell type- solid type with areas of clear cells without palisading
Basosquamous type- admixed areas of squamoid differentiation

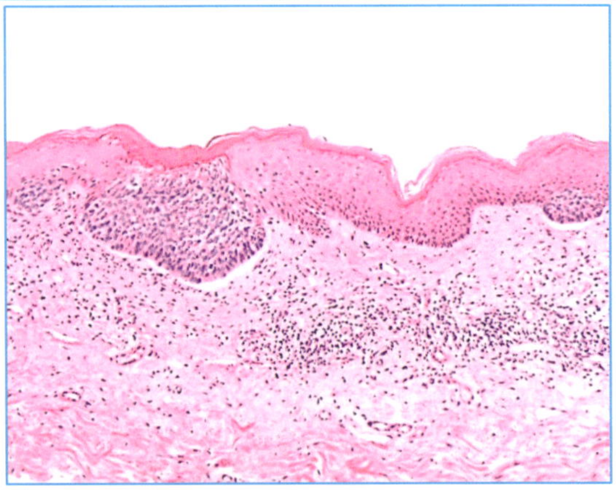
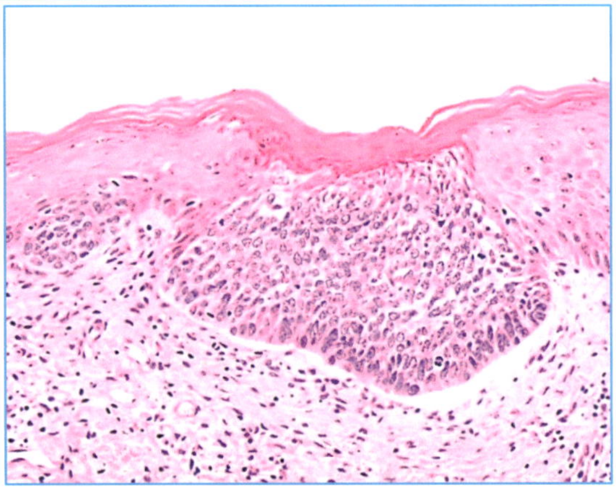

Superficial type BCC with basaloid nests at epidermo-dermal junction showing palisading of peripheral tumor cells and stromal retraction

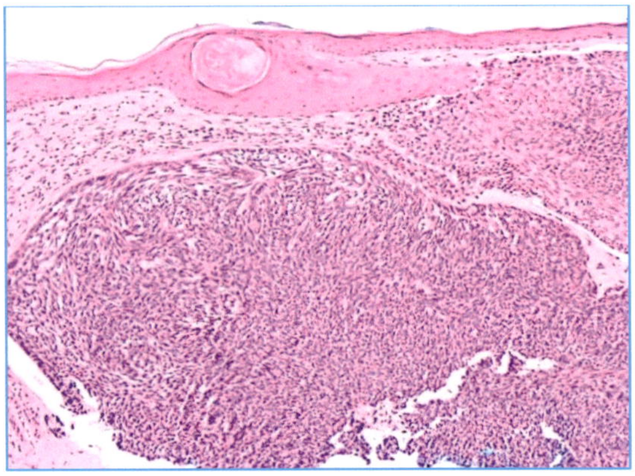
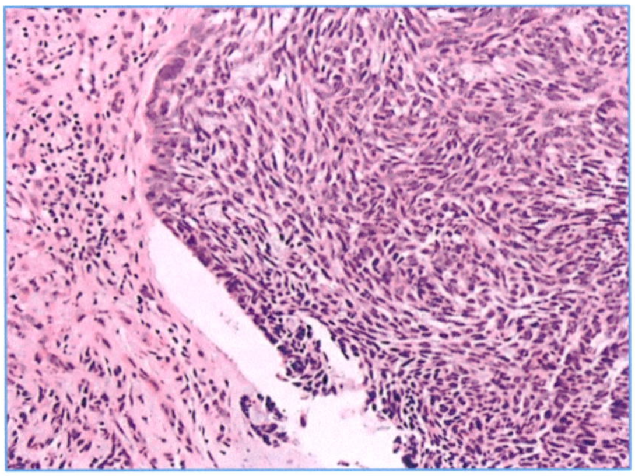

Nodular BCC with large basaloid nodules with peripheral palisading and stromal retraction

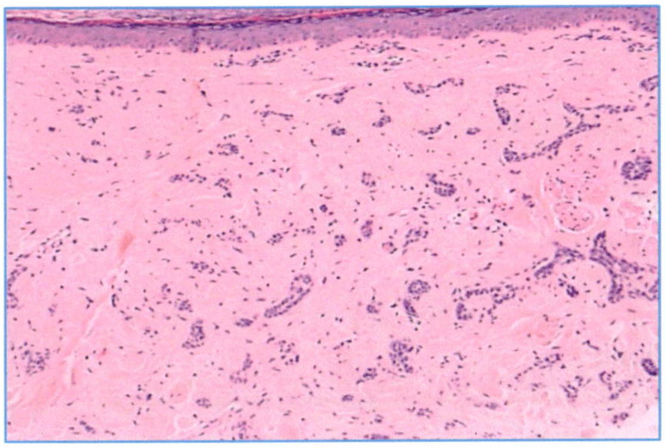

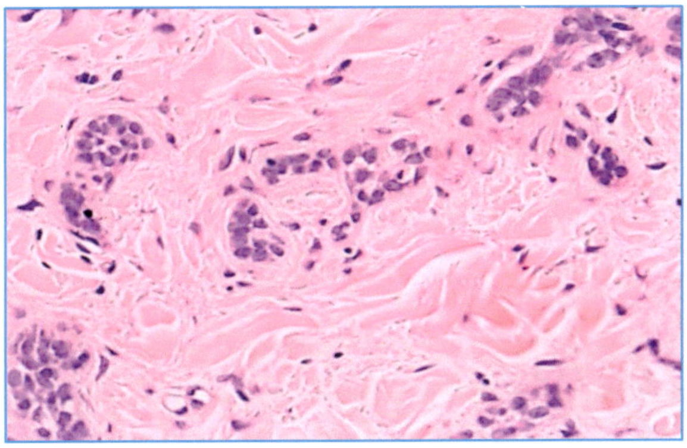

Morpheaform type BCC with narrow strands of basaloid cells in dense dermal stroma

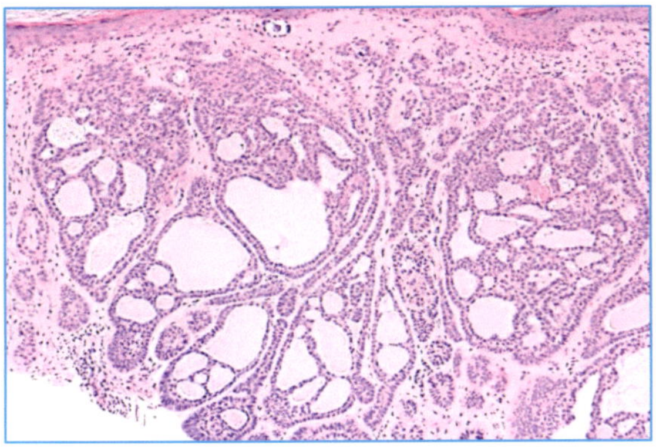

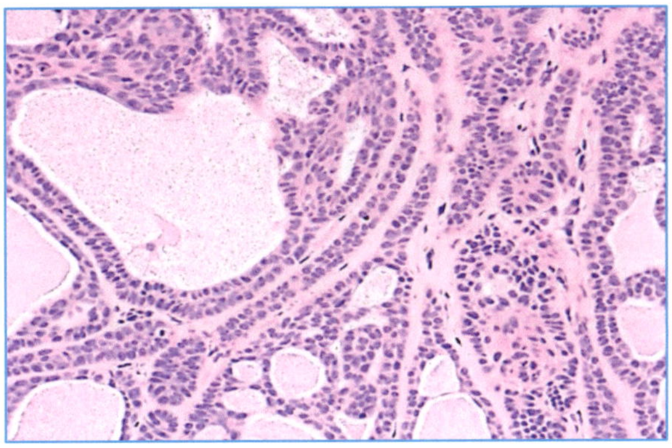

Infundibulocystic BCC with solid and cystic spaces made of basaloid cells

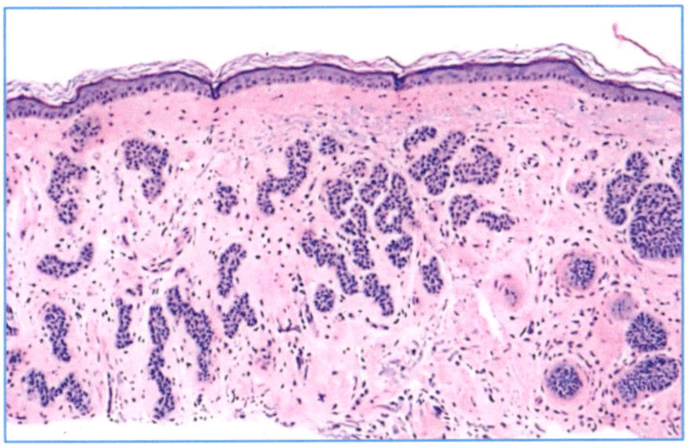

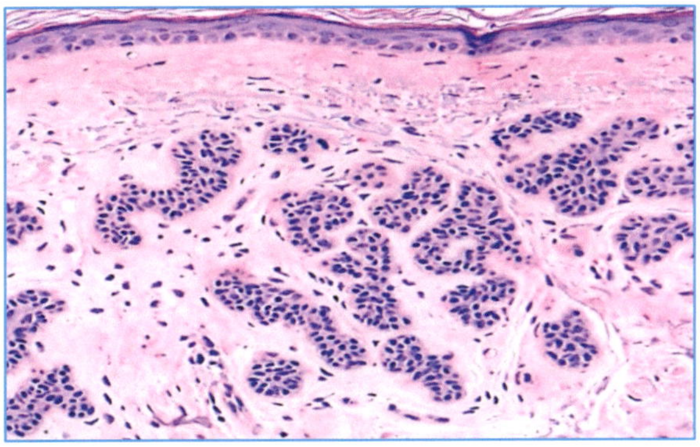

Micronodular BCC made of numerous small nests made of basaloid cells

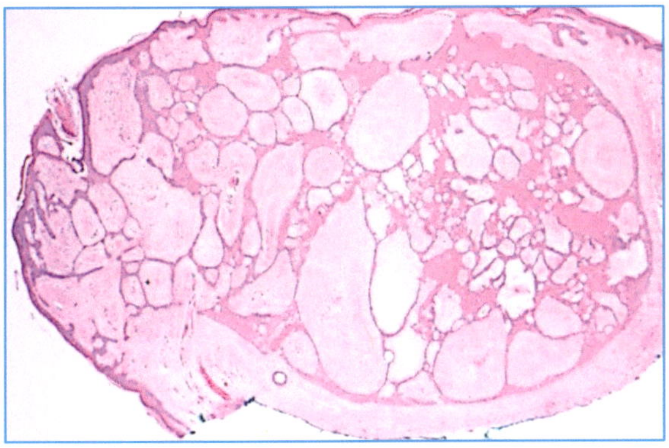

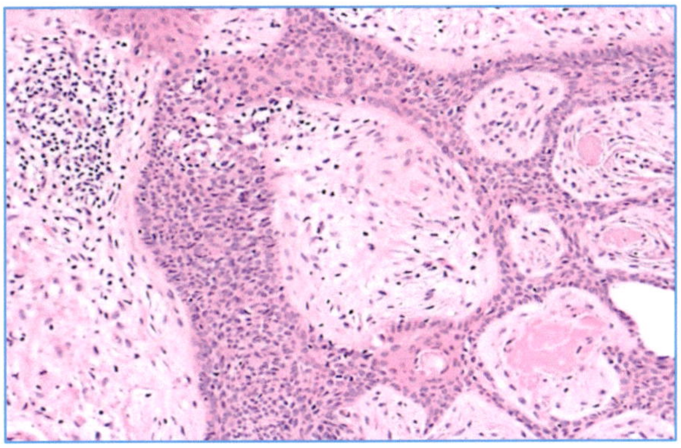

Polypoid fibroepithelioma of Pincus BCC with irregular "net-like" architecture

Epidermal tumors

ACTINIC KERATOSIS/ACTINIC CHEILITIS

-precancerous skin lesion (actinic keratosis) resulting from chronic sun exposure
-called actinic cheilitis when mucosa of lips is involved
-presents as pink brown hyperkeratotic macules, plaques
-in some cases, a hard, "wart-like" surface (one of the causes of a cutaneous horn)
-minority progress to SCC

Histopathology

Actinic keratosis

-**atypical keratinocytes** confined to the **lower 2/3rd of the epidermis**
-keratinocytes have irregular shape with enlarged nuclei, hyperchromasia, and prominent nucleoli
-mitosis can be seen
-dermal solar elastosis is prominent
-dermal lymphocytic inflammation present

Variants of actinic keratosis

Hypertrophic
-prominent orthokeratosis and focal parakeratosis
Atrophic
-flat rete ridges and thinning of the epidermis
Lichenoid
-with "band-like" dermal lymphocytic infiltrate
Acantholytic
-separation of atypical, acantholytic keratinocytes in the lower part of the dermis
Pigmented
-hyperpigmentation of basal layer keratinocytes

Actinic cheilitis

-histomorphology resembles hypertrophic actinic keratosis but changes involve squamous mucosa (absence of granular layer)

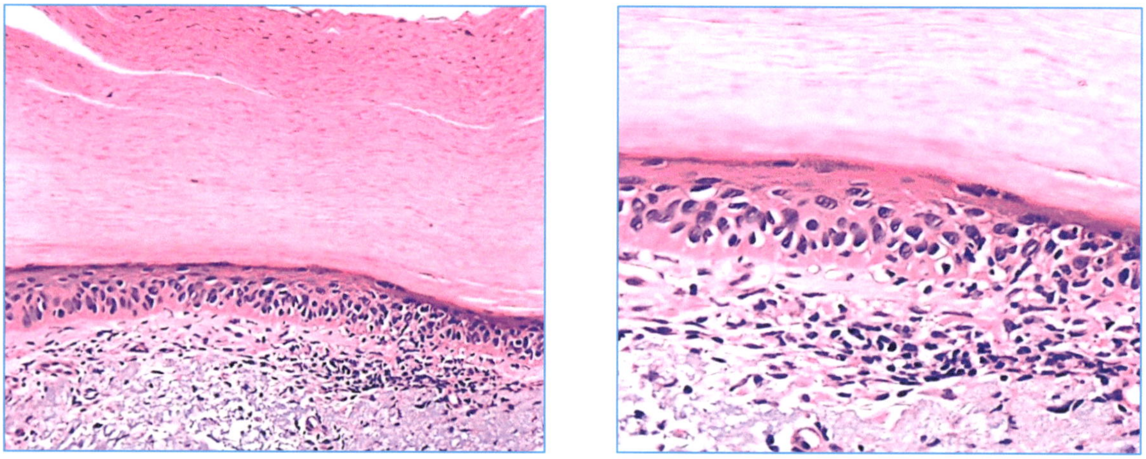

Atrophic actinic keratosis with flat, thin epidermis and atypia of keratinocytes in the lower portion

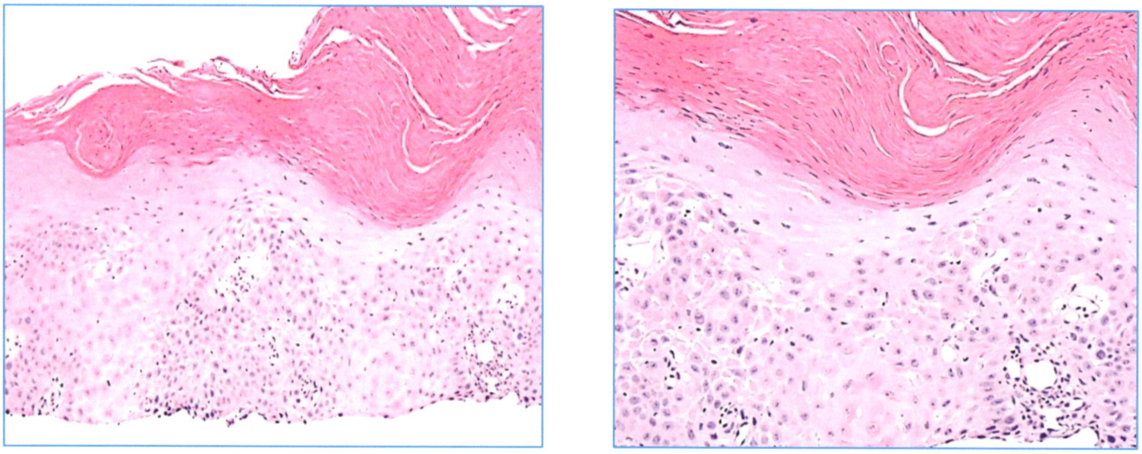

Actinic cheilitis on mucosal surface without granular layer and atypia of keratinocytes in the lower 2/3rd of the epithelium

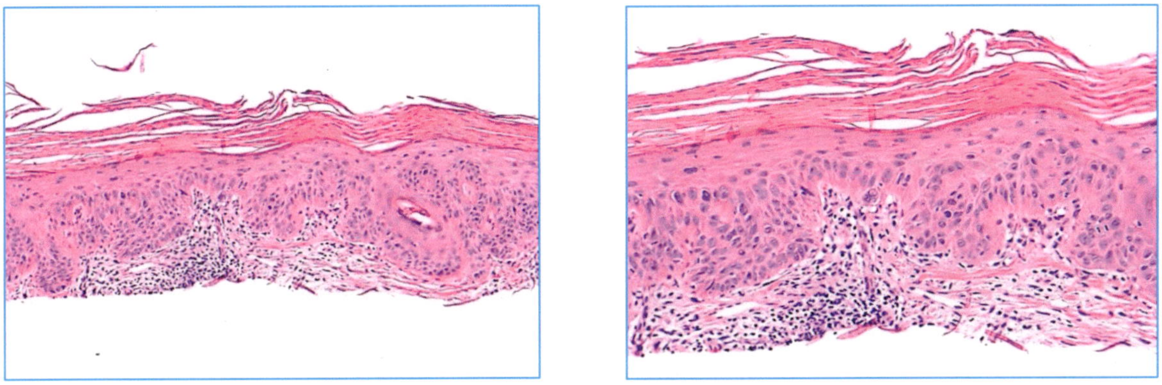

Hypertrophic actinic keratosis with prominent hyperkeratosis and focal parakeratosis

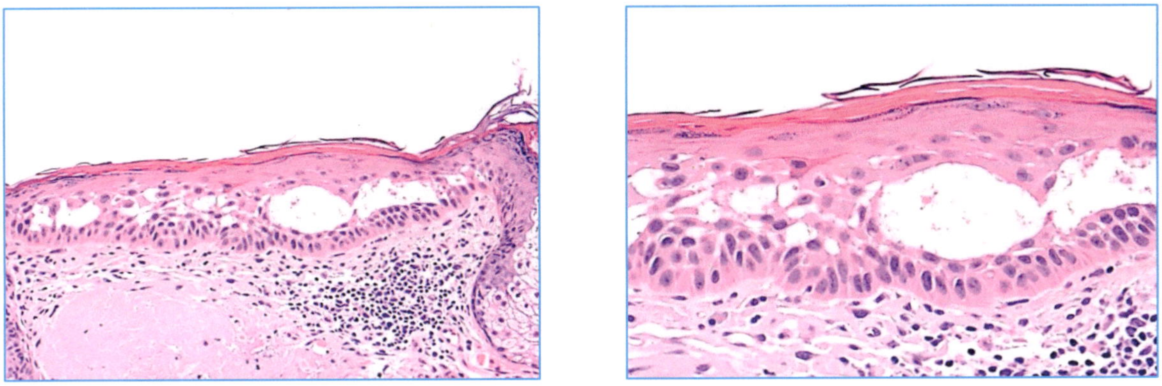

Acantholytic actinic keratosis with separation of atypical keratinocytes in the lower portion of the epidermis

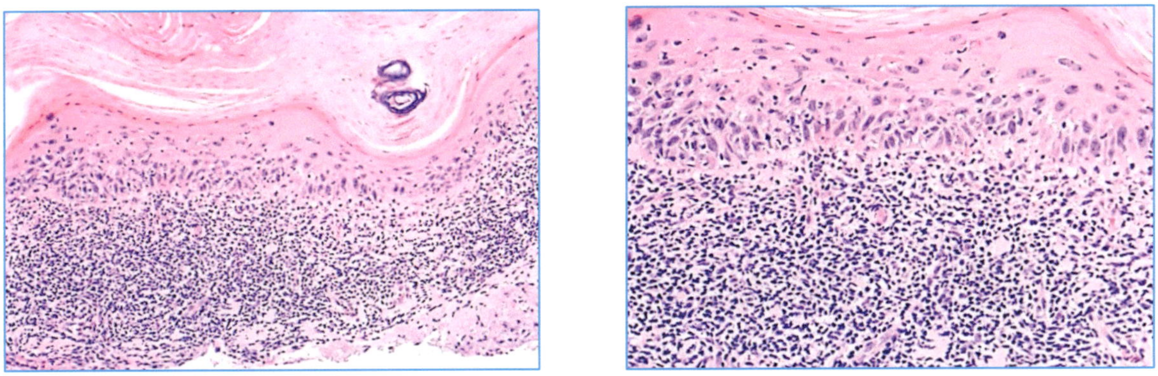

Lichenoid actinic keratosis with dermal “band-like” lymphocytes and atypical keratinocytes in the lower portion of the epidermis

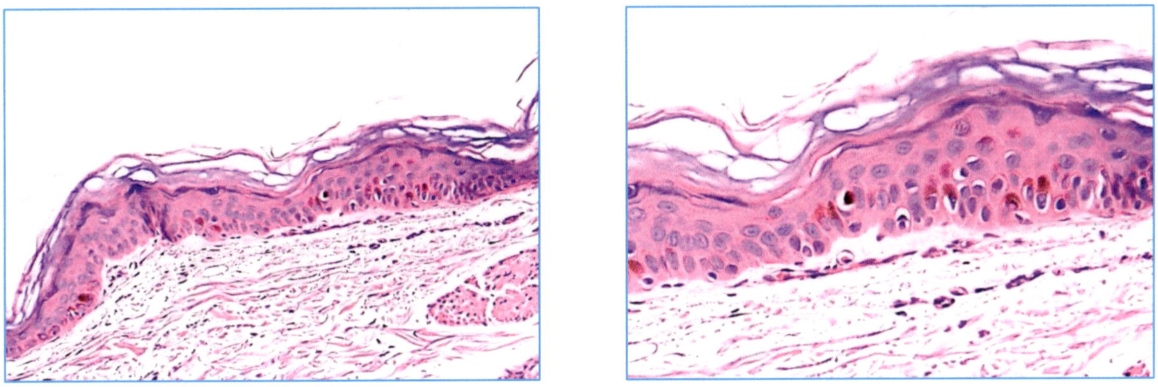

Pigmented actinic keratosis with atypical pigmented keratinocytes

Epidermal tumors

VERRUCA VULGARIS

-benign epidermal growth caused by *Human Papilloma Virus (HPV),* see more details in the chapter on viral infections
-various types of *HPV* cause different clinical manifestation (described in detail in the chapter on viral infections)
-verruca vulgaris (common wart) is caused by *HPV-1 HPV-2, HPV 4*
-flesh-colored, hyperkeratotic papules with a rough surface
-can occur anywhere but especially common on hands

Histopathology
-exophytic epidermal kyperkeratosis, papillomatosis, and hypergranulosis
-columns of epidermal parakeratosis
-koilocytes (HPV infected keratinocytes) in the upper part of the epidermis
-**koilocytes** have **small, dark, "raisin-shaped" nuclei** surrounded by **clear cytoplasm**

PAGET'S DISEASE

Mammary type
-in women with breast cancer where it starts in mammary ducts and extends into the epidermis
-eczematous, pink-red plaque on the nipple or breast
Extramammary type
-in elderly men and women
-at any site with high density of apocrine glands
-in women 80% arise in or around the vulva
-in men 40% present at the scrotum
-present as well defined erythematous red plaques

Histopathology
-epidermal infiltrate of **cells with abundant pale cytoplasm**
-cells are **scattered at all levels** of epidermis in **"buckshot"** pattern (unlike melanoma that favors lower part of the epidermis)
-cells have large vesicular nuclei with sometimes prominent nucleoli
-**cytoplasm is pale** with bluish hue (**mucin**)
-dermal mammary ducts involved with tumor cells
-tumor cells are cytokeratin 7, EMA, and CEA positive

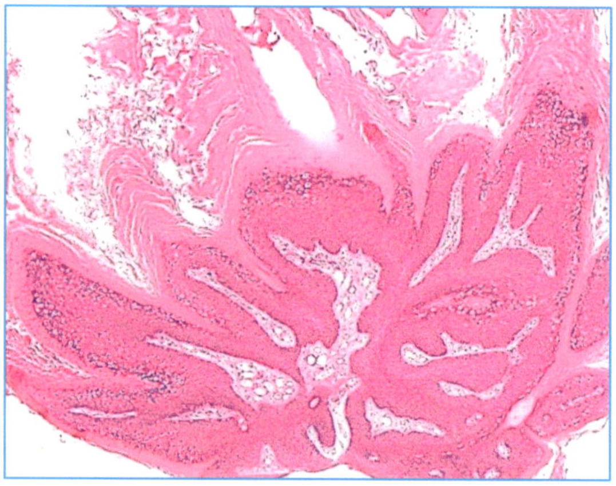
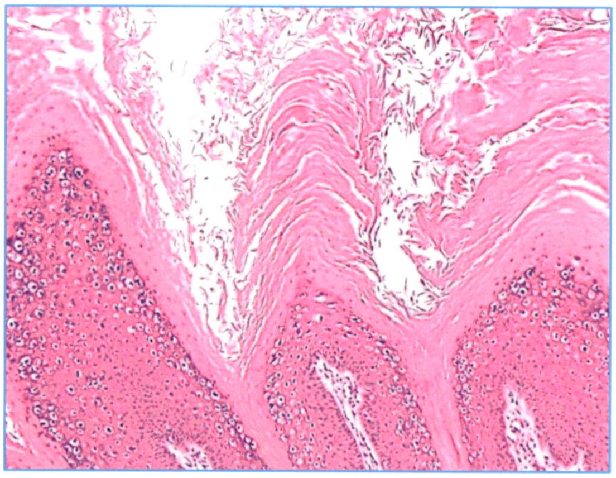

Exophytic lesion of verruca vulgaris with epidermal koilocytes and columns of parakeratosis

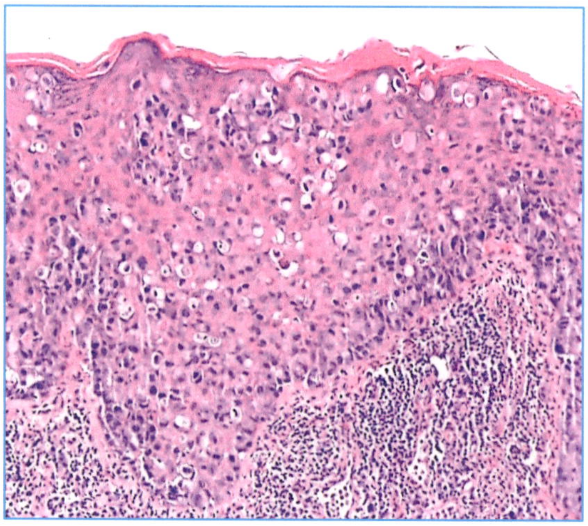
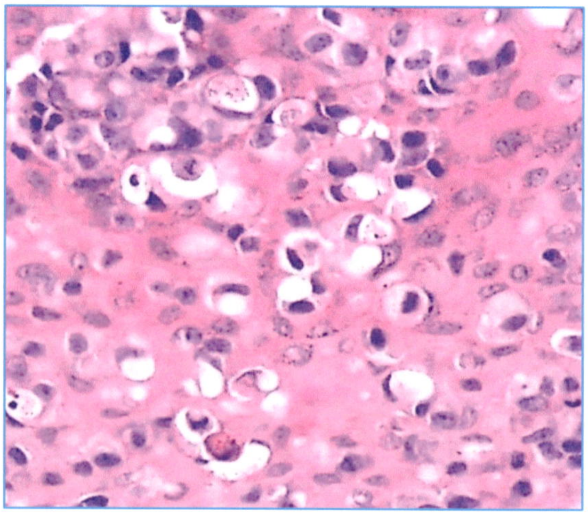

Paget's disease with malignant cells with pale/clear cytoplasm randomly scattered at all levels of the epidermis

Chapter 26

SQUAMOUS CELL CARCINOMA IN SITU (BOWEN'S DISEASE)

-malignancy arising from squamous epithelium, confined to the epidermis
-predilection for sun-exposed areas but can occur at any site
-slowly enlarging erythematous, scaly plaque

Histopathology
-acanthotic epidermis with **full thickness atypia** of keratinocytes
-keratinocytes do not mature as they approach epidermal surface and have **"wind-blown"** architecture
-keratinocytes are enlarged with irregular hyperchromatic nuclei
-mitoses and apoptotic bodies are scattered throughout the epidermis

BOWENOID PAPULOSIS

-premalignant pigmented verrucous papules
-classically on the body of the penis but can occur anywhere on genital skin
-associated with human papillomavirus, usually *HPV 16*
-although most cases are benign, a small percentage may transform into invasive squamous cell carcinoma

Histopathology
-focal or more frequently full thickness epidermal atypia
-**atypia is relatively uniform** among all affected keratinocytes
-nuclei are prominent with increased nuclear to cytoplasmic ratio
-keratinocytes do not mature
-scattered necrotic keratinocytes
-some keratinocytes may show HPV associated, koilocytic changes
-overall, similar to in situ SCC but more uniform atypia

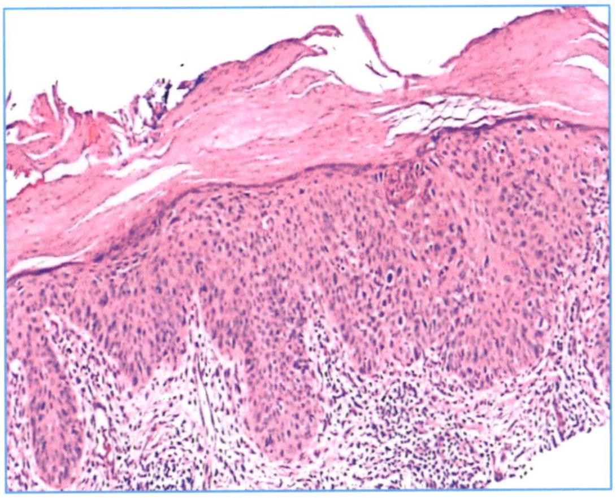

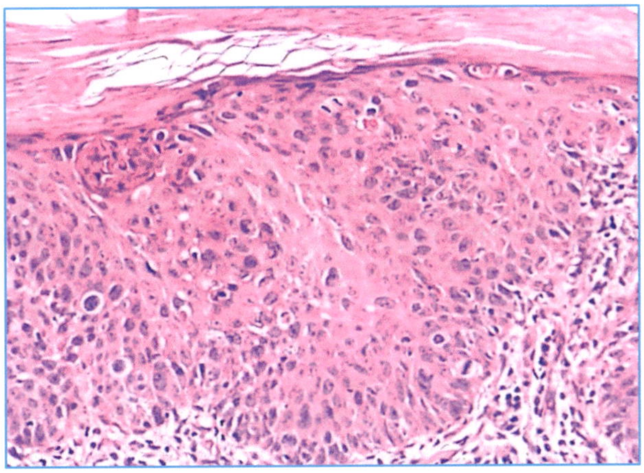

Squamous cell carcinoma in situ with full thickness irregular atypia of epidermal keratinocytes in "wind-blown" pattern

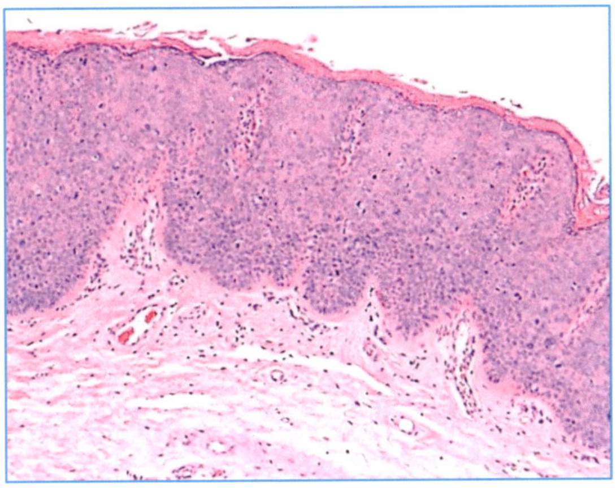

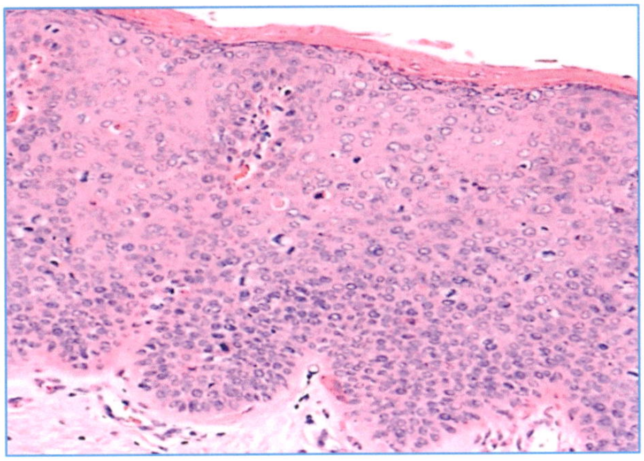

Bowenoid papulosis with full thickness, relatively uniform epidermal atypia

Epidermal tumors

SQUAMOUS CELL CARCINOMA

-second most common form of skin cancer
-usually found on areas of chronic UV exposure
-SCC is a fairly slow-growing skin cancer though it can be locally invasive or metastatic if left untreated
-usually presents as a pink indurated papule, plaque, or nodule with thick keratotic scale
-commonly erodes or ulcerates
-common at sites of old scars, burns, chronic ulcers
-increased risk in transplant patients

Histopathology

-proliferation of **atypical epithelial pink cells** starting in epidermis and invading into dermis
-invasion of dermis is infiltrative with smaller irregular strands and nests of tumor
-atypical keratinocytes have **abundant eosinophilic cytoplasm** and large irregular nuclei
-**keratinization** and formation of **squamous pearls** commonly present
-mitoses are also commonly seen

Acantholytic variant

-squamous cell carcinoma nests with central, atypical, separated, acantholytic keratinocytes

Spindle cell variant

-composed entirely of spindle cells or have a variable component of typical SCC
-spindle cells have large vesicular nuclei and scanty cytoplasm with indistinct borders

Signet cell variant (very uncommon)

-cells have displaced nuclei with "signet" ring shape

Clear cell variant

-over 50% of keratinocytes with clear cell cytoplasm

Keratoacanthoma like variant

-"crater-like" shape with dermal invasion at the base

KERATOACANTHOMA

-controversy persists if keratoacanthoma is a form of SCC or a different benign entity
-gene array analysis suggests two separate entities
-rapidly growing, painful papulonodule with central keratin core that reaches a large size within days or weeks
-if untreated, it becomes necrotic, sloughs, and heals with scarring within several weeks/months
-most commonly appears as solitary lesion, however multiple lesions can appear in Ferguson–Smith syndrome or Muir-Torre syndrome
-generalized eruptive keratoacanthoma of Grzybowski, a rare variant characterized by hundreds of tiny follicular keratotic papules over the entire body

Histopathology

-**"flask-shaped", crateriform**, symmetrical lesion with central keratin-filled epithelial invagination
-keratinocytes have **ground glass appearance** and are well differentiated
-tumor infiltrate dermis with **broad pushy borders** but do not infiltrate with smaller proliferating strands
-mild lymphocytic infiltrate abuts the lesion base

Note: if tumor base contains proliferating epithelial strands infiltrating into dermal stroma it is more consistent with SCC-KA type and should be excised

COLLISION TUMOR

-coexistence of two cancers in the same anatomical site
-most commonly basal cell carcinoma and squamous cell carcinoma

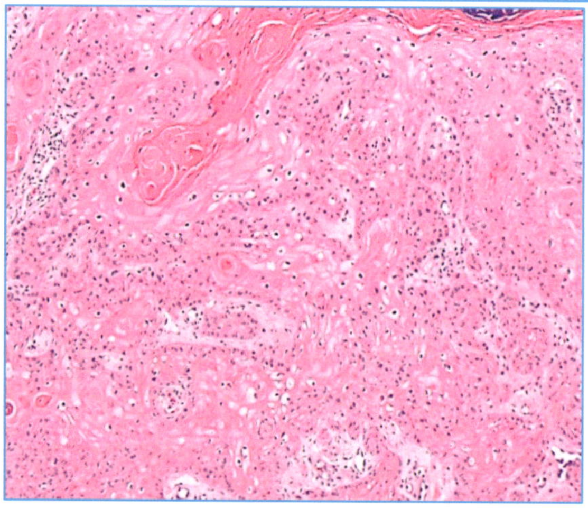

SCC made of atypical epithelial pink cells

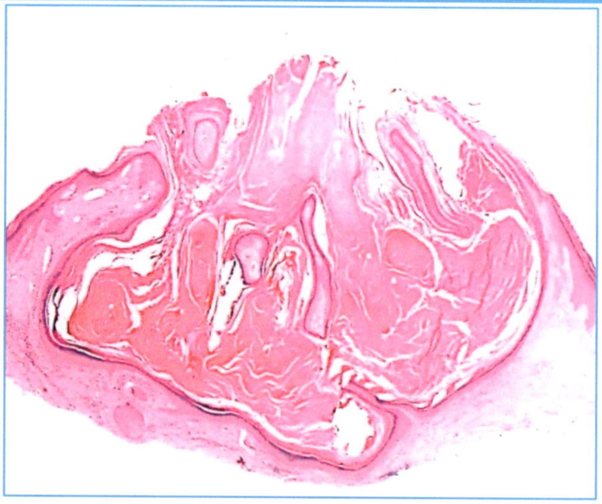

Keratoacanthoma with "crater-like" shape

Chapter 26

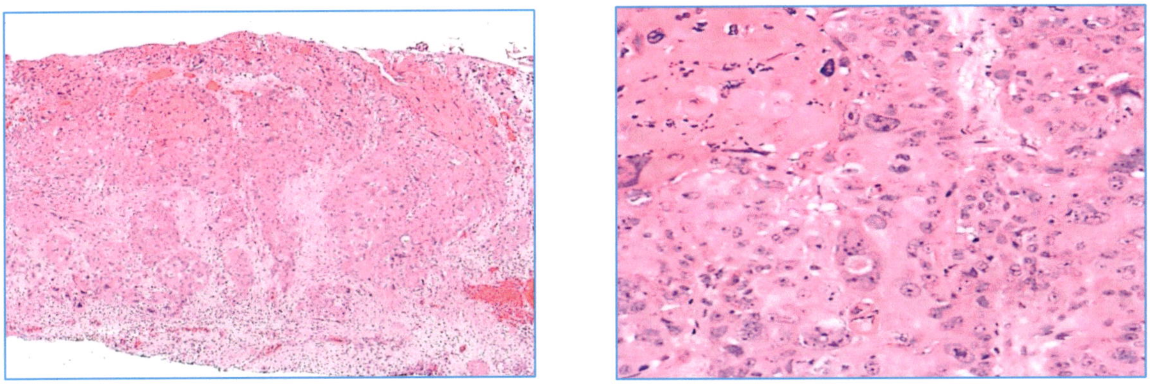

Moderately differentiated SCC with atypical, keratinizing, pink epithelioid cells

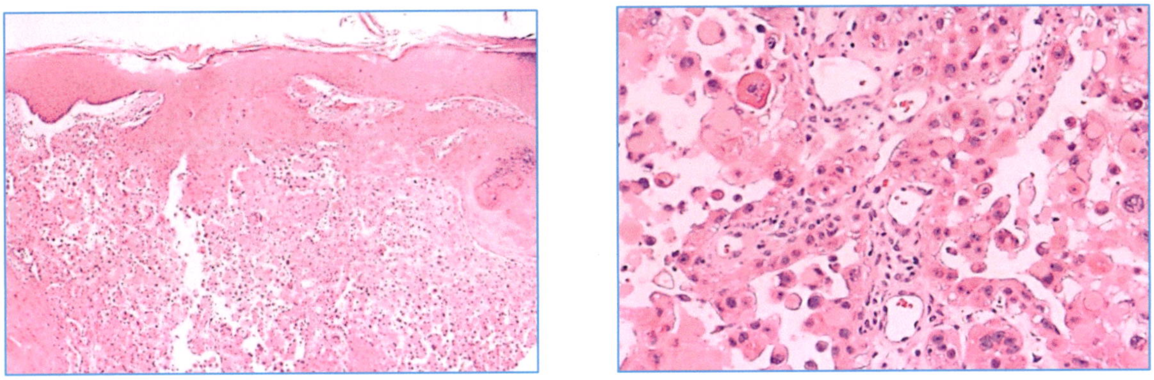

Acantholytic SCC with atypical epithelioid cells separated from each other

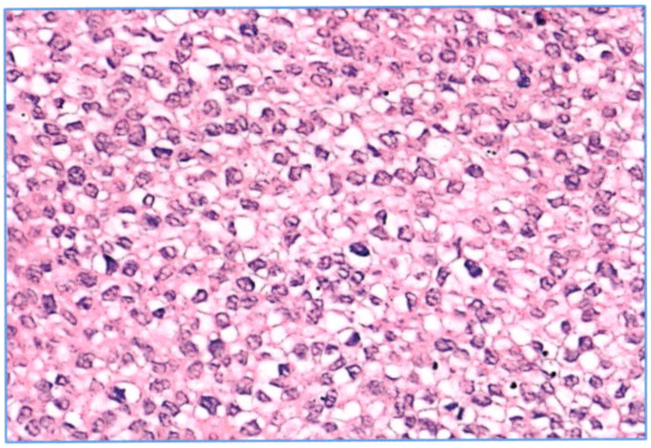

Clear cell SCC with atypical clear pink cells

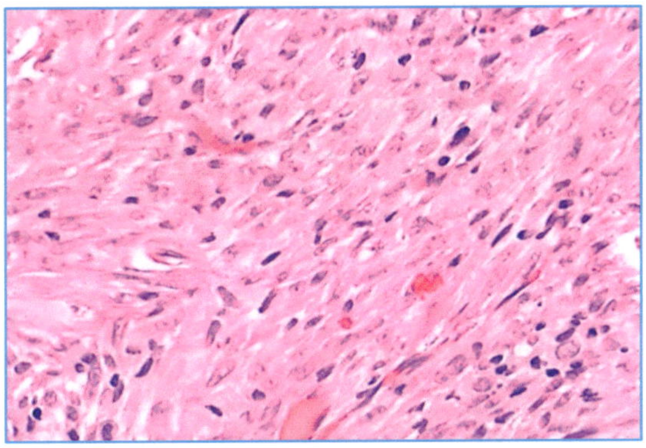

Spindle cell SCC with atypical, pink, elongated cells

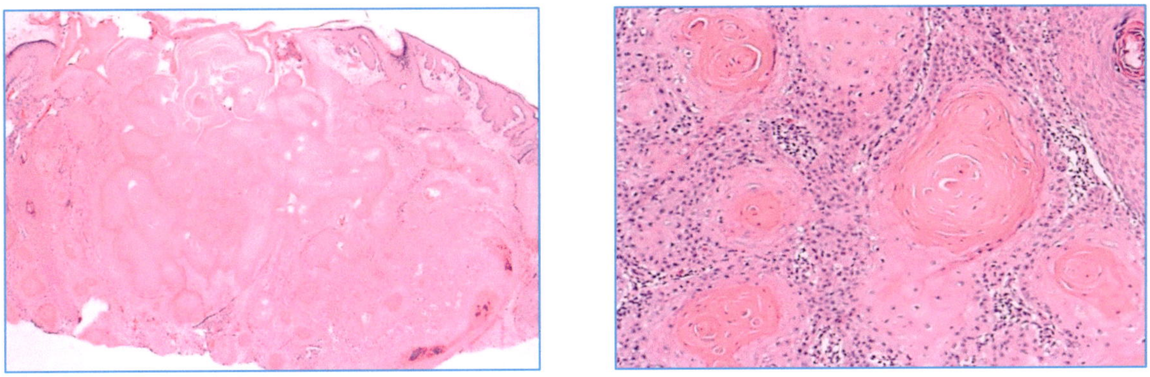

SCC, keratoacanthoma type, with crateriform silhouette and atypical invading epithelial nests

Epidermal tumors

LYMPHOEPITHELIOMA–LIKE CARCINOMA

-very rare skin tumor
-controversial whether it is inflamed squamous cell carcinoma or represents a tumor of adnexal origin
-most frequently occurs on the sun-exposed skin of the head and neck in elderly
-histologically resembles the nasopharyngeal tumor of the same name

Histopathology
-dense lymphocytic infiltrate
-atypical nested **epithelioid cells** with enlarged nuclei and vesicular chromatin, **hidden in lymphocytic infiltrate**
-**no** evidence of **keratin formation**
-adnexal differentiation can be seen

VERRUCOUS CARCINOMA

-elevated solitary nodular polypoid mass with papillary verrucous surface
-slowly growing tumor
-no HPV association
-favor oral cavity (*oral florid papillomatosis*), feet (*epithelioma cunniculatum*), and penis/perianal area (*Buschke-Loweinstein tumor*)

Histopathology
-**exophytic and endophytic** epidermal proliferation
-large, irregular, **hyperkeratotic, exophytic papillae**
-**blunt, endophytic, downward pushing rete ridges**
-**well-differentiated** squamous **epithelium** with **minimal cytological atypia**
-occasional mitosis but no necrosis
-**no** evidence of **koilocytes** despite the name

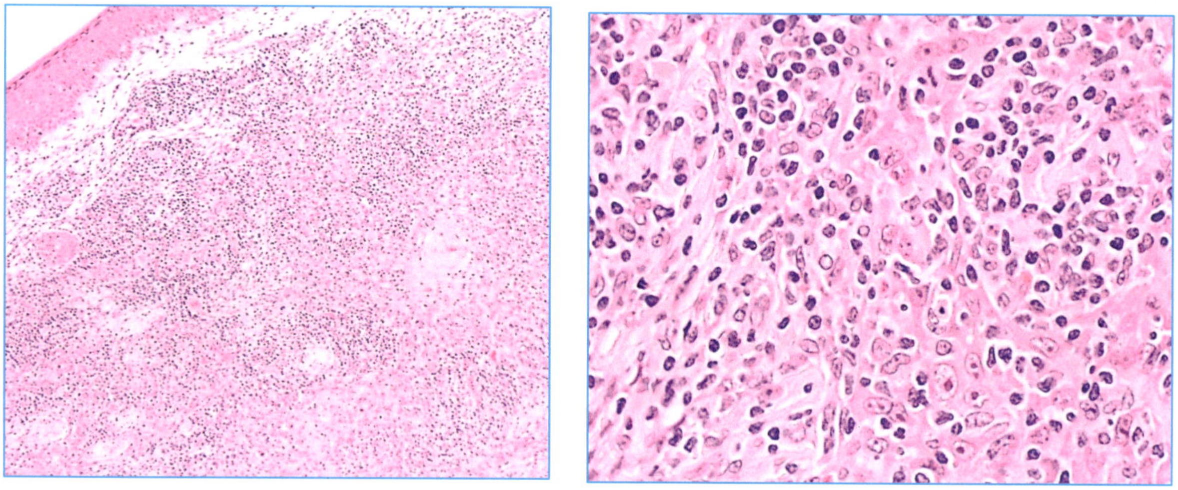

Lymphoepithelioma-like carcinoma with diffuse dermal infiltrate of pale epithelioid cells admixed with lymphocytes

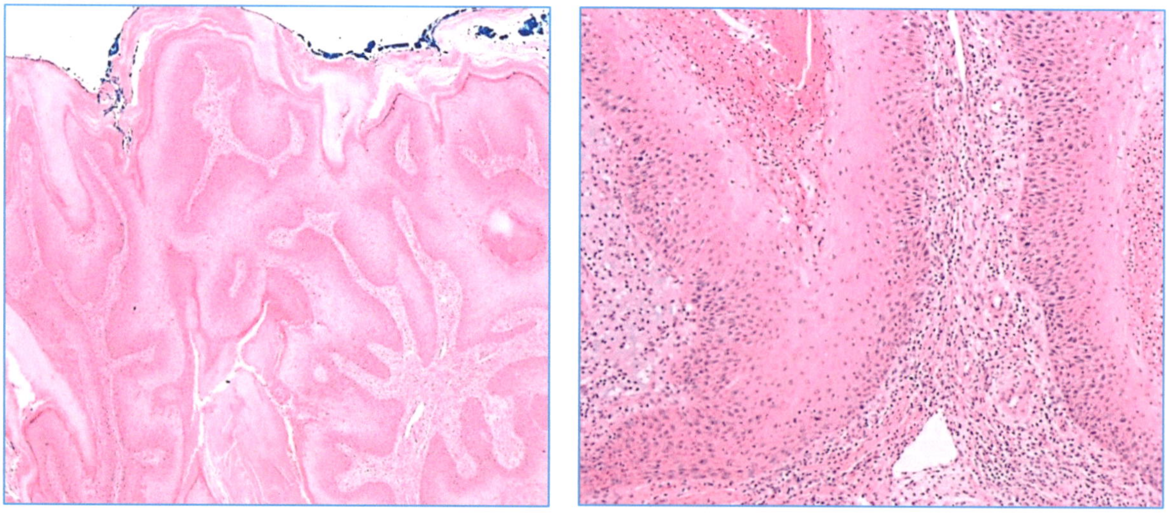

Verrucous carcinoma with exophytic and endophytic proliferation of minimally atypical epidermis

Chapter 26

HOW TO APPROACH EPITHELIAL TUMORS

IF EPIDERMIS DEMONSTRATES INTRAEPIDERMAL CLEFTING

-acantholytic acanthoma		flat or mildly indented epidermis
-warty dyskeratoma		"cup shaped" epidermis

IF EPIDERMIS IS RETICULATED (WITH THIN PAPILLAE)

-acanthosis nigricans	"box-lik"e papillomatosis in the upper dermis
-epidermal nevus	irregular papillomatosis present from childhood
-CARP	"finger-like" papillomatosis in the upper dermis
-reticulated SK	complex ("reticulated") epidermal strands that invades deeper dermis

IF EPIDERMIS SHOW IRREGULAR PAPILLOMATOSIS (WITH THICK PAPILLAE)

-prurigo nodularis		"dome-shaped"
-pseudoepitheliomatous hyperplasia		flat-topped
-halogenoderma		microabscesses common

IF EPIDERMIS IS VERRUCIFORM WITH "GOTHIC CHURCH SPIRES"

-verruca vulgaris		koilocytes
-epidermolythic acanthoma		no koilocytes with pink and blue granules
-granular parakeratosis	bordeaux red stratum corneum	prominent parakeratosis and granules
-acrokeratosis veruciformis	"SK-like" but with no cysts	present at birth
-seborrheic keratosis	horn pseudocysts	
-stucco keratosis	"SK-like" but with no cysts	small papules on ankle, feet

IF EPIDERMIS IS VERRUCIFORM BUT ALSO ENDOPHYTIC

-verrucous carcinoma	no koilocytes	minimal atypia + pushing borders

IF EPIDERMAL KERATINOCYTES ARE ENLARGED BUT NOT ATYPICAL

-large cell acanthoma	epidermis is usually flat

IF EPIDERMAL KERATINOCYTES ARE ATYPICAL

-actinic keratosis	up to bottom 2/3rd of epidermis is atypical
-SCC in situ	full thickness epidermal atypia
-Bowenoid papulosis	more uniform full thickness epidermal atypia on penis

IF EPIDERMIS IS THICK, PUSHING INTO DERMIS, BUT NOT ATYPICAL

-clear cell acanthoma	clear keratinocytes and neutrophils rimmed with dark keratinocytes
-seborrheic keratosis	uniform keratinocytes and horn pseudocysts
-inverted follicular keratosis	endophytic lesion with numerous squamous eddies

IF PALE CELLS ARE SCATTERED THROUGHOUT EPIDERMIS

-Paget's disease	randomly scattered clear cells with hint of bluish mucin

IF ATYPICAL EOSINOPHILIC (PINK) KERATINOCYTES INVADE DERMIS

-SCC

IF ATYPICAL BASOPHILIC (BLUE) KERATINOCYTES INVADE DERMIS

-BCC	stromal retraction + mucinous stroma + palisading

IF EPIDERMIS IS ENDOPHYTIC, "CRATER-LIKE", AND FILLED WITH KERATIN

-keratoacanthoma	pushing deep border
-SCC-KA type	infiltrating deep edge

Epidermal tumors

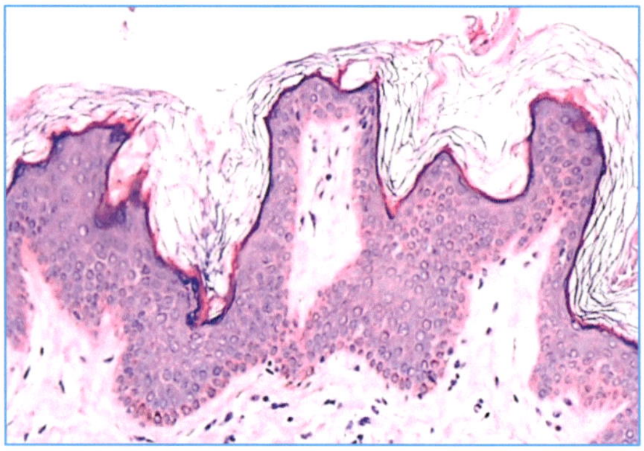

Acanthosis nigricans with "boxy" papillomatosis

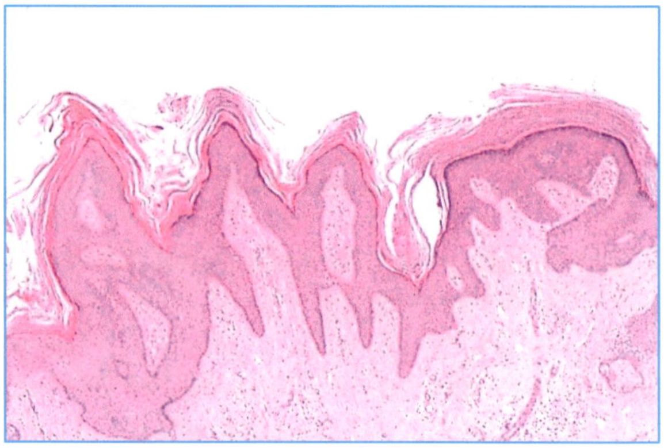

Epidermal nevus with irregular papillomatosis

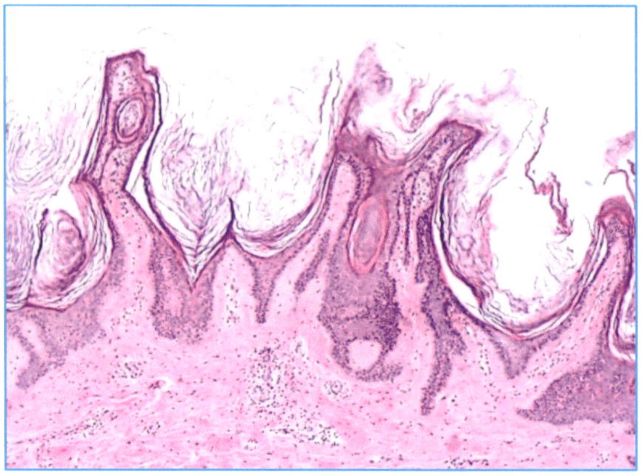

CARP with "fingers-like" epidermal protrusions

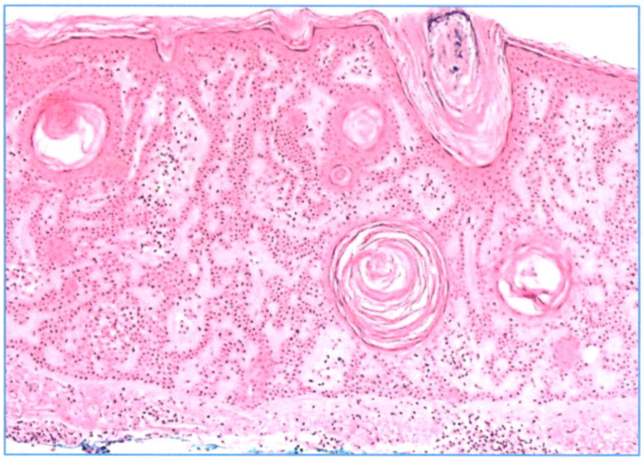

Reticulated SK with pseudocysts

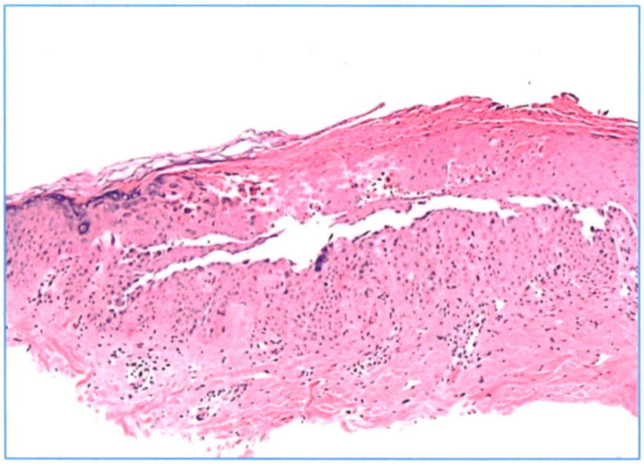

Acantholytic acanthoma is
flat lesion with intraepidermal acantholysis

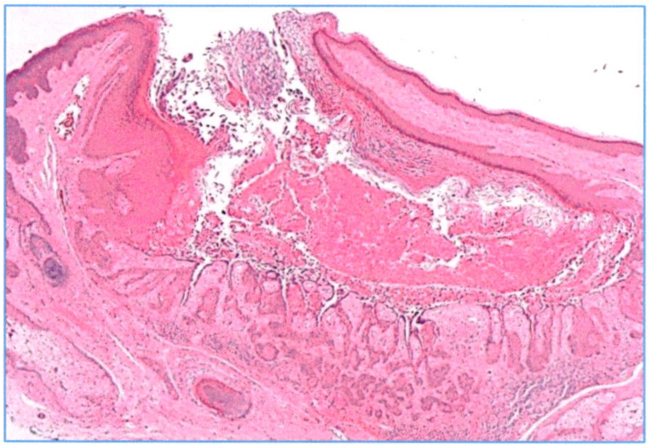

Warty dyskeratoma is
"cup-shaped" lesion with intraepidermal acantholysis

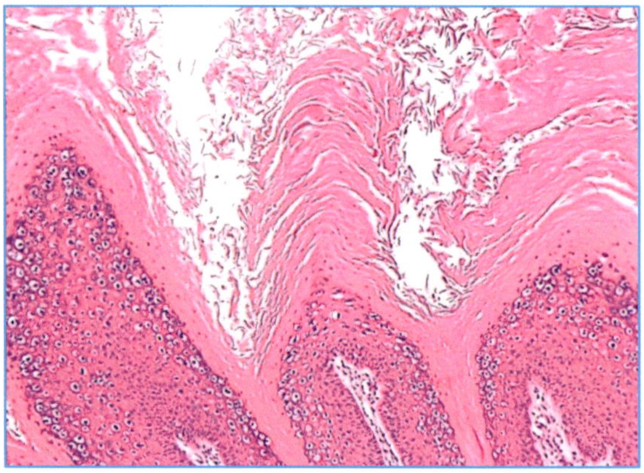

Verruca vulgaris with "gothic spires" and koilocytes

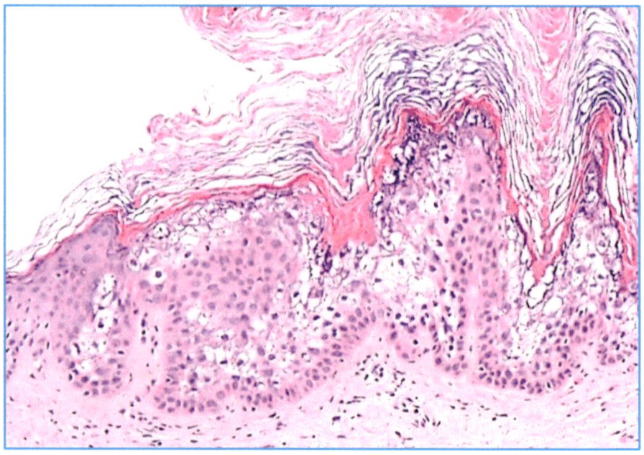

Epidermolytic acanthoma with pink and blue granules

Chapter 26

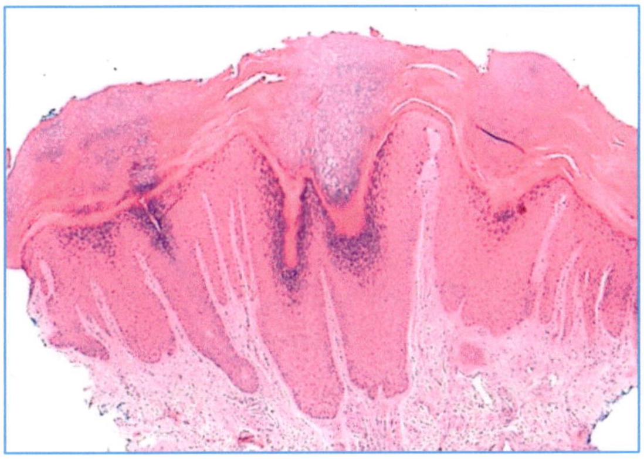

Prurigo nodularis with "dome-shaped" papillomatosis

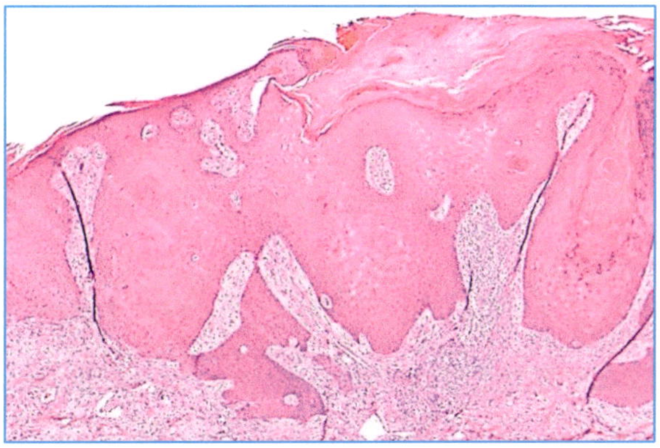

Pseudoepitheliomatous hyperplasia with irregular papillomatosis

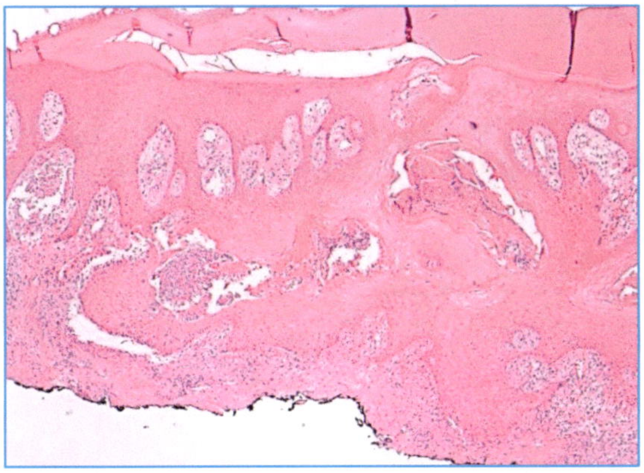

Halogenoderma with irregular epidermis with microabsesses

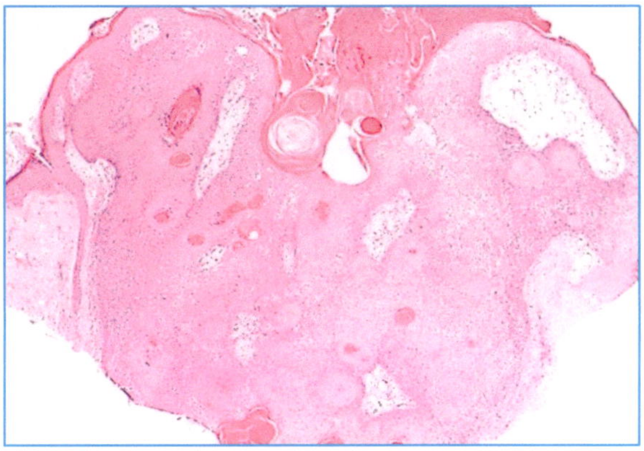

Inverted follicular keratosis is endophytic lesion with squamous eddies

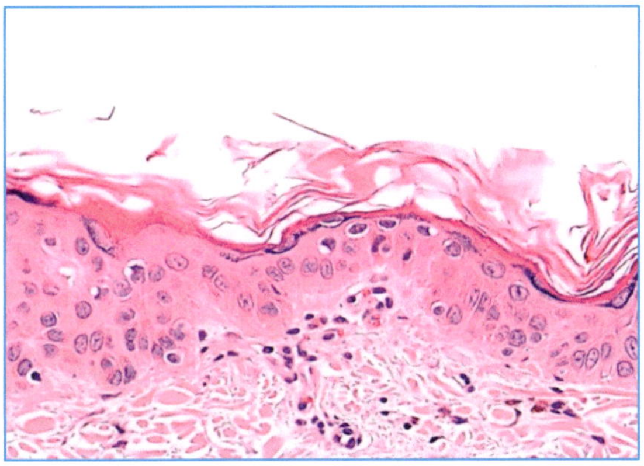

Large cell acanthoma with enlarged but not atypical keratinocytes

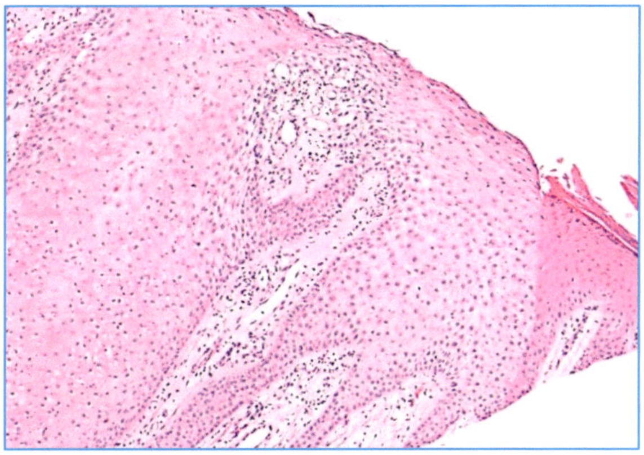

Clear cell acanthoma with clear keratinocytes with neutrophils

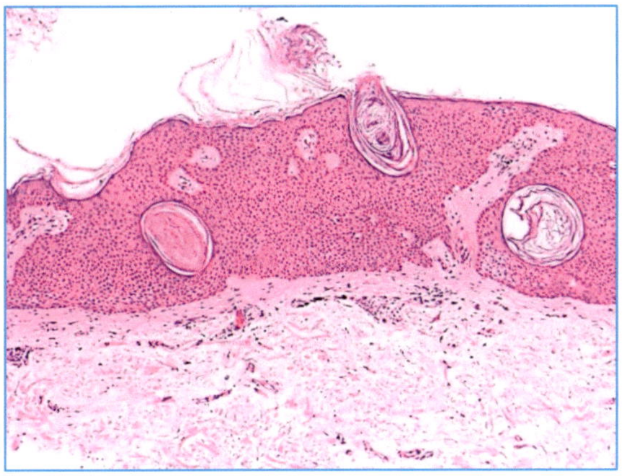

SK, acanthotic type, made of uniform cells with pseudocysts

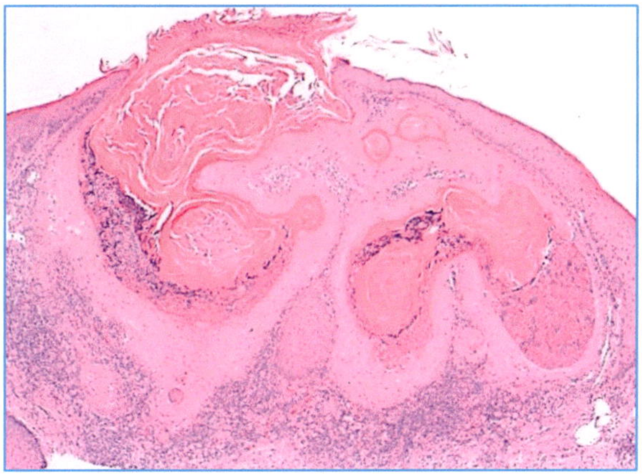

Keratoacanthoma with "volcano-like" lesion

Epidermal tumors

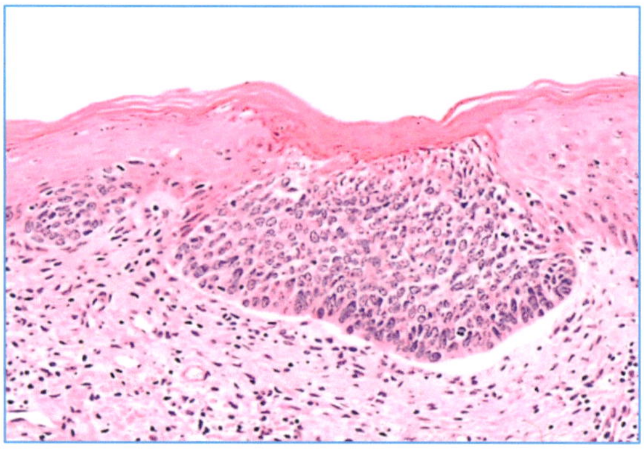

BCC, superficial type, with palisading and stromal retraction

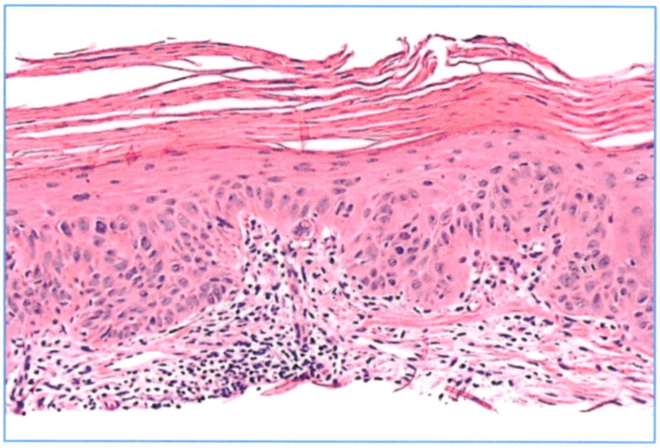

Hypertrophic AK with atypia in lower 2/3rd of the epidermis

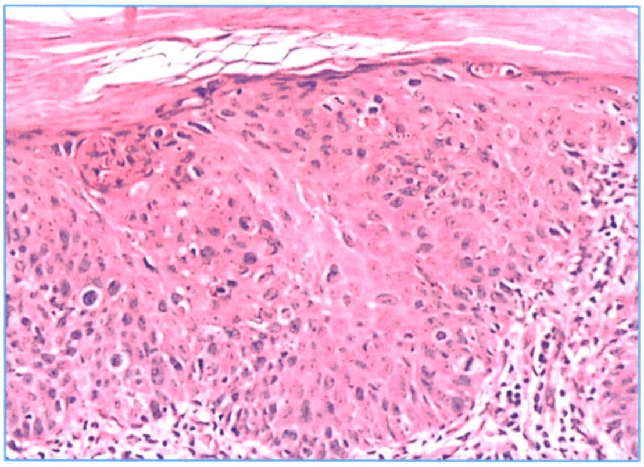

In situ SCC with full thickness irregular atypia

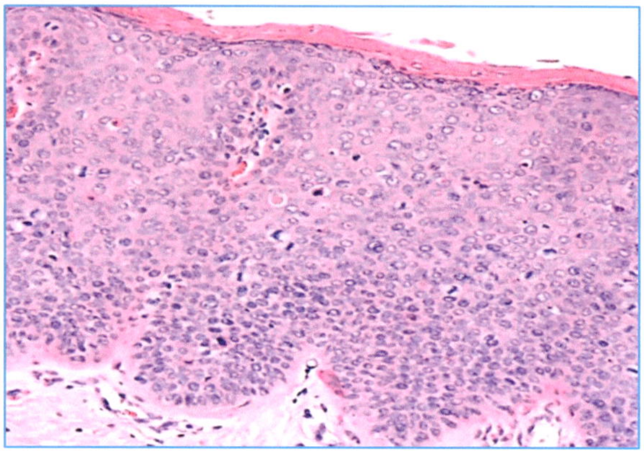

Bowenoid papulosis with more uniform full thickness atypia

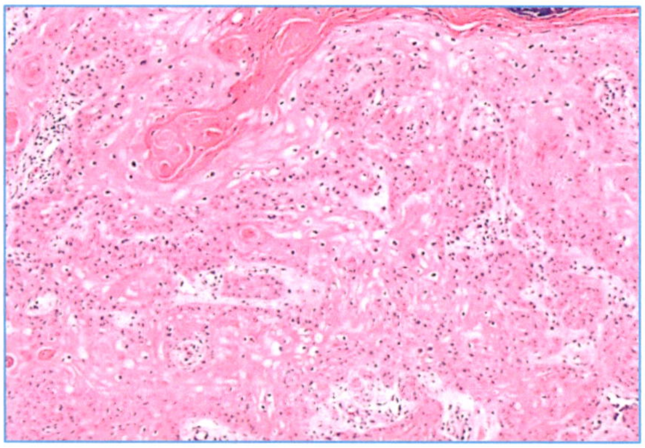

SCC with atypical epithelial cells invading dermis

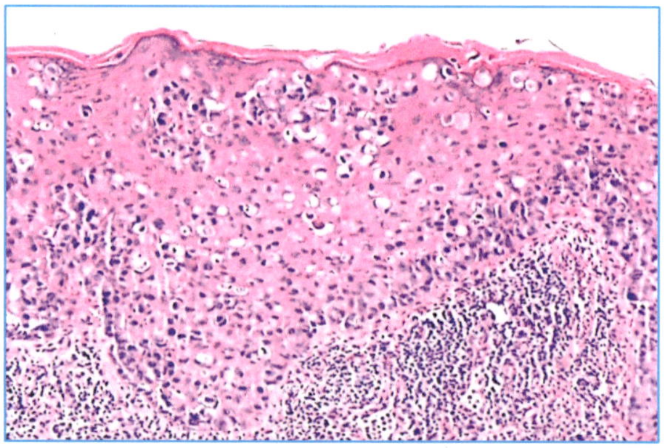

Paget's disease with scattered pale mucinous cells in epidermis

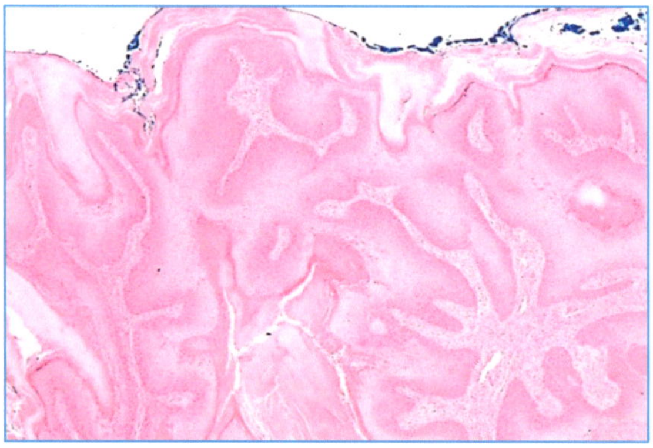

Verrucous carcinoma is
exophytic and endophytic lesion with minimal atypia

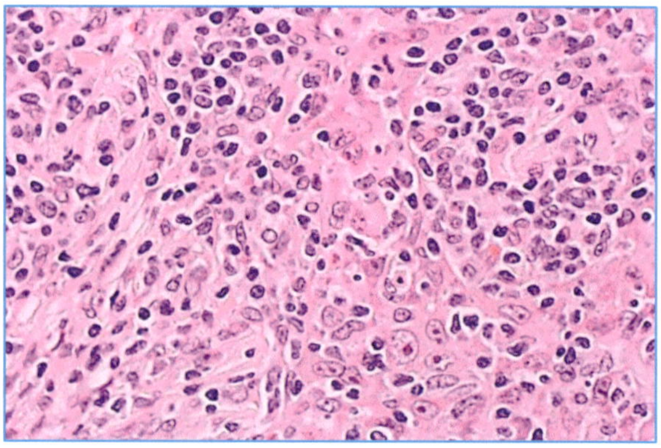

Lymphoepithelioma-like carcinoma with
atypical epithelioid cells hidden by lymphocytes

Chapter 27

FOLLICULAR TUMORS

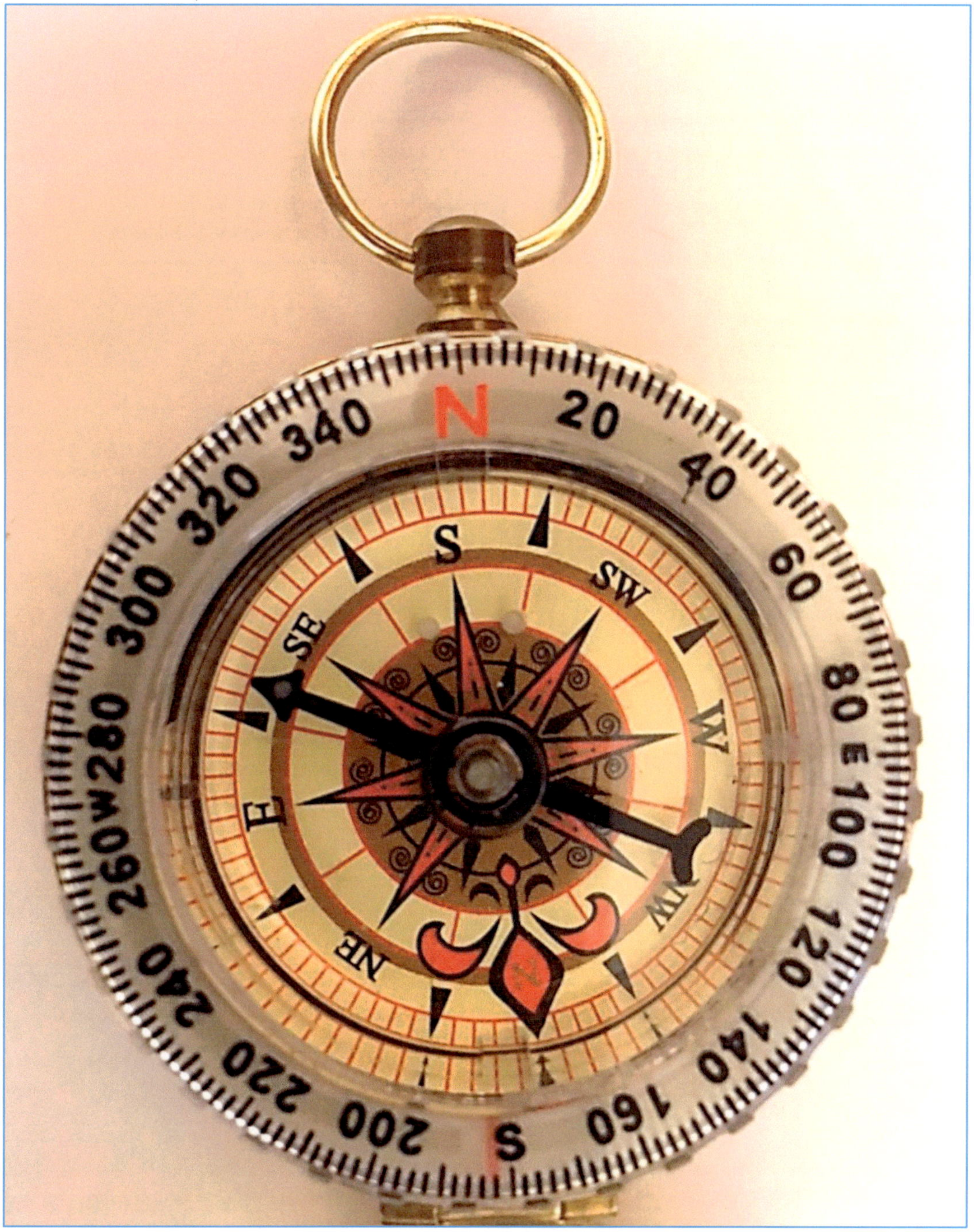

Follicular tumors

TRICHOEPITHELIOMA

-solitary benign hair follicle tumor in adults or multiple tumors in children
-it presents as a skin-colored papule (regular TE) or as "doughnut shaped", skin-colored papule with raised margins and depressed center (desmoplastic TE)
-it is associated with Brooke-Spiegler syndrome (mutation in *CYLD* gene) along with cylindroma, spiradenoma, ungual fibroma, basal cell carcinoma
-lesions favor the central face

Histopathology

-basaloid dermal tumor, only occasionally connected to the epidermis
-multiple dermal islands of basaloid cells separated by collagenous hypocellular stroma
-**no mucin in the stroma (unlike BCC)**
-peripheral palisading but **no stromal retraction**
-focal primordial follicles are seen (**"mesenchymal papillary bodies"**)
-small keratinizing **microcysts are present**
-calcification is common

Desmoplastic variant

-**cords or small nests of basaloid cells** in **dense collagenous stroma**
-**keratin cysts with common calcifications**
-no stromal retraction or mucinous stroma

TRICHOBLASTOMA

-small benign hair follicle tumor
-thought to be a **variant of trichoepithelioma**
-presents as a solitary, skin-colored to brown or blue-black papule or nodule, favoring head (#1 scalp)

Histopathology

-circumscribed basaloid dermal tumor
-located in the middle to lower dermis, **without epidermal connection**
-cords, nests, lobules of basaloid cells
-fibrotic stroma with **no stromal retraction**
-**"papillary mesenchymal bodies"** (primordial hairs) are present but **keratin cysts absent**

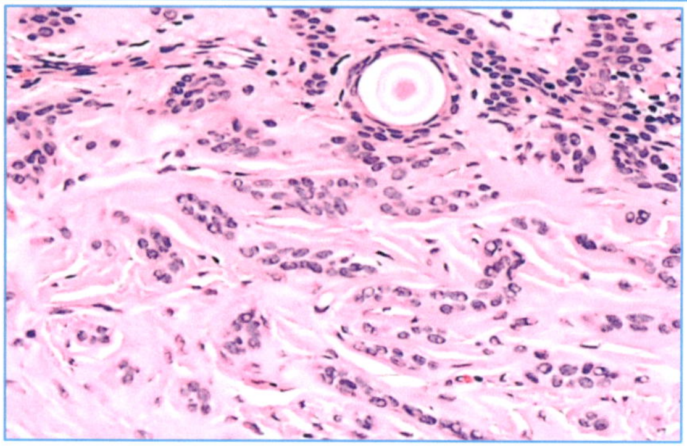

Desmoplastic TE with cords of basaloid cells in dense stroma

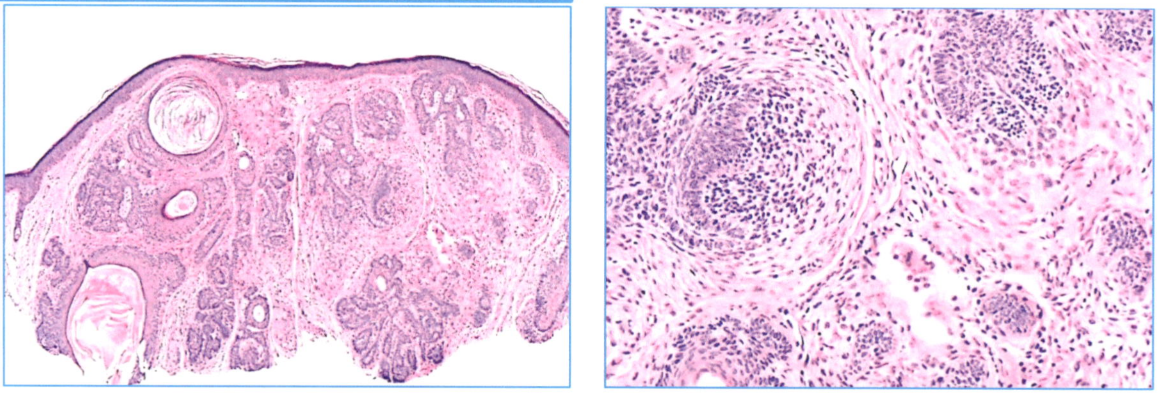

Trichoepithelioma with dermal basaloid cells, mesenchymal bodies, and multiple keratin cysts in dense stroma

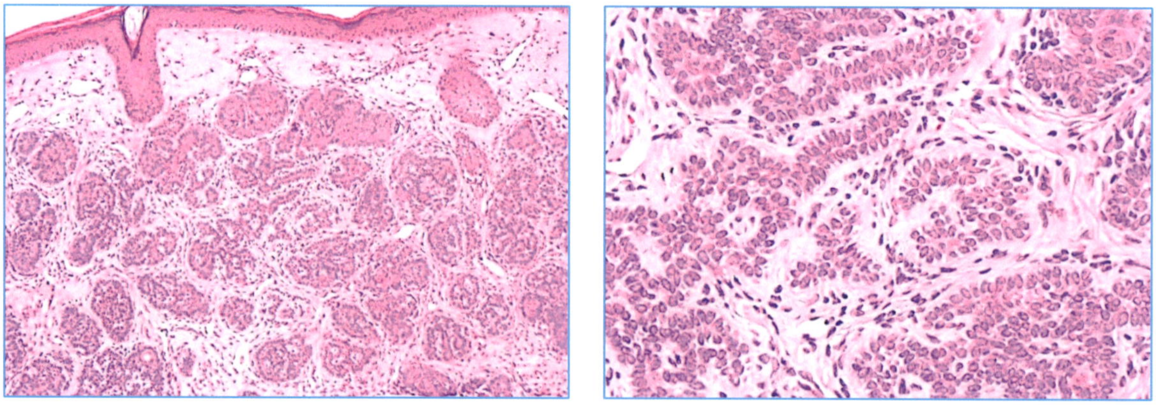

Trichoblastoma is dermal basaloid tumor with mesenchymal bodies in dense stroma. No keratin cysts or epidermal connection.

Chapter 27

CUTANEOUS LYMPHADENOMA

-probably variant of trichoblastoma
-presents as a solitary, small, flesh-colored, non-ulcerated, asymptomatic nodule
-adult males are affected more often than females
-most cases occur on the head, especially the cheek, forehead, eyelid, and temple

Histopathology

-well-circumscribed lesion in deep dermis
-irregularly shaped nests made of **peripheral basaloid** cells, **central pale** cells, and characteristic lymphocytes scattered over tumor cells
-nests are embedded in dense stroma
-absence of tumor stromal retraction

TUMOR OF FOLLICULAR INFUNDIBULUM

-rare tumor of head, neck, upper chest
-presents as solitary papule and clinically resembles superficial basal cell carcinoma
-associated with Cowden's syndrome and nevus sebaceous

Histopathology

-shallow **"plate-like"** (flat bottom) subepidermal tumor with **anastomosing basaloid strands**
-**multiple connections** to epidermis
-peripheral palisading of nuclei but no significant stromal retraction
-**trichilemmal cysts** are present

BASALOID FOLLICULAR HAMARTOMA

-presents as single or multiple, skin-colored to brown papules
-solitary lesions favor the face, scalp, and trunk
-multiple lesions also seen on extremities
-solitary basaloid follicular hamartoma may be congenital or acquired
-multiple basaloid follicular hamartomas are hereditary (autosomal dominant) or acquired (associated with myasthenia gravis, systemic lupus erythematosus)

Histopathology

-anastomosing strands of basaloid cells forming well defined dermal tumor with **a single connection** to the overlying epithelium **("tree roots-like")**
-no evidence of stromal retraction or atypia
-**small trichilemmal cysts present**

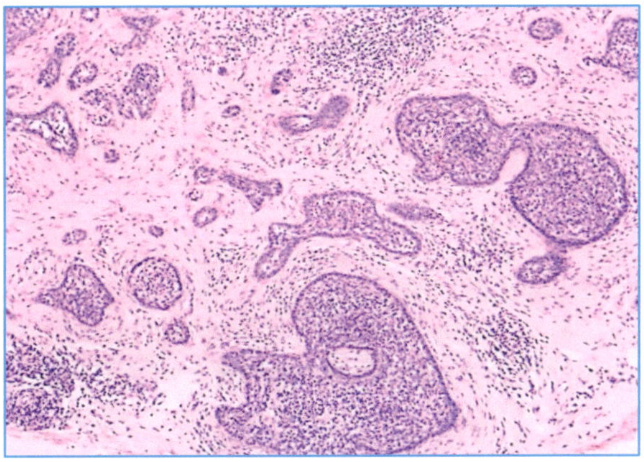

Cutaneous lymphadenoma with peripheral basaloid cells, central pale cells, and scattered lymphocytes

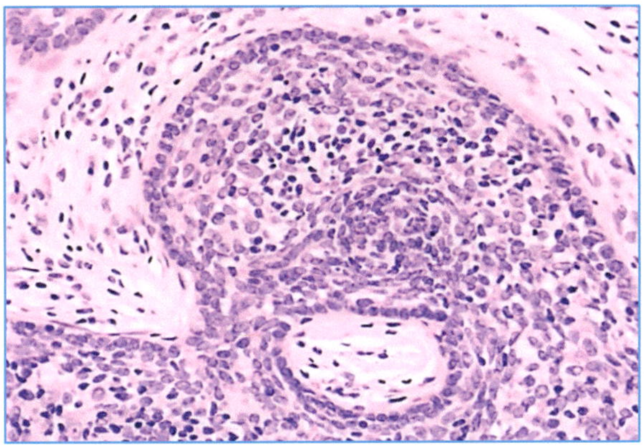

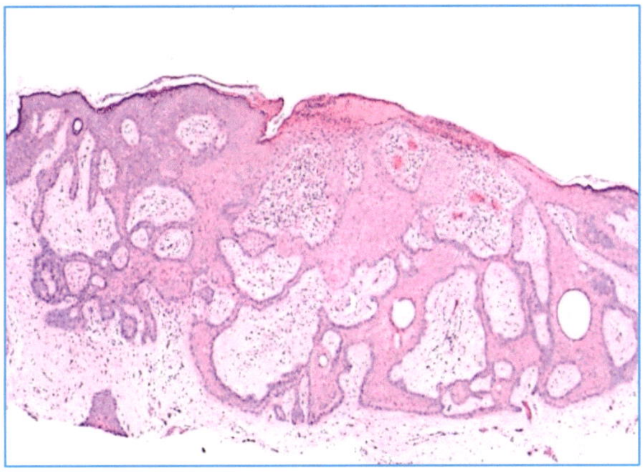

"Plate-like" tumor of follicular infundibulum

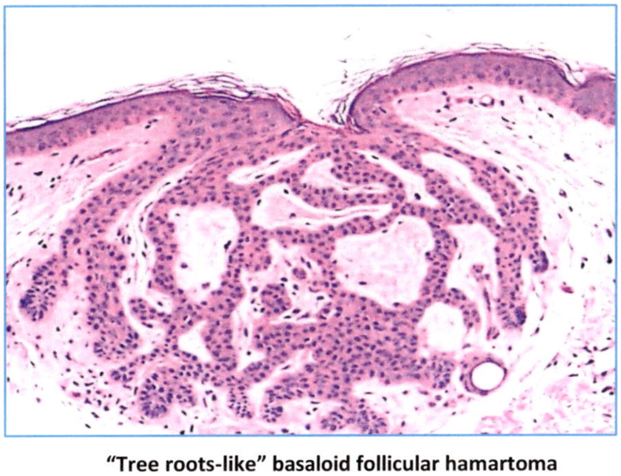

"Tree roots-like" basaloid follicular hamartoma

Follicular tumors

TRICHOADENOMA (OF NIKOLOWSKI)

-presents as skin-colored nodule mostly in adults
-typically found on either the face or buttocks

Histopathology
-well-defined dermal tumor consisting of **numerous clustered** cysts and **small basaloid epithelial strands/islands in between cysts**
-**cysts lined by flattened squamous epithelium** with a granular layer
-cysts are filled with flaky keratin
-occasional trichilemmal differentiation can be present

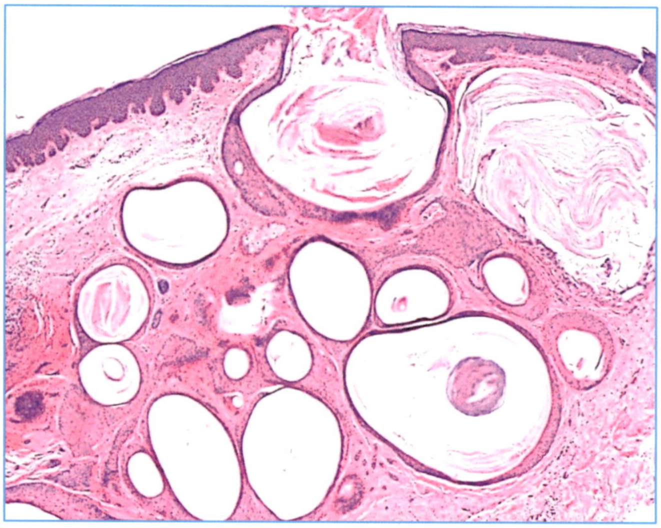

Trichoadenoma with numerous clustered cysts filled with keratin

TRICHOFOLLICULOMA

-favors central part of face
-solitary skin-colored papule or nodule
-central indentation filled with keratin and hair

Histopathology
-**central dilated hair follicles ("mother follicle")**
-**multiple smaller hair follicles** branch out from the central follicle **("baby follicles")**
-secondary follicle are at various stages of development
-sebaceous glands can be attached to the follicles

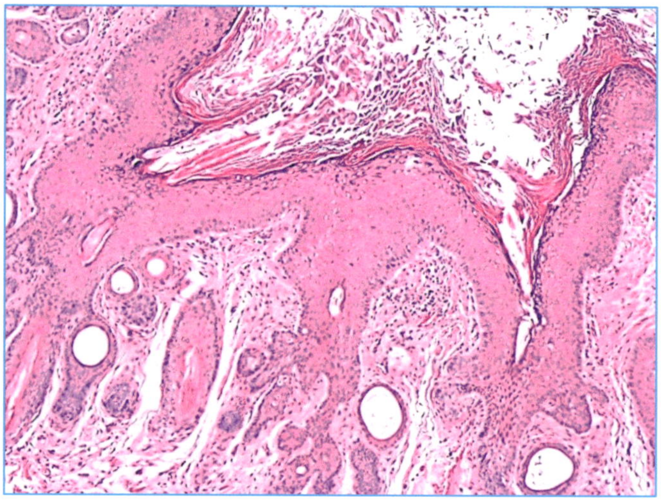

Trichofolliculoma with central dilated "mother follicle" and multiple attached "baby follicles"

NEVUS COMEDONICUS/ FAVRE-RACOUCHOT DISEASE

Nevus comedonicus
-closely grouped, open comedones present in childhood or early adulthood
-favors face, neck, trunk, arms

Favre-Racouchot disease
-multiple open comedones on sun damaged skin in elderly
-especially common under the eyes and on lateral malar cheeks

Histopathology
-**multiple cystically dilated hair follicles (comedones)** filled with compact keratin
-in Favre-Racouchot disease, cysts are set in sun damaged dermis (solar elastosis)

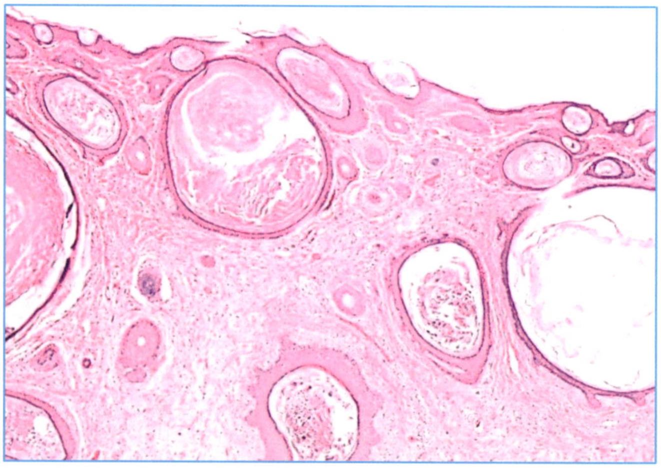

Favre-Racouchot disease with multiple dilated comedones in sun damaged dermis

Chapter 27

PILOMATRICOMA

-solitary cutaneous firm tumor nodule associated with mutations in *CTNNB1,* gene that encodes β catenin
-60% occur in the first two decades of life
-classically scalp (#1), face, and upper extremities
-"**tent sign"** (angles and facets seen with stretched skin)

Histopathology

-well circumscribed dermal/subcutaneous tumor with frequent **calcifications**
-consists of 3 components in different ratios
- -small uniform **basaloid cells** with small dark nuclei
- -**pink keratinocytic remnants ("ghost cells")**
- -keratin **foreign body cell reaction**

TRICHILEMMOMA

-solitary or multiple skin-colored keratotic papules
-multiple are associated with Cowden's syndrome (*PTEN* gene mutation)
-favors face, particularly lip

Histopathology

-lobular or multilobular tumor growing from epidermis into dermis
-lobules have pushing border and prominent eosinophilic basement membrane (**"eyeliner"** sign)
-**center** is composed of **clear**, uniform **squamoid cells** (containing glycogen)
-**peripheral cells are darker** and show **palisading**
-overlying epidermis is hyperkeratotic

Desmoplastic variant

-periphery appears like regular trichilemmoma
-**center stroma is hyalinized/desmoplastic** with embedded smaller group of tumor cells

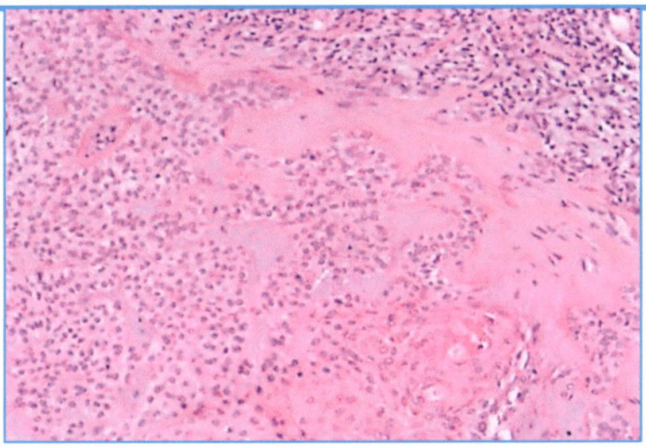

Desmoplastic trichilemmoma with hyalinized stroma

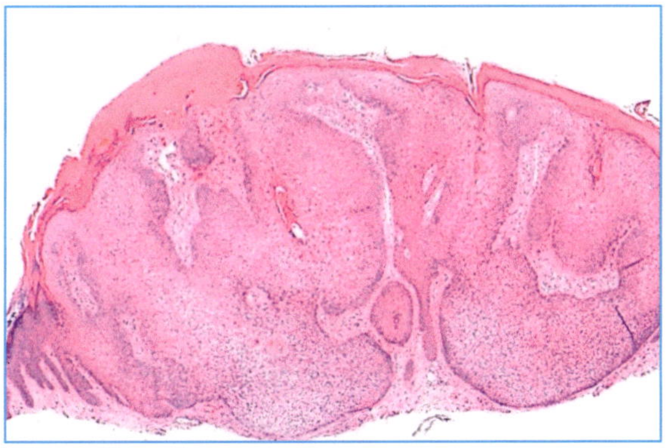

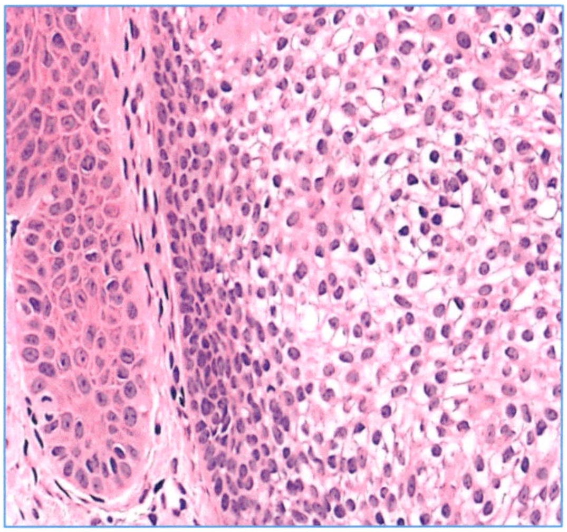

Trichilemmoma with multiple lobules made of pale central cells, peripheral darker cells, and prominent basement membrane

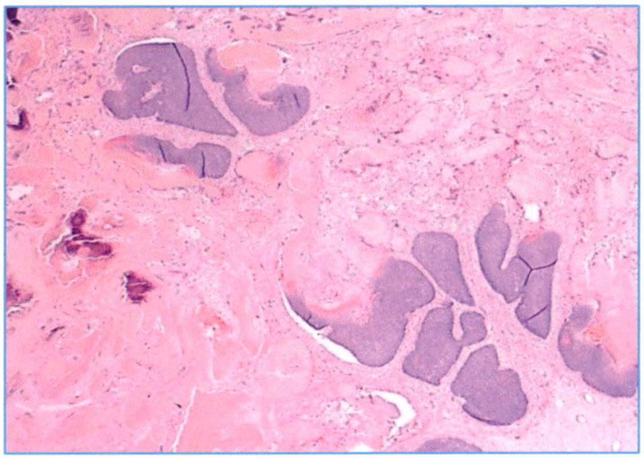

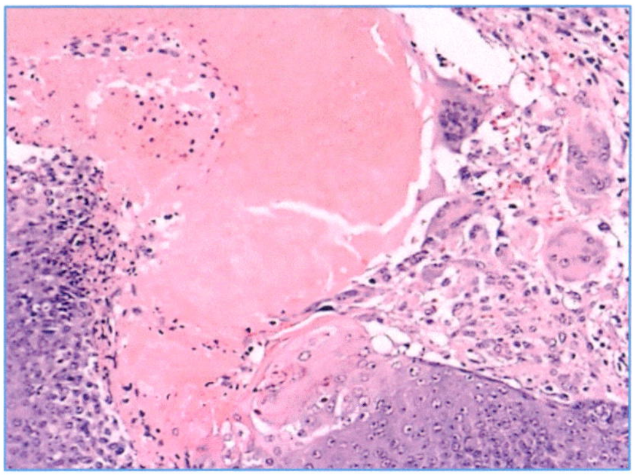

Focally calcified pilomatricoma with dark basaloid cells, pink "ghost" cells, and foreign body giant cell reaction

Follicular tumors

PANFOLLICULOMA

-very rare benign tumor that favors head or trunk
-presents as a solitary, asymptomatic, skin-colored nodule

Histopathology

-three variants based on architectural outline (nodular, superficial, and cystic)
-all variants have **differentiation toward all segments of hair follicle**: the infundibulum, stem, and bulb/papilla
-tumor is overall **basaloid** with focal pale cells of outer root sheath epithelium, and abortive hair shafts

TRICHOGERMINOMA

-very rare cutaneous adnexal neoplasm of the hair germ cells
-presents as solitary, slowly growing, dermal or subcutaneous nodule without any clinical symptoms
-mainly affects elderly people with no body site predilection

Histopathology

-well-circumscribed dermal/subcutaneous tumor
-multiple lobules separated by dense stroma
-lobules made of **central pale "cell balls"** with peripheral condensation

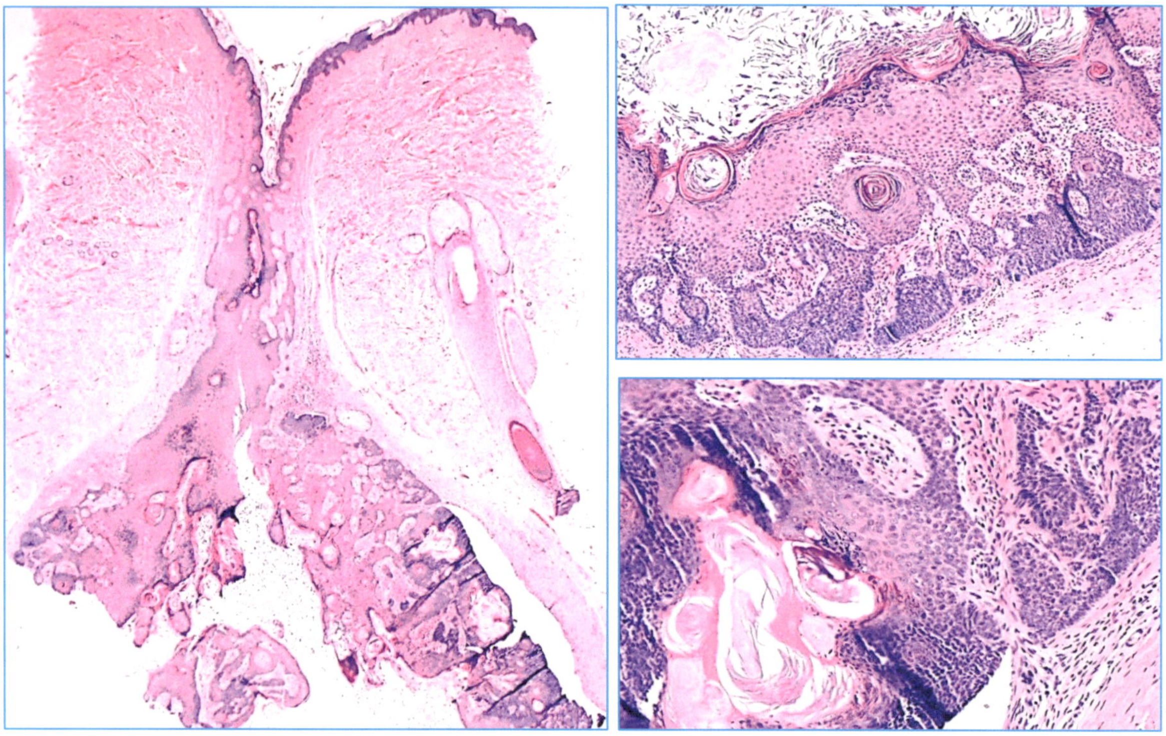

Cystic panfolliculoma with lining showing differentiation toward all elements of hair follicle

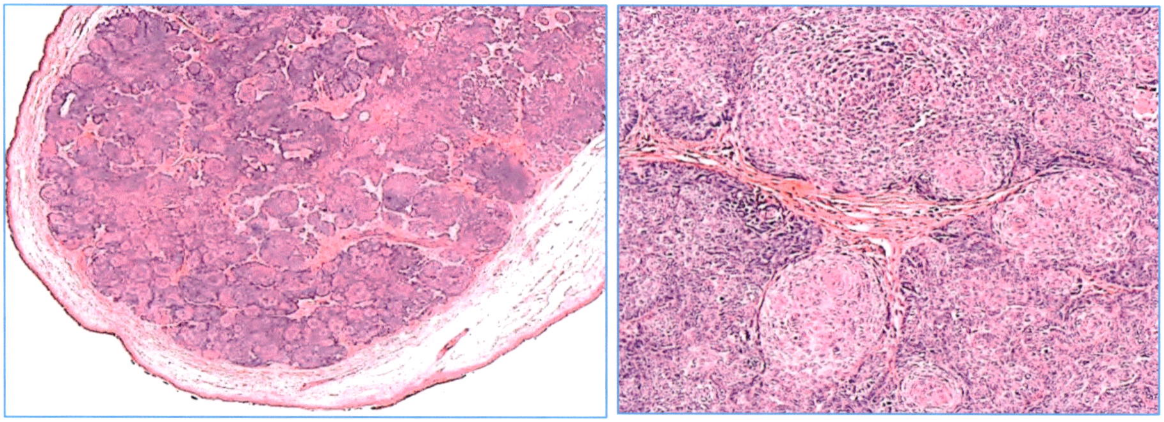

Trichogerminoma with central pale "cell balls" surrounded with basaloid cells

Chapter 27

FIBROFOLLICULOMA

-presents as asymptomatic, small, yellow to skin-colored papule(s)
-favors head, neck, chest, back, popliteal and antecubital fossa
-can be solitary or multiple
-multiple are part of Birt Hogg Dube syndrome (*FLCN* gene)

Histopathology
-dilated, distorted hair follicle filled with keratin debris
-**epithelial cords** proliferate from and swirl around hair follicle (**"octopus-like")**
-follicle surrounded by proliferation of loose connective tissue

TRICHODISCOMA

-small skin-colored papules
-favor face and upper trunk
-multiple lesions may occur in isolation or represent part of Birt Hogg Dube syndrome

Histopathology
-"**disc-like"** proliferation of hyalinized **connective tissue**
-mildly increased number of fibroblasts
-fibrous plate on either side is **bordered by hair follicle**
-commonly hair follicles have features of fibrofolliculoma (distortion, epithelial cords)

These two entities are probably the same, but histology differ based on the position of biopsy site relative to the hair follicles

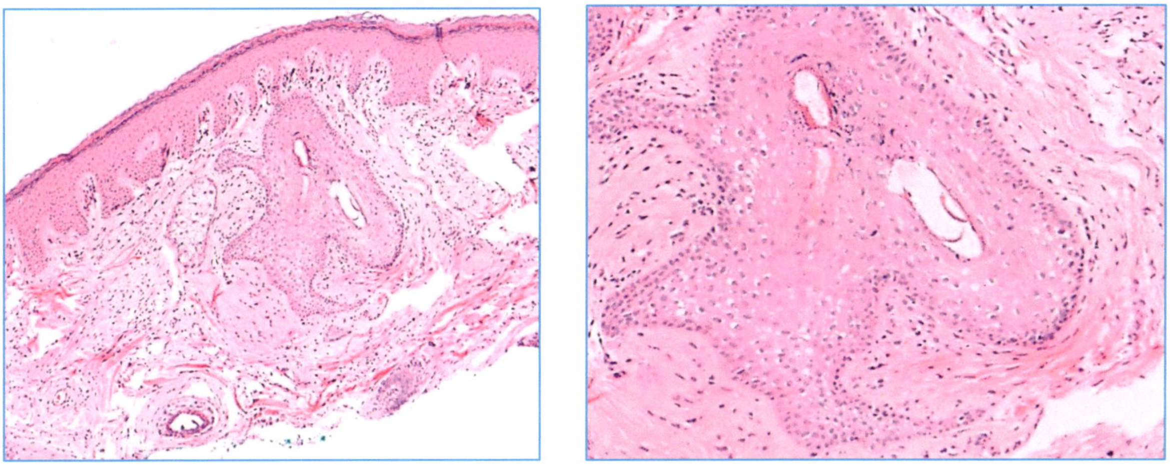

Fibrofolliculoma with "octopus-like" distorted follicle

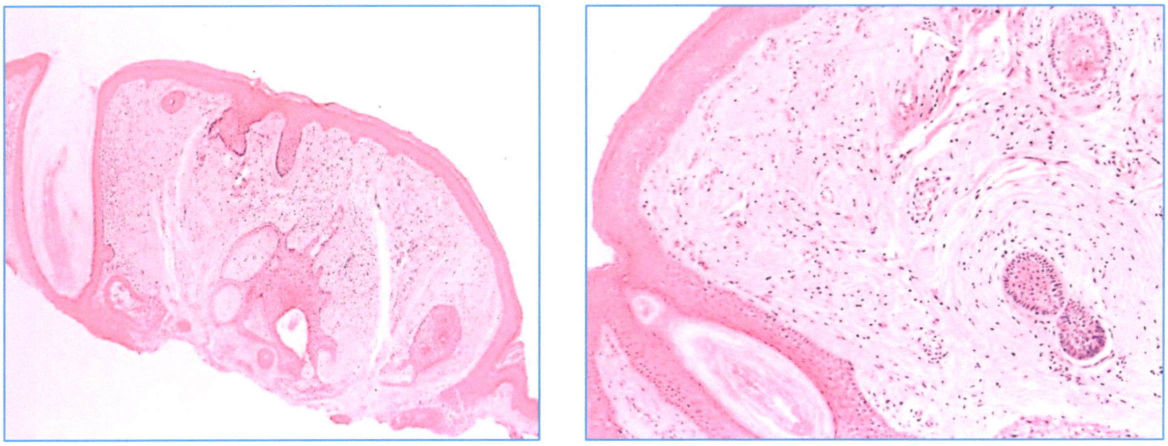

Trichodiscoma with dermal "disc-like" connective tissue abutted by distorted hair follicles

Follicular tumors

DILATED PORE OF WINER

-solitary or multiple lesions with large "comedo-like" appearance
-favors upper trunk

Histopathology
-**dilated follicular pore**
-filled with keratin debris
-squamous epithelium is acanthotic with **"finger-like" projections**

PILAR SHEATH ACANTHOMA

-small, solitary papule with central keratin filled depression or opening
-on face and head of middle-aged people
-upper cutaneous lip is the most favorite site

Histopathology
-**dilated follicle** filled with loose keratin
-pore epithelium lining is acanthotic and has **wide endophytic lobular proliferation** with pushing borders (wider than in dilated pore of Winer)

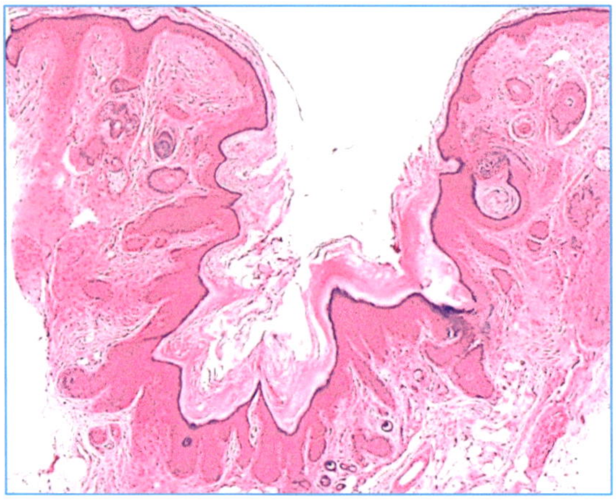

Dilated pore of Winer with "finger-like" projections

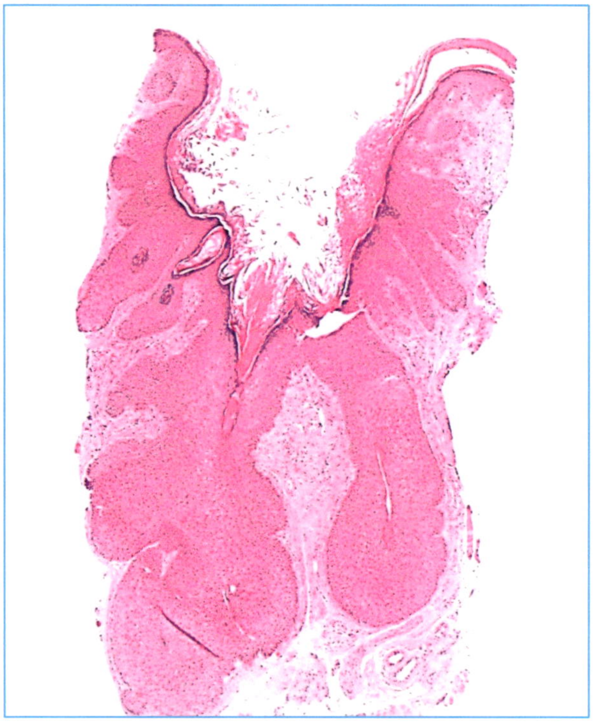

Pilar sheath acanthoma with dilated follicle and wide epidermal projections

PERIFOLLICULAR FIBROMA

-small, flesh-colored, "dome-shaped" papules
-head and neck are favored sites
-may be single or multiple
-associated with nevus lipomatosus cutaneous superficialis

Histopathology
-mildly dilated hair follicle
-concentric perifollicular fibrosis

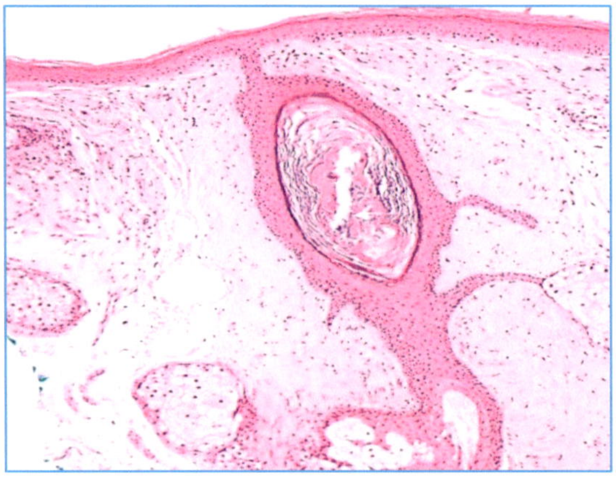

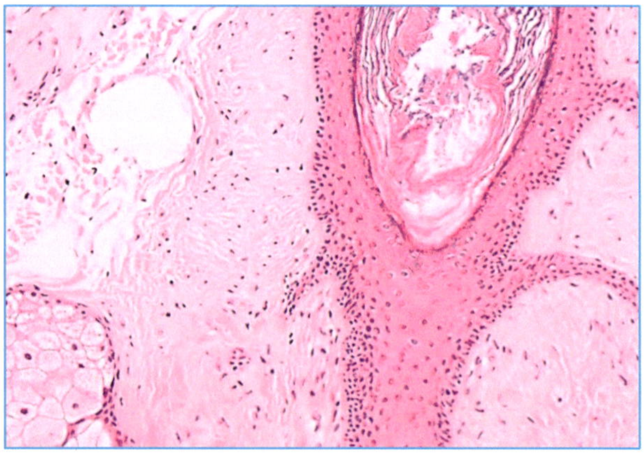

Perifollicular fibroma with dermal fibrosis around dilated follicle

Chapter 27

HOW TO APPROACH TUMORS OF FOLLICULAR ORIGIN

IF YOU SEE A SINGLE LARGE DILATED FOLLICLE

-pilar sheath acanthoma	broad projections from the follicle
-dilated pore of Winer	"finger-like" projections from the follicle
-trichofolliculoma	multiple small hairs attached to the central follicle
-perifollicular fibroma	perifollicular fibrosis

IF YOU SEE MULTIPLE LARGE DILATED FOLLICLES

-trichoadenoma	multiple cysts (comedones) with solid tumor nests in between
-nevus comedonicus	multiple cysts (comedones) only
-Favre-Racouchot	multiple cysts (comedones) + solar elastosis

IF YOU SEE DISTORTED HAIR FOLLICLE WITH SCAR

-trichodiscoma	two distorted follicles with fibrosis in between
-fibrofoliculoma	single distorted follicle with fibrosis around
-perifollicular fibroma	dilated but not distorted follicle with fibrosis

IF YOU SEE WEBBED, "NET-LIKE" TUMOR

-tumor of follicular infundibulum	"plate-like" with multiple epidermal connection
-basaloid follicular hamartoma	"tree root-like" with single epidermal connection

IF TUMOR LOOKS LIKE NODULAR OR MICRONODULAR BCC BUT WITHOUT ATYPIA, EPIDERMAL CONNECTION, STROMAL RETRACTION, OR MUCINOUS STROMA

-trichoepithelioma	superficial tumor with small cysts and calcification
-trichoblastoma	deeper tumor with no cysts or calcifications
-cutaneous lymphadenoma	similar to trichoblastoma with clear cells and lymphocytes
-trichogerminoma	balls of pale cells within tumor nodules
-panfolliculoma	multiple stages of hair follicle differentiation seen within tumor

IF TUMOR NODULE(S) ARE BROADLY CONNECTED TO EPIDERMIS WITH CLEAR CELLS AND NO ATYPIA

-trichilemmoma	clear cells with thick pink BMZ ("eyeliner" sign)

IF TUMOR IS PINK AND BLUE WITH NO OBVIOUS HAIR DIFFERENTIATION

-pilomatricoma	dark blue cells, pink "ghost" cells, inflammation

WORD OF CAUTION

-benign trichilemmoma and pilomatricoma have exceedingly rare malignant variants called trichilemmal carcinoma and pilomatrix carcinoma
-they are believed to occur from a malignant transformation of long standing benign trichilemmoma or pilomatricoma and not de novo
-histologically, usually a portion of benign tumor or tumor resembling benign tumor is present
-additionally, malignant areas are found characterized by areas of necrosis, cytological atypia, and presence of mitoses

Follicular tumors

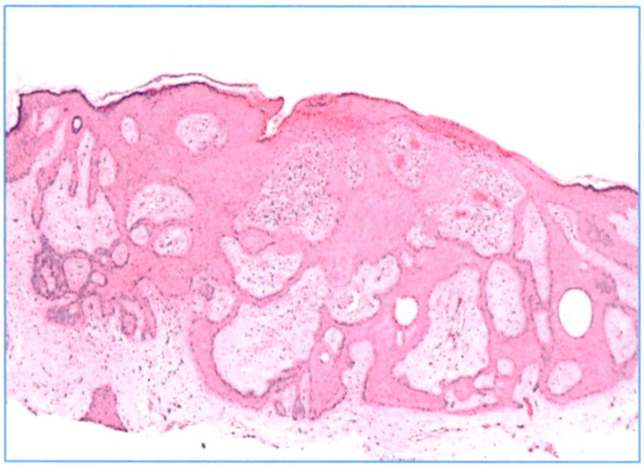

Tumor of follicular infundibulum is a "plate-like" lesion with multiple epidermal connections

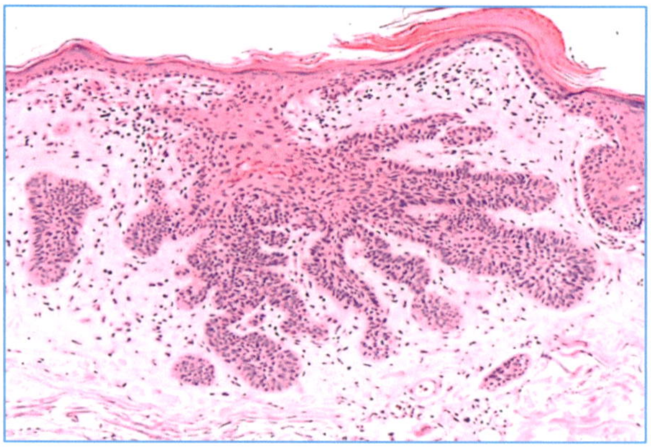

Basaloid follicular hamartoma is shaped as tree root with single epidermal attachment

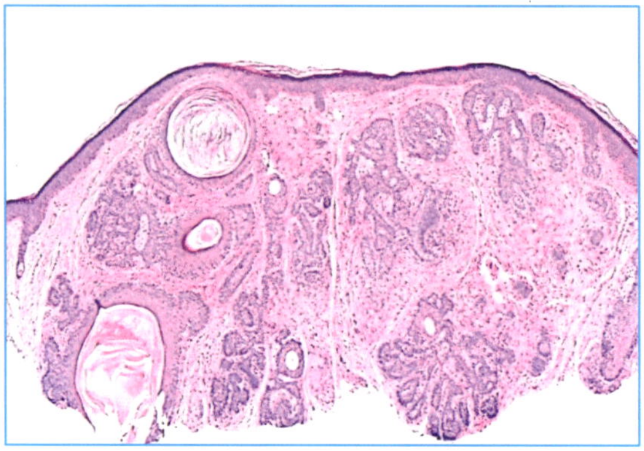

Trichoepithelioma is basaloid tumor with mesenchymal bodies and cysts but no myxoid stroma or retraction

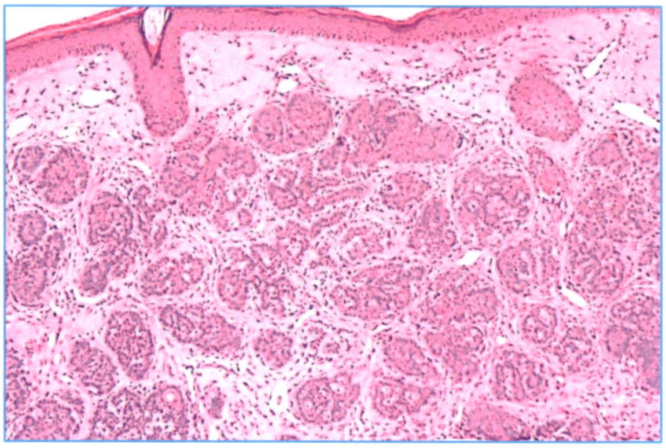

Trichoblastoma is basaloid tumor with mesenchymal bodies but no cysts and no myxoid stroma or retraction

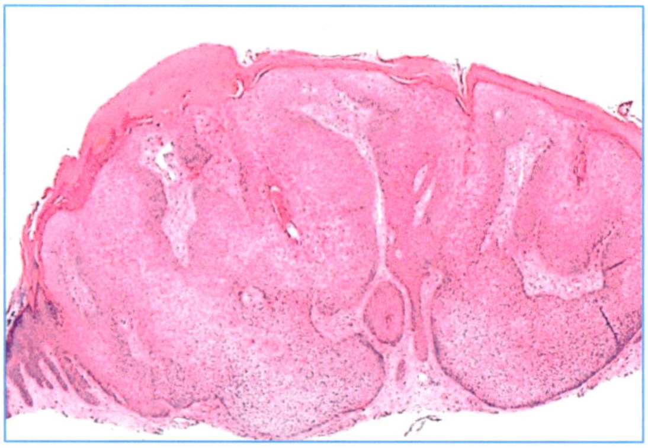

Trichilemmoma with lobules of clear cells with "eyeliner"

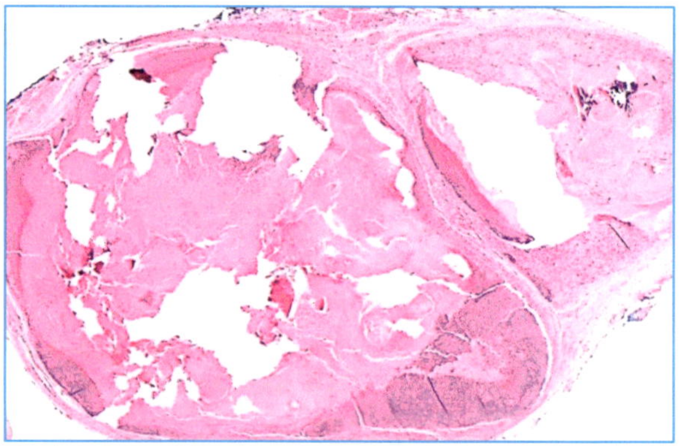

Pilomatricoma with dark blue and pink "ghost" cells

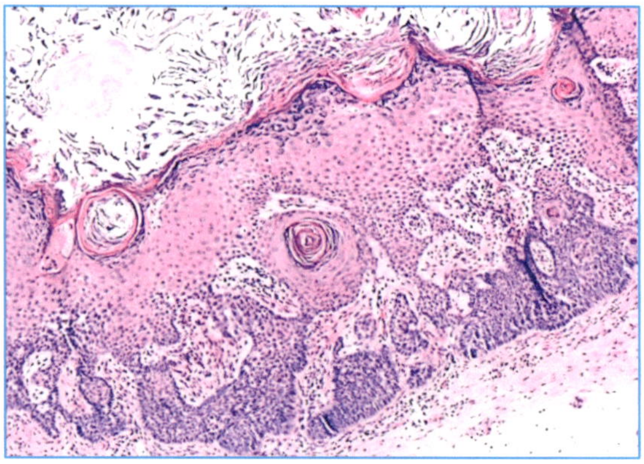

Panfolliculoma is made of multiple elements of differentiating hair follicle

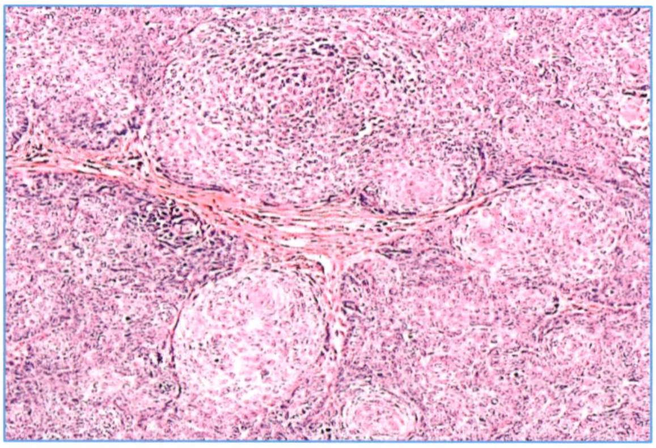

Trichogerminoma is basaloid tumor with balls of pale cells

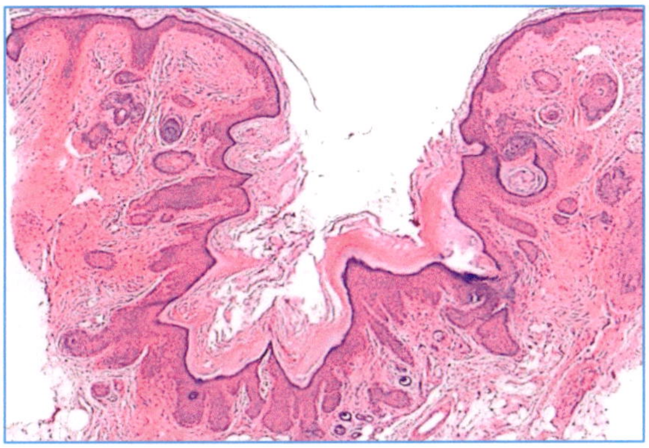

Dilated pore of Winer with "finger-like" projections

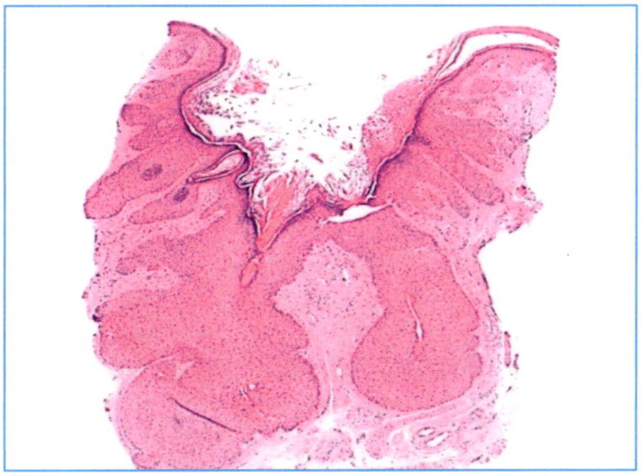

Pilar sheath acanthoma with broad projections

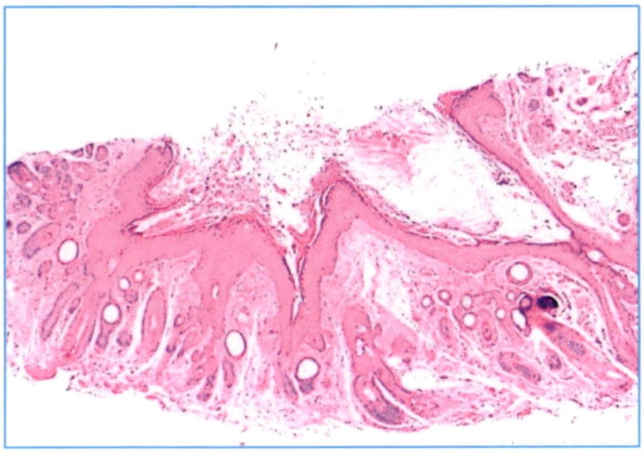

Trichofolliculoma with
multiple hairs attached to central dilated hair follicle

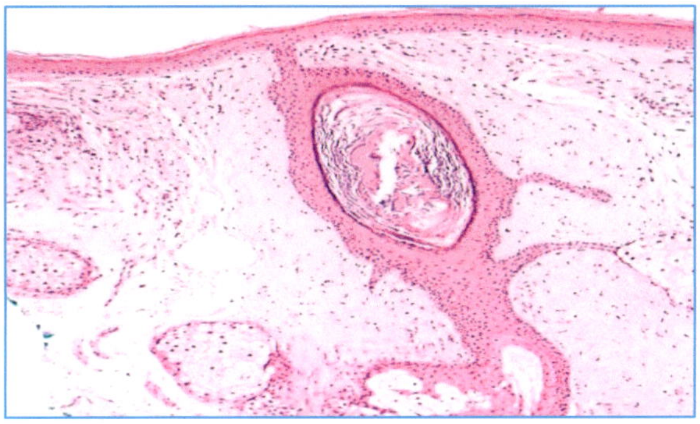

Perifollicular fibroma with dilated follicle with circular fibrosis

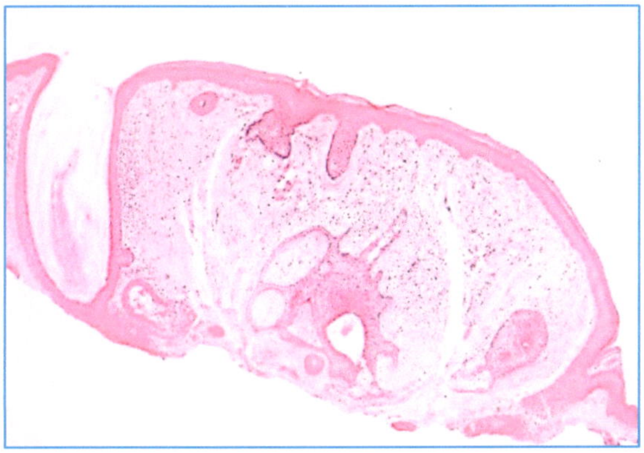

Trichodiscoma with fibrous plate between 2 distorted follicles

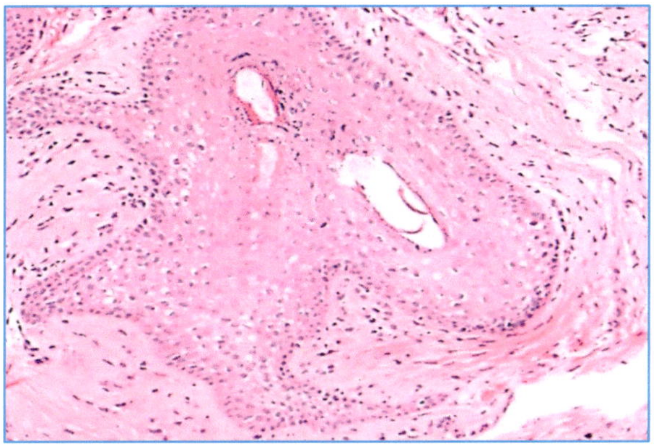

Fibrofolliculoma with distorted follicle and perifollicular fibrosis

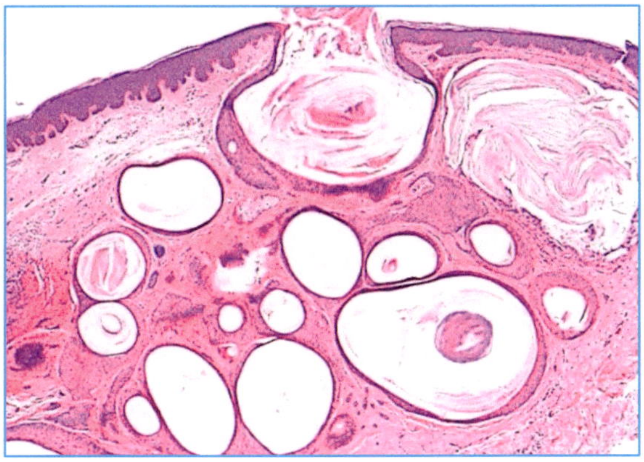

Trichoadenoma with multiple cysts and solid tumor in between

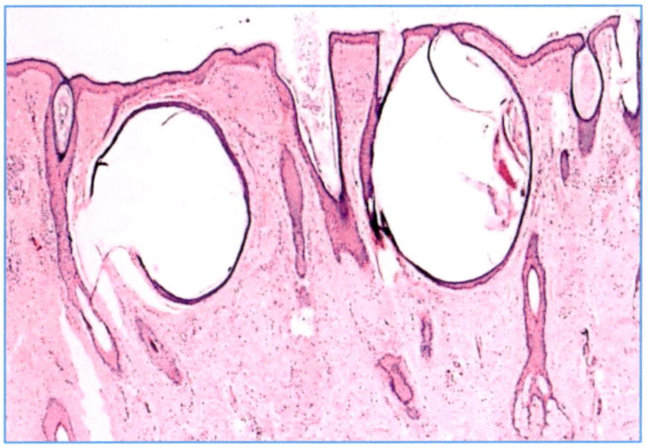

Nevus comedonicus with multiple comedones

Follicular tumors

Chapter 28

SEBACEOUS TUMORS

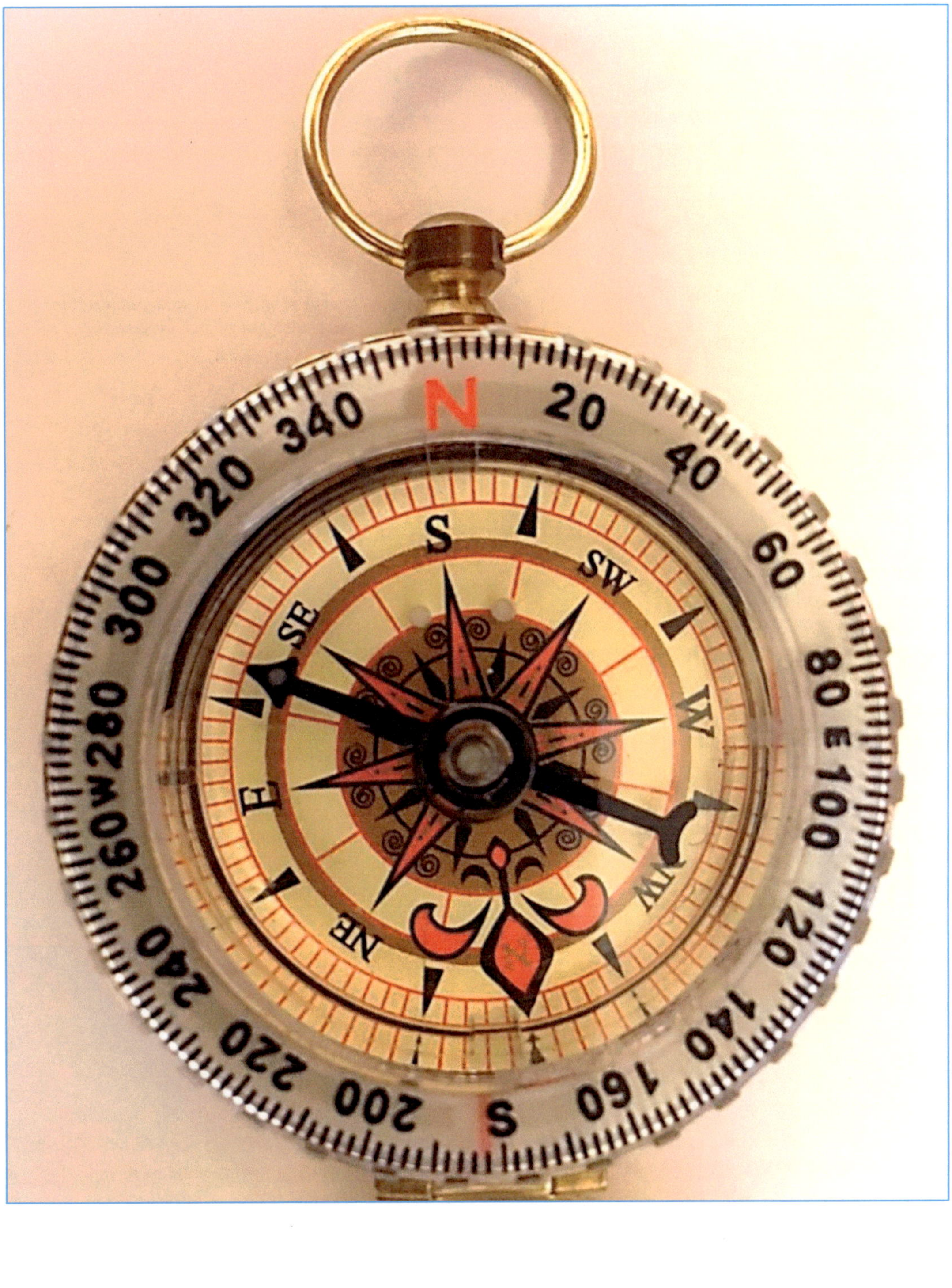

Sebaceous tumors

NEVUS SEBACEOUS OF JADASSOHN

-congenital malformation of sebaceous differentiation
-presents at birth or in infancy
-scalp is favored site
-initially presents as a hairless, yellow-orange plaque, typically on the scalp
-typically becomes more verrucous around puberty
-numerous secondary tumors listed below may arise within nevus sebaceous
-trichoblastoma (most common), syringocystadenoma papilliferum, trichilemmoma, sebaceoma, sebaceous adenoma, proliferating pilar tumor, and basal cell carcinoma (rare)

Histopathology

-**hyperkeratotic, acanthotic epidermis** with **irregular papillomatosis**
-**immature sebaceous glands in infants** and young children that become **hyperplastic at or after puberty** and again regress with older age
-**hair follicles are decreased in number** and are immature with **primitive germs**
-**apocrine glands can be prominent** in deeper dermis after puberty

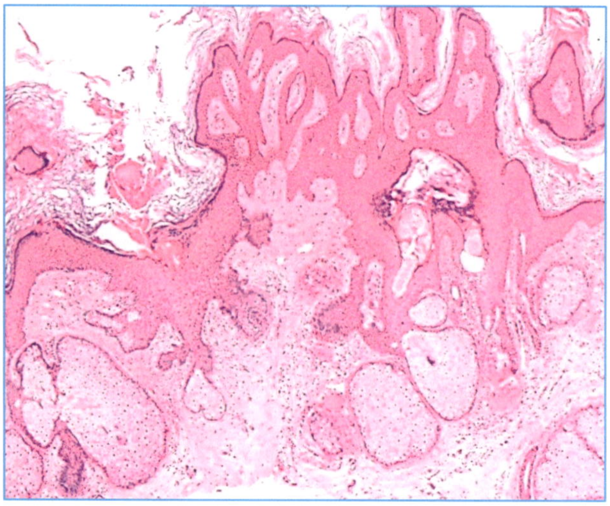

Nevus sebaceous with epidermal proliferation and prominent sebaceous glands

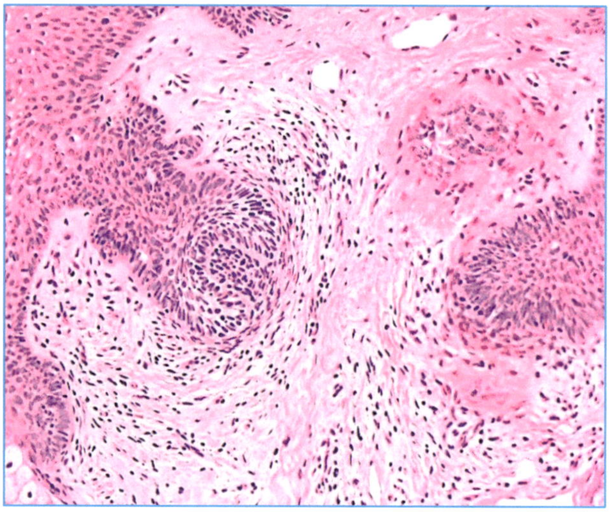

Immature hair follicle in nevus sebaceous

FOLICULOSEBACEOUS CYSTIC HAMARTOMA

-rare cutaneous hamartoma
-presents as asymptomatic firm dermal nodule
-predilection for the central face and scalp

Histopathology

-**radiating mature sebaceous lobules attached to central dilated follicle**
-stroma is usually fibrotic

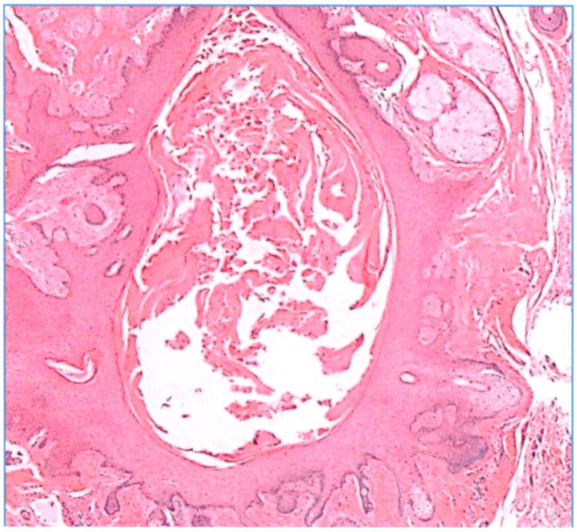

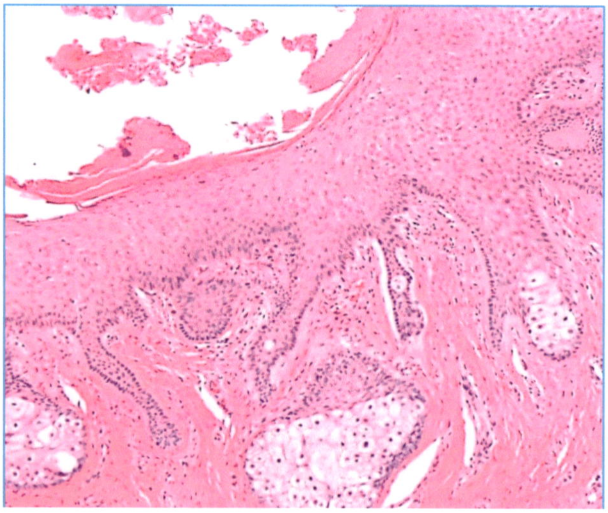

Folliculosebaceous cystic hamartoma with multiple sebaceous glands attached to dilated central follicle

Chapter 28

SEBACEOUS HYPERPLASIA

-benign sebaceous proliferation
-presents as small, yellow papule with a small, central dell, most commonly on the face
-telangiectasias can be present, raising suspicion for BCC, which prompts biopsy

Histopathology
-nodular shape
-hyperplasia of mature sebaceous glands
-**multiple sebaceous glands** (four or more) **attached to a central infundibulum**

FORDYCE SPOTS (FORDYCE GRANULES)

-ectopic sebaceous glands
-present as tiny yellow papules along vermillion border of the lip or on the oral mucosa

Histopathology
-**normal sebaceous glands not associated with hair follicle** and **without communication with epithelial surface**

SEBACEOUS ADENOMA

-benign sebaceous cutaneous tumor
-presents as yellow, tan, pink or skin-colored papules
-favors the head and face, with the nose and cheek most frequently affected
-associated with Muir-Torre syndrome (MTS)
-lesions that develop in patients with MTS more commonly occur on the trunk and extremities
-loss of expression of *MSH-1, MLH-2, MSH-6* in lesion is associated with MTS

Histopathology
-well circumscribed sebaceous lesion attached to the epidermis
-lobules are **composed of mature sebocytes** (vacuolated cytoplasm) centrally and germinative basaloid cells at the periphery
-**basaloid cells always make up less than half of the tumor cell volume**
-this key feature distinguishes the lesion from sebaceoma in which basaloid cells represent more than half the tumor cell volume

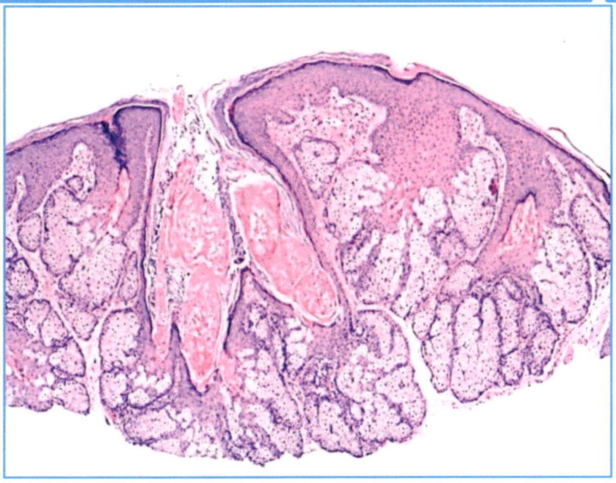
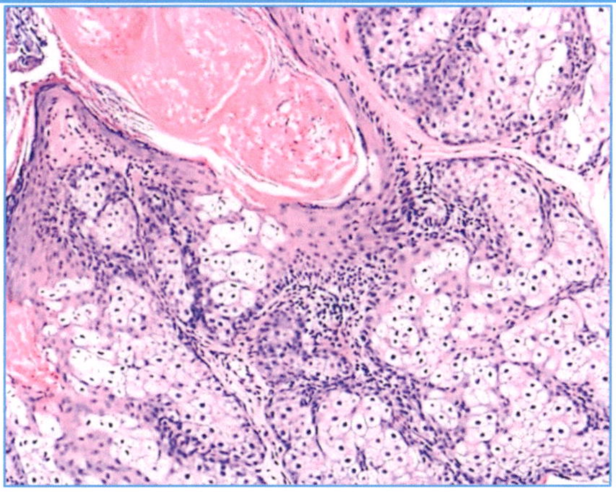

Sebaceous hyperplasia with multiple normal sebaceous glands attached to the central follicle

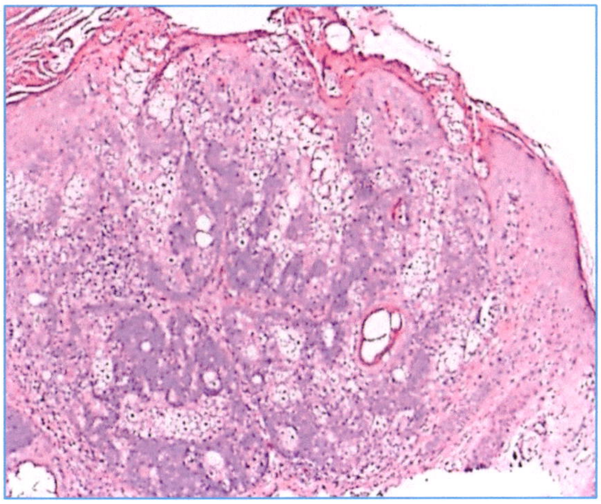
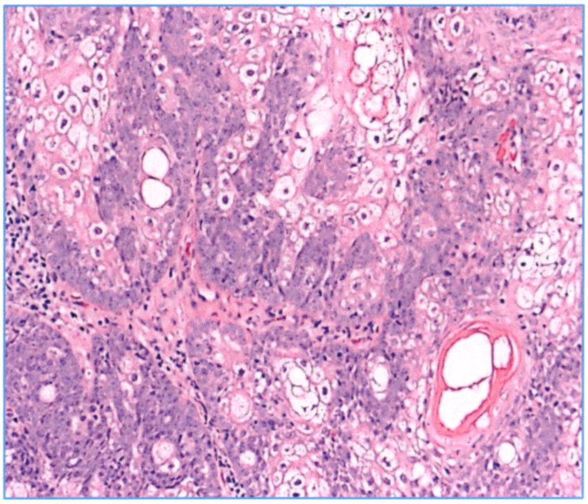

Sebaceous adenoma forming tumor nodule with basaloid cells making less than half of the tumor

Sebaceous tumors

SEBACEOMA (SEBACEOUS EPITHELIOMA)

-benign sebaceous tumor of the skin
-solitary, yellow-orange papules or nodules
-can arise in a pre-existing nevus sebaceous
-favors the face and scalp and less frequently the chest, back and neck
-associated with Muir-Torre syndrome but less frequently than sebaceous adenoma

Histopathology
-well-circumscribed, relatively symmetrical lesion with smooth borders
-lobulated, nodular basaloid tumor islands with epidermal connection
-the **basaloid component comprises greater than 50% of the tumor** with mature clear sebocytes forming less than 50% of the tumor
-cytologic atypia is minimal and mitoses are few and not atypical

SEBACEOUS CARCINOMA

-malignant sebaceous tumor of the skin
-presents as a yellow-orange plaque or nodule
-favors face, particularly the eyelid, and scalp
-associated with Muir-Torre syndrome

Histopathology
-invasive multilobular basaloid tumor
-usually connected to the epidermis
-**sebaceous cells with varying levels of atypia** scattered among **basaloid or squamoid cells**
-sebaceous cells in the center of lobules are more differentiated (look like normal sebocytes) while cell at the periphery are less differentiated
-cells are cytologically atypical with multivacuolated cytoplasm and large nuclei
-necrosis and mitosis are commonly present

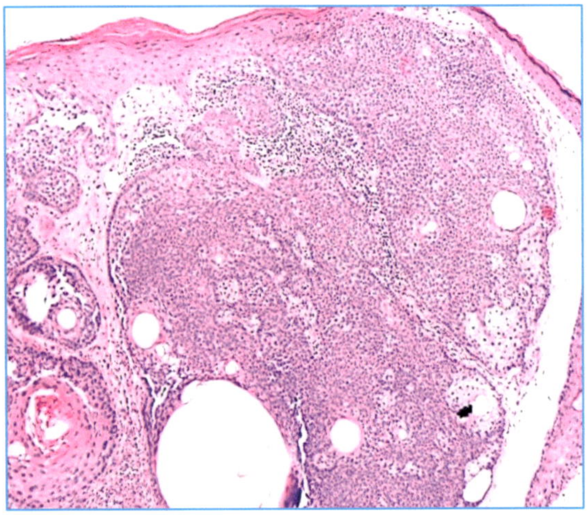
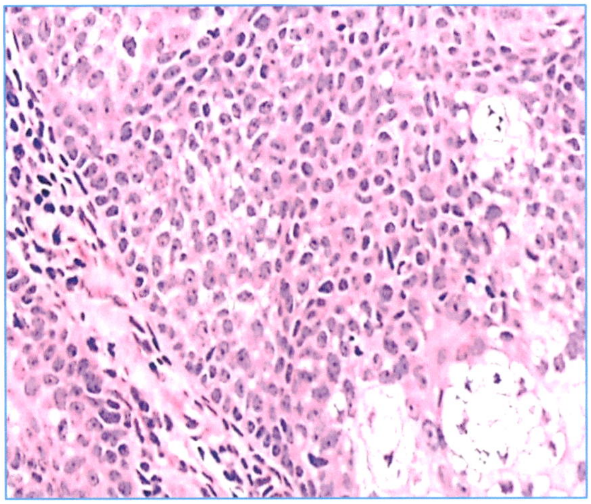

Sebaceoma forming tumor nodule with predominant basaloid cell and scattered clear sebocytes without atypia

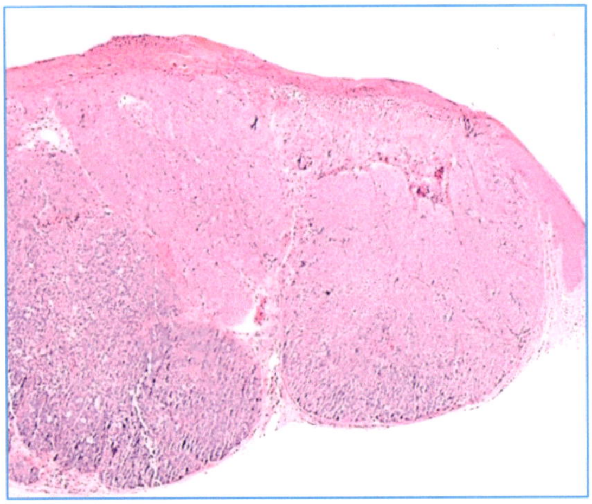
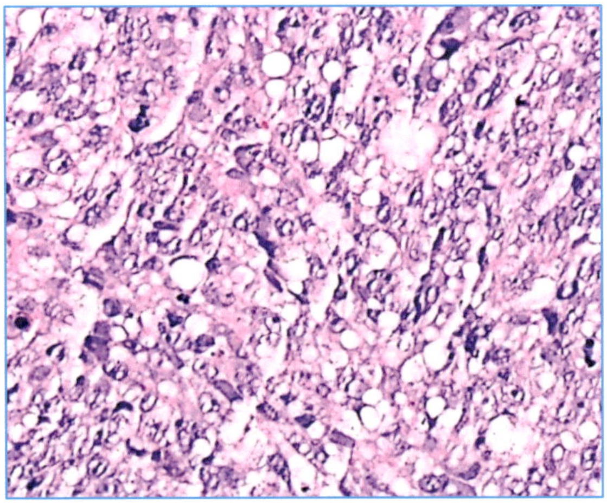

Sebaceous carcinoma consisting of irregular basaloid cells admixed with atypical pale sebocytes and scattered mitoses

Chapter 28

HOW TO APPROACH SEBACEOUS LESIONS

DETERMINE IF LESION HAS SEBACEOUS ORIGIN

SEBACEOUS GLANDS APPEAR NORMAL

-Fordyce spot	normal sebaceous glands without hair follicle
-sebaceous hyperplasia	normal sebaceous tissue with too many glands
-nevus sebaceous	normal sebaceous glands with epidermal proliferation
-folliculosebaceous cystic hamartoma	dilated follicle with attached normal sebaceous glands

SEBACEOUS GLANDS FORM TUMOR WITH MILD ATYPIA

-sebaceous adenoma	>50% mature clear sebaceous cells
-sebaceoma	<50% mature clear sebaceous cells

MALIGNANT APPEARING TUMOR WITH ONLY A HINT OF SEBACEOUS DIFFERENTIATION

-sebaceous carcinoma

NOTE: TUMORS WITH CLEAR CELL CHANGES THAT CAN BE MISTAKEN FOR SEBACEOUS TUMOR

-clear cell squamous cell carcinoma
-clear cell basal cell carcinoma
-clear cell hidradenoma
-renal cell carcinoma
-granular cell tumor
-trichilemmoma

Sebaceous tumors

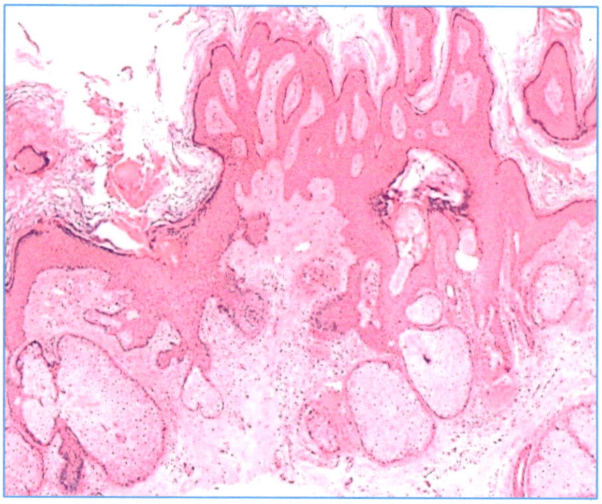

Nevus sebaceous with epidermal proliferation and prominent sebaceous glands

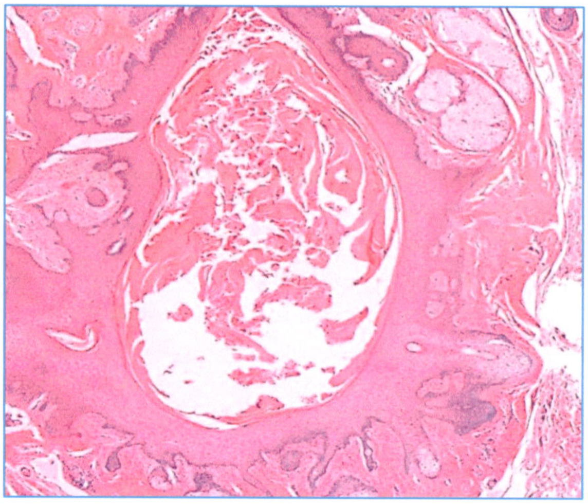

Folliculosebaceous cystic hamartoma with multiple sebaceous glands attached to dilated central follicle

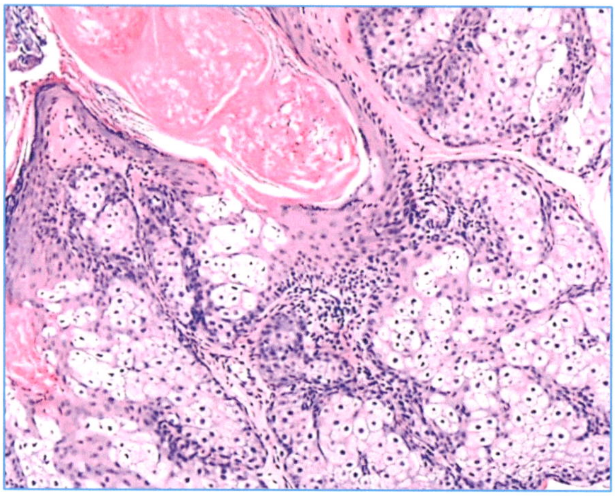

Sebaceous hyperplasia with multiple normal sebaceous glands attached to the central follicle

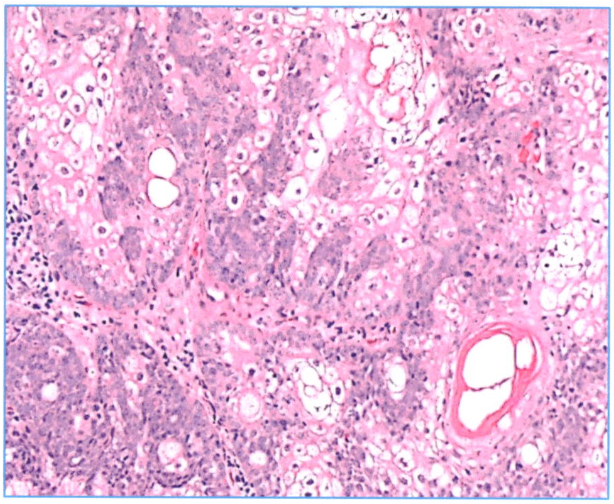

Sebaceous adenoma forming tumor nodule with basaloid cells making up less than half of the tumor

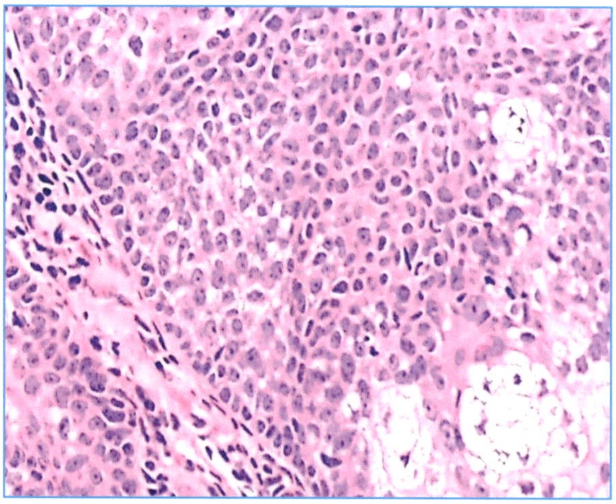

Sebaceoma forming tumor nodule with predominant basaloid cell with scattered clear sebocytes without atypia

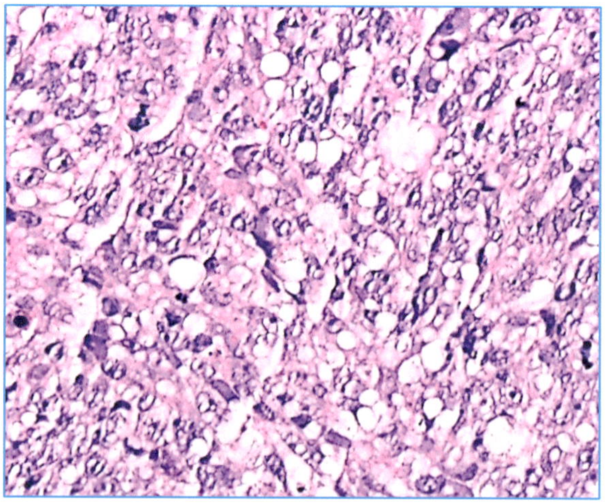

Sebaceous carcinoma invades dermis and consists of atypical basaloid cells and atypical pale sebocytes

Chapter 29

SWEAT GLAND TUMORS

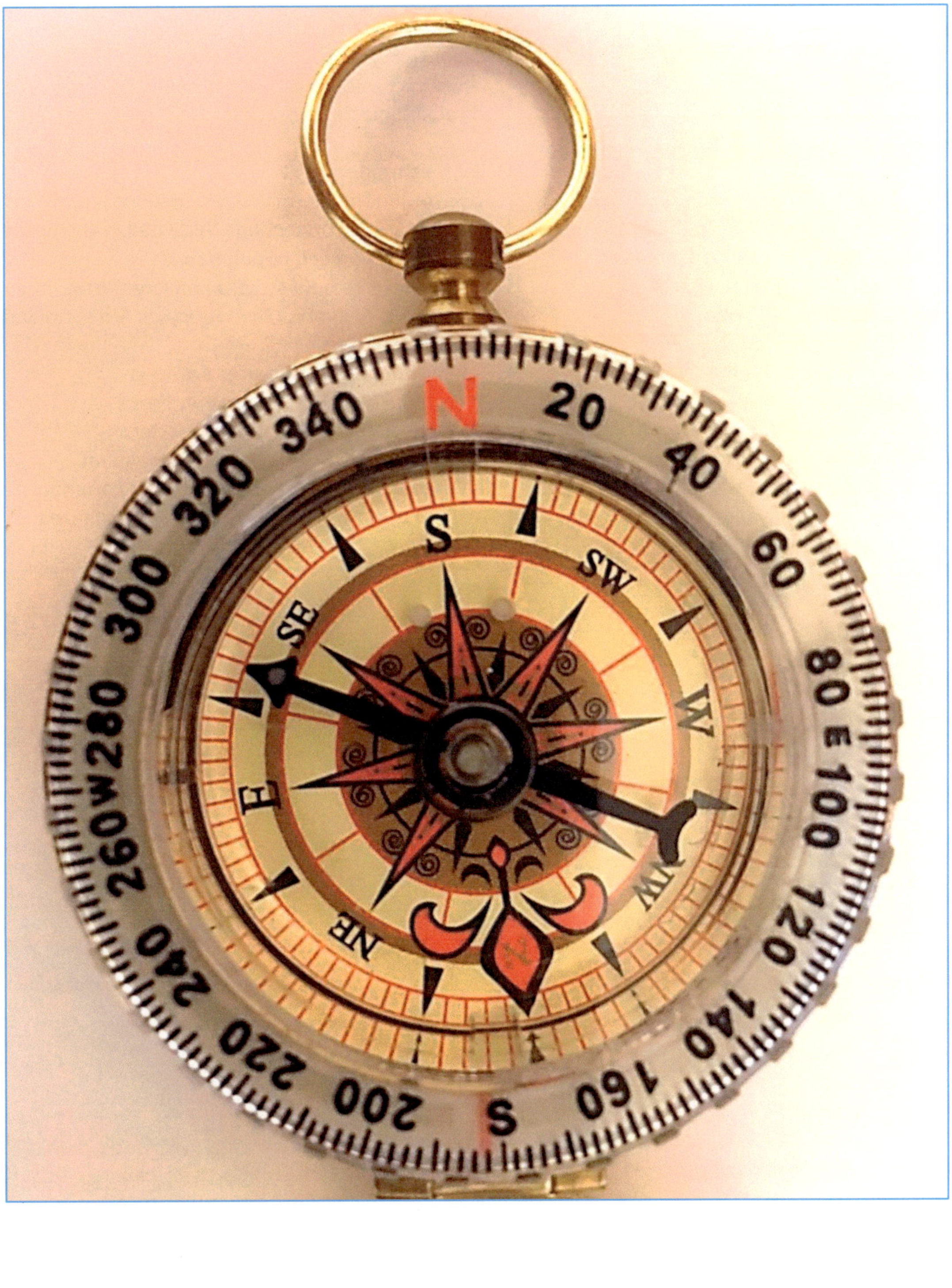

Sweat gland tumors

CYLINDROMA

-benign sweat gland tumor
-skin-colored, reddish or bluish nodule(s) ranging from a few mm to several cm
-located on the scalp, head or neck and may form multinodular plaque ("turban tumor")
-more common in women
-mostly incidental and solitary
-multiple tumors are usually part of Brooke-Spiegler syndrome (*CYLD* mutation)

Histopathology

-dermal nodule **not connected to the epidermis**
-multiple small, irregularly shaped lobules
-lobules form a mosaic **"jigsaw puzzle" pattern**
-tumor consists of **two cell population**, not always easily separated
-mostly peripheral cells with dark nuclei, scant cytoplasm, and palisading
-more centrally located larger cells with vesicular nuclei and more cytoplasm
-scattered small ducts can be seen
-prominent eosinophilic **hyaline stroma** is seen in between and within tumor lobules

SPIRADENOMA

-benign sweat gland tumor
-skin-colored, blue, or pink solitary nodule
-nodule is typically painful, well demarcated, and has a spongy or cystic feel
-usually less than 1 cm in size
-favor the upper trunk or extremities
-multiple tumors may be a sign of Brooke-Spiegler syndrome (*CYLD* mutation)

Histopathology

-one or multiple dermal/subcutaneous nodules with no epidermal connection **("blue ball in the dermis")**
-consists of **two cell population**
-smaller darker outside cells and larger paler inner cells
-on close examination, **lymphocytes are sprinkled** over tumor cells
-small "duct-like" structures are seen
-if multiple nodules are present, they form **pseudo "jigsaw puzzle"** pattern
-if only single nodule is present prominent **dilated vessel at tumor periphery** is common
-stroma around and inside nodule is hyalinized

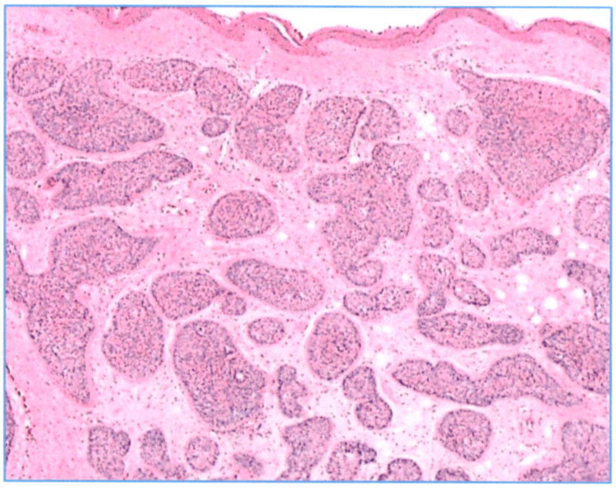

Cylindroma forming "jigsaw puzzle" pattern

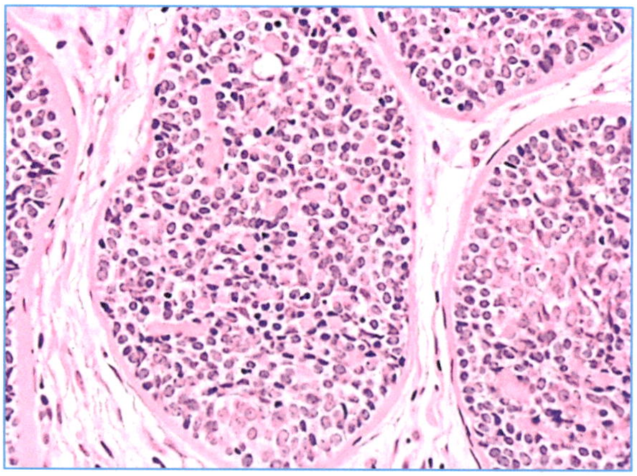

Cylindroma made of darker and paler cells in pink stroma

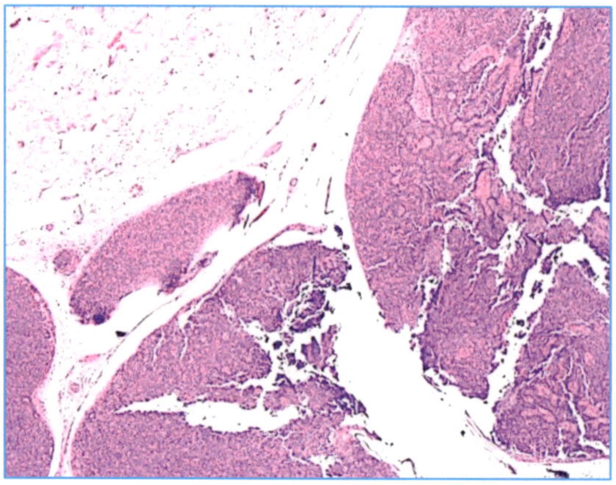

Spiradenoma with irregular "pseudo jigsaw puzzle" pattern

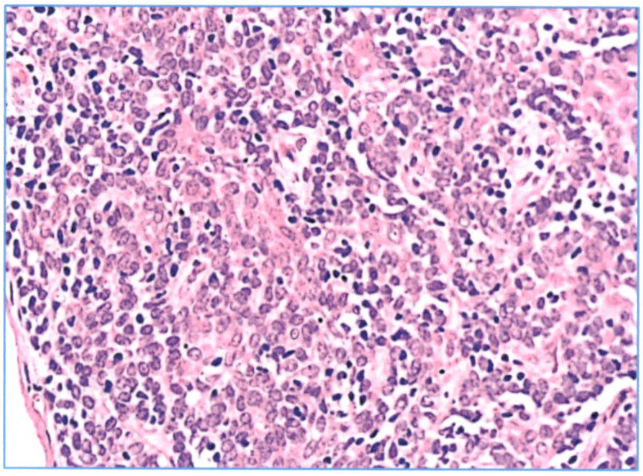

Spiradenoma with sprinkled lymphocytes

POROMA, DERMAL DUCTAL TUMOR, HIDROACANTHOMA SIMPLEX

-benign sweat gland tumors
-solitary pink to reddish papule or nodule
-mostly in middle-aged adults
-favors plantar and palmar skin but can also appear anywhere on the extremities

Histopathology

All three tumors are similar and only differentiated by their histological location:

Hidroacanthoma simplex (epidermis)
-epidermal proliferation of **monotonous, uniform, basaloid cells (poroid cells)** that broadly push into the papillary dermis
-**small "duct-like" structures** are present
-no peripheral palisading or stromal retraction (unlike BCC)

Poroma (epidermis + dermis)
-nodular well circumscribed tumor with **multiple epidermal connections**
-made of very **uniform poroid cells** forming broad columns extending into the dermis
-some cells can be pale due to the glycogen giving squamoid appearance
-no evidence of cytological atypia or mitosis
-small "duct-like" structures are present

Dermal duct tumor (dermis)
-**dermal islands of uniform, poroid, basaloid cells** within the dermis
-**no epidermal connection**
-small "duct-like" structures are present

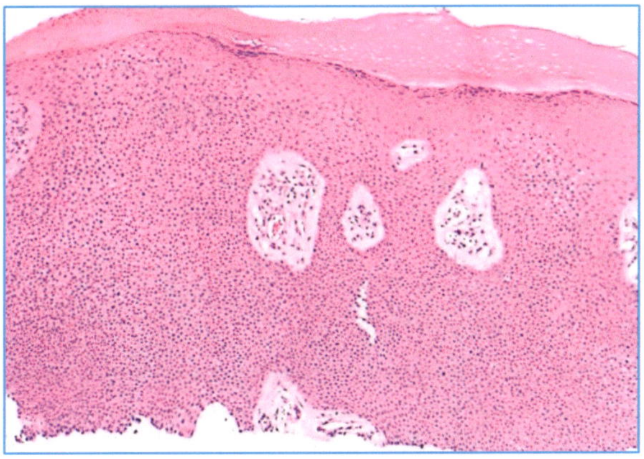

Poroma made of uniform cells with multifocal epidermal connection

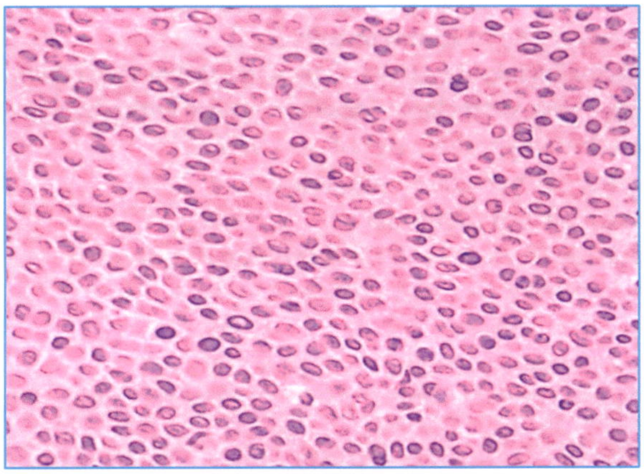

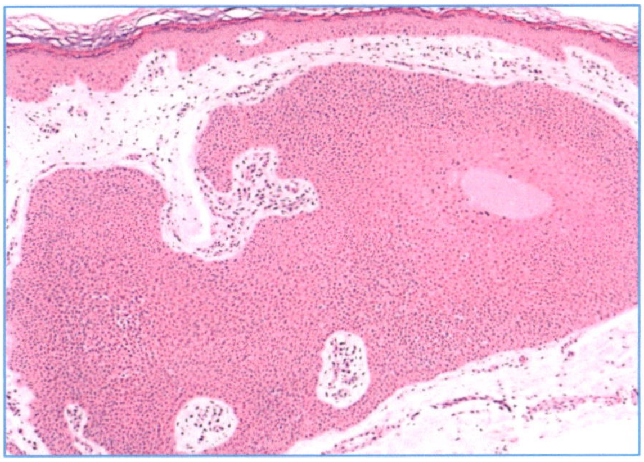

Dermal duct tumor with dermal nodule made of monotonous cells with scattered small ducts

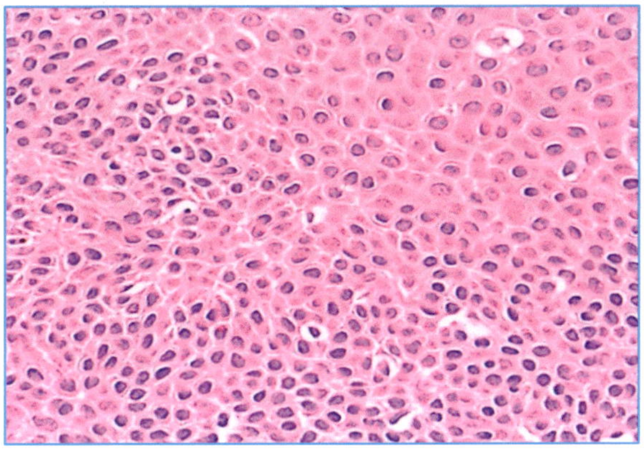

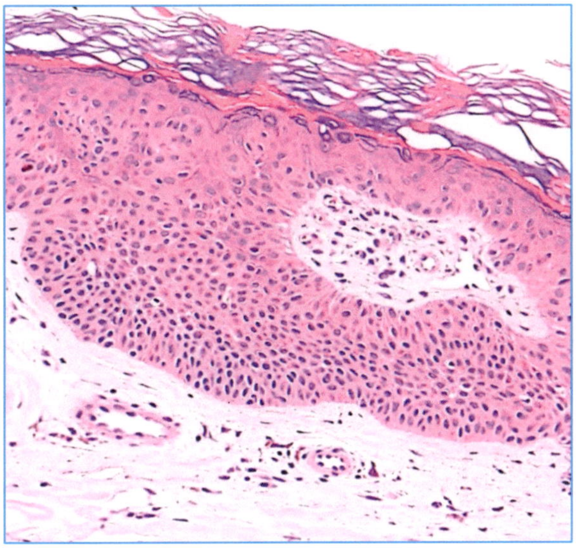

Hidroacanthoma simplex made of uniform poroid cells entrapping small ducts

Sweat gland tumors

NODULAR HIDRADENOMA (ECCRINE ACROSPIROMA, SOLID-CYSTIC HIDRADENOMA, CLEAR CELL HIDRADENOMA)

-benign sweat gland tumor
-painless, solitary, solid or partially cystic skin-colored nodule
-slight preponderance in females of middle age with no site predilection

Histopathology
-deep, circumscribed, non-encapsulated tumor occasionally connected to the epidermis
-it can be primarily **solid, cystic, or solid and cystic** giving different names
-usually made of **2 kind of cells**
-**smaller basaloid** (poroid) cells with darker cytoplasm
-**larger cells with clear cytoplasm** (filled with glycogen)
-ratio between two types of cells varies
-**if clear cells predominate, it is called clear cell hidradenoma**
-occasionally scattered **third cell population** with squamoid or mucinous differentiation
-**stroma** in between cells is **hyalinized**
-small ductal structures are frequently seen

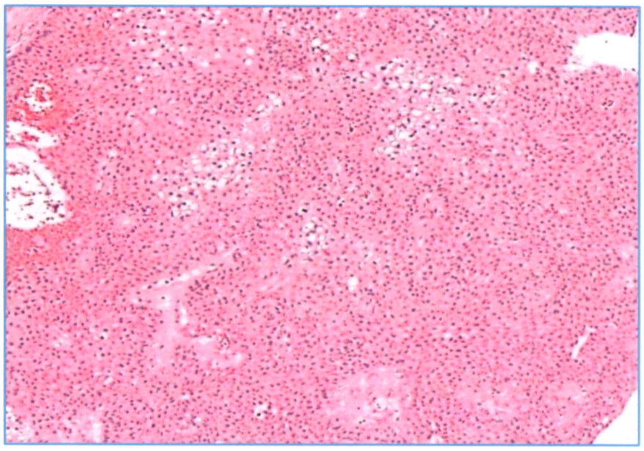

Nodular hidradenoma with two cells population

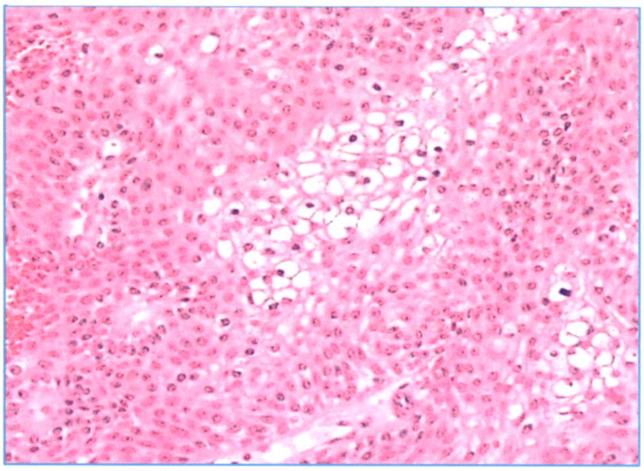

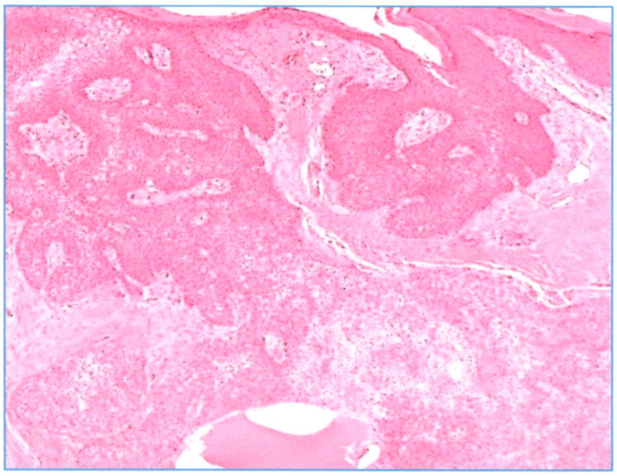

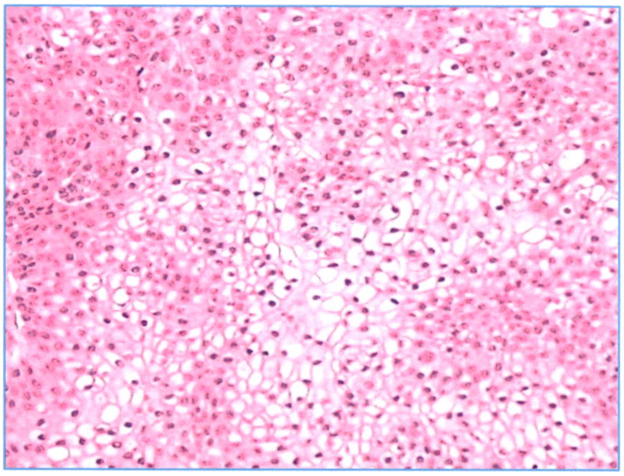

Clear cell hidradenoma with predominant clear cells

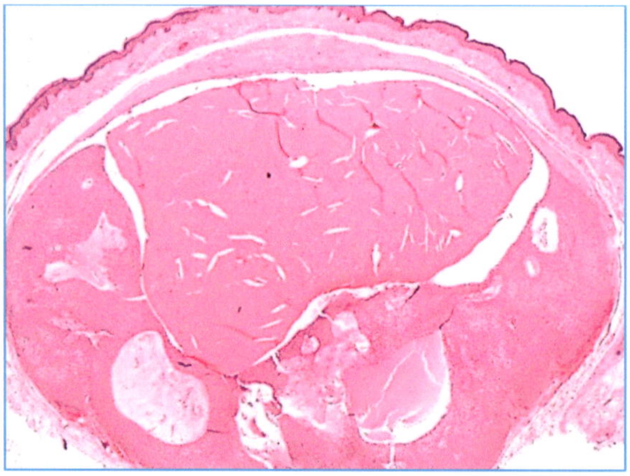

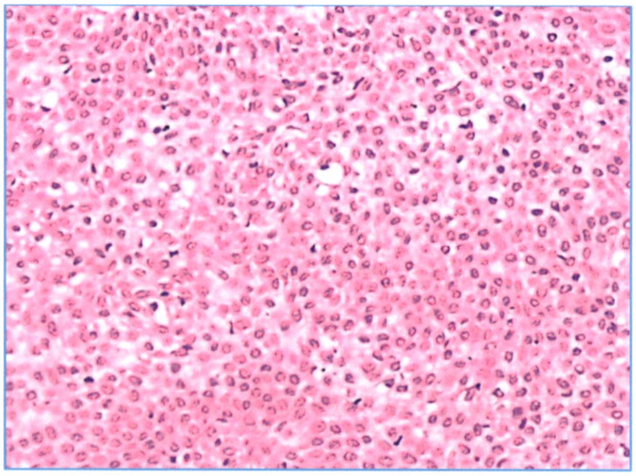

Solid-cystic hidradenoma with large cystic area and nodular areas made of clear and dark uniform cells

HIDRADENOMA PAPILLIFERUM

-clinical appearance is not specific
-may present as a slow-growing, skin-colored nodule
-almost exclusively presents at vulvar and perianal areas in adult women

Histopathology

-well-circumscribed dermal nodule **without a connection to the epidermis**
-**complex "maze-like"** papillary glandular structures
-**papillae lined by two layers of cells**
-inner columnar or cuboidal secretory epithelium with **apical snouts** and outer myoepithelial cells
-**papillary stroma is sclerotic** and **hypocellular**

SYRINGOCYSTADENOMA PAPILLIFERUM

-majority of tumors present at birth or in childhood
-multiple clinical presentations, all highly associated with nevus sebaceus

Solitary type

-skin-colored or brown nodule with crusted verrucous surface
-favors shoulder, axilla, and genital area

Plaque type

-hairless, yellow brown papule, plaque on scalp

Linear type

-yellow brown papules in linear pattern
-favors neck and face

Histopathology

-tumor is **always connected to the epidermis**
-"cup-shaped", nodular, cystic invagination
-irregularly-shaped broad papillae
-**papillae are lined with two cell layers** with the inner layer showing apocrine snouts
-**papillary core/stroma contains** characteristic **numerous plasma cells**

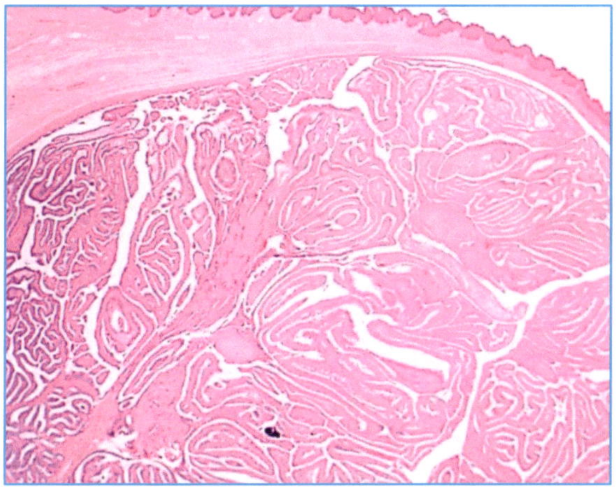

Hidradenoma papilliferum presents as "maze-like" structure not connected to epidermis

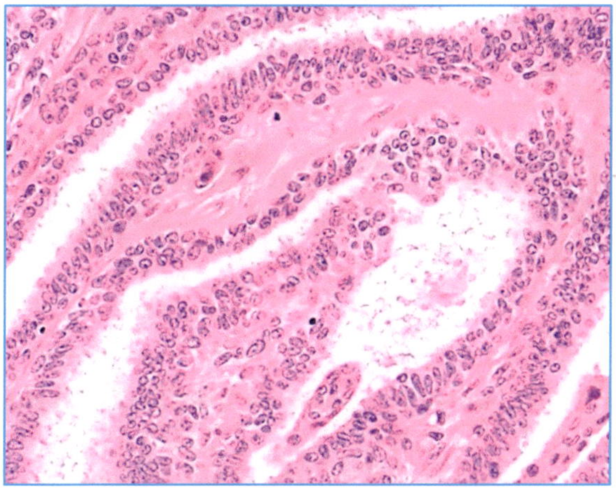

Hidradenoma papilliferum is lined with 2 cells lining with inner cells containing apocrine snouts

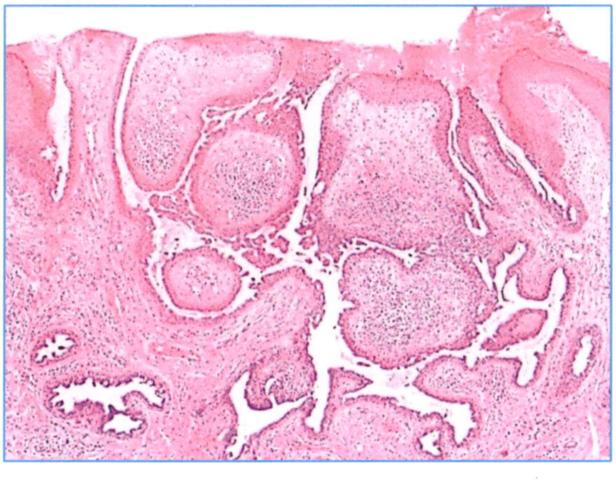

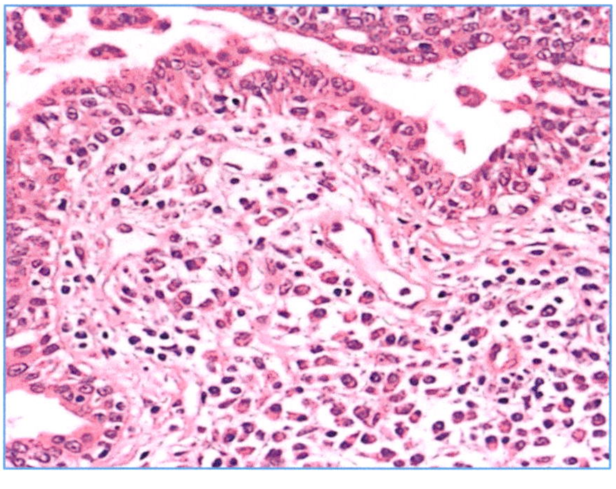

Syringocystadenoma papilliferum is connected to epidermis, lined with 2 cells layer, and contains stromal plasma cells

Sweat gland tumors

HIDROCYSTOMA	APOCRINE PAPILLARY CYSTADENOMA
-solitary, small, "dome shaped", translucent papule -slow-growing and painless -favors head and neck area with periorbital site being the most common site Histopathology -originates from eccrine or apocrine glands -cyst has a corrugated outline and usually an empty lumen -lined with **two layers of cells** -**outer flat myoepithelial cells** and **inner cuboidal cells** -if **apocrine in origin** cytoplasmic **snouts are present** -if of **eccrine origin**, cuboidal cells **do not have snouts**	-variant of apocrine hidrocystoma with similar clinical presentation Histopathology -**multiple "hidrocystoma-like" cysts** predominate -in addition, **solid and papillary projections** from the cyst wall are present -**papillae are small** with fibrovascular core covered with several layers of cuboidal cells -inner layer of cells have apocrine snouts -focal cytological atypia and increased mitotic activity can be present -excise with negative margins

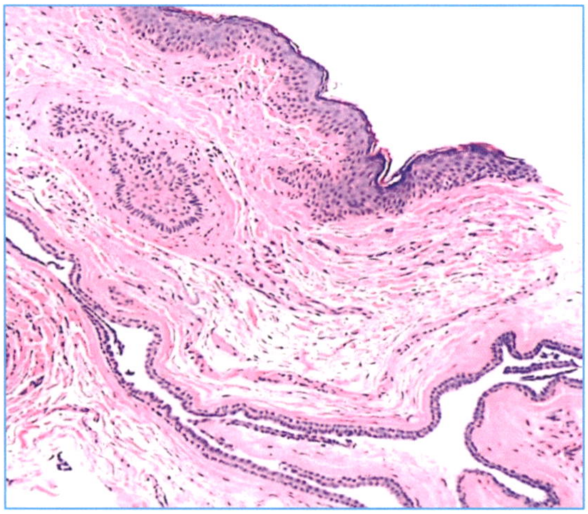

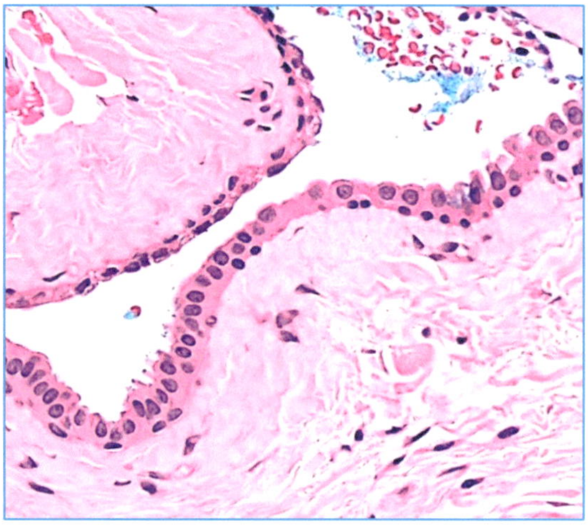

Apocrine hidrocystoma with corrugated cyst lined with two cells layer of which inner layer has apocrine snouts

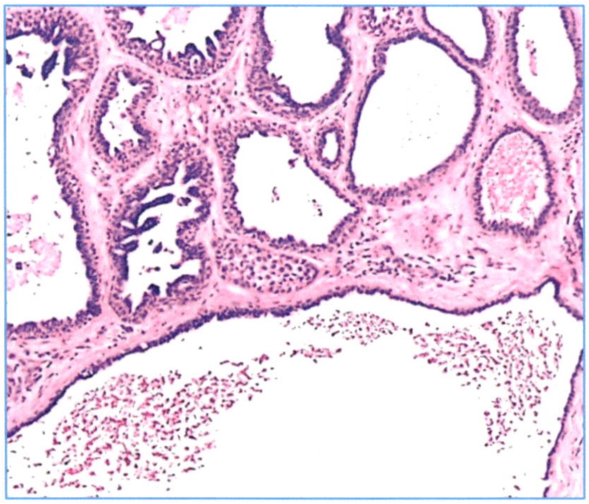

Apocrine papillary cystadenoma with multiple "hidrocystoma-like" cysts

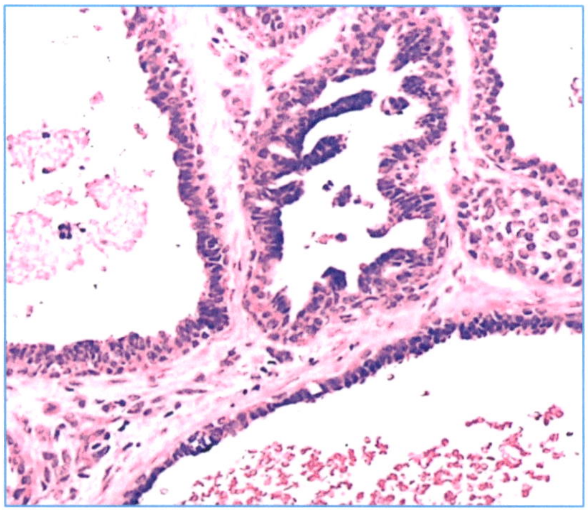

Apocrine papillary cystadenoma with papillary proliferations arising from cyst wall

TUBULAR APOCRINE ADENOMA

-slow growing, painless subcutaneous nodule
-favors the scalp and is more common in women
-associated with nevus sebaceus of Jadassohn and syringocystadenoma papilliferum

Histopathology
-typically scalp specimen
-well circumscribed dermal tumor that may extend into subcutis
-multiple, **variably sized, cystic tubular structures** with **two cell layers** in fibrous stroma
-inner layer shows **snouts** of apocrine secretion (“**decapitation” secretion**)
-**pseudopapillae** are common

PAPILLARY ECCRINE ADENOMA

-slowly growing subcutaneous nodule
-favors acral surfaces or legs and is more common in African Americans

Histopathology
-well-circumscribed dermal tumor
-made of **cystic, “duct-like” structures** in dense fibrous stroma
-ducts are **lined by 2 layer**s (focally more) of bland **epithelial cells with eosinophilic cytoplasm**
-**snouts** of secretion are **absent**
-**intraluminal papillae** are present and focal cribriform ducts can be seen
-no significant atypia is present

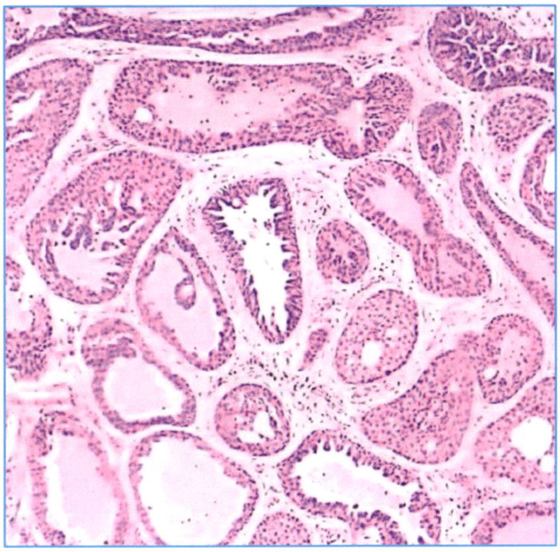

Tubular apocrine adenoma with tubular structures covered with 2 or multiple cells layer

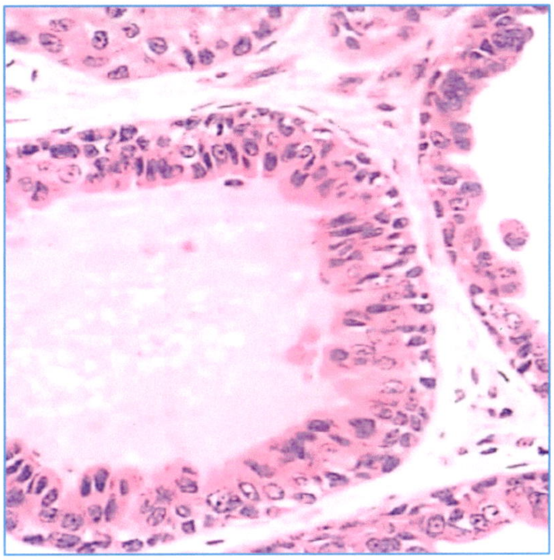

Tubular apocrine adenoma with pseudopapillae and apocrine snouts

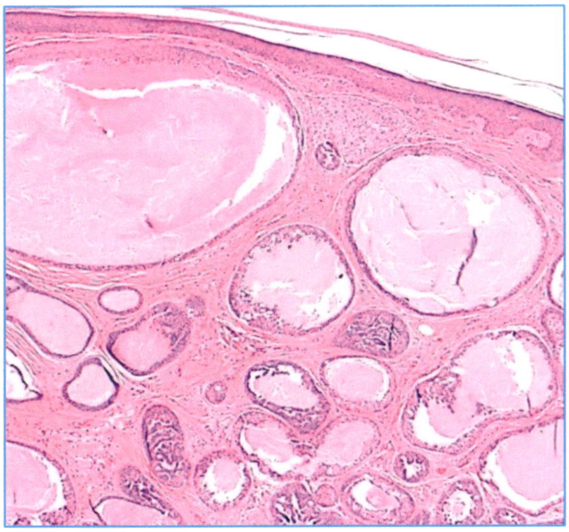

Papillary eccrine adenoma with more cystic structures comparing to tubular structures of apocrine adenoma

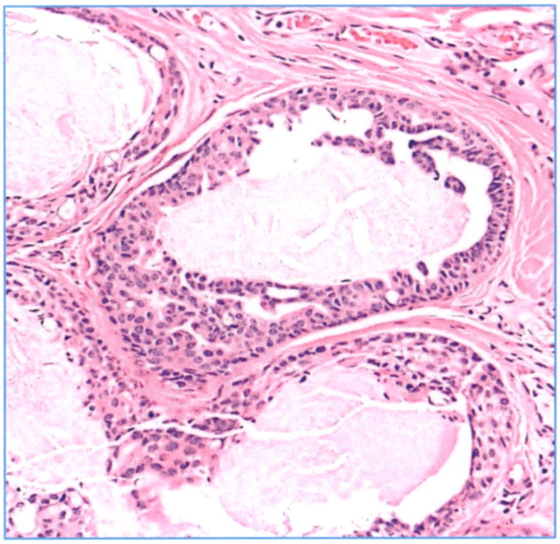

Papillary eccrine adenoma with intraductal papillae and absent snouts of secretion

Sweat gland tumors

SYRINGOMA

-skin-colored or yellowish firm papules with smooth surface and symmetrical distribution
-periorbital area is a favored site
-eruptive form typically presents on the anterior chest, abdomen, neck, and arms
-more common in Asians and females
-associated with Down, Brooke-Spiegler and Nicolau-Balus syndromes
-diabetes mellitus is strongly associated with clear cell variant of syringoma

Histopathology

-**small irregular ducts and tubules** within the **superficial dermis**
-some ducts have characteristic **"tadpole" or "comma" appearance**
-overall creates a **"paisley tie" appearance**
-ducts are lined with two layers of cells
-**infiltrative growth and atypia are absent** (unlike MAC)
-in **clear cell variant, lining cells have clear cytoplasm**
-clear cell changes can be only focal

CHONDROID SYRINGOMA (MIXED TUMOR OF SKIN)

-present as a solitary, slow-growing, painless firm nodule
-most often seen in middle-aged men
-favors the nose, followed by the cheek and upper lip

Histopathology

-well-circumscribed dermal tumor with **no epidermal connection**
-tumor is **biphasic** with **epithelioid cells** in a prominent **myxoid, chondroid stroma**
-ratio of epithelium and stroma is variable
-epithelial component consists of small and large cell clusters and ductal structures
-**ductal structures have various shapes** some being syringoid ("tadpole" shaped)
-ducts are lined with two layers of cuboidal cells
-focal squamous, sebaceous, trichilemmal, eccrine/apocrine differentiation can be seen

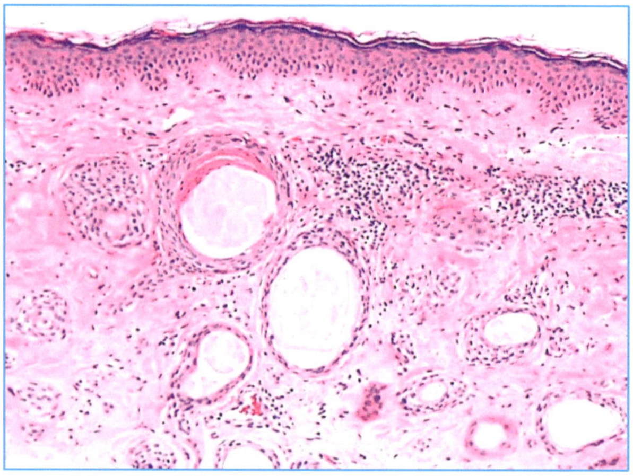

Syringoma with dermal ducts in "paisley tie" appearance

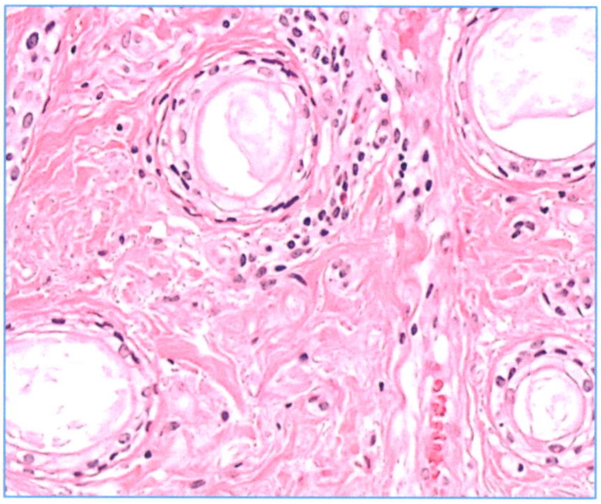

Clear cell syringoma with ducts lined with clear cells

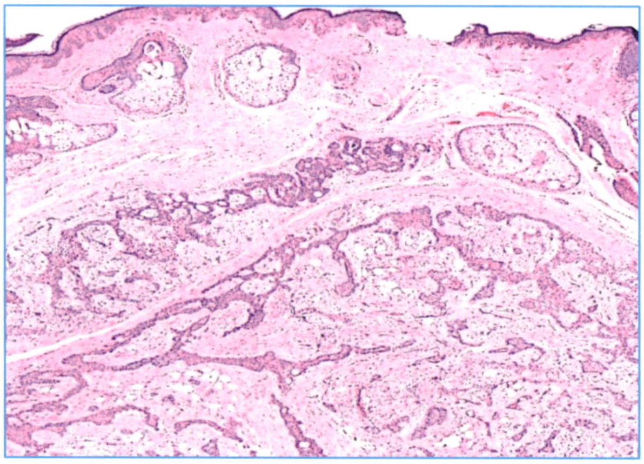

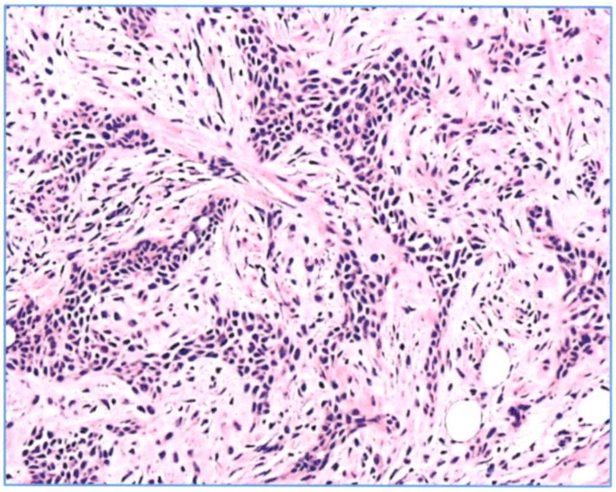

Chondroid syringoma with irregular ductal structures in myxoid, "chondroid-like" stroma

Chapter 29

SYRINGOFIBROADENOMA

-rare benign cutaneous tumor with eccrine differentiation
-varied clinical manifestations
-can present as a solitary nodular lesion or as multiple papules, nodules, and plaques
-associated with hidrotic ectodermal dysplasia, Schöpf-Schulz-Passarge syndrome, and chronic stasis dermatitis
-present usually on the extremities of the elderly

Histopathology
-**anastomosing cords and strands** of cuboidal epithelial cells in fibrovascular mucinous stroma
-**arises from epidermis at multiple points**
-well-formed **sweat ducts are present within the strands**

MUCOEPIDERMOID CARCINOMA

-malignant tumor of the minor salivary glands
-presents as a deep subcutaneous, skin-colored nodule on the face of middle-aged or elderly people

Histopathology
-tumor is made of **mucous secreting "goblet" cells and epithelioid cells**
-mucous cells are large with pale cytoplasm
-epithelioid cells are large atypical cells with vesicular, hyperchromatic nuclei
-extravasation of mucin into the stroma can induce a foreign body reaction

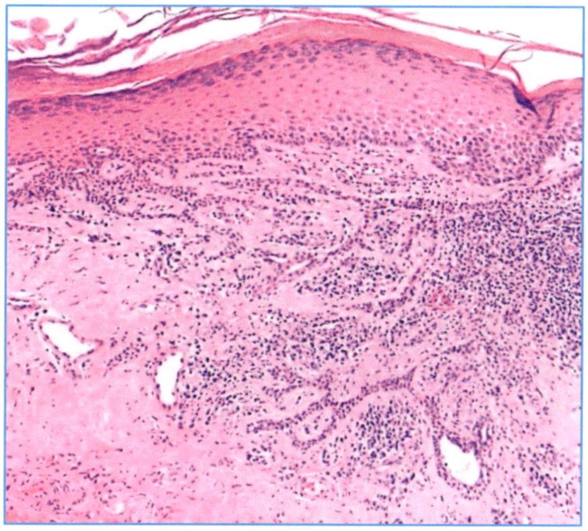

Syringofibroadenoma with multiple strands arising from epidermis

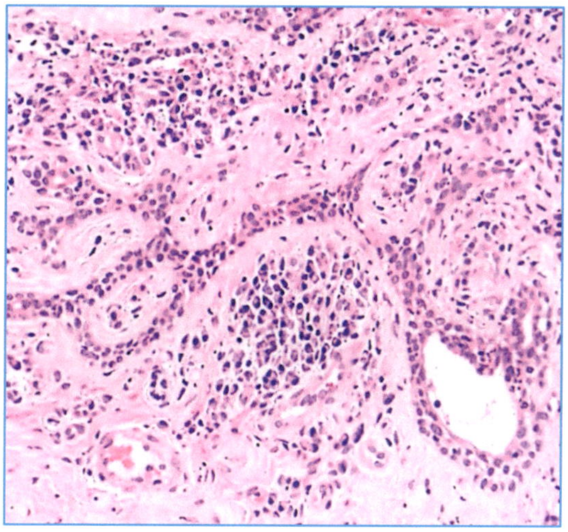

Syringofibroadenoma with ducts present within epithelial strands

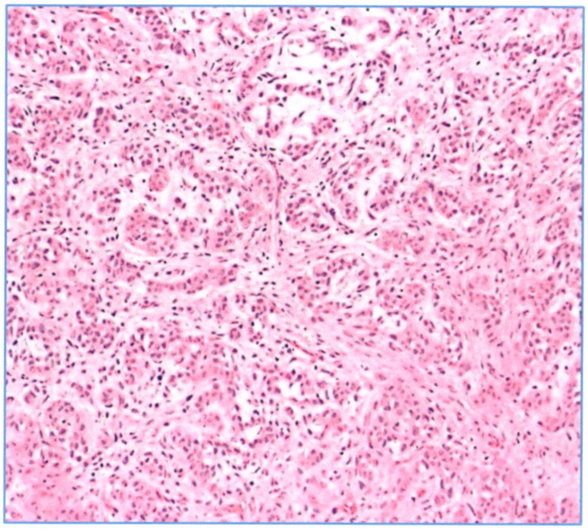

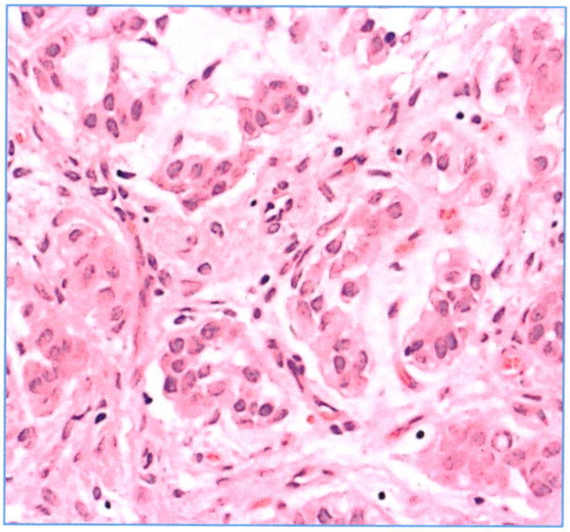

Mucoepidermoid carcinoma made of epithelial and mucin producing cells in mucinous stroma

Sweat gland tumors

MICROCYSTIC ADNEXAL CARCINOMA

-slow growing, flesh-colored or yellowish plaque or nodule
-favors the face (upper lip) and axilla of adults
-locally aggressive with a high recurrence rate
-rarely metastatic

Histopathology

-tumor **involves the dermis and subcutis** (unlike syringoma)
-superficial dermal part consists of **solid islands and strands** of basaloid and squamous cells alternating with small **keratinous cysts**
-focal calcification can be present
-**ductal structures are present** within epithelioid strands and can have resemblance to syringoid "tadpoles"
-**deeper component** consists of **infiltrating solid strands and cords of cells in a sclerotic stroma with no cysts**
-cytological atypia is minimal and mitoses are uncommon
-malignancy is suggested mainly by infiltrative nature

SYRINGOID ECCRINE CARCINOMA

-slow growing, flesh-colored or yellowish plaque or nodule
-favors the scalp and face of the elderly
-locally aggressive but rarely metastatic

Histopathology

-infiltrating dermal and subcutaneous tumor
-**no keratocysts** (unlike MAC)
-made of **infiltrating strands and cords** of basaloid cells with lumen formation
-they form ductal, cystic, and "tadpole-like" structures like syringoma
-differs from syringoma by its cellularity and deep invasiveness

Note:
Syringoid eccrine carcinoma is probably a variant of microcystic adnexal carcinoma without keratocysts

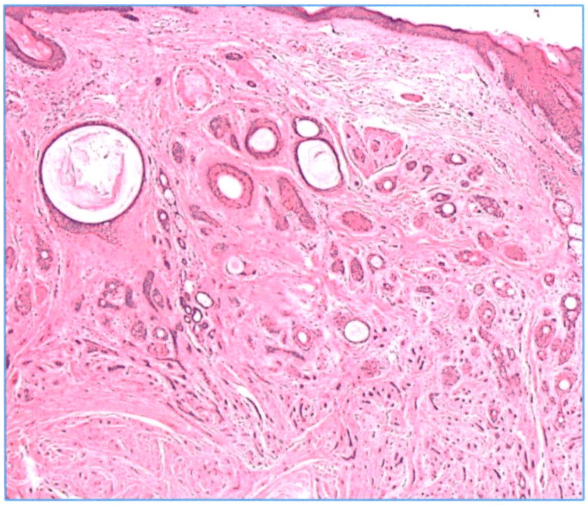

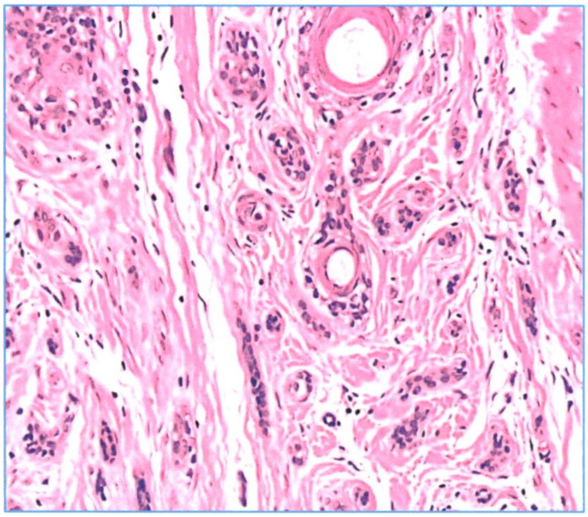

MAC with keratocysts, "tadpoles-like" ducts, and infiltrating ductal structures

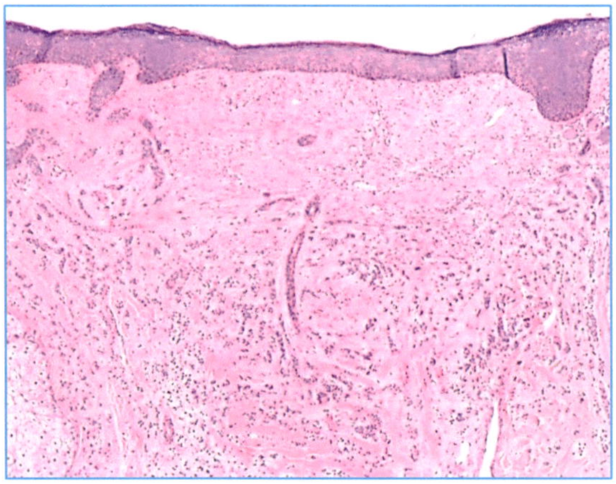

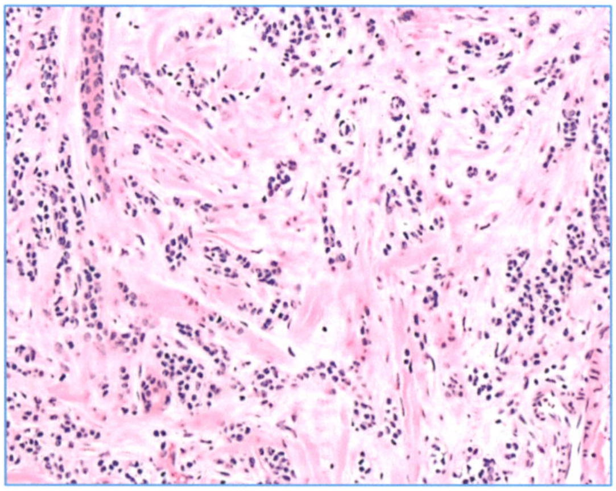

Syringoid eccrine carcinoma with deep infiltrating cords and strands of basaloid cells

(AGGRESSIVE) DIGITAL PAPILLARY ADENOCARCINOMA

-rare, slow-growing, painless tumor
-presents as solitary papule or nodule
-favors the distal portion of the fingers and toes
-rapidly metastasize

Histopathology

-dermal, multinodular, cystic tumor
-**solid and cystic components** with closely aggregated back-to-back glandular architecture
-tumor cells are smaller, cuboidal in shape with nuclear hyperchromasia
-**papillary projections** in cystic area are lined by cuboidal or columnar atypical cells
-cytologic atypia and mitoses are present but are variable

SQUAMOID ECCRINE DUCTAL CARCINOMA

-slow-growing, solitary nodular plaque on the scalp, arms, legs, or trunk
-in middle-aged and elderly individuals
-half are misdiagnosed as squamous cell carcinoma on the incisional biopsy

Histopathology

-infiltrating tumor with poorly defined edges
-prominent **superficial squamous differentiation with atypical squamoid cells** that looks like SCC (thus many are misdiagnosed as SCC on superficial shave biopsy)
-in the central and **deep areas of the tumor, the neoplastic aggregates consist of infiltrating basaloid cells**
-they form **angulated, irregular ductal tubular structures** that resemble syringoma or MAC

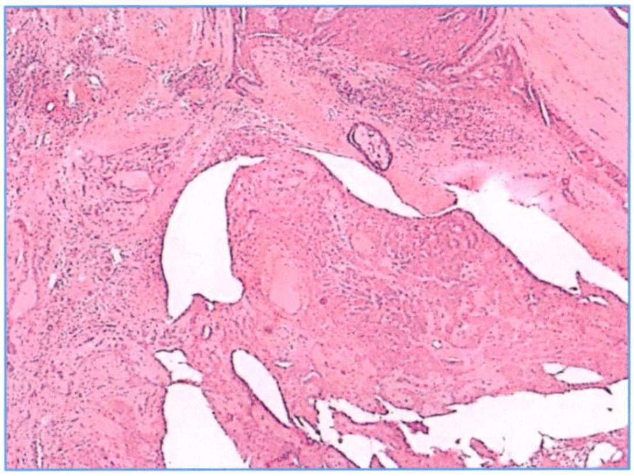
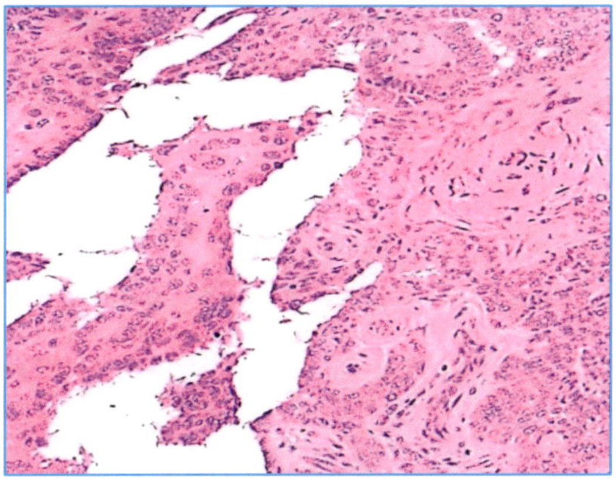

Digital papillary adenocarcinoma with solid and cystic areas and papillary projections of atypical cells

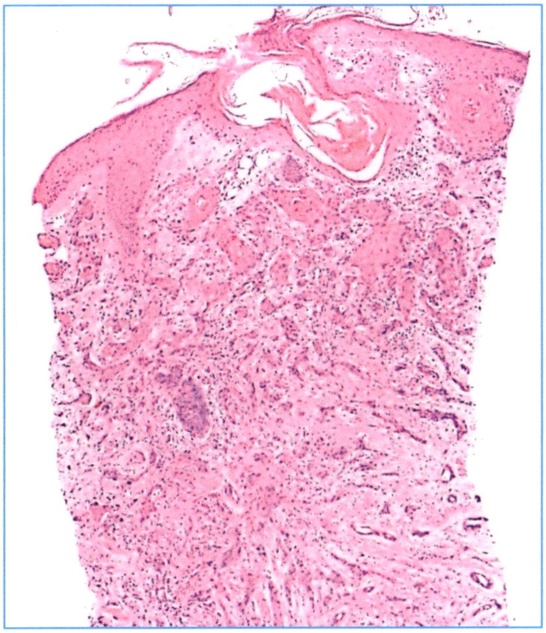
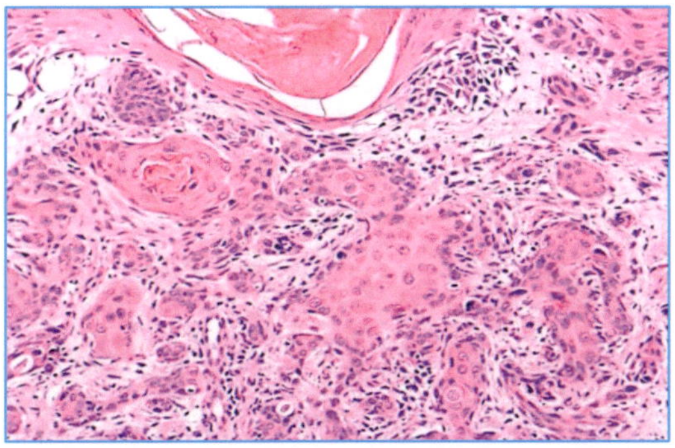
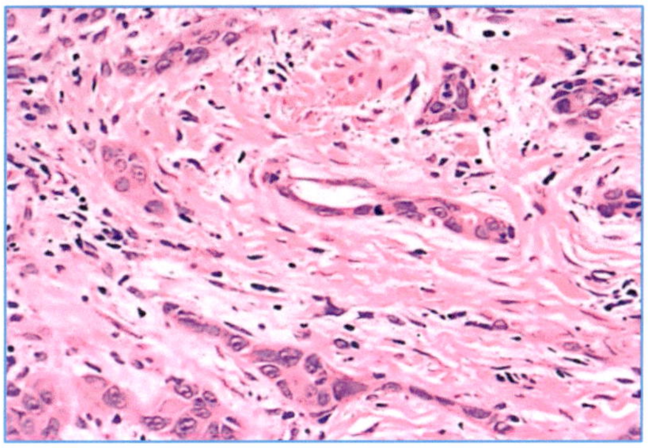

Squamoid eccrine ductal carcinoma with superficial portion resembling SCC and middle and deep portion resembling MAC

Sweat gland tumors

ADENOID CYSTIC CARCINOMA

-rare tumor that presents as a subcutaneus slow growing nodule
-may arise as a cutaneous metastasis from the salivary gland
-predilection for the scalp and chest
-indolent course and local aggressive behavior in primary cutaneous cases

Histopathology

-dermal and subcutaneous tumor without epidermal connection
-tumor made of small basaloid cells arranged in solid and cribriform pattern
-**cribriform areas** have **"Swiss cheese-like" appearance**
-**round open spaces are filled with mucin**
-perineural invasion is very common

PRIMARY CUTANEOUS MUCINOUS CARCINOMA

-very rare primary malignant sweat gland tumor
-slow growing papule/nodule
-mostly in elderly individuals
-favors the face (especially eyelids), scalp, axilla

Histopathology

-well-circumscribed dermal and subcutaneous tumor with pushing borders
-**large pools of mucin** separated by fibrous tissue
-**malignant epithelial cells** forming solid and cribriform nests **floating in mucin** lakes
-metastatic mucinous carcinoma (GI, ovary, breast) can look identical
-clinical correlation and immunostaining is required to exclude metastasis

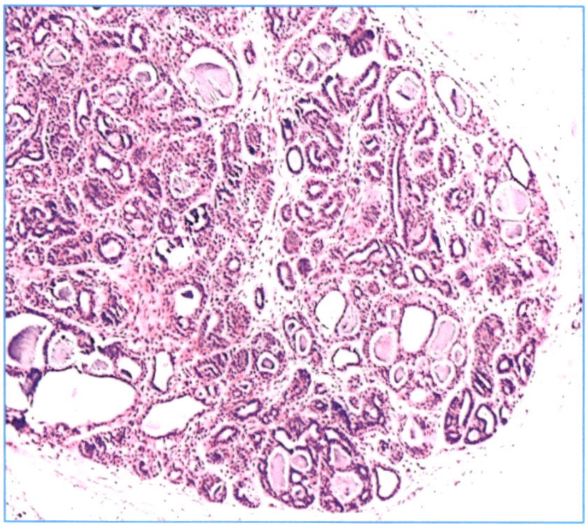
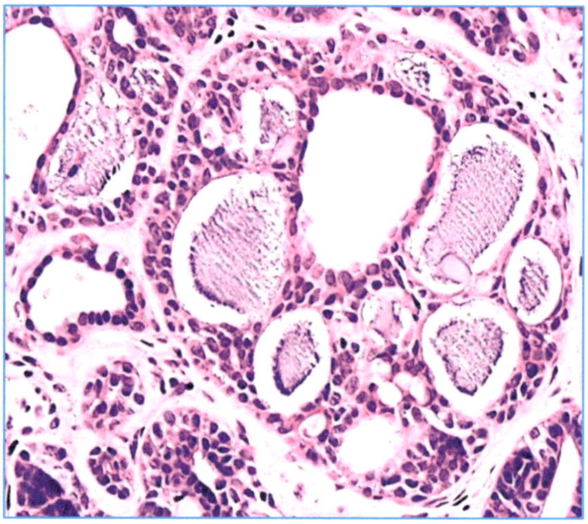

Adenoid cystic carcinoma with "Swiss cheese-like" appearance and round open spaces filled with mucin

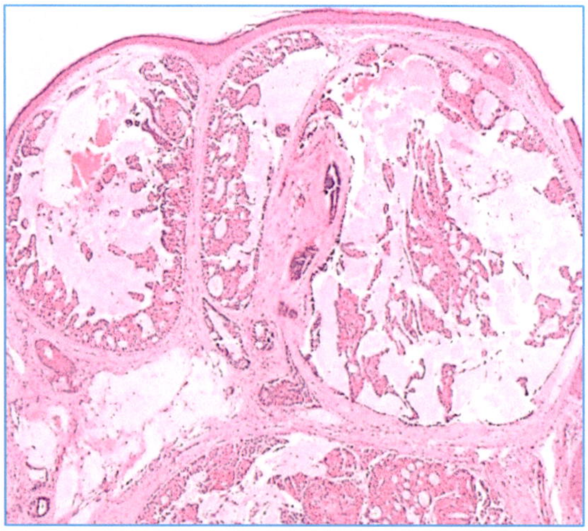
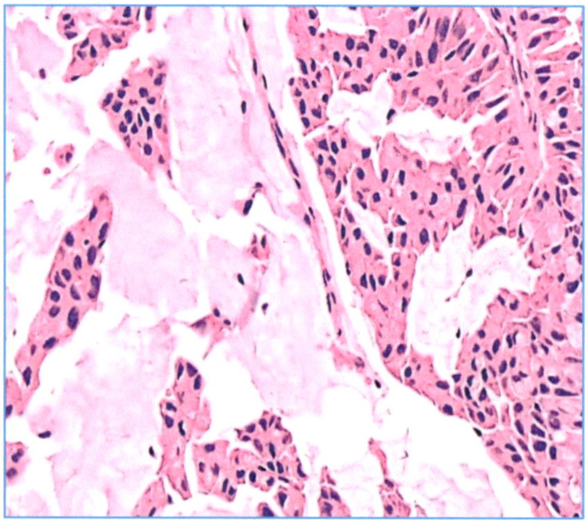

Mucinous carcinoma with large pools of mucin containing atypical epithelial cells

APOCRINE CARCINOMA

-rare adnexal carcinoma that occurs in middle-aged adults
-favors the axilla and the anogenital region but has also been described on the eyelid, ear, chest
-clinical findings vary but typically presents as erythematous, slow-growing, firm or cystic nodule

Histopathology
-dermal and subcutaneous poorly circumscribed tumor
-**infiltrating tubular, papillary and/or micronodular glandular structures**
-cells are atypical, hyperchromatic with **abundant eosinophilic cytoplasm**
-apocrine snouts present only in low grade neoplasms
-mitoses present with variable necrosis
-histology and IHC staining mirrors those seen in mammary ductal carcinoma
-therefore, metastatic breast cancer should always be clinically excluded

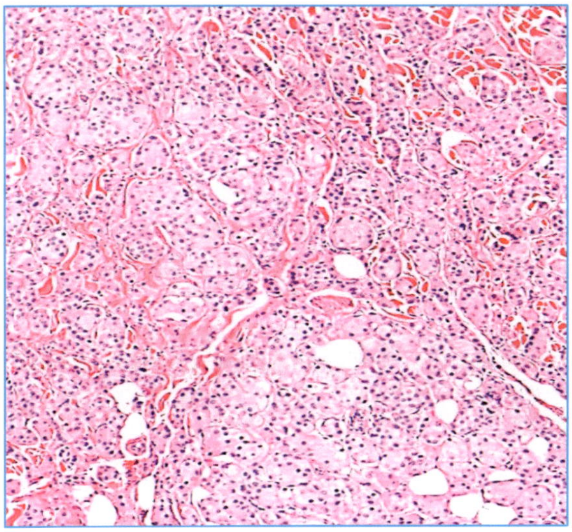
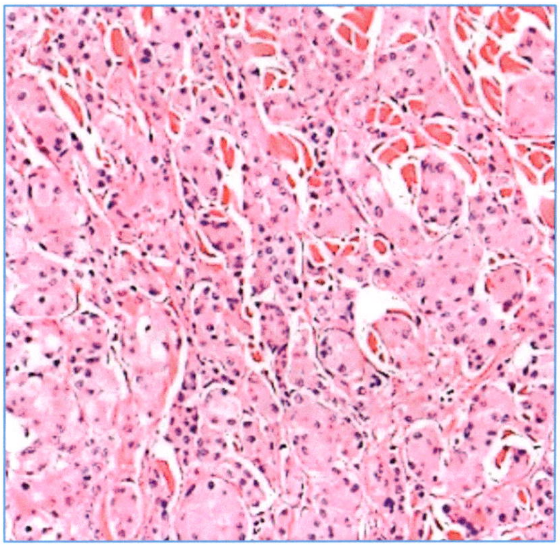

Moderately differentiated apocrine carcinoma with glandular structures made of cells with eosinophilic cytoplasm

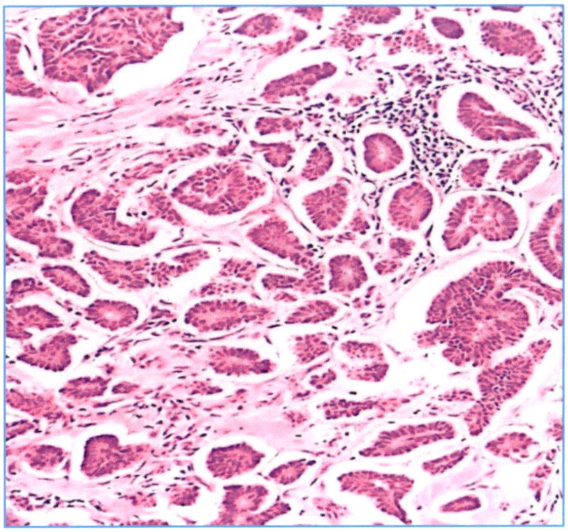
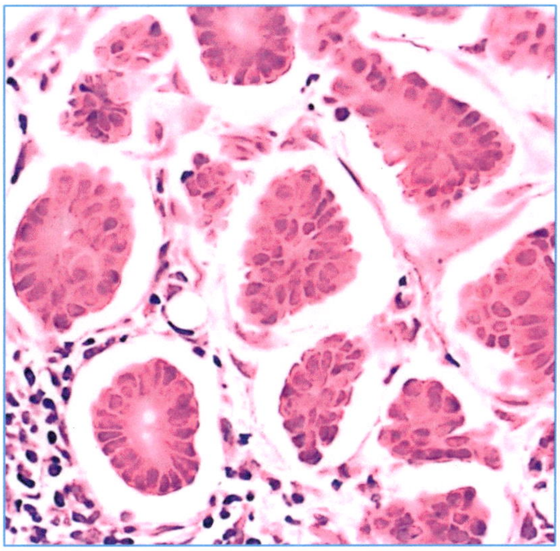

Well-differentiated apocrine carcinoma with irregular ducts made of cells with dark nuclei and eosinophilic cytoplasm with snouts

Sweat gland tumors

HOW TO APPROACH SWEAT GLAND TUMORS

DETERMINE IF TUMOR IS PREDOMINANTLY NODULAR, DUCTAL, OR CYSTIC/PAPILLARY

IF NODULAR AND APPEARS BENIGN

Tumor has 1 uniform cell population

-poroma	epidermal and dermal proliferation
-dermal duct tumor	dermal proliferation
-hidroacanthoma simplex	epidermal proliferation

Tumor has 2 cells population

-cylindroma	smaller tumor islands forming "jigsaw puzzle" with smaller pieces
-spiradenoma	large nodule "blue ball in the dermis" or multiple larger nodules forming "jigsaw puzzle" with large pieces + sprinkled lymphocytes
-nodular hidradenoma	no "jigsaw puzzle" + frequent 3rd type of cells (squamoid, mucinous, clear) + commonly cystic

IF NODULAR AND APPEARS MALIGNANT

-apocrine carcinoma	resembles breast carcinoma
-adenoid cystic carcinoma	"Swiss cheese" pattern with mucin
-prim. cutaneous mucinous ca.	large lakes of mucin
-mucoepidermoid carcinoma	atypical epithelioid cells with focal mucin

IF DUCTAL AND APPEARS BENIGN

-syringoma	"tadpole" shaped ducts only in the superficial dermis
-chondroid syringoma	chondroid stroma with syringoid ductal structures
-syringofibradenoma	strands arising from the epidermis and forming ducts

IF DUCTAL AND APPEARS MALIGNANT

-microcystic adnexal carcinoma	cysts in the upper dermis + infiltrating strands in the deep dermis
-syringoid eccrine ca.	"MAC-like" but with no cysts
-squam. eccrine ductal carcinoma	top looks like SCC

IF CYSTIC/PAPILLARY AND APPEARS BENIGN

-tubular apocrine adenoma	large cystic ducts + apocrine snouts + small papillae
-papillary eccrine adenoma	large cystic ducts + no snouts + larger papillae
-hidrocystoma	cyst lined with two cell layers + no papillae
-apocrine papil. cystadenoma	hidrocystoma + papillary/solid area
-solid-cystic hidradenoma	nodular and cystic tumor with two or three cell types
-hidradenoma papilliferum	complex papillary lesion + no epidermal connection
-syringocystadenoma papill.	complex papillary lesion with epidermal connection + plasma cells in papillary stroma

IF CYSTIC/PAPILLARY AND APPEARS MALIGNANT

-microcystic adnexal ca.	cysts in the upper dermis + infiltrating strand in deep dermis
-digital papillary adenoca.	acral lesion with nodular and cystic/papillary areas

Note: Any benign sweat gland tumor (e.g. cylindroma, spiradenoma, acrospiroma, poroma) has its malignant variant. They are very rare and usually arise in long standing benign tumors. Histologically, all are characterized by the presence of necrosis and increased mitotic activity in the background of a benign tumor.

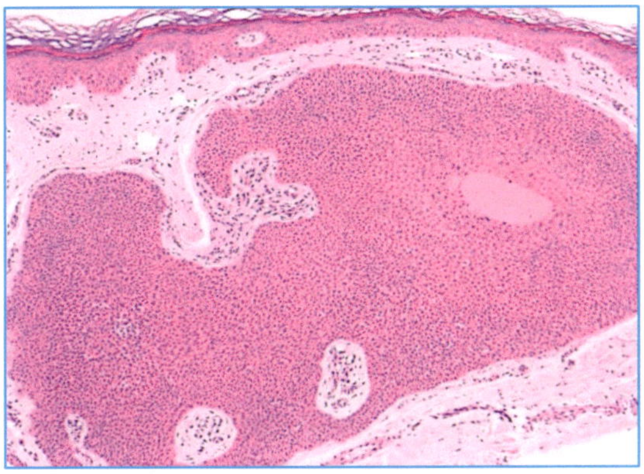

Dermal duct tumor with uniform, poroid cells in dermis

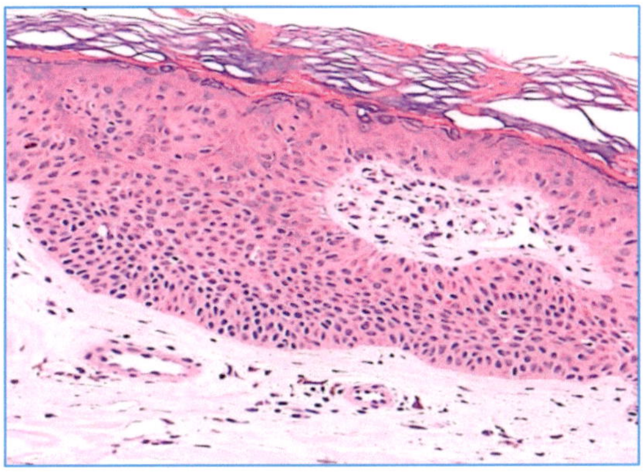

Hidroacanthoma simplex with uniform, poroid cells in epidermis

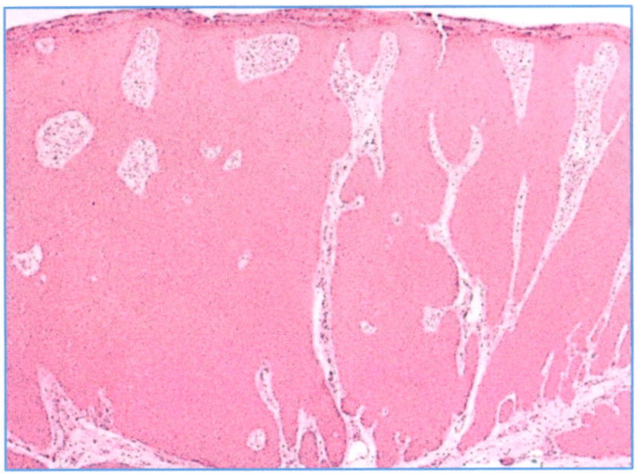

Poroma with uniform epidermal and dermal cells

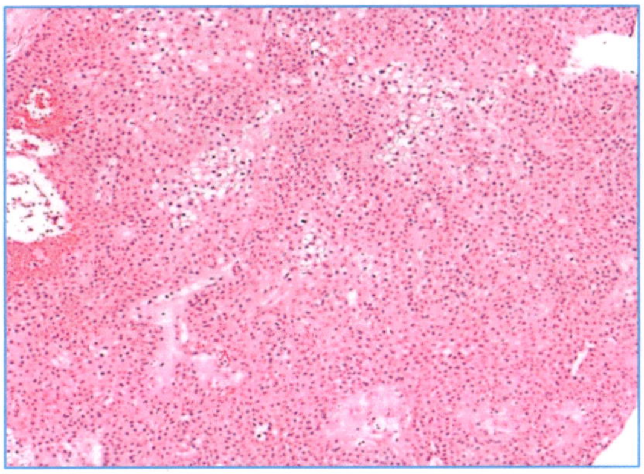

Acrospiroma with two cell populations forming a nodule

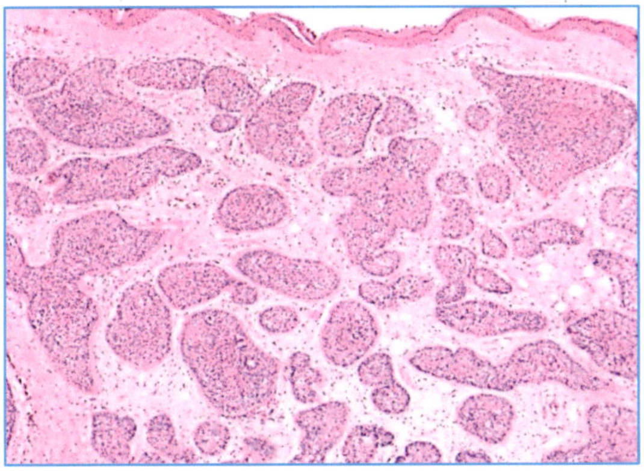

Cylindroma with small lobules forming "jigsaw puzzle"

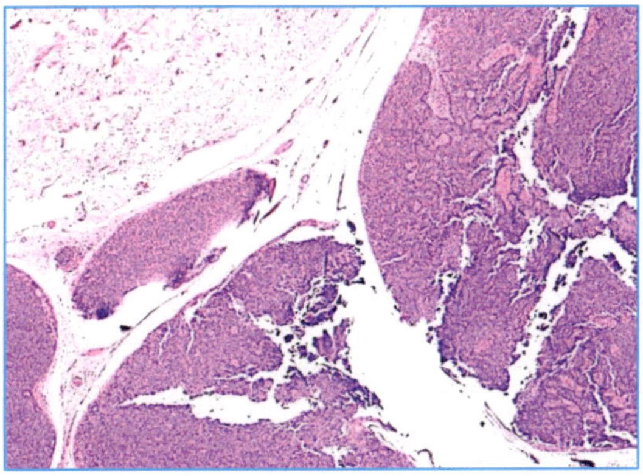

Spiradenoma with large nodules forming "pseudo-puzzle"

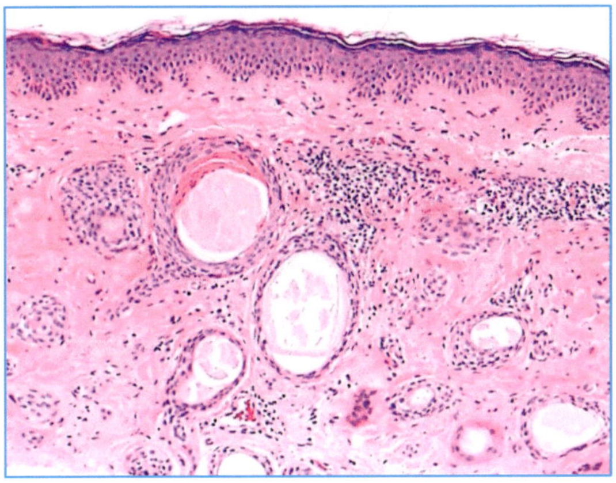

Syringoma with dermal "tadpole-shaped" ducts

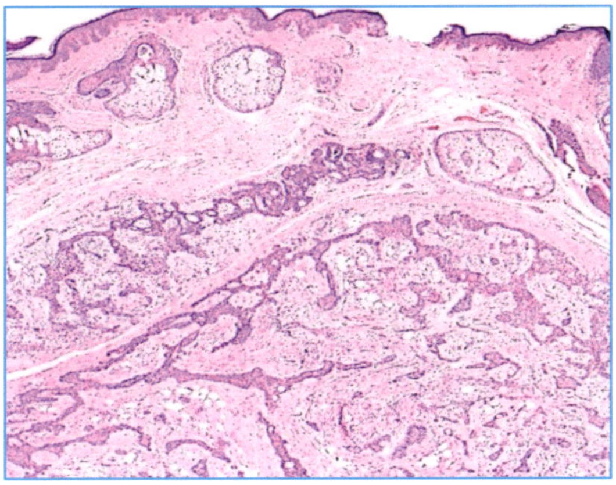

Chondroid syringoma with irregular ducts in chondroid stroma

Sweat gland tumors

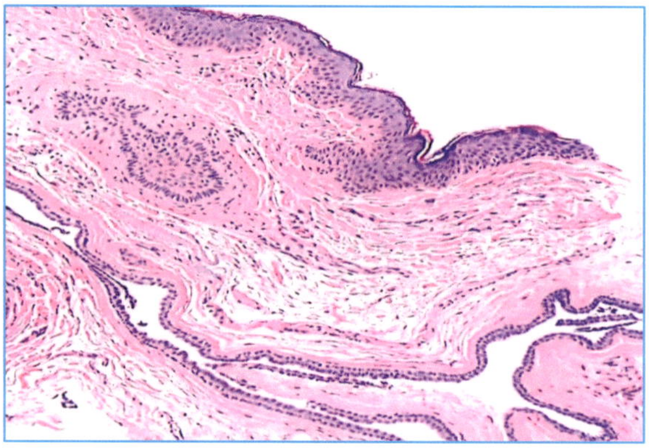

Hidrocystoma with cyst lined with two cells layer

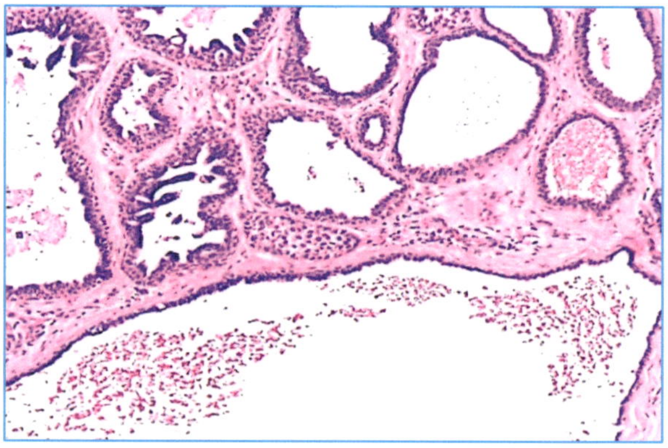

Apocrine papillary cystadenoma is hidrocystoma with papillary/cystic areas

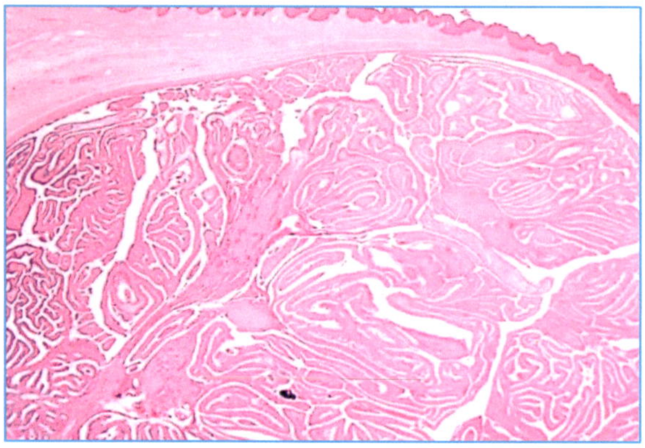

Hidradenoma papilliferum complex "maze-like" papillae without epidermal connection

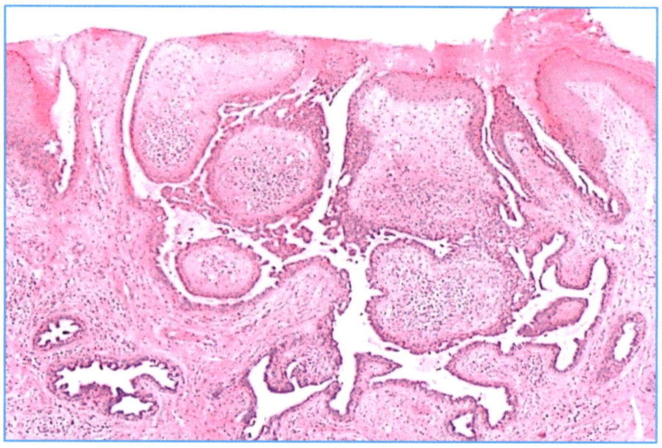

Syringocystadenoma papilliferum is papillary lesion connected to epidermis with stromal plasma cells

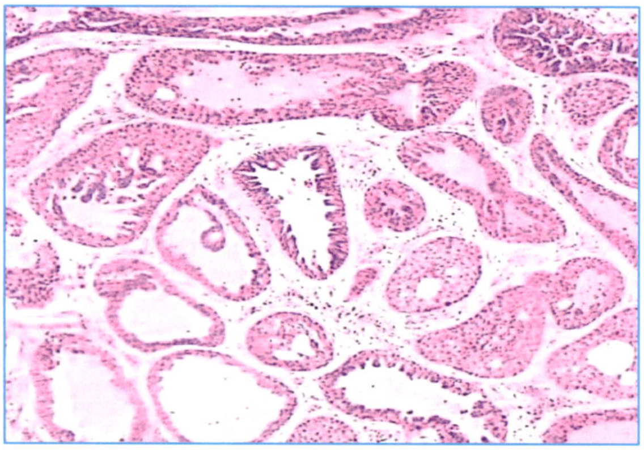

Tubular apocrine adenoma with apocrine snouts present

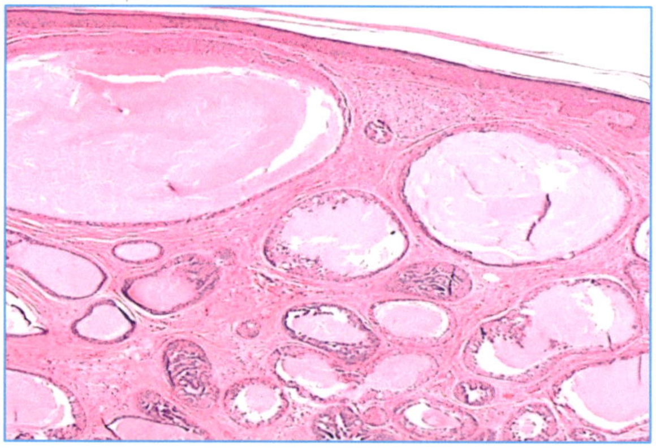

Papillary eccrine adenoma with absent snouts

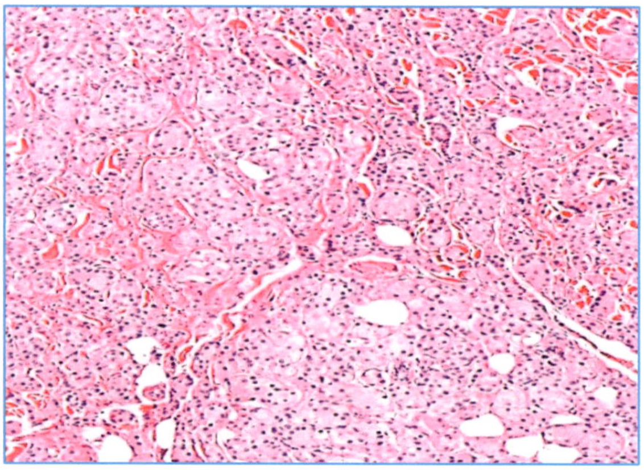

Apocrine carcinoma with atypical eosinophilic ducts

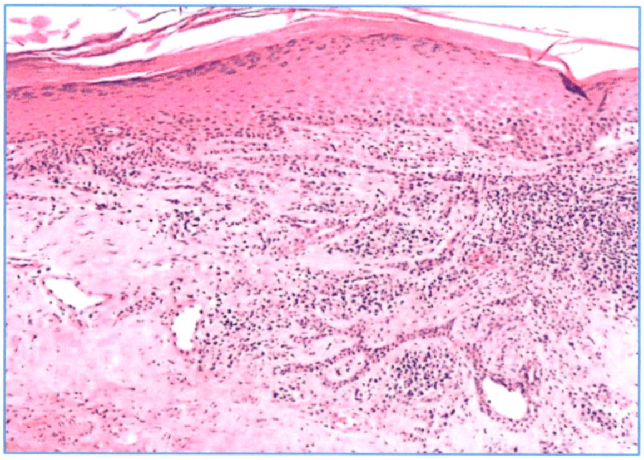

Syringofibroadenoma with retiform ducts infiltrating dermis

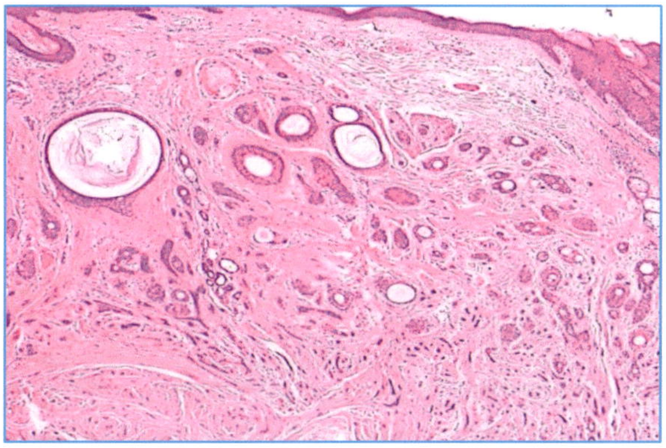

MAC with superficial cysts and deep infiltrating ducts

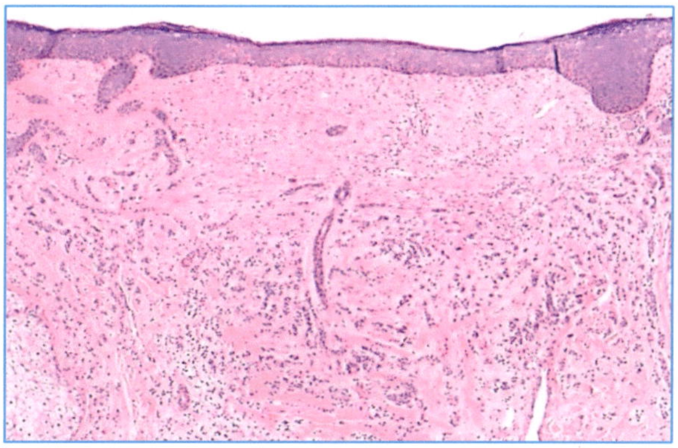

Syringoid eccrine carcinoma with only infiltrating ducts

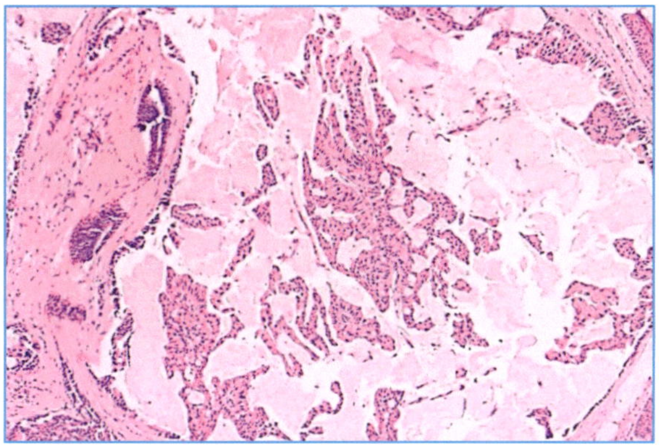

Mucinous carcinoma with tumor cells in lakes of mucin

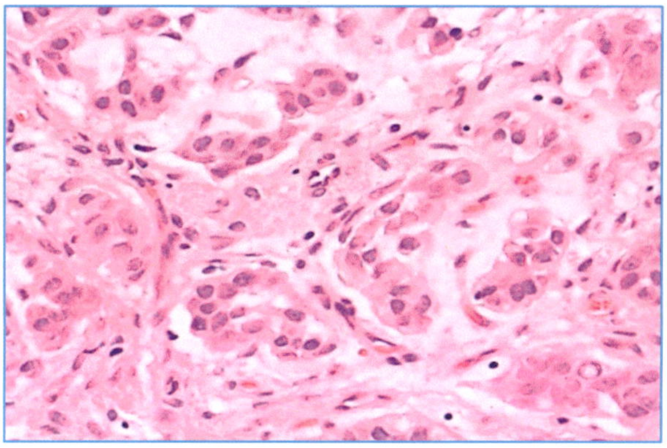

Mucoepidermoid carcinoma with atypical epithelioid cells and focal mucin

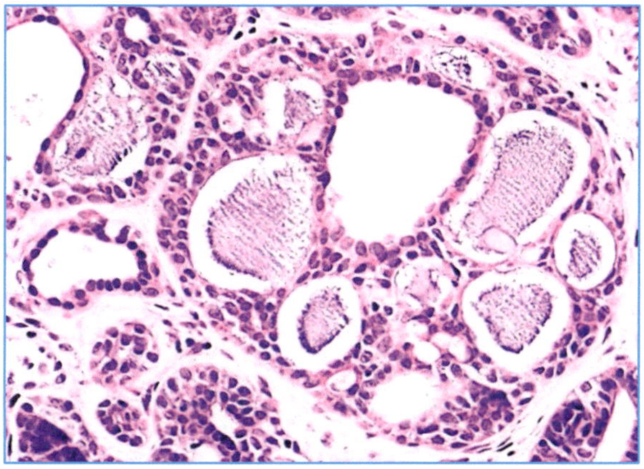

Adenoid cystic carcinoma with “Swiss cheese” appearance

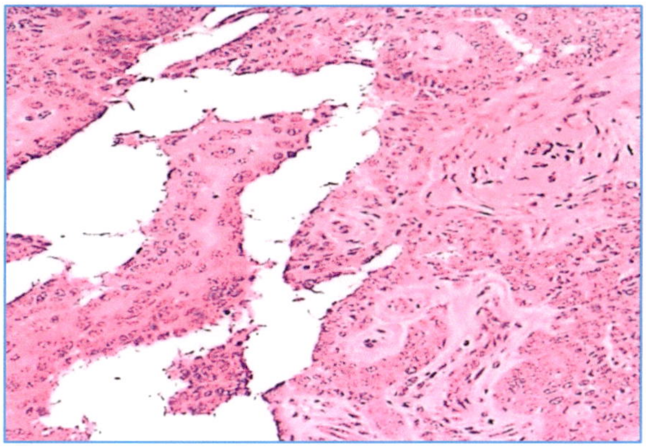

Digital papillary adenocarcinoma with papillary and solid areas

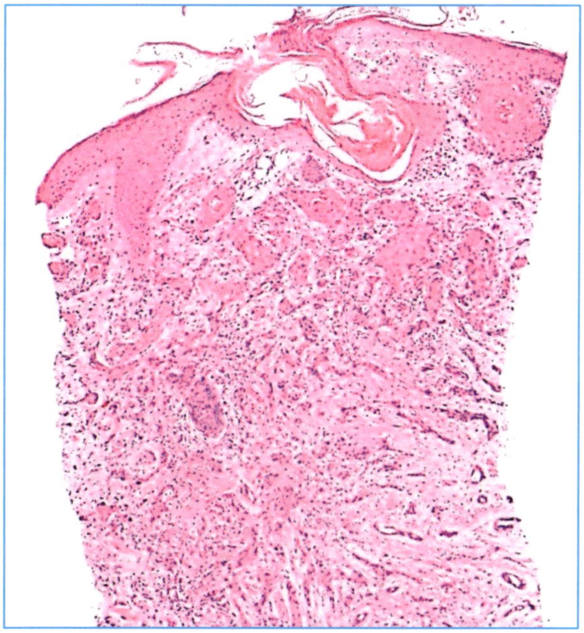

Squamoid eccrine ductal carcinoma with superficial SCC appearance and deep infiltrating ducts

Sweat gland tumors

Chapter 30

MELANOCYTIC TUMORS

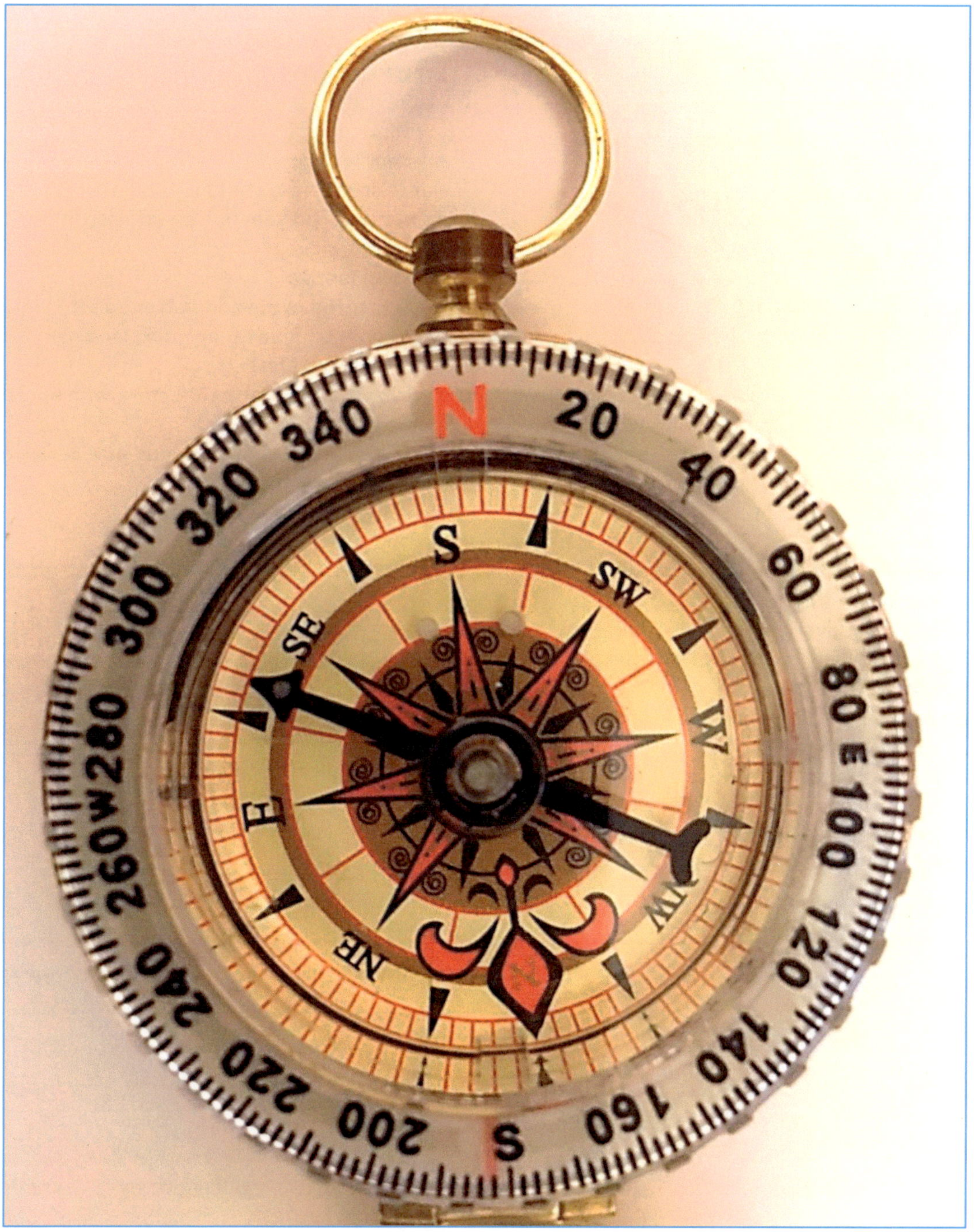

Melanocytic tumors

LENTIGO

-evenly pigmented, light brown macules with a variety of clinical presentations

Solar lentigo

-caused by chronic sun exposure
-common in fair skinned people over age 40
-appears on sun-exposed areas of the body (face, hands, shoulders, and arms)

Lentigo simplex

-clinically similar to solar lentigo but **not** caused by sun exposure
-can occur anywhere on the body
-often starts at birth or during childhood
-the spots can go away over time
-multiple can be seen in various syndromes (Bannayan- Riley-Ruvalcaba, Cowden, Noonan, Peutz- Jeghers, Xeroderma pigmentosum)

Ink spot lentigo

-variant of solar lentigo characterized by very dark color and a beaded or wiry, markedly irregular outline
-appears after a sunburn in people who have lighter pigmented skin

Mucosal lentigo

-light brown macules on mucosal surfaces
-lower lip is a favored site

Ephelides (freckles)

-numerous small tan or light brown macules on sun-exposed skin
-common on the face of redheaded or blonde, fair-skinned individuals
-produced by exposure to ultraviolet light and typically fade in the winter

PUVA, tanning bed and radiation lentigines

-appear after these exposures

Histopathology

Solar lentigo

-**elongated "club shaped" rete ridges**
-**hyperpigmentation** of basal layer of keratinocytes
-appearance of **"dirty socks hanging on a clothesline"**
-mildly increased number of dermal melanocytes
-dermal **solar elastosis is present**

Lentigo simplex

-the same histology as solar lentigo but **without dermal solar elastosis**

Ink spot lentigo

-similar to solar lentigo but more pigmented
-pigmentation is present at rete but also in between rete ridges

Mucosal lentigo

-**hyperpigmented, wide and flattened rete** ridges of epithelium with **no granular layer**

Ephelides (freckles)

-normal wavy epidermal architecture with epidermal hyperpigmentation
-rete ridges are not prominent, and number of melanocytes is normal
-no significant solar elastosis

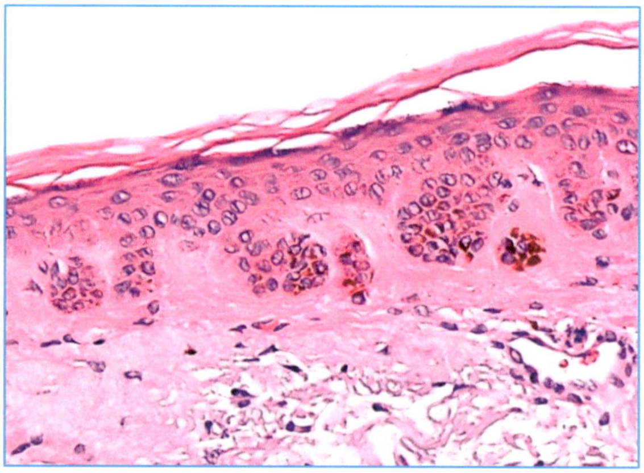

Solar lentigo with "dirty socks" appearance and solar elastosis

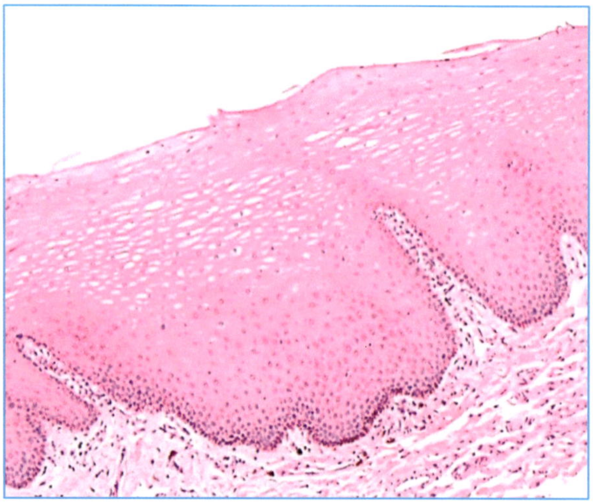

Mucosal lentigo with wide hyperpigmented rete ridges

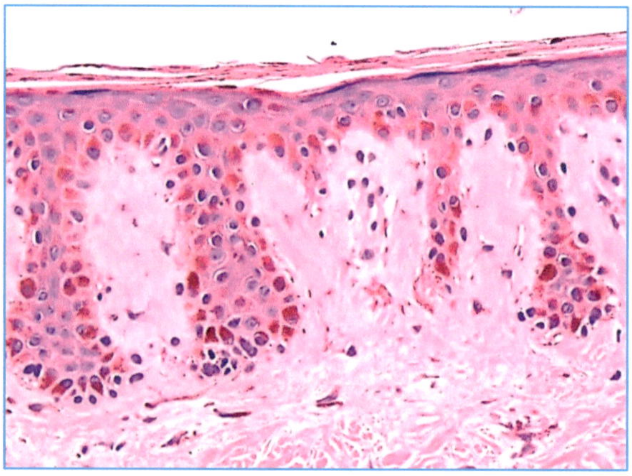

Lentigo simplex with "dirty socks" appearance and no solar elastosis

Chapter 30

ACQUIRED MELANOCYTIC NEVI

-benign proliferation of melanocytes not present at birth
-most develop in childhood and adolescence and number of nevi peaks by the 3rd decade of life

Junctional nevus
-brown, tan, flat or only slightly elevated macule or papule
-round/oval, with smooth borders and uniform color

Compound nevus
-slightly raised, pink, tan-brown papule
-round/oval, smooth borders, and uniform color
-may grow "bristle-like" hair

Dermal nevus
-raised, "dome shaped", pink or brown papule
-round/oval, smooth borders, and uniform color
-may grow course hair

Histopathology

Junctional nevus
-nests of nevus cells at the epidermo-dermal junction
-nests are relatively uniform and located at the tips of rete ridges
-cells do not show cytological atypia or variability
-no individual epidermal melanocytes with pagetoid spread
-no dermal inflammation or significant fibrosis

Dermal nevus
-**symmetrical lesion** with only dermal melanocytes
-**cells mature** with increased depth (**become smaller and less nested**)
-**superficially, type A** (epithelioid) cells that are **larger and form nests** are seen
-cells have abundant pink cytoplasm and round nuclei that can have small nucleoli
-they have **tendency to produce melanin**
-**deeper, type B** cells that are smaller, **not forming groups** are present
-they **resemble lymphocytes** and rarely produce melanin
-**at the bottom, type C** cells that **resemble fibroblasts or Schwann cells** are seen
-mitoses are usually not present and if present they are in the superficial portion of the lesion

Compound nevus
-combination of junctional and dermal nevus
-junctional component does not extend laterally for more than 3 rete ridges relative to dermal component (no "shouldering")

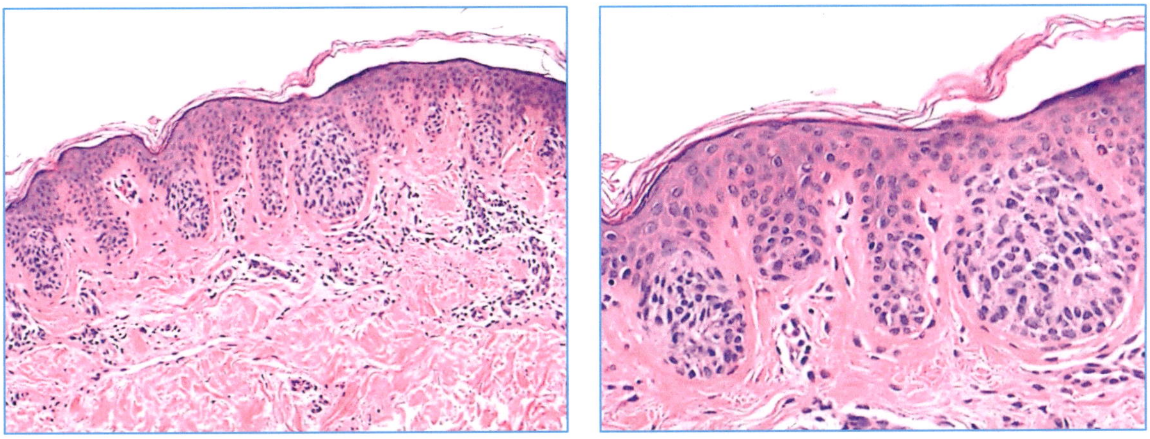

Junctional nevus with nests of uniform melanocytes at the tips of the rete ridges

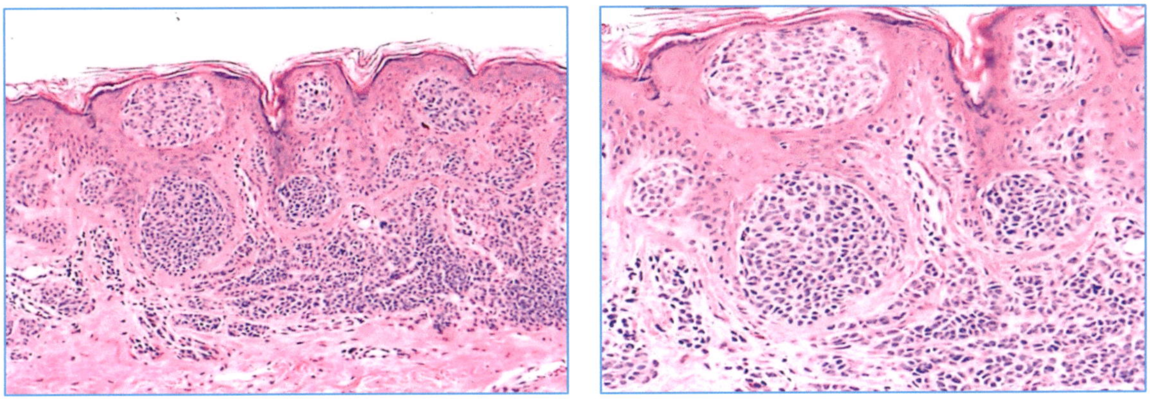

Compound nevus with junctional melanocytic nests with underlying dermal maturing melanocytes

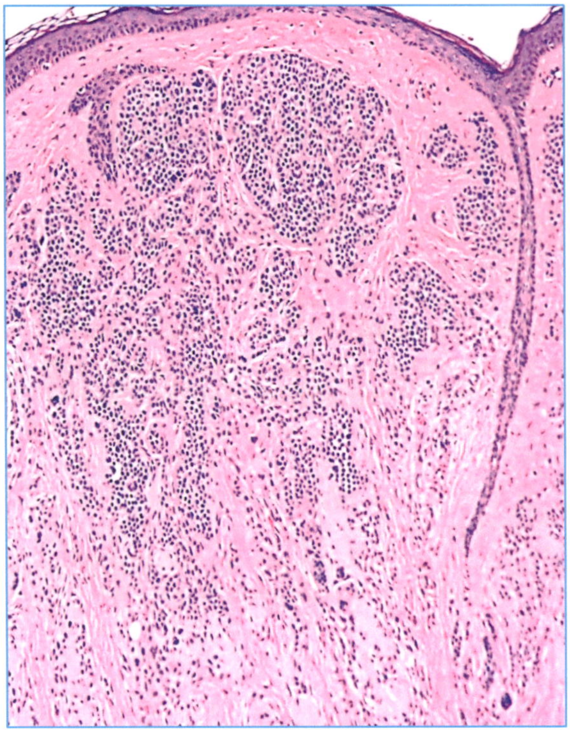

Dermal nevus demonstrates maturation from top to bottom

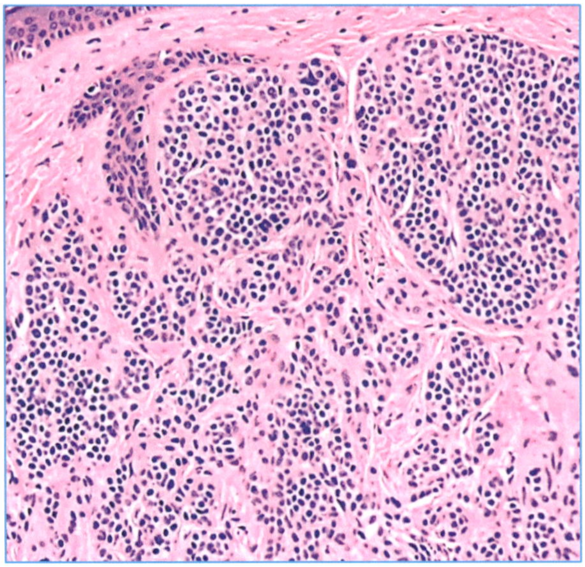

Type A (top) and type B nevus cells (bottom)

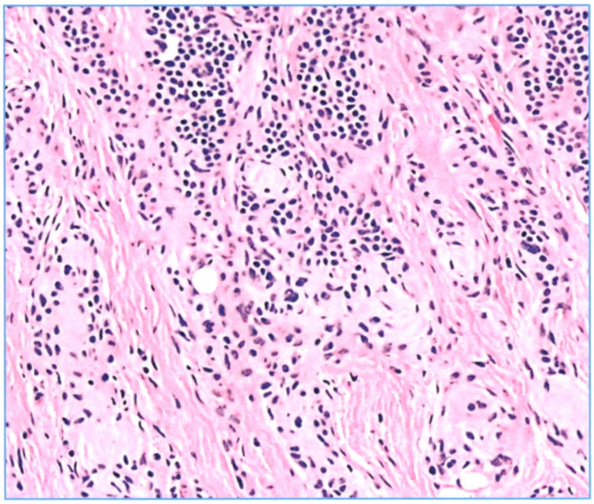

Type B (top) and type C nevus cells (bottom)

HALO NEVUS (SUTTON'S NEVUS)

-presents as an ordinary nevus encircled by halo of sharply marginated depigmentation
-favors the back of younger individuals
-may herald vitiligo, or rarely melanoma at the distant site

Histopathology

-lesion is symmetrical with numerous **dermal lymphocytes mingling with nevus cells ("cocktail party")**
-ordinary junctional, compound, or dermal nevus is hiding within the inflammation
-nevus cells mature normally, and atypia is minimal
-there is a well-defined inferior border of the lesion

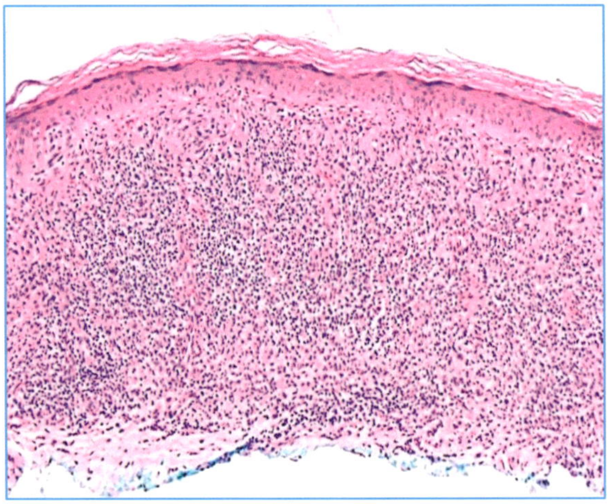

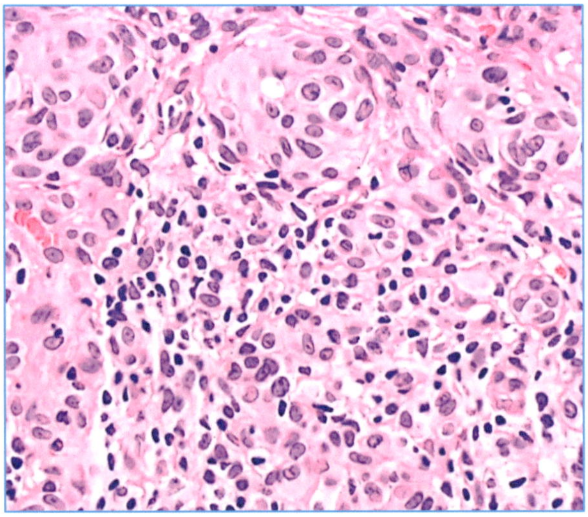

Halo nevus with nevus cells among numerous lymphocytes

Chapter 30

CONGENITAL NEVUS

-variably-sized, brown papule or plaque with regular or slightly irregular borders present at birth
-coarse hair often grows from the lesion
-mostly single but occasionally also multiple
-present in about 1% of newborns
-divided by size into small (<1.5 cm), medium (1.5-20cm) and large (>20 cm)
-large congenital nevi can be seen in conjunction with neurocutanous melanosis (*NRAS* gene mutation)
-can develop proliferative nodules within them

Histopathology

-**compound or dermal nevus**
-melanocytes mature and no atypia is seen
-characteristic **periadnexal, perivascular and perineural** single cell **nevoid infiltrate**
-**nests of nevus cells** can be found **within pilar muscle and adnexal structures**
-can be heavily pigmented and number of terminal hairs can be increased

SPECIAL SITE NEVUS

-benign melanocytic nevi located on special body sites that demonstrate unusual histopathological features
-originally described on acral sites and genitalia
-but occur also on ears, scalp, breast, flexural skin, legs, shoulder

Histopathology

-asymmetrical lesion with **poor lateral circumscription** (nests can trail off)
-**junctional melanocytic nests are enlarged** and **irregularly nested** (at tips, sides, and between rete ridges)
-**clefting** between junctional melanocytes and keratinocytes is common
-epidermal pagetoid spread is common in the center of the lesion
-mitosis can be seen, but not atypical

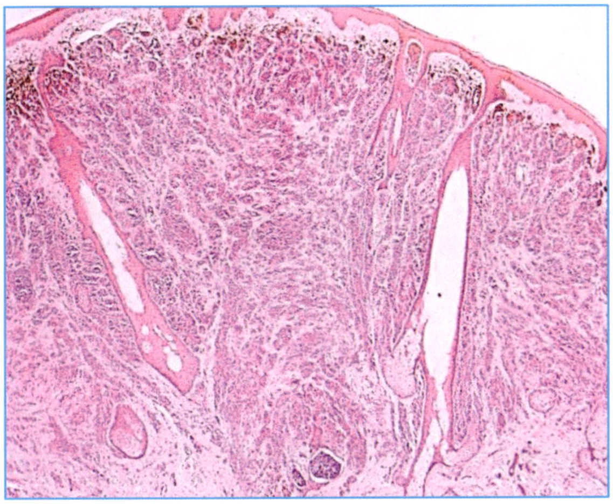

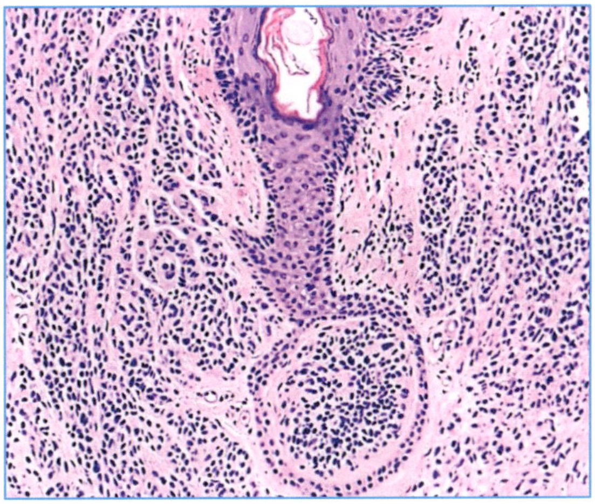

Congenital nevus surrounds adnexal structures with nevus nest present within hair follicle

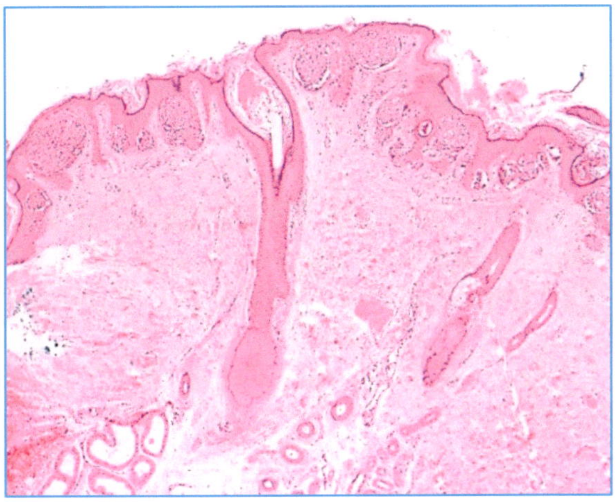

Axillary special site nevus with large nests and poor lateral circumscription

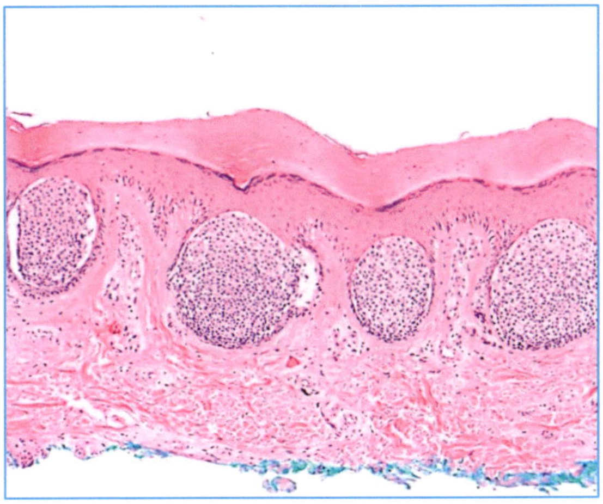

Acral special site nevus with large junctional nests

Melanocytic tumors

BLUE NEVUS

-occurs due to arrest of melanocytes in the dermis
-firm, dark-blue to gray-black, sharply defined macule or papule
-usually round or oval in shape and less than 1 cm in diameter
-favorite sites are scalp, sacrum, hands, and feet
-frequently exhibit activating mutations in *GNAQ* or *GNA11* genes

Histopathology
-most commonly in the **upper dermis**
-**elongated, pigmented dendritic melanocytes** present in between **thickened hyalinized collagen bundles**
-variable number of pigmented melanophages
-**dendritic melanocytes like to surround adnexal and neurovascular structures** in whorled pattern

CELLULAR BLUE NEVUS

-solitary, blue-black, smooth nodule
-usually at least 1 cm in diameter
-favorite sites are buttocks and scalp

Histopathology
-dermal and subcutaneous pigmented tumor with **"dumbbell"** shape
-**biphasic tumor** with pushing margins composed of:
-**heavily pigmented dendritic melanocytes** (as in blue nevus) with dermal fibrosis and melanophages and **cellular area of epithelioid and spindle cells with clear or finely pigmented cytoplasm** with **minimal** amount of **melanin**
-no or minimal atypia and no or rare mitotic figures

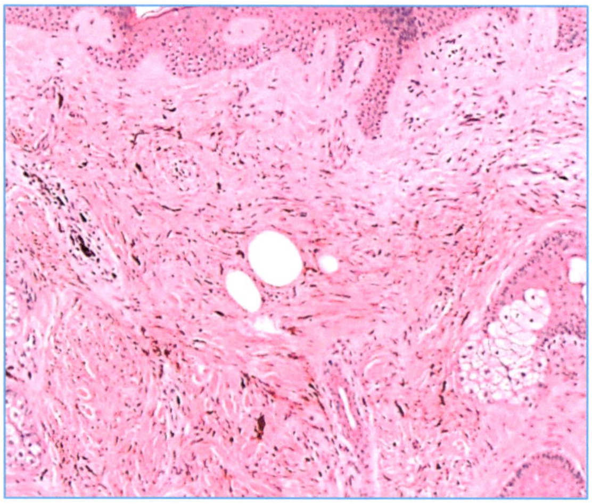
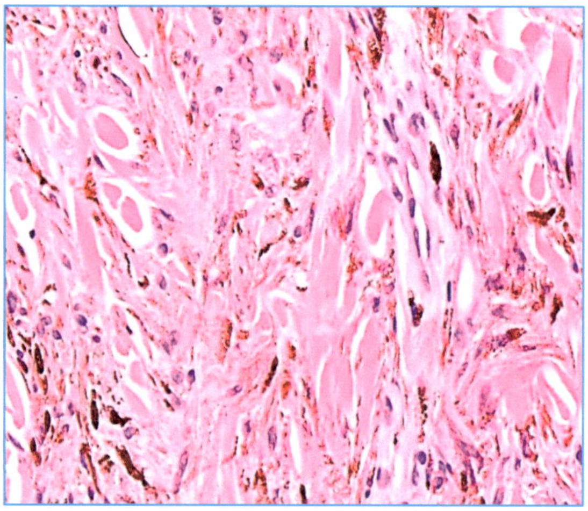

Blue nevus with elongated pigmented melanocytes in between prominent collagen bundles

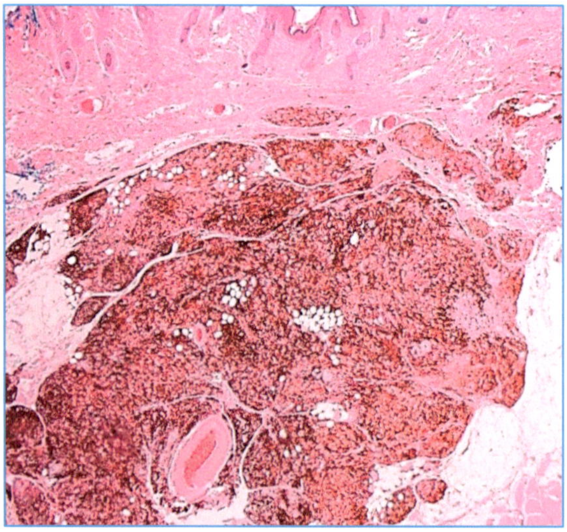
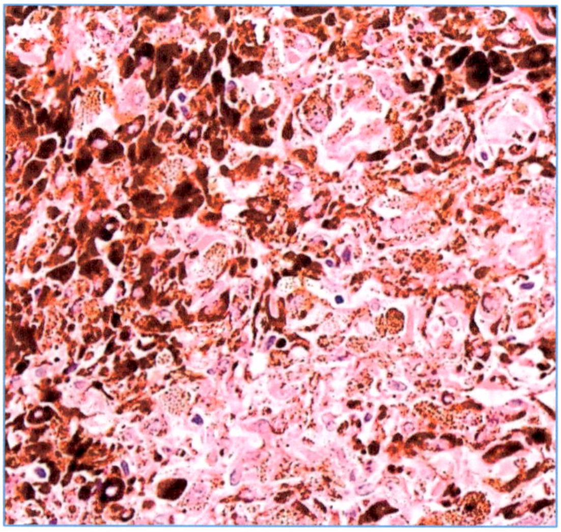

"Dumbbell shaped" cellular blue nevus with heavily pigmented melanocytes admixed with lightly pigmented epithelioid melanocytes

DEEP PENETRATING NEVUS	INVERTED TYPE A NEVUS
-subtype of benign melanocytic nevus -presents as a dark blue to black papule -may appear asymmetrical and unevenly pigmented -generally, presents between the second and third decades of life -shows a slight female predominance -favor head and neck, followed by the extremities and trunk Histopathology -**"V-shaped" lesion** that extends into the deep dermis and subcutis -lesion is **wrapping around adnexal structures** (follicles, vessels, nerves, sweat glands) -composed of **vertically oriented heavily pigmented spindle cells** and/or **pale epithelioid cells in nests admixed with macrophages** -mitoses are rare	-subtype of benign melanocytic nevus -presents as a clinically normal-appearing dermal or compound nevus -typically uniform in color -sometimes has an eccentric area of nested darker pigmentation Histopathology -pigmented **type A nevus cells** (epithelioid, nested) are **found in the middle or close to the bottom** of otherwise normal dermal or compound nevus -deep type A cells are clustered and surrounded by type B and C cells -deep area usually contains numerous melanophages -no evidence of mitoses or cytological atypia

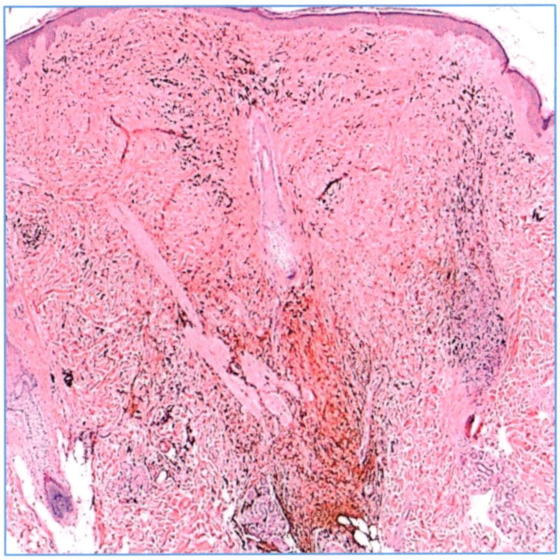
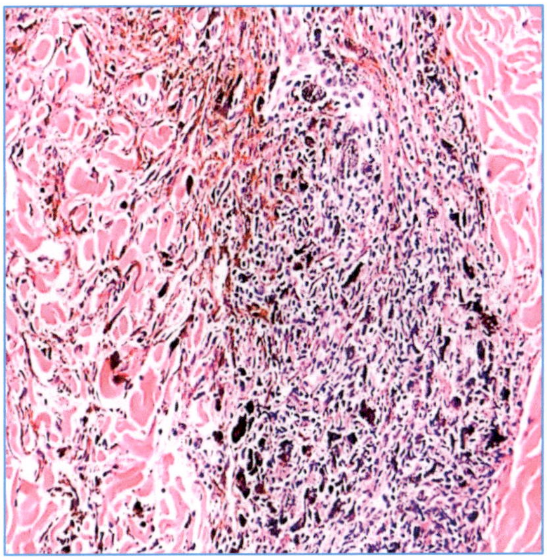

Deep penetrating nevus wrapping around adnexal structures and consisting of pigmented spindle cells and lighter epithelioid cells

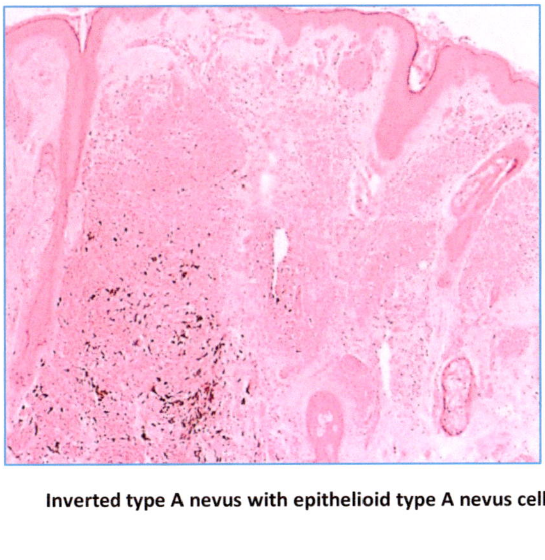
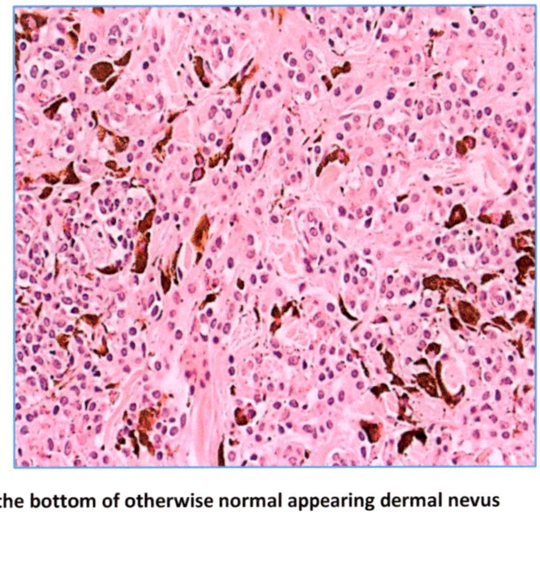

Inverted type A nevus with epithelioid type A nevus cells at the bottom of otherwise normal appearing dermal nevus

Melanocytic tumors

SPITZ NEVUS

-benign acquired nevus associated with mutation in *HRAS* gene
-usually solitary, symmetric, well-circumscribed papule or nodule uniform in color
-sometimes they erupt as multiple lesions
-tends to grow very rapidly (reaching a size of approximately 1 cm within 6 months) and thereafter remaining static
-most commonly (70%) seen in children and adolescents
-favors the face, neck, and legs
-on dermoscopy, Spitz nevus displays uniform rounded structures with prominent punctate or rounded blood vessels

Histopathology
-symmetrical, well-circumscribed lesion with **hypertrophic epidermis**
-can be junctional, dermal or compound
-proliferation of **epithelioid and/or spindle cells**
-cells have **abundant cytoplasm** with **large nuclei** and **prominent lilac-colored nucleoli**
-junctional nests demonstrate focal separation from the epidermis (**"clefting"**)
-cells form junctional nests organized in "**teardrops"** shape (appear to be "**raining down**")
-focal pagetoid spread can be seen but only in center of the lesion
-eosinophilic hyaline globules (**Kamino bodies**) at epidermo-dermal junction
-dermal cells mature with descent
-no atypia or atypical mitoses

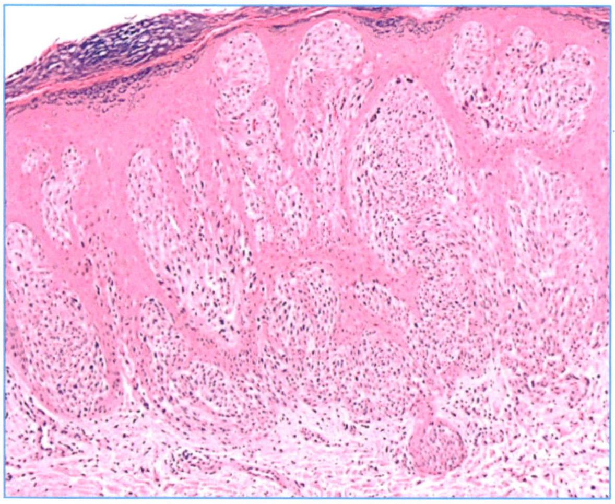

Compound Spitz nevus with reactive proliferative epidermis

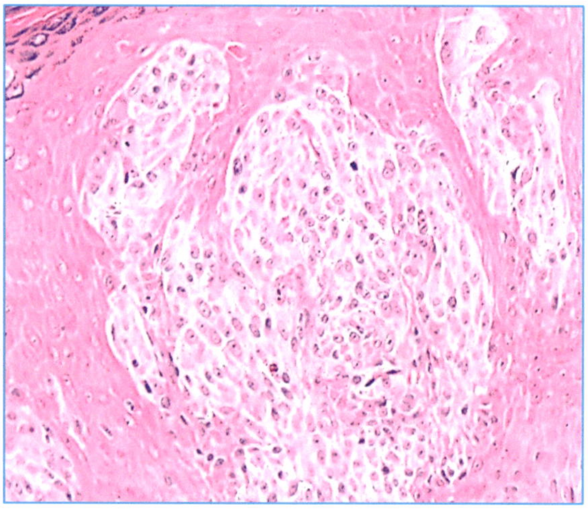

Compound Spitz nevus with "raining down" junctional nests made of pink spindle cells

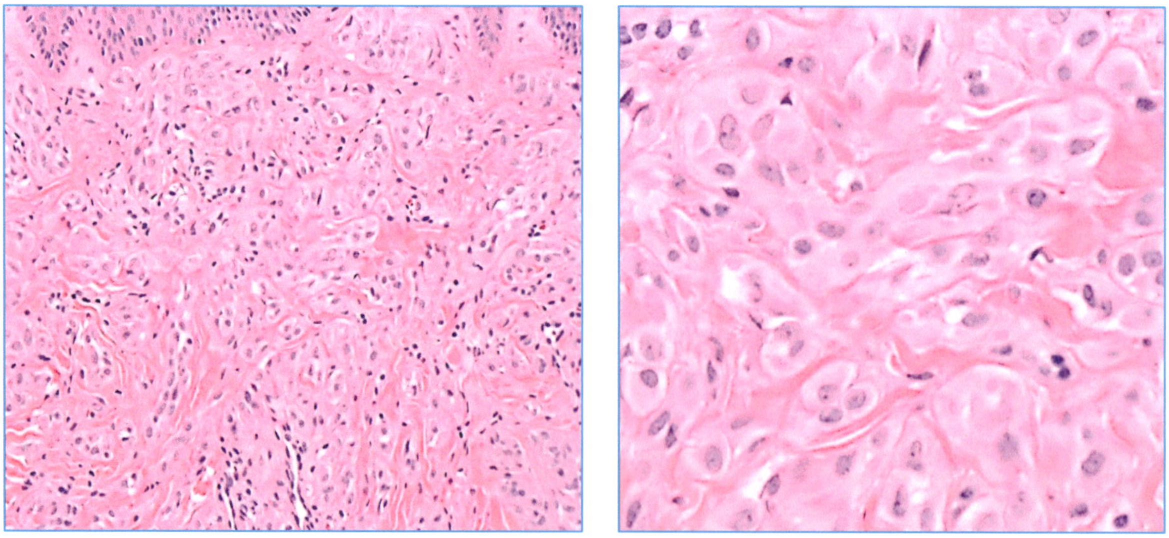

Dermal Spitz nevus made of epithelioid cells with abundant pink cytoplasm and prominent nuclei

PIGMENTED SPINDLE CELL NEVUS OF REED

-considered a pigmented variant of Spitz nevus
-presents as evenly-pigmented, symmetrical, black/dark brown, "dome-shaped" papule/nodule
-generally found on the trunk or lower extremities of young women
-characteristically shows a starburst pattern on dermoscopy with radial pseudopods around the perimeter

Histopathology

-**mostly junctional** or less frequently superficial compound melanocytic proliferation with a hyperkeratotic epidermis
-melanocytes are predominantly or exclusively **spindled and pigmented**
-laterally symmetrical, well-defined lesion
-junctional nests are formed from **vertically oriented spindle cells**
-spindle cells have **"tear drop" appearance** with **focal "clefting"** from the epidermis
-**abundant pigment** is seen within and outside of cells
-**dermal component is absent or shallow**
-numerous dermal melanophages can be present
-mitoses and cytological atypia are rare

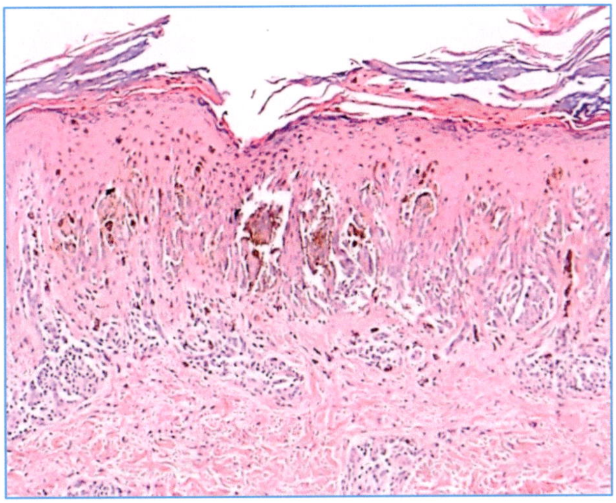

Reed's nevus with junctional melanocytic proliferation

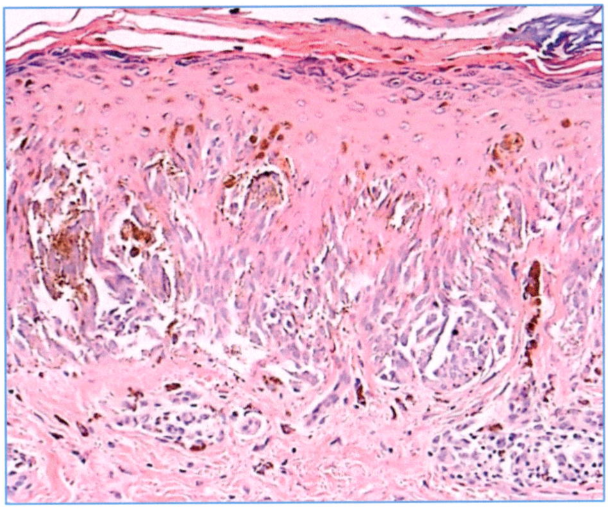

Reed's nevus with pigmented, clefted junctional nests and dermal melanophages

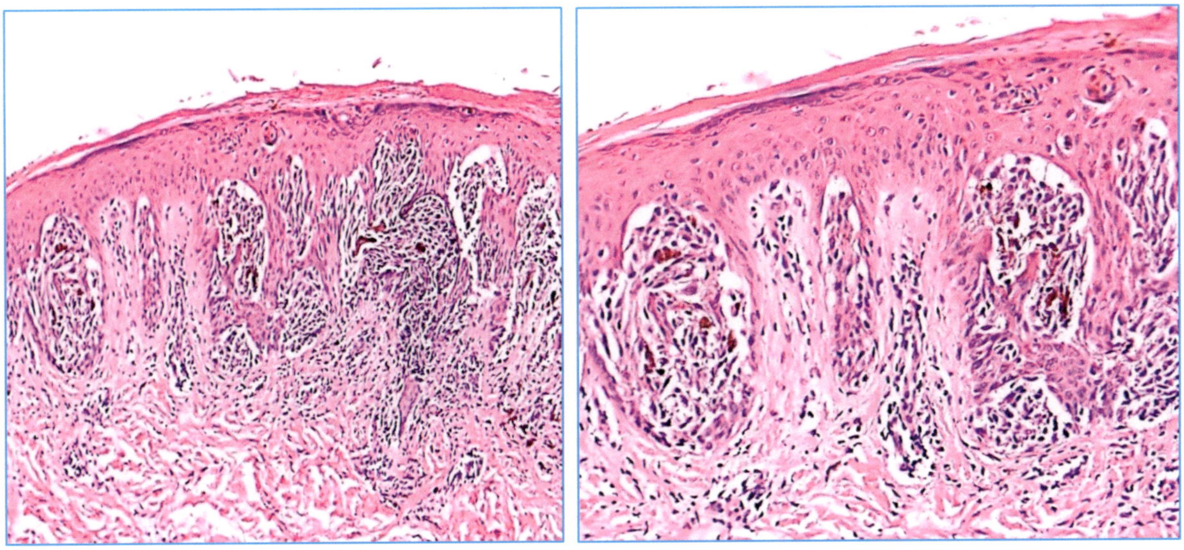

Junctional Reed's nevus with "tear drop-like" pigmented junctional melanocytic nests

RECURRENT NEVUS

-nevus recurring at the site of a previous biopsy or inadequate excision of a nevus
-appears usually within a year of previous surgery
-may present as hyperpigmented macule or papule within the previous scar
-may have irregular borders

Histopathology
-atrophic **flat epidermis** with underlying **dermal scar**
-variably atypical **melanocytic proliferation in the epidermis limited to area above the scar**
-maturing **dermal nevus cells underneath the scar**

COMBINED NEVUS

-benign melanocytic nevus composed of two histologically distinct nevus cell populations
-favored sites are the trunk, head, and neck
-usually seen in middle-aged men
-presents as brown, black papule and can display irregular pigmentation

Histopathology
-**two types of melanocytic proliferations** in the same pigmented lesion
-most common combination is **blue nevus and dermal nevus**
-any combination can occur

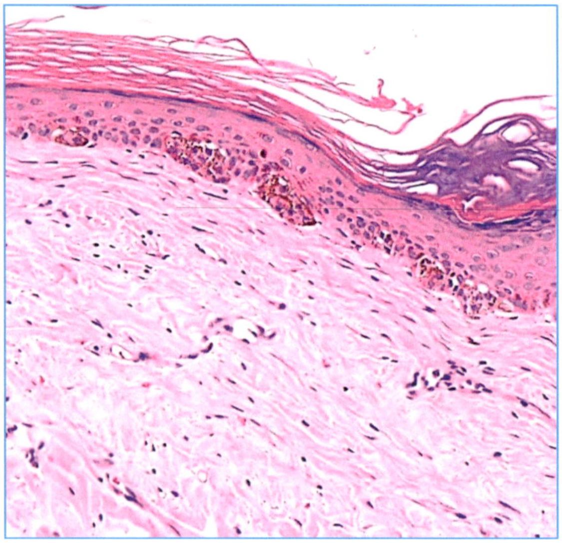

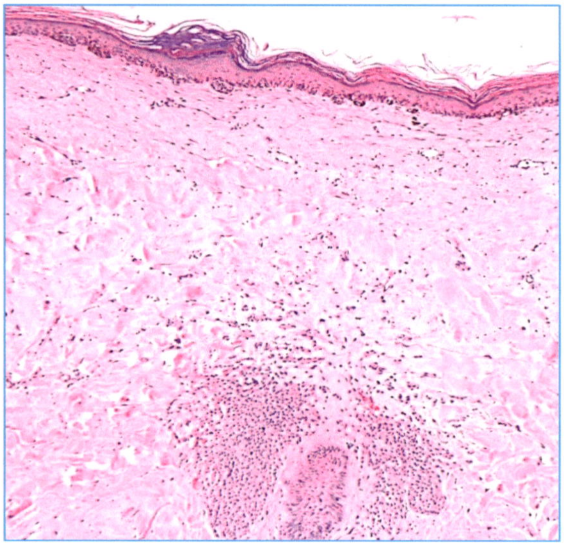

Recurrent nevus with junctional melanocytes above and dermal melanocytes below dermal scar

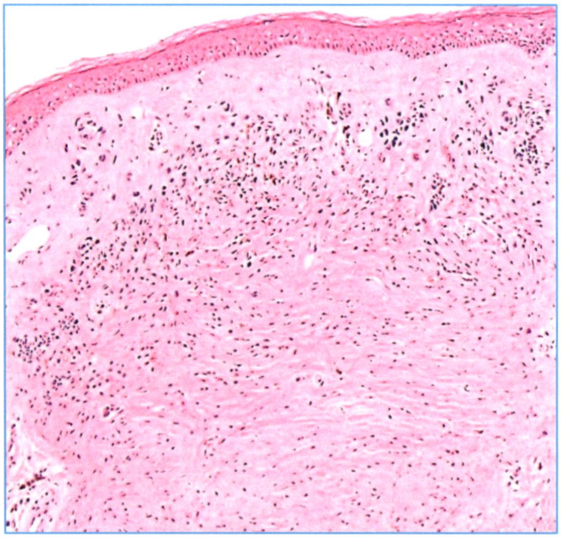

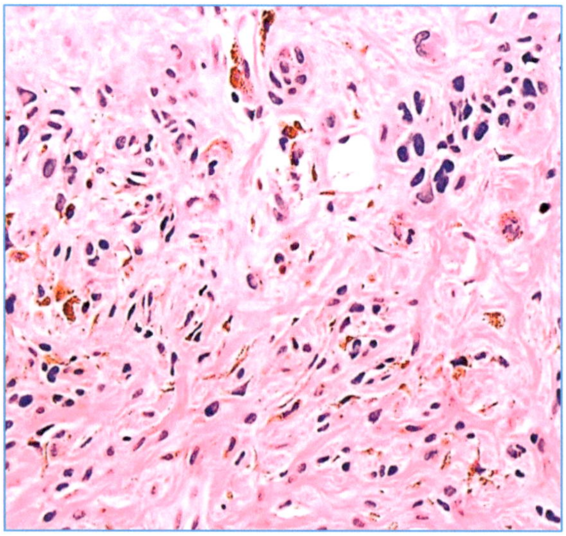

Combined dermal nevus above and blue nevus below

BAPOMA
BRCA1-associated protein (*BAP1*) inactivated melanocytic tumor (BIMT)

-benign atypical Spitzoid tumor characterized by a mutation in the *BAP-1* gene
-"dome-shaped" or pedunculated pink to light brown asymptomatic papule
-mostly sporadic, solitary, or rarely multiple (in 2nd-3rd decade of life) as part of a syndrome with germline *BAP-1* mutation
-syndrome is associated with history of uveal and cutaneous melanoma and mesothelioma

Histopathology

-**"dome-shaped"** lesion with a mostly dermal melanocytic proliferation and two histological patterns:
-one pattern has two cell population; **conventional nevus cells and larger epithelioid cells**
-the second pattern consists of **only epithelioid cells**
-in both patterns **prominent lymphocytic inflammation** can be present at the periphery
-epithelioid cells have vesicular chromatin and abundant amphophilic cytoplasm with some pleomorphism but mitotic activity is low
-they show **loss of nuclear BAP-1** staining and **frequent BRAF mutation**, unlike Spitz tumors

DERMAL MELANOCYTOSIS

-group of conditions often present at birth that is due to arrest of melanocytes in embryogenesis and includes nevus of Ito, nevus of Ota, and slate gray nevus

Nevus of Ito and nevus of Ota

-mostly unilateral (95%) blue-gray irregular patches
-stable over time
-nevus of Ota is in periocular location and can affect sclera (follows V1/V2 of the trigeminal nerve)
-patients with nevus of Ota have higher risk of developing glaucoma
-nevus of Ito is confined to the neck, shoulder, and proximal arm regions
-nevus of Ito and nevus of Ota can be seen in isolation or together

Slate gray nevus (Mongolian spot)

-slate gray patches usually on lower back and buttocks
-present in darker-skinned babies at birth
-normally disappears by three to five years of age

Histopathology

-**resembles** a subtle **blue nevus** but **less cellular without dermal sclerosis**
-**sparse spindle dendritic melanocytes** (easy to miss on low magnification)
-in **nevus of Ito and Ota**, cells are in the **mid dermis**
-in **slate gray nevus, cells are in the deeper dermis**

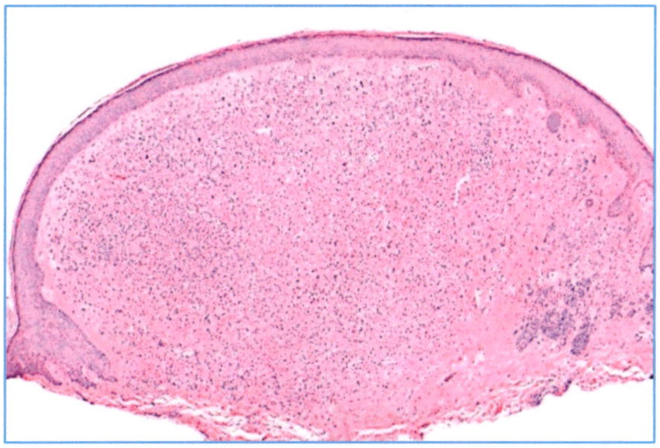

BAPoma is "dome-shaped" dermal lesion

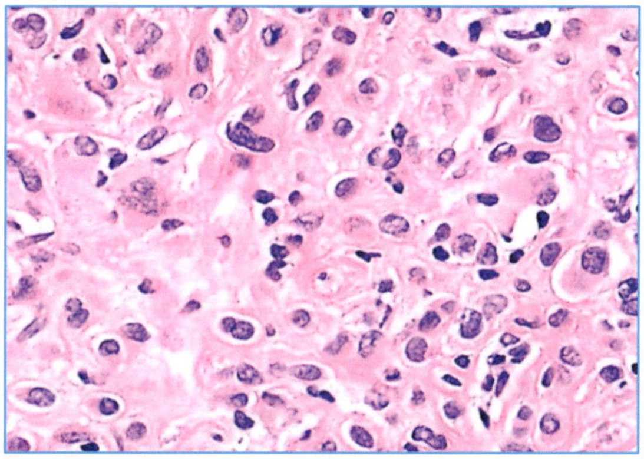

BAPoma with large epithelioid cells admixed with normal nevus cells

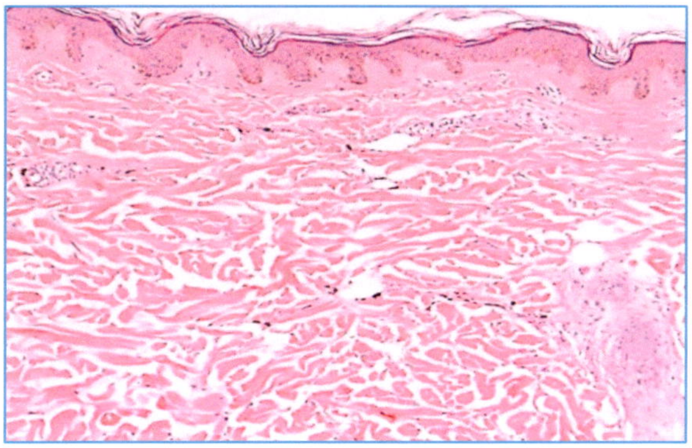

Nevus of Ito appears as normal skin at low magnification

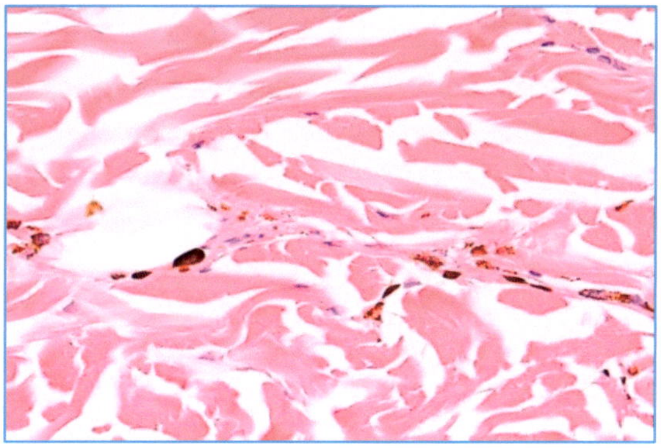

Nevus of Ito with slender pigmented melanocytes

Melanocytic tumors

DYSPLASTIC NEVUS (CLARK'S NEVUS)

-melanocytic lesion with atypical histological and clinical features present in 5% of Caucasians
-while benign, considered a risk factor for melanoma as 20% of melanomas arise in dysplastic nevi
-asymmetric, variably pigmented lesions that are often larger than ordinary nevi
-may be seen in FAMM (familial atypical mole and melanoma) syndrome (AD mutation in the *CDKN2A* gene)

Histopathology

-architectural and/or cytological atypia (dysplasia)
-lentiginous melanocytic proliferation with disarray and **fusion of junctional nests ("bridging")**
-variation in nest size and shape and extension of junctional component 3 rete ridges over the dermal component (**"shouldering")**
-melanocytes with ample gray cytoplasm
-melanocytic **nuclei are same or larger size than keratinocytes of the spinous layer**
-nuclear pleomorphism with occasional cells with hyperchromatic irregular nuclei, prominent nucleoli
-epidermal pagetoid scatter of melanocytes limited to the center of the lesion (unlike melanoma)
-fibroplasia of the papillary dermis

CLEAR CELL SARCOMA (MALIGNANT MELANOMA OF SOFT PARTS)

-rare tumor primarily affecting young adults between 20 to 40 years old
-deep subcutaneous mass on the extremities, trunk, or limb girdle
-tends to occur near tendon, fascia, or aponeuroses

Histopathology

-deep dermal and subcutaneous tumor
-can be attached to tendon
-made of uniform cells with **clear to eosinophilic cytoplasm**
-nuclei are round with vesicular chromatin and prominent nuclei
-characteristic **fibrous septae separate fascicles of tumor cells**
-melanin pigment frequently present
-tumor expresses melanocytic markers (S-100, Melan-A, HMB45, SOX10 positive)
-characteristic translocation t(12;22)(q13;q12): *ATF1-EWS* is present that is not seen in regular melanomas

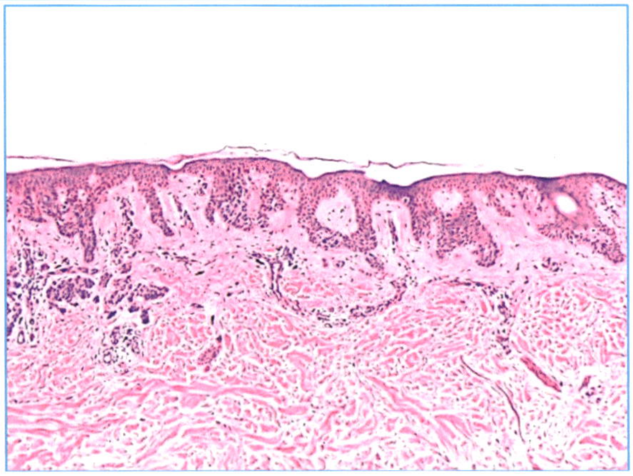

Dysplastic nevus with lateral extension of junctional melanocytes ("shouldering)

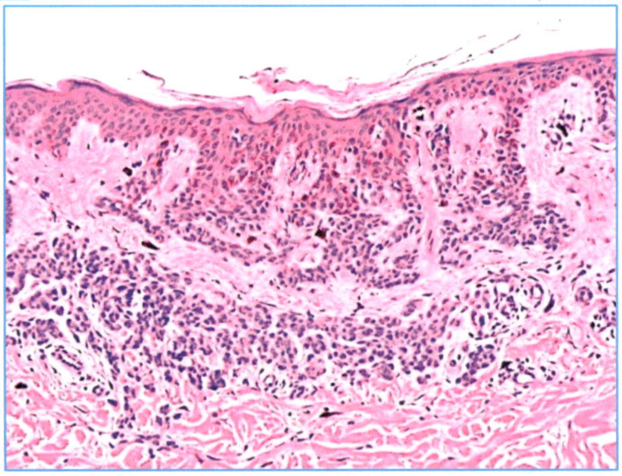

Dysplastic nevus with fusion of junctional melanocytes nests ("bridging") and dermal fibroplasia

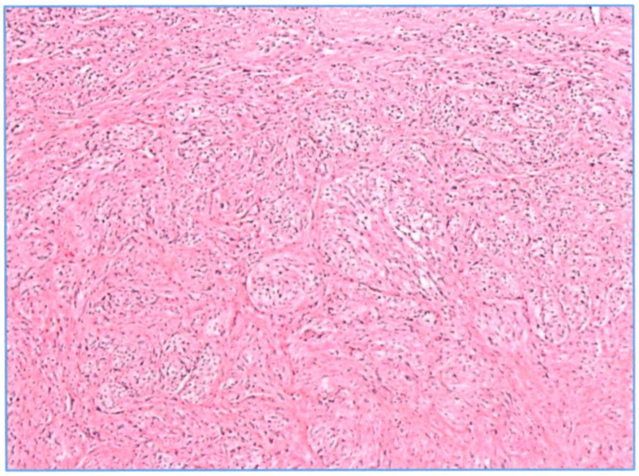

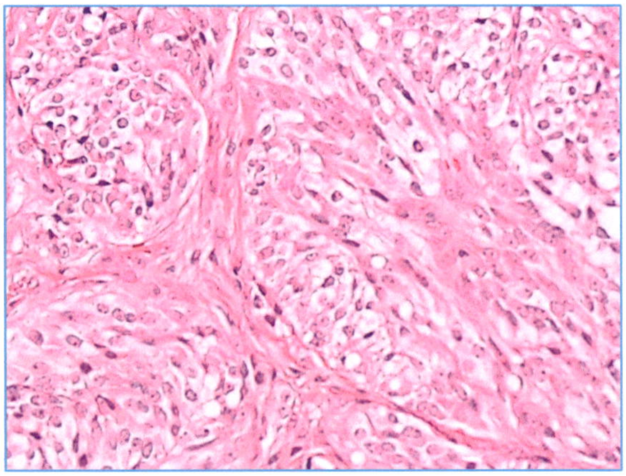

Clear cell sarcoma with cluster of clear cells separated by fibrous septae

Chapter 30

MELANOMA

Malignant tumor of melanocytes with multiple clinical presentations/subtypes:

Superficial spreading melanoma
- most common subtype
- favors the back in males and legs in females
- macule, papule, or plaque that may progress to a nodule
- classically asymmetrical shape with irregular borders and variation in color

Lentigo maligna melanoma
- classically in older patients, on sun-exposed skin
- flat macule or patch with irregular borders and shape
- variation of hues of tan brown and black

Nodular melanoma
- typically, a rapidly growing dark, brown-black nodule
- color and borders are more regular than in other types of melanoma
- commonly bleed and ulcerate

Acral lentiginous melanoma
- more common in darker skin types
- brown-black macule or patch with irregular borders and variation in color on the soles, palms, fingers, toes
- pigment involves the ridges and the furrows of skin
- can be subungual, in which case present as longitudinal melanonychia with Hutchinson's sign

Nevoid melanoma
- challenging to diagnose because it looks a lot like a benign nevus
- it can be any color, including brown, black, blue, or red and tends to be "dome-shaped"

Pigmented epithelioid melanocytoma ("animal type" melanoma)
- distinct, low-grade variant of melanoma
- all age groups, with preponderance in young adult
- "dome-shaped" irregularly pigmented dark papule
- can be associated with Carney complex

Histopathology

Superficial spreading melanoma
- proliferation of **confluent atypical melanocytes** at all levels of epidermis (**pagetoid spread**)
- cells are **single or in irregular nests**
- when limited to the epidermis term **melanoma in situ** is used
- eventually atypical melanocytes invade the dermis **(invasive melanoma)**
- level of invasion is determined by **Breslow level** (measured from epidermal granular layer to the deepest dermal melanoma cells)
- invading malignant melanocytes form confluent nests or sheets of dermal cells that **do not mature** (unlike nevus)
- scattered mitoses, dermal inflammation, and irregularly scattered melanin pigment are commonly present

Lentigo maligna melanoma
- **atrophic epidermis** with loss of rete ridges
- atypical melanocytes, mostly single or in small nests form **a confluent band, replacing basal layer keratinocytes**
- malignant melanocytes involve the follicular epithelium
- dermis shows solar elastosis, pigment incontinence, and mild chronic inflammation
- if melanoma invades the dermis it does not show maturation and tends to show spindle cell features

Nodular melanoma
- **predominantly dermal proliferation**
- dermal nodule(s) made of atypical melanocytic cells with scattered mitosis
- **no evidence of melanocytic maturation**
- pigment is unevenly distributed
- **epidermal melanoma component** is usually **limited to epidermis above dermal nodule**

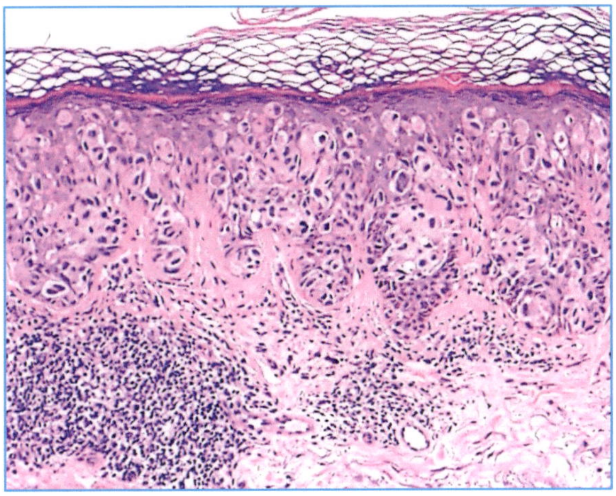

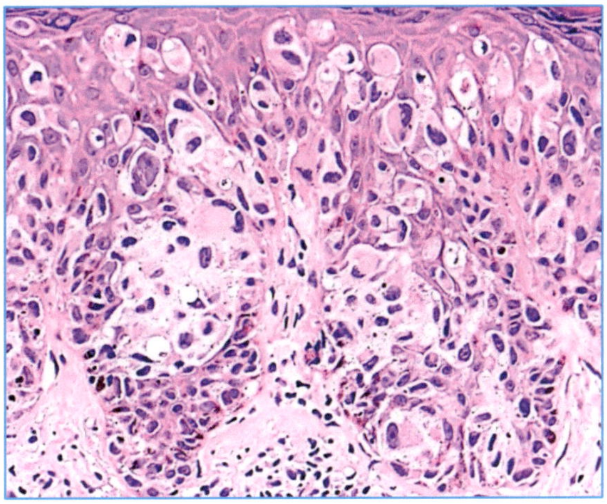

Melanoma in situ with atypical epidermal melanocytes, either single or in small irregular groups, consuming epidermis

Melanocytic tumors

Desmoplastic melanoma
-variant of nodular melanoma
-ill-defined dermal tumor **resembling a scar**
-**dermal lymphocytic aggregates** are present
-malignant **spindle-shaped melanocytes** are present in a **sclerotic stroma**
-cells are **S100 and SOX 10 positive** and **HMB-45 and Melan-A negative**
-overlying in situ melanoma is usually present

Acral lentiginous melanoma
-**hyperkeratotic acral epidermis** with **lentiginous confluent growth of atypical melanocytes**
-pagetoid appearance can be pronounced
-atypical melanocytes can be heavily pigmented
-dermal invasion of atypical epithelioid melanocytes commonly present

Nevoid melanoma
-"dome-shaped" lesion **resembling architecturally dermal nevus** (pseudomaturation of nevoid cells) on low magnification
-on higher magnification cells are atypical
-mitotic figures are found in deeper portion of the tumor
-HMB45 stains deep tumor portion confirming a lack of maturation

Pigmented epithelioid melanocytoma
-heavily-pigmented dermal tumor that extends into the subcutis in infiltrative pattern
-tumor commonly induces epidermal hyperplasia
-junctional component is usually lacking but intraepidermal melanophages are common
-tumor consists of **three kinds of cells**: **spindle,** "blue nevus-like" melanocytes, **medium size epithelioid cells that are heavily pigmented**, and **large epithelioid melanocytes that are usually less pigmented** or have "dot-like" melanin granules distributed at the periphery of the cell
-cells do not show significant atypia and mitotic activity is low

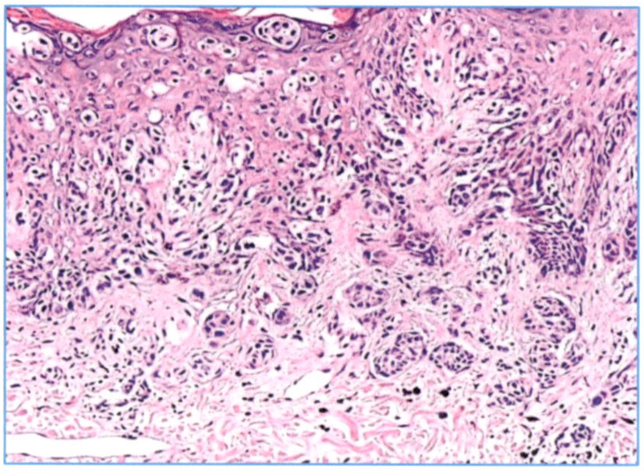

Superficial spreading melanoma invading dermis

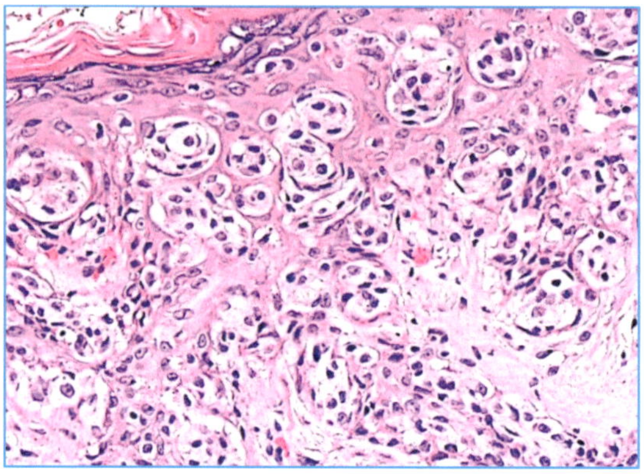

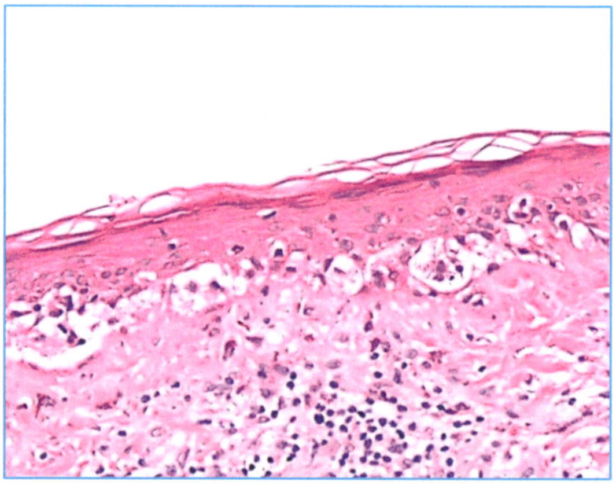

Lentigo maligna melanoma with linear band of atypical melanocytes replacing basal layer keratinocytes

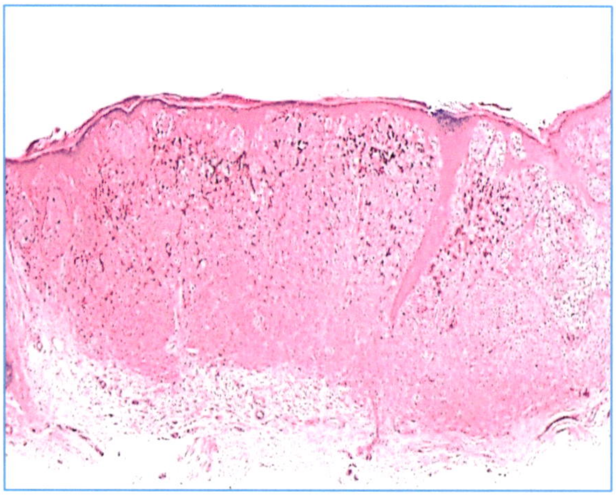

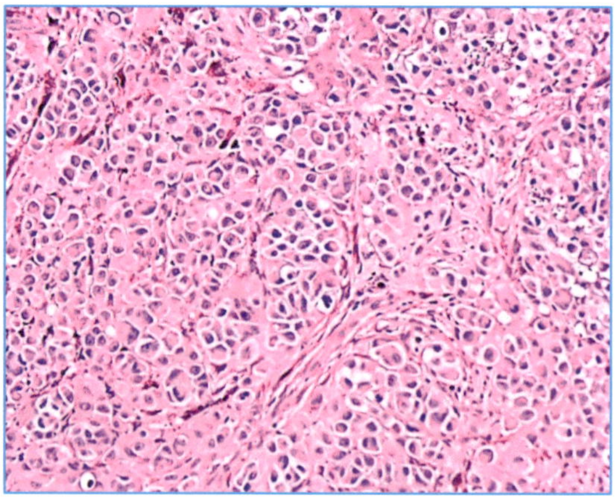

Nodular melanoma with "dome-shaped" dermal proliferation of atypical melanocytes that don't mature with descent

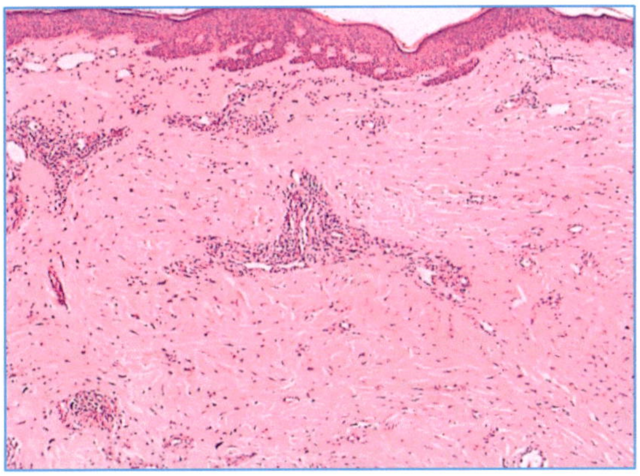

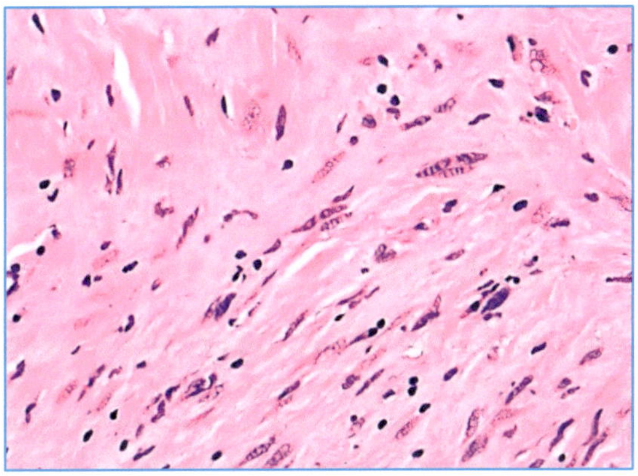

Desmoplastic melanoma with spindled malignant melanocytes in "scar-like" stroma with peripheral lymphocytic aggregates

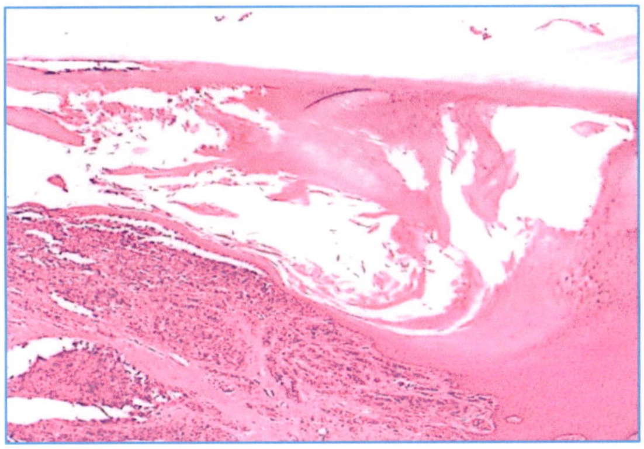

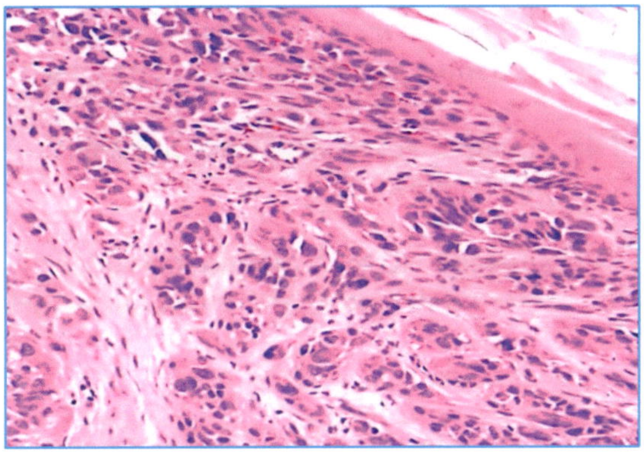

Subungual acral melanoma with non-maturing, invading, atypical melanocytes

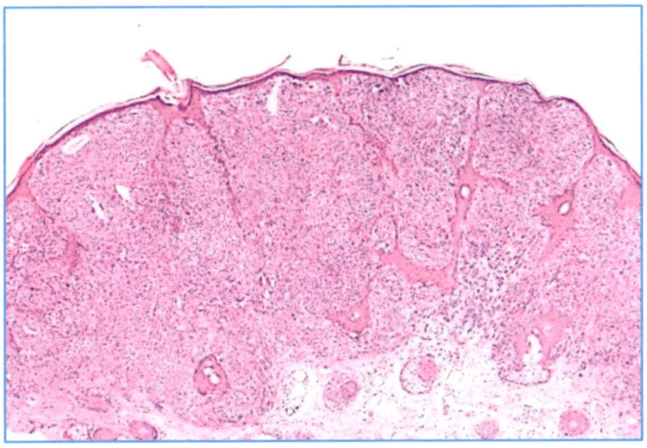

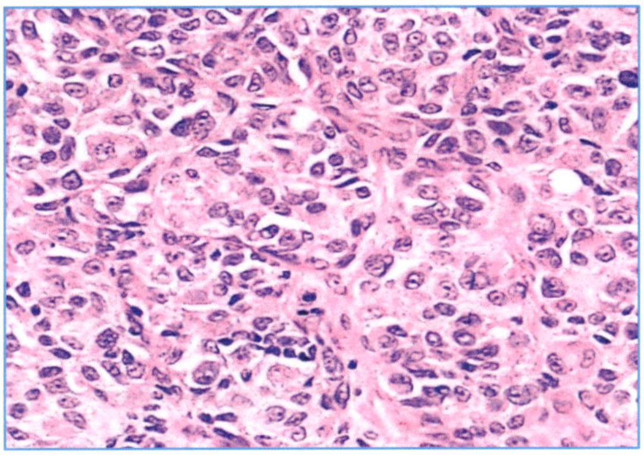

Nevoid melanoma that architecturally resemble nevus, but melanocytes are cytologically atypical

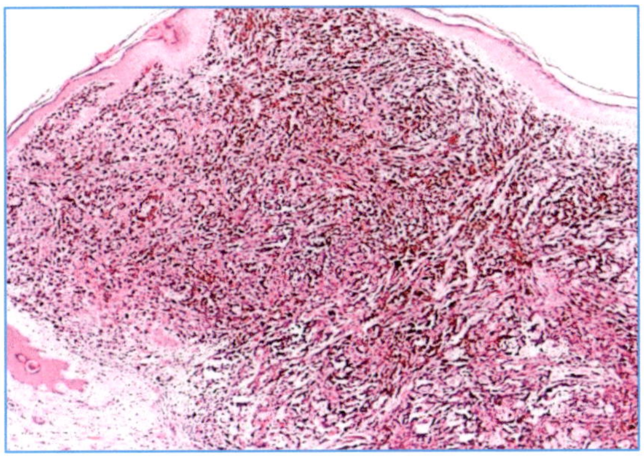

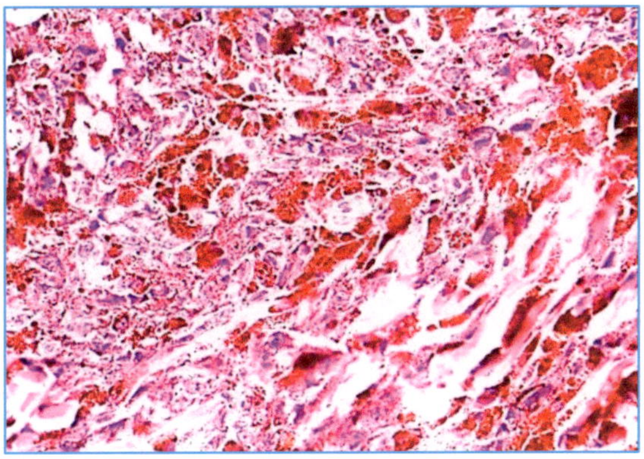

Pigmented epithelioid melanocytoma with mixture of heavily pigmented melanocytes and paler larger epithelioid melanocytes

Melanocytic tumors

HOW TO APPROACH MELANOCYTIC LESIONS

IF EPIDERMAL MELANIN IS INCREASED BUT NUMBER OF MELANOCYTES APPEARS NORMAL

-solar lentigo	"club" shaped rete ridges + increased melanin + solar elastosis
-lentigo simplex	"club" shaped rete ridges + increased melanin + no solar elastosis
-freckle	normal wavy epidermis with increased melanin
-ink spot lentigo	"solar lentigo-like" with extensive epidermal melanin

IF THERE IS EPIDERMAL AND/OR DERMAL MELANOCYTIC PROLIFERATION

DECIDE IF YOU ARE CONCERNED ABOUR MALIGNANCY BASED ON 5 QUESTIONS:

A. **Do junctional melanocytes demonstrate architectural atypia (bridging, shouldering, pagetoid spread)?**
B. **Are melanocytes cytologically irregular/atypical?**
C. **Is there any epidermal pagetoid spread of melanocytes?**
D. **Do dermal melanocytes demonstrate maturation?**
E. **Is dermal pigment unevenly distributed?**

If the answer is YES to all of these questions

-melanoma

If the answer is NO to all of these questions

-acquired or congenital nevus (junctional, dermal, compound)

If the answer to A, B, and C is YES

-melanoma in situ	epidermal melanocytes are confluent + wide pagetoid spread
-dysplastic nevus	no melanocytic confluence + pagetoid spread only in the center

If the answer to A, B, and C is YES but you are not sure

-Spitz nevus	cells are epithelioid and/or spindled and irregular but not atypical pagetoid spread only present in the center of the lesion
-nevus of Reed	cells are spindled and irregular but not atypical + prominent pigment pagetoid spread only present in the center of the lesion
-special site nevus	resembles mildly dysplastic nevus on a special site of the body

If the answer to A and B is YES and dermal scar is present

-recurrent nevus	atypia is limited to area above the scar

If the answer to D is difficult to give because of numerous dermal lymphocytes

-halo nevus

If the answer to D is maybe YES and answer to E is YES:

-inverted type A nevus	type A melanocytes/pigment underneath type B melanocytes
-deep penetrating nevus	pigmented spindle/epithelioid cells wrapping adnexa

IF DERMAL ELONGATED PIGMENTED DENDRITIC MELANOCYTES ARE PRESENT

-blue nevus	numerous pigmented spindled melanocytes in hyalinized collagen
-nevus of Ota/Ito	sparse pigmented spindled melanocytes in upper dermis
-slate gray nevus	sparse pigmented spindled melanocytes in deeper dermis

IF LESION APPEARS AS EXUBERANT BLUE NEVUS WITH "DUMBBELL" SHAPE

-cellular blue nevus	blue nevus cells admixed with epithelioid cells with less pigment

IF BLUE NEVUS IS ADMIXED WITH DERMAL OR COMPOUND NEVUS

-combined nevus

Chapter 30

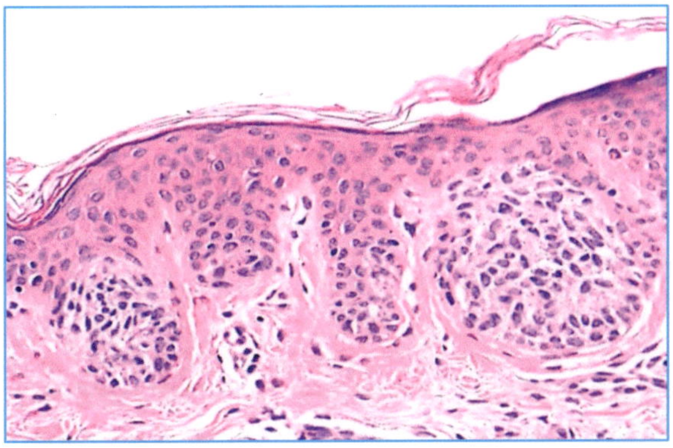

Junctional nevus with nests of melanocytes at rete ridges tips

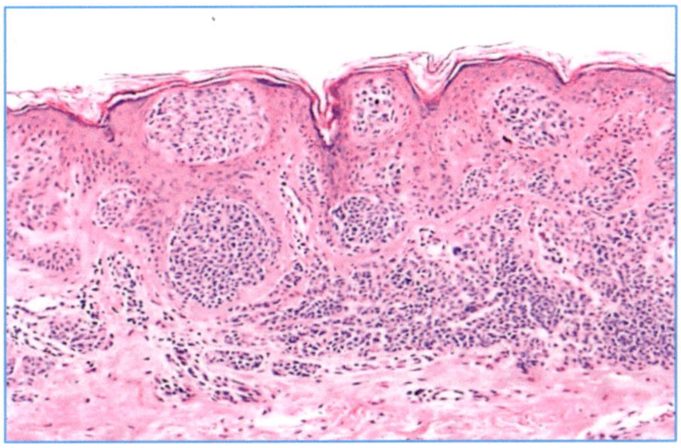

Compound nevus with junctional and dermal melanocytes

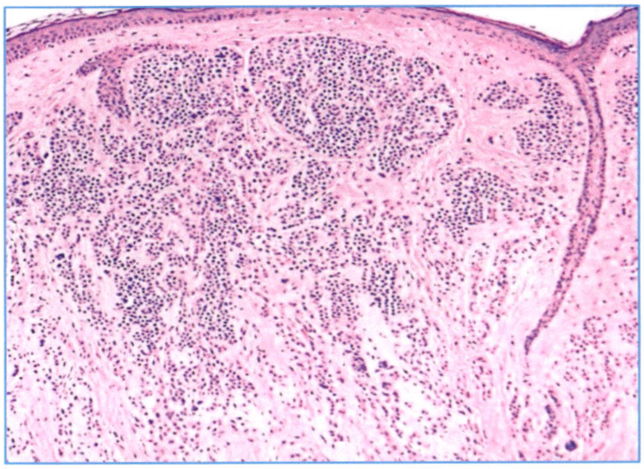

Dermal nevus with type A, B, and C maturing melanocytes

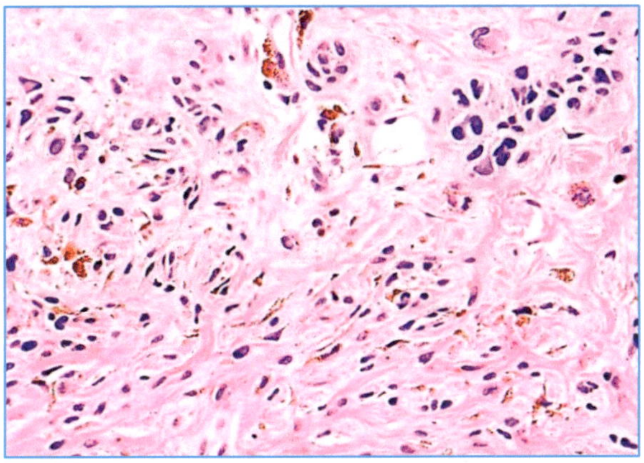

Combined nevus with dermal nevus (top) and blue nevus (bottom)

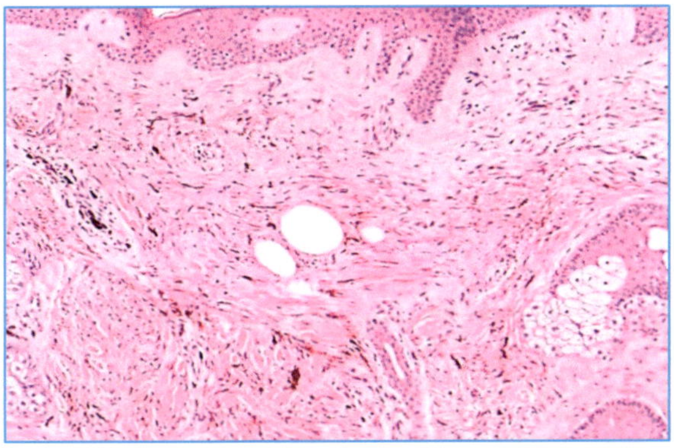

Blue nevus with pigmented spindle cells
surrounding adnexae in prominent hyalinized stroma

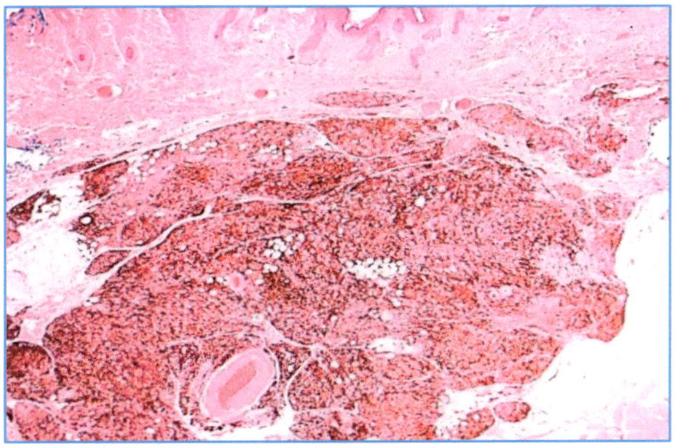

Cellular blue nevus with pigmented deep nodule made of
blue cells and pale, epithelioid, lightly pigmented nests

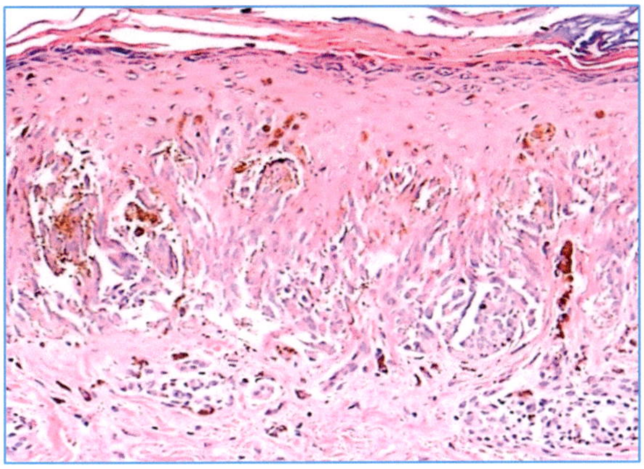

Reed nevus with junctional pigmented spindle cell nests

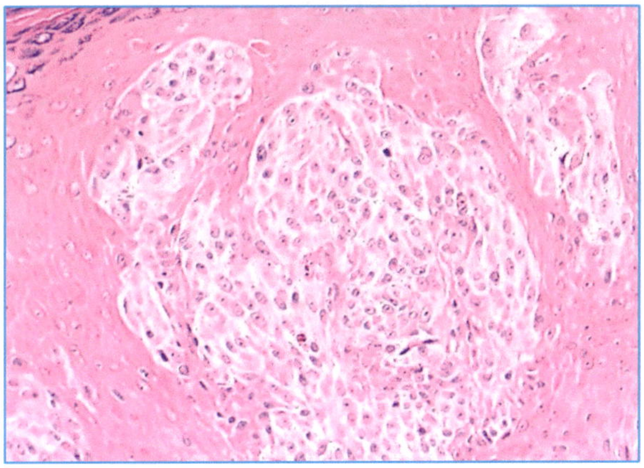

Spitz nevus with epithelioid nests and Kamino bodies

Melanocytic tumors

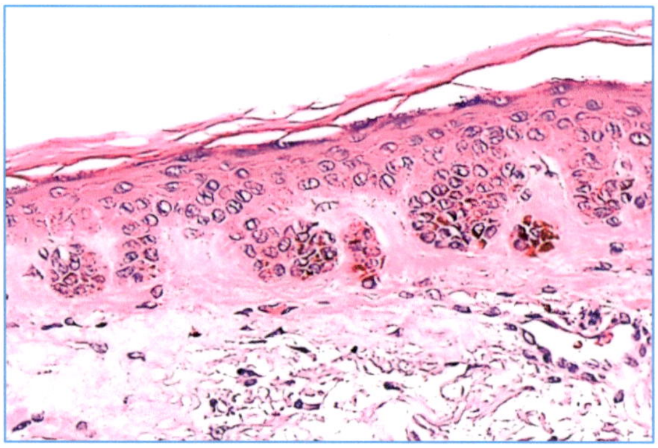

Solar lentigo with elongated rete ridges with melanin

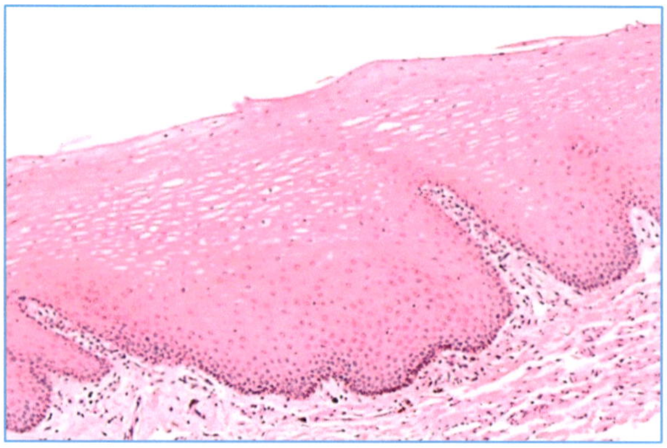

Mucosal lentigo with broad, pigmented rete ridges

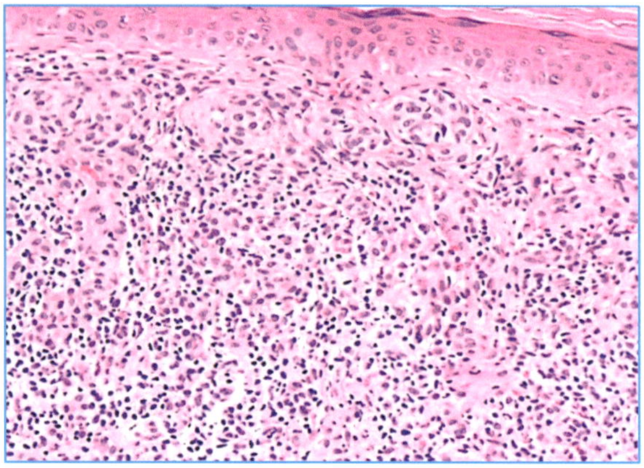

Halo nevus with dermal nevus cells hidden among lymphocytes

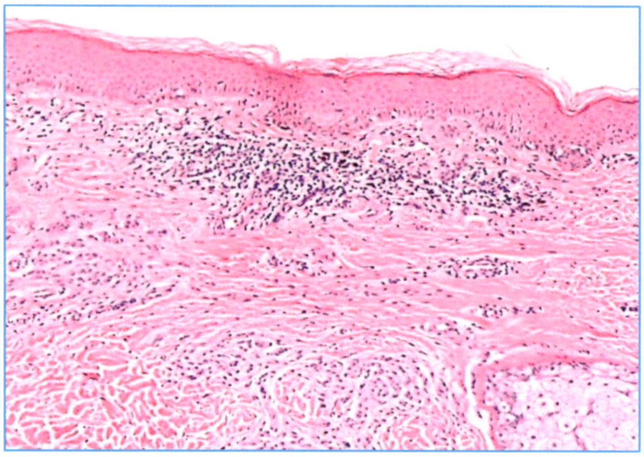

Recurrent nevus with melanocyte above and below scar

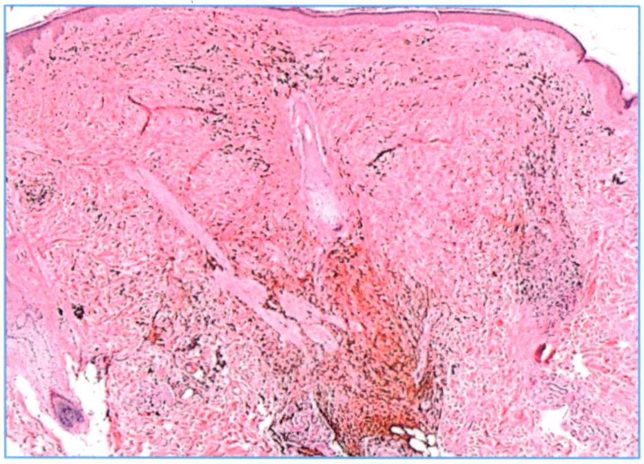

Deep penetrating nevus with
pigmented lesion following adnexal structures

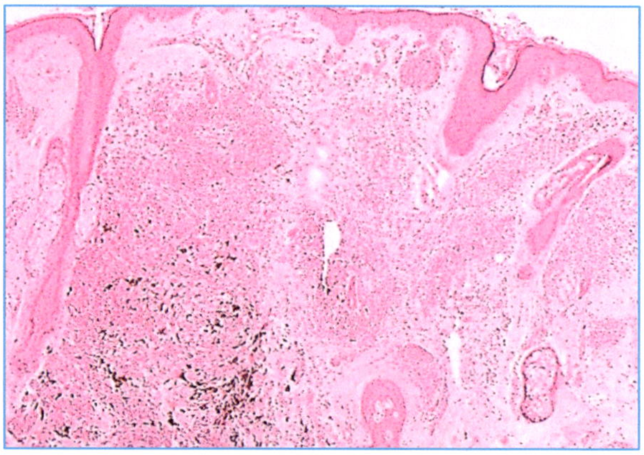

Inverted type A nevus with
deep pigmented type A nevus cells

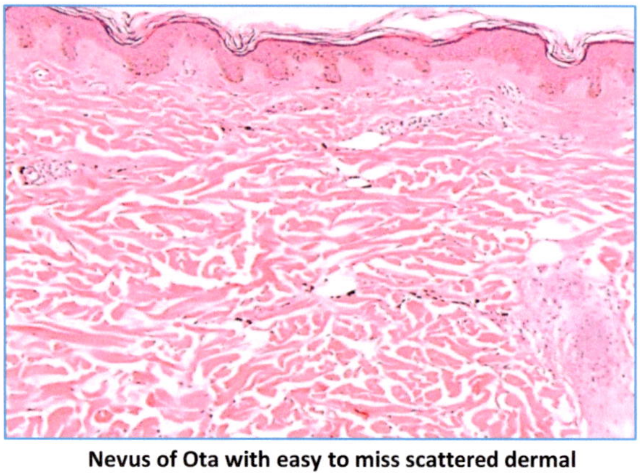

Nevus of Ota with easy to miss scattered dermal
pigmented spindle cells

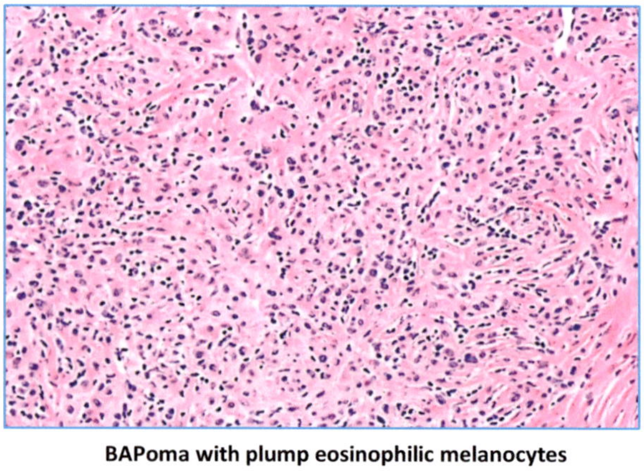

BAPoma with plump eosinophilic melanocytes
with no maturation

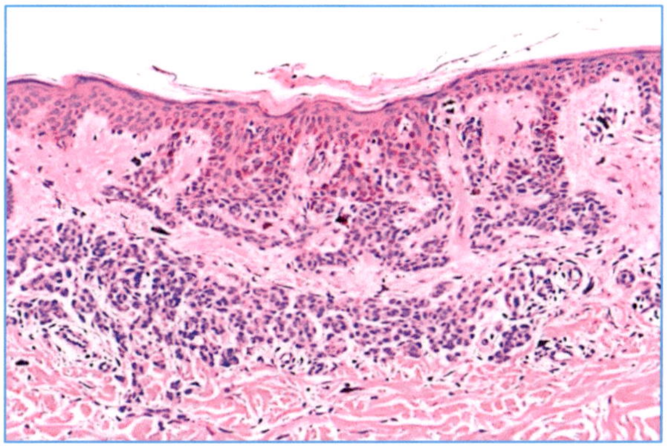

Dysplastic nevus with bridging of epidermal nests

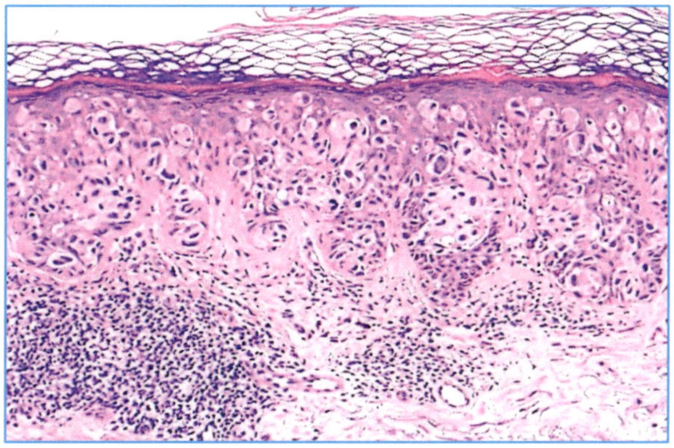

Melanoma in situ with confluent epidermal melanocytes

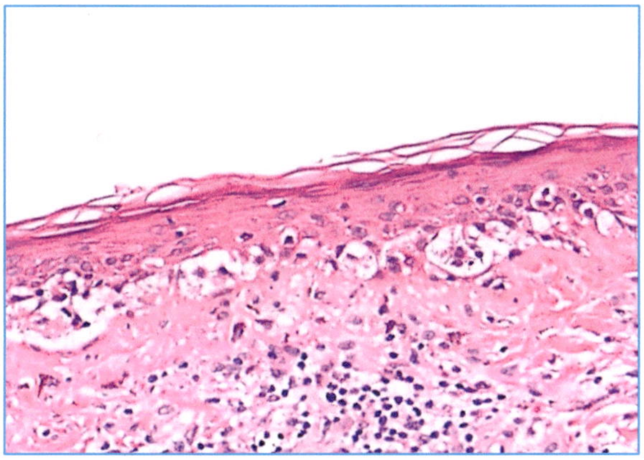

Lentigo maligna melanoma with atrophic epidermis
and epidermal line of atypical melanocytes

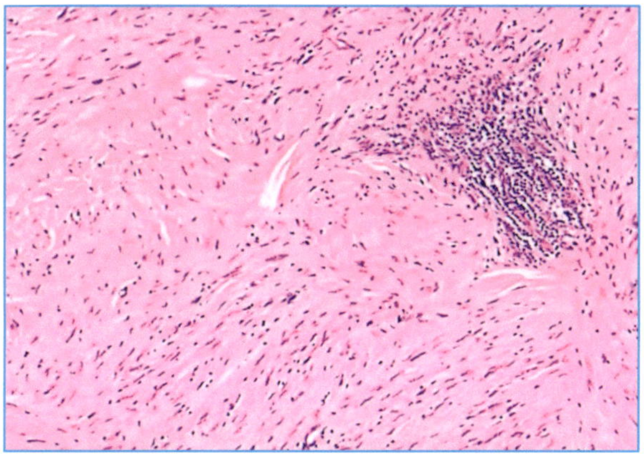

Desmoplastic melanoma with "scar-like" lesion with peripheral
lymphocytic aggregates and atypical spindle cell melanocytes

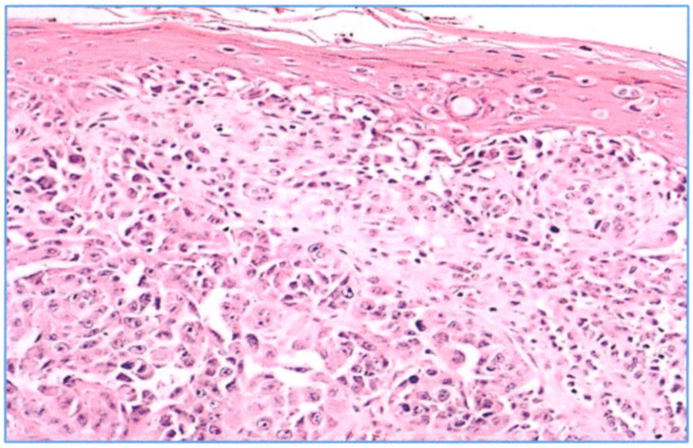

Melanoma, superficially invasive,
with confluent atypical melanocytes

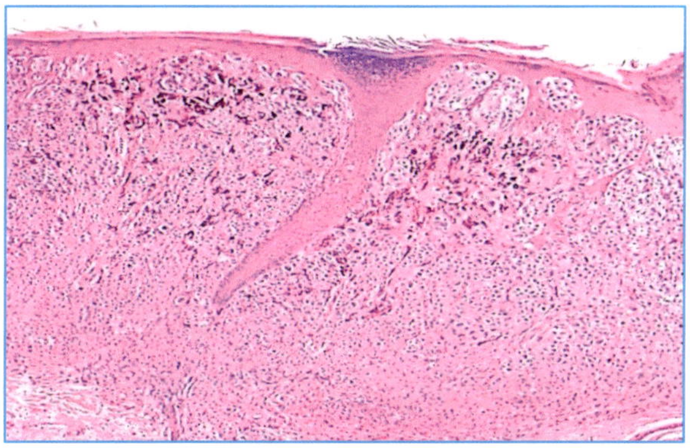

Nodular melanoma with non-maturing atypical melanocytes

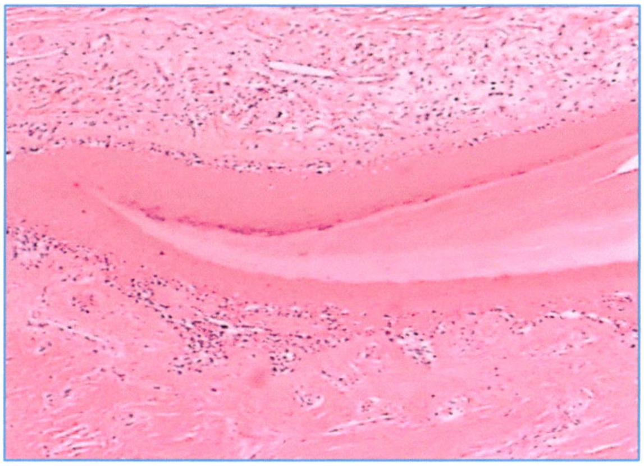

Subungual melanoma with junctional confluent melanocytes

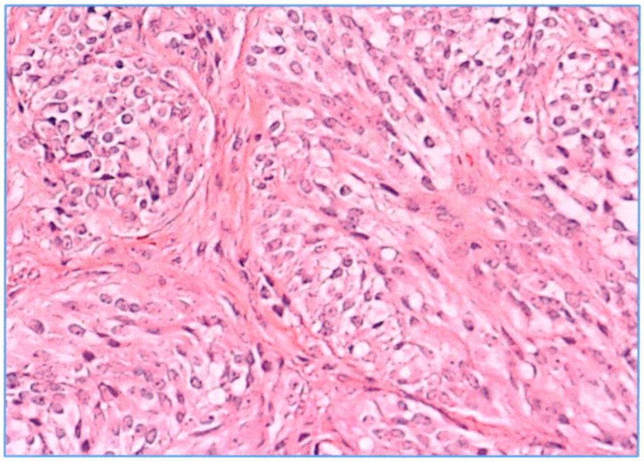

Clear cell sarcoma with clear cells separated by fibrous stroma

Melanocytic tumors

Chapter 31

FIBROUS TUMORS

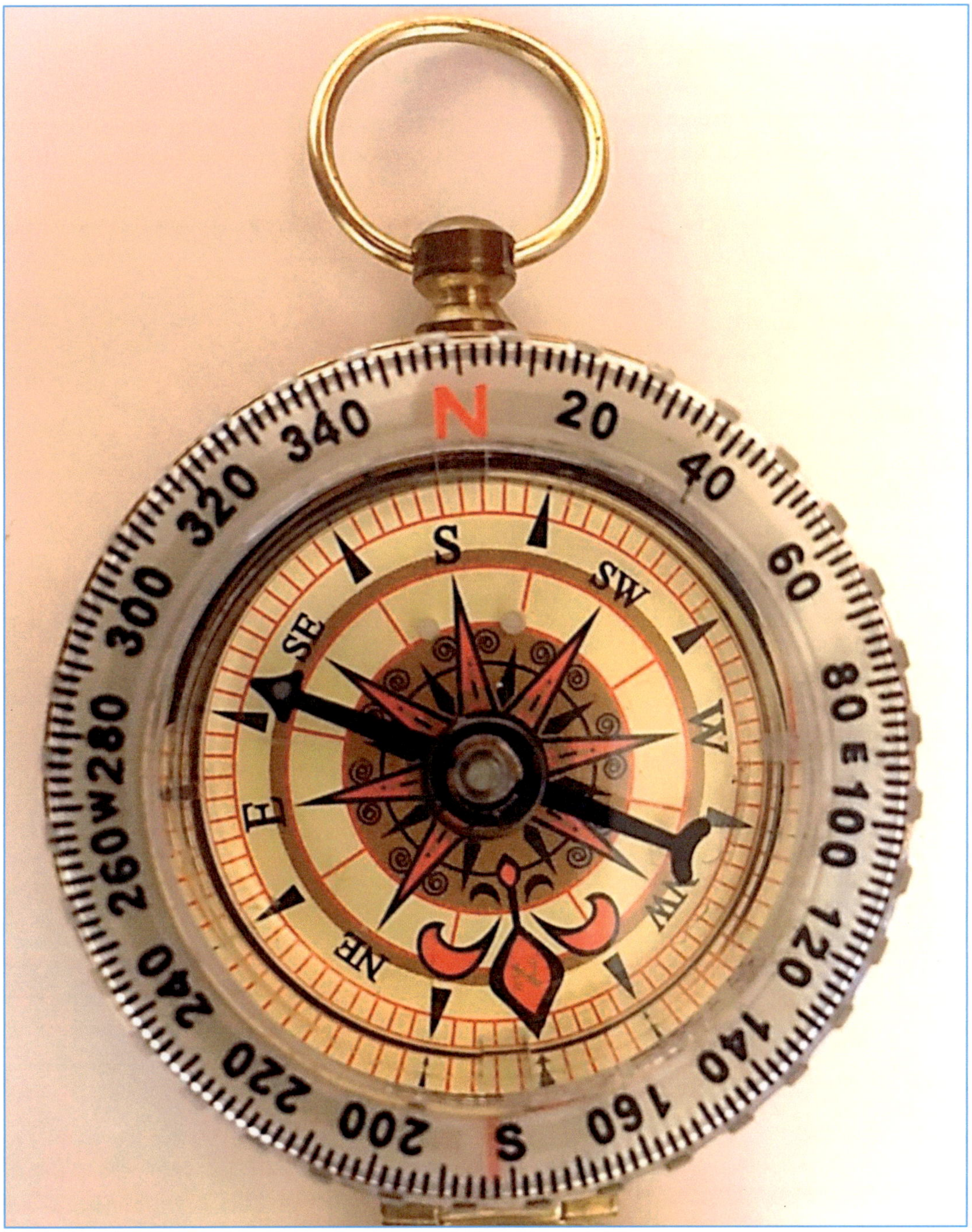

Fibrous tumors

DERMATOFIBROMA
(BENIGN FIBROUS HISTIOCYTOMA)

-"dome-shaped" pink to brown papule or nodule
-usually darker in the center
-slow growing and painless
-lateral compression produces depression, known as "dimple sign"
-favors the lower leg
-more common in younger and middle-aged women

Cellular dermatofibroma

-typically, a nodule on the cheeks of younger adults

Histopathology

-epidermis is acanthotic, with irregular papillomatosis and hyperpigmentation of basal layer **("dirty socks")**
-proliferation of **dermal, spindle to oval fibroblasts and round to oval histiocytic cells**
-scattered **Touton giant cells** (giant cells with **"wreath-like"** nuclei)
-stroma appears hyalinized with prominent **collagen trapping**

Variants

Cellular dermatofibroma

-deeper and more cellular lesion
-cells are rounder (epithelioid) and occasional mitoses can be seen
-more likely to recure after incomplete excision

Aneurysmal dermatofibroma

-cellular lesion; abundant hemosiderin and RBCs

Clear cell (lipidized) dermatofibroma

-many clear, foamy cells in the background of ordinary dermatofibroma

Epithelioid cell histiocytoma

-characteristic **epidermal collarette**
-tumor cells have **abundant eosinophilic cytoplasm** with vesicular nuclei and prominent nucleoli
-only variant with **ALK1 positive cells**
-frequent inflammatory infiltrate

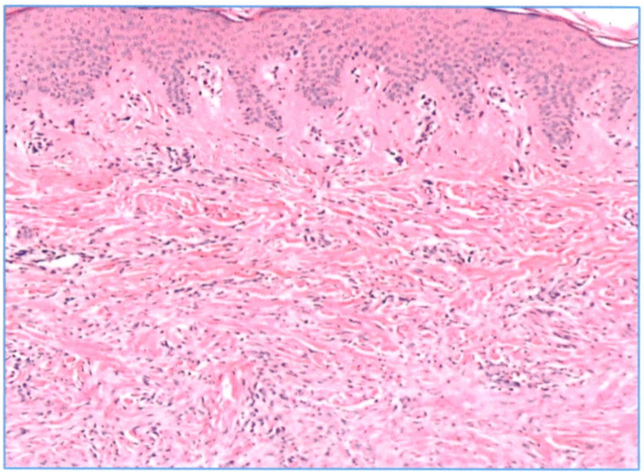

DF with fibrohistiocytic cells and trapped hyalinized collagen

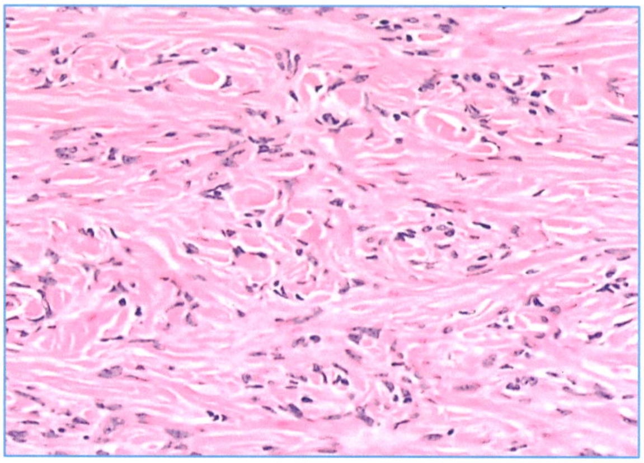

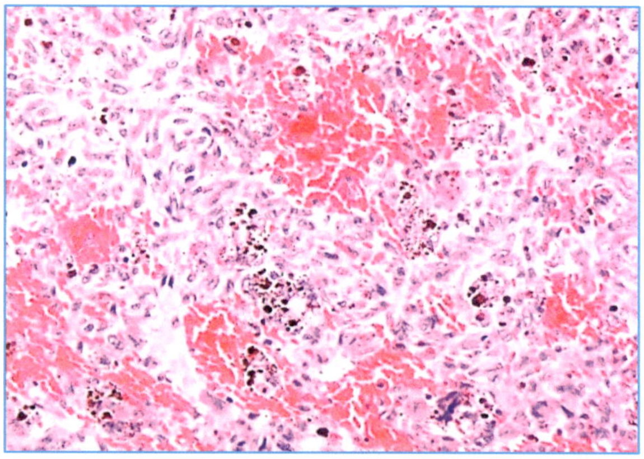

Aneurysmal DF with RBCs and hemosiderin

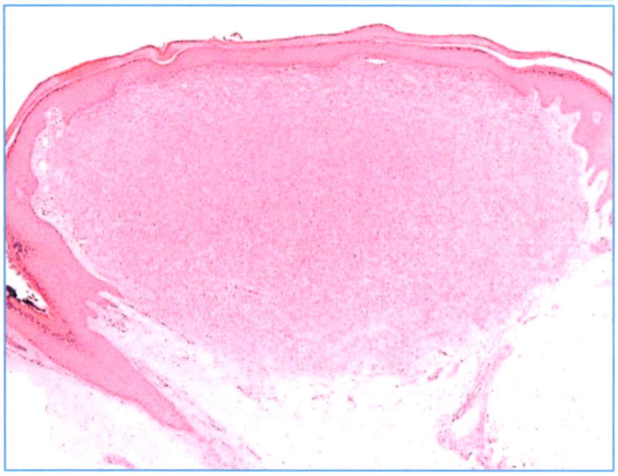

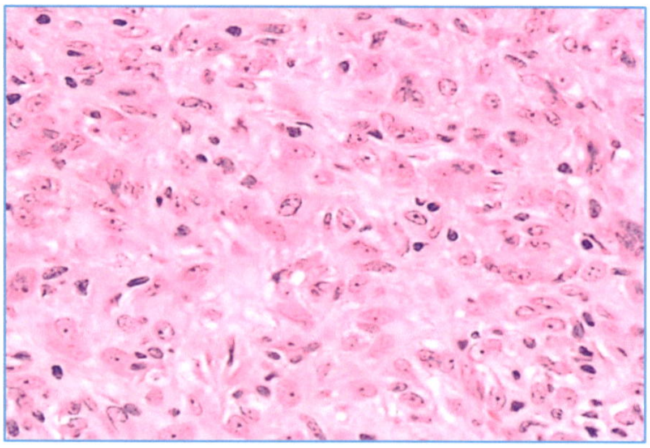

Epithelioid cell histiocytoma with characteristic collarette and rounded epithelioid cells

DERMATOMYOFIBROMA

-firm red-brown plaque, or less frequently nodule, resembling a large DF
-favors the upper trunk, upper arms, axillae, or neck
-more common in young adults with female predominance

Histopathology
-dermal spindle cell proliferation
-uniform cells are predominantly **oriented parallel to surface, "plaque-like"**
-cells have **myoid appearance** (spindled cells with **eosinophilic cytoplasm and more blunt ends**)
-no extension into subcutis
-no cytological atypia or mitoses
-tumor cells are SMA positive and factor XIII and CD34 negative

MYOFIBROMA

Two clinical variants
Infantile form
-the most common fibrous tumor of infancy (60% are congenital)
-most commonly presents as multiple purple nodules
-favors the head and is more common in females
-can involve internal organs and bones
Adult form
-presents as solitary nodule with purple color resembling vascular neoplasm
-more common on head and neck
-is benign and does not involve internal organs

Histopathology
-circumscribed deep dermal/subcutaneous nodule
-tumor appears **biphasic**
-parts have **myxoid or hyalinized stroma** with admixed **spindle cells with short plump nuclei** and overall **chondroid or chondromyxoid appearance**
-other parts are more **cellular with more round or polygonal cells around branching vessels** with "**hemangiopericytoma-like**" appearance
-areas of calcification can often be seen
-tumor cells are **SMA positive**

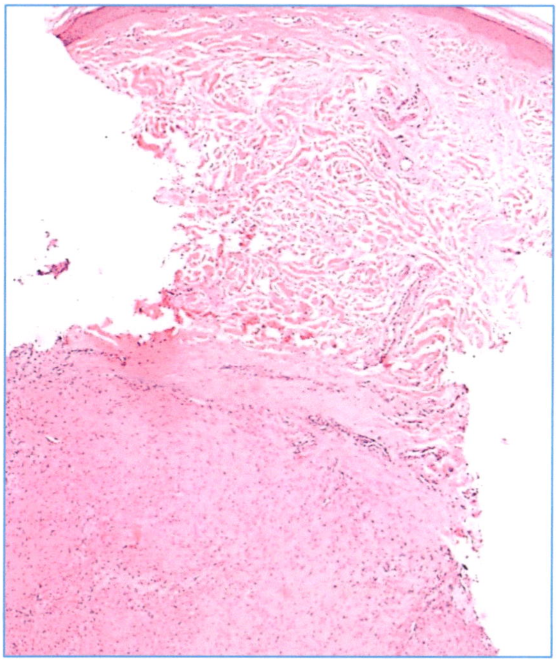
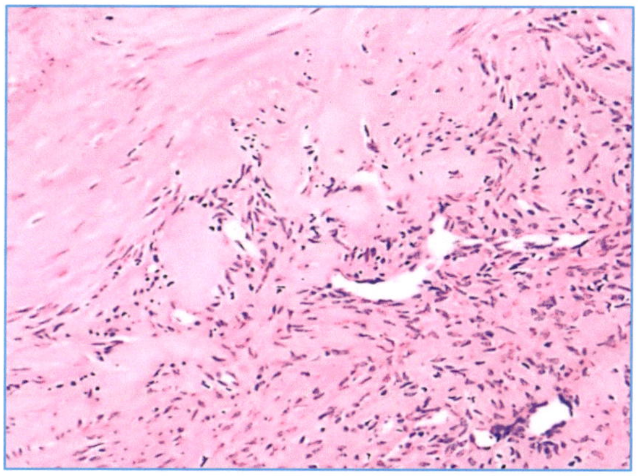

Myofibroma is biphasic subcutaneous tumor made of "cartilage-like" cell poor areas and cell rich, "hemangiopericytoma-like areas"

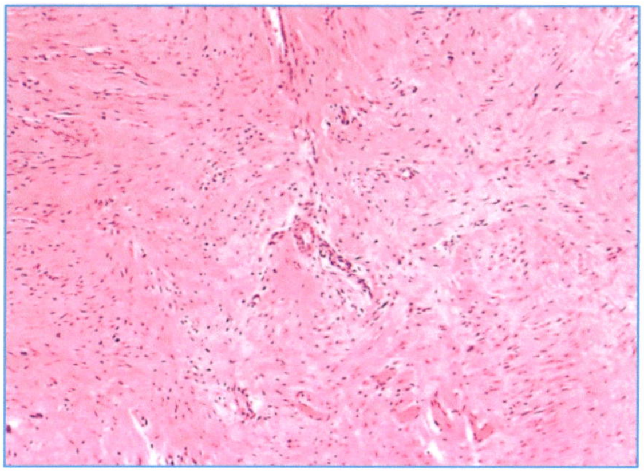
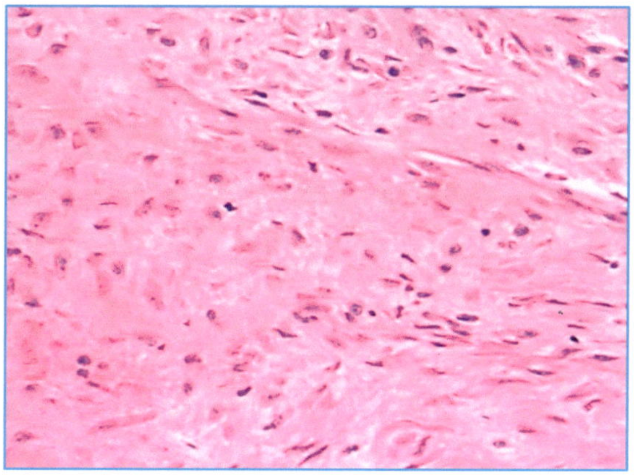

Dermatomyofibroma with "muscle-like" appearance of eosinophilic spindled cells with blunt ends

Fibrous tumors

MYXOMA (SUPERFICIAL ANGIOMYXOMA)

-solitary or multiple flesh-colored nodules on the face, trunk, or extremities
-may occur as the first sign of Carney complex

Histopathology
-vaguely circumscribed, dermal, nodular or multilobulated tumor
-**mucinous stroma** with **stellate or spindled fibroblasts**
-there is **often a proliferation of blood vessels** (hence the term superficial angiomyxoma)

SUPERFICIAL ACRAL FIBROMYXOMA

-presents as a slow-growing, solitary, fleshy tumor
-favors the hands and feet, with a predilection for the periungual region of fingers and toes
-mostly asymptomatic, but may be uncomfortable with pressure or occasionally painful
-more common in males

Histopathology
-non-encapsulated dermal tumor
-Grenz zone often separates the epidermis and the tumor
-tumor is composed of **stellate and spindled fibroblastic cells in** a random pattern in a **myxoid or myxoid/collagenous matrix (fibromyxoid stroma)**
-mast cells are common
-spindle cells are **CD34 and CD99 positive**

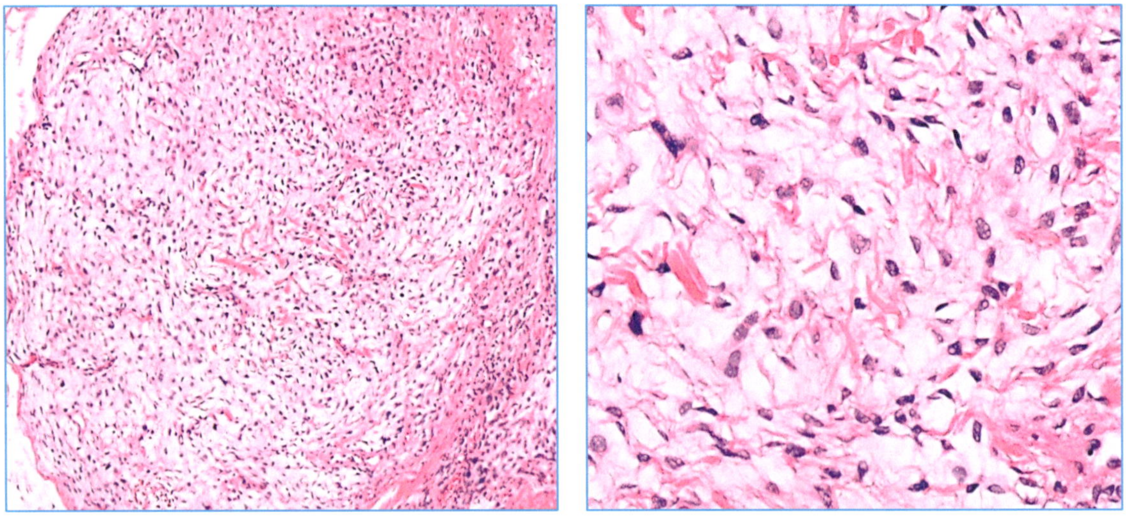

Myxoma with stellate fibroblasts in myxoid stroma and an increased number of capillaries

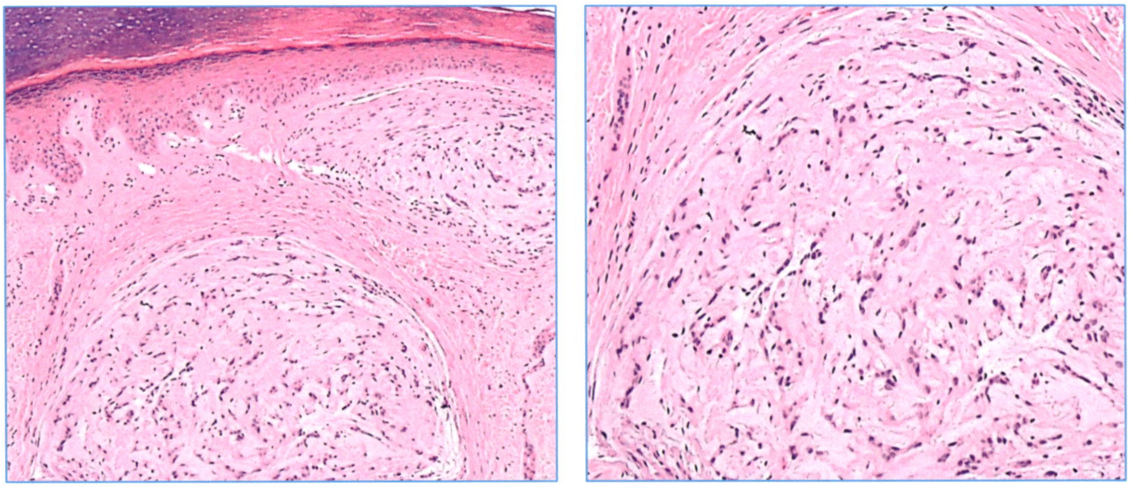

Superficial acral fibromyxoma with spindled fibroblasts in fibromyxoid stroma

PLEOMORPHIC FIBROMA

-skin-colored, polypoid, slow growing lesion
-usually occurs in middle aged adults

Histopathology
-polypoid, "**skin tag-like" lesion**
-**fibrotic stroma**
-enlarged, multinucleated cells with bizarre, smudged, hyperchromatic nuclei, so called **"floret giant cells"**
-cells are **CD34 positive**
-no mitoses

SCLEROTIC FIBROMA (CIRCUMSCRIBED STORIFORM COLLAGENOMA)

-solitary, skin-colored, dermal nodule
-favors the head, neck, and upper extremities
-generally seen in adults
-associated with Cowden syndrome

Histopathology
-well-circumscribed, non-encapsulated dermal nodule
-**hypocellular hyalinized collagen** bundles in storiform pattern
-"**cleft-like" spaces** in between collagen bundles giving a "**woodgrain" appearance**
-tumor cells are **CD34 positive**

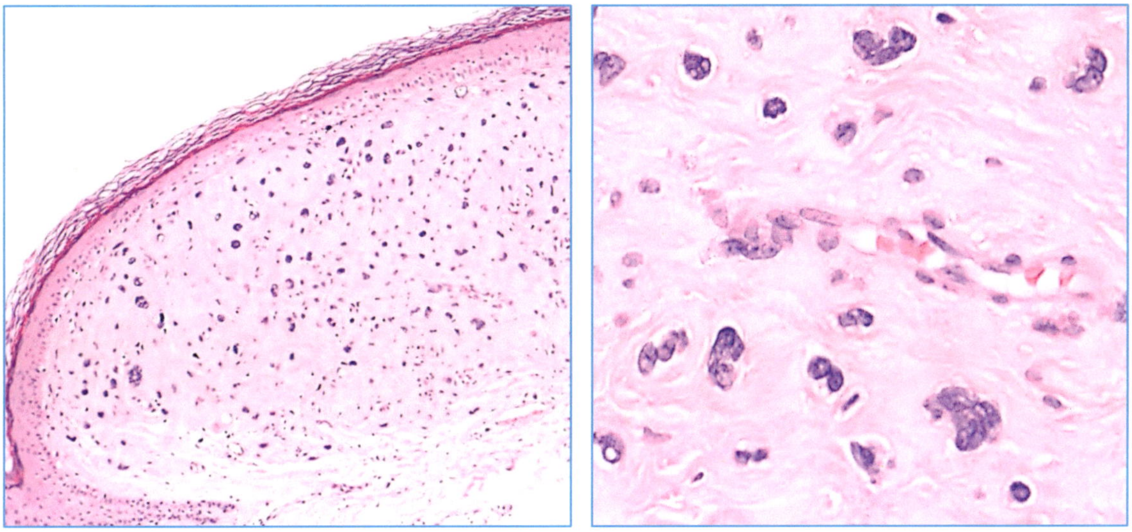

Pleomorphic fibroma appears as "skin tag-like" lesion with "floret giant cells" in fibrotic stroma

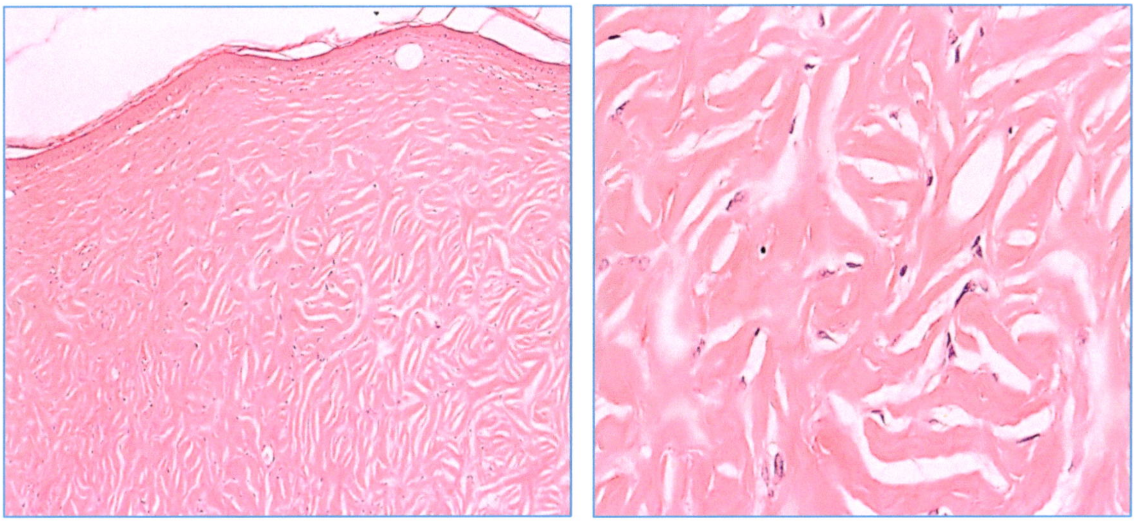

Sclerotic fibroma with hyalinized collagen with a "woodgrain" appearance

Fibrous tumors

ANGIOFIBROMA
(ADENOMA SEBACEUM, FIBROUS PAPULE OF NOSE, PEARLY PENILE PAPULE)

-various clinical presentations:

Fibrous papule of nose

-solitary, small papule on the nose

Pearly penile papule

-small papules on the coronal margin and sulcus of the penis

Adenoma sebaceum

-multiple papules and nodules in mid face, particularly the nasolabial fold

-multiple angiofibromas are associated with tuberous sclerosis, MEN1, and NF2

Histopathology

-"**dome-shaped"** dermal lesion

-**dilated thin dermal vessels**

-spindled and **irregular stellate fibroblasts**

-multinucleated fibroblast can be present

-**dense collagenous stroma**

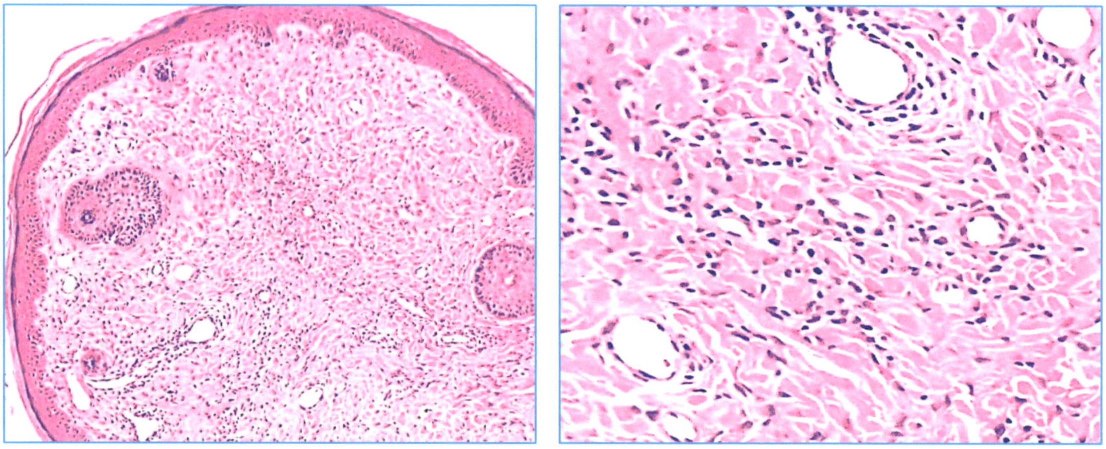

Angiofibroma is a "dome-shaped" lesion with an increased number of dilated capillaries

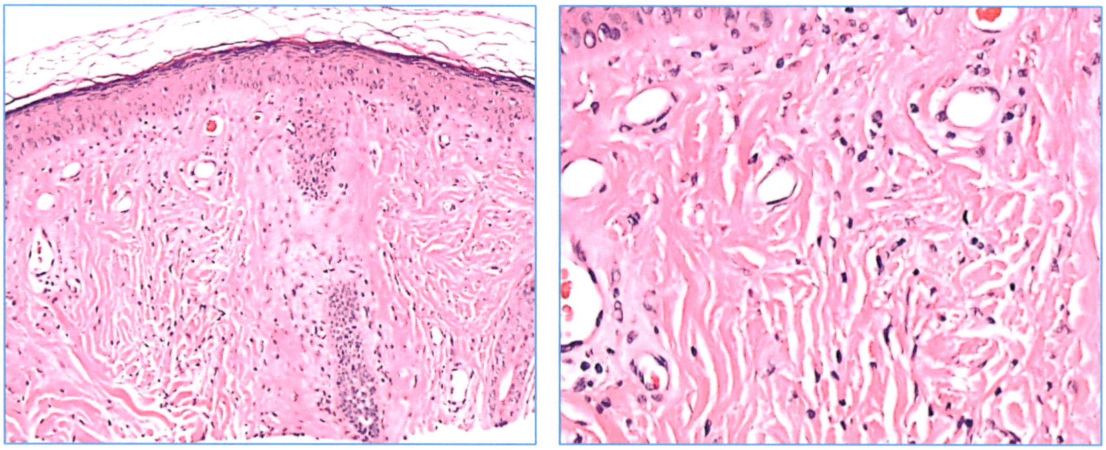

Angiofibroma with fibrotic stroma and scattered irregular stellate fibroblasts

Chapter 31

DIGITAL FIBROMAS:
ACRAL FIBROKERATOMA (ACQUIRED DIGITAL FIBROKERATOMA), PERIUNGUAL FIBROMA, CELLULAR DIGITAL FIBROMA

Acral fibrokeratoma and cellular digital fibroma
-present as solitary, painless, skin-colored, small, "horn-like" nodule in an adult located on the fingers, toes, palms, or feet

Periungual fibroma (Koenen tumor)
-pink nodules arising from the nail fold
-associated with tuberous sclerosis

Cellular digital fibroma
-present as small, skin-colored papule on the fingers or toes

Histopathology

Acral fibrokeratoma
-polypoid lesion with hyperkeratotic, acanthotic epidermis (acral skin)
-lesion is **hypocellular** with **thickened collagen** bundles
-superficial **capillaries** can be **dilated**

Periungual fibroma
-similar to acral fibrokeratoma but may have multinucleated giant cells and stellate, "ganglion-like" cells

Cellular digital fibroma
-dense cellular proliferation of uniform **CD34 positive**, **CD99 negative** cells in a **myxoid background**

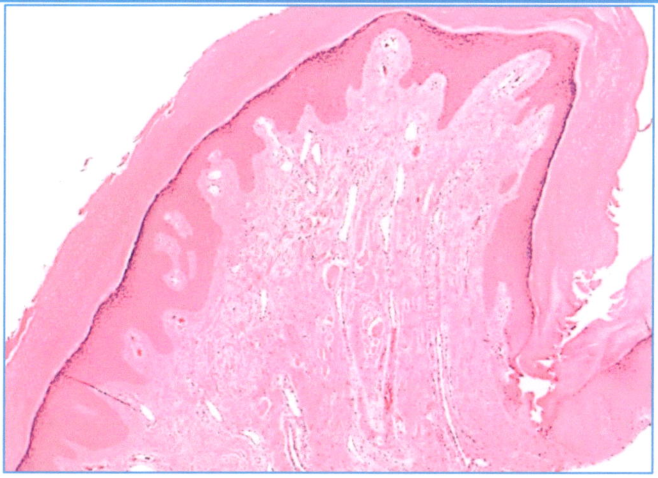

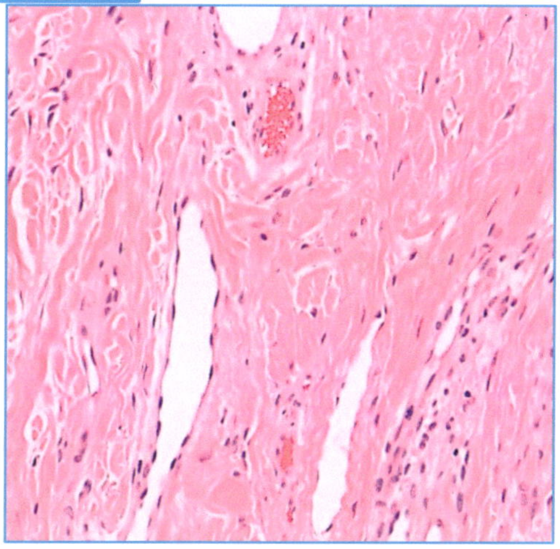

Acral fibrokeratoma is a polypoid lesion with dense fibrotic stroma with dilated capillaries and only scattered fibroblasts

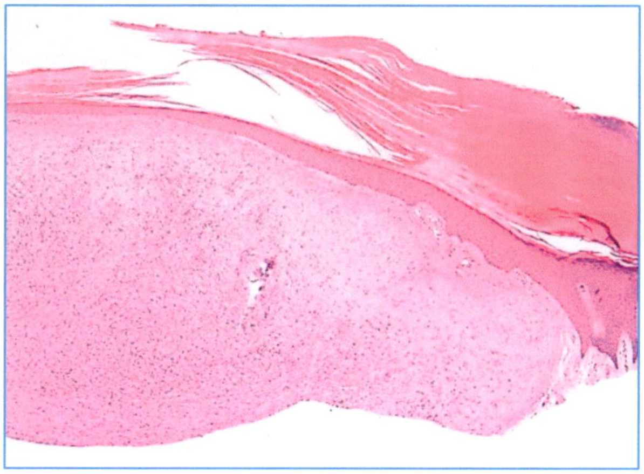

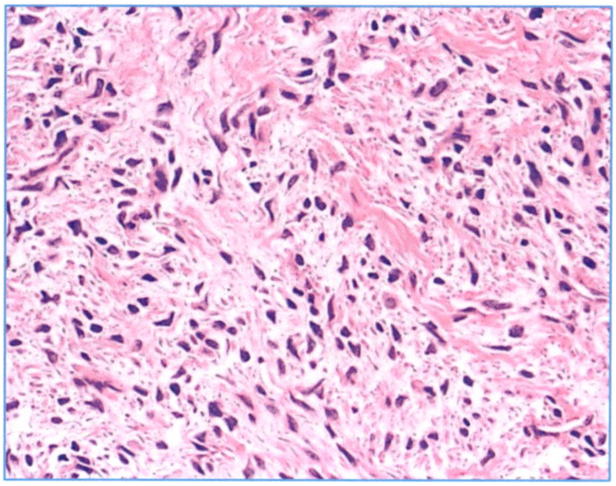

Cellular digital fibroma with uniform cells in myxoid stroma

Fibrous tumors

CALCIFYING APONEUROTIC FIBROMA

-benign calcifying fibrous tumor
-presents as slowly growing subcutaneous nodule
-favors hands and feet with male predominance
-most tumors occur in the first decade of life
-tumor is often closely related to aponeuroses, tendons, or fascia

Histopathology
-infiltrative fibrous growth that extends into surrounding tissue
-**plump fibroblasts** with round or ovoid nuclei within a **dense collagenous stroma**
-central **foci of calcification** surrounded by **"chondrocyte-like" cells**

FIBRO-OSSEOUS PSEUDOTUMOR OF THE DIGITS

-rare benign tumor
-favors proximal phalange of fingers
-presents as rapidly growing digital nodule that is slightly mobile
-can occur at any age but has predisposition for young adult women

Histopathology
-ill-defined dermal/subcutaneous tumor
-proliferation of **spindle shaped myofibroblasts** (calponin and SMA positive) in myxoid stroma
-large deposits of **pinked osteoid** rimmed by **uniform osteoblasts**
-mitotic figures and giant cells can be present

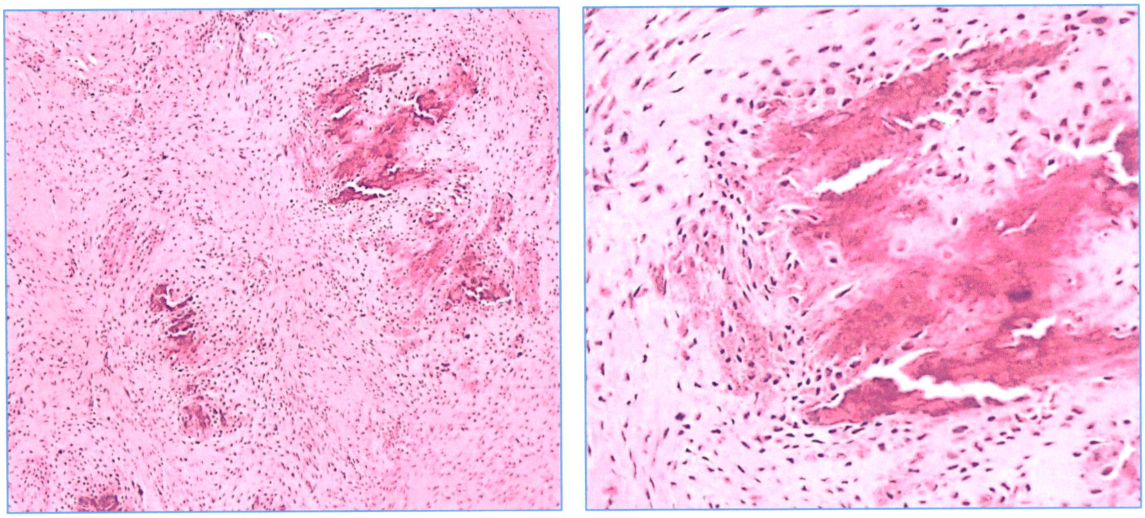

Calcifying aponeurotic fibroma with scattered foci of calcification in dense stroma with plump fibroblasts

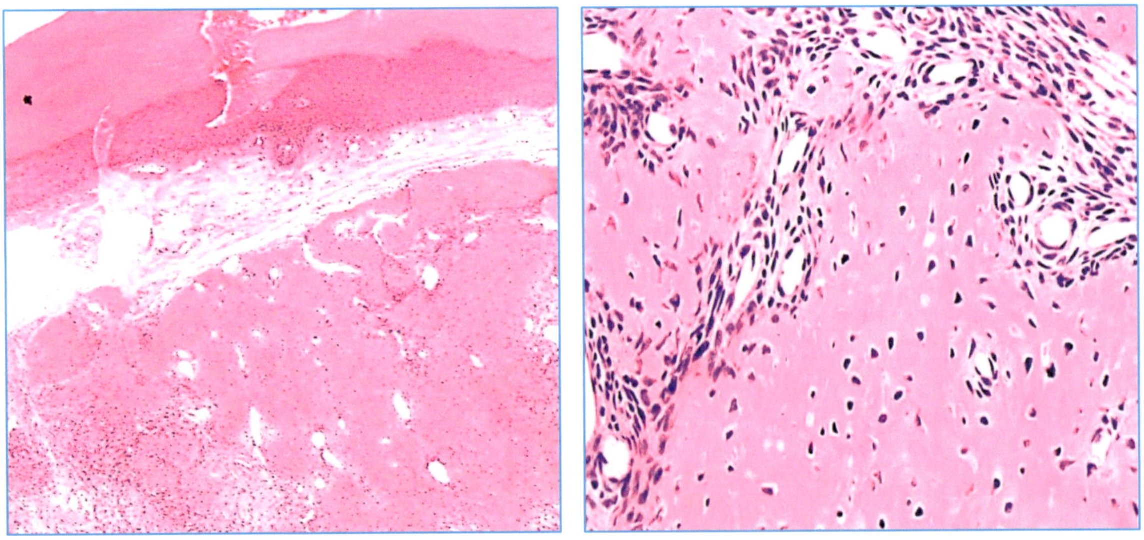

Fibro-osseous pseudotumor of the digits with pink osteoid rimmed with myofibroblasts and osteoblasts

FIBROUS HAMARTOMA OF INFANCY

-rapidly growing, painless, ill-defined subcutaneous or intradermal nodule
-mostly solitary and rarely multiple lesions
-mostly occurs in children younger than 2 years of age (20% are congenital)
-favors axillae and upper part of extremities

Histopathology
-poorly defined subcutaneous lesion
-characteristic triphasic morphology:
-fibroblastic fascicles
-mature adipose tissue
-primitive myxoid mesenchyme

INFANTILE DIGITAL FIBROMATOSIS (INCLUSION BODY FIBROMATOSIS)

-single or multiple subcutaneous nodule on the dorsal and lateral aspects of the fingers or toes
-nodules are pinkish, gelatinous or firm
-occur in infants less than 1 year of age (30% are congenital)

Histopathology
-uniform dermal and subcutaneous myofibroblastic proliferation
-interlaced "spindle-shaped" cells and collagen fibers
-characteristic **pink-red, globular cytoplasmic inclusions** that at first glance **resemble RBCs**
-inclusions are SMA, calponin, desmin positive

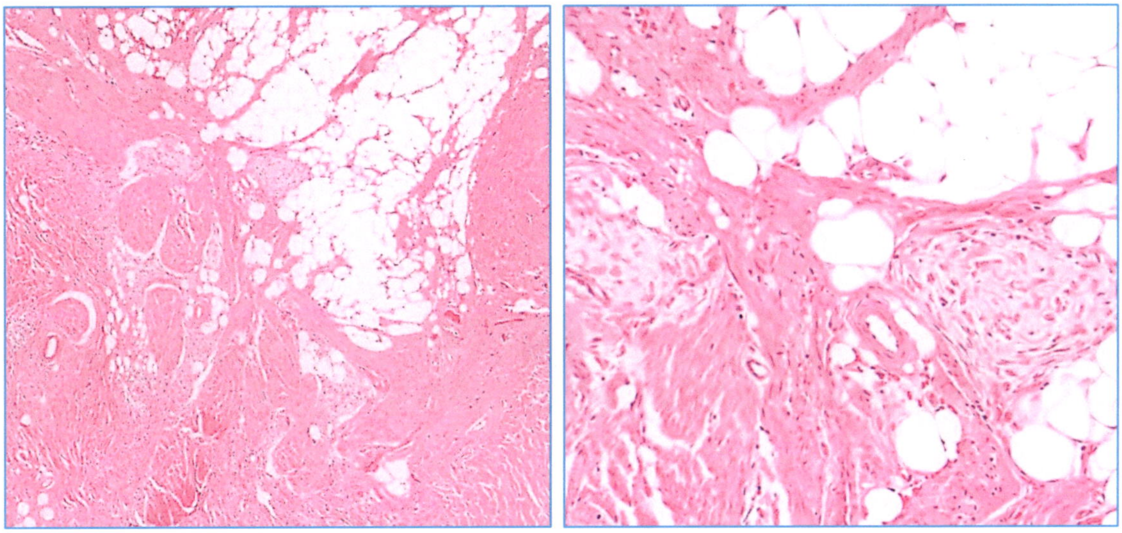

Fibrous hamartoma of infancy composed of adipocytes, myxoid mesenchyme, and fibroblastic fascicles

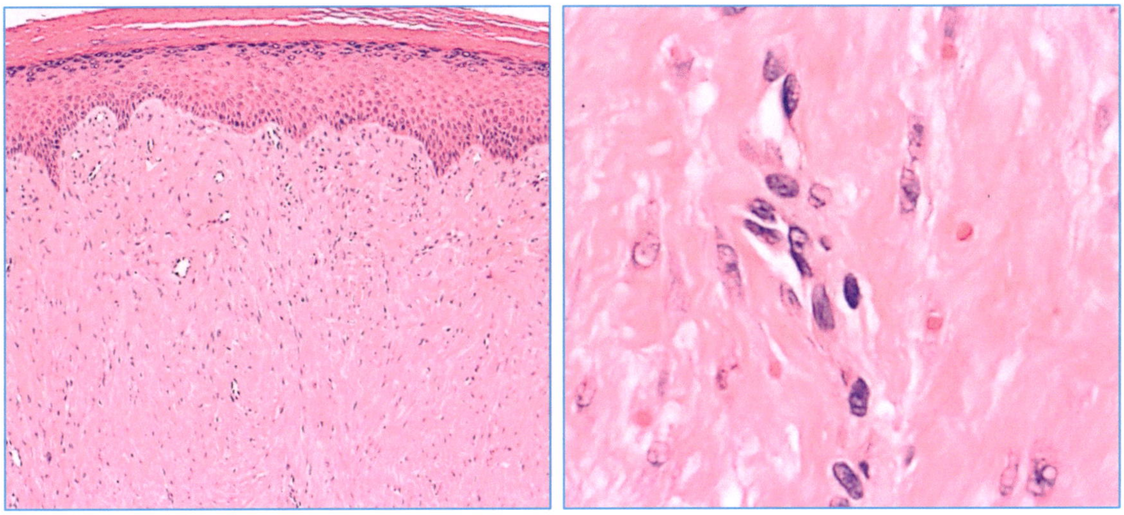

Infantile digital fibromatosis of acral skin with characteristic pink-red inclusions resembling RBCs

Fibrous tumors

FIBROMATOSIS

Can be divided into:

Superficial (fascial)

-palmar (Dupuytren's), plantar (Ledderhose), penile (Peyronie's), and knuckle pad
-slow growing nodule
-cause contracture
-almost half of palmar/plantar are bilateral

Deep (musculoaponeurotic)

-also called desmoid tumor
-deep fibromatosis can compress vital organs and be life-threatening

Histopathology

-**long subcutaneous fascicles** of **uniform, bland myofibroblasts** of variable cellularity
-no cellular atypia
-uniformly distributed collagen
-growth along fascia, aponeuroses, and tendons

HYALINE FIBROMATOSIS

-very rare autosomal recessive disorder caused by mutations in *ANTXR2* gene
-the severity of the symptoms falls along a spectrum
-in milder cases (previously called juvenile hyaline fibromatosis), symptoms begin in childhood
-in severe cases (previously called infantile systemic hyalinosis), symptoms are present at birth or begin within the first few months
-milder form is characterized by multiple, very painful, slow-growing cutaneous nodules
-lesions favor hands, neck, scalp, ears, and nose
-in severe form nodules are also in muscle and internal organs

Histopathology

-ill-defined dermal and subcutaneous lesion
-amorphous **hyalinized eosinophilic stroma**
-scattered bland **plump to spindled fibroblasts**

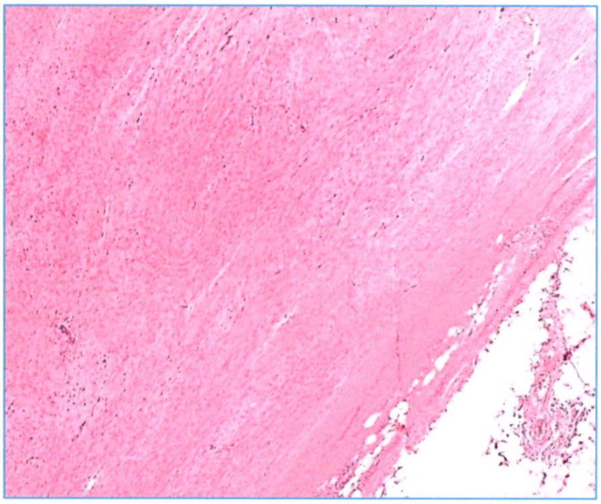
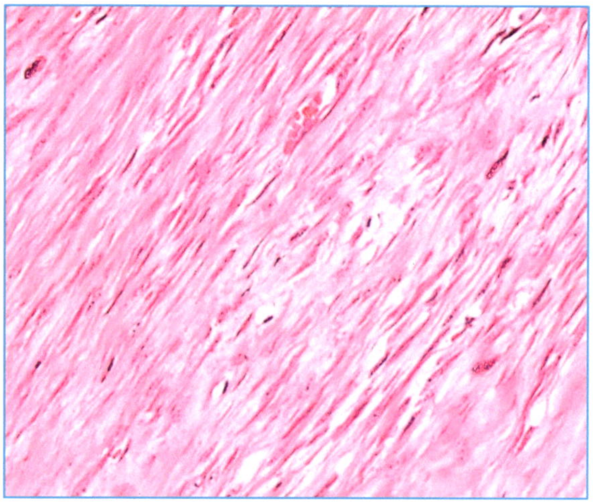

Fibromatosis with long parallel fascicles made of uniform elongated myofibroblasts

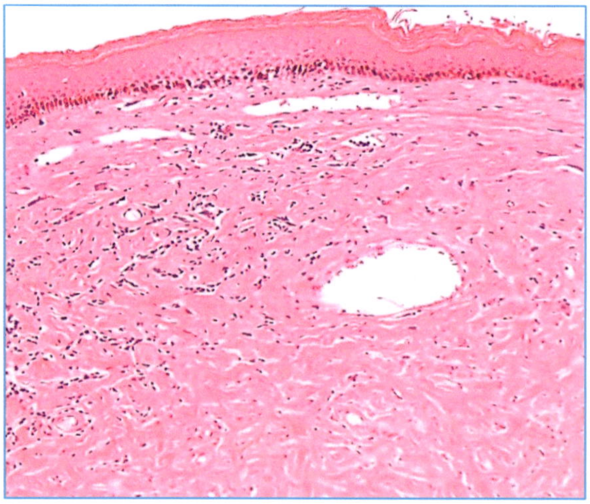
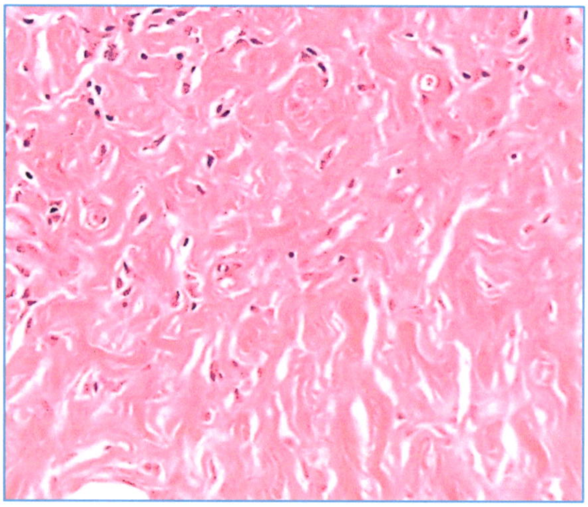

Hyaline fibromatosis with dense hyalinized stroma and plump round fibroblasts

ELASTOFIBROMA

-rare, slow-growing benign tumor
-present as subcutaneous swelling, commonly bilateral
-favor the subscapular area in elderly women
-often attached to the periosteum of the ribs
-Xq12-q22 translocation in one third of the cases

Histopathology

-ill-defined, eosinophilic, dermal/subcutaneous tumor interdigitated into adipose tissue
-made of **hyalinized collagen** bundles admixed with **thick elastic fibers**
-characteristic **"beaded" elastic fibers** with **"pipe cleaner-like" appearance**

FIBROMA OF TENDON SHEATH

-uncommon, slow-growing benign tumor
-well circumscribed, nodular tumor attached to tendon or tendon sheath
-favor fingers, hands or wrist

Histopathology

-well circumscribed nodule
-made of **hyalinized eosinophilic stroma** with compressed capillaries and **scattered spindled cells (SMA+)**

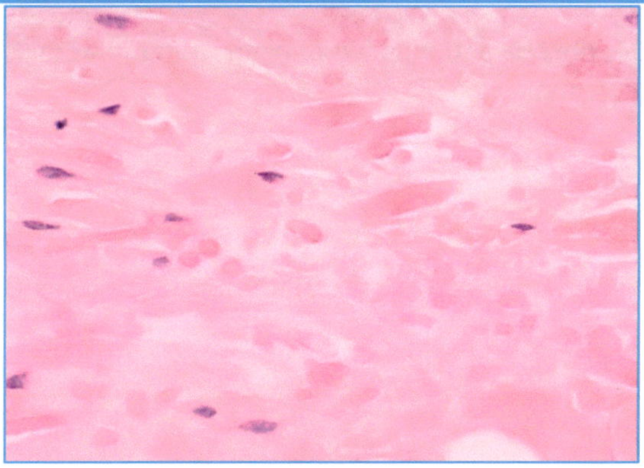

Elastofibroma with thick elastic fibers among hyalinized collagen

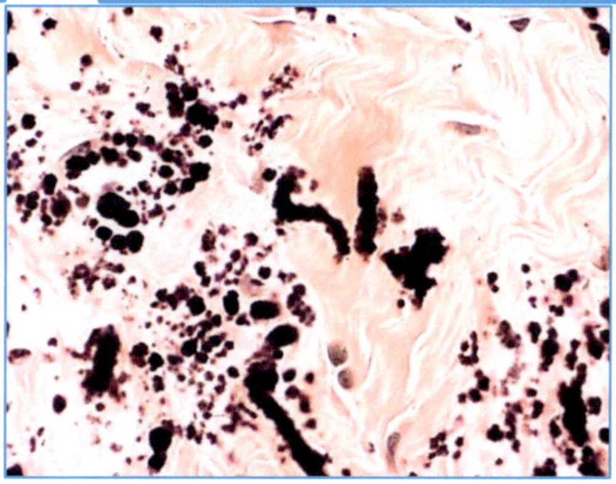

Elastofibroma with "beaded" elastic fibers with "pipe cleaner" appearance (VVG stain)

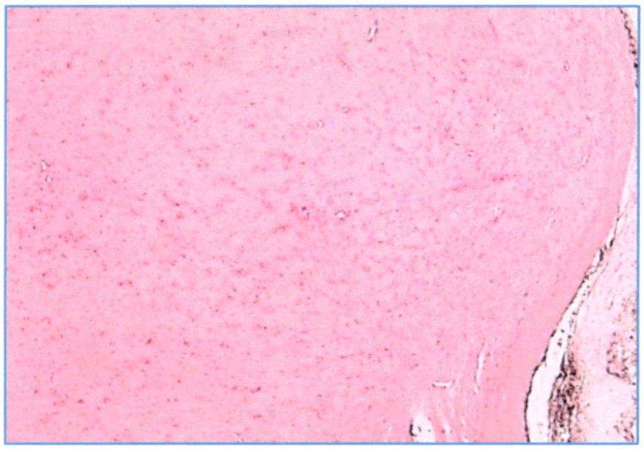

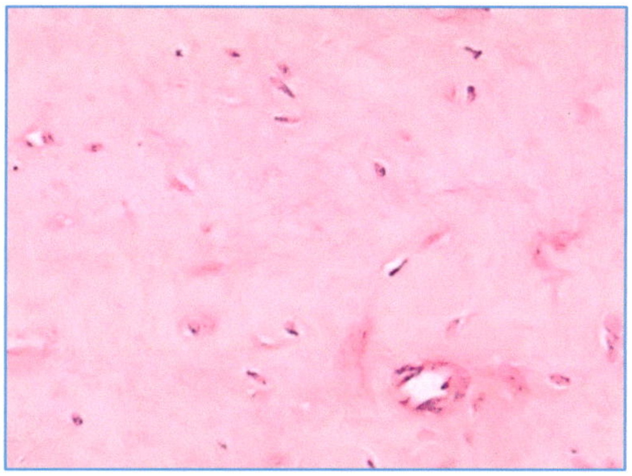

Fibroma of tendon sheath form deep nodule with hyalinized stroma and scattered spindled cells

SOLITARY FIBROUS TUMOR

-rare painless subcutaneous tumor
-favor head and thigh

Histopathology

-well circumscribed, histologically variable tumor
-uniform, **epithelioid, oval or spindled cells in collagenous stroma**
-focal **"hemangiopericytoma-like" vessels**
-tumor cells are **CD34, CD99 and bcl-2 positive**

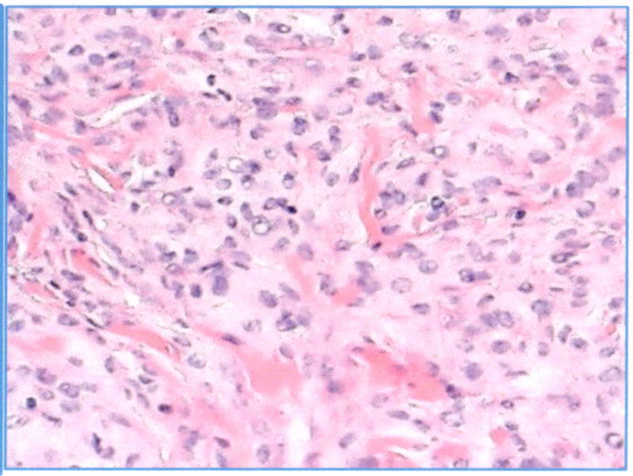

Fibroma of tendon sheath with epithelioid oval cells

Fibrous tumors

GIANT CELL TUMOR OF TENDON SHEATH

-uncommon benign tumor
-favors young adults and is more common in females
-slowly growing, painless nodule
-predilection for the dorsal surface of the fingers (distal interphalangial joint is the most common site)
-tumor is fixed to underlying tendon
-recurrence is common if not completely excised

Histopathology
-circumscribed, multinodular tumor in the deep dermis or subcutis
-it can be attached to tendon
-composed of **"osteoclast-like" giant cells** (giant cells with variable size and variable number of nuclei), variable xanthoma cells, and chronic inflammatory cells
-**eosinophilic fibrous stroma**

MULTINUCLEATE CELL ANGIOHISTIOCYTOMA

-rare disease
-it is debated whether it is neoplastic or a non-neoplastic reactive process
-predominantly on the extremities of middle-aged and elderly women
-presents with an insidiously developing group of asymptomatic red brown papules and plaques with central atrophy

Histopathology
-proliferation of **haphazardly arranged capillaries** and small venules in superficial to mid reticular dermis
-**irregular multinucleated giant cells** scattered in the dermis
-**stroma is fibrotic** and mild lymphocytic inflammation is usually present

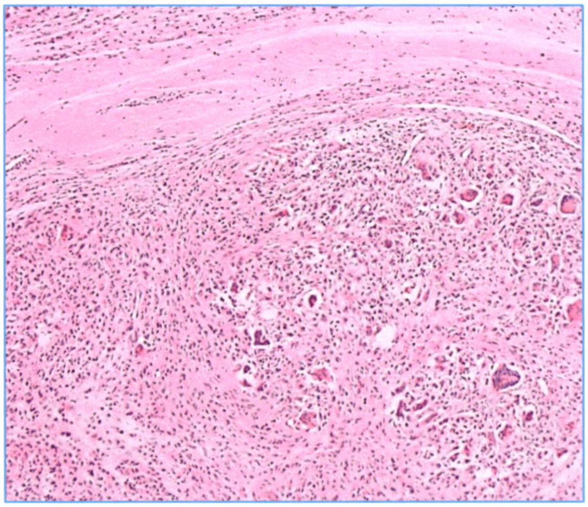
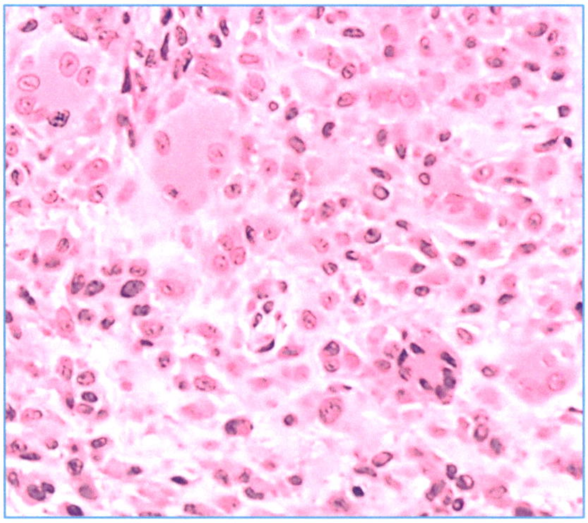

Giant cell tumor of tendon sheath with numerous "osteoclast-like" giant cells admixed with histiocytes and lymphocytes

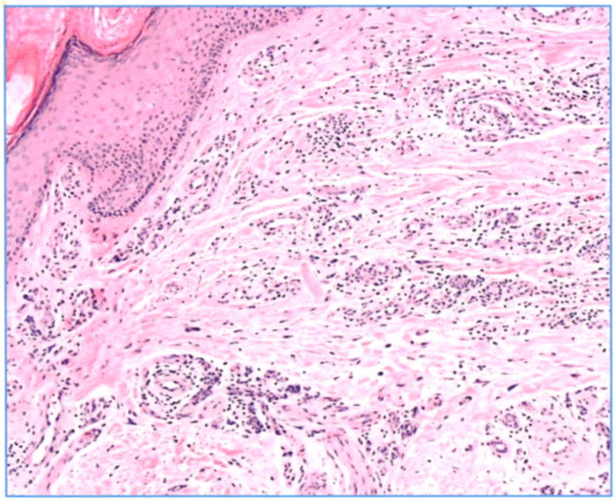
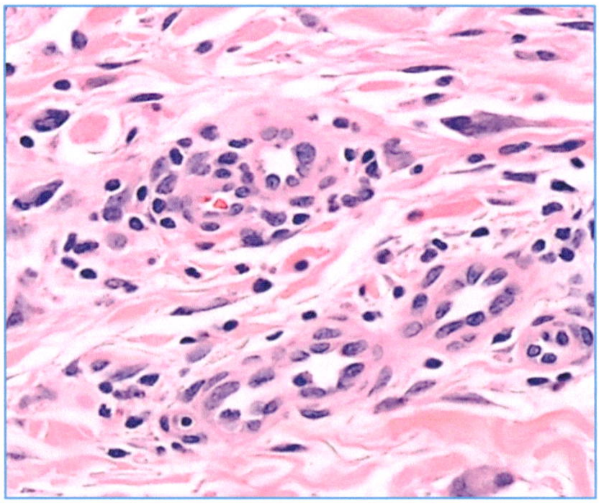

Multinucleate cell angiohistiocytoma with numerous capillaries in sclerotic stroma containing scattered, irregular giant cells

ANGIOMYOFIBROBLASTOMA

-rare subcutaneous nodular tumor
-occurs almost exclusively in the vulvovaginal area of women
-tumors grow slowly and are painless
-it has low tendency for local recurrence

Histopathology

-hypocellular and hypercellular areas in the background of **edematous stroma**
-**abundant vessels** of various wall thickness
-stroma consists of **spindled and ovoid stromal cells**
-no mitotic figures or significant nuclear atypia is seen
-tumor cells are desmin, SMA, estrogen, and progesterone receptor positive

ONYCHOMATRICOMA

-benign fibroepithelial tumor of the nail matrix
-predominantly affects the fingernails
-peak incidence is in the fifth decade of life
-clinically characterized by thickened, yellowish nail plate
-transverse or longitudinal over curvature of the nail plate, splinter hemorrhage, and multiple holes in the nail plate when viewed from the free margin

Histopathology

-**epithelial digitations** originating from the matrix epithelium
-**projections lack a granular layer** as is typical for normal nail matrix
-they are **surrounded by dense stroma** that is commonly hypercellular
-pleomorphic fibroblasts are occasionally present

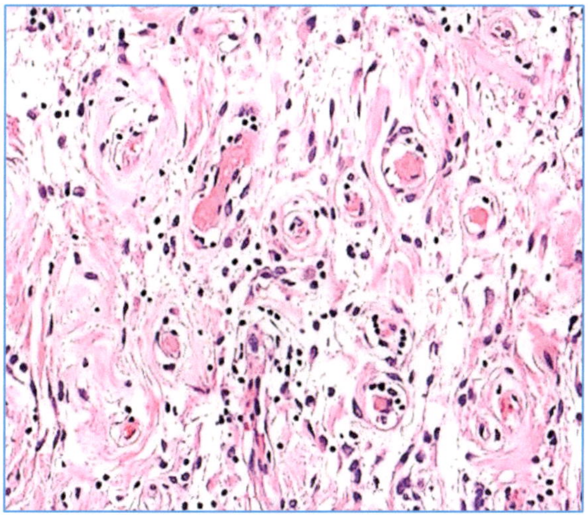
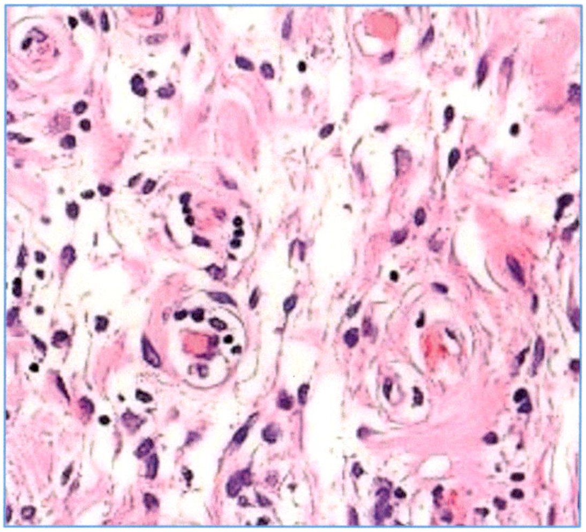

Angiomyofobroblastoma with numerous small vessels in edematous stroma with ovoid stromal cells

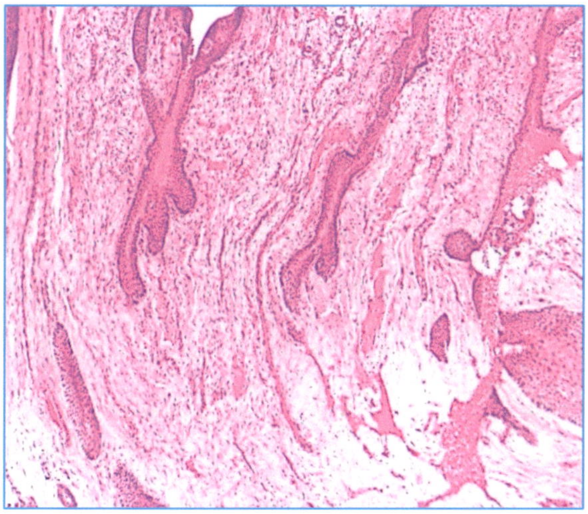
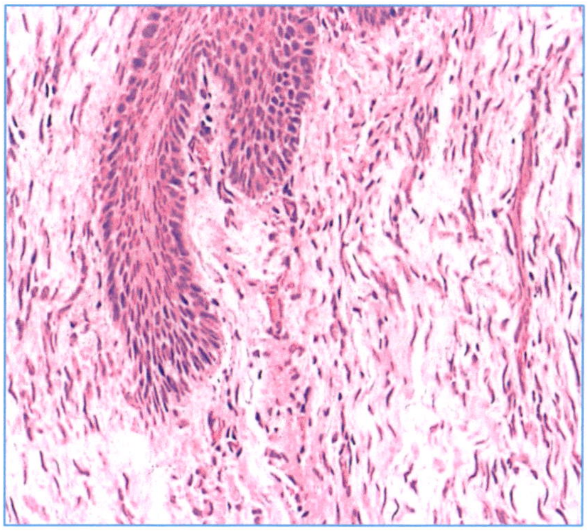

Onychomatricoma with "finger-like" epithelial protrusions surrounded by fibrous stroma

Fibrous tumors

NODULAR FASCIITIS/ CRANIAL FASCIITIS/PROLIFERATING FASCIITIS

-benign, rapidly growing subcutaneous or deep soft tissue mass
-sometimes associated with prior trauma
-occurs in children and young to middle-aged adults
-forearm is favored site in adult and head/neck in children
-**cranial fasciitis** is a **variant** that occurs in infants and involves the scalp and skull

Histopathology

-well-circumscribed deep subcutaneous tumor
-often associate with fascia
-**variable cellularity** with **hyper and hypocellular areas** and focal **myxoid stroma**
-made of uniform **SMA positive fibroblasts**
-haphazard or focally **storiform pattern (“tissue culture” appearance)**
-**extravasated RBCs** can be present
-**mitoses are common but not atypical**
-**proliferating fasciitis** is a **variant with “ganglion-like” giant cells**

MYOEPITHELIOMA

-rare benign tumor that occurs in young adults with a male preponderance
-favors the extremities
-presents as dermal/subcutaneous nodule

Histopathology

Two presentations:

-solid tumor with **ovoid/round, pink epithelioid cells** with **minimal or no stroma**
-***or*** epithelioid, plasmocytic, or spindle **cells in reticular pattern in myxoid stroma**
-minimal atypia although malignant variant with atypia has been described
-tumor cells are **EMA, S-100, and calponin positive** and variably pancytokeratin positive

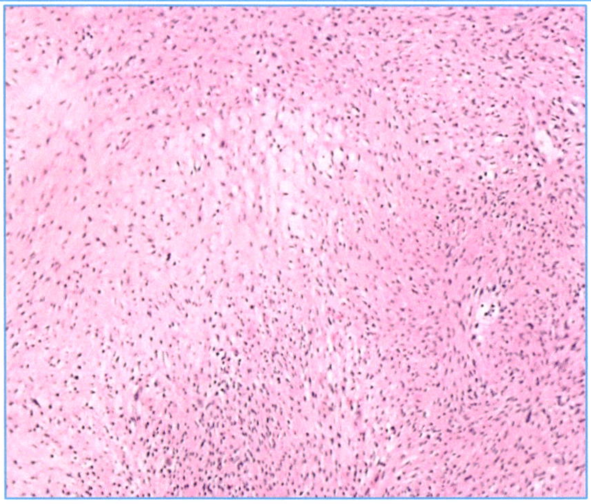
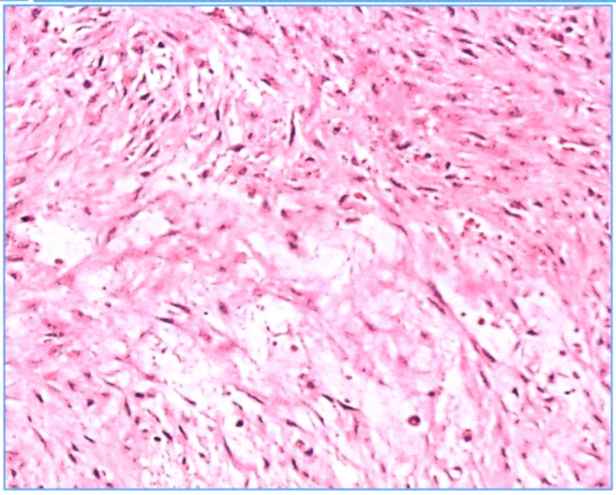

Nodular fasciitis with variation in tumor cellularity, focal presence of myxoid stroma, and scattered RBCs

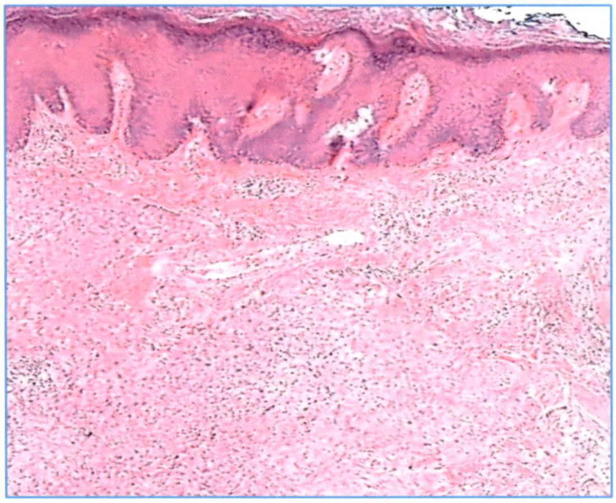
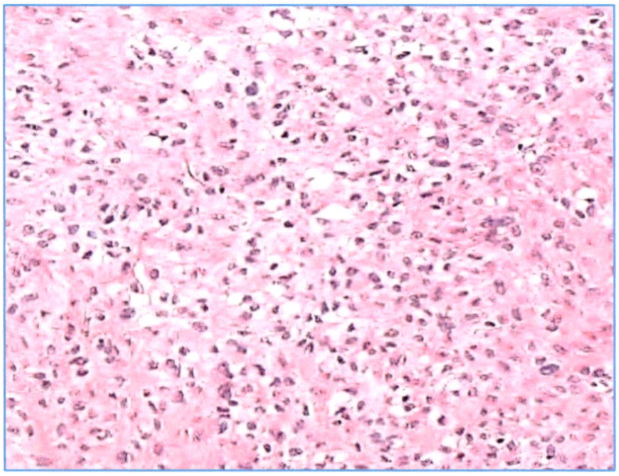

Myoepithelioma with uniform epithelioid cells with minimal stroma

Chapter 31

ATYPICAL FIBROXANTHOMA

-low-grade malignant sarcoma
-presents as a solitary rapidly enlarging ulcerated nodule
-appears on the head or neck of the elderly
-highly favors sun-damaged skin

Histopathology

-epidermis is frequently excoriated
-superficial dermal proliferation of atypical spindle cells
-prominent polymorphism with **very atypical, bizarre cells ("big ugly" cells)**
-mitoses can be numerous
-prominent dermal solar elastosis
-usually **does not invade the subcutis**
-cells are **CD10 and factor XIII positive**

UNDIFFERENTIATED PLEOMORPHIC SARCOMA (MALIGNANT FIBROUS HISTIOCYTOMA)

-usually occurs as deep subcutaneous nodules
-favors the arms and legs of elderly men
-UNPS is diagnosis of exclusion of malignant sarcomas that cannot be more precisely categorized

Histopathology

-infiltrating **deep** dermal and subcutaneous tumor
-manifests a broad range of histological appearances
-most common type is **pleomorphic type**
-histologically **resembles AFX** (many bizarre cells) but with deep invasion
-made of **bizarre pleomorphic fibroblastic cells**
-**numerous atypical mitoses** and common necrosis
-if pleomorphic type has more than 50% of myxoid area it is called **myxoid type**
-if pleomorphic type has numerous "osteoclast-like" giant cells it is called **giant cell type**
-if pleomorphic type has extensive inflammation and xanthoma cells it is called **inflammatory type**

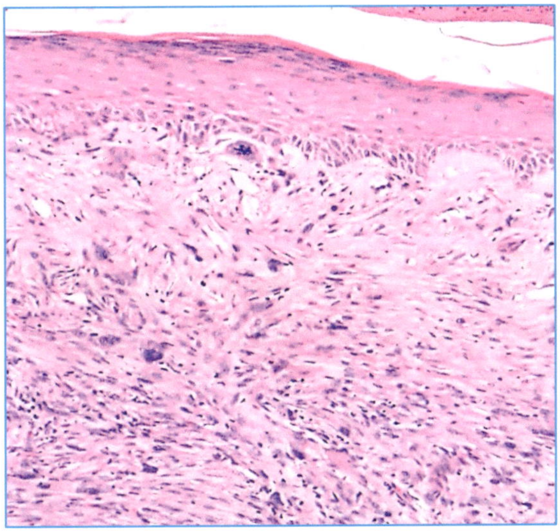
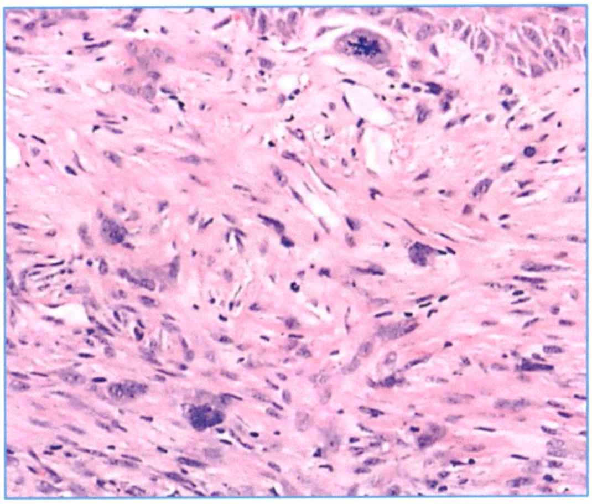

AFX with dermal proliferation of very atypical, bizarre cells in the background of solar elastosis

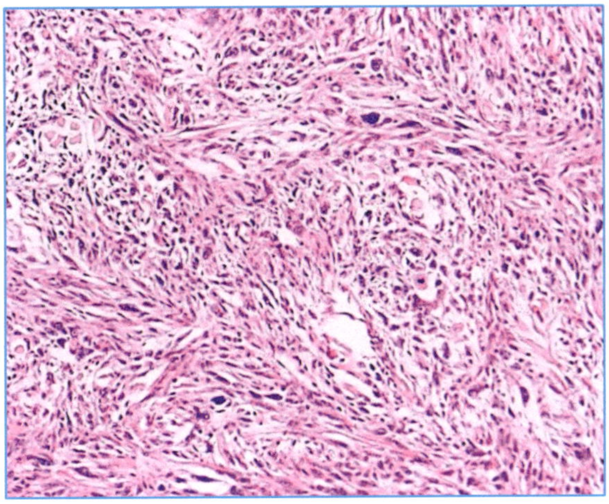
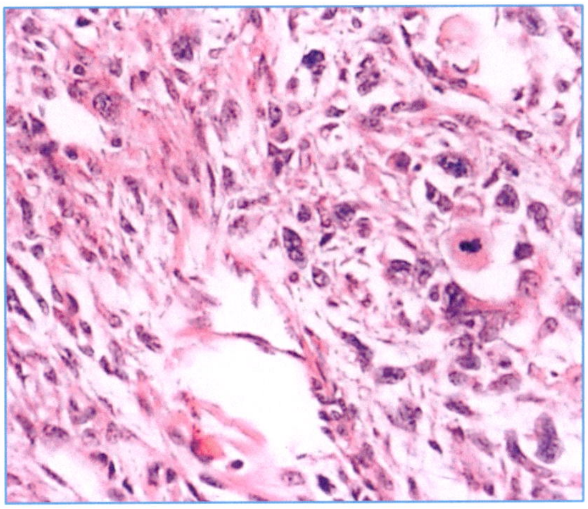

UNPS is histologically indistinguishable from AFX but the tumor is much deeper

Fibrous tumors

DERMATOFIBROSARCOMA PROTUBERANS	FIBROSARCOMA
-malignant fibrohistiocytic tumor -predilection for torso and proximal extremities -favors young and middle-aged adults -presents with solitary, slow-growing nodules arising in an indurated plaque -90% have the chromosomal translocation t(17;22) fusing *COL1A1* and *PDGFβ* genes Histopathology -deep dermal tumor that invades subcutis -homogenous, **bland appearing spindle cells** (despite being malignant) arranged in uniform storiform pattern -cells **diffusely infiltrate fat in "honeycomb" pattern** -some tumors contain scattered dendritic melanin-containing cells (**Bednar tumor**) -tumor cells are diffusely CD34 positive and factor XIII negative	-malignant fibrohistiocytic tumor with two clinical subtypes **Adult type** -deep seated, slow-growing, sometimes painful mass favoring lower extremities **Congenital and infantile type** -children 1 year of age or less -20% are congenital -favors distal extremities -nodule is located more superficially -majority of congenital infantile cases have translocation between chromosomes 12 and 15 forming the fusion gene *ETV6-NTRK3* Histopathology -it is diagnosis of exclusion -**uniform fibroblasts** organized **in fascicles** -fascicles are arranged in acute angles to each other **("herringbone" pattern)** -**mitoses commonly seen**

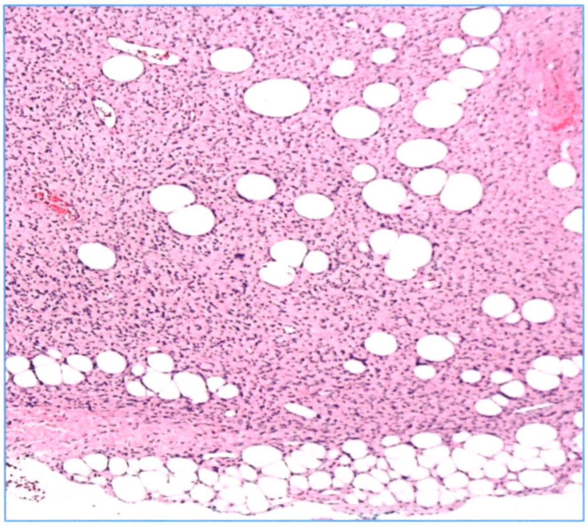

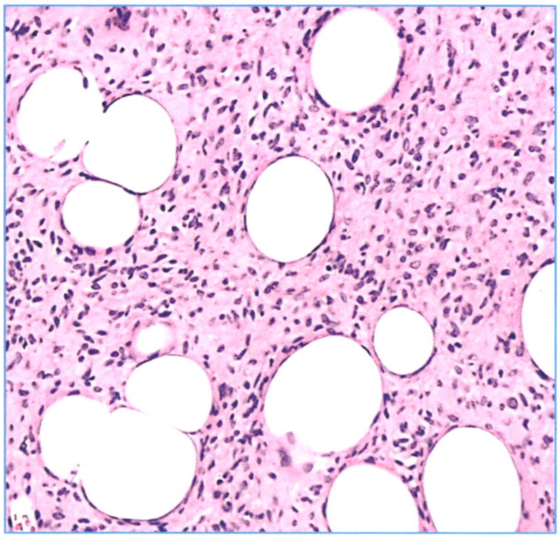

DFSP with uniform cells invading fat in "honeycomb" pattern

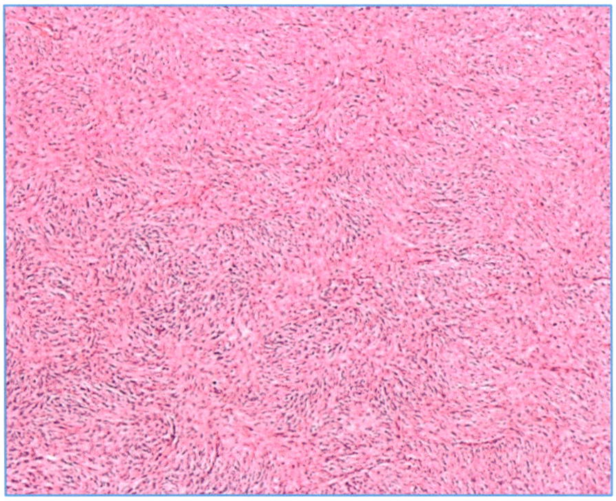

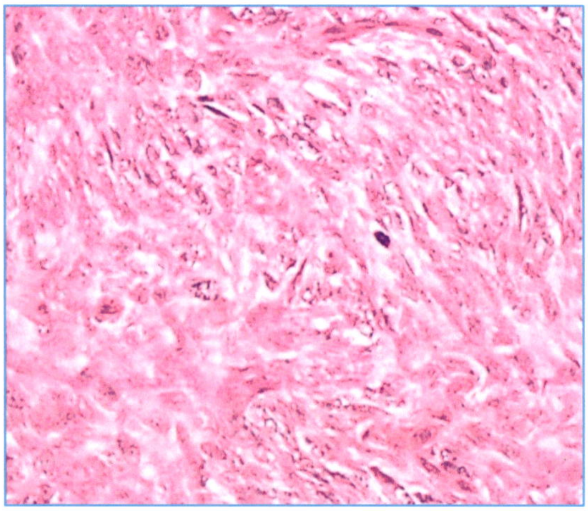

Fibrosarcoma with elongated cells forming fascicles arranged in "herringbone" pattern. Mitoses are present.

EPITHELIOID SARCOMA

-slow-growing malignant dermal or subcutaneous nodular tumor
-occurs in adolescents and young adults and favors the distal extremities, particularly the hand and wrist
-may ulcerate when superficial or can be attached to tendons or fascia when deep

Histopathology
-can **simulate a granulomatous process**, with or without necrosis (pseudogranulomatous morphology)
-central **necrosis surrounded** by uniform **epithelioid small to medium-sized cells with eosinophilic cytoplasm**
-cells are pancytokeratin and EMA positive
-spindle cells can also be identified but usually at the periphery of a nodule
-variable mitotic activity and cytological atypia

SUPERFICIAL LOW GRADE FIBROMYXOID SARCOMA

-superficial variant accounts for about 15% of all low grade fibromyxoid sarcomas
-slow-growing, subcutaneous, painless tumor
-favors the lower limbs of younger male adults
-presence of *FUS* and *CREB3L2* (or *CREB3L1*) gene fusion is a characteristic feature

Histopathology
-relatively circumscribed, low/moderately cellular, subcutaneous proliferation of spindle cells
-cells are bland with minimal atypia
-**alternating fibrous and myxoid stroma in whorled pattern**
-40% of tumors have more epithelioid cells and collagen rosettes
-characteristically, **MUC4 stain is positive**

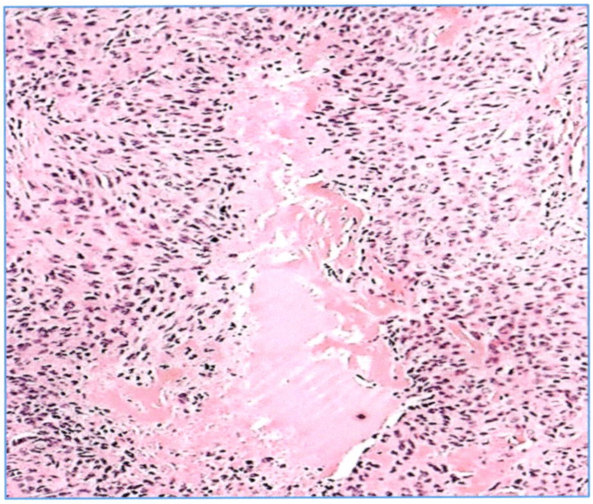

Epithelioid sarcoma with irregular necrosis surrounded by epithelioid eosinophilic cells

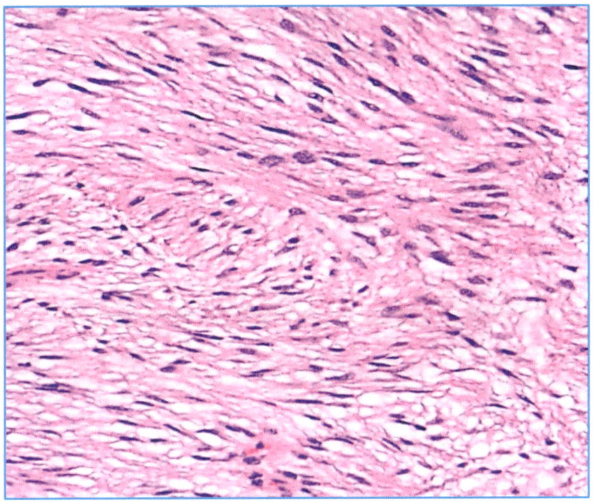

Low grade fibromyxoid sarcoma with spindle cells in whorled pattern in myxoid stroma

MYXOFIBROSARCOMA

-malignant, slow-growing, painless nodule on the leg or arm mainly seen in the elderly
-it is myxoid variant of **undifferentiated pleomorphic sarcoma**

Histopathology
-dermal/subcutaneous multinodular tumor
-variable tumor cellularity with **curvilinear vessels**
-tumor consists of two cell types
-elongated, **spindle-shaped "fibroblast-like" cell** with enlarged, hyperchromatic nuclei and **larger atypical "histocyte-like" cells** embedded in **myxoid material**
-more cellularity indicates a higher tumor grade

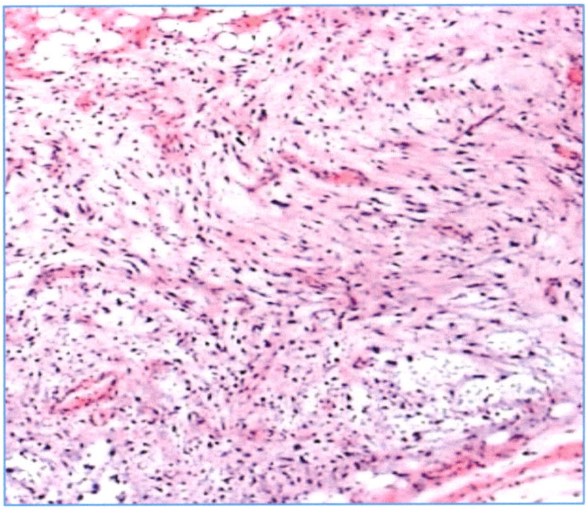

Myxofibrosarcoma made of spindled and histiocytic cells with curvilinear vessels in myxoid stroma

Fibrous tumors

HOW TO APPROACH FIBROHISTIOCYTIC TUMORS

EXCLUDE TUMORS OCCURING MOSTLY IN CHILDREN

-fibrous hamartoma of infancy	fibroblasts + adipose tissue + myxoid mesenchyme
-infantile digital fibromatosis	pink cytoplasmic inclusions resembling RBCs
-hyaline fibromatosis	scattered fibroblasts in pink hyalinized stroma
-calcifying aponeurotic fibroma	multiple foci of calcification

IF TUMOR IS HYPERCELLULAR OR OF NORMAL CELLULARITY

-dermatofibroma	epidermal "dirty socks" + trapped collagen
-dermatomyofibroma	"DF-like" appearance with "muscle-like" cells + no trapped collagen
-myofibroma	deep nodule made of hyper/hypocellular areas + variably myxoid stroma
-fibromatosis	fascicles of uniform fibroblasts in unidirectional orientation
-nodular fasciitis	deep hyper/hypocellular nodule + tissue culture appearance
-myoepithelioma	epithelioid pink cells with minimal stroma in solid or reticulated pattern
-pleomorphic fibroma	skin tag appearance with "monster" cells

IF TUMOR IS HYPOCELLULAR

-sclerotic fibroma	"woodgrain" appearance
-acral fibrokeratoma	acral skin + polypoid hypocellular lesion + dilated capillaries

IF VESSELS ARE VERY PROMINENT

-multinucleate cell angiohistiocytoma	dermal capillaries + irregular giant cells
-angiomyofibroblastoma	capillaries in edematous stroma + spindled stromal cells

IF VESSELS ARE PRESENT BUT LESS PROMINENT

-angiofibroma	dome shaped + dilated capillaries + stellate fibroblasts
-acral fibrokeratoma	acral skin + polypoid hypocellular lesion + dilated capillaries
-periungual fibroma	as acral fibrokeratoma + may have occasional giant cells

IF TUMOR IS MYXOID AND APPEARS BENIGN

-myxoma	extensive mucinous stroma with stellate fibroblasts
-super. acral fibromyxoma	CD34+, CD99+ spindled fibroblasts+ variably myxoid background
-myofibroma	deep biphasic tumor + variably myxoid background
-cellular digital fibroma	CD34+, CD99- plump fibroblasts + variably myxoid background

IF PROMINENT GIANT CELLS ARE PRESENT

-giant cell tumor of tendon sheath	deep lesion + mixed inflammation + giant cells
-multinucleate cell angiohistiocytoma	vessels are more prominent than giant cells

IF MATURE BONE OR CALCIFICATIONS ARE PRESENT

-fibro-osseous pseudotumor of the digits	bone and osteoclasts
-calcifying aponeurotic fibroma	calcifications and "chondrocytes-like" cells

IF FIBROUS TUMOR IS SUBUNGUAL

-onychomatricoma	epithelial "finger-like" projections + fibrous stroma
-periungual fibroma	like acral fibrokeratoma + may have occasional giant cells

IF LESION APPEARS MALIGNANT

-AFX	superficial lesion with extensive cytological atypia
-MFH/UNPS	deep lesion similar to AFX
-DFSP	CD34+ deep lesion with "honeycomb" pattern
-fibrosarcoma	atypical fibroblasts in "herringbone" pattern
-epitheliod sarcoma	granulomatous appearance with central necrosis
-myxofibrosarcoma	atypical fibrohistiocytic cells + myxoid stroma + curvilinear vessels
-low grade fibromyxoid sarcoma	atypical fibroblasts in alternating fibrous and myxoid stroma

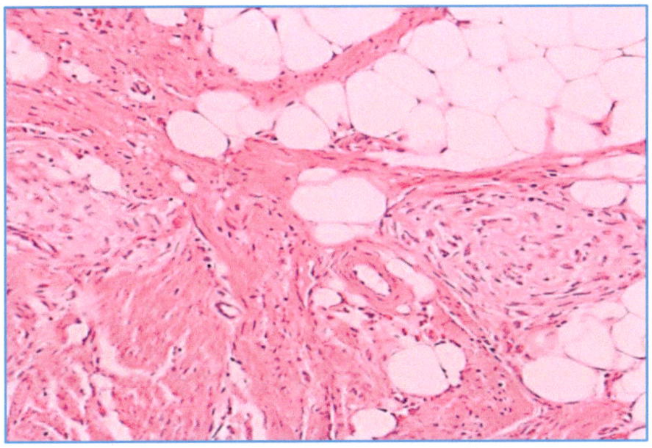

Fibrous hamartoma of infancy consists of adipocytes, fibroblasts, mesenchymal tissue

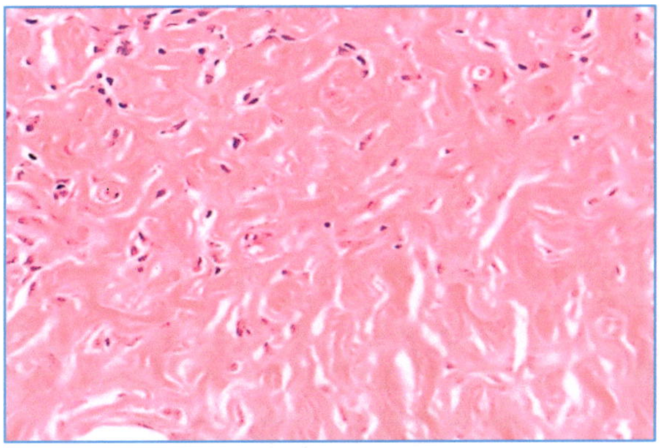

Hyaline fibromatosis is hypocellular lesion with pink hyalinized stroma

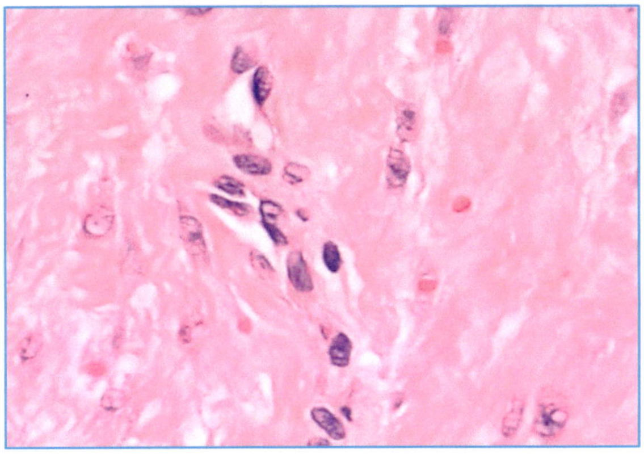

Infantile digital fibromatosis with "RBC-like" inclusions

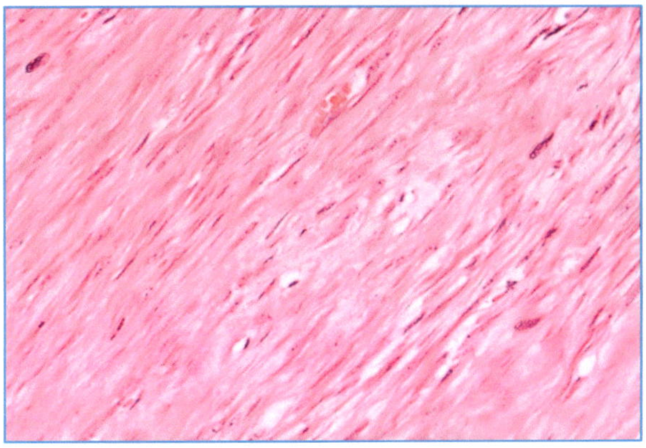

Fibromatosis with uniform fascicles of fibroblasts

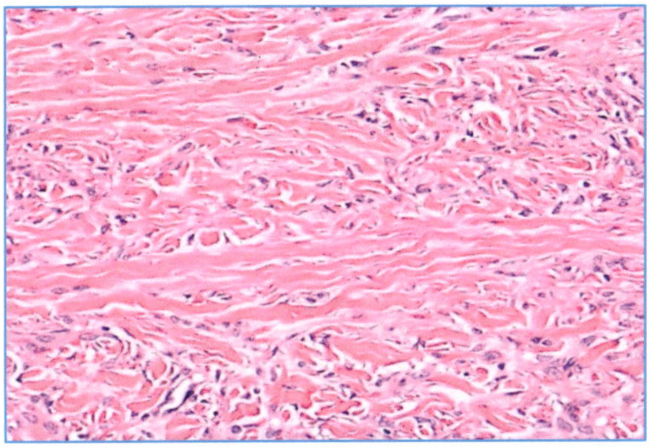

DF with fibroblasts in between trapped prominent collagen

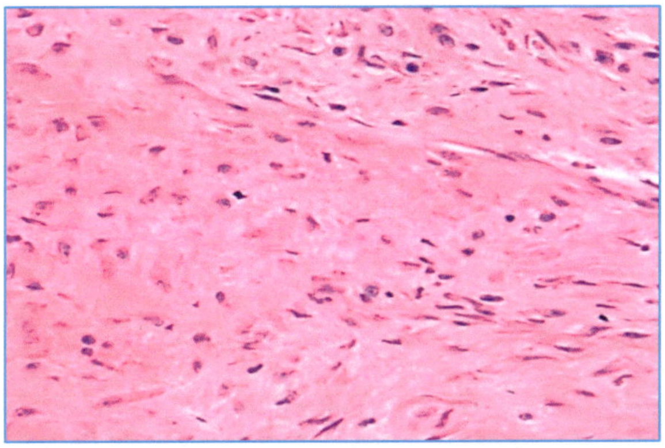

Dermatomyofibroma is "DF-like" with pink muscle appearance

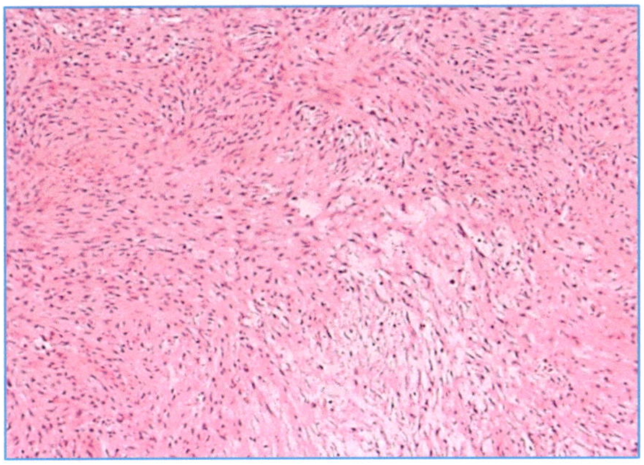

Nodular fasciitis with fibroblast tissue culture appearance

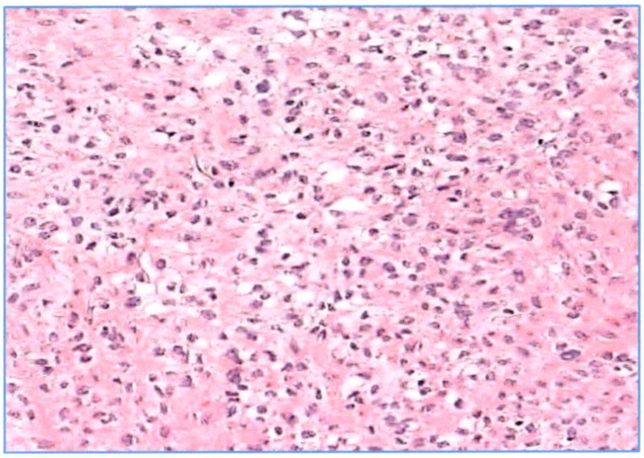

Myoepithelioma with epithelioid cells

Fibrous tumors

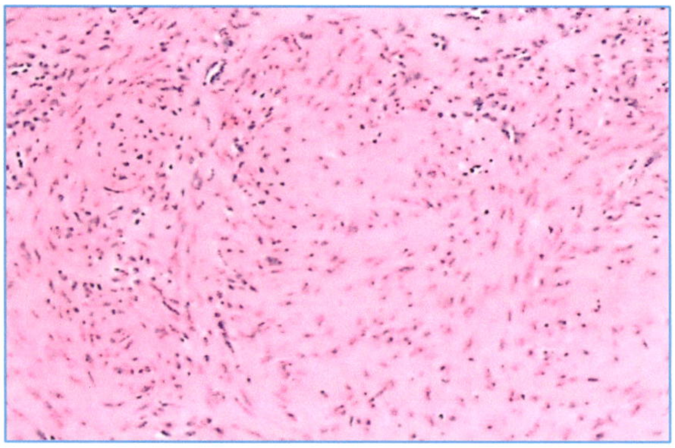

Myofibroma with hyper and hypocellular areas in myxoid stroma

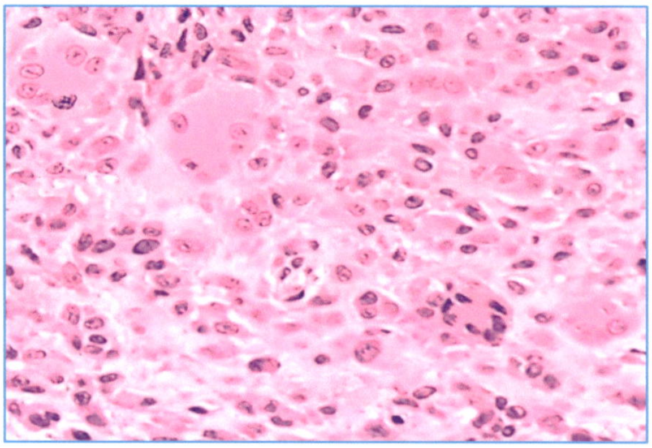

Giant cell tumor of tendon sheath with "osteoclast-like" giant cells

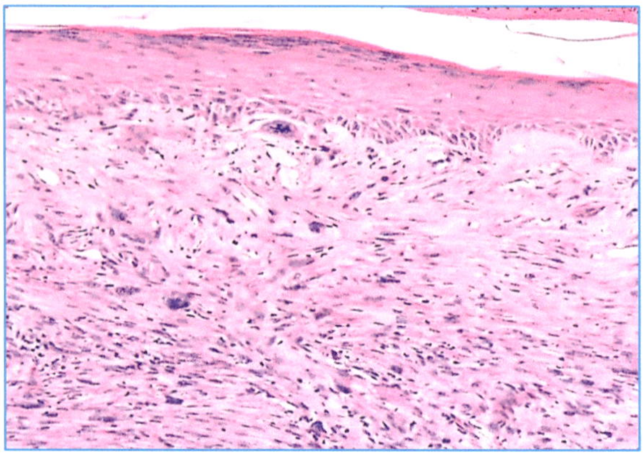

AFX is superficial cellular lesion with bizarre cells

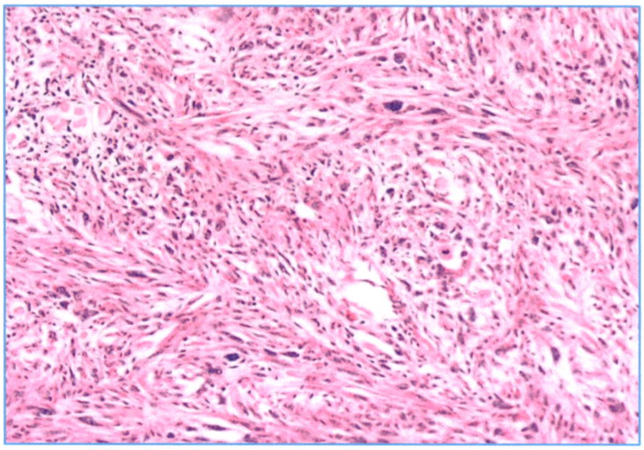

UNPS is deep cellular lesion with bizarre cells

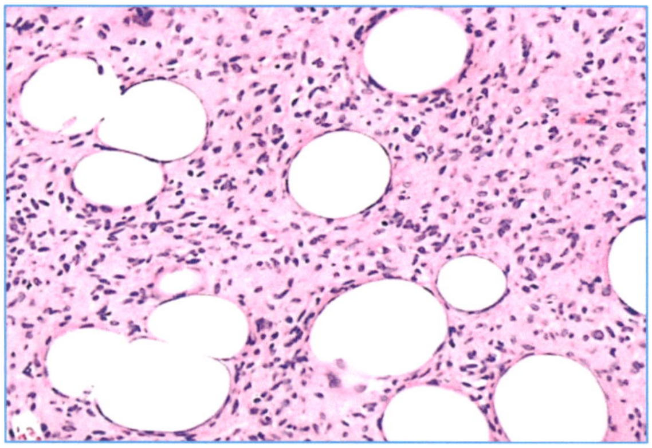

DFSP with spindle cells infiltrating fat in "honeycomb" pattern

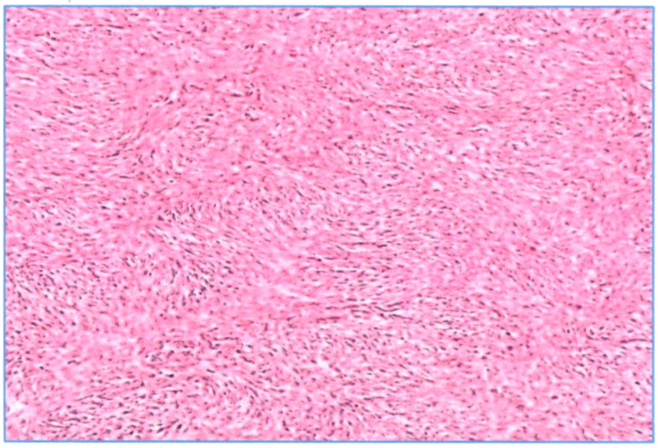

Fibrosarcoma with fascicles in "herringbone" pattern

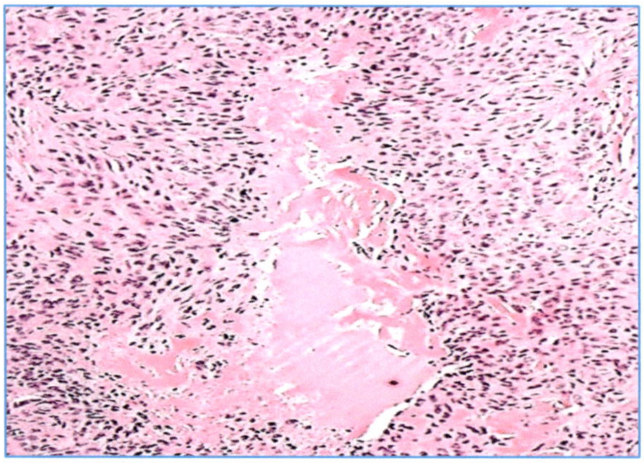

Epithelioid sarcoma with necrotic, granulomatous appearance

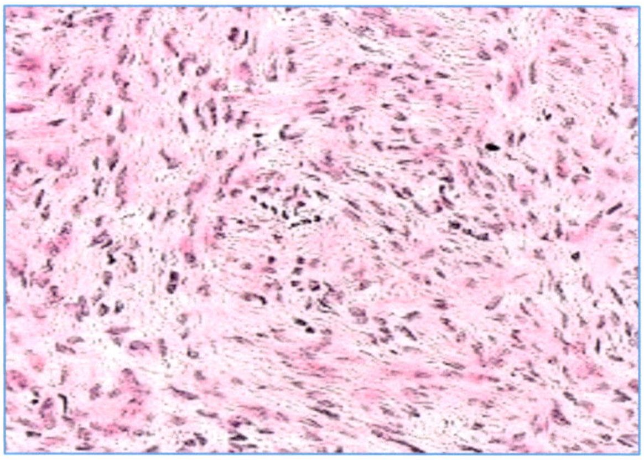

Low grade fibromyxoid sarcoma with whorled pattern in myxoid stroma

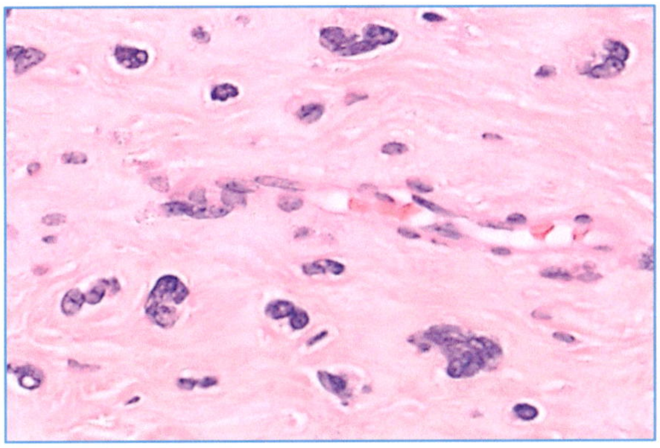

Pleomorphic fibroma with "floret giant cells"

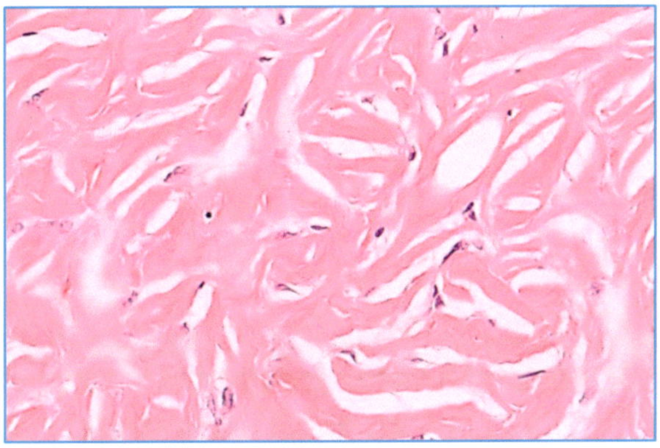

Sclerotic fibroma with "wood grain" appearance

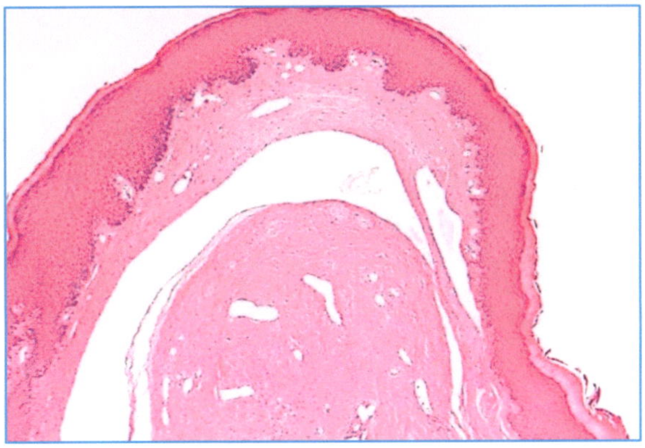

Acral fibrokeratoma is
hypocellular fibrotic lesion with dilated vessels

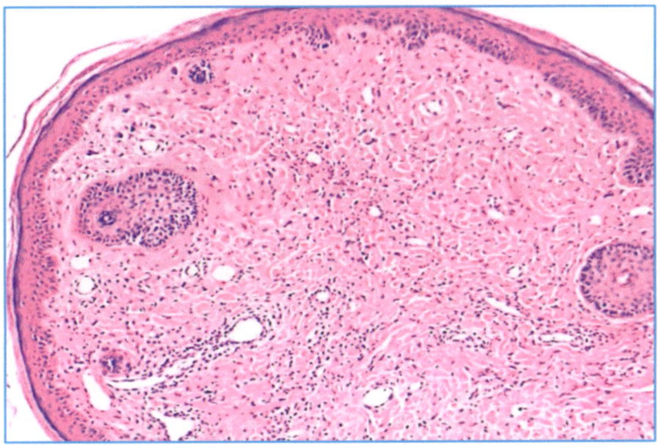

Angiofibroma with dilated capillaries and stellate fibroblasts

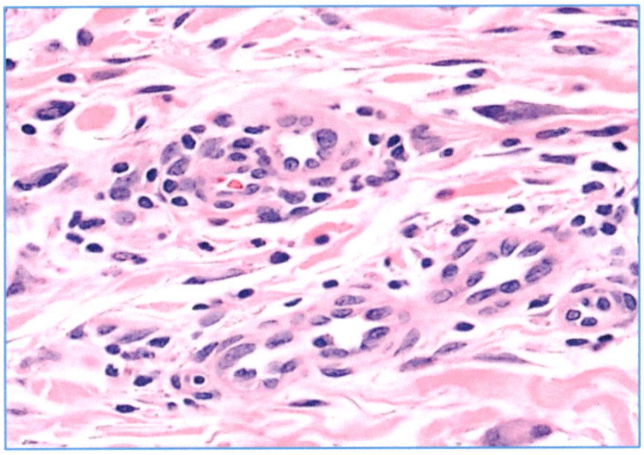

Multinucleate cell angiohistiocytoma is
vascular lesion with irregular giant cells

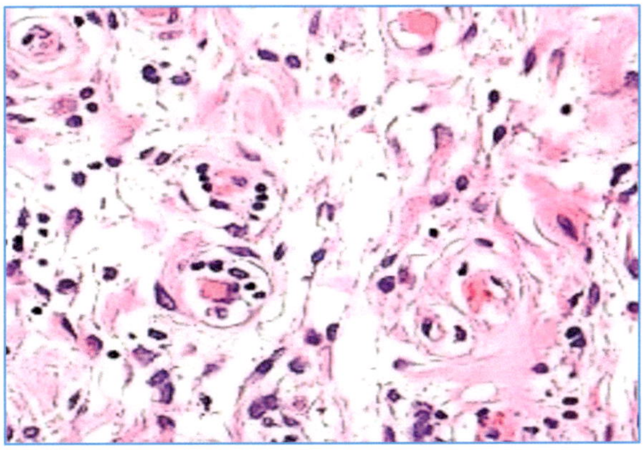

Angiomyofibroblastoma is
vascular lesion with myofibroblasts

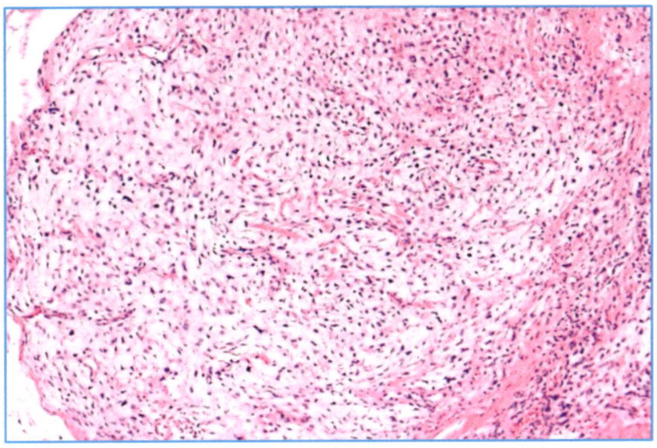

Myxoma with myxoid nodule and scattered fibroblasts

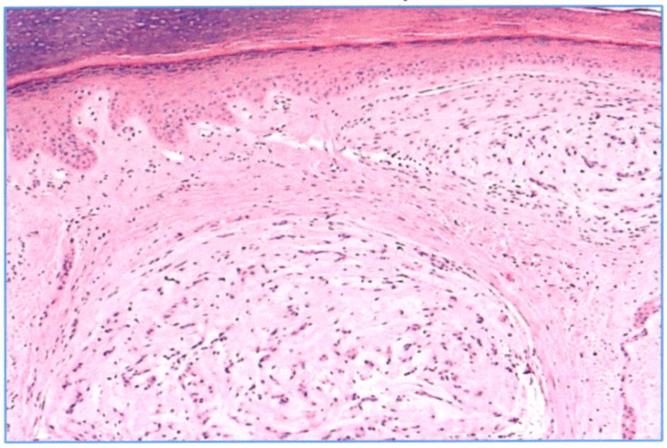

Superficial acral fibromyxoma with
spindle cells in myxoid nodules at acral site

Fibrous tumors

Chapter 32

HISTIOCYTIC TUMORS

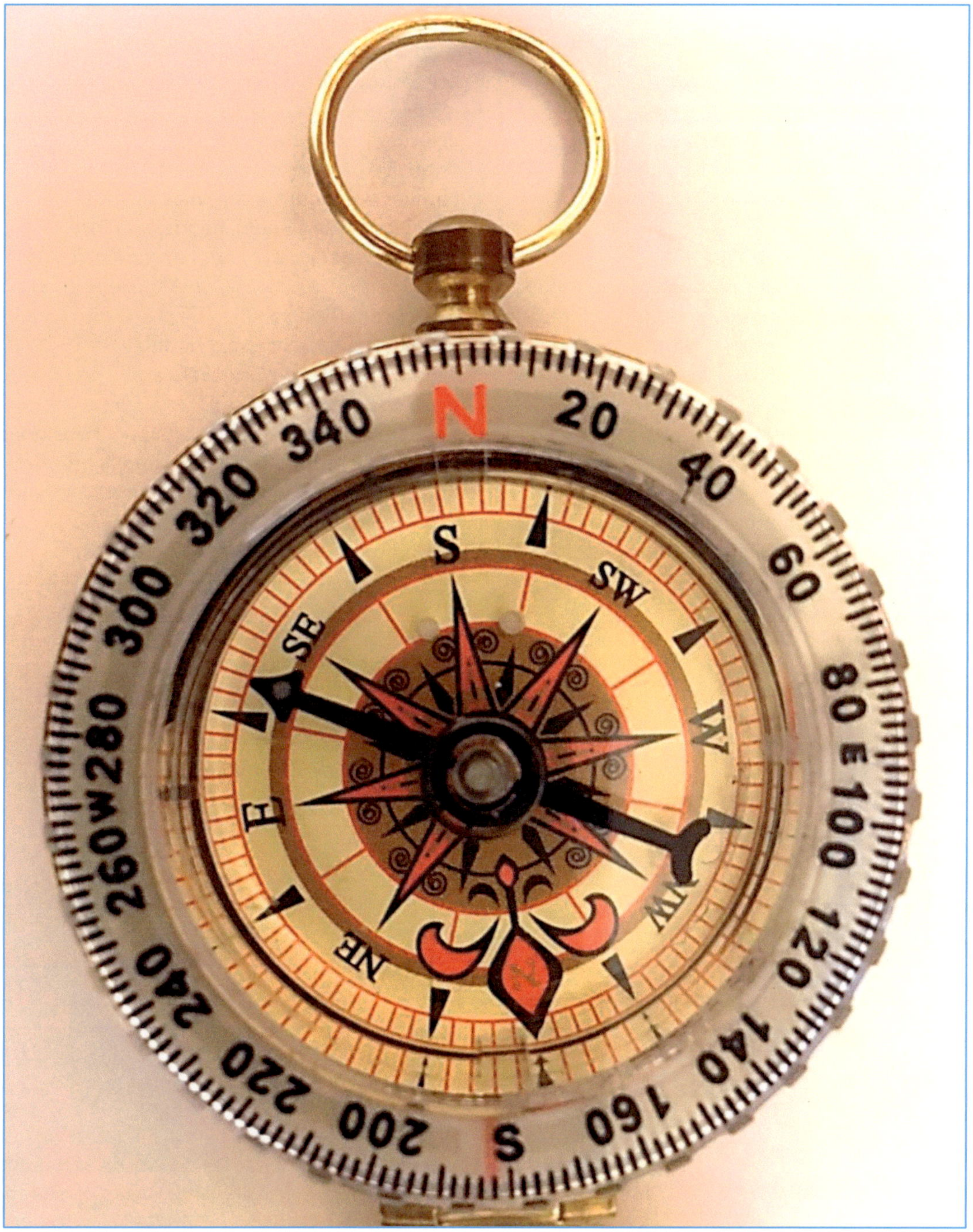

Histiocytic tumors

JUVENILE XANTHOGRANULOMA (XANTHOGRANULOMA)

-most common non-Langerhans cell histiocytosis
-mostly children (median age 22 months) but can be seen in adults
-20% are congenital
-10x more common in Caucasians
-solitary (80%) or multiple, red-brown, firm, rubbery dermal nodules
-predilection for head, neck, upper trunk, proximal part of limbs

Histopathology
-non-encapsulated dermal nodule
-**histiocytic proliferation** with **admixed lymphocytes** and **scattered eosinophils**
-many histiocytes have foamy cytoplasm (**xanthoma cells**)
-scattered **Touton giant cells** (giant cells with **"wreath-like"** nuclei and foamy xanthomatous cytoplasm)

Note: xanthoma disseminatum and **benign cephalic histiocytosis** have same histology

RETICULOHISTIOCYTOMA (LIPOID DERMATOARTHRITIS)

Solitary reticulohistiocytoma
-solitary, dermal nodule in adult men; rarely children
-predilection for trunk and extremities

Multicentric reticulohistiocytoma
-middle-aged adults (peak 50 years of age)
-skin lesions with destructive polyarteritis
-1/3 present with only skin lesions, 1/3 with only arthritis, and 1/3 with both
-extensive (few to few hundreds) red brown papules and nodules that may ulcerate
-predilection for fingers, hands, and face
-characteristic "coral beads" around nail folds

Histopathology
-non-encapsulated dermal nodule
-nodule consists of **histiocytes** and **multinucleated giant cells**
-**giant cells** have eosinophilic glassy **"two-toned" cytoplasm** with darker center and lighter rim
-small number of lymphocytes and neutrophils accompany histiocytic cells
-**xanthoma cells are absent** (unlike JXG)

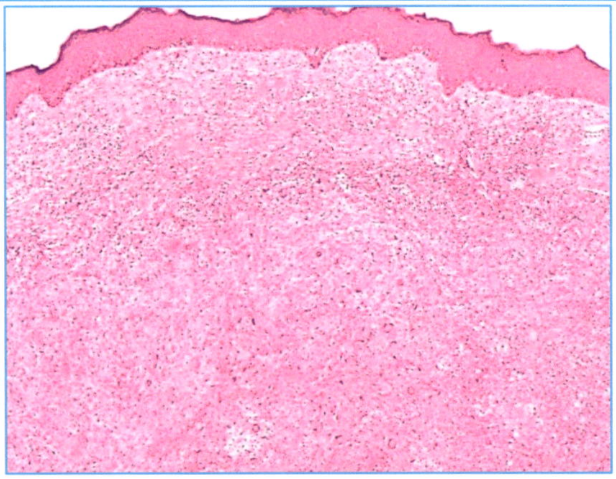

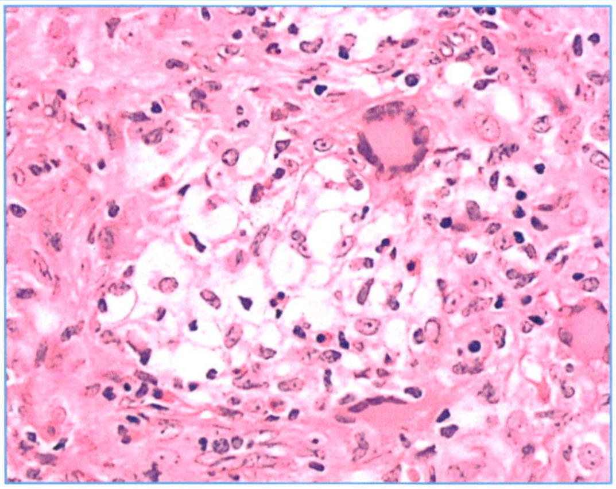

JXG with mixed inflammation containing histiocytes, xanthoma cells, eosinophils, and Touton giant cells

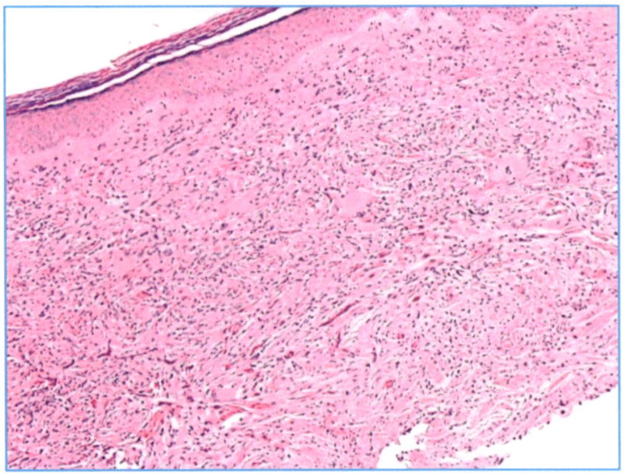

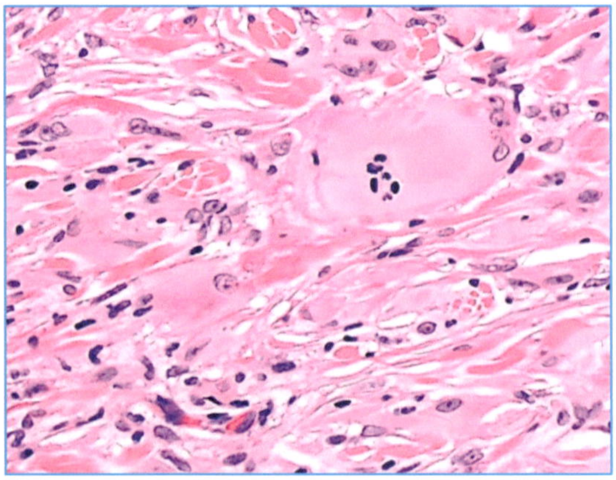

Reticulohistiocytoma with "two-toned" giant cells and no xanthoma cells

MALAKOPLAKIA

-chronic inflammatory disease due to macrophages' inability to kill ingested *E.coli*
-affects urogenital tract of older individuals
-rarely occurs in the perianal/periuretral skin

Histopathology

-diffuse superficial and deep histiocytic infiltrate with scattered lymphocytes and plasma cells
-histiocytes have abundant PAS+ eosinophilic cytoplasm
-laminated **calcopherites** inclusions (**Michaelis-Gutmann bodies**) within histiocytes are characteristic
-inclusion stain for iron and calcium and contain non-digested *E.coli*

ROSAI-DORFMAN DISEASE

-usually occurs in the first two decades of life
-cervical lymphadenopathy with fever and leukocytosis
-one third of patients, usually middle-aged, will have skin involvement
-yellow-red papules, plaques, and nodules
-eyelids and malar area are favored sites
-majority of lesions spontaneously resolve

Histopathology

-dense dermal **infiltrate of large histiocytes** with **abundant eosinophilic cytoplasm**
-**admixed lymphocytes, plasma cells, and neutrophils**
-characteristic phagocytosis of lymphocytes and plasma cells by **"bean bag"** histiocytes (**emperipolesis**)
-histiocytes are **CD68 and S100 positive** and **CD1A negative**

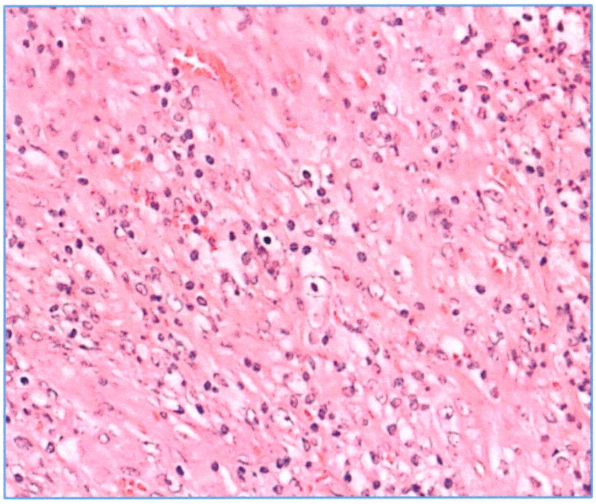

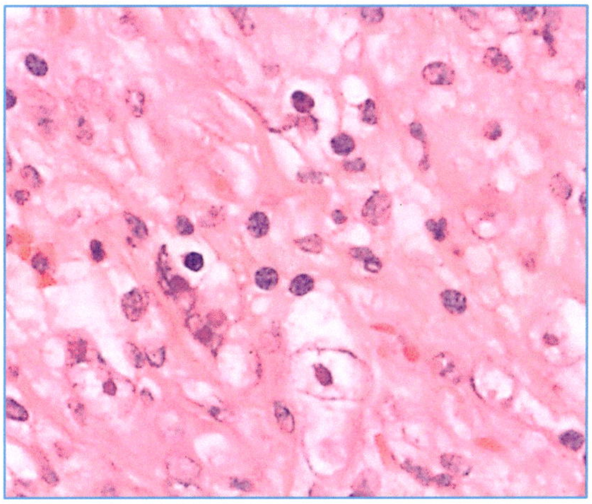

Malakoplakia with diffuse histiocytes with calcopherites inclusions

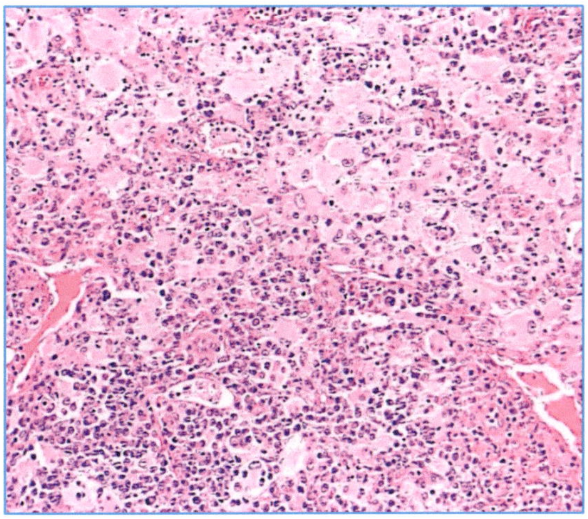

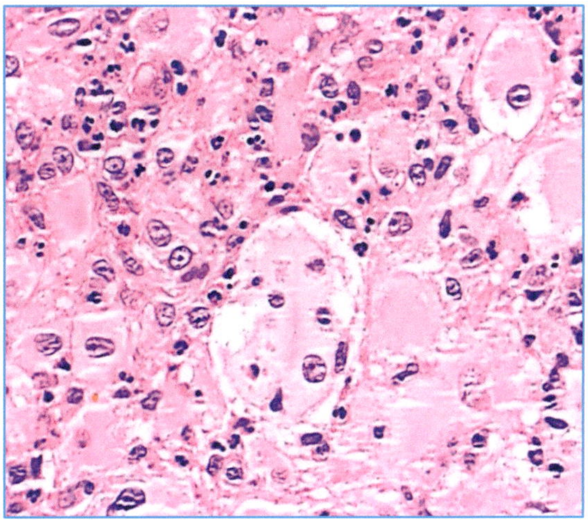

Rosai-Dorfman disease with "bean bag" histiocytes

Histiocytic tumors

XANTHOMAS

Various clinical presentations, some associated with hyperlipidemia due to genetic defect or abnormal metabolism

Xanthelasma

-plane xanthoma of periorbital area
-only half of the patients have hyperlipidemia

Eruptive xanthoma

-numerous eruptive yellow papules
-extensor surfaces, buttock, intertriginous area
-oral lesions common
-seen in patients with uncontrolled diabetes, alcoholism, or patients that are on oral retinoids
-associated with type I, IV, V hyperlipidemia

Tendinous xanthoma

-lobulated yellow nodules along the course of tendons (Achilles, extensor tendons of fingers)
-associated with type II hyperlipidemia

Tuberous xanthoma

-yellow pink nodules on elbows, knees
-associated with type II and III hyperlipidemia

Diffuse plane xanthoma

-predilection for trunk and neck
-associated with multiple myeloma with no lipid abnormalities

Verruciform xanthoma

-solitary flat plaque or warty papule
-oral cavity and genital area are favored sites

Papular xanthoma

-very rare disease
-yellow-red papules on face, trunk, and rarely oral

Planar xanthoma

-yellow soft plaques and macules divided based on location into:

Intertriginous xanthoma and Xanthoma striatum palmaris

-associated with type II hyperlipidemia (homozygous familial hypercholesteremia)

Histopathology

Xanthelasma

-groups or sheets of **uniform xanthoma cells** (foamy macrophages) with **no inflammation**

Eruptive xanthoma

-dermal infiltrate consisting of **xanthoma cells** with **admixed lymphocytes, histiocytes, neutrophils**
-presence of intracellular and **extracellular dermal lipid**

Tuberous and tendinous xanthoma

-histologically identical
-dermal **"sheet-like" infiltrate of xanthoma cells**
-**minimal or no lymphocytic inflammation**
-**extracellular lipid can be present**
-**fibrosis** particularly in older lesion

Diffuse plane xanthoma and planar xanthoma

-have identical histology
-**xanthoma cells** with **few scattered lymphocytes**

Verruciform xanthoma

-**verruciform appearance** with epidermal hyperkeratosis, papillomatosis, acanthosis
-tips of **dermal papillae contain xanthoma cells**

Papular xanthoma

-dermal infiltrate of xanthoma cells with variable number of giant cells

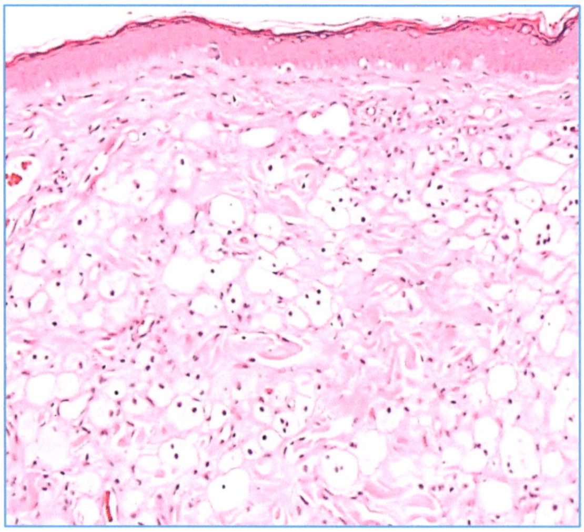

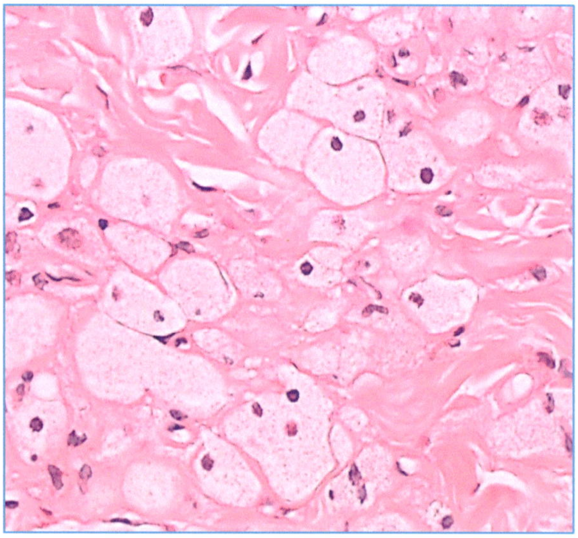

Xanthelasma made of foamy xanthoma cells with no inflammation

Chapter 32

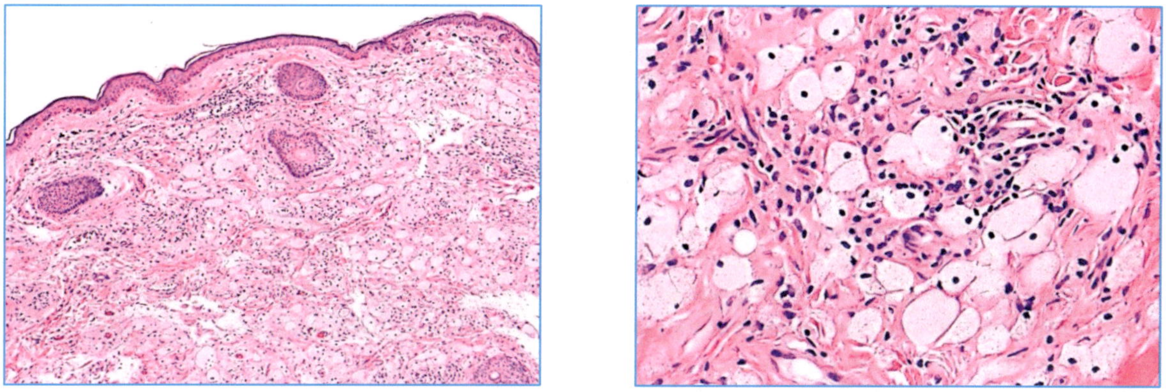

Diffuse plane xanthoma with xanthoma cells and scattered lymphocytes

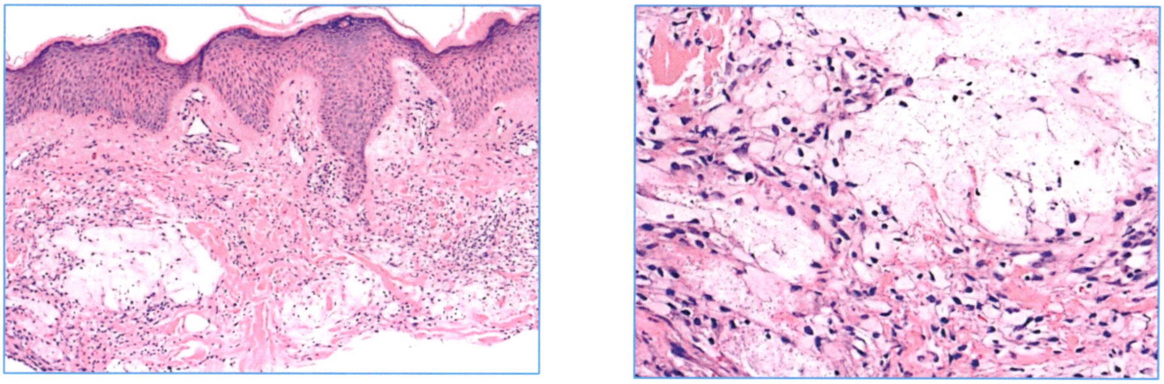

Eruptive xanthoma with xanthoma cells, lymphocytes, and extracellular lipid

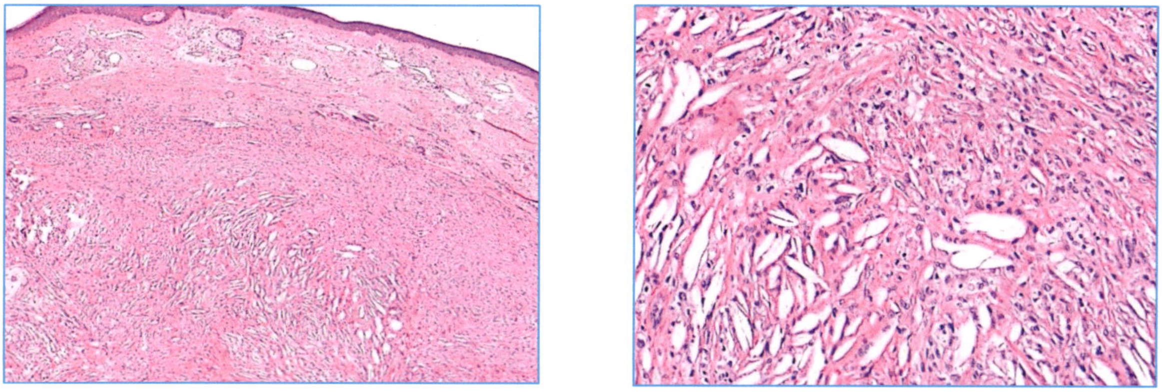

Tuberous xanthoma with extracellular lipid and fibrosis

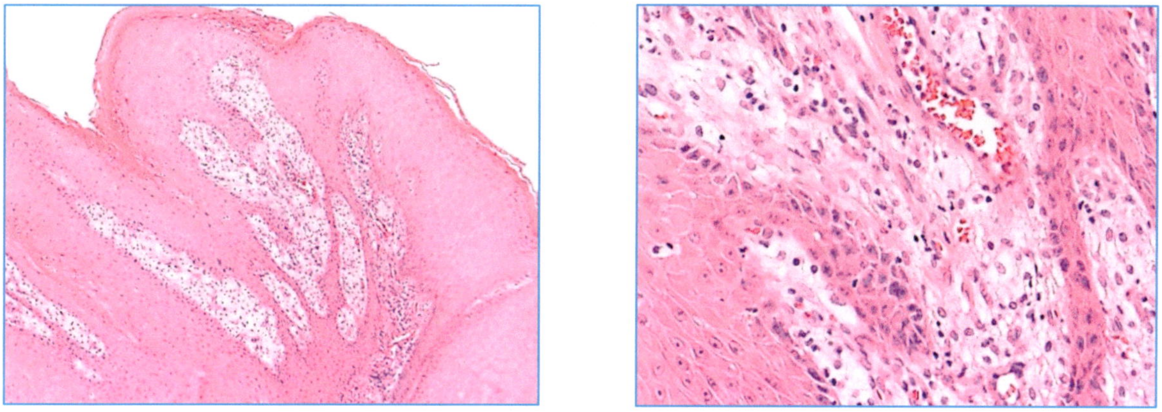

Verruciform xanthoma with xanthoma cells in papillary dermis

Histiocytic tumors

LANGERHANS CELL HISTIOCYTOSIS (HISTIOCYTOSIS X)

-rare histiocytic disorder with highest incidence before age 1
-new classification is based on number of organs (or systems) involved

Unifocal group

-in children with proliferation in one organ
-most common focus is in bone (called **eosinophilic granuloma** in old nomenclature)
-if present in skin it is called **cutaneous single system LCH**
(previously called **congenital self-healing reticulohistiocytosis or Hashimoto-Prizker disease)**
-solitary or multiple red or purple brown papules or nodules that can ulcerate
-spontaneous regression within 3 months

Multifocal unisystem group (previously called **Hand-Schuller-Christian disease**)

-children with fever, bone lesion, and diffuse skin eruption on scalp and ear canal
-skin lesions present as crops of pink yellowish macule and papules
-almost half develop diabetes insipidus and exophtalmus

Multifocal multisystemic group (previously called **Letterer-Siwe disease**)

-disease of infancy with acute course with poor prognosis
-disseminated visceral, lymph node, bone marrow, and skin lesions

Histopathology

-diffuse dermal and subcutaneous **infiltrate of histiocytes**
-abundant eosinophilic cytoplasm and some have **"reniform"** or **"coffee-bean"** shaped nuclei
-epidermal invasion can be seen
-admixed are **scattered lymphocytes and occasional eosinophils**
-giant cells can be present but are generally rare
-**tumor cells are CD1A, S100 and Langerin (CD207) positive and contain Birbeck granules**
(seen by electron microscopy)
-*BRAF V600E* mutation is present in 60% of patients and is predictive of poor prognosis

INDETERMINATE CELL HISTIOCYTOSIS

-very rare disease and usually limited to skin
-appears at any age as pink to red, variably sized, non-itchy, painless papules or nodules
-same histological features as Langerhans cell histiocytosis but unique IHC pattern
-cells are S100 and CD1A positive but Langerin (CD207) negative and there are no Birbeck granules

ERDHEIM-CHESTER DISEASE

-rare multisystem disease of adults with high mortality
-affects long bones, heart, and CNS with frequent exophthalmos and diabetes insipidus
-skin involved in one third of cases
-it represents extracutaneous systemic form of JXG although it can also present with clinical presentation and histology of LCH, diffuse xanthoma/xanthelasma, or reticulohistiocytoma

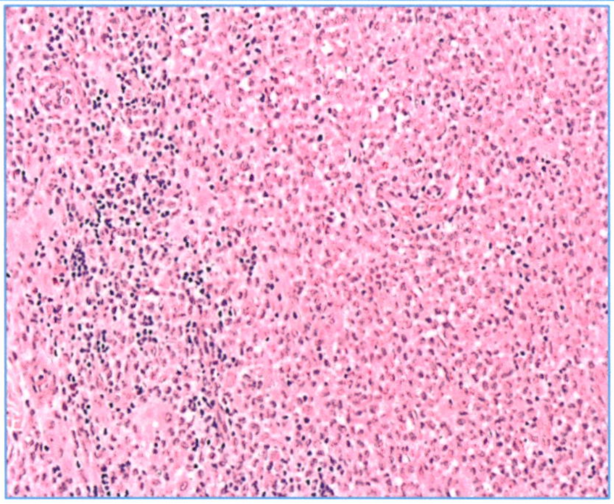
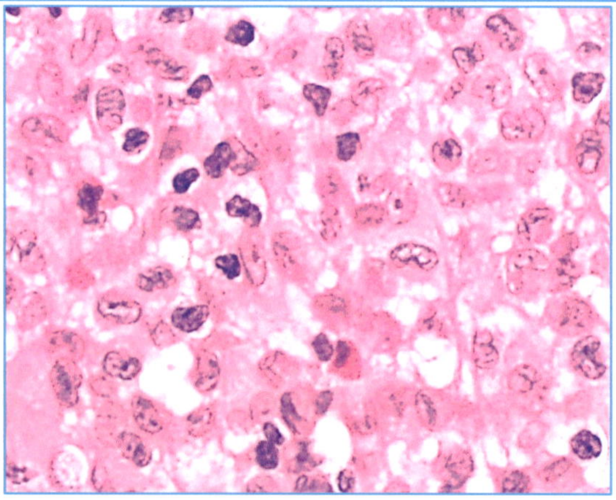

Langerhans cell histiocytosis with diffuse infiltrate of histiocytes, some with "coffee-bean" shaped nuclei, and eosinophils

MASTOCYTOSIS

-heterogenous collection of disorders
-can be divided in cutaneous and systemic

Cutaneous mastocytosis with four variants

Urticaria pigmentosa/maculopapular cutaneous mastocytosis
-most common type
-favor trunk and limbs
-more common in infants and young children
-it can occur in adults but systemic mastocytosis should be excluded
-yellowish red to yellowish brown urticarial macules and papules
-raised and erythematous when stroken **(Darier's sign)**

Diffuse cutaneous mastocytosis
-less common
-almost exclusively in childhood
-diffusely thickened skin, **"orange peel",** with no individual lesions

Mastocytoma of skin
-single lesion almost exclusively in children
-without predilection for site

Telangiectasia macularis eruptiva perstans (TMEP)
-variant that is **not officially listed in WHO classifications** of mastocytosis
-commonly seen in dermatology practice
-widespread itchy rash with telangiectatic macules on erythematous base
-can occur at any age but favor young adults

Systemic mastocytosis
-adult with multifocal bone infiltrates of mast cells
-cutaneous red brown macules, papules, nodules

Histopathology
All types (except TMEP) have similar histological features
-diffuse dermal/subcutaneous infiltrate
-round, uniform cells with centrally located nucleus (**"fried egg"**)
-mast cells stain with mast tryptase, CD117, Giemsa and toluidine blue
Telangiectasia macularis eruptiva perstans
-dermal telangiectasis with increased number of perivascular mast cells (>10 in high power field)

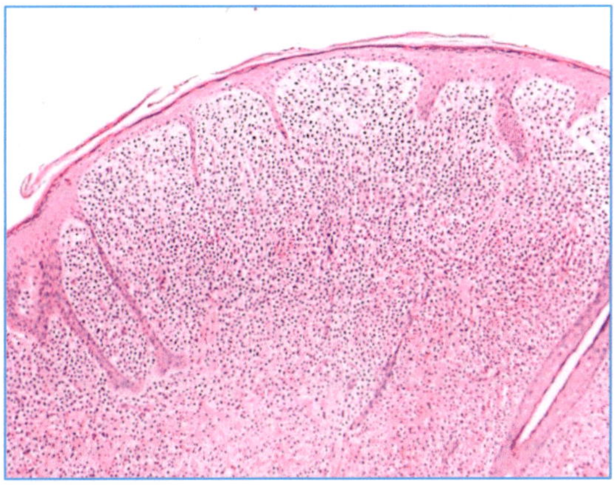

Mastocytosis with diffuse infiltrate of uniform "fried egg" mast cells

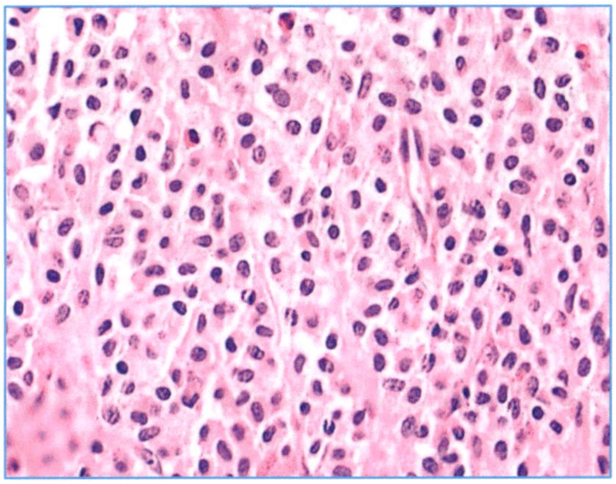

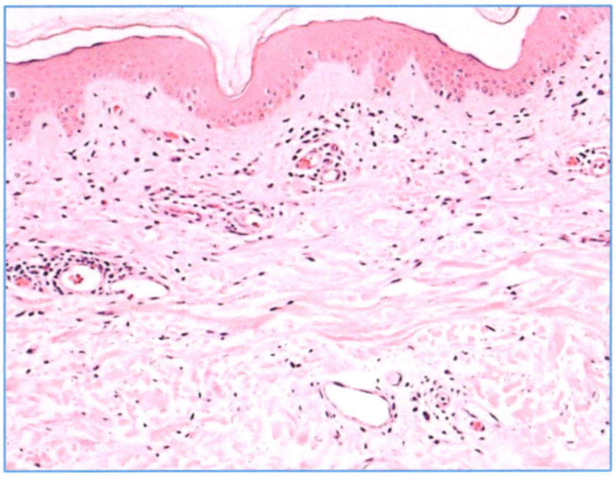

TMEP with dermal telangiectasias and increased number of perivascular mast cells

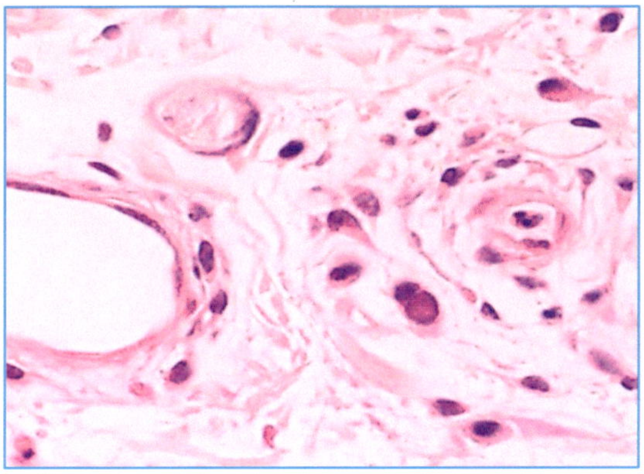

Histiocytic tumors

HOW TO APPROACH DIFFUSE HISTIOCYTIC OR XANTHOMATOUS PROCESS

IF YOU SEE NUMEROUS XANTHOMA CELLS

only xanthoma cells	**-xanthelasma**	periorbital
	-tuberous xanthoma	elbow, knee variable extracellular lipid and fibrosis
	-tendinous xanthoma	Achilles variable extracellular lipid and fibrosis
xanthoma cells + few lymphocytes	**-plane xanthoma**	trunk
	-intertriginous xanthoma	folds
	-palmar xanthoma	palms
xanthoma cells + lymphocytes + neutrophils +extracellular lipid	**-eruptive xanthoma**	numerous papules
xanthoma cells + variable giant cells	**-papular xanthoma**	
verrucous epidermis + xanthoma cells in dermal papillae	**-verruciform xanthoma**	

IF YOU SEE HISTIOCYTES, EOSINOPHILS, TOUTON GIANT CELLS, AND SOME XANTHOMA CELLS

-xanthogranuloma	solitary
-xanthoma disseminatum	numerous lesions + mucosa
-benign cephalic histiocytosis	numerous lesions in infants

IF YOU SEE HISTIOCYTES WITH "TWO TONED" PINK GIANT CELLS AND NO XANTHOMA CELLS

-reticulohistiocytoma

IF YOU SEE DIFFUSE HISTIOCYTES AND NO XANTHOMA CELLS

-Rosai-Dorfman disease	pale histiocytes, lymphocytes and neutrophils with emperipolesis
-malakoplakia	lymphocytes and histiocytes with calcopherites
-Langerhans cells histiocytosis	"kidney-shaped" histiocytes, lymphocytes and eosinophils

"HISTIOCYTES-LIKE" CELLS WITH FINE GRANULAR CYTOPLASM

-cutaneous mastocytosis	diffuse mastocytic infiltrate
-TMEP	dermal telangiectasia with perivascular mast cells

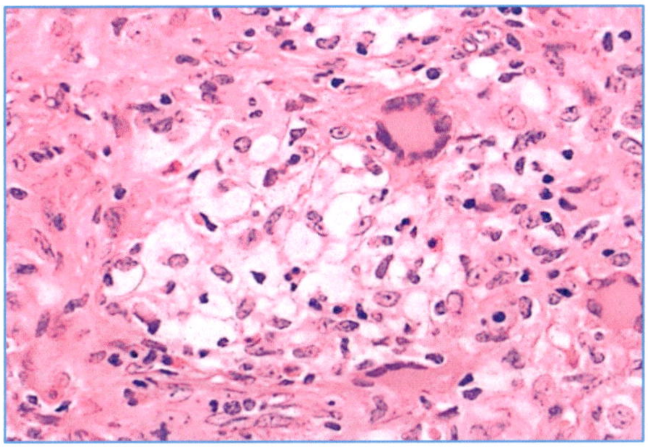

Xanthogranuloma with Touton giant cells

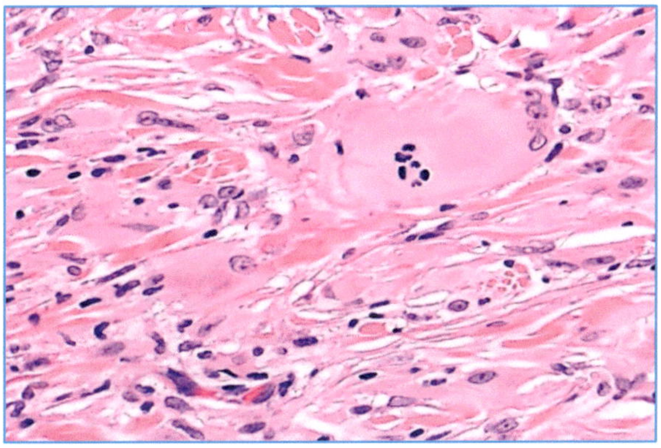

Reticulohistiocytoma with giant cell with pink cytoplasm

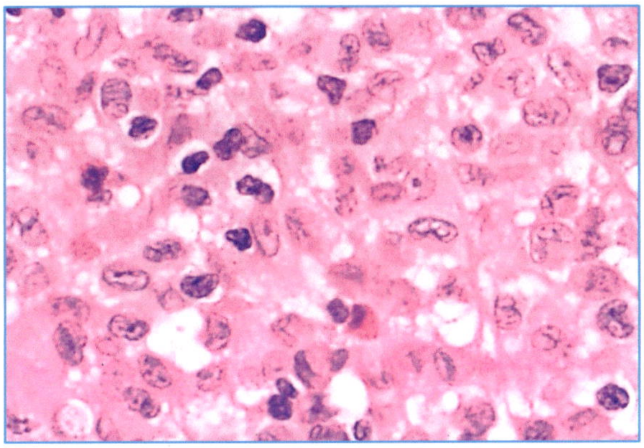

Langerhans cell histiocytosis with "kidney shaped" histiocytes and eosinophils

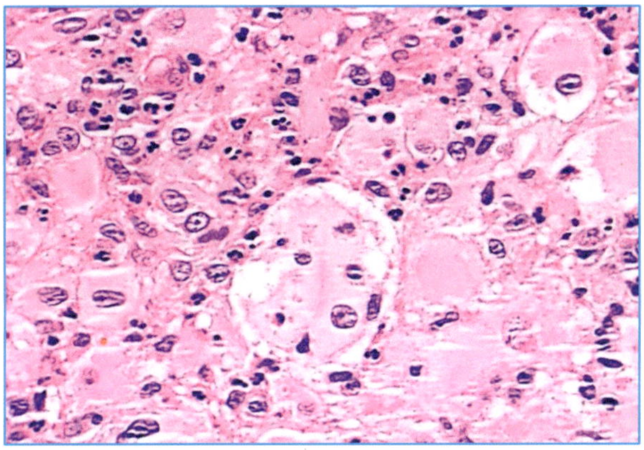

Rosai Dorfman disease with emperipolesis

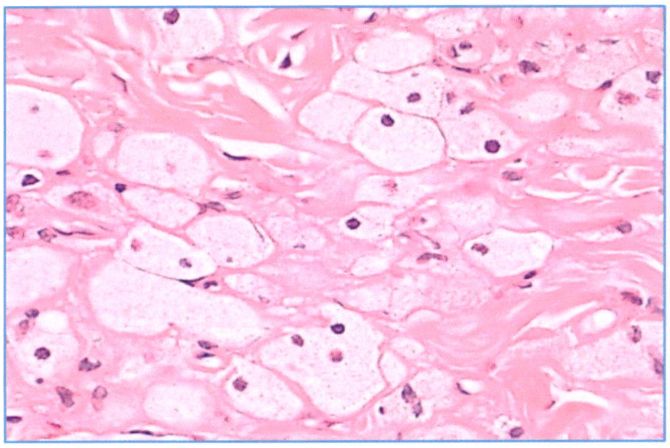

Xanthelasma with plane xanthoma cells

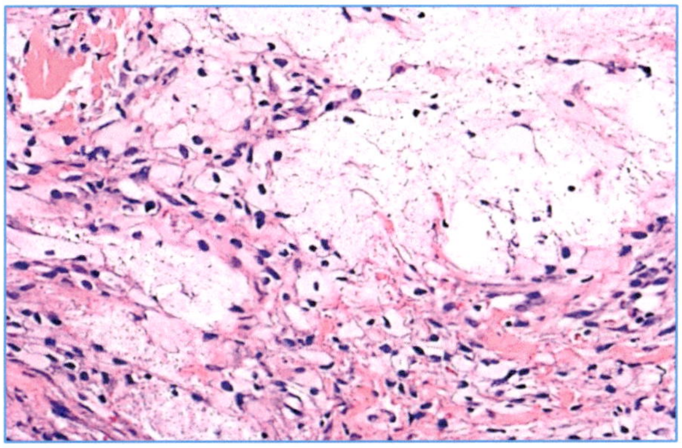

Eruptive xanthoma with xanthoma cells, mixed inflammation, and extracellular lipid

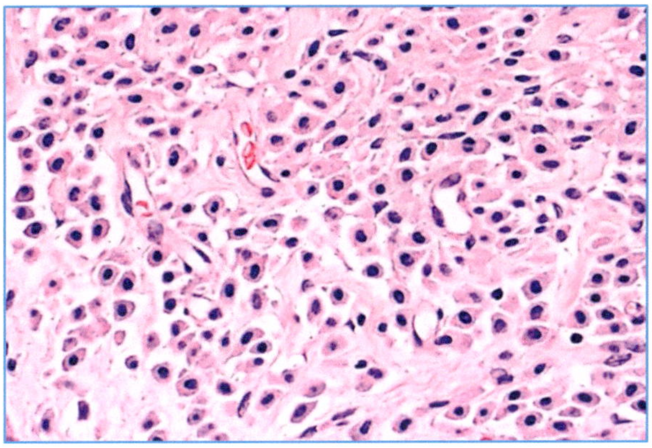

Urticaria pigmentosa with "fried egg" mastocytes

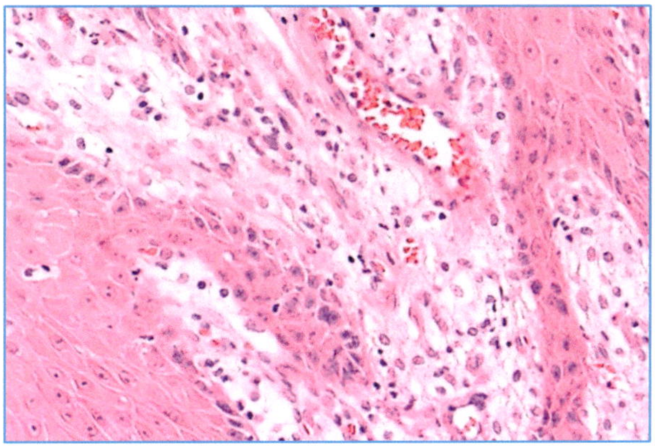

Verruciform xanthoma with xanthoma cells in dermal papillae

Histiocytic tumors

Chapter 33

LYMPHOPROLIFERATIVE TUMORS

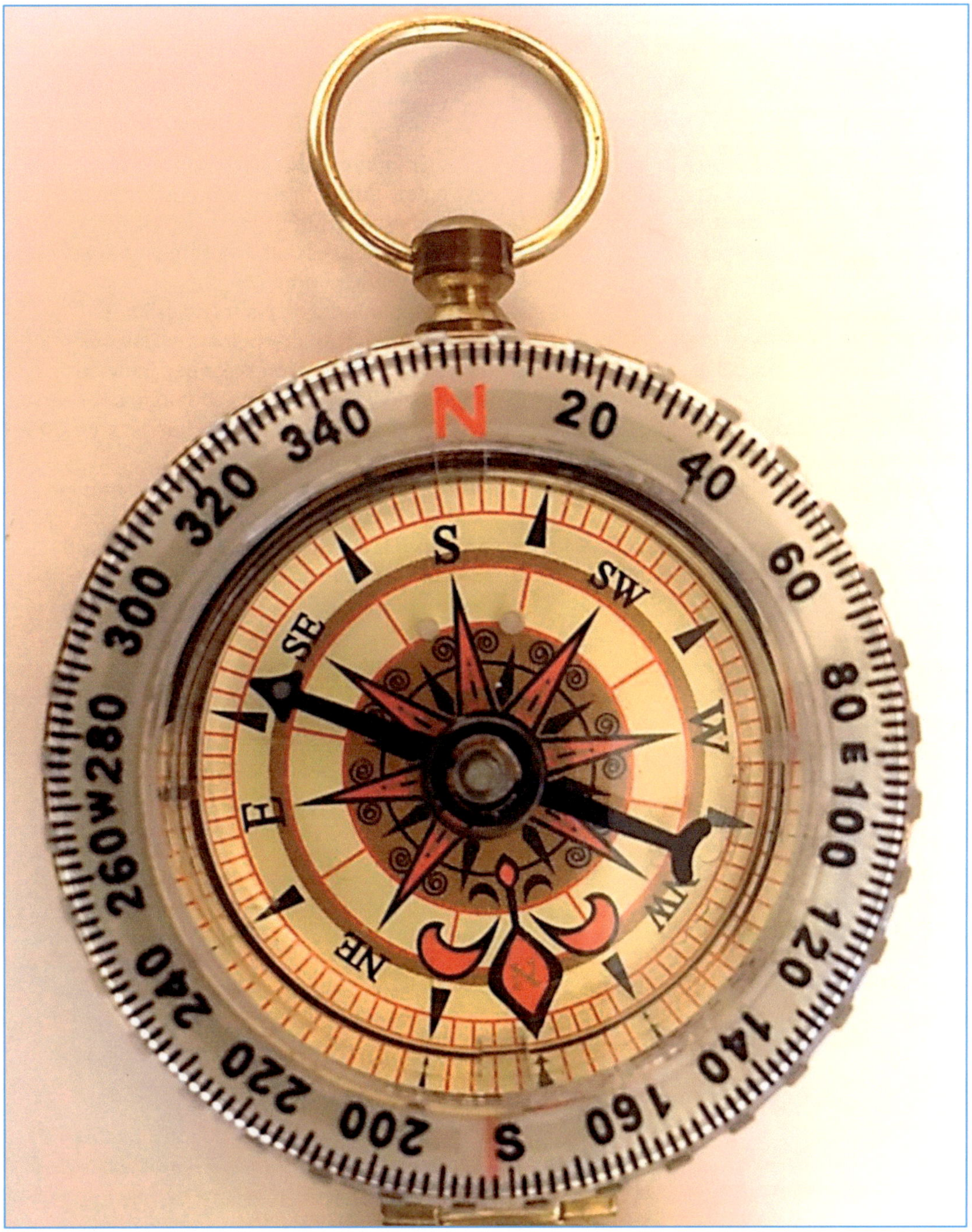

Lymphoproliferative tumors

MYCOSIS FUNGOIDES
(CUTANEOUS T-CELL LYMPHOMA)

-most common cutaneous T-cell lymphoma with indolent clinical course
-more common in middle-aged and elderly men
-lesions most commonly occur on the buttock, hips, and thigh ("double covered area")
-progresses through patch, plaque, and finally tumor stage
-initially presents as patch stage with irregular, ill-defined, large, pink-brown patch (>3cm)
-later, lesions may become thickened forming red to violaceous plaques (plaque stage) or progress to nodule (tumor stage)
-erythroderma can develop at any stage

Histopathology

-tumor cells of classical MF type are **CD3, CD5, CD4 positive and CD8 negative**

Patch stage

-lymphocytic epidermotropism (lymphocytes scattered in the epidermis and in a linear array along the epidermo-dermal junction)
-lymphocytes have dark nuclei and perinuclear clear halo ("lumps of coal on a pillow")
-few dermal lymphocytes and dermal fibrosis

Plaque stage

-**epidermotropism is more pronounced**
-lymphocytes are more atypical
-intraepidermal collection of atypical lymphocytes **(Pautrier's microabscesses**) are characteristic but are seen only in a minority of cases
-epidermis can show psoriasiform proliferation
-there is **denser "band-like" dermal infiltrate** with reactive and malignant lymphocytes
-dermal eosinophils and plasma cells can be seen

Tumor stage

-epidermal epidermotropism can be extensive but can be also lost
-**dense dermal atypical lymphocytic infiltrate**
-infiltrate appears monomorphic

Less common MF variants:

Folliculotropic

-associated with alopecia; can cause leonine facies
-atypical lymphocytes infiltrate the hair follicles and often spare the epidermis
-mucin is commonly seen in the hair follicle

Pagetoid reticulosis

-presents as psoriasiform plaque on the arm or legs
-hyperplastic epidermis infiltrated by numerous lymphocytes in pagetoid pattern
-cells are CD4+/CD8- or CD4-/CD8+

Granulomatous slack skin

-extremely rare with development of hanging skin folds in axilla/groin
-dermal granulomatous infiltrate with CD4+ cells

Hypopigmented MF

-hypopigmented patches solely or in combination with erythematous patches
-more common in darker-skinned individuals
-appears in younger adults with indolent course
-histology like patch stage MF but cells are **CD4-/CD8+**

Sézary syndrome

-pruritic erythroderma with lymphadenopathy and and **Sézary cells** in the blood, skin, lymph nodes
-Sézary cells are neoplastic CD4+ T cells with **cerebriform nuclei**

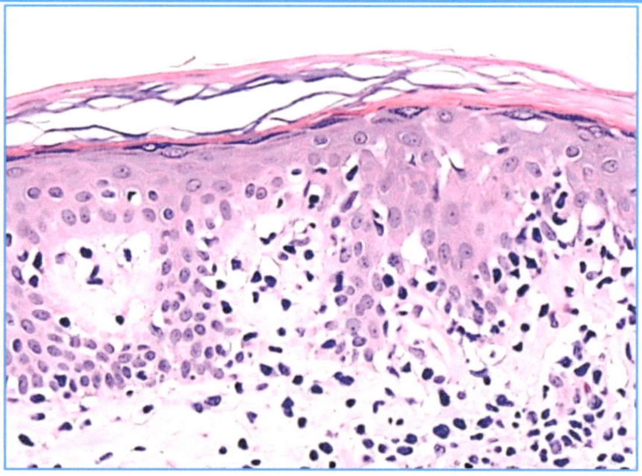

Patch stage MF with epidermal lymphocytes

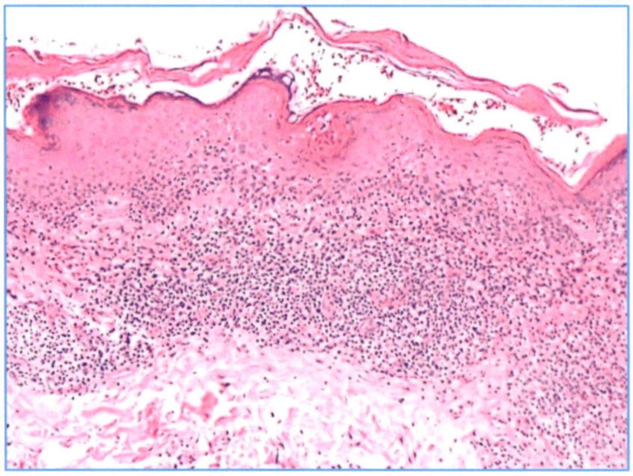

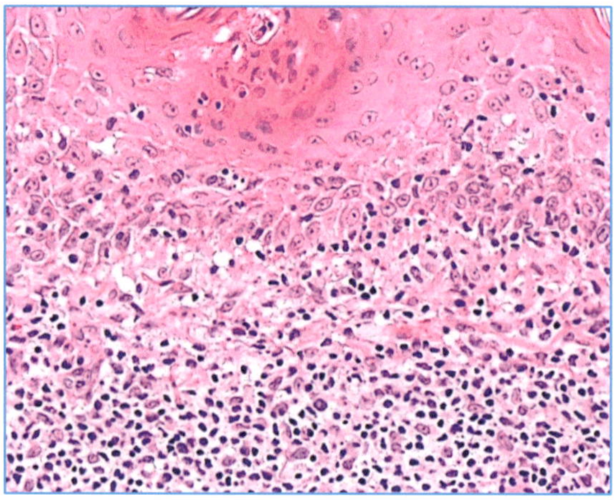

Plaque stage MF with lichenoid dermal lymphocytic infiltrate and scattered epidermal lymphocytes

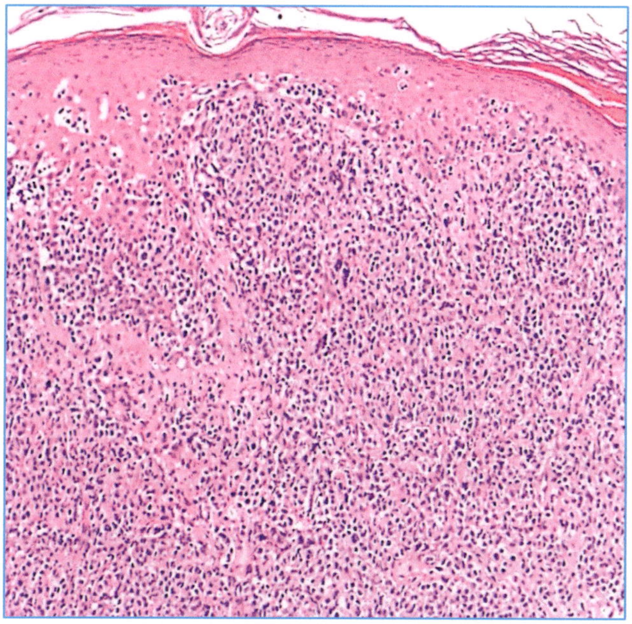
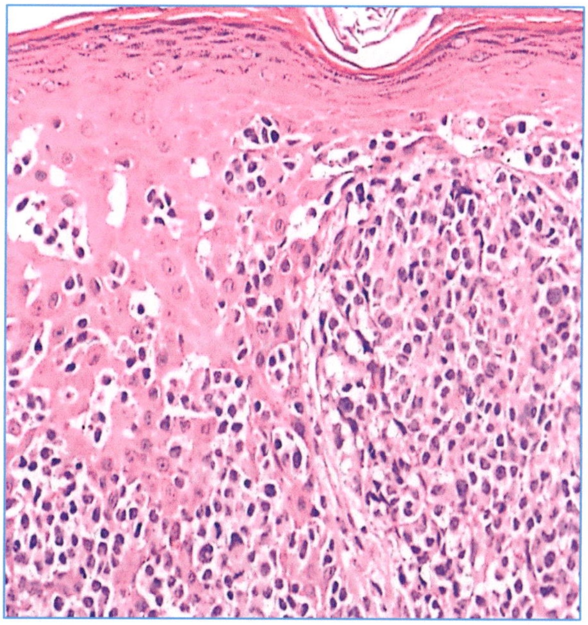

Tumor stage MF with dense dermal lymphocytic infiltrate and lymphocytic epidermotropism

LYMPHOMATOID PAPULOSIS (LYP)

-recurrent crops of red-brown ulcerating papules
-crops vary in number from a few to more than hundred
-spontaneously heal leaving scars
-favors the trunk and extremities
-more common in middle-aged men
-considered low-grade malignancy with good prognosis
-10-20 % have or will develop another lymphoma

Histopathology

-five types characterized by CD30+ cells (except type B)
-usually less than 30% of cells are CD30+ with exception of type C with majority of CD30+ cells

Type A (most common; 80%)

-"**wedge-shaped"** infiltrate of lymphocytes, some neutrophils and/or eosinophils
-scattered or small clusters of **large atypical** cells that are **CD30 positive but CD15 negative**
-they are also CD4 positive and CD8 negative
-large cells resemble Reed Sternberg cells of Hodgkin diseases (those are CD30 and CD15 positive)
-epidermotropism can be seen

Type B (rare: <5%)

-resembles early stage of MF (CD4+/CD8-/**CD30-**)

Type C (~10%)

-resembles anaplastic CD30+ large cell lymphoma
-cells are CD4+/CD8- and **most of them are CD30+**

Type D (rare: <5%)

-epidermotropic CD4-/CD8+ lymphocytes

Type E (rare: <5%)

-angiocentric and angiodestructive infiltrate of CD4-/CD8+ lymphocytes

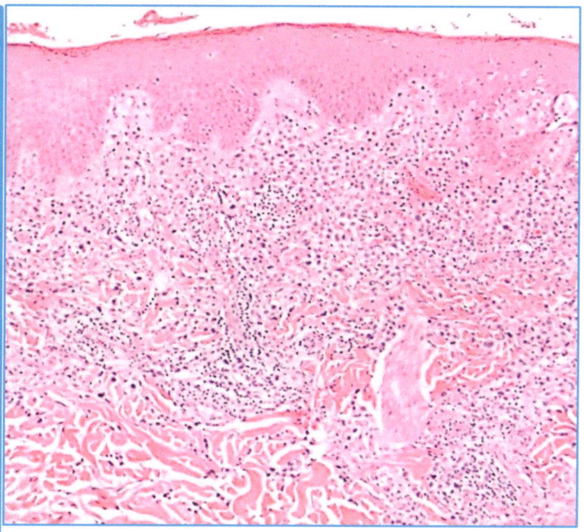

LyP, type A, with "wedge-shaped" infiltrate of large, atypical lymphocytes admixed with small lymphocytes and neutrophils

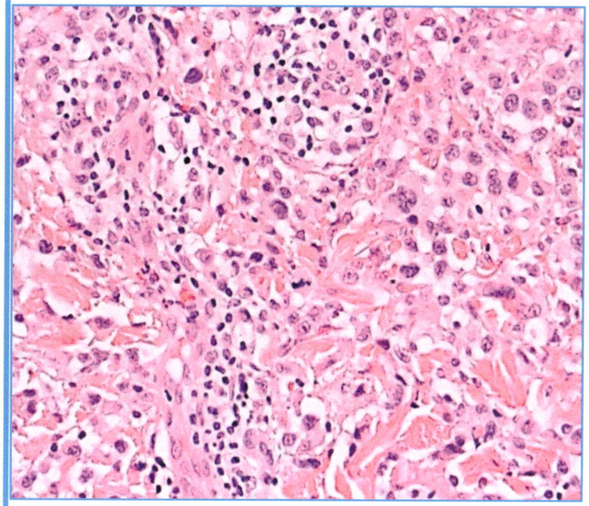

Lymphoproliferative tumors

PRIMARY CUTANEOUS ANAPLASTIC LARGE CELL LYMPHOMA (PCALCL)

-presents as a solitary, large, pink-violaceous, ulcerated nodule
-occurs on normal-appearing skin

Histopathology
-epidermotropism is variable
-there is diffuse dermal and subcutaneous infiltrate
-**cells are large, pleomorphic** with irregular nuclei
-by definition, **more than 75% of cells are CD30 positive**
-cells are also CD4 positive with variable loss of CD3, CD5
-majority are ALK negative, unlike the systemic form of ALCL that is ALK positive

SUBCUTANEOUS PANICULITIS-LIKE T CELL LYMPHOMA (SPTCL)

-subcutaneous painless nodules
-favors legs and trunk of adults
-tumor rarely ulcerates
-excellent prognosis

Histopathology
-diffuse, mostly **lobular lymphocytic infiltrate of adipose tissue**
-**lymphocytic rimming of adipocytes**
-lack of patchy germinal centers
-lymphocytes are CD3+ and mostly CD4-/CD8+

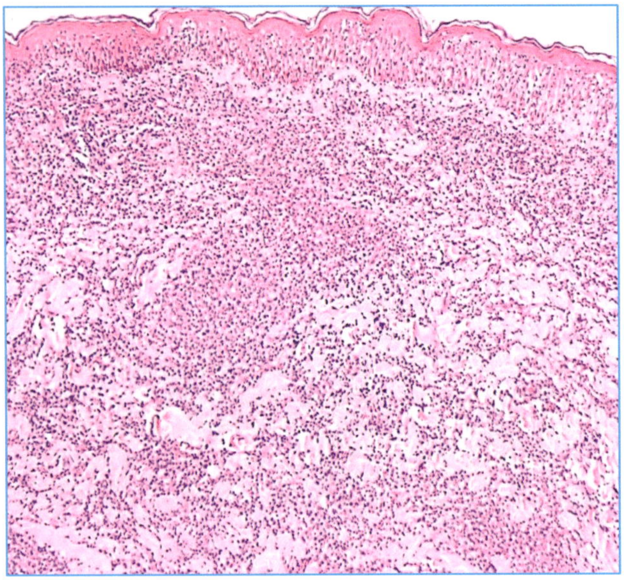

PCALCL with diffuse dermal and subcutaneous infiltrate

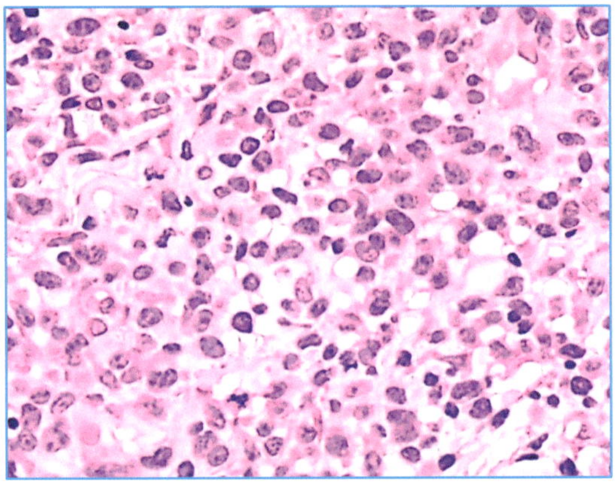

PCALCL with large, pleomorphic lymphocytes

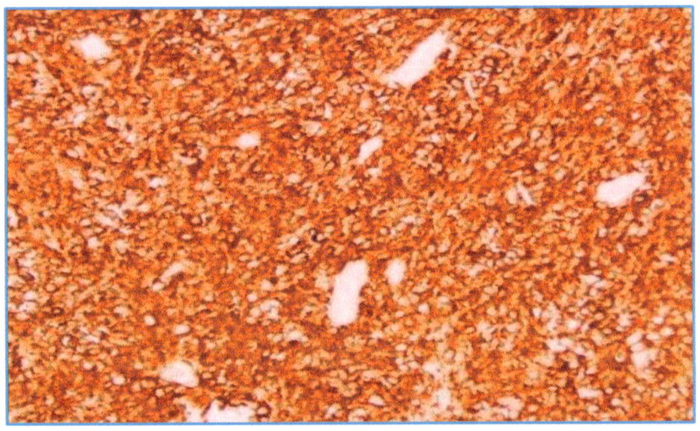

PCALCL stains strongly and diffusely with CD30 stain

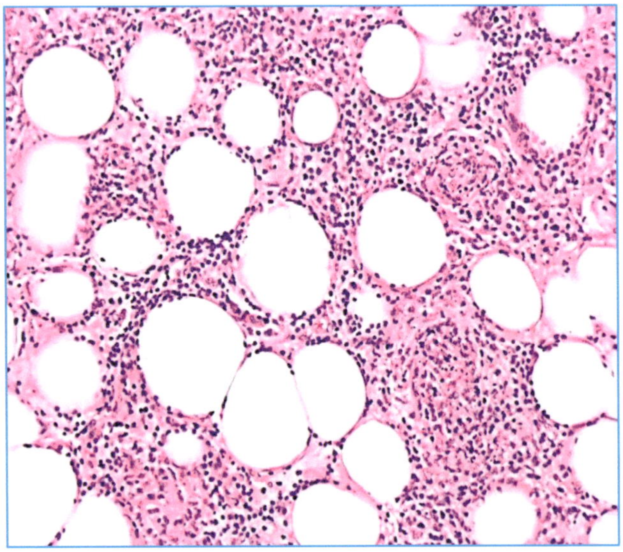

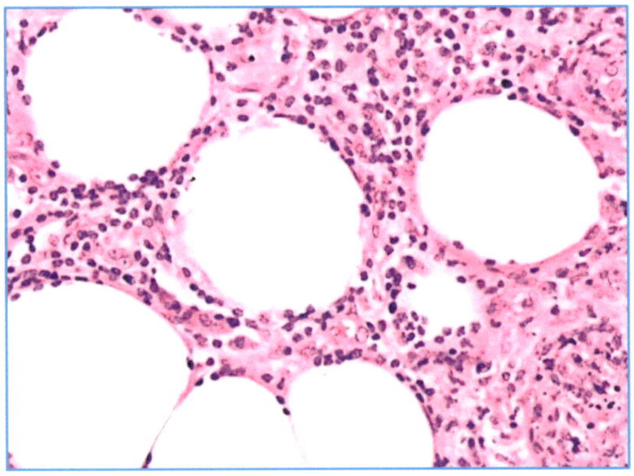

SPTCL with lymphocytes diffusely infiltrating subcutaneous lobules and rim adipocytes

ADULT T-CELL LEUKEMIA/LYMPHOMA

-rare disease endemic to Japan, the Caribbean, and central Africa
-linked to the prevalence of *HTLV-1*
-characterized by leukemia, widespread lymph nodes involvement, and hypercalcemia
-skin is involved in half of patients
-can present erythematous patches, papules and nodules

Histopathology

-perivascular (most common), nodular, or diffuse dermal infiltrate
-**epidermotropism** is common with "Pautrier-like" microabscesses , **similar to MF**
-**"floret" or "clover-leaf" shaped T cells can be present**
-cells are CD3 and CD25 positive
-most but not all are CD4+/CD8-
-***HTLV-1* is integrated** in the lymphocytes

EXTRANODULAR NK/T CELL LYMPHOMA, NASAL TYPE (ANGIOCENTRIC LYMPHOMA)

-rare disease
-more common in middle aged Asians and Central Americans
-strongly associated with EBV
-presents with symptoms of nasal obstruction or as a destructive necrotic midfacial lesion (lethal midline granuloma)

Histopathology

-involves epidermis, dermis, and subcutis
-diffuse infiltrate of tumor cells with prominent **angiocentricity and/or angiodestruction**
-extensive **necrosis is present**
-tumor cells are CD2, CD56, granzyme B, perforin positive
-CD3, CD4, CD5, and CD8 stains are negative

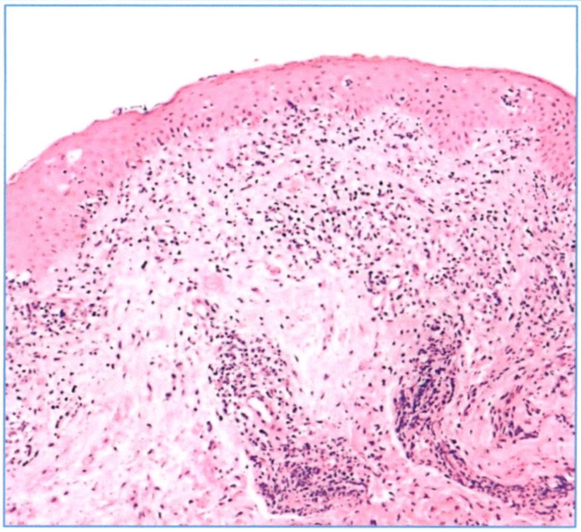
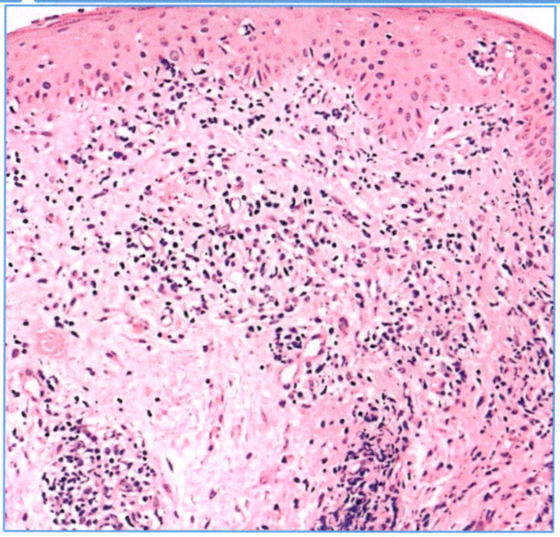

Adult T-cell leukemia/lymphoma resembling MF with epidermal lymphocytes and "Pautrier-like" microabscesses

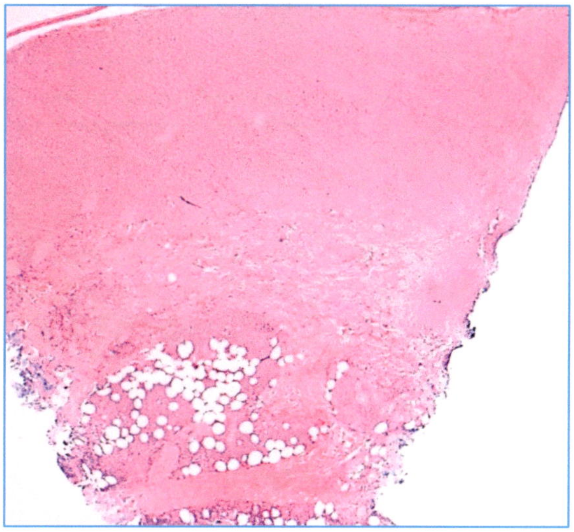
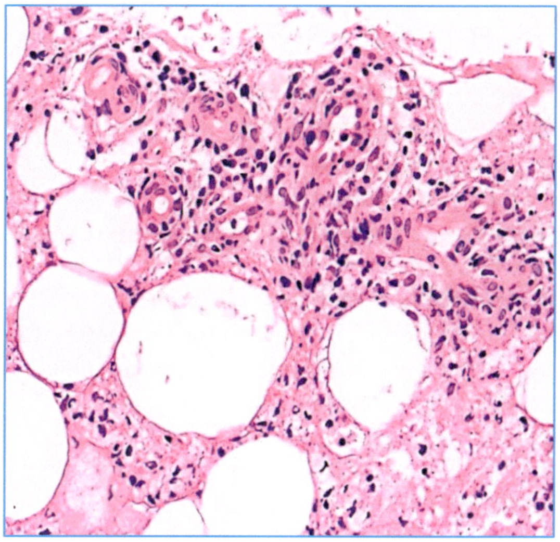

Extranodular NK/T cell Lymphoma, nasal type with necrosis and atypical lymphocytes around damaged vessels

PRIMARY CUTANEOUS PERIPHERAL T-CELL LYMPHOMA, RARE SUBTYPES

PRIMARY CUTANEOUS GAMMA DELTA T-CELL LYMPHOMA

-rare, rapidly fatal lymphoma, with most cases in adults
-favors extremities and presents with ulcerated plaques and nodules

Histopathology

-usually, a superficial dermal infiltrate with variable epidermotropism
-less frequently, a subcutaneous nodule with rimming of adipocyte similar to subcutaneous panniculitis-like T cell lymphoma
-tumor cells have **gamma/delta phenotype** and are **CD2, CD3, CD56, granzyme, perforin positive**
-CD4, CD8, and β-F1 negative

PRIMARY CUTANEOUS CD8+ AGGRESSIVE EPIDERMOTROPIC CYTOTOXIC T-CELL LYMPHOMA (PCAE-CTCL)

-aggressive clinical course
-disseminated eruptive hemorrhagic papules and nodules
-common ulceration and epidermal necrosis

Histopathology

-usually lichenoid dermal infiltrate with marked epidermotropism
-cells are **CD3, CD8, perforin positive**
-CD4 and CD30 are negative

PRIMARY CUTANEOUS ACRAL CD8+ T-CELL LYMPHOMA

-indolent clinical course
-most common in middle-aged men
-presents as a solitary reddish papule
-favors the ear (60%), followed by nose and feet

Histopathology

-dense, monotonous dermal infiltrate of medium size lymphocytes
-minimal epidermotropism
-tumor cells are **CD3, CD8, and TIA1 positive**
-CD4 and **perforin** are **negative**

PRIMARY CUTANEOUS CD4+ SMALL/MEDIUM T-CELL LYMPHOMA (PSM-TCL)

-solitary plaque or nodule
-favors face, neck, upper trunk
-by definition, no patches typical of mycosis fungoides

Histopathology

-**indistinguishable from tumor stage MF**
-needs clinical correlation (**lack preceding patches**)
-diffuse, dense dermal infiltrate of small/medium size uniform lymphocytes
-mild epidermotropism
-tumor cells are CD3, CD4 positive
-CD8 and CD30 stains are negative

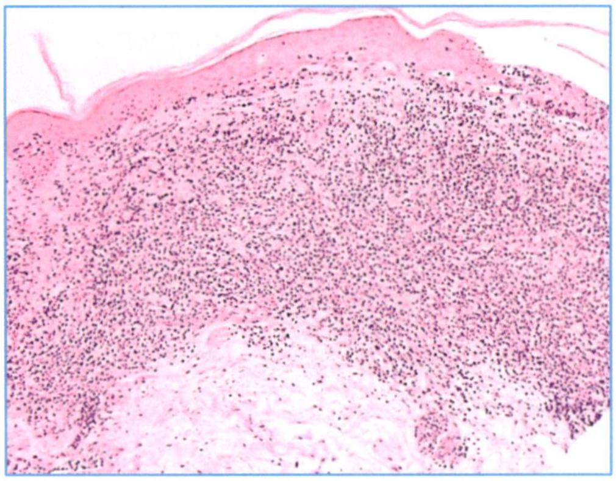

PCAE-CTCL with lichenoid infiltrate and extensive epidermotropism

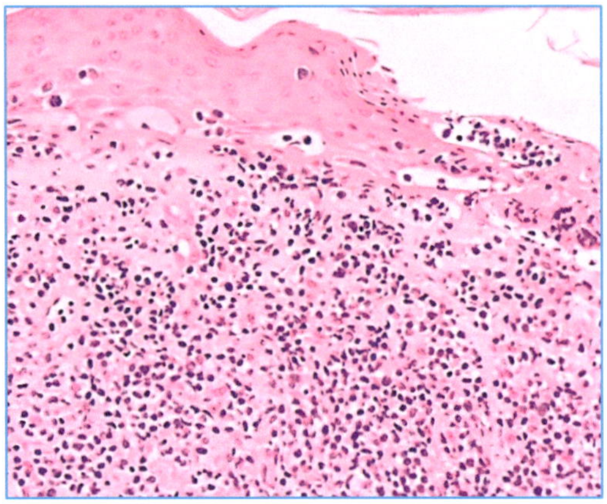

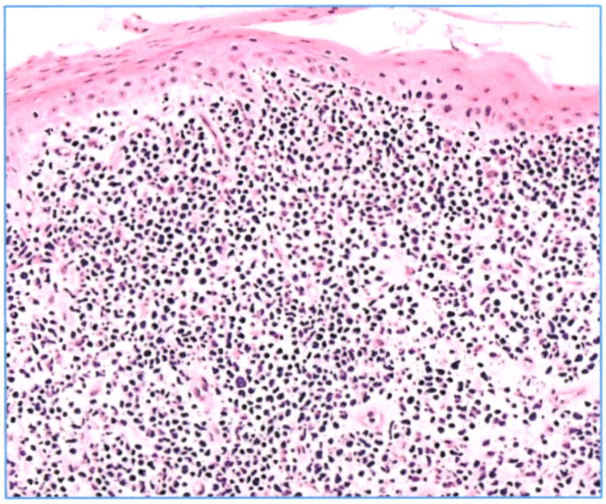

PCSM-TCL with small/medium lymphocytes and focal epidermotropism

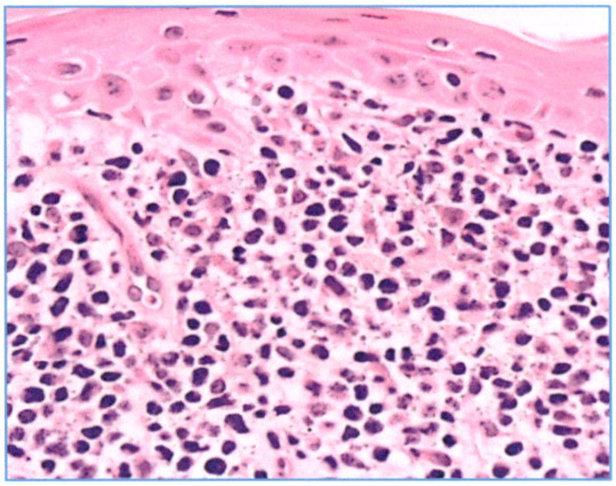

Chapter 33

LEUKEMIA CUTIS (CHLOROMA)

-localized or disseminated skin infiltration by leukemic cells
-any leukemia can cause it but most commonly occurs with acute myelomonocytic leukemia (M4) and acute monocytic leukemia (M5)
-sudden onset of pink-violaceous, small papules, nodules, or plaques

Histopathology
-poorly defined diffuse dermal/subcutaneous lesion with **Grenz zone**
-on gross cross sections the tumor can have a greenish color (chloroma) due to the presence of myeloperoxidase which oxidize after exposure to air
-made of **large myeloblasts** with atypical appearance (high nucleus to cytoplasm ratio) of "cells that do not belong to the skin"
-immunophenotype of leukemic cells depends on the type of leukemia
-**lysozyme and myeloperoxidase stains usually positive**

EXTRAOSSEOUS PLASMACYTOMA

-cutaneous manifestation of multiple myeloma
-constitutes only 1% of plasma cell neoplasms
-favors head and neck region of middle-aged men
-present as pink red plaques or nodules

Histopathology
-diffuse or nodular subcutaneous infiltrate of **malignant plasma cells** with eccentric nuclei
-**Dutcher bodies** (pink mass of immunoglobulin within plasma cell) can be present
-epidermis is not involved and **Grenz zone** is commonly present
-cytology varies from well differentiated to poorly differentiated
-tumor cells are **CD38, CD79a, and CD138 positive** and **CD20, PAX-5 negative**

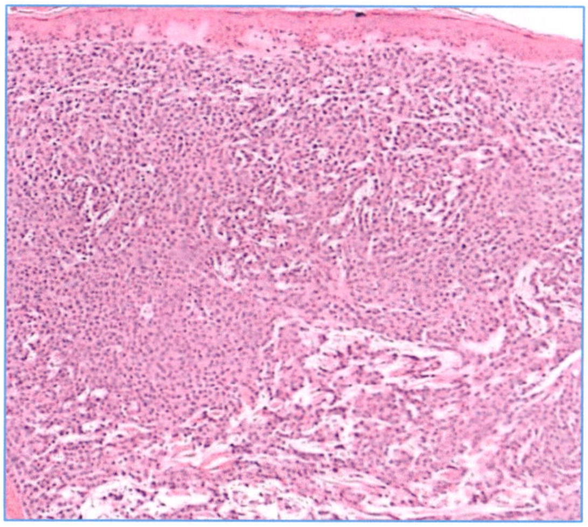

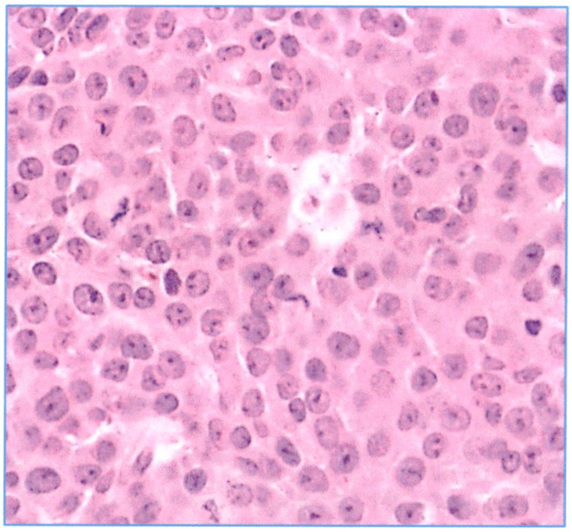

Leukemia cutis, AML M4, with diffuse sheet of atypical myoblasts with scattered mitoses

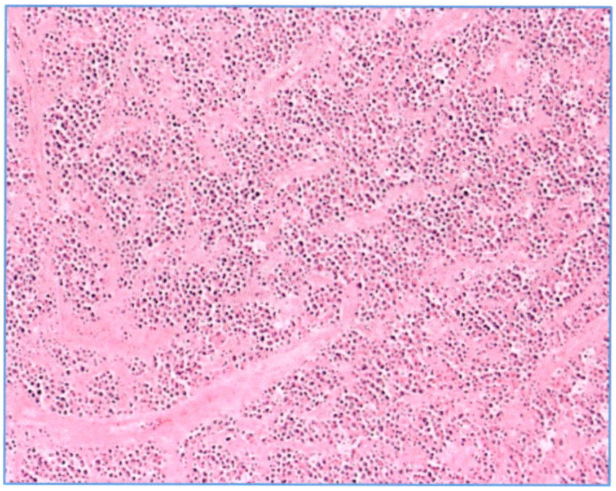

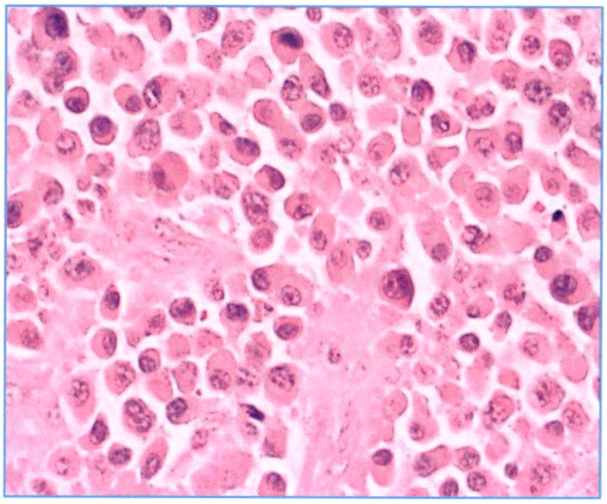

Extraosseous plasmacytoma with diffuse infiltrate of atypical plasma cells with eccentric nuclei

Lymphoproliferative tumors

CUTANEOUS B-CELL LYMPHOMA

There are multiple cutaneous B-cell neoplasms but all present with similar, nonspecific, violaceous plaques or nodules. Also, histopathology of all of them is similar with the exception of intravascular large B-cell lymphoma. There is sparing of the epidermis and extensive dermal lymphocytic infiltrate. Size of the cells and presence or absence of lymphoid follicles can give a hint about the subtype. However, **special stains are always needed to determine the type.** Multiple markers can be tested but these five need to be used first.

	CD20	CD10	BCL2	BCL6	MUM-1
PCFCL	+	+/-	-	+/-	-
PCMZL	+	-	-	-	-
PCMCL	+	-	+	-	+/-
DLBCL	+	-	+	+/-	+

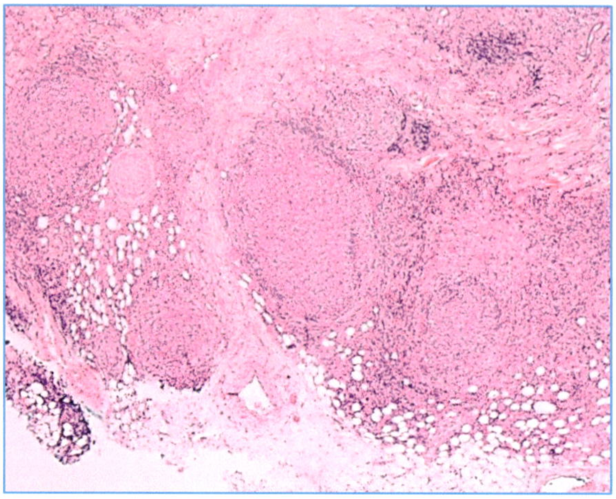

PCFCL with follicular growth pattern made of central larger pale and outer smaller darker lymphocytes

PRIMARY CUTANEOUS FOLLICLE CENTER LYMPHOMA (PCFCL)

-accounts for 50% of primary cutaneous B-cell lymphomas
-affects middle-aged adults with slight male preponderance
-favors the scalp, forehead, and trunk
-presents as erythematous plaque or nodule

Histopathology
-sparing of the epidermis
-shows a follicular or diffuse growth pattern
-follicle made of two kind of cells normally found in the germinative follicle
-**small to medium cells (centrocytes) and large lymphocytes (centroblasts) admixed with some normal small lymphocytes**
-tumor cells are CD20, CD79a positive
-Bcl-6 and CD10 are +/-
-CD5, CD43, Bcl-2, cyclin D1 are negative

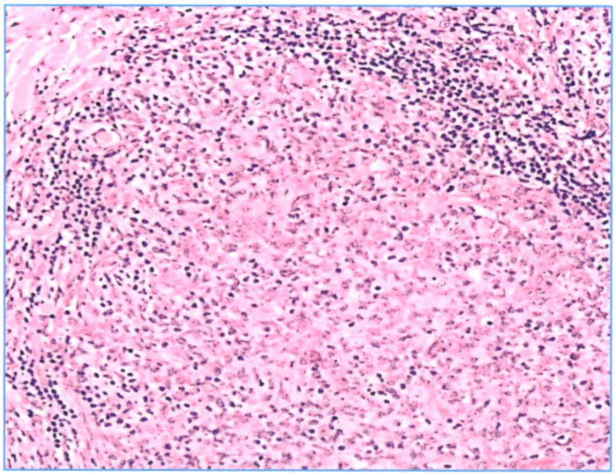

PRIMARY CUTANEOUS MANTLE CELL LYMPHOMA (PCMCL)

-primary tumors are extremely rare and most cases represent cutaneous manifestation of the systemic disease
-mostly in middle-aged and older individuals with a male predominance

Histopathology
-no lymphocytic epidermotropism
-diffuse dermal/subcutaneous infiltrate
-**small to medium sized lymphocytes** with irregular nuclei
-cells are CD5, CD20, cyclin D1, Bcl-2 positive
-Bcl-6, CD10, CD23 are negative

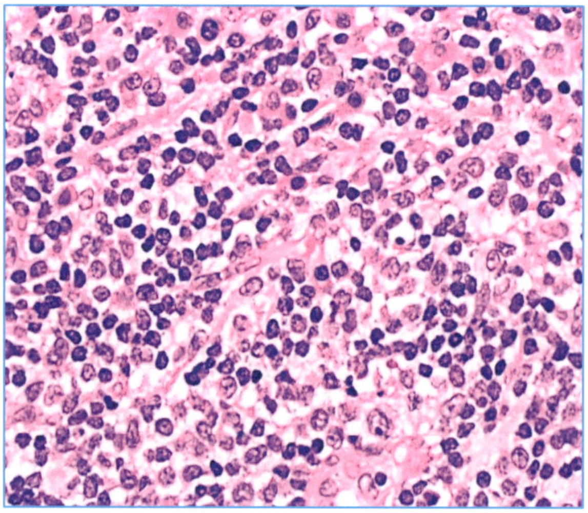

PCMCL with small to medium size lymphocytes

Chapter 33

INTRAVACULAR LARGE B-CELL LYMPHOMA

-very rare aggressive neoplasm of the elderly
-widely-disseminated extranodal tumor involvement
-skin and nervous system are most affected
-interestingly, lymph nodes are usually spared
-presents as purple patches or/and plaques
-lesions favor legs (particularly the anterior inner aspect of the thighs) and trunk

Histopathology

-large, **atypical lymphocytes within dilated dermal vessels**
-tumor cells express CD20, Bcl-2, MUM1

PRIMARY CUTANEOUS DIFFUSE LARGE B-CELL LYMPHOMA, LEG TYPE (DLBCL)

-presents as a red/violaceous, rapidly growing skin nodule
-occurs mostly in elderly females (male to female ratio in 1:3.5) and affects mostly the lower legs

Histopathology

-dermal/subcutaneous **sheet of large monotonous cells with irregular nuclei**
-infiltrate is sparing epidermis
-very few reactive lymphocytes
-mitoses are easily identified
-tumor cells are CD20+, CD79a+, Bcl-2+, MUM1+, MYC+, Bcl-6 +/-, CD10-

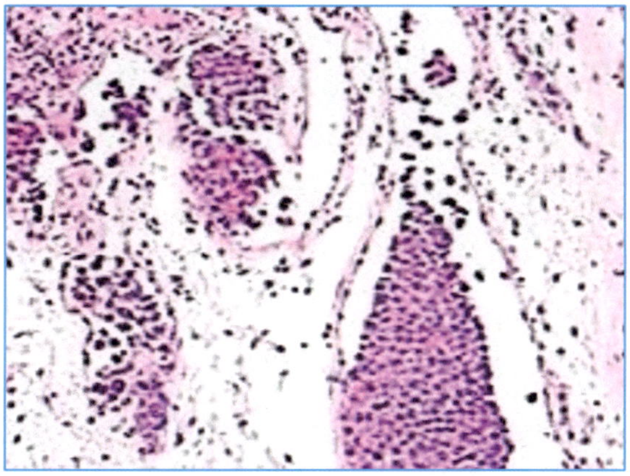

Intravascular large B-cell lymphoma with balls of atypical lymphocytes within dilated dermal vessels

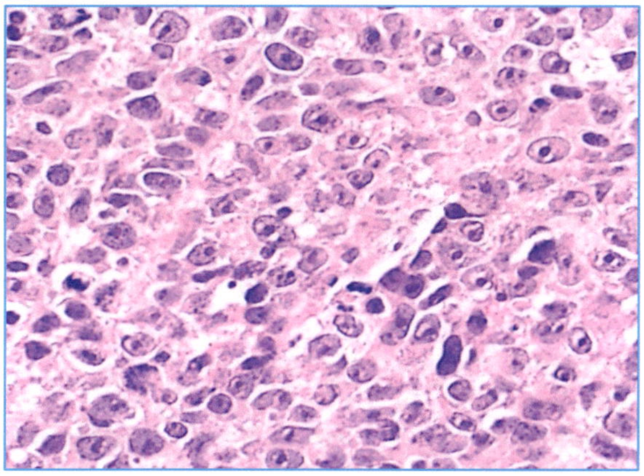

DLBCL with sheet of large, monotonous, atypical cells

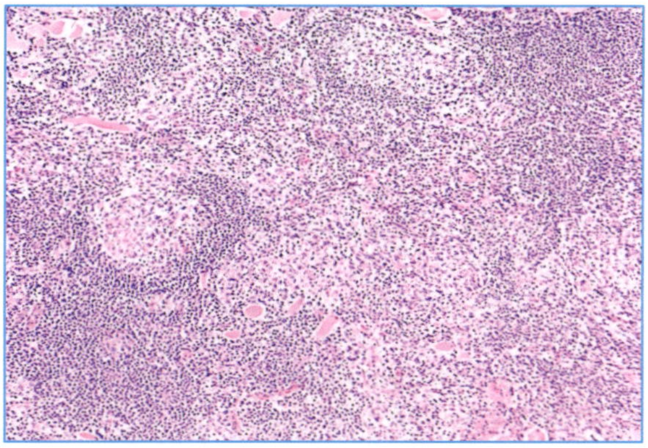

PCMZL with pale germinal centers surrounded by small lymphocytes

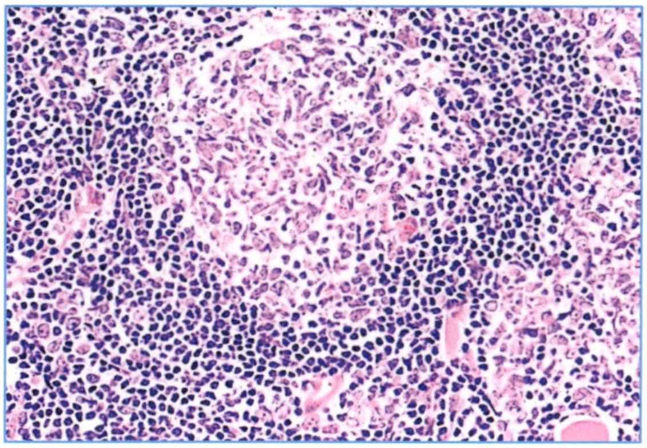

PRIMARY CUTANEOUS MARGINAL ZONE LYMPHOMA (PCMZL)

-the second most common cutaneous B-cell lymphoma
-in newest WHO classification it is not a separate entity but part of extranodal marginal zone lymphoma of mucosa associated lymphoid tissue (MALT lymphoma)
-MALT lymphoma presents most commonly as gastric lymphoma (50%)
-about 9% of MALT lymphomas are skin primary

Histopathology

-dense nodular infiltrate with **vague pale germinal centers** sparing epidermis
-they are surrounded by dark small lymphocytes and more peripherally with pale neoplastic marginal zone lymphocytes
-neoplastic cells are CD20, CD79a positive and Bcl-2, Bcl-6, CD5, CD10 negative

Lymphoproliferative tumors

HOW TO APPROACH TUMORS OF LYMPHOPROLIFERATIVE ORIGIN

IF LYMPHOCYTES INFILTRATE THE EPIDERMIS AND DERMIS

-T-cell lymphomas	lymphocytic infiltrate
-lymphomatoid papulosis	mixed cell population with CD30 positive cells

IF CELLS INFILTRATE THE DERMIS BUT NOT THE EPIDERMIS

-B-cell lymphoma	lymphocytic infiltrate
-lymphomatoid papulosis	mixed cell population with CD30 positive cells
-rare T-cell lymphoma	extremely rare, need IHC stains
-plasmacytoma	plasmacytoid cells with eccentric nuclei
-leukemia cutis	history of systemic leukemia

THEN DETERMINE

IF LYMPHOCYTES ARE IN THE EPIDERMIS WITH A MILD DERMAL INFILTRATE

-patch stage MF	patch

IF LYMPHOCYTES ARE IN THE EPIDERMIS WITH A MODERATE DERMAL INFILTRATE

-plaques stage MF	plaque
-adult T-cell leukemia/lymphoma	skin rash, endemic, HTLV-1 associated

IF LYMPHOCYTES INFILTRATE THE EPIDERMIS AND DERMIS

-tumor stage MF	few CD30 positive cells
-anaplastic large cell lymphoma	majority of cells are CD30 positive

IF DERMAL MIXED INFLAMMATION AND VARIABLE EPIDERMOTROPISM ARE PRESENT

-lymphomatoid papulosis	large CD30+ cells (<20%) with neutrophils, histiocytes, and eosinophils

IF MOSTLY LYMPHOCYTIC PANNICULITIS IS PRESENT

-subcutaneous panniculitis-like T cell lymphoma	diffuse proliferation unlike lupus that is patchy

IF THERE IS EPIDERMAL, DERMAL, SUBCUTANEOUS LYMPHOCYTIC INFILTRATE WITH PROMINENT VASCULAR DAMAGE

-extranodal NK/T cell lymphoma

IF THERE IS DIFFUSE DERMAL LYMPHOCYTIC INFILTRATE WITH NORMAL EPIDERMIS

-primary cutaneous follicle center lymphoma (#1 B-cell lymphoma)	larger follicles or diffuse growth
-primary cutaneous marginal zone lymphoma (#2 B-cell lymphoma)	smaller vague follicles
-mantle cell lymphoma (rare)	diffuse uniform lymphocytes
-diffuse large B-cell lymphoma, leg type	large atypical cells on the leg

IF BALLS OF LYMPHOCYTES ARE WITHIN DILATED DERMAL VESSELS

-intravascular large B-cell lymphoma

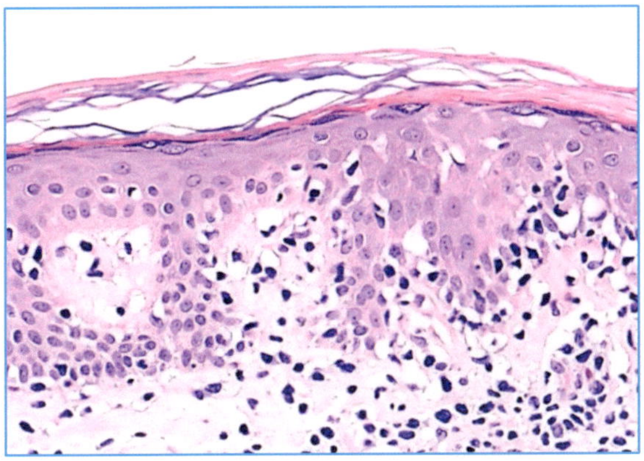

MF, patch stage, with epidermal lymphocytes

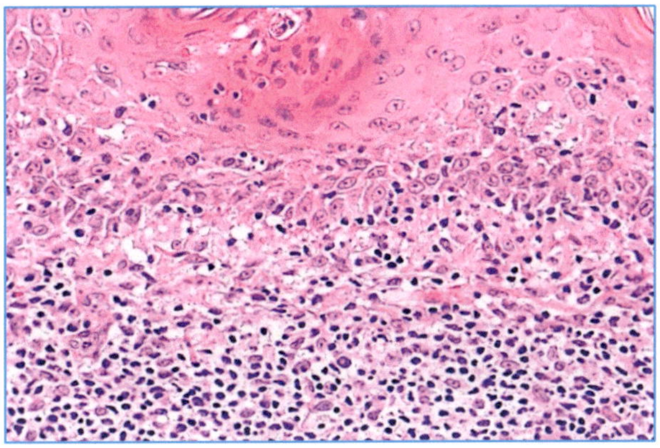

MF, plaque stage, with epidermal and dermal lymphocytes

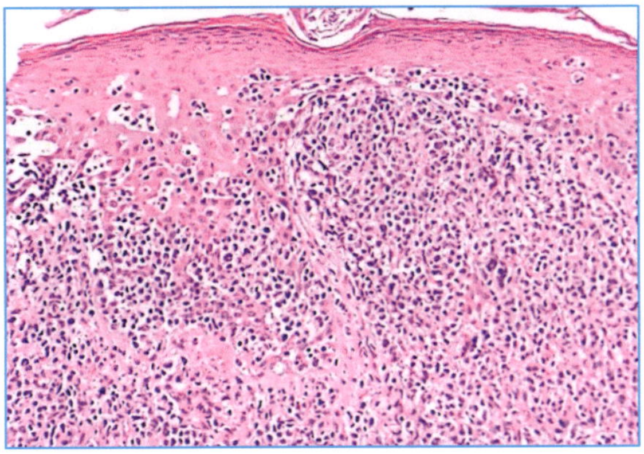

MF, tumor stage, with atypical lymphocytes forming nodule

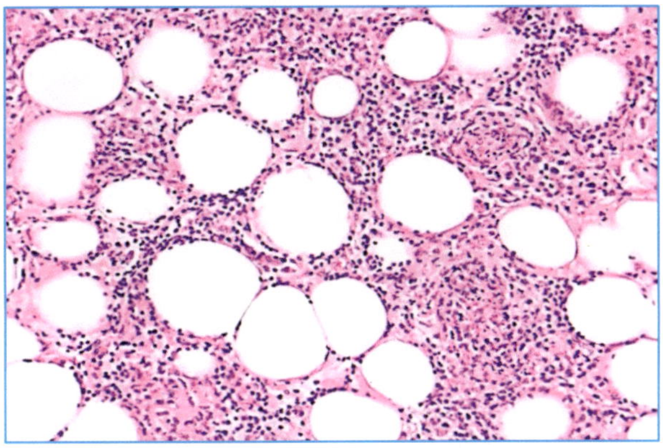

Subcutaneous panniculitis-like T cell lymphoma with lymphocytes infiltrating fat and rimming adipocytes

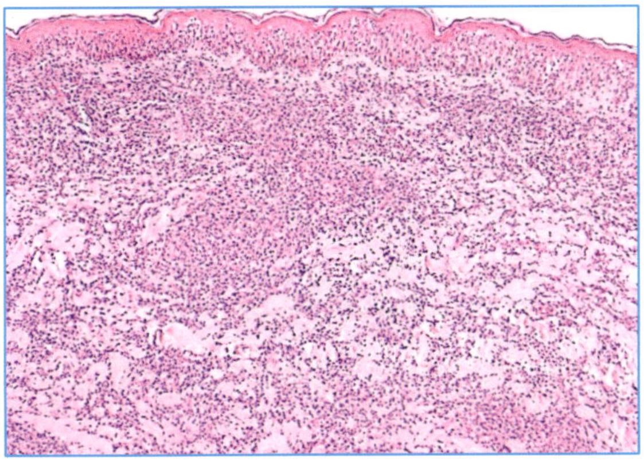

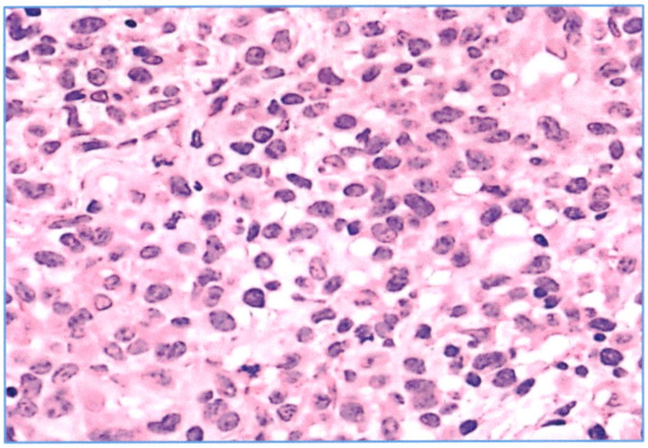

Anaplastic large cell lymphoma with diffuse infiltrate of atypical large cells

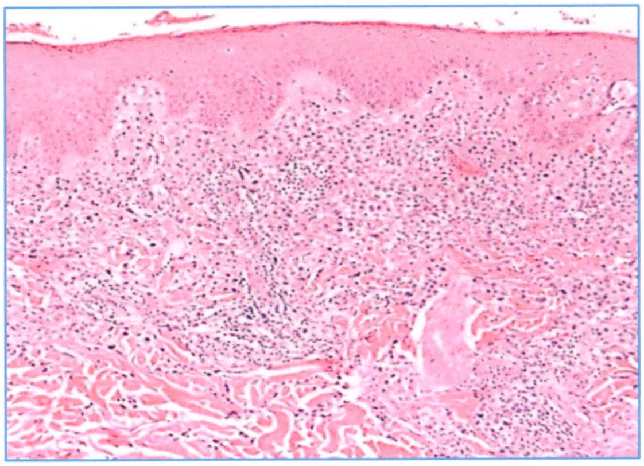

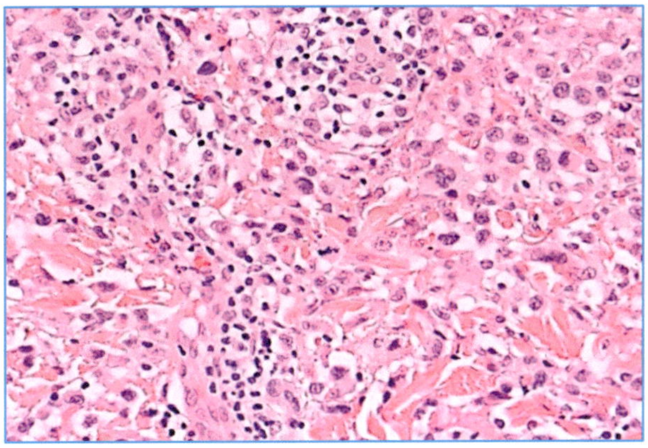

Lymphomatoid papulosis with mixed cell population with some large cells

Lymphoproliferative tumors

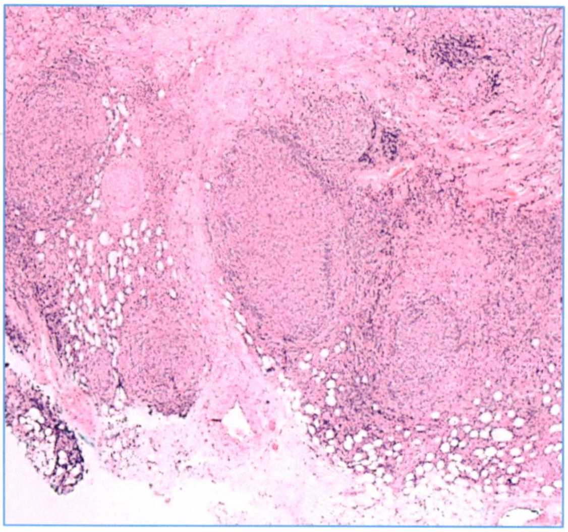

Follicle center lymphoma with large, poorly defined follicles

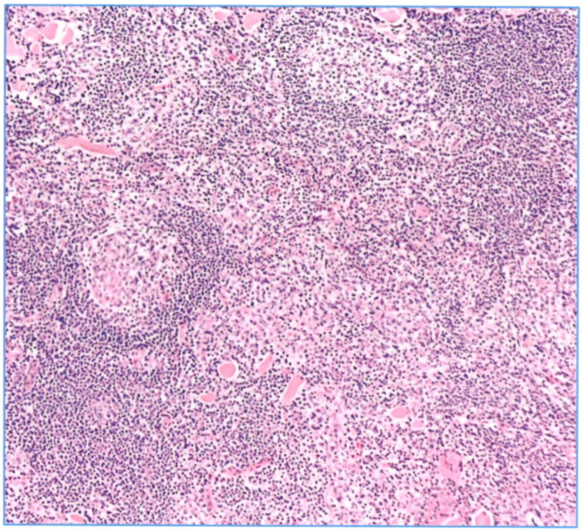

Marginal zone lymphoma with small, poorly defined follicles

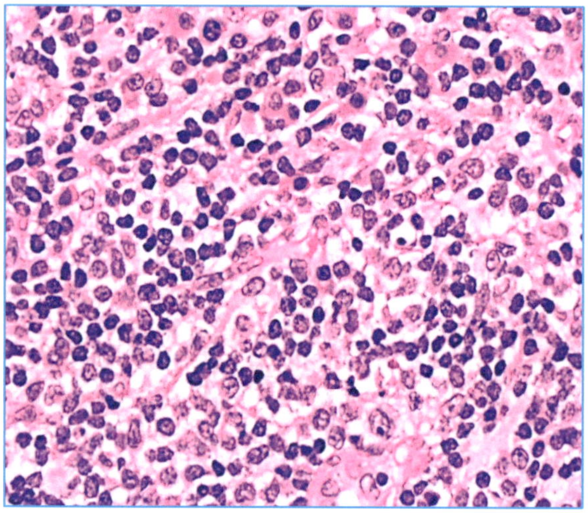

Mantle cell lymphoma with a sheet of small uniform lymphocytes

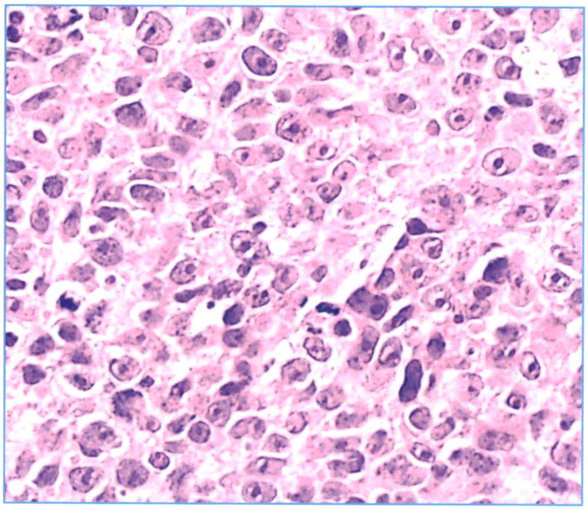

Diffuse large B-cell lymphoma, leg type, with a sheet of large, atypical lymphocytes

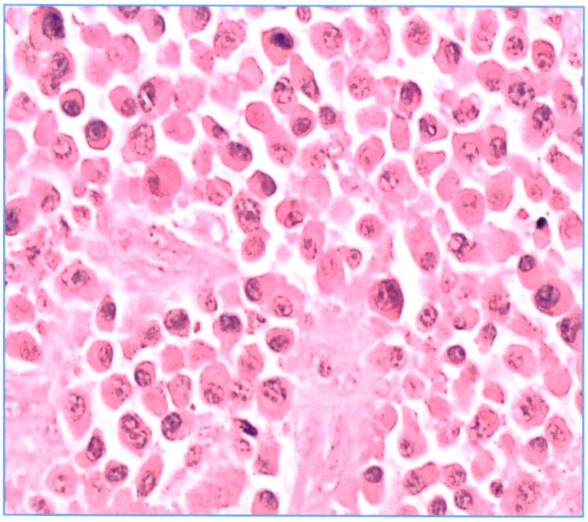

Plasmacytoma with plasma cells with eccentric nuclei

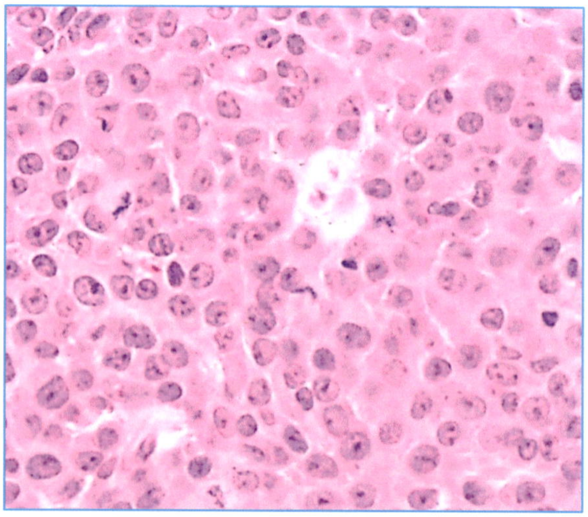

Leukemia cutis with atypical myeloid blast cells

Chapter 34

VASCULAR TUMORS

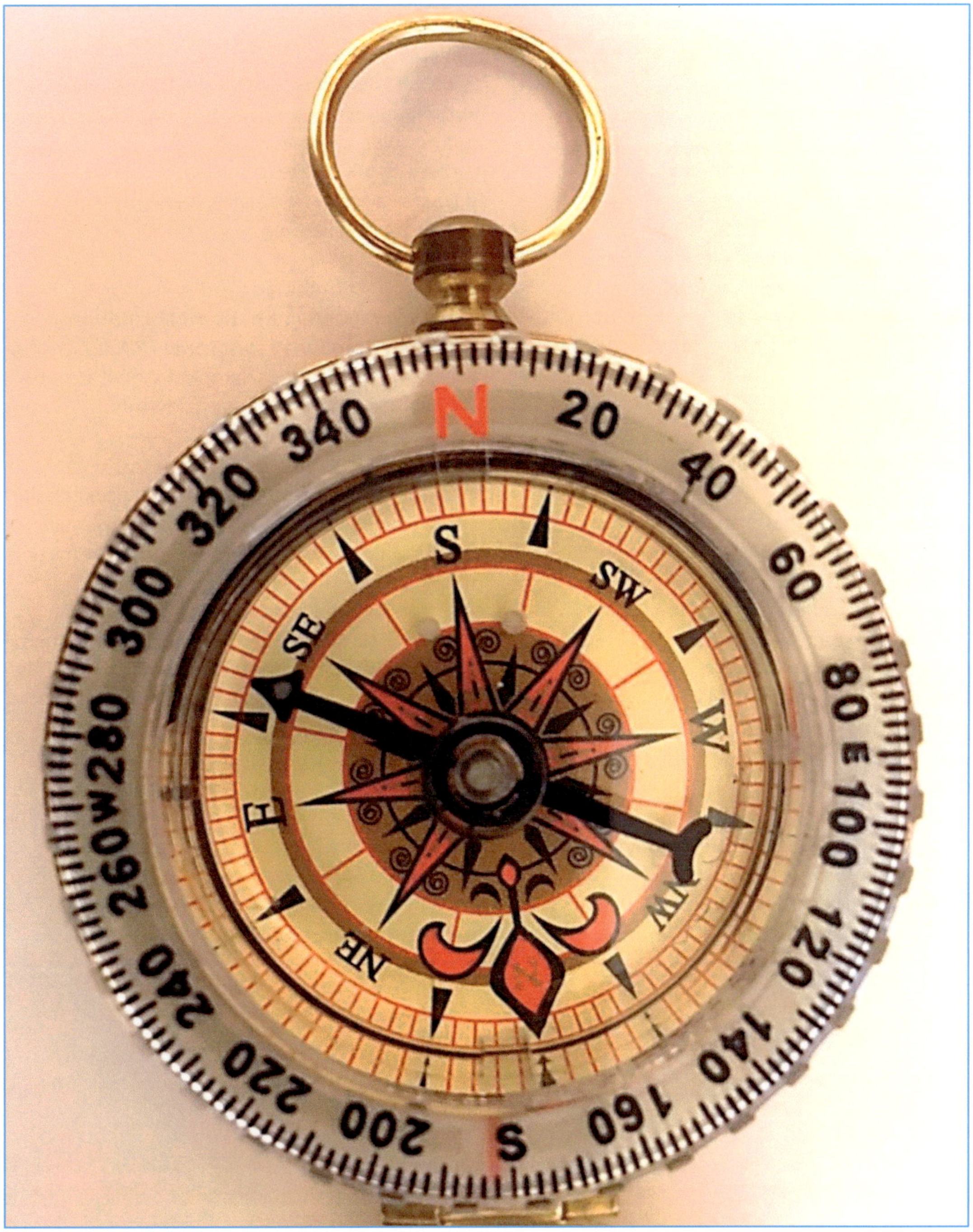

Vascular tumors

VASCULAR MALFORMATIONS

-group of congenital vascular malformations
-can be capillary, venous, arteriovenous, or mixed

Capillary malformations

Nevus simplex (salmon patch, stork bite)
-pink-red, blanchable patches present at birth
-usually midline and symmetrical
-favors nape of neck and glabella
-typically becomes lighter as child ages

Port wine stain (nevus flammeus)
-dark, red-purple patches present at birth
-most often on the face and neck
-as the child ages, the lesion will deepen in color and sometimes thicken and develop bumps

Sturge-Weber syndrome (*GNAQ* mutation)
-port wine stains involving ophthalmic branch of trigeminus
-soft tissue/muscle hypertrophy under malformation
-ocular and neurological complications

Arteriovenous malformations

Cobb's syndrome (sporadic)
-spinal AV malformation
-cutaneous capillary malformation ("port wine stain-like") of the same dermatome
-common neurological abnormalities

Parkes-Weber syndrome (*RASA 1* mutation)
-AV malformation of the lower extremities with fast AV shunts (unlike slow-flow malformation in Klippel-Trenaunay syndrome)
-associated venous and lymphatic malformation causing soft tissue and bony hypertrophy
-lytic bone lesions can be seen
-common high output cardiac failure

Venous malformations

Maffucci syndrome (*IDH1 and IDH2* mutation)
-deep venous malformation of hands and feet
-multiple hemangiomas and enchondroma with short stature and fractures
-high risk for chondrosarcoma

Blue rubber bleb nevus syndrome (sporadic)
-multiple blue, rubbery, compressible papules and nodules present at birth
-involves trunk and extremities
-GI tract malformations with small intestine blebs and common bleeding

Combined capillary/venous/lymphatic malformations

Klippel-Trenaunay syndrome (*PIK3CA* mutation)
-mixed capillary/venous/lymphatic malformation of lower extremity with overgrowth of soft tissue and bone
-common venous varicosities with thrombophlebitis and high-output cardiac failure

Proteus syndrome (*AKT1* mutation)
-mixed capillary/venous/lymphatic malformation of lower extremity with overgrowth of soft tissue and bone
-characteristic cerebriform connective tissue nevi, organomegaly, impaired intelligence

Histopathology
-in all forms vascular **lesions are broad**
-depending on the variant, numerous dilated capillaries, arteries, veins, and lymphatics are present
-in **salmon patch** capillaries are **restricted to the dermis**
-in **port wine stain** capillaries are present in the **dermis and subcutis**

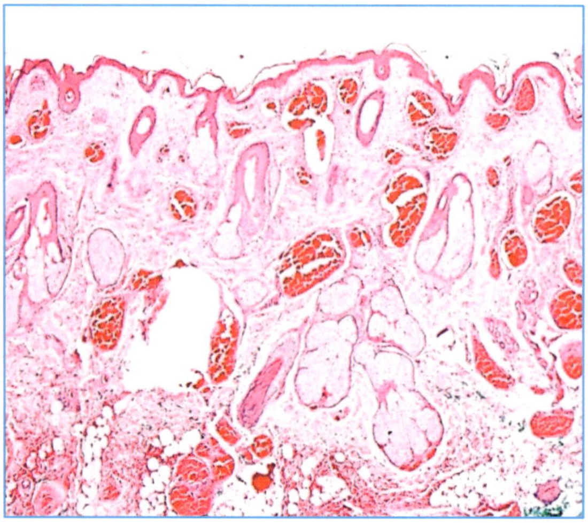

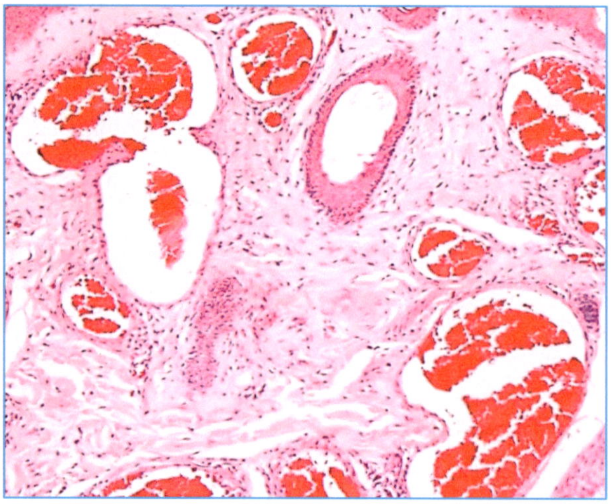

Port wine stain with numerous dermal and subcutaneous dilated capillaries

ARTERIOVENOUS HEMANGIOMA

-solitary red, purple papule, usually less than 1 cm in size
-more common in older individuals
-head and neck are favored sites

Histopathology
-well circumscribed dermal nodule
-**mixture of thick and thin-walled vessels**
-wall of thicker vessels has prominent muscle (arteries) whereas thinner vessels (veins) have thinner muscle in the wall
-no evidence of cytological atypia

CAVERNOUS HEMANGIOMA

-usually becomes apparent in childhood
-blue to purple plaques and nodules
-favors head and neck area

Histopathology
-located in deeper dermis or subcutis
-multinodular appearance with **large dilated and congested vascular channels**
-**walls of the vessels are thin** and covered with flat endothelial cells
-closely resemble venous malformation that has thicker walls

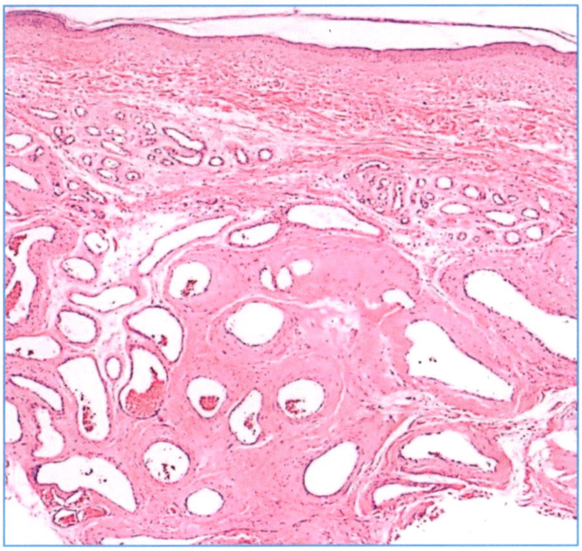

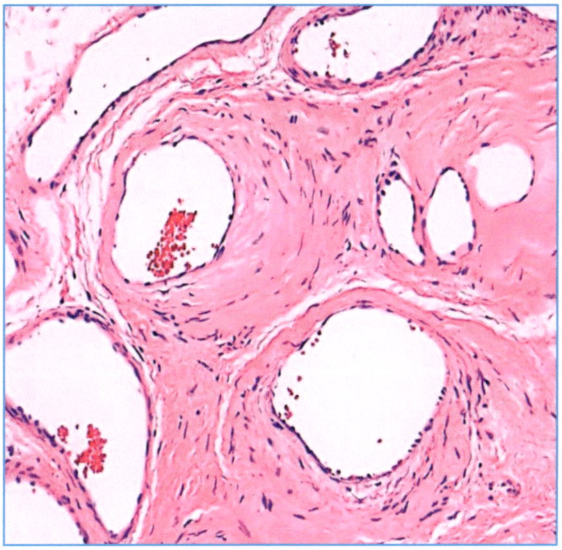

AV hemangioma with thick and thin vessels

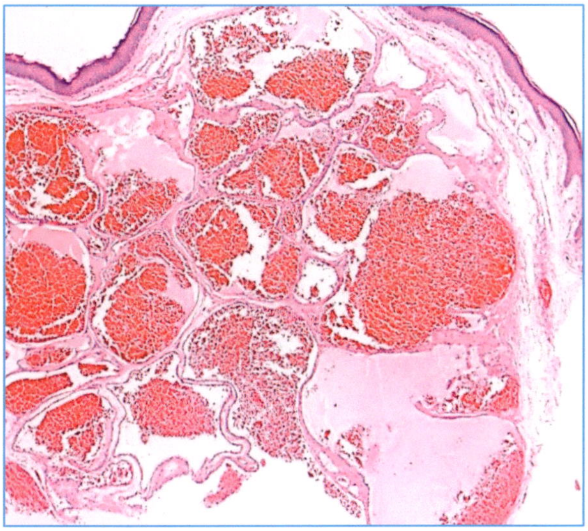

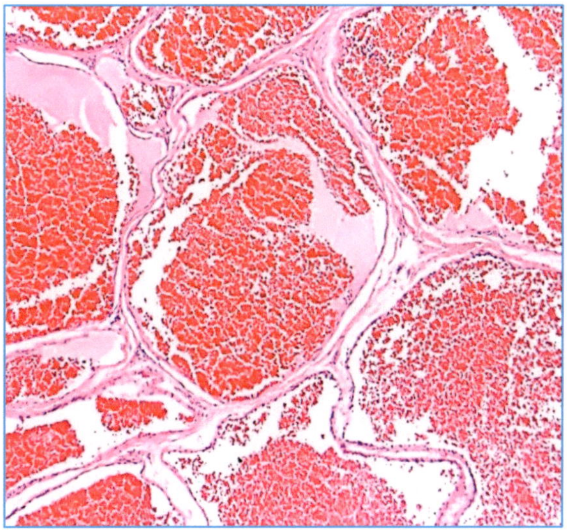

Cavernous hemangioma with dilated vessels with very thin wall

Vascular tumors

INFANTILE (STRAWBERRY) HEMANGIOMA

-most common hemangioma of childhood
-occurs in up to 5% of children and presents during the first four weeks of life
-head and neck are the most common sites
-presents as bright red, blanched papules/plaques or deeper, blue-purple nodules
-grows rapidly in first 6 months and then shrinks in size slowly over the next few years
-skin changes often remain following involution

Histopathology
-type of **capillary hemangioma**
-dermal/subcutaneous tumor with multilobular architecture
-vascular proliferation with inconspicuous vascular lumina in early immature lesions
-in older lesions lumina are more prominent
-**GLUT-1 staining is positive** (negative in vascular malformations)

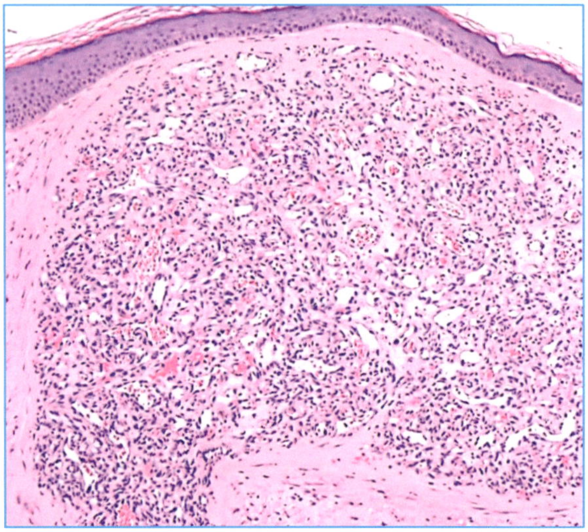

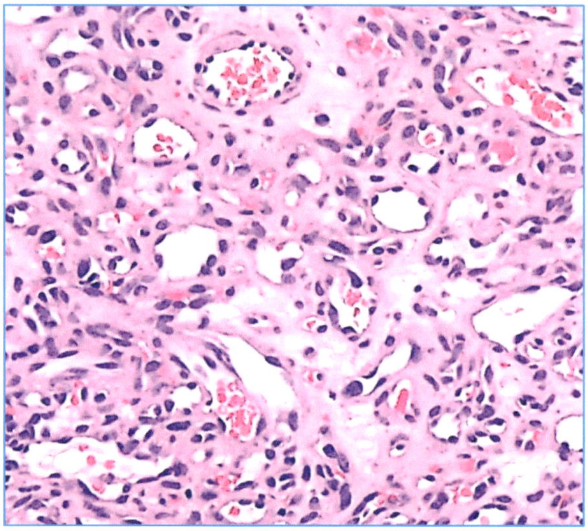

Infantile hemangioma with proliferation of small capillaries

SPIDER ANGIOMA

-present in 10-15% of normal adults
-can be associated with liver disease, thyrotoxicosis, pregnancy, and hormonal contraception
-rarely occurs below the umbilicus
-appears as a central blanchable red dot with circumferential arborizing vessels ("spider legs")

Histopathology
-**vertical dermal artery** that gives rise to **small branching vessels**

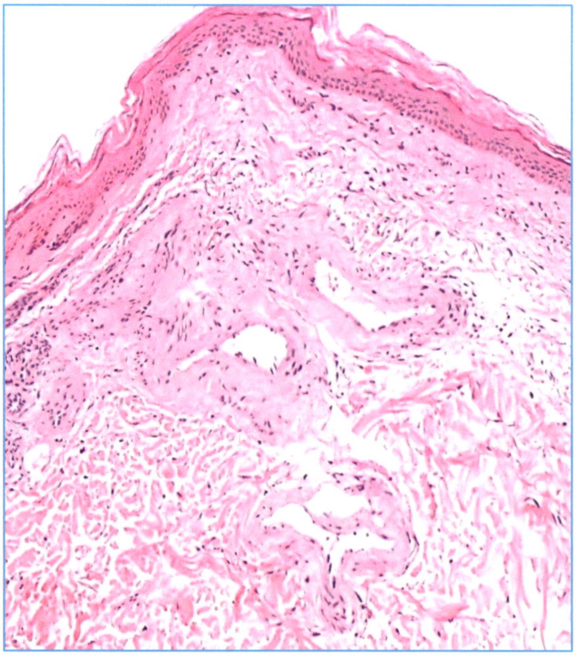

Spider angioma with vertical dermal vessel branching at the top

CHERRY ANGIOMA

-common benign vascular tumor
-presents as small, cherry red, circular or oval papule
-trunk is favored site
-more common after 3rd decade of life

Histopathology
-**"dome-shaped"** dermal lesion
-**epidermal collarettes** surround a dermal vascular proliferation of vessels of various sizes
-tumor is made of **dilated congested vascular channels** separated by stroma
-no evidence of atypia

PYOGENIC GRANULOMA (LOBULAR CAPILLARY HEMANGIOMA)

-rapidly growing, friable, red papule or nodule that bleeds easily
-presents in children and young adults
-also common in pregnant women
-fingers, face, scalp, and gingiva are favored sites

Histopathology
-polypoid, **frequently ulcerated lesion**
-an **epidermal collarette** is commonly seen
-dermal and subcutaneous proliferation of **capillaries forming multiple lobules**
-endothelial cells are plump but cytologically bland
-RBCs extravasation is common

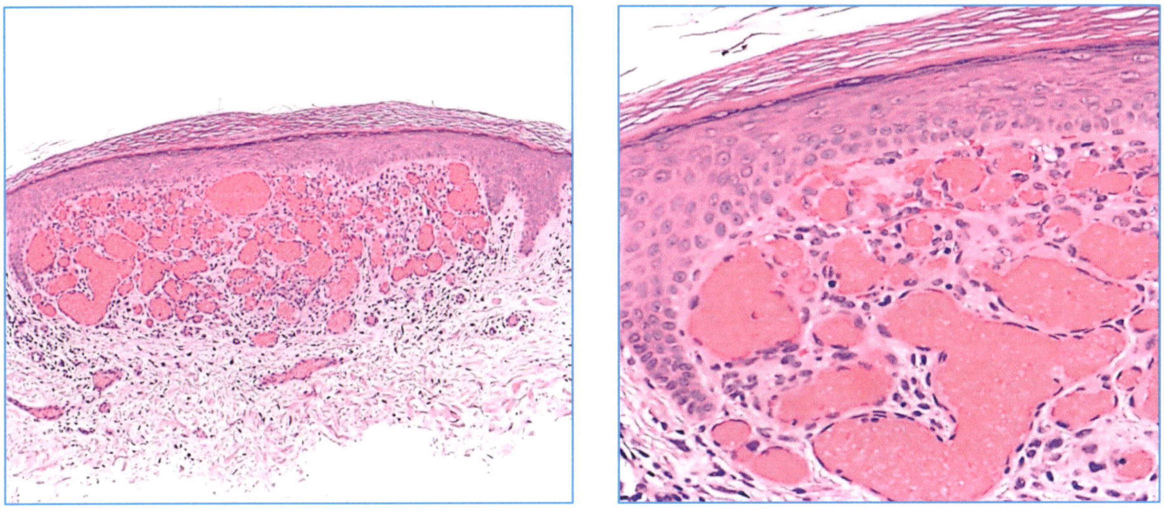

Cherry angioma with epidermal collarette surrounding benign appearing dermal vessels of various sizes

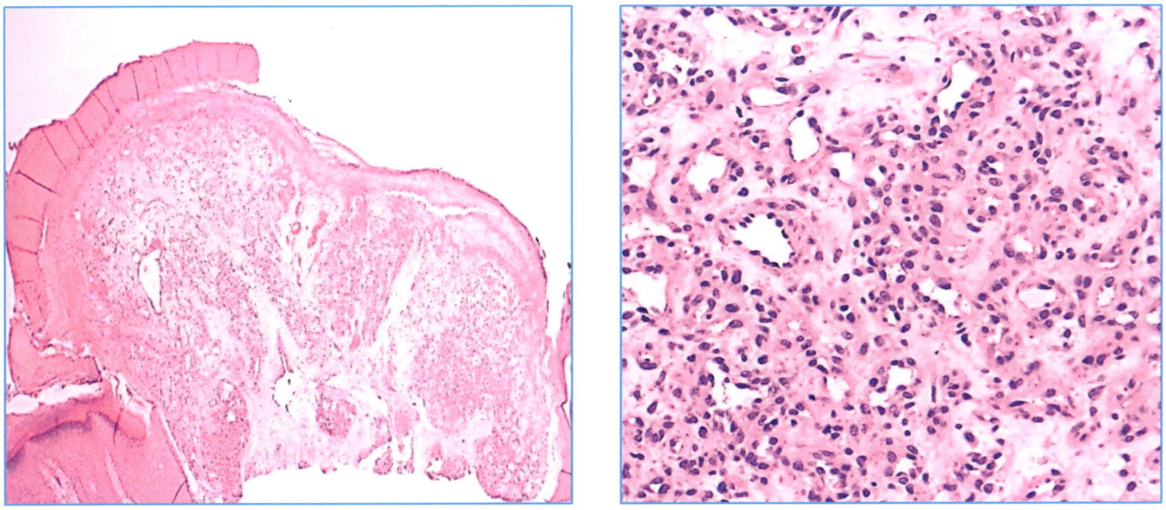

Ulcerated pyogenic granuloma made of multiple lobules of benign capillaries

Vascular tumors

GLOMERULOID HEMANGIOMA

-rare vascular tumor associated with POEM syndrome (**p**olyneuropathy, **o**rganomegaly, **e**ndocrinopathy, **M**-protein, skin changes)
-presents with multiple violaceous papules
-favors trunk and proximal extremities
-more common in Asian population and women

Histopathology
-well-circumscribed cluster of dilated dermal vascular channels
-channels are filled with **vascular loops similar to renal glomeruli**
-**eosinophilic globules** are present within endothelial cells

TUFTED HEMANGIOMA

-uncommon benign vascular tumor
-presents as a slowly enlarging red macule or plaque
-favors neck, shoulder, or upper trunk
-most commonly noted in early childhood but occasionally might be congenital
-some consider it mild variant of Kaposiform hemangioendothelioma
-can be associated with Kasabach-Merritt phenomenon (consumptive coagulopathy)

Histopathology
-poorly-defined dermal vascular proliferation that can extend into the subcutis
-**scattered "cannon ball-like" dermal capillary proliferations**
-**vascular "tufts" in dilated vascular spaces**
-endothelial cells are rounded to "spindle-shaped"
-surrounding stroma is fibrotic and contains **"cleft-like" capillary spaces**

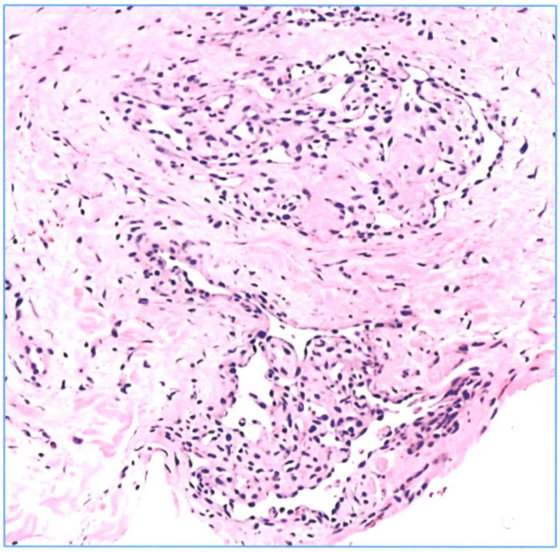
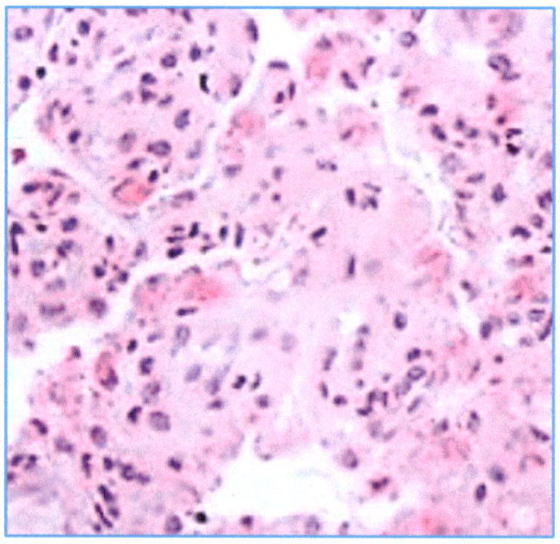

Glomeruloid hemangioma with vascular spaces resembling kidney glomeruli and characteristic eosinophilic globules

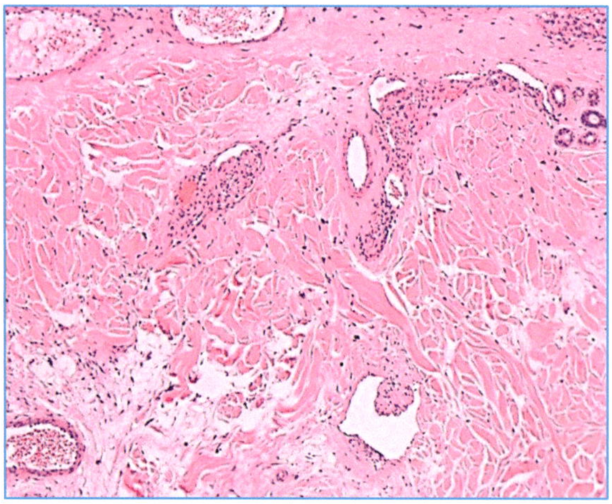

Tufted hemangioma with scattered "cannon ball" appearance

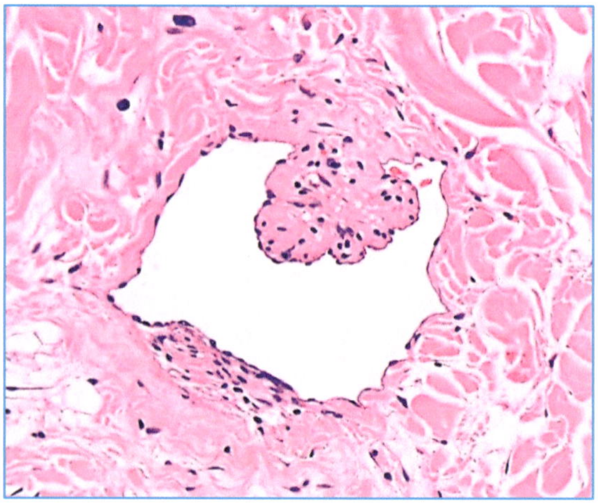

Tufted hemangioma with vascular "tufts"

MICROVENULAR HEMANGIOMA

-small, reddish, painless papules in young to middle-aged adults
-favored sites are the arms and trunk

Histopathology
-**poorly-defined** dermal lesion resembling patch stage of Kaposi sarcoma
-**branching capillaries and small venules**
-vessels with **collapsing narrow lumina**
-no endothelial atypia or spindle cells (unlike KS)
-dermal sclerosis
-HHV8 negative

SPINDLE CELL HEMANGIOMA

-slowly growing, solitary or multiple, skin-colored dermal or subcutaneous nodules
-preference for the distal extremities and more common in young adults
-multiple lesions can be associated with Klippel-Trenaunay and Maffucci syndromes

Histopathology
-well-circumscribed nodule
-tumor is **"biphasic"** in nature
-spindle cells form solid areas that abut cavernous thin walled vascular spaces
-**resemble KS** but cells are HHV8 negative

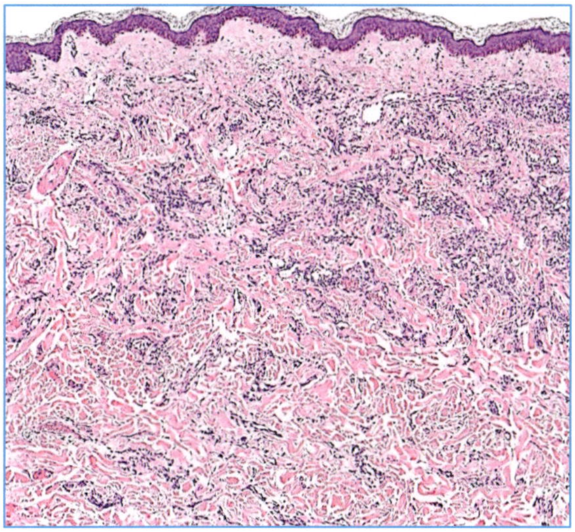

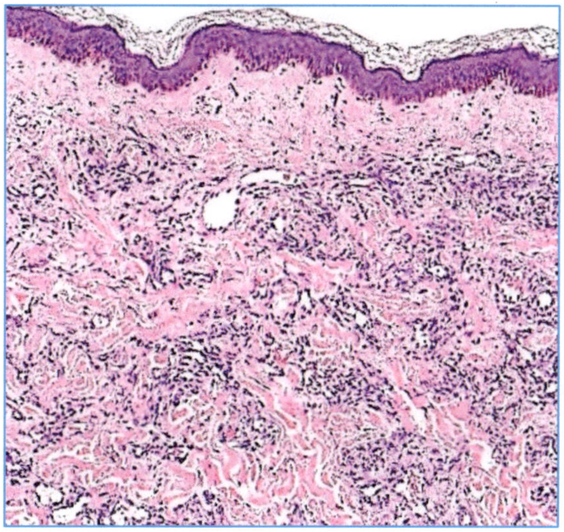

Poorly defined lesion of microvenular hemangioma with branching capillaries with collapsed vessel wall

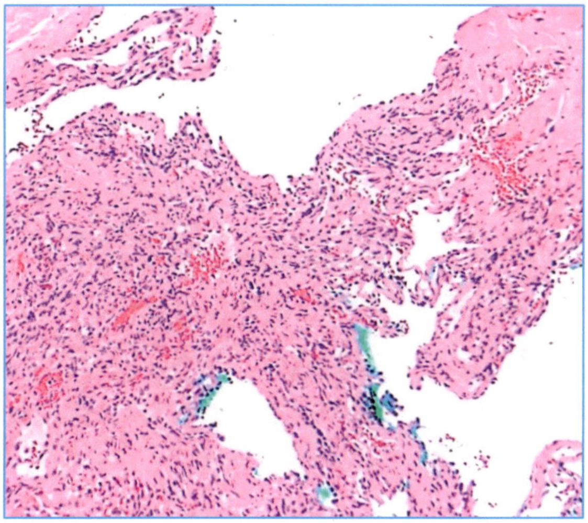

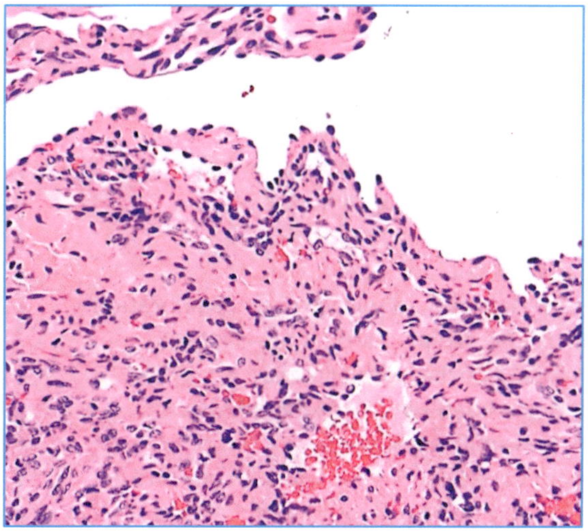

Spindle cell hemangioma with cavernous spaces surrounded by solid areas made of uniform spindled endothelial cells

Vascular tumors

ACQUIRED ELASTOTIC HEMANGIOMA

-slow-growing lesion associated with sun exposure in older individuals
-favors the forearm and neck
-presents as a flat or raised, red to violaceous, irregular, solitary plaque

Histopathology
-proliferation of **small, benign-appearing vessels** in the upper dermis
-**vessels are organized parallel to the epidermis**
-**significant dermal solar elastosis**

VENOUS LAKE

-dark blue compressible papule or nodule
-typically presents on the face, particularly lip or ear, of elderly adults

Histopathology
-**widely dilated dermal vessel**
-vessel has a thin wall and is filled with blood
-background dermal solar elastosis

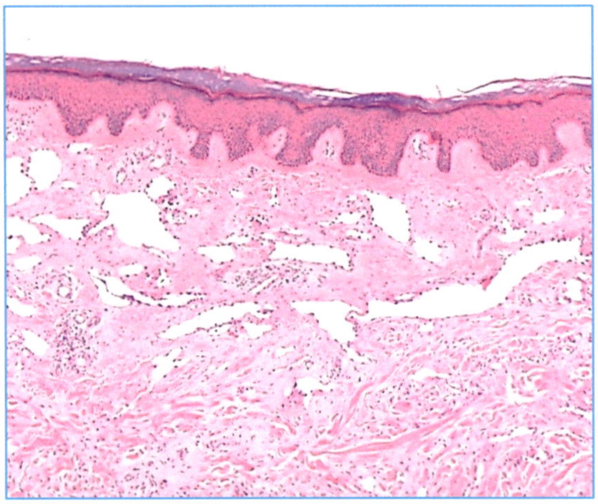

Acquired elastotic hemangioma with prominent solar elastosis and dermal capillaries parallel to the epidermis

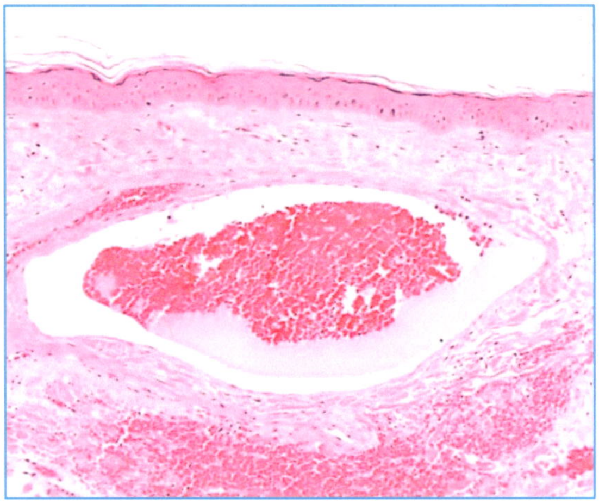

Widely dilated dermal vessel forming venous lake

HOBNAIL HEMANGIOMA (TARGETOID HEMOSIDEROTIC HEMANGIOMA)

-classically presents as a targetoid lesion consisting of a small red-purple papule surrounded by pale area and peripheral hemorrhagic ring
-in older lesions, the halo and surrounding ring often disappear and resolve
-favors the extremities, especially lower, of young to middle-aged adults

Histopathology
-“**wedge-shaped”** dermal vascular proliferation
-superficial vascular channels are dilated with focal papillary projections
-vessels are **lined with endothelial cells with “hobnail”** appearance
-deeper vessels can invade the subcutis and are smaller and more collapsed with flat endothelial cells
-hemosiderin is prominent in older lesions

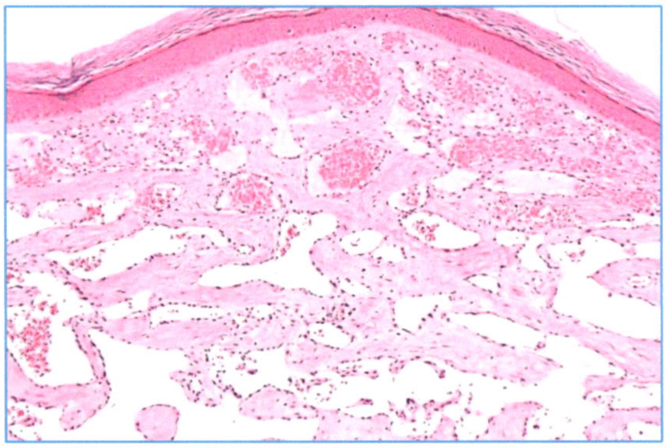

Wedge-shaped hobnail hemangioma

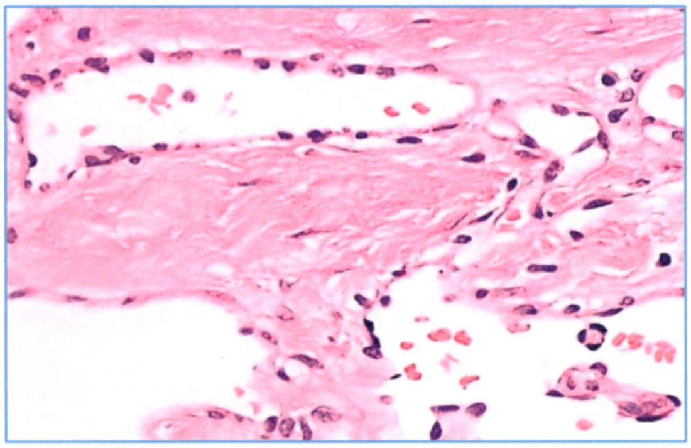

Endothelial cells with “hobnail” appearance

ANGIOKERATOMA

-several clinical variants with solitary or multiple red-purple, sometimes hyperkeratotic papules

Solitary angiokeratoma

- favors extremities with wide age range

Angiokeratoma of Mibelli

-usually in children/adolescents
-multiple, warty, blue-purple lesions over the bony prominences of the hands and feet

Angiokeratoma of Fordyce

-clustered lesions on the scrotum or vulva in elderly patients

Angiokeratoma circumscriptum

-usually in children, females > males
-hyperkeratotic, red-purple papules coalescing into plaques

Angiokeratoma corporis diffusum

-widespread, red-purple papules, frequently in clusters on the trunk, in childhood
-associated with Fabry's disease, fucosidosis, and beta-galactosidase deficiency

Histopathology

-irregular epidermal acanthosis and hyperkeratosis
-**irregularly dilated vascular channels in the papillary dermis**
-**vascular channels are pushing against epidermis**, which appears elevated

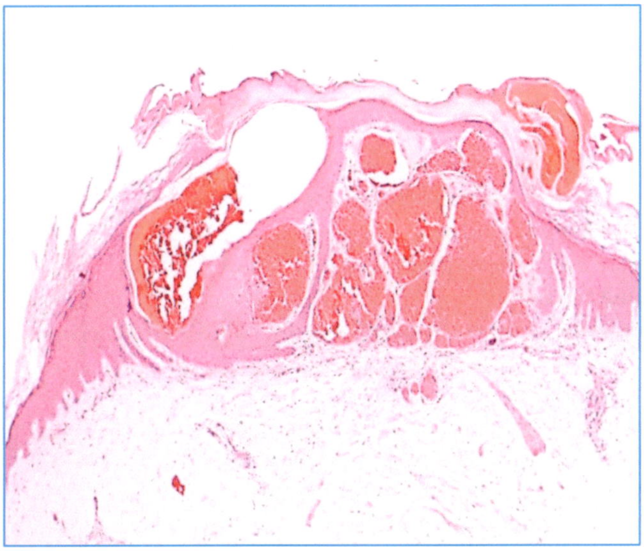

Angiokeratoma with irregular hyperkeratotic epidermis

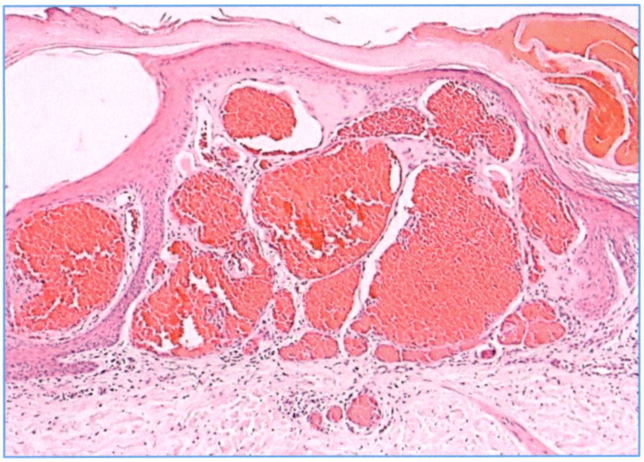

Angiokeratoma with large vessel pushing against epidermis

VERRUCOUS HEMANGIOMA

-macular purple lesion with a verrucous surface
-presents at birth or soon after
-probably represents a vascular malformation
-may be single or grouped and most commonly on extremities

Histopathology

-acanthotic, **hyperkeratotic epidermis with verruciform architecture**
-larger dilated vascular channels, filed with blood, are present in the papillary dermis
-larger vascular spaces are pushing against epidermis (as in angiokeratoma)
-**small capillaries are present in the reticular dermis** (unlike angiokeratoma)

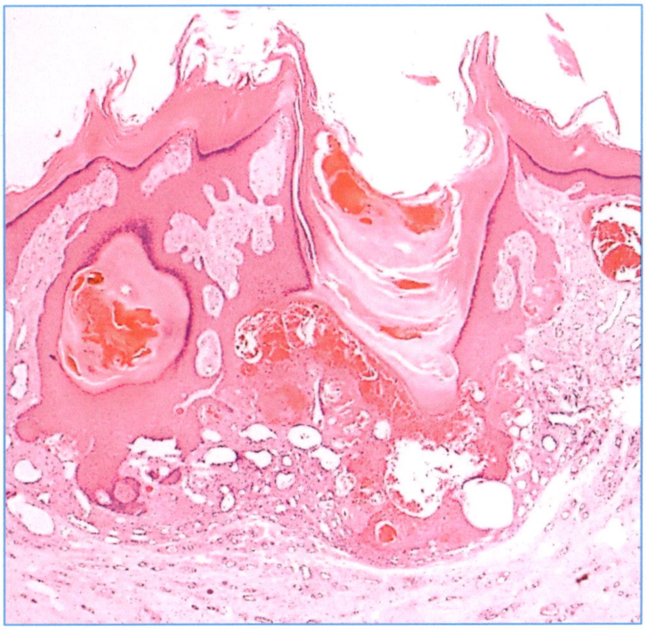

Verrucous hemangioma with larger vessels in papillary dermis and small capillary proliferation in reticular dermis

EPITHELIOID HEMANGIOMA (ANGIOLYMPHOID HYPERPLASIA WITH EOSINOPHILIA)

-benign vasoproliferative condition characterized by single or multiple red-brown papules or plaques
-can be painful or itchy
-usually on the head (scalp, ear) or neck of young adults
-peripheral blood eosinophilia may be noted

Histopathology
-dermal collection of vessels of variable size
-vessel's lumen can be collapsed or open
-vessels are lined with plump, enlarged, or "hobnail" shaped endothelial cells
-cytoplasmic vacuoles can be seen in some endothelial cells
-**perivascular fibrosis with an "onion skin"** appearance is characteristic
-stromal inflammatory infiltrate varies in intensity
-consist of mostly lymphocytes, sometimes with formation of lymphoid follicles
-**variable number of eosinophils** from many to very few or none

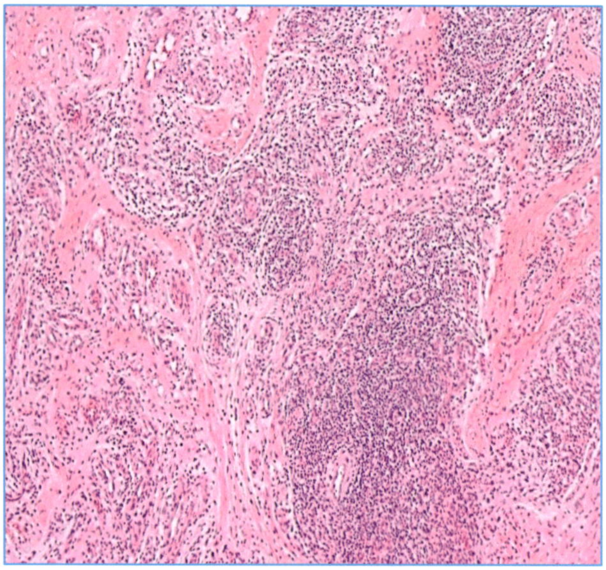

Epithelioid hemangioma with vascular and lymphocytic proliferation

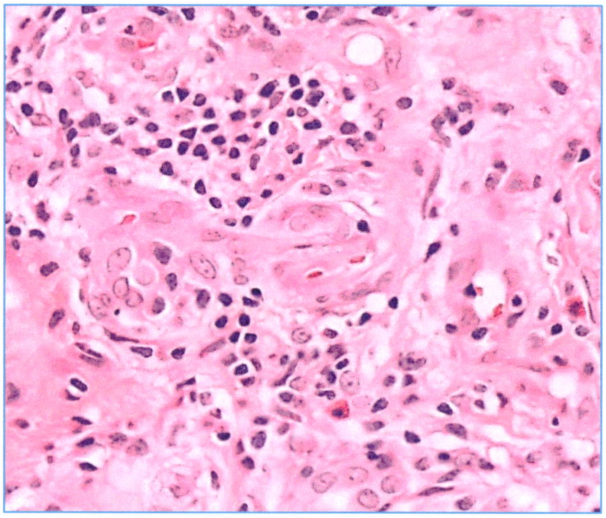

Capillaries are lined with plump endothelial cells and surrounded by lymphocytes and eosinophils

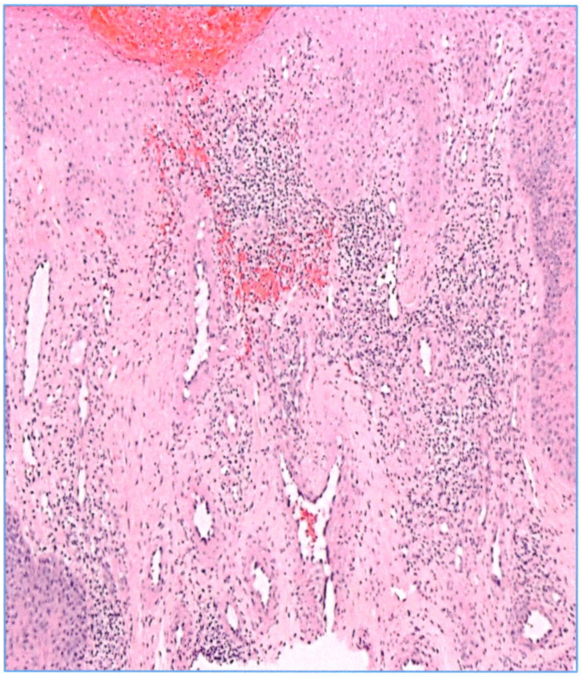

Vascular and lymphocytic hyperplasia

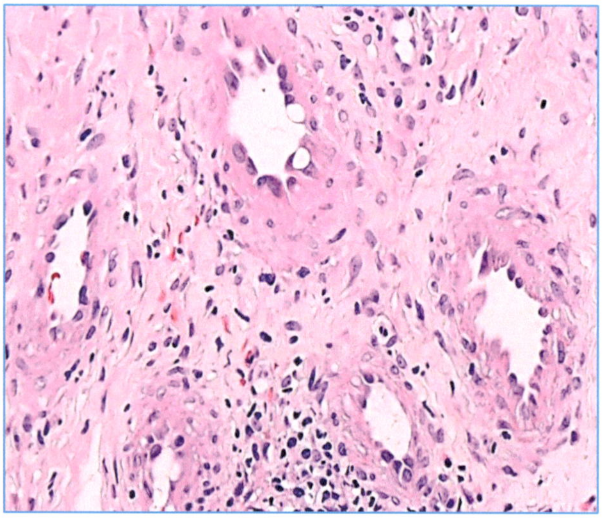

Perivascular fibrosis with "onion skin" appearance

INTRAVASCULAR PAPILLARY ENDOTHELIAL HYPERPLASIA (MASSON'S TUMOR)

-skin-colored to blue, firm, deep subcutaneous nodule, sometimes painful
-favors fingers, head (lip, tongue), neck, trunk
-female predominance

Histopathology
-probably represents an unusual variant of organizing thrombus or traumatized angioma
-**intravascular circumscribed** tumor
-**organizing fibrin thrombus** in vascular spaces with **hyalinized stroma**
-numerous **papillae and anastomosing irregular intravascular channels**
-lined by **plump endothelial cells**

LYMPHANGIOMA

-most cases are developmental defects
-majority are present at birth or in early childhood with two variants

Superficial lymphangioma (lymphangioma circumscriptum)
-cluster of clear/blue vesicles on the buttock or trunk, said to resemble "frog spawn"
-may discharge a clear fluid

Deep lymphangioma (cystic hygroma)
-favors neck and axilla
-large, single or multiloculated, fluid-filled cavities
-associated with hydrops fetalis and fetal death
-common in Turner, Noonan, and Maffucci syndromes

Histopathology
-dermal (circumscriptum) or subcutaneous (cystic hygroma) **ectatic lymphatic channels**
-lined with flat, bland endothelial cells
-**lymphatic flaps protruding to the lumen**
-lymphatic channels can be empty or **filled with lightly pink acellular lymph**
-occasional red blood cells can be seen

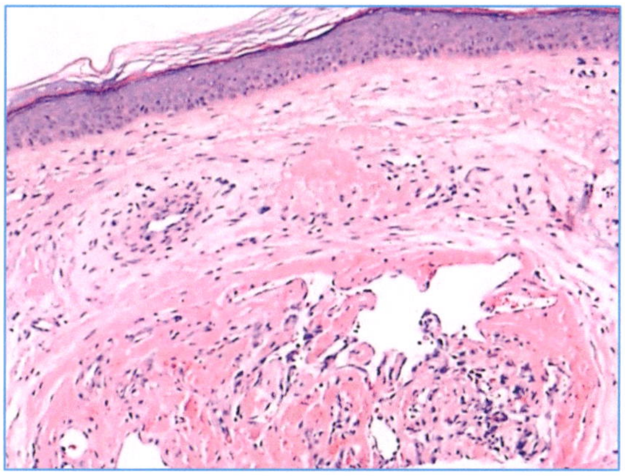

Masson's tumor arising in thrombosed vessel

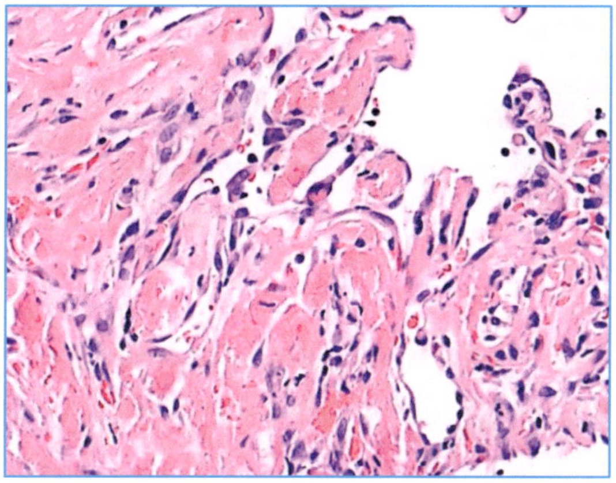

Masson's tumor with numerous papillae in hyalinized stroma

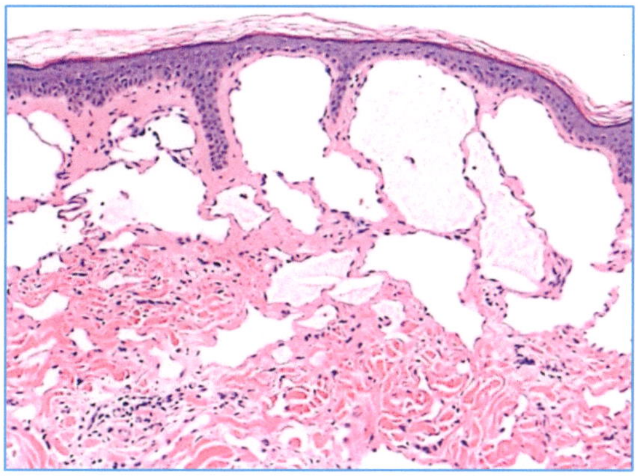

Lymphangioma with large channels filled with pink lymph

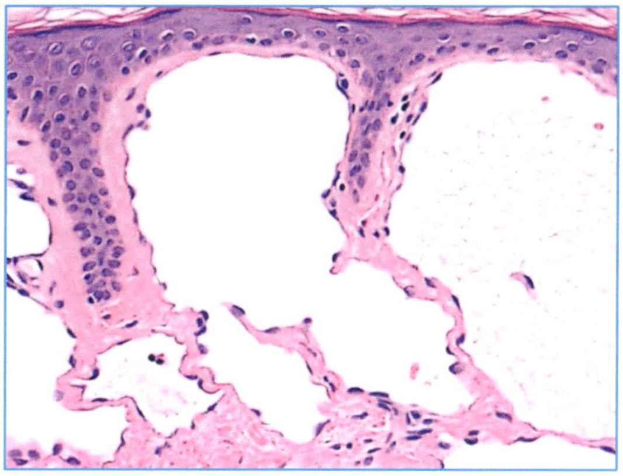

Lymphatic spaces with characteristic lymphatic flaps

Vascular tumors

CUTANEOUS COLLAGENOUS VASCULOPATY	REACTIVE ANGIOENDOTHELIMATOSIS
-rare microangiopathy of dermal blood vessels -most often occurs in middle-aged to older adults -etiology remains unknown -presents as blanchable, non-urticating macules -typically begins on the lower extremities and then spread to the trunk and upper extremities -clinical similarity to generalized essential telangiectasia Histopathology -**dilated capillaries** and post-capillary venules -**thickened vessel wall with marked collagen deposition** (PAS positive) -no inflammation	-rare angioproliferative condition -presents with multiple erythematous macules or plaques that can ulcerate -propensity to involve limbs -associated with severe systemic diseases such as antiphospholipid syndrome, sarcoidosis, cryoglobulinemia, chronic infections and immunosuppression in kidney transplant and cancer patients Histopathology -scattered and focally clustered dermal small vessels poorly marginated -lined by **plump endothelial cells** with no atypia -dermal **hemosiderin** commonly present -**mild lymphocytic inflammation** is present

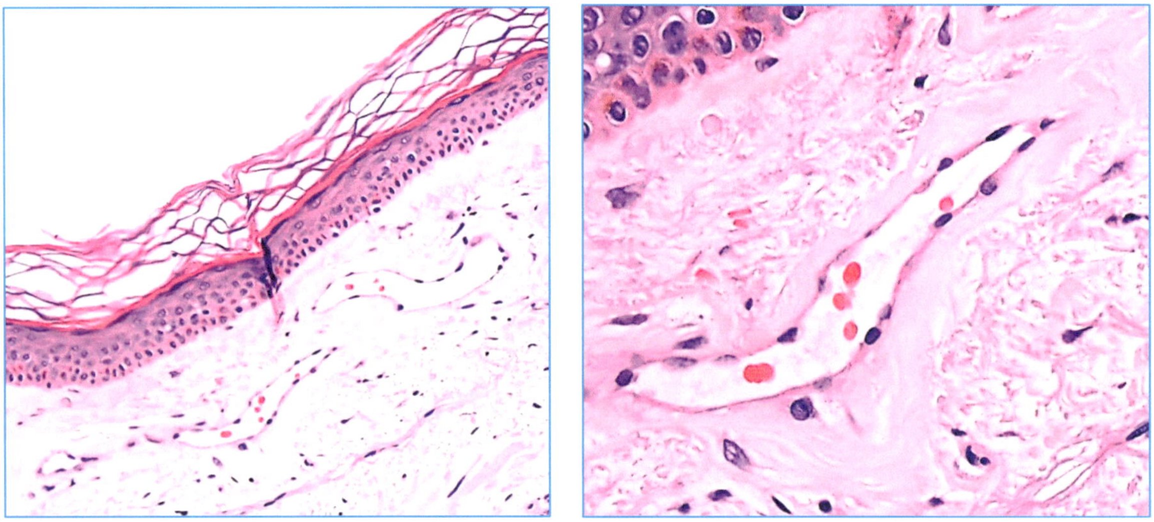

Cutaneous collagenous vasculopathy with dermal telangiectasias with pink thickened vessel wall

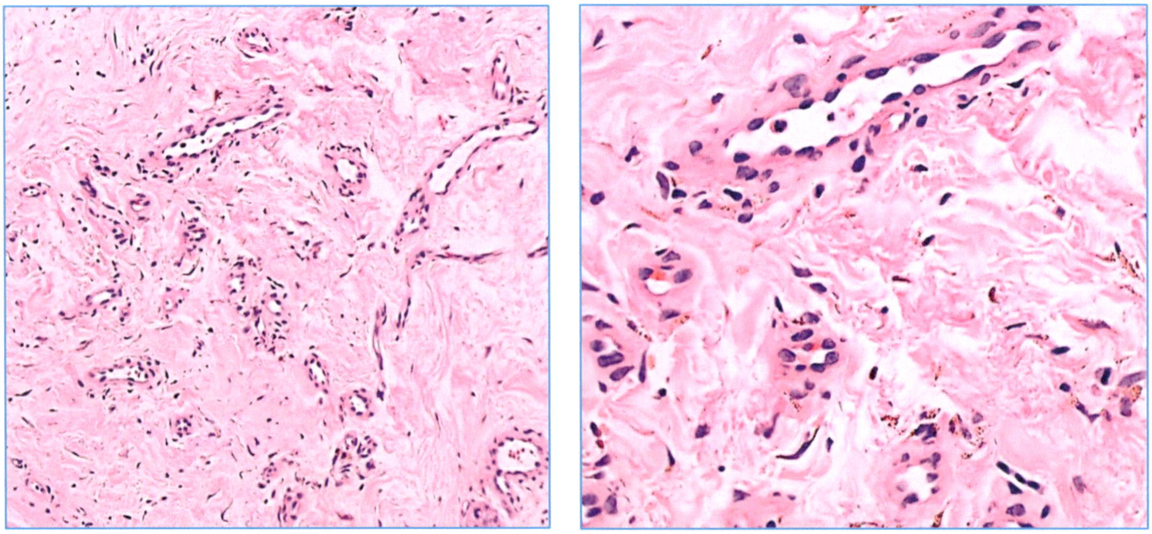

Reactive angioendotheliomatosis with proliferation of dermal capillaries lined with bland plump endothelial cells. Scattered dermal hemosiderin and few lymphocytes are present.

GLOMUS TUMOR/ GLOMUVENOUS MALFORMATION

-benign tumors derived from the Sucquet-Hoyer canal of the glomus body and divided in two variants

Glomus tumor
-solitary, **painful**, purple dermal nodule
-favors fingertips and subungual location
-usually in young adults

Glomuvenous malformation (glomangioma)
-lately considered malformation rather than neoplasm
-presents in infancy or childhood
-**painless** dermal nodule
-favor lower extremities but usually not fingers
-small subset of them are multiple and are part of familial glomus tumor syndrome (*GLMN* gene)

Histopathology

Glomus tumor
-solid nests and sheets of **"glomus-like" cells** surrounding inconspicuous vessels
-**cells are uniform, with dark nuclei and pale eosinophilic cytoplasm**
-**vessels are small, compressed, and not conspicuous**
-lack of polymorphism

Glomuvenous malformation (glomangioma)
-**prominent large, dilated vessels**
-**surrounded by uniform cells usually** made of **2-4 layers** of uniform **"glomus-like" cells**
-no cytological atypia or mitoses
-**"glomus-like" cells are SMA positive**

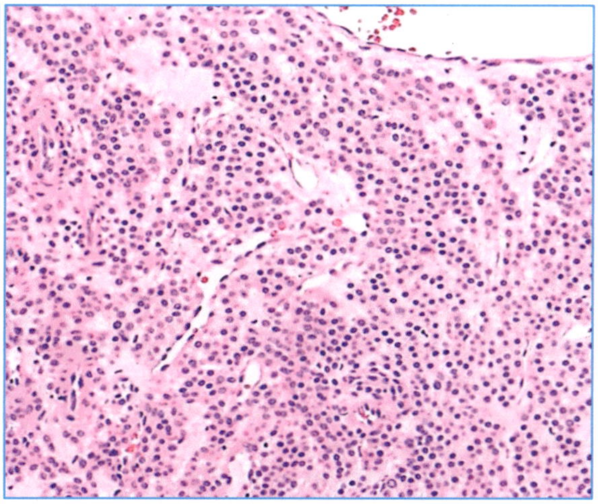

Glomus tumor made of uniform cells with dark nuclei and pink cytoplasm

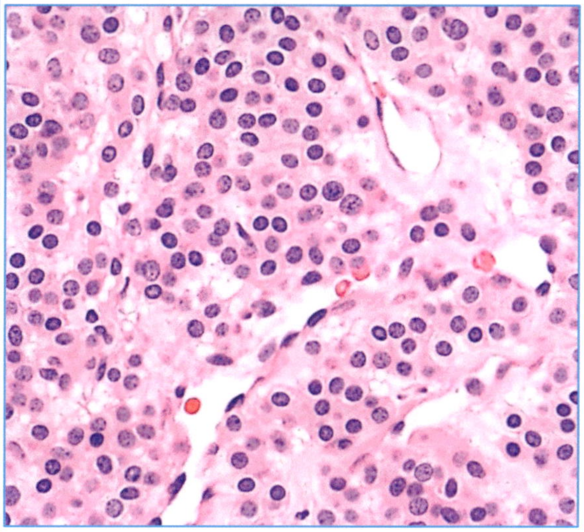

Glomus tumor with compressed vessels surrounded by uniform cells

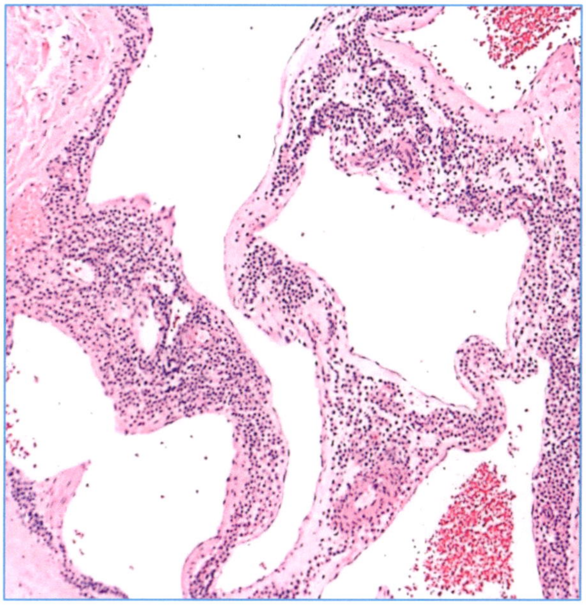

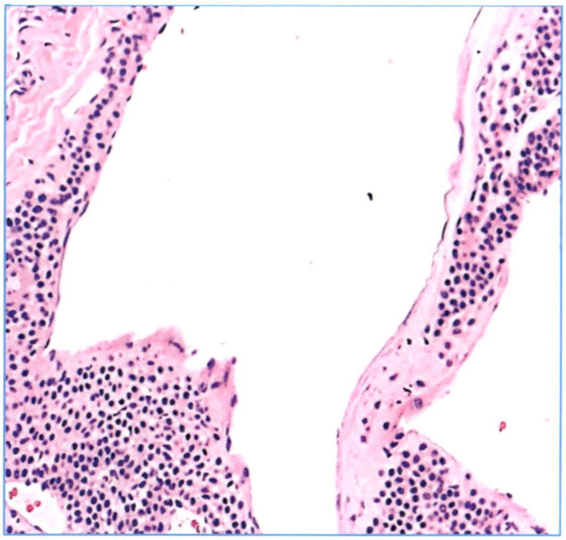

Glomuvenous malformation with several layers of uniform cells surrounding prominent dilated vascular channels

Vascular tumors

STASIS DERMATITIS

-consequence of longstanding venous insufficiency
-swelling of lower legs and feet with skin hyperpigmentation and dry scales
-purple papules and nodules can be present
-more common in elderly and obese individuals

Histopathology

-epidermal acanthosis and hyperkeratosis
-proliferation of **small benign dermal vessels in lobular pattern** resembling capillary hemangioma
-vessels have round lumina and plump endothelial cells
-red blood cell extravasation can be present

ACROANGIODERMATITIS (PSEUDO-KAPOSI SARCOMA)

-benign vascular disorder with several clinical variants

Mali type

-exaggerated stasis dermatitis seen in elderly
-bilateral and associated with chronic venous insufficiency
-purple-blue to brown papules and plaques on malleoli of both legs

Stewart—Bluefarb syndrome

-secondary to congenital arteriovenous malformation (AV shunts) of the lower leg

Gravity purpura (dermite ocre of Favre)

-presents as purpura on lower legs over site of venous varicosities during the first pregnancy

Histopathology

-dermal **round and elongated small vascular channels** arranged in vague nodular pattern
-**vascular spaces are aligned back-to-back and surrounded with prominent hemosiderin**
-no "slit-like" vascular channels or stromal spindle cells (unlike KS)

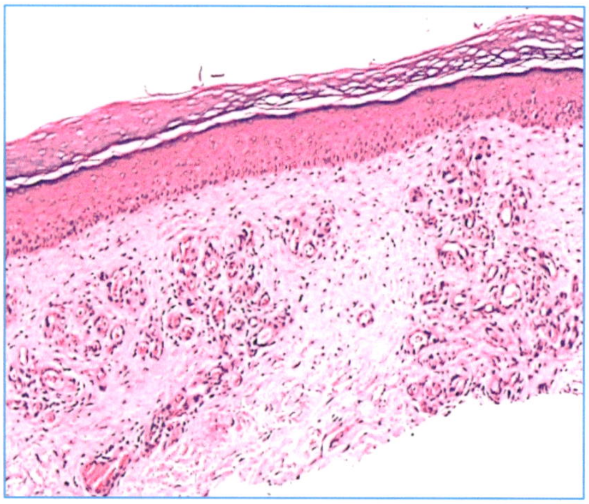

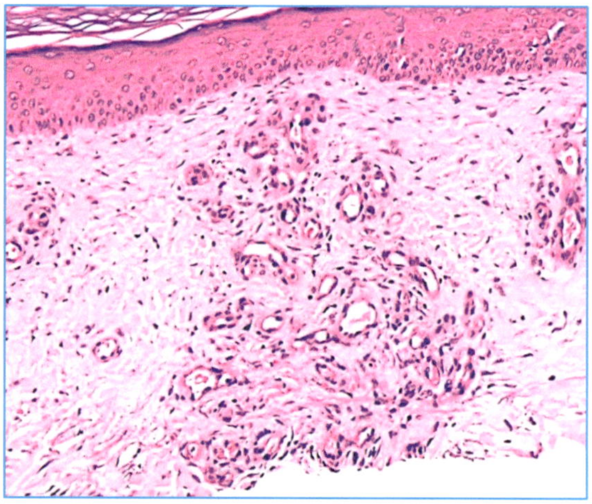

Stasis dermatitis with proliferation of capillaries in lobular pattern

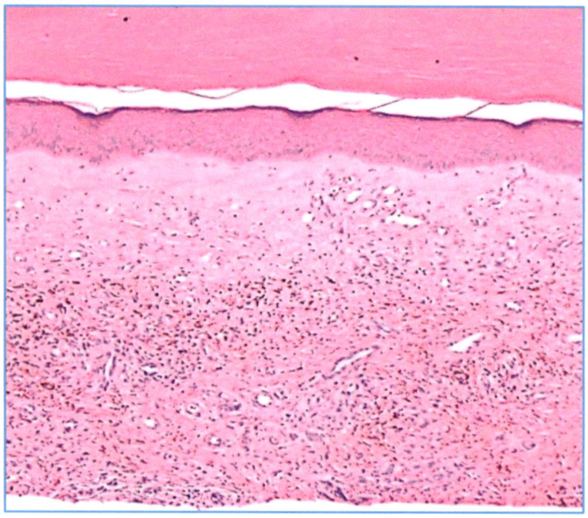

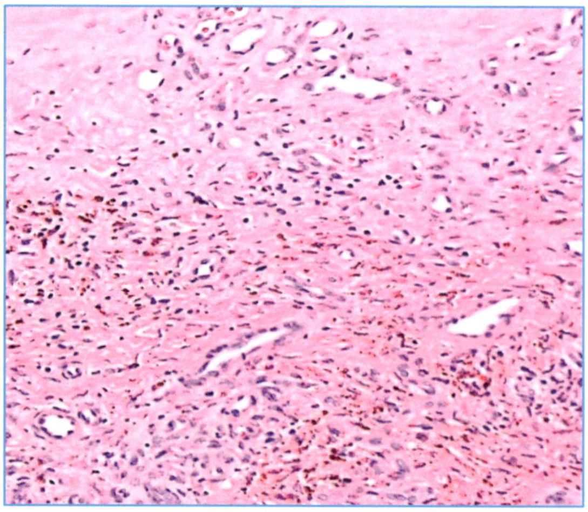

Acroangiodermatitis with extensive dermal capillary proliferation and dermal hemosiderin

HEMANGIOPERICYTOMA

-rare, low grade cutaneous vascular tumor

Adult type

-deeply-seated tumor with preference for the thigh, pelvis, or retroperitoneum

-can cause hypoglycemia

Infantile type

-solitary subcutaneous nodule present at birth or in the first year of life

Histopathology

Adult type

-well-circumscribed, vaguely lobulated dermal tumor

-made of numerous **tightly packed thin-walled vessels**

-characteristic **"staghorn" branching pattern** of blood vessels

-**endothelial cells are uniformed**, small, ovoid to "spindle-shaped"

-number of mitoses varies

Infantile type

-similar to adult form but with satellite nodules and more **multilobular** architecture

-cells are also more polymorphic

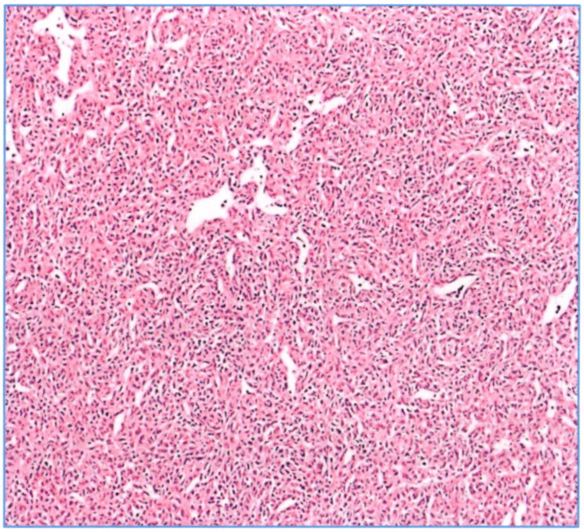

Hemangiopericytoma made of uniform endothelial cells with "staghorn" branching pattern of blood vessels

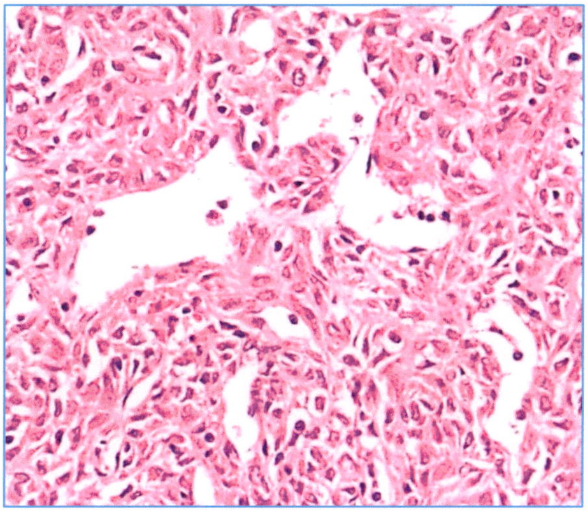

ANGIOMATOSIS

-progressive swelling of soft tissue with pain or discoloration of the affected area

-presents in infancy or childhood

-most often on the lower extremity or trunk

-difficult to treat with high recurrence rate

Histopathology

-**deep dermal and subcutaneous** benign appearing **vascular proliferation**

-nests of **proliferating capillaries arranged in a lobular pattern**, displacing adjacent fat

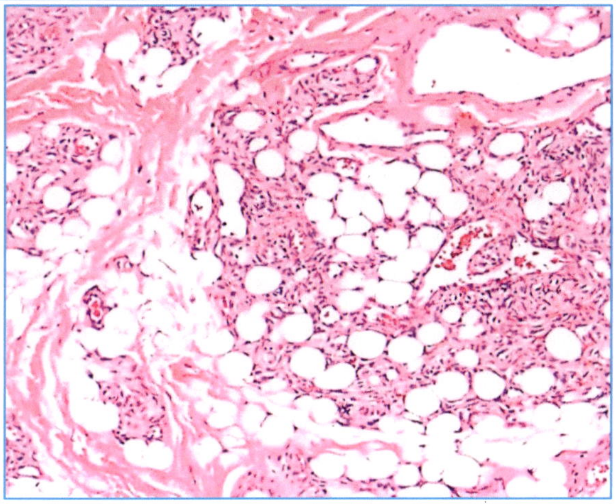

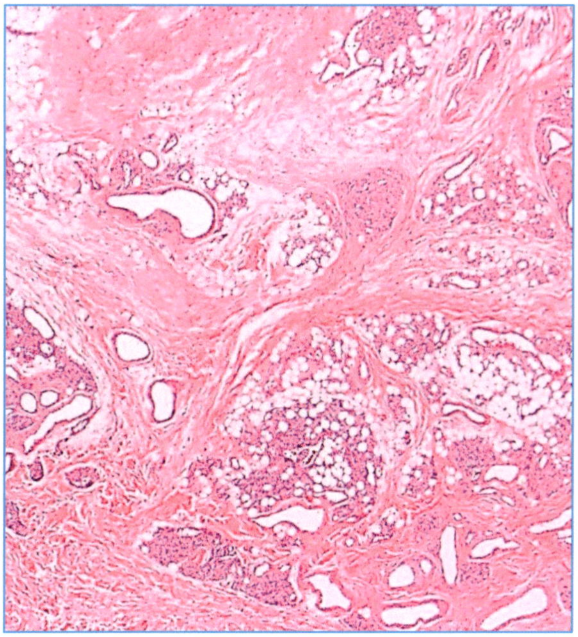

Deep subcutaneous angiomatosis with lobular proliferation of capillaries displacing subcutaneous fat

Vascular tumors

EPITHELIOID HEMANGIOENDOTHELIOMA

-rare, intermediate-grade vascular tumor of middle-aged individuals
-usually arises in the soft tissue
-skin involvement is extremely rare
-typically presents as a solitary, slightly painful erythematous papule, nodule, plaque or non-healing ulcer

Histopathology
-**poorly circumscribed** dermal/subcutaneous tumor
-aggregates of oval to polygonal cells with **abundant eosinophilic cytoplasm and round nuclei**
-vesicular nuclear chromatin and frequent prominent nucleoli
-nuclear pleomorphism is minimal
-**intracytoplasmic vacuolization are regular features**
-well-defined vessels are not present
-stroma is hyalinized or myxoid

RETIFORM HEMANGIOENDOTHELIOMA

-rare, low-grade vascular neoplasm
-presents as a red-purple subcutaneous plaque or nodule on the distal extremities or trunk of young adults
-may recur locally but rarely metastasizes
-associated with chronic lymphedema and radiotherapy

Histopathology
-dermal or subcutaneous proliferation of **arborizing elongated vascular channels (reminiscent of normal rete testis)**
-vessels are lined **by monomorphic "hobnail" endothelial cells**
-associated with a variably prominent lymphocytic infiltrate in approximately 50% of cases
-there is focal presence of papillae within the vessels

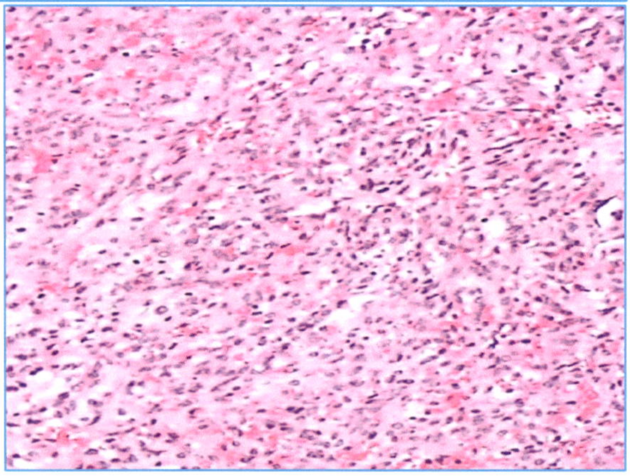
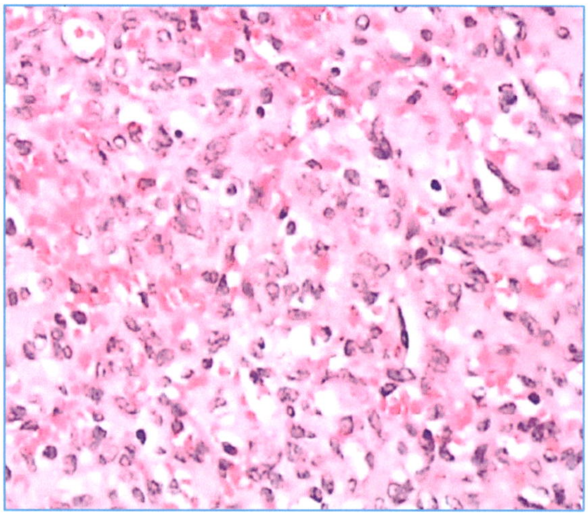

Epithelioid hemangioendothelioma with oval cells with dark nuclei and prominent cytoplasm with intracytoplasmic vacuoles

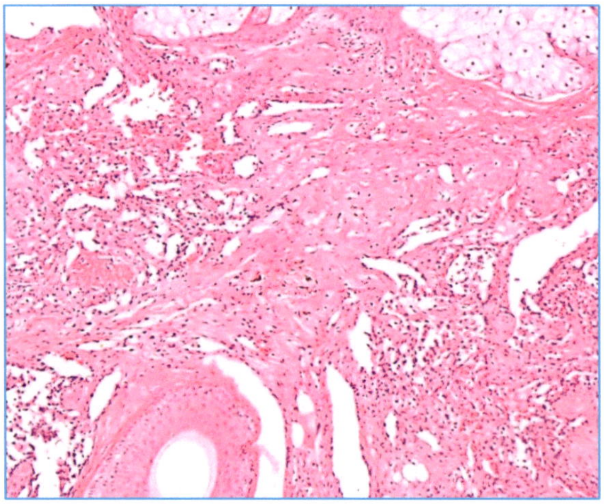
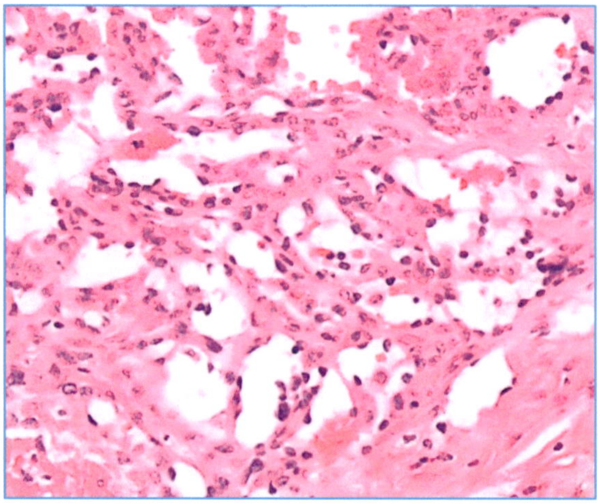

Retiform hemangioendothelioma with arborizing vascular channels lined with endothelial cells with prominent dark nuclei

Chapter 34

BACILLARY ANGIOMATOSIS

-reactive process caused by *Bartonella henselae* or *B. quintana*
-mostly in AIDS patients or immunosuppressed patients
-presents as solitary or multiple "dome-shaped" reddish papules, patches, or nodules
-older lesions have a friable surface resembling pyogenic granuloma

Histopathology

-**proliferation of vessels with plump endothelial cells** and open lumina
-**neutrophils with nuclear dust** in between small vascular channels
-**hemorrhage is common**
-bacteria in areas rich with neutrophils, best detected with **Warthin-Starry silver stain**
-for more details see the chapter on bacterial infections

PECOMA

-rare mesenchymal tumors consisting of perivascular epithelioid cells (PECs)
-can occur in any part of the human body and occasionally in skin
-presents as subcutaneous nodule
-strong female preponderance (80-90%)

Histopathology

-poorly defined dermal/subcutaneous tumor
-**delicate capillary network** surrounded by **epithelioid cells with pale, clear, or granular pink cytoplasm arranged in nests**
-tumor is usually benign with no cytological atypia and no infiltrative growth
-cells stain for muscle markers (SMA, desmin)
-melanocytic markers Melan-A, MITF, HMB45 are positive, but S-100 is negative

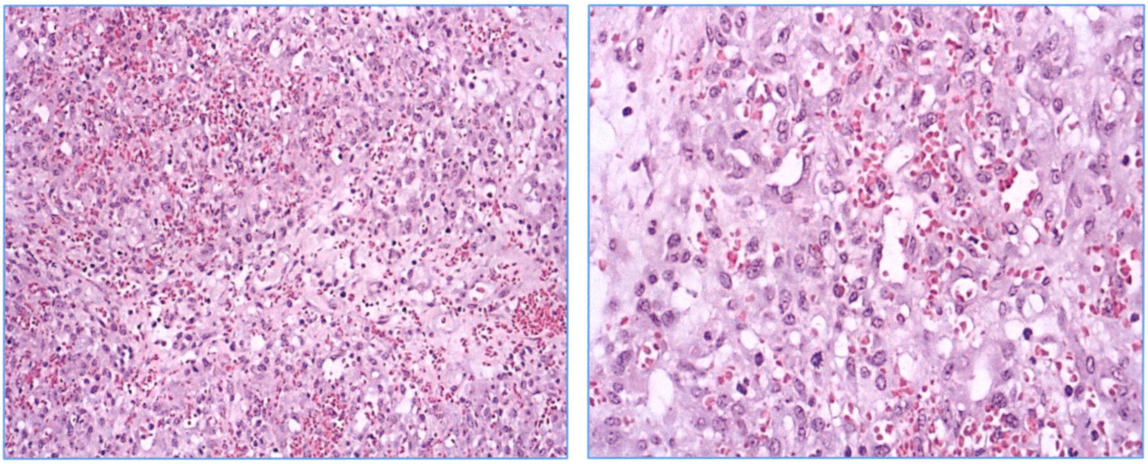

Bacillary angiomatosis with plump endothelial cells surrounded with neutrophilic nuclear dust and hemorrhage

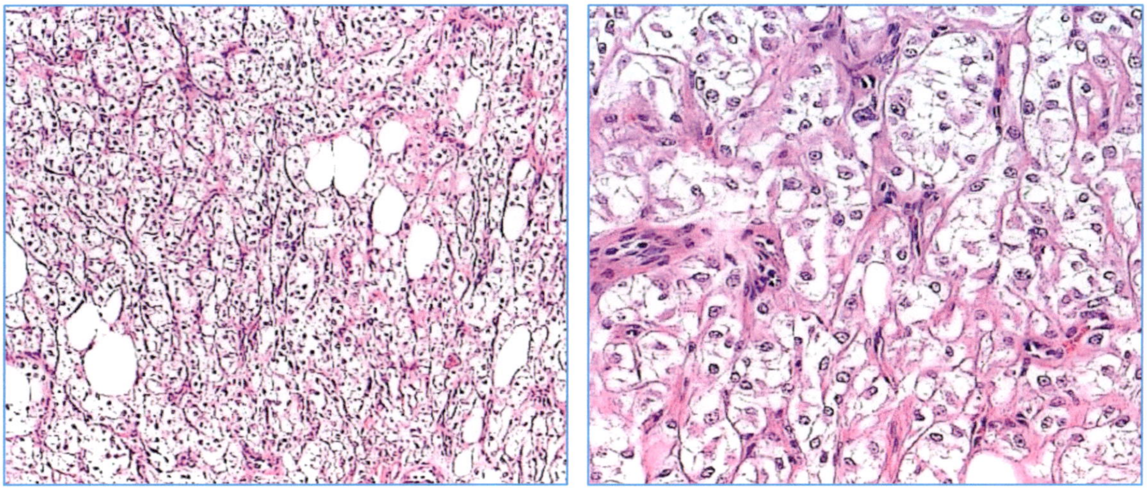

PEComa with nests of clear cells surrounded by delicate capillaries

Vascular tumors

ANGIOSARCOMA

-aggressive vascular malignancy of the skin and soft tissue
-presents as a bluish or violaceous nodule, plaque, or patch
-twice as common in men
-in men favors the scalp and face and is associated with arsenic and polyvinyl chloride exposure
-in women most common on breast post radiation for breast cancer or on upper extremities in area of chronic lymphedema (Stewart-Treves syndrome)

Histopathology
-**infiltrative**, poorly circumscribed tumor
-anastomosing, irregular, **dilated vessels dissecting collagen in "staghorn" pattern**
-plump **endothelial cells with "hobnail" appearance**
-endothelial cells are atypical and can be **multilayered**
-mitoses ae commonly present
-some areas have "cleft-like" spaces, resembling Kaposi's sarcoma, but without spindle cells in between
-radiation induced tumors are ***c-MYC* positive**

ATYPICAL VASCULAR PROLIFERATION

-vascular proliferation that develops on average 3 years after radiation for breast cancer
-single or multiple erythematous papules or patches on breast/chest
-benign lesion but may progress to angiosarcoma

Histopathology
Lymphatic type
-thin walled anastomosing lymphatic channels in superficial dermis
Vascular type (more common)
-relatively well-circumscribed
-small dermal, dilated, **irregularly shaped capillaries**
-vessels **dissect collagen** in "slit-like" pattern but do not infiltrate deep (unlike KS)
-endothelial cells lack cytological atypia or multilayering
-overall similar to angiosarcoma but differs by well-circumscribed nature and **absence of extension into subcutaneous tissue**
-also, there is **lack of multilayering, mitoses, and hemorrhage**
-***c-MYC* stain is negative** unlike positivity seen in radiation induced angiosarcoma

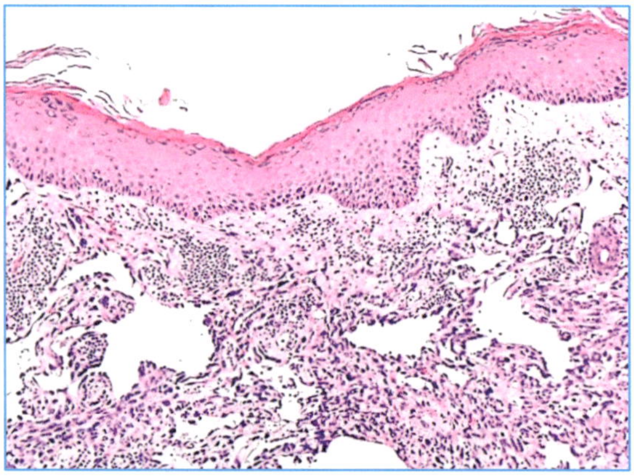

Angiosarcoma with dilated vessels in staghorn pattern

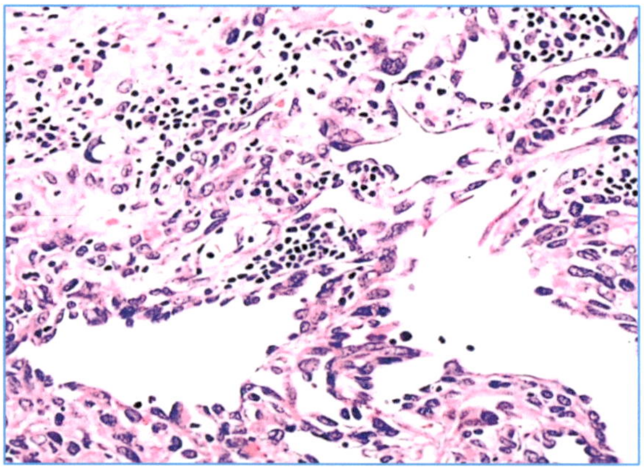

Angiosarcoma with atypical endothelial cells with hobnailing

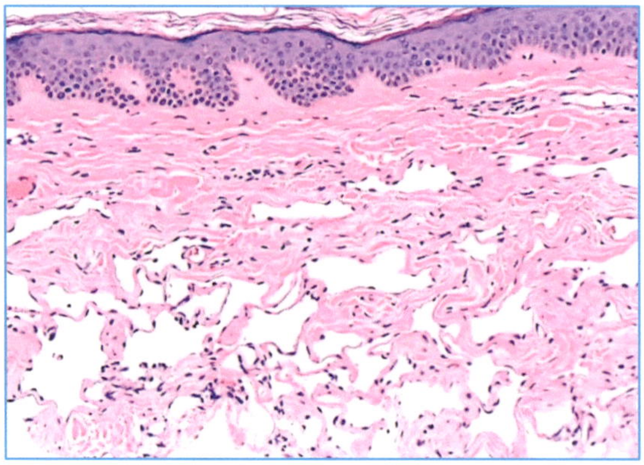

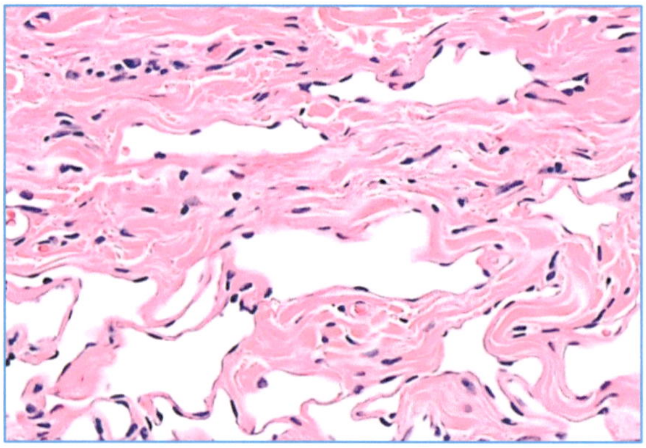

Atypical vascular proliferation with irregularly shaped capillaries without atypia of endothelial cells

KAPOSI'S SARCOMA

-*HHV-8* associated vascular malignancy
-clinically presents as violaceous macules, patches, papules, plaques, or nodules
-four characterisic variants

Classic Kaposi's sarcoma

-typically, in elderly men of Mediterranean or Jewish origin
-lesions predominantly on the distal part of legs
-associated with a second malignancy (usually hematological) in one third of patients

African endemic Kaposi's sarcoma

-endemic to parts of Africa with various presentations
Nodular type- like classic form
Florid type- more aggressive with deeper subcutaneous extension
Infiltrative type- even more aggressive with mucocutaneous and visceral involvement
Lymphoadenopathic type- in children and it involves lymph nodes usually without cutaneous involvement

AIDS associated Kaposi's sarcoma

-in HIV positive patients
-solitary or multiple violaceous lesions favoring face and trunk

Iatrogenic immunocompromised Kaposi's sarcoma

-seen in immunosuppressed patients (transplant and chemotherapy patients) and autoimmune diseases

Histopathology

Patch stage

-dermal, ill-defined lesion that is easy to miss histologically
-**subtle proliferation of small, "capillary-like", vascular channels**
-vessels are compressed between thick collagen, around larger, irregular vessels and around adnexa
-minimal red blood cell extravasation

Plaque stage

-increased, more easily detected dermal vascular proliferation
-numerous **"slit-like" or "sieve-like"** vascular spaces with **spindle endothelial cells**
-**red blood cell extravasation** with lymphocytes and **plasma cells**

Nodular stage

-diffuse **nodular proliferation of atypical spindle endothelial cells**
forming fascicles with **"slit-like" spaces** in between
-red blood cell extravasation

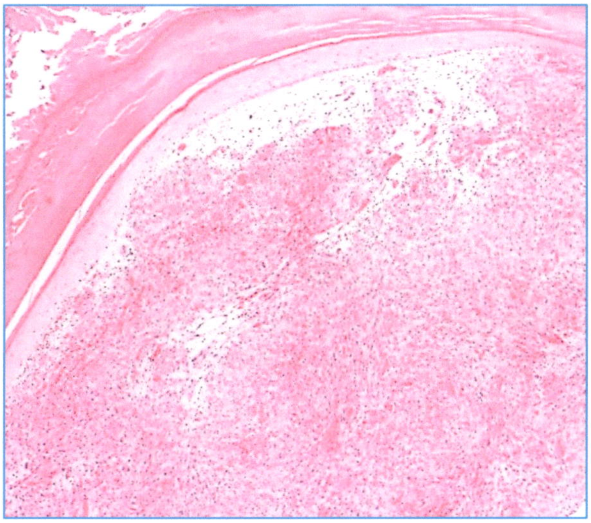

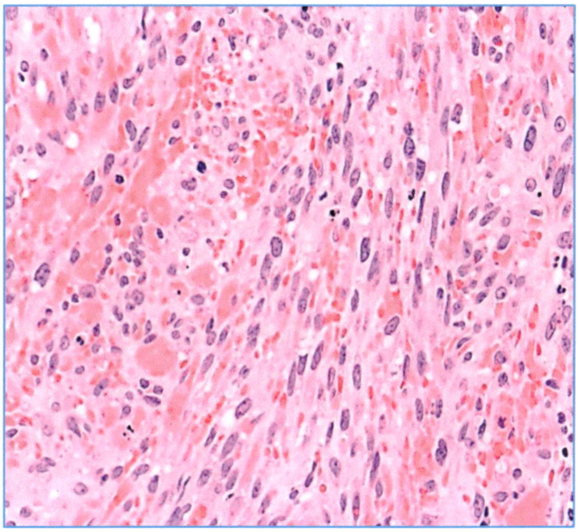

Kaposi's sarcoma, nodular stage, with spindle cells forming "slit-like" spaces and RBCs extravasation

Vascular tumors

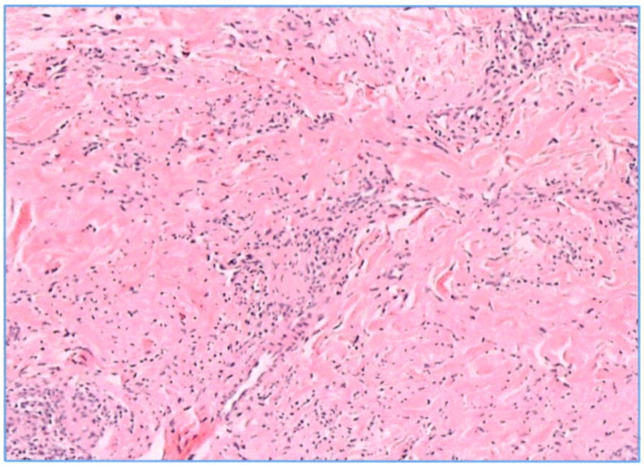
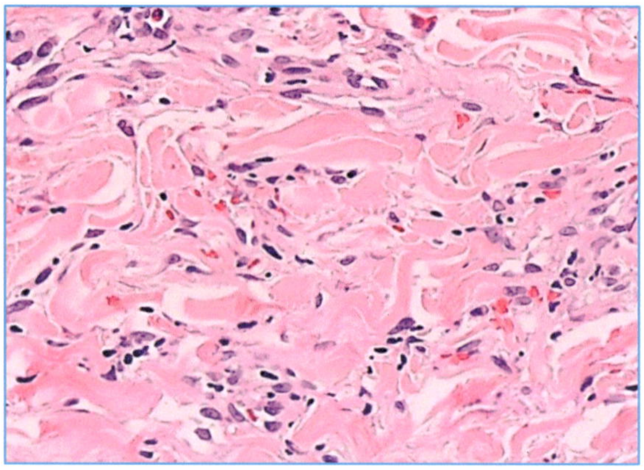

Kaposi's sarcoma, patch stage, with subtle proliferation of "slit-like" vessels

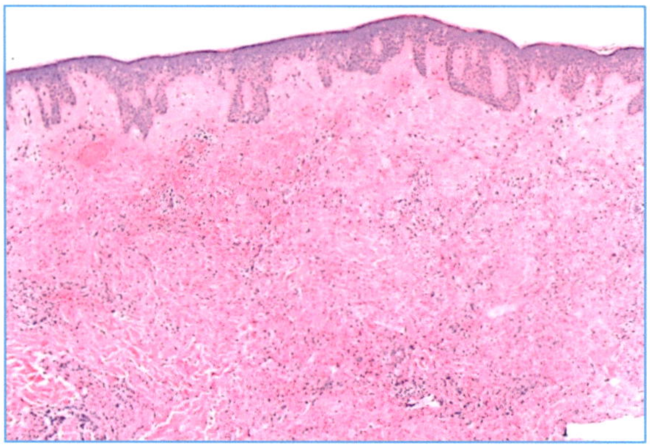
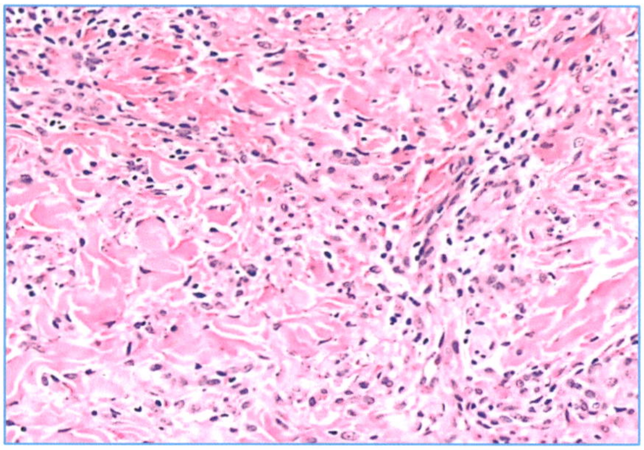

Kaposi's sarcoma, plaque stage, with prominent spindle cells and hemorrhage

KAPOSIFORM HEMANGIOENDOTHELIOMA

- -soft tissue mass or subcutaneous nodule usually in children less than 10 years old
- -usually on the upper extremities but also in retroperitoneum and intrathoracic
- -associated with Kasabach-Merritt phenomenon

Histopathology

- -dermal/subcutaneous multinodular tumor
- -spindle endothelial cells with "slit-like" spaces and RBCs form nodules **resembling nodular stage KS**
- -peripheral area consists of small blood vessels **resembling a capillary hemangioma**
- -tumor is **HHV8 negative**

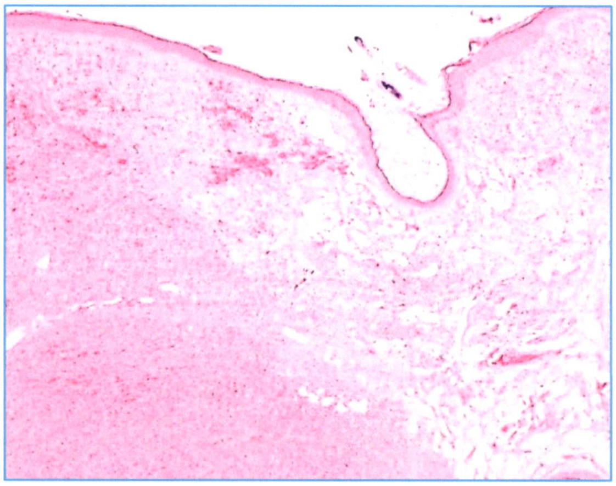

Kaposiform hemangioendothelioma

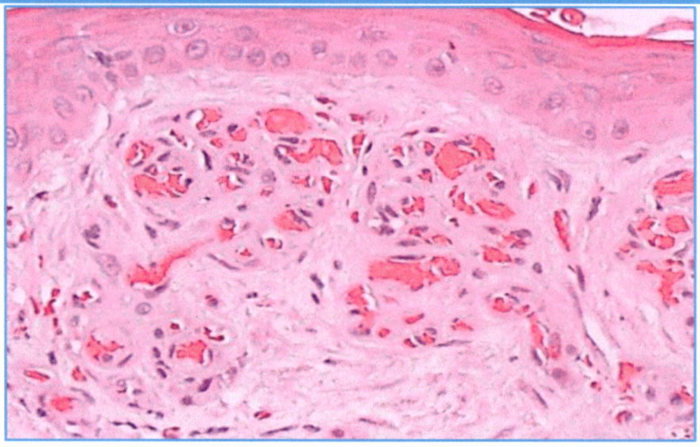
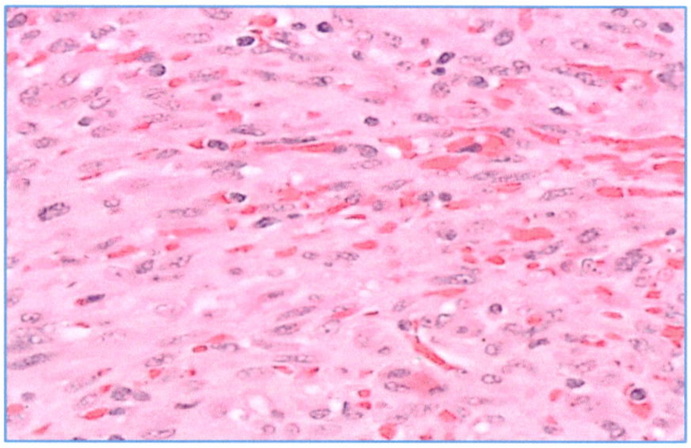

Kaposiform hemangioendothelioma with "capillary hemangioma-like" area (left) and "KS-like" area (right)

Chapter 34

HOW TO APPROACH VASCULAR TUMORS

LESION IS MADE OF LARGE NUMBER OF NORMAL VESSELS

-benign vascular tumors

DETERMINE PATIENT'S AGE

NEWBORN		
-infantile hemangioma	capillary proliferation	GLUT-1 positive
-nevus simplex	widely dilated capillaries	GLUT-1 negative
CHILDHOOD		
-vascular malformations		
-tufted hemangioma	"cannon balls" with vascular tufts	
-glomeruloid hemangioma	glomeruloid vascular proliferation	POEMs syndrome
-cavernous hemangioma	large, thin walled vessels	
-pyogenic granuloma	excoriated lobular capillary proliferation with collarette	
-angiomatosis	deep, infiltrating capillary proliferation	
-verrucous hemangioma	verruciform epidermis	
-angiokeratoma	dilated thin walled vessels elevating epidermis	
-lymphangioma	lymphatic channels with flaps	
ADULT		
-cherry angioma	epidermal collarettes encircle small vessels	
-spider angioma	vertical vessel with few dilated vascular channels	
-arterio-venous hemangioma	thick and thin walled vessels	
-pyogenic granuloma	eroded lobular capillary proliferation with collarette	
-Masson's tumor (IPEH)	thrombosed vessels + papillae	
-angiokeratoma	dilated thin walled vessels elevating epidermis	
-venous lake	single, large, thin walled vessel	
-acquired elastotic hemangioma	irregular capillaries + extensive solar elastosis	
-hobnail hemangioma	wedge shaped capillary lesion with "hobnail" endothelial cells	
-microvenular hemangioma	poorly defined lesion with collapsed capillaries	
-spindle cell hemangioma	biphasic lesion: cystic and spindled area	
-stasis dermatitis	lobular capillary proliferation on lower legs	

VASCULAR PROLIFERATION SURROUNDED BY UNIFORM CELLS

-glomus tumor	compressed, subtle vascular spaces
-glomuvenous malformation	dilated, obvious vascular channels

VASCULAR PROLIFERATION WITH NEUTROPHILIC DEBRIS

-bacillary angiomatosis	"KS-like" with neutrophils

VASCULAR PROLIFERATION WITH MIXED INFLAMMATION

-epithelioid hemangioma	vessels with "onion skin" + eosinophils

LESION IS MADE OF ATYPICAL VASCULAR CHANNELS

-angiosarcoma	irregularly shaped vessels dissecting collagen
-atypical vascular proliferation	irregular vessels only in the superficial dermis
-Kaposi's sarcoma	"slit-like" vascular channels and spindle cells
-Kaposiform hemangioendothelioma	"KS-like" + "capillary hemangioma-like" areas
-acroangiodermatitis	lobular pattern with hemosiderin and no spindle cells

NOT SURE IF THE LESION IS VASCULAR

-hemangiopericytoma	spindle cells with staghorn empty spaces
-epithelioid hemangioendothelioma	epithelioid cells with intracytoplasmic vacuoles
-retiform hemangioendothelioma	arborizing vessels with "hobnails"

Vascular tumors

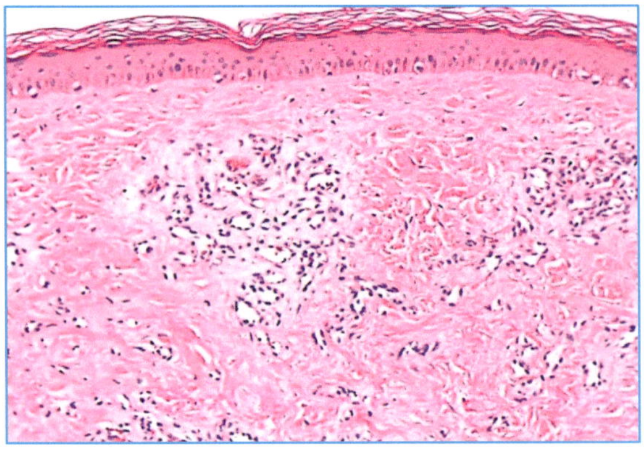

Infantile hemangioma with capillary proliferation

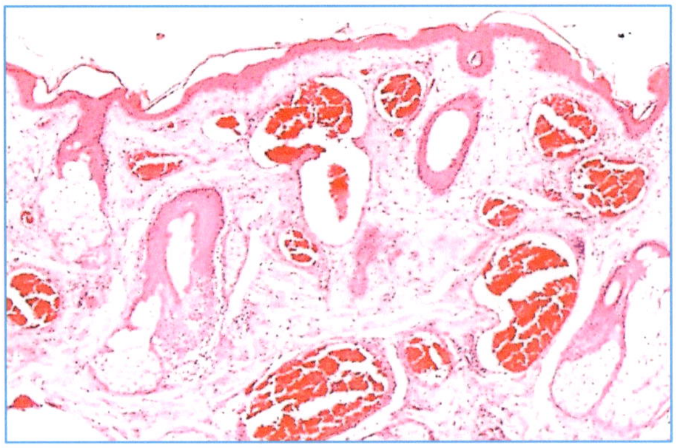

Port wine stain is broad lesion with dilated vessels

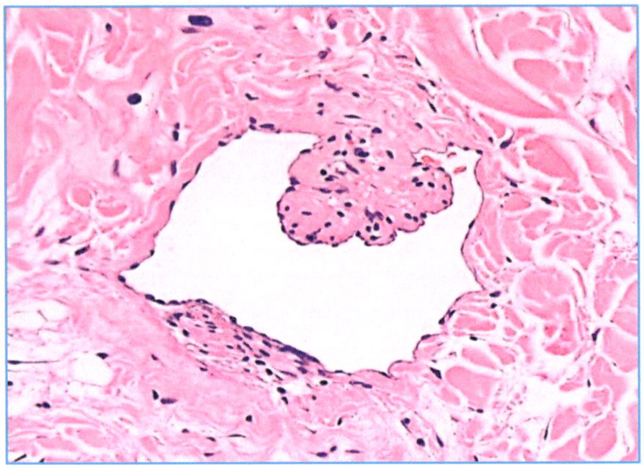

Tufted hemangioma with vascular tuft

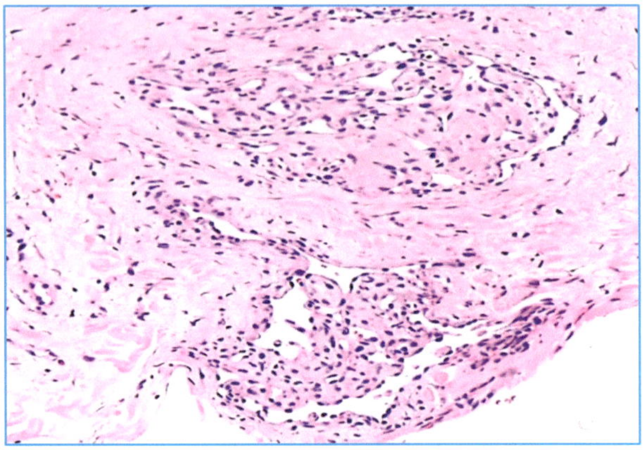

Glomeruloid hemangioma resembles kidney glomeruli

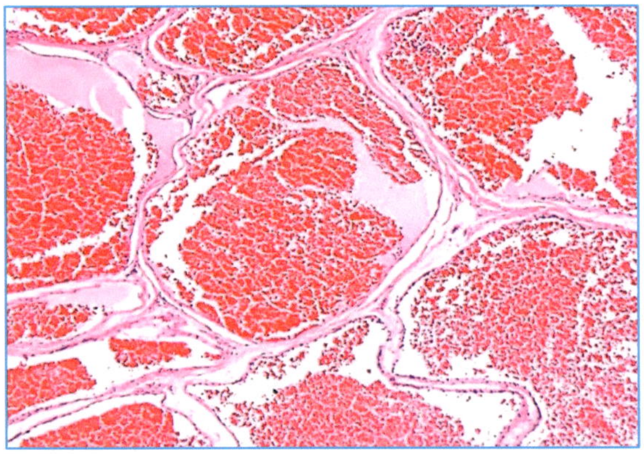

Cavernous hemangioma with thin-walled dilated vessels

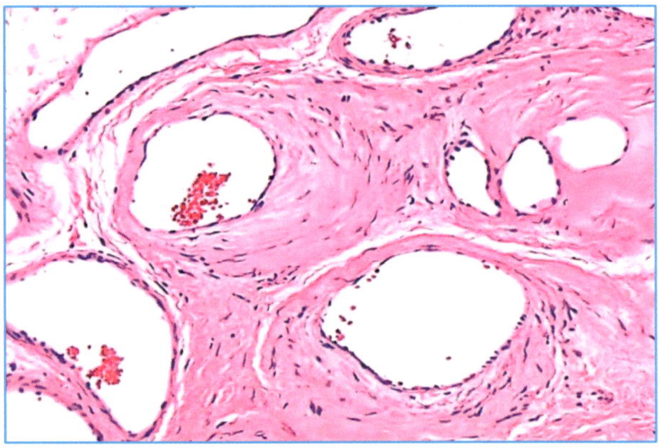

AV hemangioma with thin and thick-walled vessels

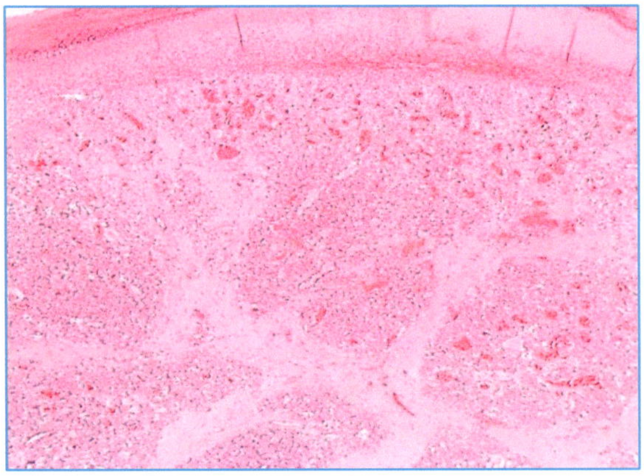

Pyogenic granuloma is excoriated lobular capillary lesion

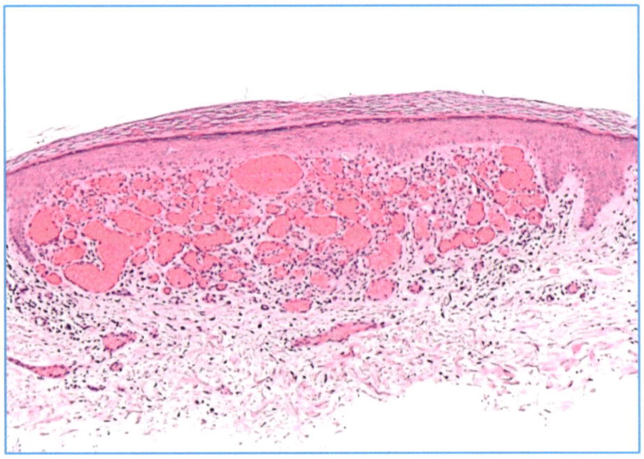

Cherry angioma with epidermal collarettes hugging vessels

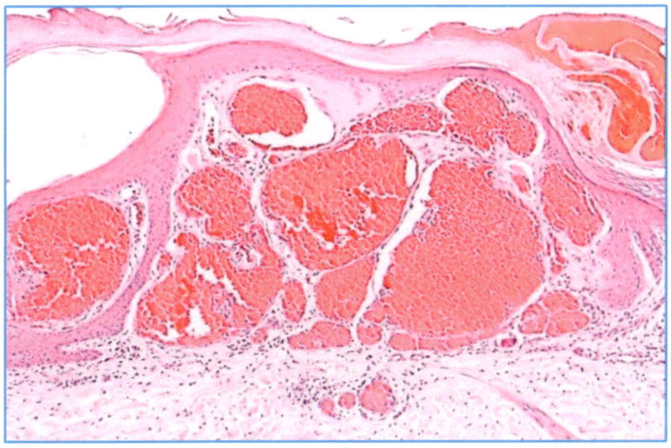

Angiokeratoma with dilated vessels lifting epidermis

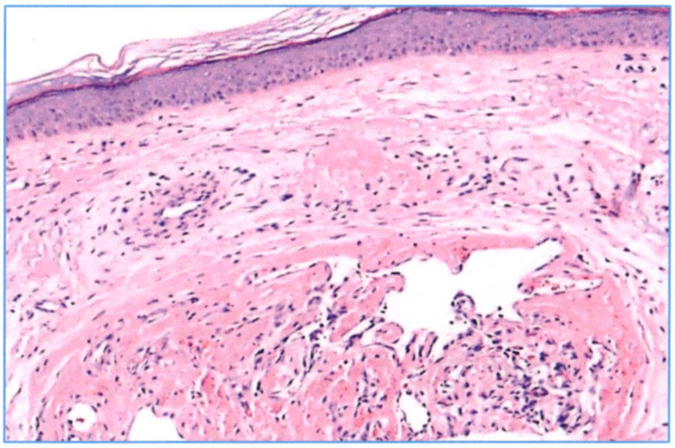

Masson's tumor with organizing thrombus in a dilated vessel

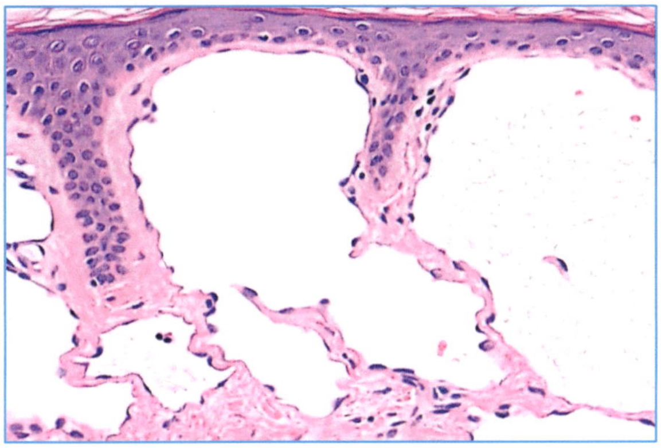

Lymphangioma with lymphatic flaps

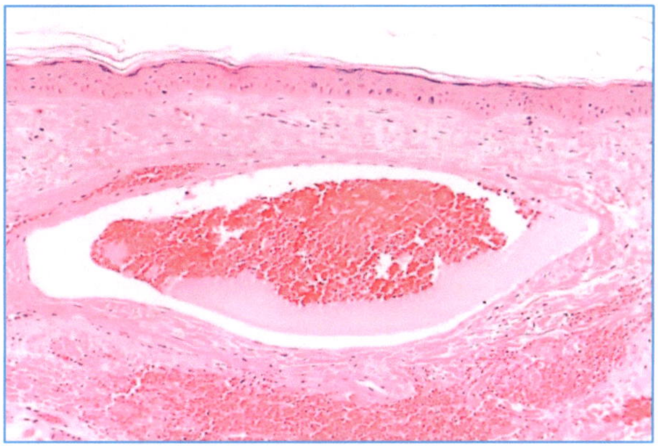

Venous lake with single widely dilated vessel

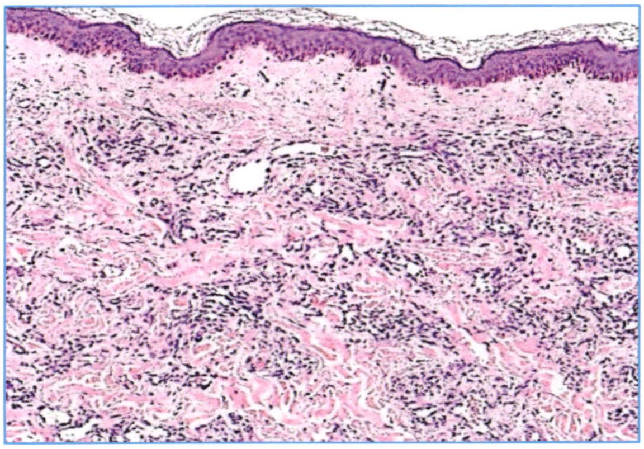

Microvenular hemangioma with collapsed vascular channels

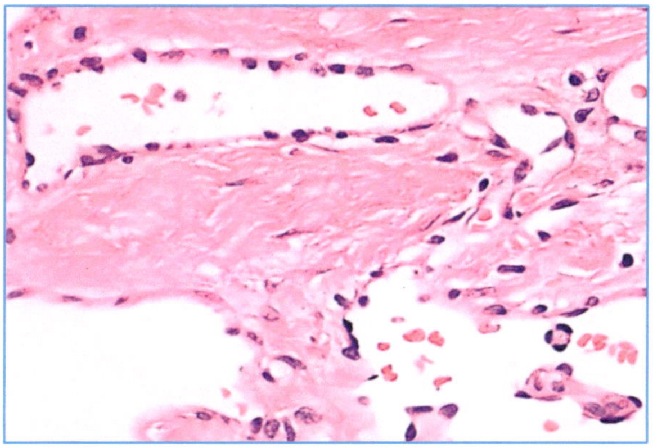

Hobnail hemangioma with prominent endothelial nuclei

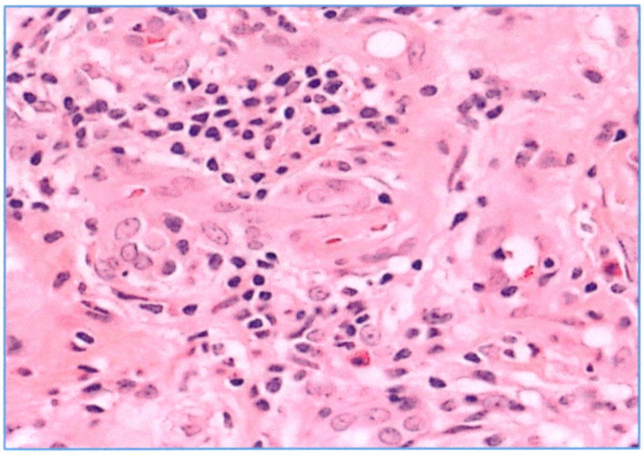

Angiolymphoid hyperplasia with eosinophilia with plump endothelial cells and mixed inflammation with eosinophils

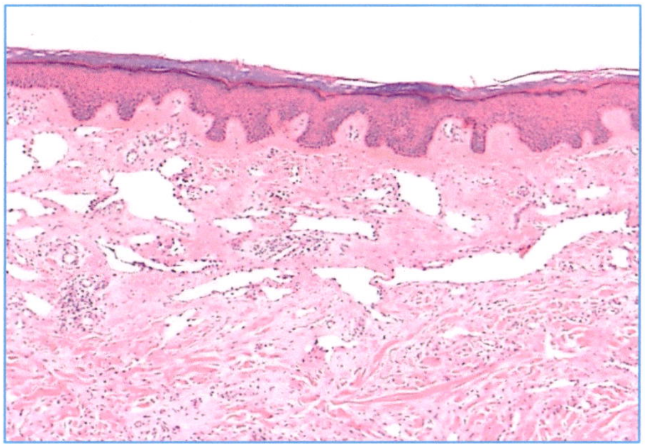

Acquired elastotic hemangioma with horizontal, shallow vascular proliferation and dermal solar elastosis

Vascular tumors

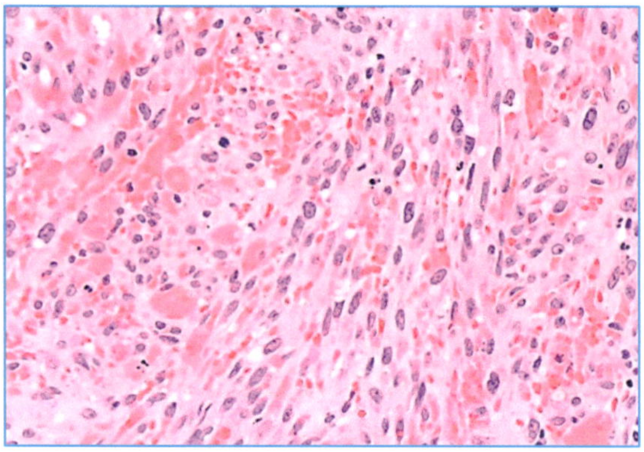

KS, nodular type, with numerous spindle cells with RBCs

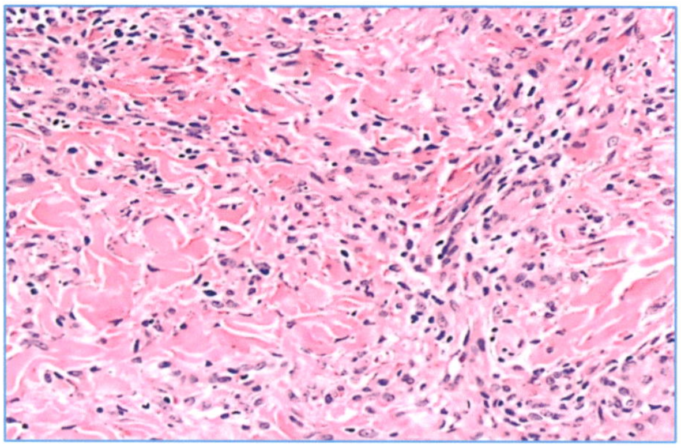

KS, plaque stage, with "slit-like" vascular channels

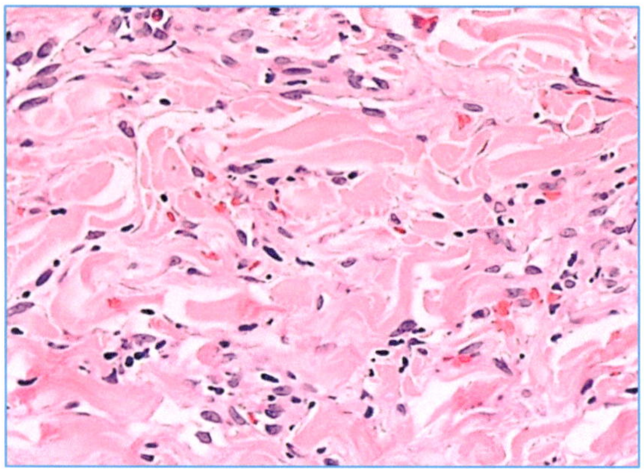

KS, patch stage, with subtle vascular slits in between collagen

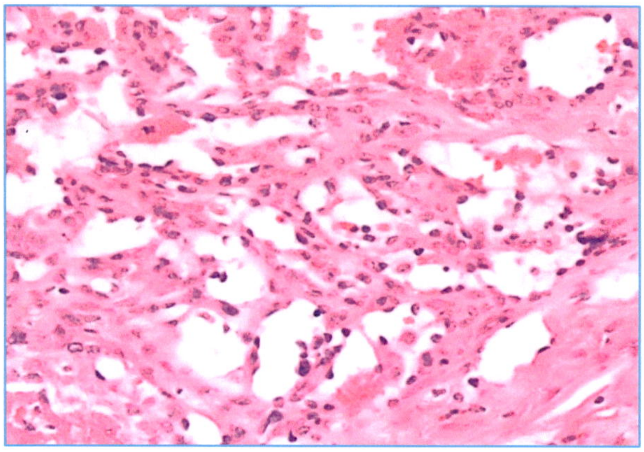

Retiform hemangioendothelioma with "rete testis-like" appearance

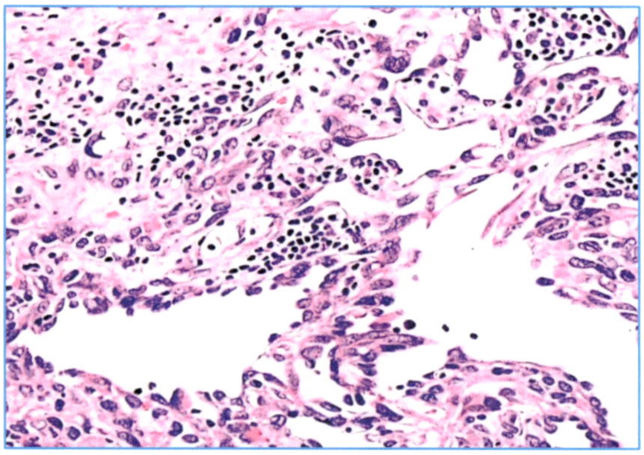

Angiosarcoma with "staghorn shaped" vessels with hobnail nuclei and no spindled cells in between channels

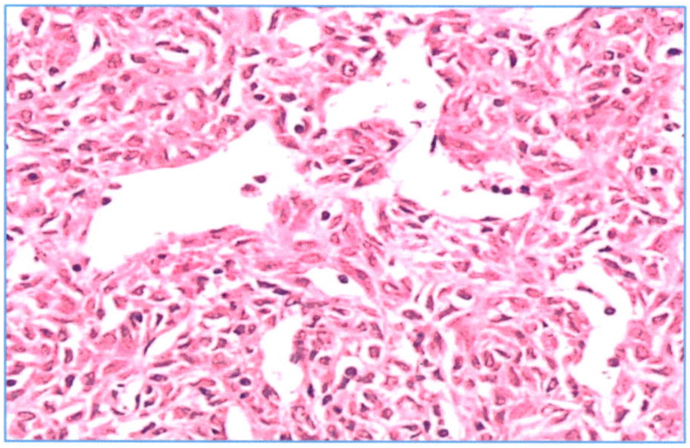

Hemangiopericytoma with "staghorn shaped" empty spaces and spindled cells in between

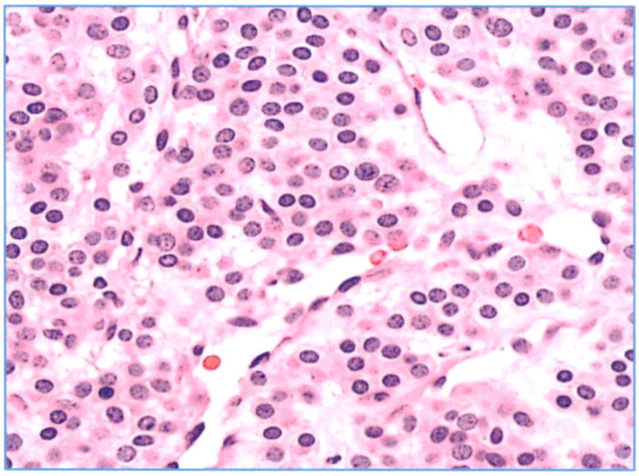

Glomus tumor with uniform cells around collapsed vessels

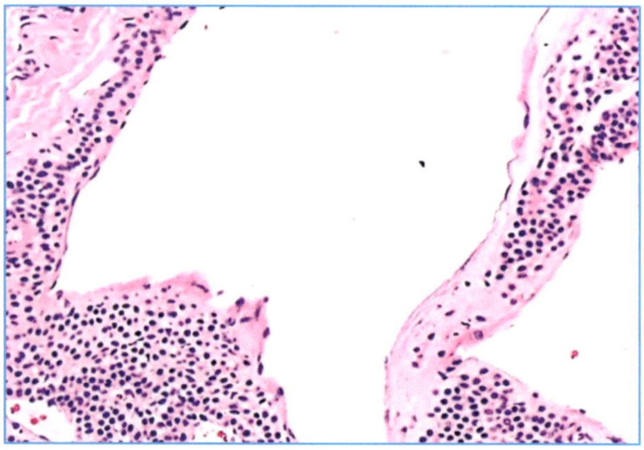

Glomangioma with dilated vessels and uniform cells around

Chapter 35

NEURAL, NEUROENDOCRINE, MUSCLE, FAT, CARTILAGE, AND BONE TUMORS

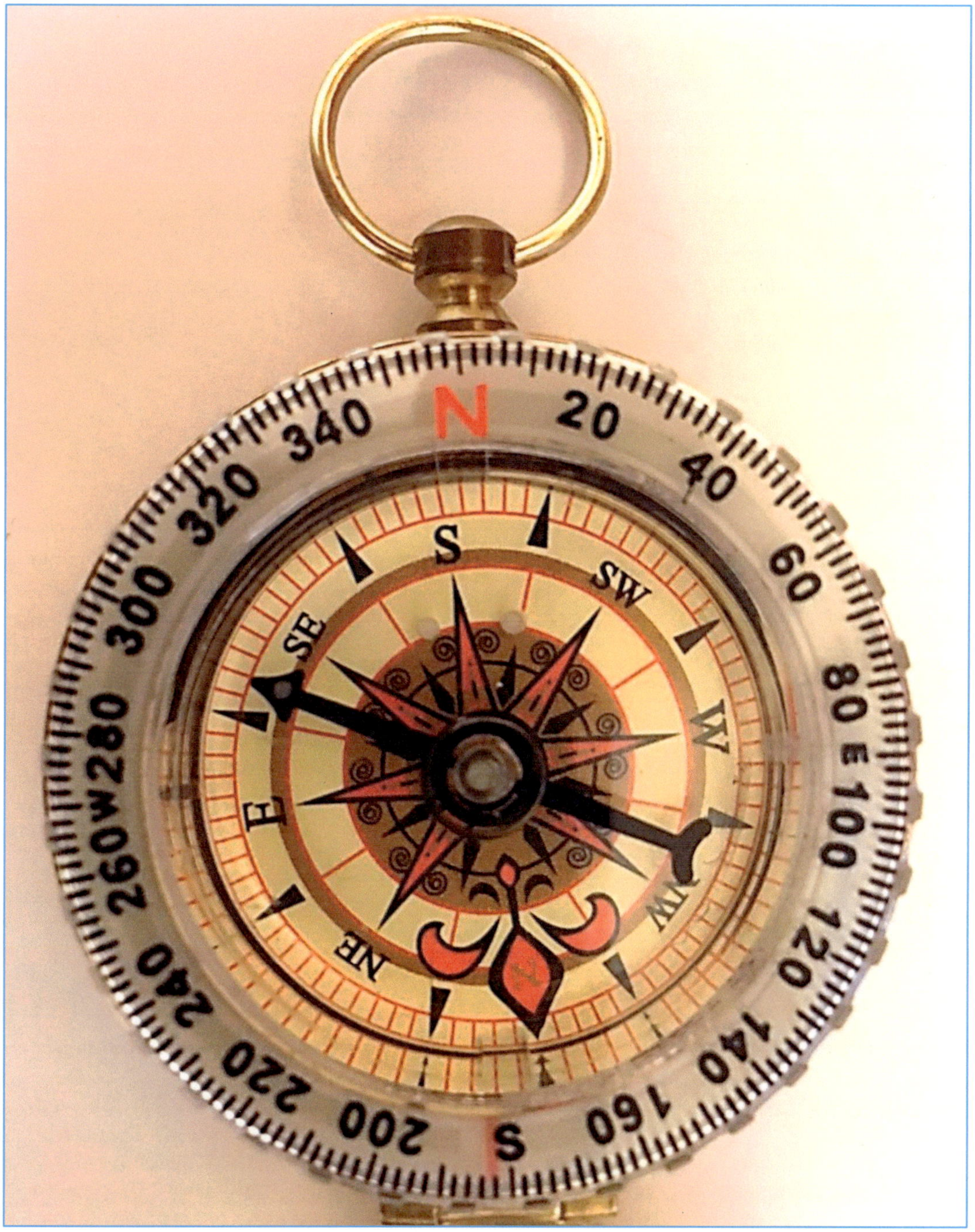

Neural, neuroendocrine, muscle, fat, cartilage, and bone tumors

NEUROFIBROMA

-benign tumor of neural origin
-usually a solitary tumor (90% of cases) but multiple lesions are seen as part of NF1
-appears as pink to skin-colored rubbery papules, (sometimes pedunculated) or nodules
-exhibits "buttonhole" sign where on palpation, the lesion retracts into the subcutis and reappear on the release of pressure

Histopathology
-**Grenz zone** separating the epidermis from a dermal/subcutaneous tumor
-tumor is poorly defined and made of **spindle cells with wavy, serpentine nuclei (S100 positive)**
-**scattered mast cells** are present
-stroma is pink and loose, **"bubble gum" stroma**
-no evidence of cytological atypia or mitoses

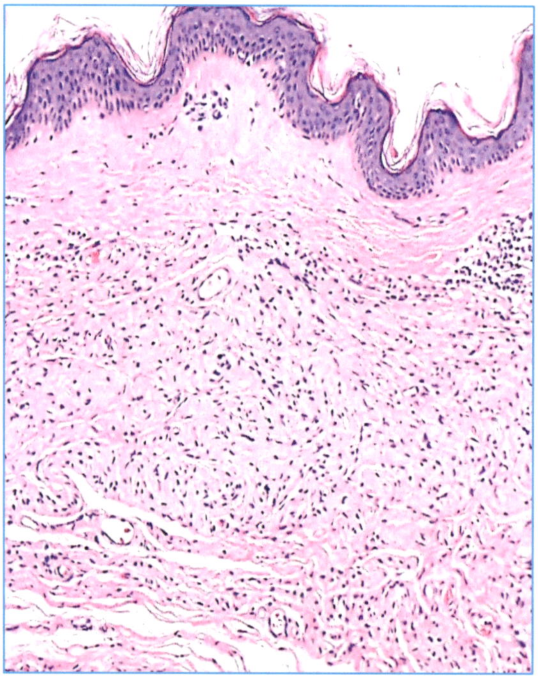

NF proliferation separated from the epidermis by Grenz zone

TRAUMATIC NEUROMA

-non-neoplastic lesion that occurs due to the body's aberrant attempt at nerve regeneration following injury, including previous surgery
-presents as small, firm, skin-colored, often painful nodules at the site of previous trauma

Histopathology
-**irregular** arrangement of **large and small neural fascicles** embedded in scar tissue

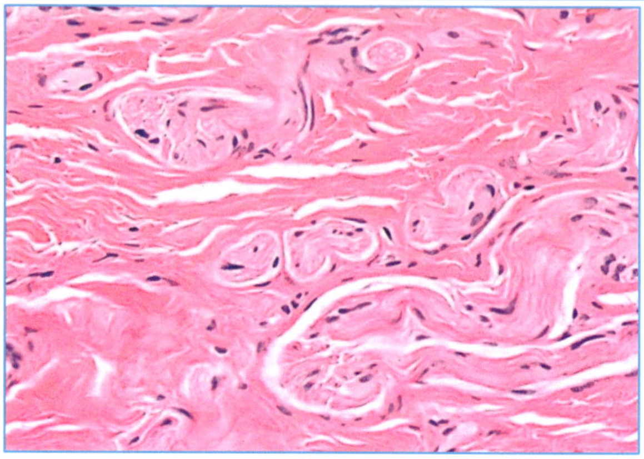

Traumatic neuroma with wavy nerves in scar tissue

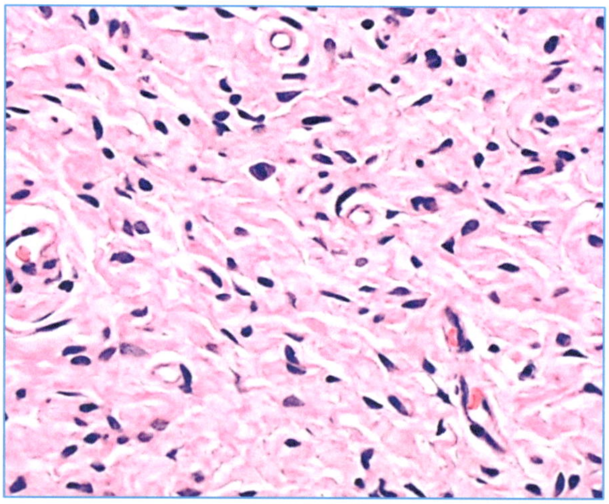

NF with spindle cells and few mast cells in "bubble gum" stroma

NEUROFOLLICULAR HAMARTOMA

-presents as a single, asymptomatic, skin-colored papule in middle-aged or older adults
-usually on the face near the nose
-resembles a fibrous papule

Histopathology
-**distorted** hyperplastic **pilosebaceous units**
-**surrounded with bland spindle cells (S100+)** that **resemble neurofibroma cells**

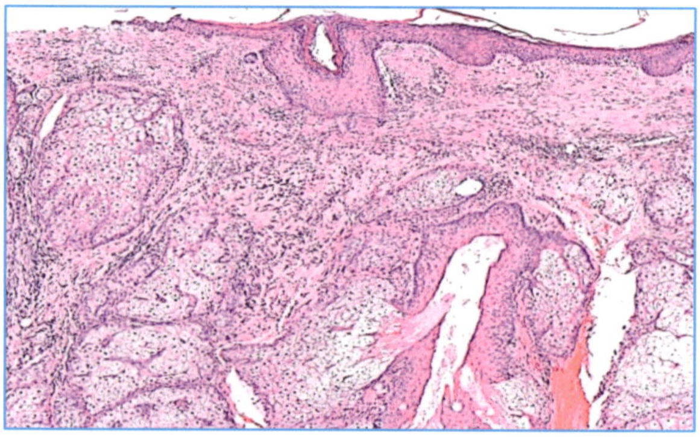

Neurofollicular hamartoma with distorted follicles and sebaceous glands surrounded with "NF-like" cells

Chapter 35

CELLULAR NEUROTHEKEOMA

-rare benign tumor of unclear but presumed fibrohistiocytic origin
-presents as a solitary, firm, pink painless papule
-typically, on the head, neck, or upper extremities of younger adult women

Histopathology
-lobulated dermal tumor based in the mid dermis, sparing the epidermis
-comprised of **fascicles and nests of plump spindle and epithelioid cells** with relatively abundant cytoplasm
-**gray-blue, loose, myxoid stromal** background
-nuclear pleomorphism varies from inconspicuous to marked
-atypical mitoses can be seen
-tumor cells are **NKI-C3**, CD10, NSE, pGp9.5 **positive** and **S-100**, SOX10 **negative**

DERMAL NERVE SHEATH MYXOMA

-benign nerve sheath tumor, formerly referred to as neurothekeoma because of similar histology
-solitary, small, painless, skin-colored papule/nodule
-mainly in young and middle-aged adults
-favors the extremities, most often the fingers

Histopathology
-dermal tumor with **multilobular appearance**
-uniform, **round to spindle cells arranged in a swirling pattern in a myxoid matrix**
-fibrous stroma separates fascicles
-mitoses can be seen
-cells are **S100 positive, NKI-C3 negative**

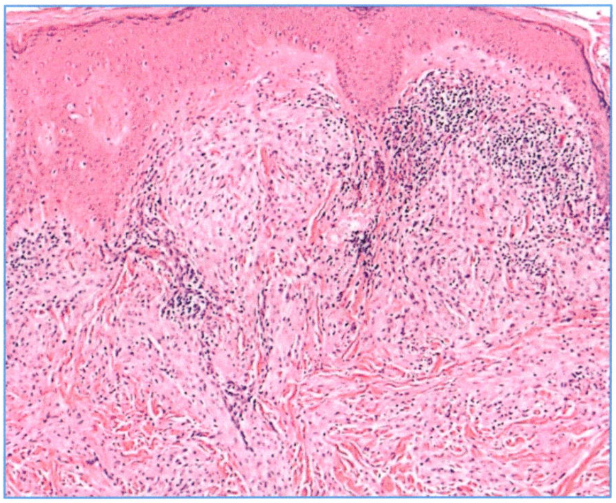
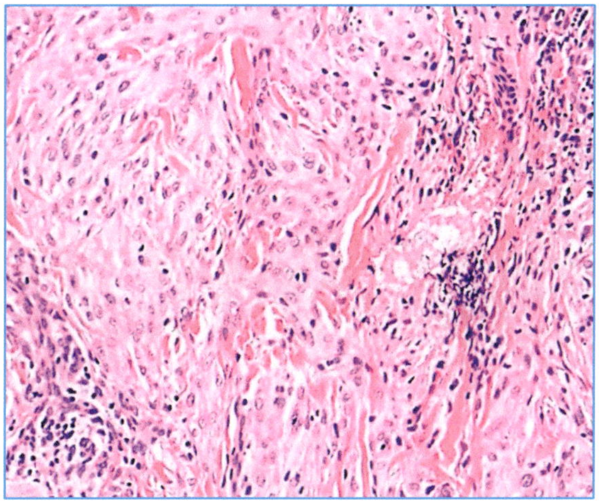

Cellular neurothekeoma with diffuse dermal proliferation of plump spindle cells in myxoid background

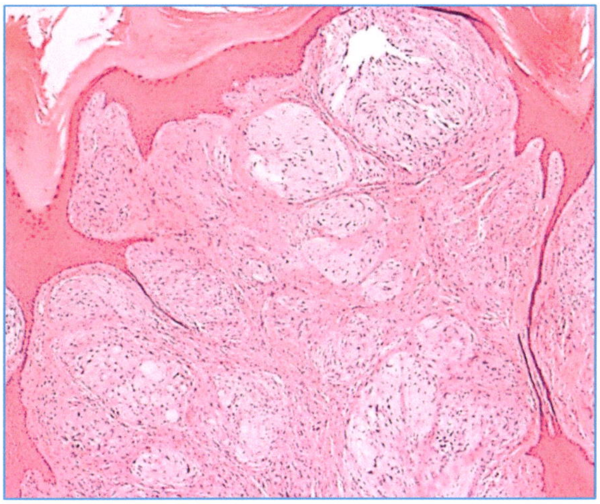
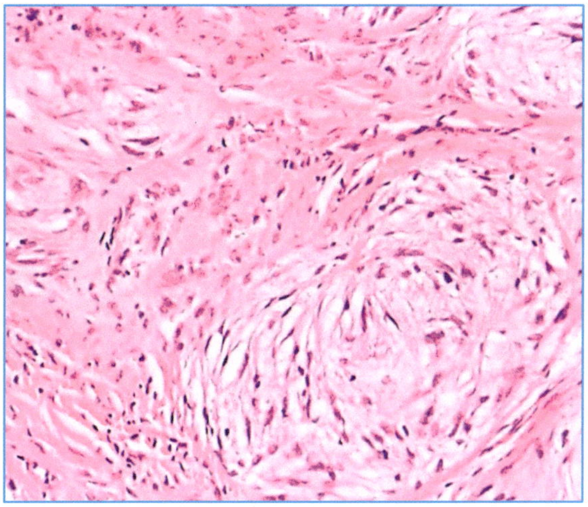

Dermal nerve sheath myxoma with multi lobular appearance made of swirling balls of spindle cells in myxoid background

Neural, neuroendocrine, muscle, fat, cartilage, and bone tumors

PALISADED AND ENCAPSULATED NEUROMA (SOLITARY CIRCUMSCRIBED NEUROMA)

-small, slowly growing, skin-colored papule
-solitary and painless
-usually on the face favoring eyelid, nose, perioral skin, and oral mucosa
-in middle-aged people favoring females

Histopathology
-well-circumscribed **dermal nodule**
-surrounded by pseudocapsule (not really encapsulated despite the name)
-formed by well-developed **fascicles of spindle cells with pointed, tapered ends** resembling endoneurium
-cells are S100 positive
-vague **alteration in cellularity** with **palisading (pseudo Verocay bodies)**
-**resembles Schwannoma, but is superficial**

SCHWANNOMA

-benign peripheral nerve sheath tumor
-solitary, pink, dermal or subcutaneous nodule
-favors flexural extremities, head and neck
-multiple lesions are associated with NF2 (bilateral acoustic neuromas) and schwannomatosis

Histopathology
-**deep, subcutaneous,** well-circumscribed tumor
-epidermis is rarely seen due to tumor depth
-made of **elongated, spindle, wavy cells with tapered ends** (S100 positive)
-alternating cellularity (**hypercellular Antoni A** areas and **hypocellular Antoni B** areas)
-characteristic nuclear palisading forming **Verocay bodies** (areas of hypercellularity enclosing an area of hypocellularity)

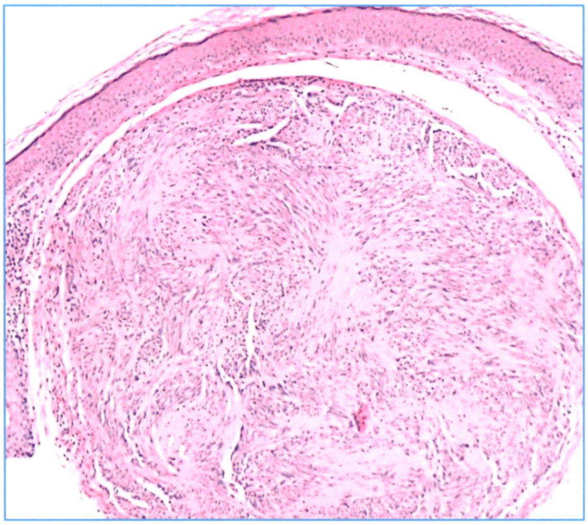
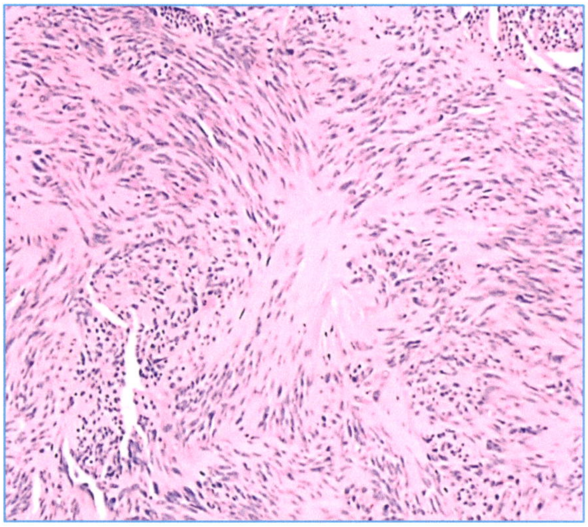

Palisaded and encapsulated neuroma is dermal tumor with hyper and hypocellular areas of elongated cells with tapered ends

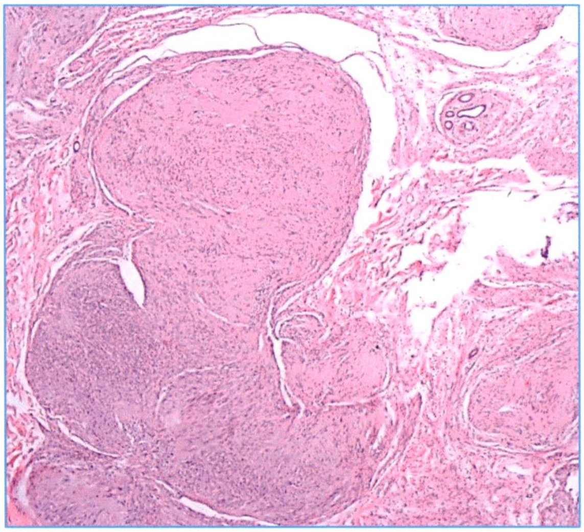
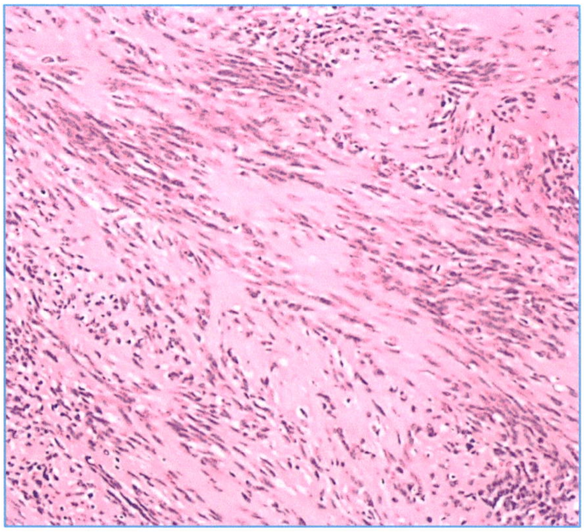

Schwannoma is deep subcutaneous tumor made of spindle cells with pointed ends forming Verocay bodies

MALIGNANT PERIPHERAL NERVE SHEATH TUMOR

-rare tumor that presents as a rapidly growing nodule in subcutis
-favors head and neck of middle-aged people
-associated with neurofibromatosis type 1 (lifetime risk is about 10%)

Histopathology
-multinodular deep dermal/subcutaneous tumor
-made of **atypical spindle cells** with **wavy nuclei forming fascicles** (S100 positive)
-cells are **pleomorphic** and some can have bizarre appearance
-vaguely **hypercellular and hypocellular areas** with nuclear palisading resembling Schwannoma
-**mitoses** and necrosis are common
-variants are myxoid (with more than 50% of myxoid cells), giant cell, and inflammatory

PERINEURIOMA

-rare benign peripheral nerve sheath tumor
-presents as intraneural and extraneural
-cutaneous lesions are extraneural and present as a firm, skin-colored papule in middle-aged adults
-favors limbs and trunk

Histopathology
-dermal/subcutaneous ill-defined tumor
-bland, **elongated**, “**neurofibroma-like” cells** organized in **parallel, whorled (“meningioma-like”), or storiform pattern**
-collagenous or myxoid stroma
-some cases show hyalinized stroma with “onion-skin” fibrosis around fascicles (**sclerosing perinerioma**)
-tumor cells are **EMA and GLUT1 positive** and **S100 negative**

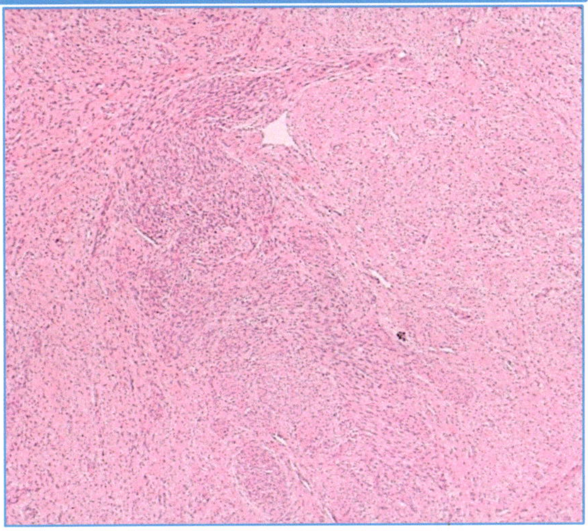

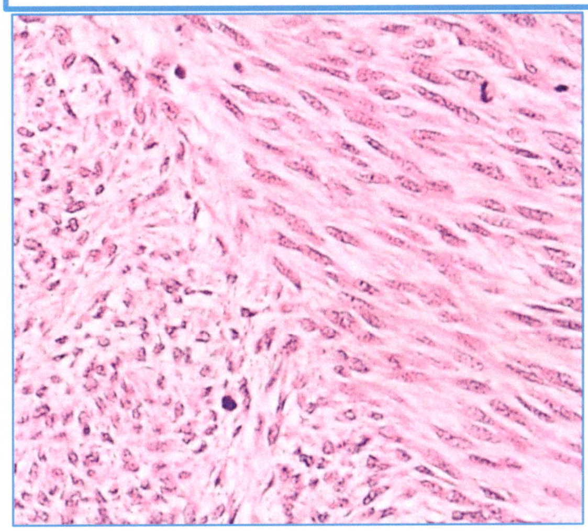

Malignant peripheral nerve sheath tumor with alternating cellularity consisting of atypical spindle cells with numerous mitoses

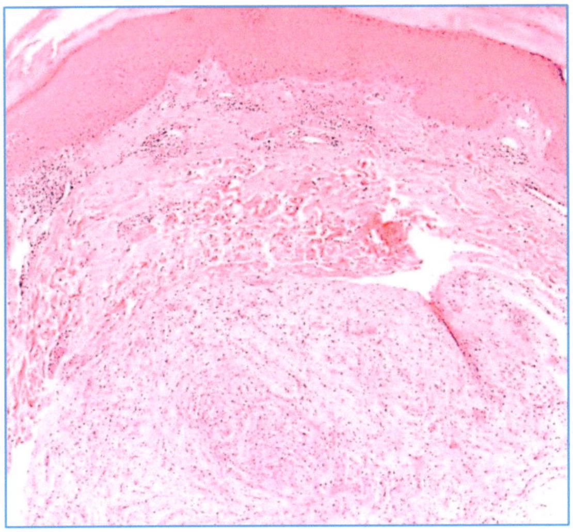

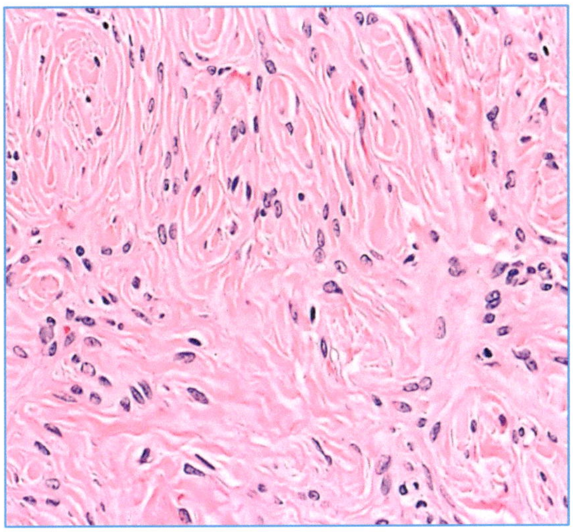

Sclerosing perineurioma with “neurofibroma-like” cells forming fascicles organized in whorled pattern

LIPOMAS

Multiple variants:

Lipoma, spindle cell lipoma, pleomorphic lipoma

-common benign fat tumors
-all are clinically similar presenting as soft, rounded, mobile, skin-colored subcutaneous nodules
-may occur at any site but spindle cell lipomas favor the posterior neck
-usually occur in middle-aged patients

Lipomatosis

-localized overgrowth of mature adipose tissue
-involves not only the subcutis but also the underlying musculature
-**diffuse type** begins in childhood and affects large area of trunk or extremities
-**cervical type** affects middle-aged men with history of alcohol consumption
-**pelvic type** more frequent in young African American women with perirectal and perivesicular overgrowth of fat

Histopathology

Lipoma

-not encapsulated mature fat with thin fibrous septa
-adipocytes stains positive with S100

Variants are:

Spindle cell lipoma

-tumor made of mature fat plus uniform, bland **spindle cells** (CD34+)
-variable myxoid background and **"ropey" collagen**
-mast cells are common

Pleomorphic lipoma

-can look **like regular or spindle cell lipoma**
-in addition, **multinucleated giant cells with dense cytoplasm** and **peripheral nuclei** (**"floret" cells**)

Lipomatosis

-mature adipose tissue in an infiltrative growth pattern

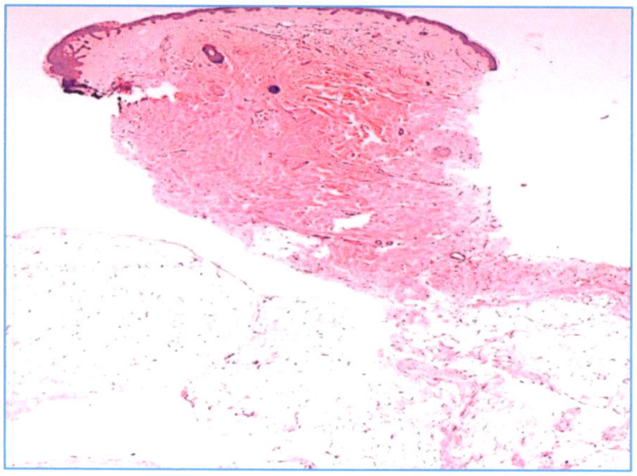

Lipoma with large nodule of mature fat

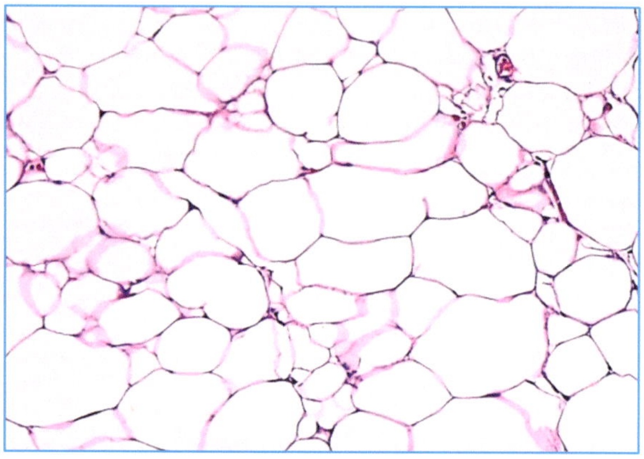

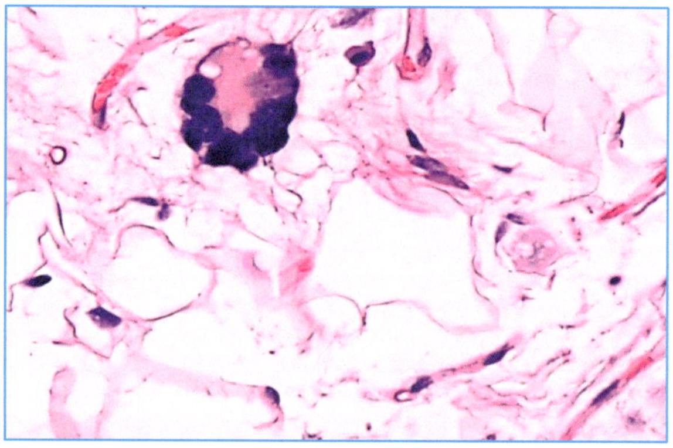

Pleomorphic lipoma with "floret" cells

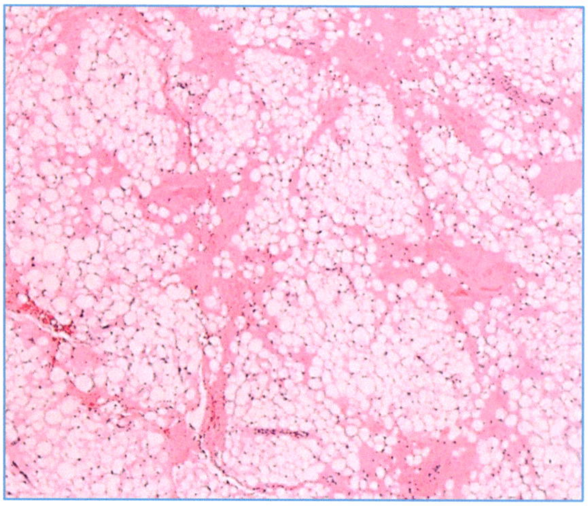

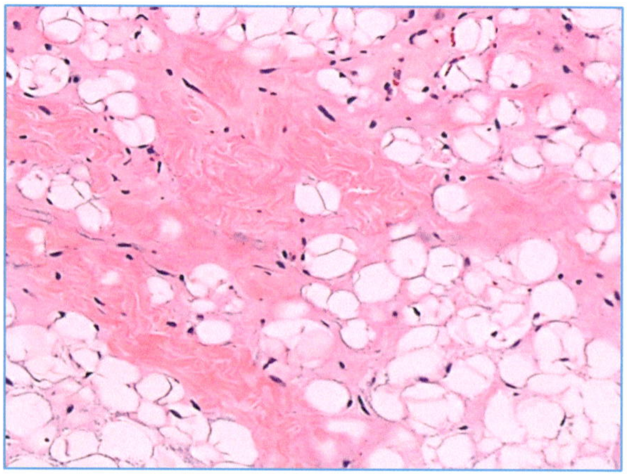

Spindle cell lipoma with adipocytes admixed with spindle cells and "ropey" collagen

Chapter 35

ANGIOLIPOMA

-solitary or more frequently multiple (2-4), painful, soft, mobile, subcutaneous nodules in young adults
-favors the extremities and trunk

Histopathology
-consists of **mature adipose tissue plus a capillary proliferation** with no evidence of atypia
-vascular component comprises more than 5% of the tumor
-capillaries are more concentrated around tumor periphery

ANGIOMYOLIPOMA

-commonly found in the kidney, where it is associated with tuberous sclerosis
-rarely presents as a subcutaneous nodule in the skin (not associated with tuberous sclerosis)

Histopathology
-bundles of **myoid "cigar-shaped" spindle cells, adipocytes, and small to medium vascular channels**
-cells are **HMB 45 positive**

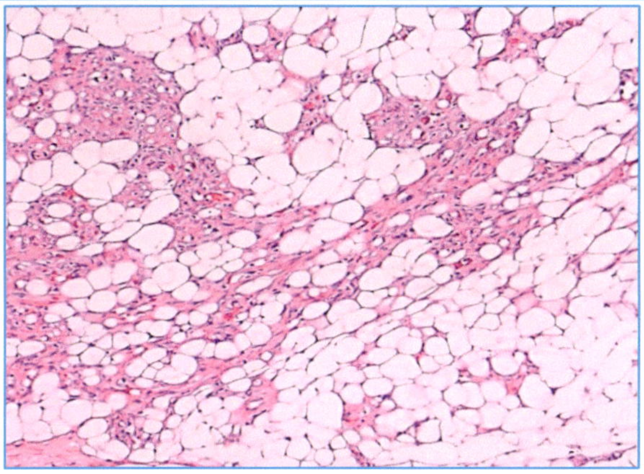
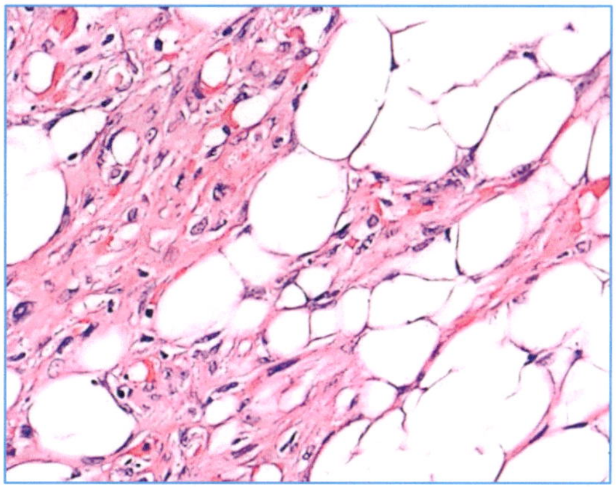

Angiolipoma with mature adipose tissue and prominent capillaries

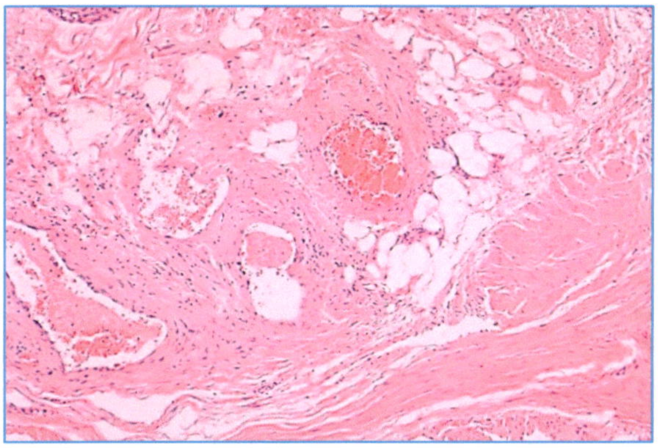
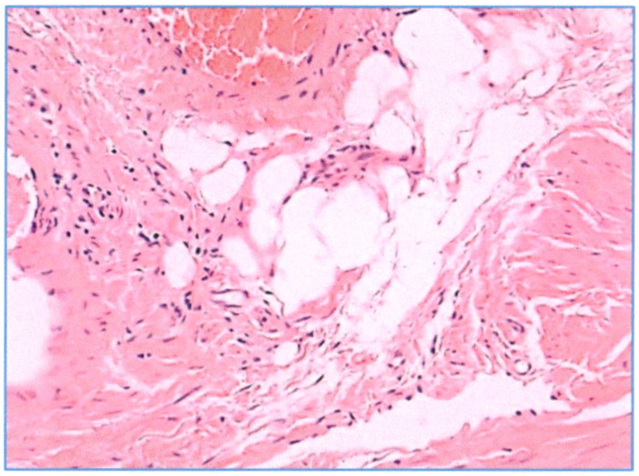

Angiomyolipoma made of fat, muscles, and vessels

NEVUS LIPOMATOSUS

-hamartoma of ectopic mature fat
-soft cerebriform pedunculated papule
-usually unilateral, on the buttock, lower back, or thigh
-usually present at birth or shows up in childhood or early adolescence

Histopathology
-**polypoid lesion** with a broad base
-**mature fat within the superficial dermis**
-adnexal structures are absent

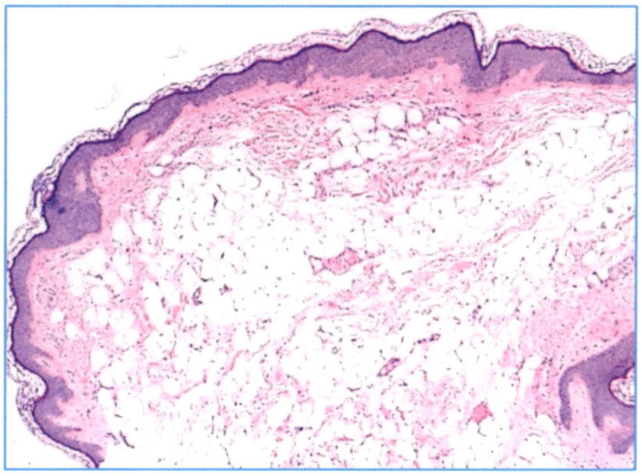

Nevus lipomatosus with adipocytes in the dermis

ATYPICAL LIPOMATOUS TUMOR/ WELL DIFFERENTIATED LIPOSARCOMA

-accounts for close to half of all liposarcomas
-mostly in middle-aged and elderly adults
-both of these tumors are morphologically and genetically identical
-variation in terminology is intended to avoid both under treatment and overtreatment
-if the tumor is located on the extremities (usually thigh), there is no risk of metastasis
-complete resection is generally curative and term atypical lipomatous tumor is preferred
-if the tumor is deep seated (retroperitoneum, mediastinum, paratesticular) the chance of achieving negative margins is significantly diminished and the risk of local recurrence and death are increased
-in these cases, the term well-differentiated liposarcoma is preferred

Histopathology
-generally composed of mature fat with **variation in size of adipocytes**
-bands of **fibrotic stroma containing cells with enlarged, hyperchromatic nuclei**
-they can form giant "floret cells"
-lipoblasts may be seen but are not needed for diagnosis
-genetic testing reveals ring or giant marker/rod chromosomes composed of material from 12q13-15
-**MDM2,** CDK4, TSPAN31 and HMGA2 genes are amplified

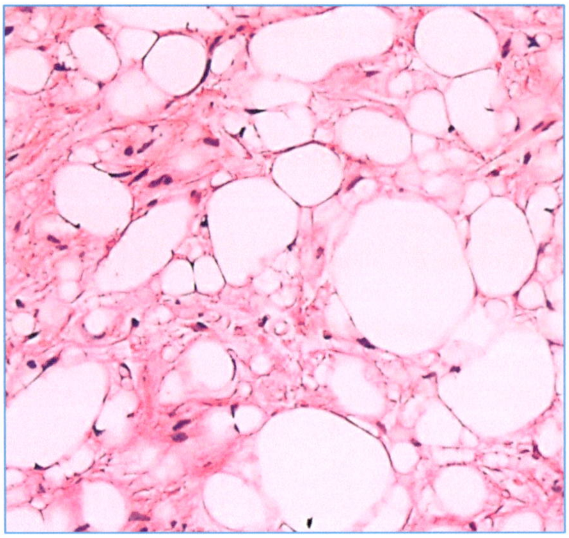

Well differentiated liposarcoma with variation in size of adipocytes and hyperchromatic stromal cells

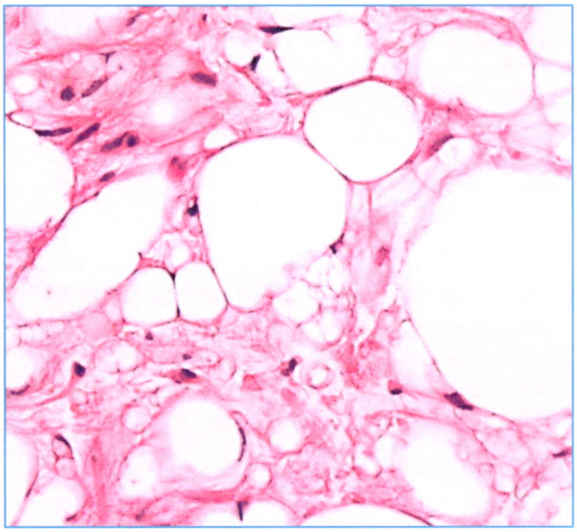

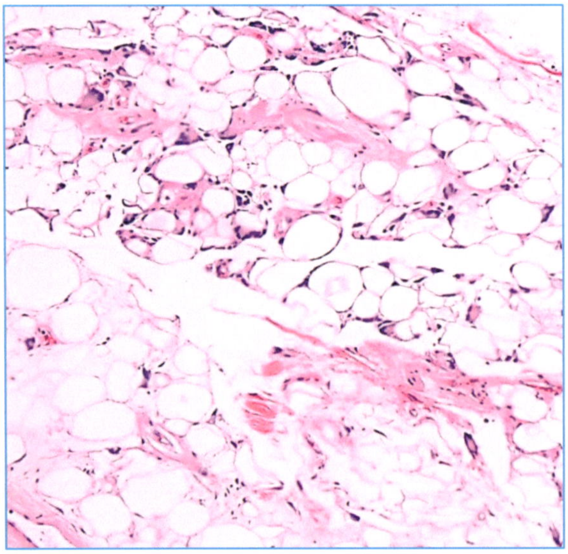

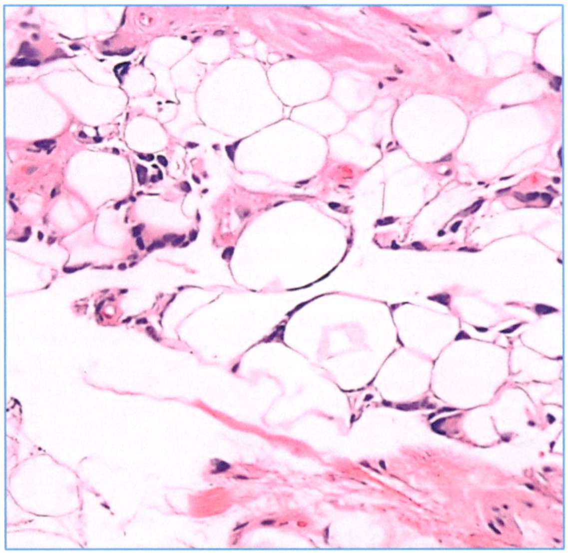

Atypical lipomatous tumor with variable adipocytes and fibrotic stroma in between with scattered dark, irregular stromal cells

LIPOSARCOMA- MYXOID/PLEOMORPHIC/DEDIFFERENTIATED

-liposarcoma is the most common soft tissue sarcoma in adults
-however, rarely occurs in the subcutaneous soft tissue
-most frequently presents as atypical lipomatous tumor/well differentiated liposarcoma
-less frequently presents as myxoid/round cell liposarcoma or even less commonly as pleomorphic liposarcoma or dedifferentiated liposarcoma
-can appear at any age as subcutaneous nodule and favors extremities and trunk
-myxoid/round cell liposarcoma is characterized by reciprocal translocation, which results in the formation of the *FUS-DDIT3* chimeric gene

Histopathology

Myxoid/round cell liposarcoma

-poorly defined subcutaneous nodule made of adipocytes of variable size in **myxoid background**
-prominent **"chicken wire-like"** capillaries
-admixed round cells can be present

Pleomorphic liposarcoma

-contains **atypical bizarre lipoblasts**
-**hyperchromatic atypical pleomorphic cells**
-common mitoses

Dedifferentiated liposarcoma

-liposarcoma with transition, either in the primary tumor or as a recurrence, to a sarcoma that is typically non lipogenic
-liposarcoma may or may not be identifiable in the background

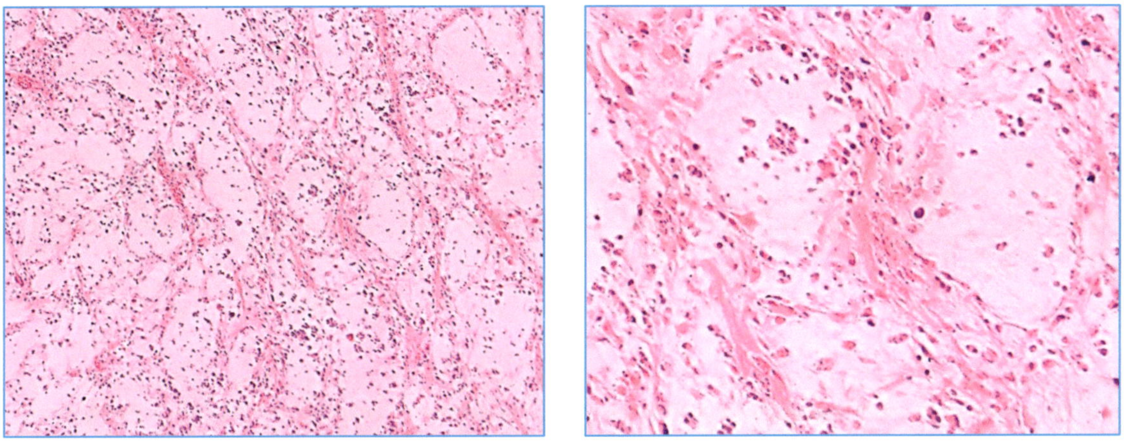

Myxoid liposarcoma with "chicken wire" vessels in myxoid stroma

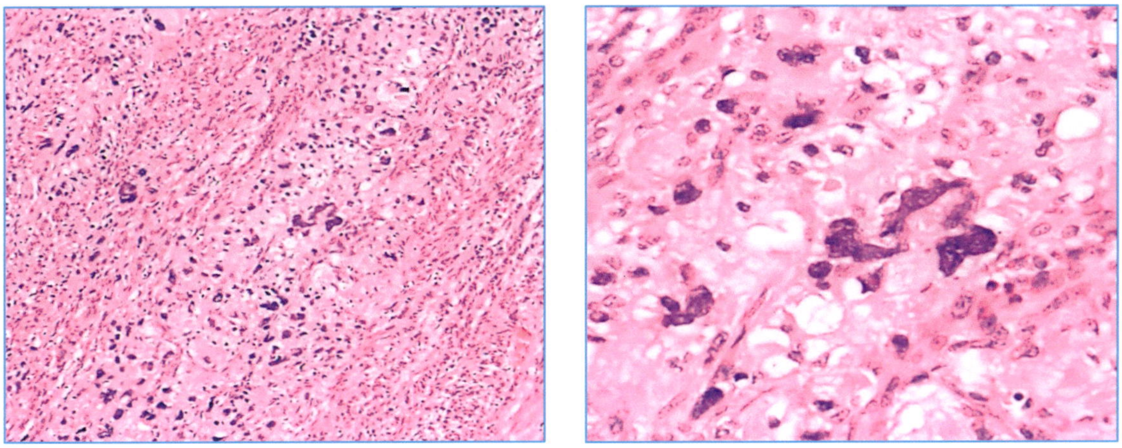

Pleomorphic liposarcoma with bizarre cells with hyperchromatic irregular nuclei

LEIOMYOMA (PILAR LEIOMYOMA)

-painful muscle tumor that presents as reddish-brown cutaneous nodules (more often multiple than solitary)
-appears early in childhood
-favors the face, back, genitals, and nipples
-multiple lesions can be part of hereditary leiomyomatosis and renal cell cancer (HLRCC), an autosomal dominant cancer syndrome caused by a mutation in the *fumarate hydratase FH* gene

Histopathology
-ill-defined dermal tumor arising from the arrector pili muscle
-made of smooth muscle spindle cells with **eosinophilic cytoplasm and oval, blunt-ended nuclei ("cigar-shaped")**
-cells form interlacing fascicles with **less stroma in between fascicles** comparing to hamartoma
-no evidence of mitoses or necrosis

SMOOTH MUSCLE HAMARTOMA

-usually present at birth or shortly after
-favor trunk (lumbosacral area) and extremities
-poorly defined indurated patch or plaques of a variable size with prominent vellus hair

Histopathology
-bundles of smooth muscles in dermis and subcutis arranged in **haphazard pattern**
-normal stroma between muscle fascicles

BECKER'S NEVUS (MELANOSIS)

-large, one-sided, brown patch on upper torso
-common hypertrichosis
-most common in young adult males

Histopathology
-elongation of rete ridges with epidermal basal layer hyperpigmentation
-dermal smooth muscle hamartoma changes

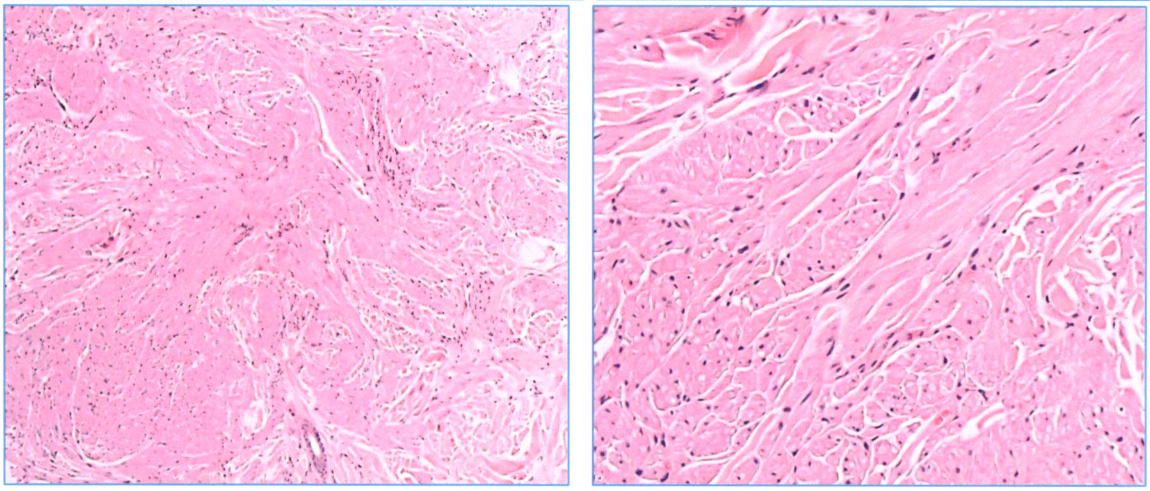

Leiomyoma with spindle eosinophils cells with "cigar-shaped" nuclei forming fascicle with minimal intervening stroma

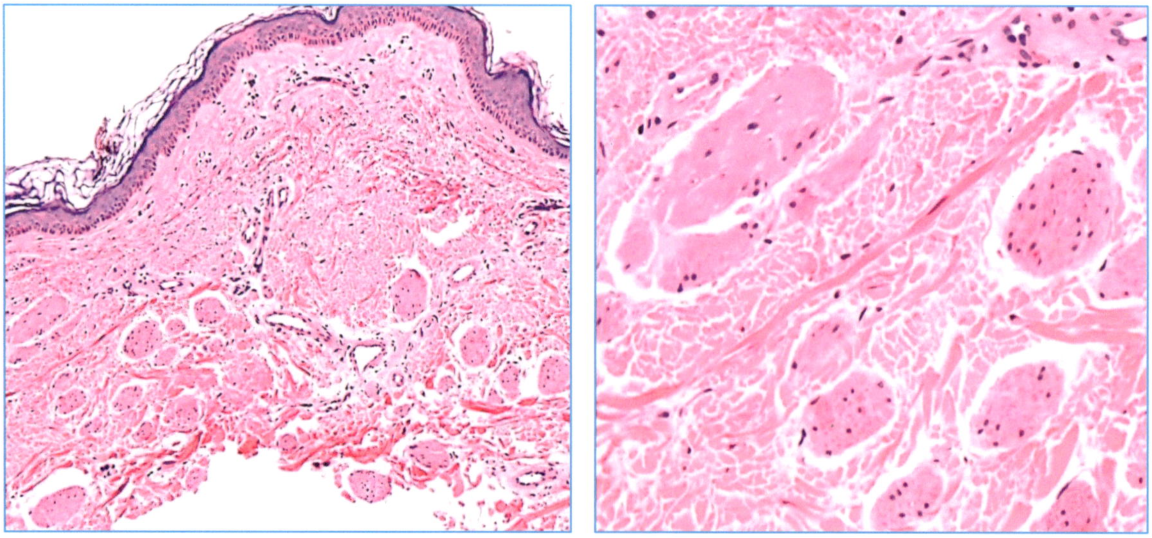

Smooth muscle hamartoma with numerous randomly oriented smooth muscle bundles separated by stroma

ANGIOLEIOMYOMA

-benign, solitary, painful, red-brown nodule or plaque
-usually on the lower extremities
-more common in women

Histopathology
-well-circumscribed tumor with fibrous pseudocapsule
-made of interlacing bundles of **pink benign appearing smooth muscle**
-numerous collapsed **vascular channels** surrounded by muscle bundles
-no cytological atypia or mitoses
-myxoid changes and calcifications can occasionally be seen in the stroma

LEIOMYOSARCOMA

-malignant tumor of the smooth muscle
Two clinical variants:
-**superficial form** arising from arrector pili muscle and **deep subfascial form** arising from vascular smooth musle
-seen in elderly patients and favors men
-may occur anywhere on the body
-presents as dermal or deep subcutaneous nodule with red-brown discoloration and possible ulceration

Histopathology
-ill-defined dermal/subcutaneous spindle cells lesion
-cells have a **myoid appearance** with **eosinophilic cytoplasm** and **oval "cigar-shaped" nuclei**
-cells form interwoven fascicles
-**mitoses are present** (3 or more per 10 hpf) and necrosis can be seen
-cells are SMA and desmin positive

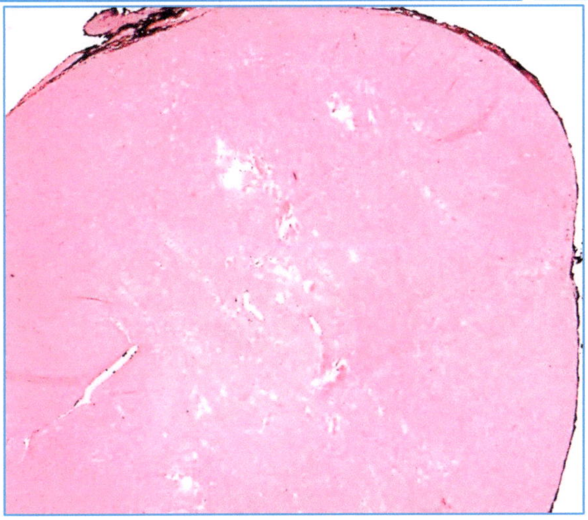

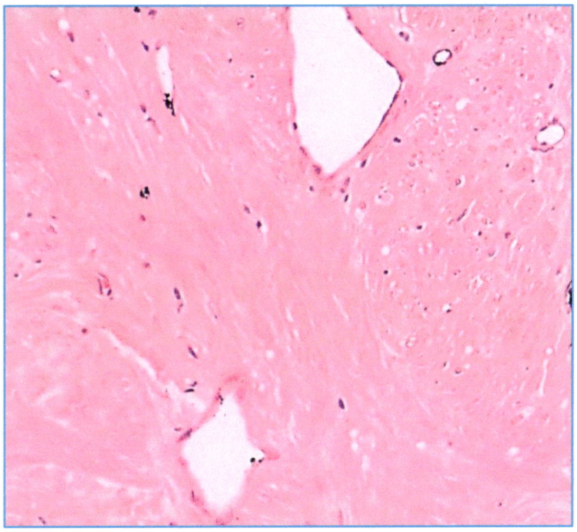

Angioleiomyoma made of pink, monomorphic muscle bundles surrounding small vessels

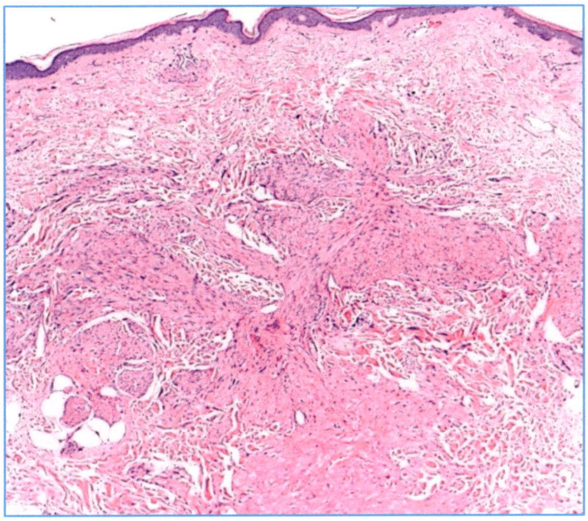

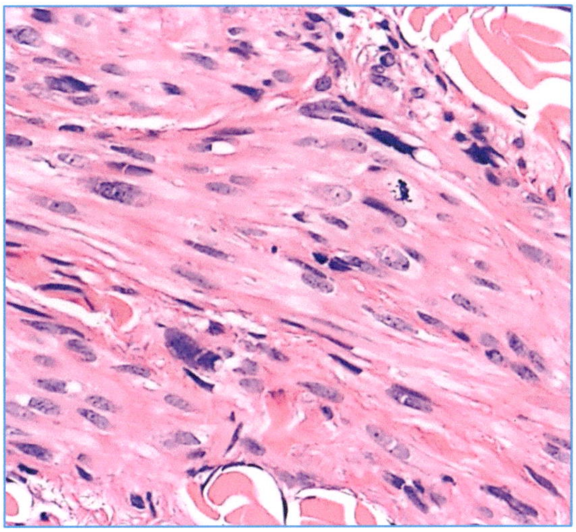

Infiltrating leiomyosarcoma made of bundles of eosinophilic cells with irregular, dark, "cigar-shaped" nuclei

RHABDOMYOMA

-very rare cutaneous tumor
-presents as a solitary subcutaneous nodule
-more common in young boys (fetal rhabdomyoma) and older men (adult rhabdomyoma)
-head and neck are favored sites
-genital type can occur in vagina (rarely vulva)

Histopathology

Adult rhabdomyoma

-well-circumscribed proliferation of **round or polygonal cells** with small **dark nuclei pushed to the side**
-**deeply eosinophilic finely granular cytoplasm**
-striation is variable

Fetal rhabdomyoma

-well circumscribed proliferation of **slender spindle cells** forming fascicles in a **myxoid stroma**
-striation is variable

RHABDOMYOSARCOMA

-very rarely a primary tumor of the skin
-the most common soft tissue sarcoma of children and adolescents
-more common in boys
-favors head, neck, and urogenital area

Histopathology

-belongs to the **"small blue cell tumor"** category

Embryonal rhabdomyosarcoma

-the most common type (75%)
-undifferentiated **small, round, blue cells** with common mitoses
-sheet of cells with **alternating hyper and hypocellular areas**
-myxoid stroma is common

Alveolar rhabdomyosarcoma

-round **small, blue cells lining prominent fibrous septae**, like pulmonary alveoli

Pleomorphic rhabdomyosarcoma

-sheets of large, atypical pleomorphic cells with eosinophilic cytoplasm

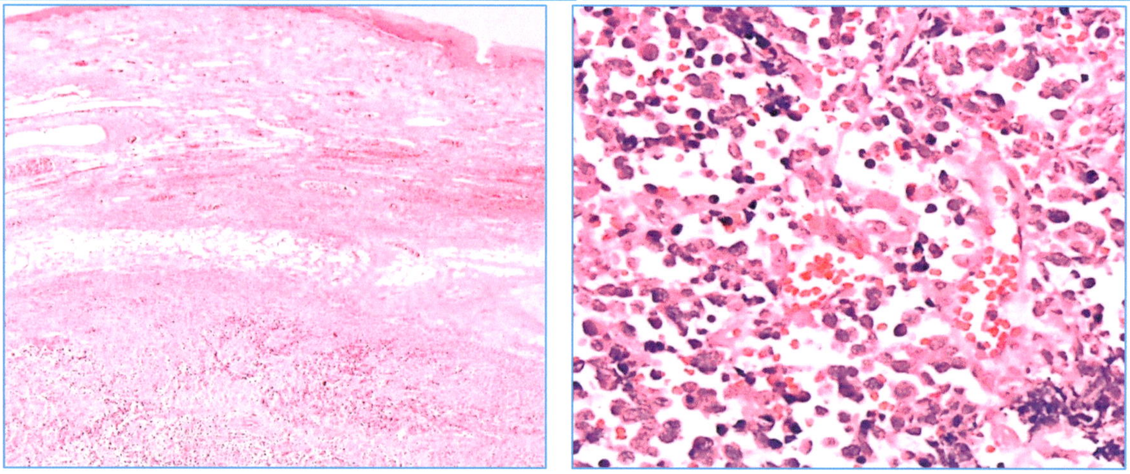

Rhabdomyosarcoma, embryonal type, with hyper and hypocellular areas containing small, round, blue cells

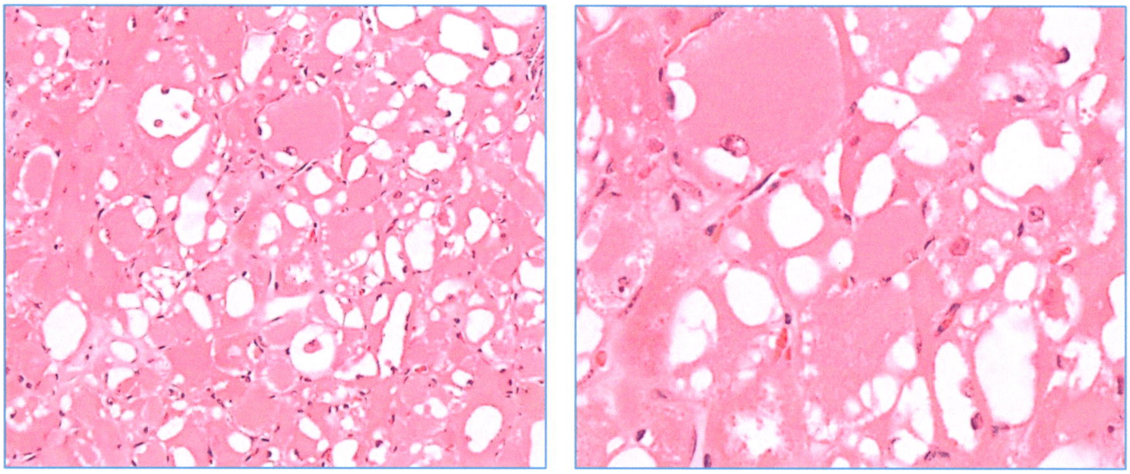

Rhabdomyoma, adult type, made of cells with large pink cytoplasm and small nuclei pushed to the side

GRANULAR CELL TUMOR

-benign tumor thought to originate from Schwann cells
-presents as slow-growing, skin colored, solitary nodule
-can develop on any skin or mucosal surface (tongue is the most common site)

Histopathology
-non-encapsulated poorly defined tumor
-epidermal pseudoepitheliomatous hyperplasia
-tumor is made of **round to oval, uniform cells** with **fine, dusty, eosinophilic cytoplasmic granules** (representing phagolysosome aggregates)
-**larger granules surrounded by a clear halo** (pustulo-ovoid bodies of Milian) are also present
-no cytological atypia and very rare mitoses
-tumor cells are S-100 positive

HIBERNOMA

-rare benign tumor arising from brown fat
-slow-growing, non-tender nodule in the subcutaneous or deep soft tissue
-primarily in scapular area but also axilla, lower neck, and thigh
-favors young women

Histopathology
-lobulated dermal/subcutaneous tumor
-round/oval **"mulberry cells"** with granular, coarsely vacuolated, eosinophilic cytoplasm ("**bubbly appearance"**)
-admixed normal adipocytes
-lipofuscin pigment commonly present
-cells are S100 positive (fat origin)

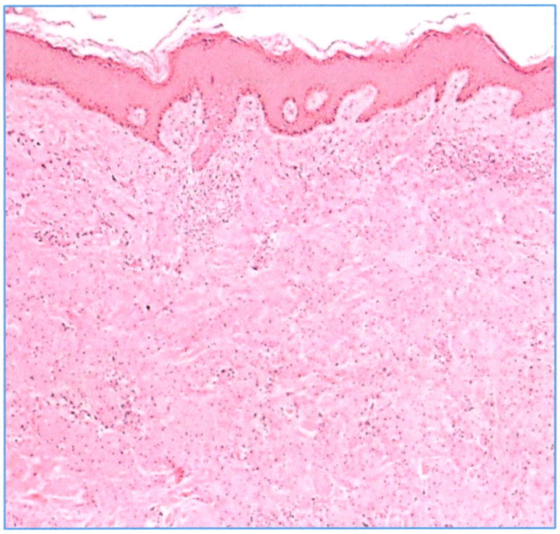
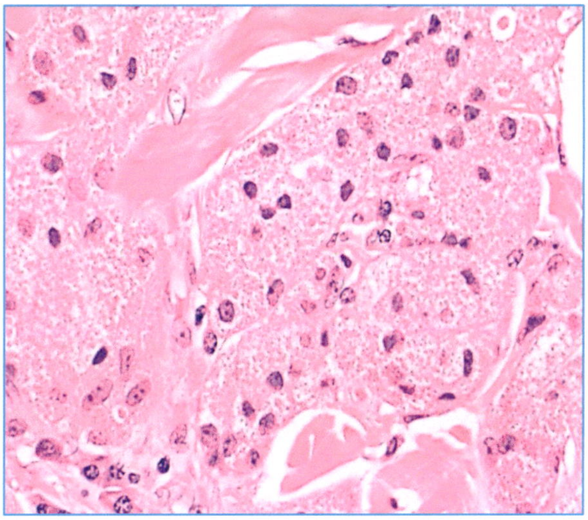

Granular cell tumor with sheet of eosinophilic cells with dusty cytoplasmic granules. Pustulo-ovoid bodies of Milian with clear halo are present.

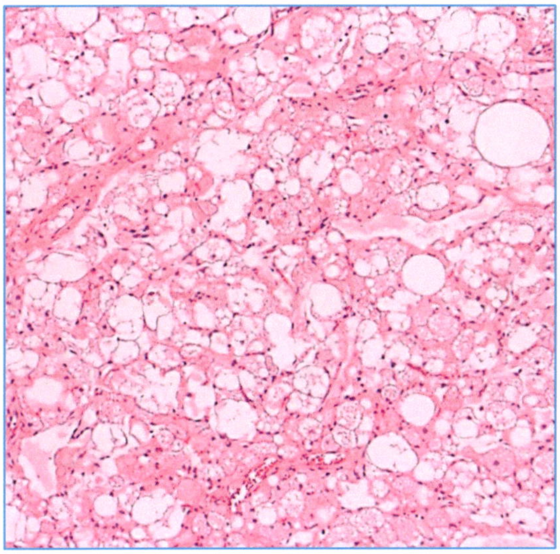
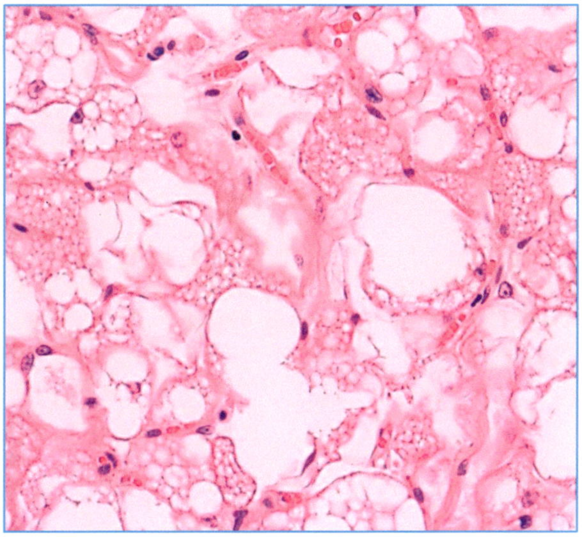

Hibernoma made of coarsely vacuolated, eosinophilic "mulberry cells"

Neural, neuroendocrine, muscle, fat, cartilage, and bone tumors

ENDOCRINE MUCIN-PRODUCING SWEAT GLAND CARCINOMA

-very rare, low-grade carcinoma
-presents as a slow-growing, painless mass
-primarily appears on the eyelid
-favors elderly Caucasian females

Histopathology

-well-circumscribed, multinodular, intradermal tumor
-consists of round-to-oval cells with round nuclei and abundant cytoplasm
-**mucinous microcysts** within the tumor
-moderate atypia and infrequent mitoses
-tumor cells are **positive with synaptophysin, chromogranin, CK7, EMA, ER and PR** but **CK20 negative**

MERKEL CELL CARCINOMA (PRIMARY NEUROENDOCRINE CARCINOMA)

-aggressive malignant neuroendocrine tumor of the skin
-presents as fast-growing firm, painless, red-purple nodule
-occurs on sun exposed areas (head, neck, distal extremities) of elderly individuals
-*Merkel cell polyomavirus* is frequently present and might contributes to pathogenesis

Histopathology

-dermal/subcutaneous basaloid tumor without an epidermal connection
-round to oval uniform cells with large nuclei and speckled, **"salt and pepper",** gray-purple chromatin
-mitoses and necrosis are common
-tumor cells are **CK20, CD56, synaptophysin, chromogranin positive**, and **CK7 negative**

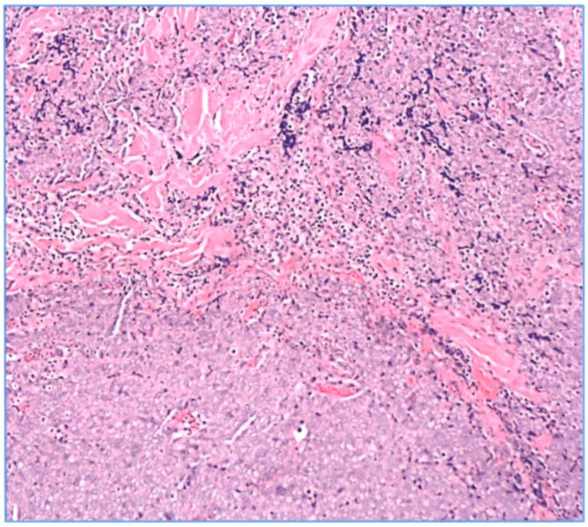
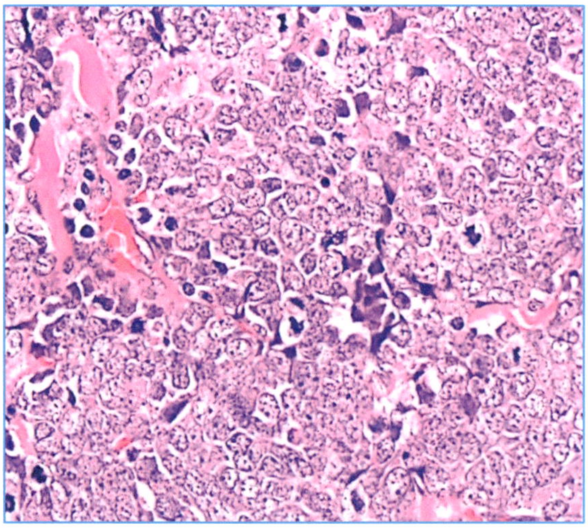

Merkel cell carcinoma made of sheet of round cells with large nuclei and gray-purple speckled chromatin

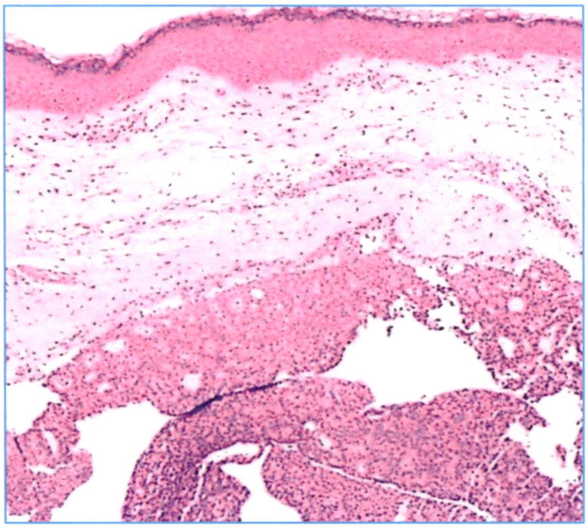
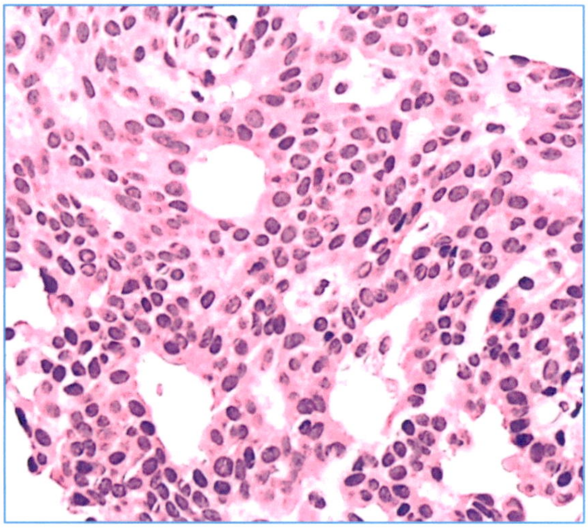

Endocrine mucin-producing sweat gland carcinoma with characteristic mucinous microcysts

EXTRASKELETAL CHONDROMA

-presents as small, painless subcutaneous nodule
-most commonly in adults on fingers, toes, ears, nose

Histopathology
-well-circumscribed lobulated tumor
-consists of **mature hyaline cartilage with normal chondrocytes**
-calcification and ossification can occur
-*HMGA2* gene is frequently rearranged

OSTEOMA CUTIS

-bone formation in the skin that can be

Primary
-part of several different hereditary disorders (e.g. Albright's osteodystrophy), all associated with *GNAS* gene mutations
-multiple, small, skin-colored or whitish, rock-hard papules that may coalesce into plaques
-occurs early in childhood with random distribution

Secondary
-the most common form
-associated with inflammatory diseases (e.g. acne), collagen vascular diseases, various neoplasm (e.g. pilomatricoma, chondroid syringoma), or trauma
-**miliary osteoma cutis of the face** is a variant usually seen in women within acne scars

Histopathology
-**lamellar normal appearing bone** present in the dermis and subcutis
-**osteoblasts and osteoclasts** are seen
-calcification and bone marrow can be present

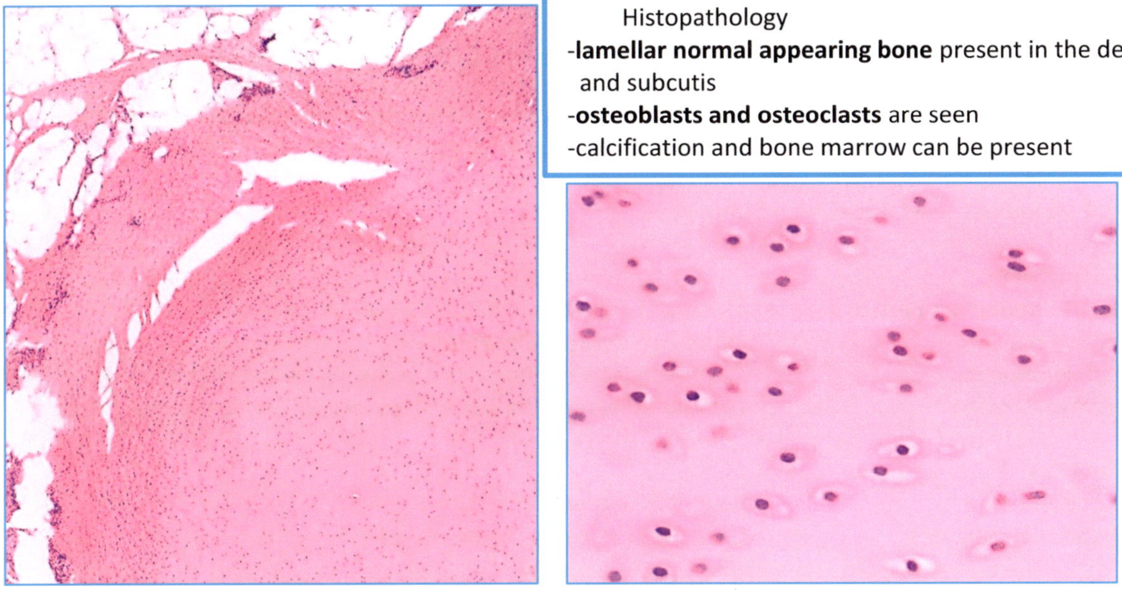

Extraskeletal chondroma with mature hyaline cartilage and normal chondrocytes

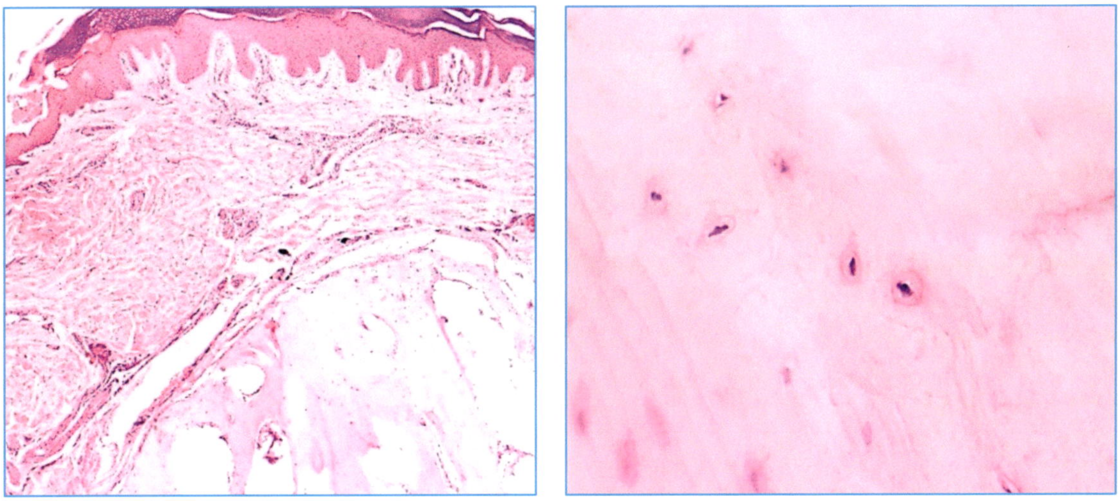

Osteoma cutis with formation of normal bone with osteocytes in the dermis

Neural, neuroendocrine, muscle, fat, cartilage, and bone tumors

HOW TO APPROACH TUMORS OF NEURAL, NEUROENDOCRINE, MUSCLE, FAT, OR BONE ORIGIN

DETERMINE PRIMARY COMPONENT OF TUMOR AND ITS ORIGIN

NEURAL (spindle shaped nuclei with pointed ends)

-Schwannoma	deep dermis/subcutis + palisading + Antony A/B areas
-neuroma (PEN)	"Schwannoma-like" nodule in superficial dermis
-neurofibroma	spindle wavy cells (S100+, EMA-) forming no pattern + mast cells + no trapped collagen + bubble gum stroma
-MPNST	atypical spindle cells vaguely reminiscent of Schwannoma
-perineuroma	"NF-like" (S100-, EMA+) cells in storiform or whorled pattern
-dermal sheath myxoma	cells (S100+, NKI-C3-) in balls of myxoid stroma
-cellular neurothekeoma	more cellular (NKI-C3+ and S100-) and less myxoid
-traumatic neuroma	large disorganized nerve bundles
-neurofollicular hamartoma	"NF-like" cells around prominent pilosebaceous units
-granular cell tumor	reactive epidermis + dusty pink round cells (S100+)

NEUROENDOCRINE (small blue cells)

-Merkel cell carcinoma	steel gray-blue nuclei (chromogranin+, CK20+, CD7-, TTF1-)
-endocrine mucin-producing sweat gland carcinoma	mucinous microcysts (chromogranin+, CK20-, CD7+)
-metastatic small cell lung ca.	more blue/less gray (chromogranin+, CK20+, CD7-, TTF1+)

MUSCLE (spindle shaped nuclei with blunt ends)

NO STRIATION

-smooth muscle hamartoma	increased dermal muscles in normal stroma
-leiomyoma	normal muscle proliferation with minimal stroma
-angioleiomyoma	normal muscle nodule with increased number of vessels
-leiomyosarcoma	resembles leiomyoma but with focal atypia and mitoses

STRIATION

-rhabdomyoma	dark pink cells with striation
-rhabdomyosarcoma	small blue cell tumor (stains needed to confirm origin)

FAT

-lipoma	nodular overgrowth of normal adipose tissue
-angiolipoma	lipoma + more than 5% of benign vascular tissue
-angiomyolipoma	lipoma + admixed muscle and vascular tissue
-spindle cell lipoma	lipoma + myxoid background and "ropey" collagen
-polymorphic lipoma	lipoma + scattered "floret" cells
-lipomatosis	diffuse overgrowth of normal adipose tissue
-nevus lipomatosus	polypoid lesion + normal fat abutting epidermis
-hibernoma	coarsely granular "mulberry cells"
-atypical lipomatous tumor	lipocytes of various size + hyperchromatic stromal cells
-myxoid liposarcoma	myxoid stroma + "chicken wire" vessels
-pleomorphic liposarcoma	atypical bizarre lipoblasts

BONE AND CARTILAGE

-osteoma	lamellar bone with osteocytes
-chondroma	mature hyaline cartilage

Chapter 35

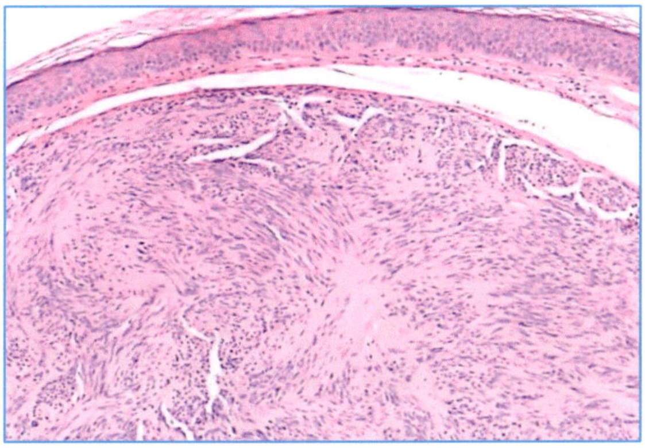

PEN is superficial lesion with alternating palisading

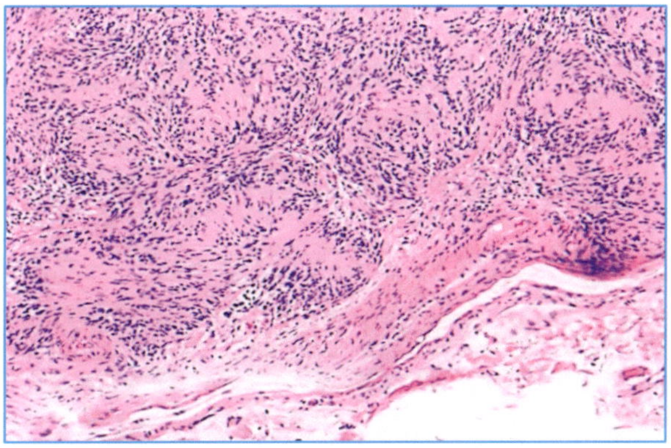

Schwannoma is deep lesion with palisaded spindle cells

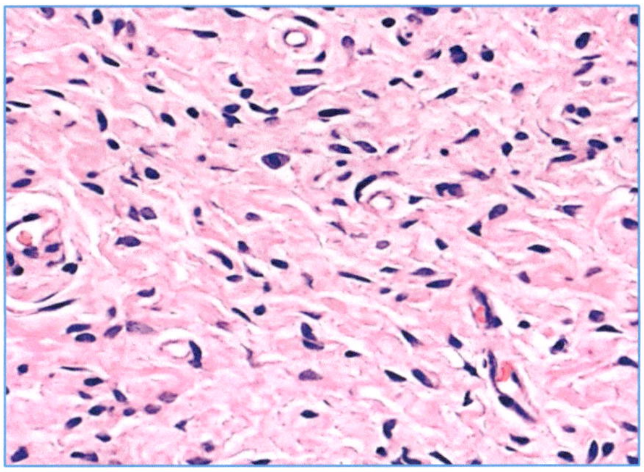

Neurofibroma with wavy cells with admixed mast cells

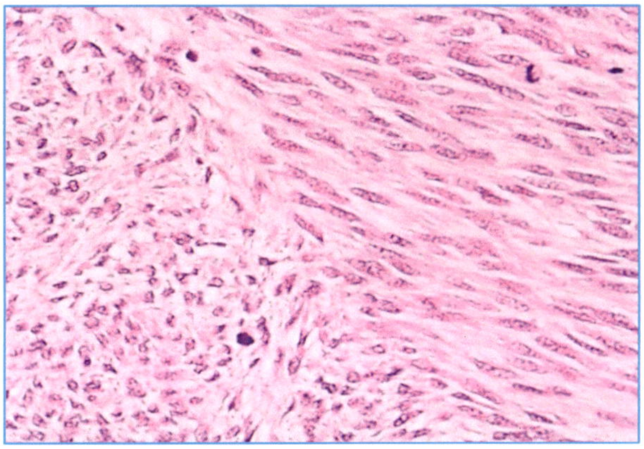

MPNST with spindle cell fascicles with mitoses and atypia

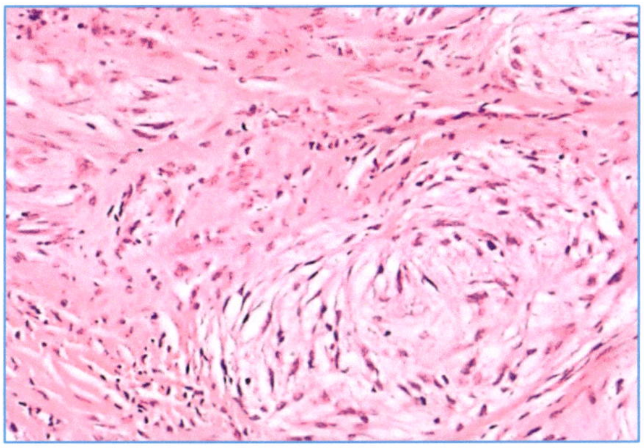

Dermal nerve sheath myxoma with
spindle cells in balls of myxoid stroma

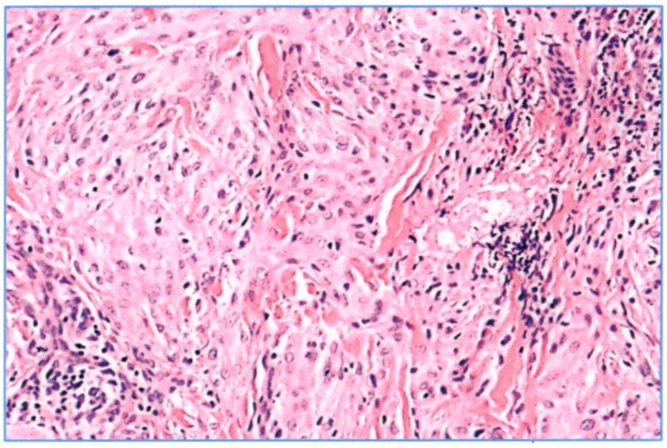

Cellular neurothekeoma with
epithelioid cells in a diffuse myxoid background

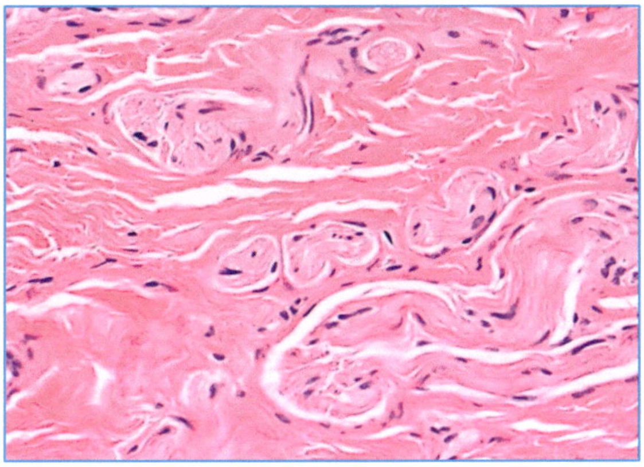

Traumatic neuroma with disorganized neural elements

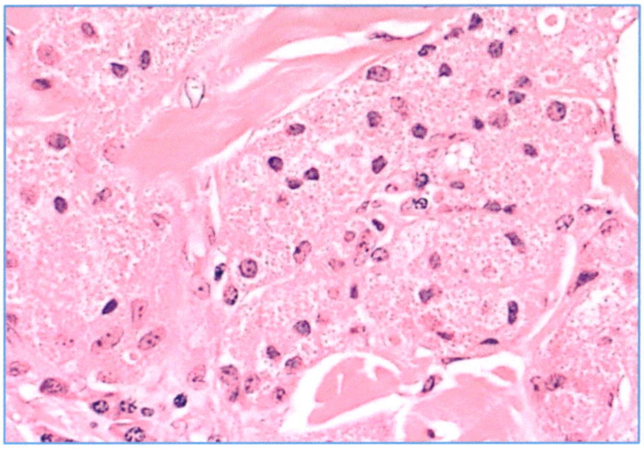

Granular cell tumor with cells with dusty pink cytoplasm

Neural, neuroendocrine, muscle, fat, cartilage, and bone tumors

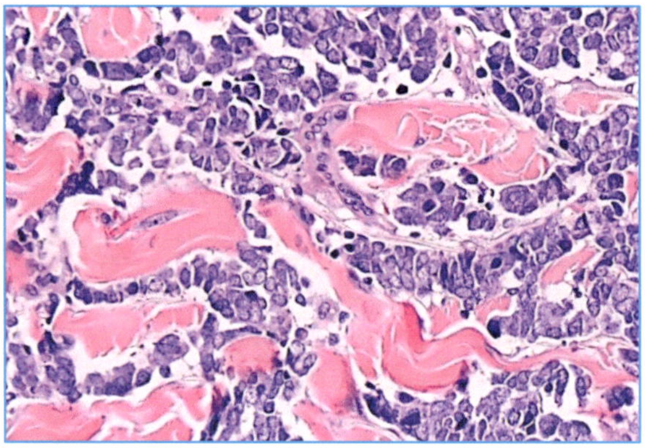

Merkel cell carcinoma with atypical steel gray blue cells

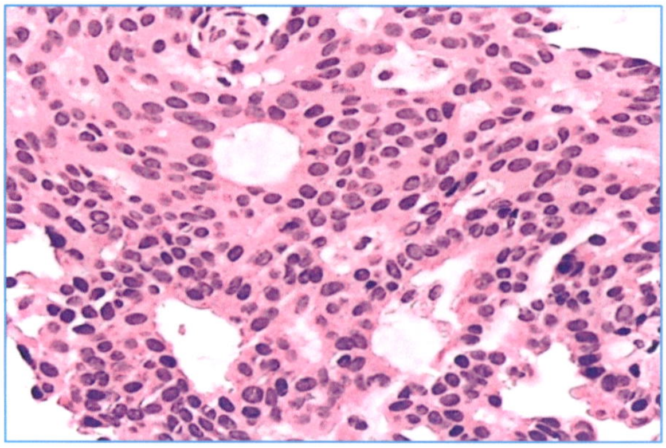

Endocrine mucin-producing sweat gland carcinoma with mucinous microcysts

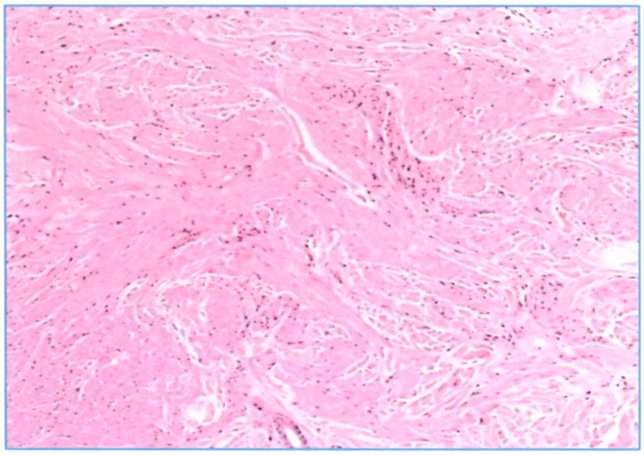

Leiomyoma with benign muscle bundles with minimal stroma

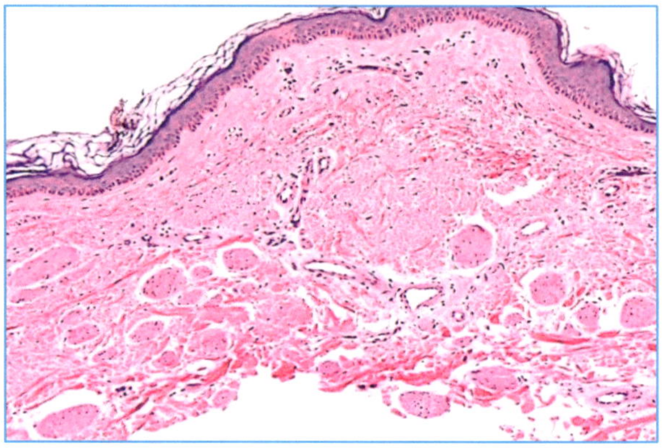

Smooth muscle hamartoma with muscle bundles separated by stroma

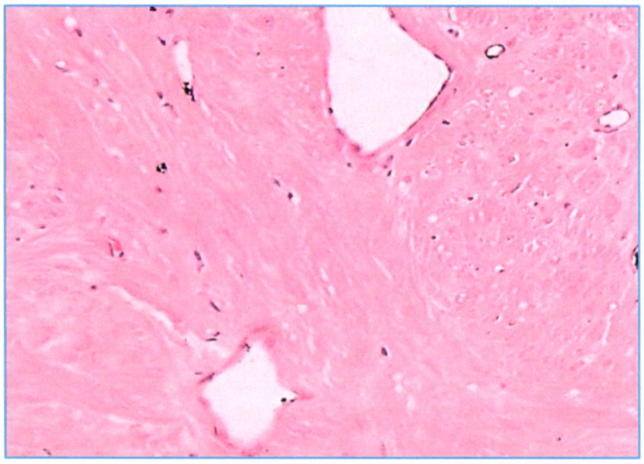

Angioleiomyoma with benign muscle and prominent vessels

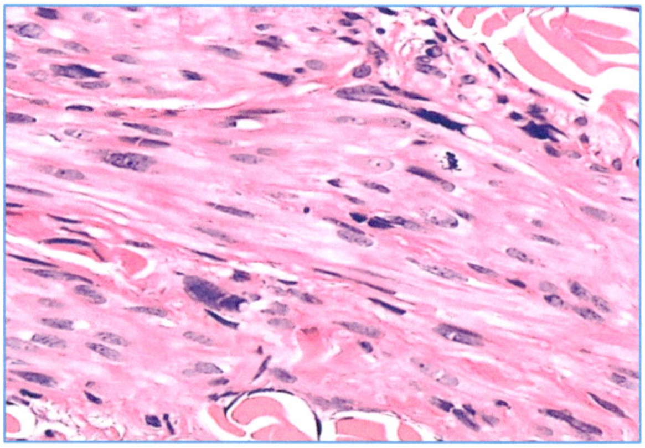

Leiomyosarcoma with fascicles with mitoses and atypia

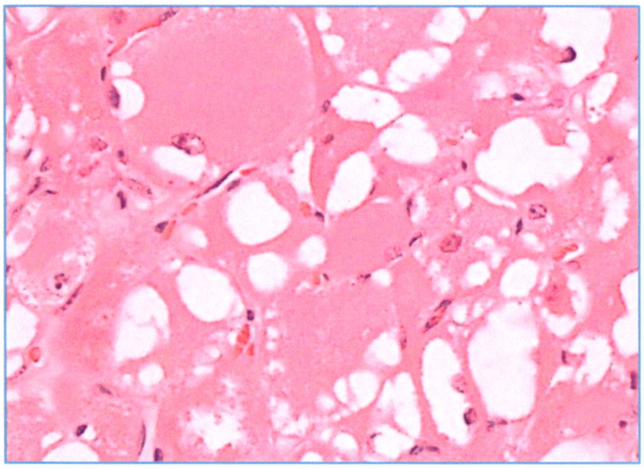

Rhabdomyoma with large dark pink cells with striation

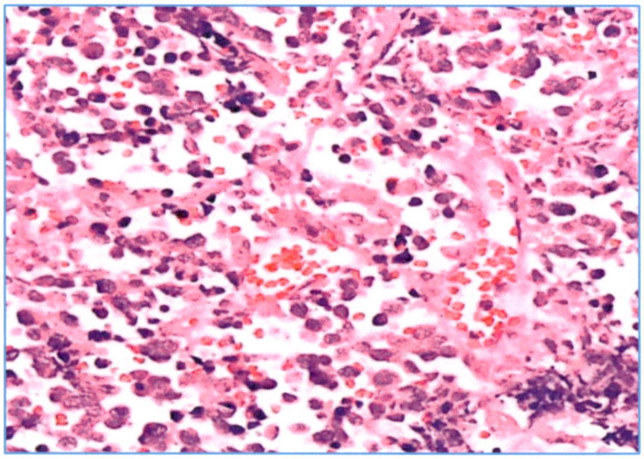

Rhabdomyosarcoma with small blue cells

Chapter 35

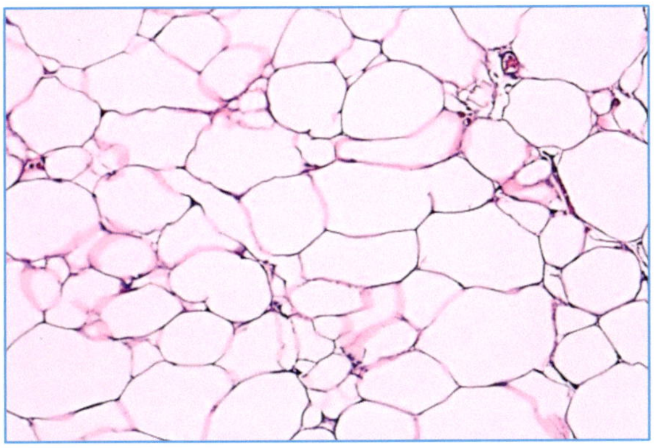

Lipoma with normal adipocytes

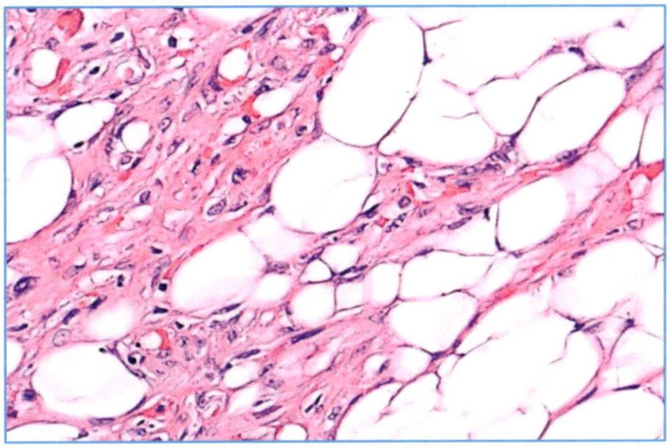

Angiolipoma with normal fat and numerous vessel

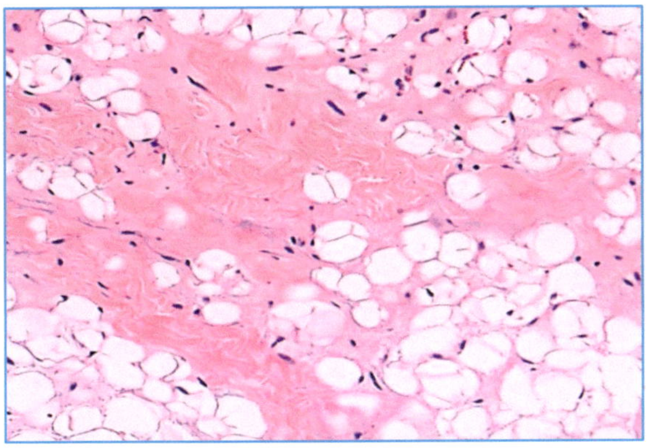

Spindle cell lipoma with myxoid stroma and "ropey" collagen

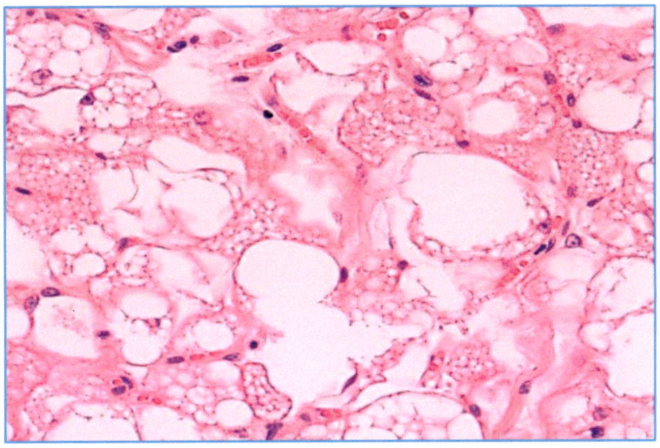

Hibernoma with "mulberry cells"

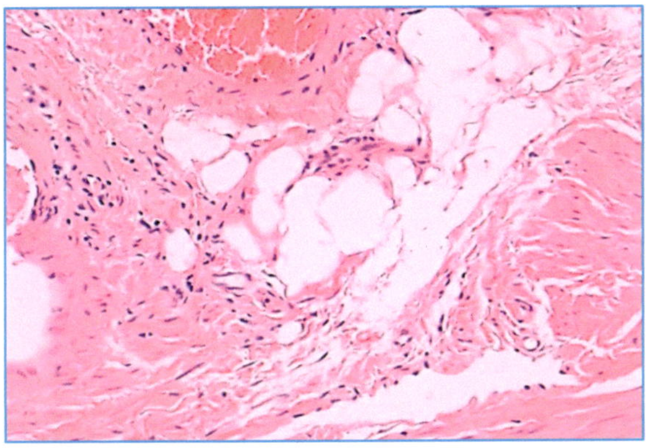

Angiomyolipoma with normal adipocytes, muscle, and vessels

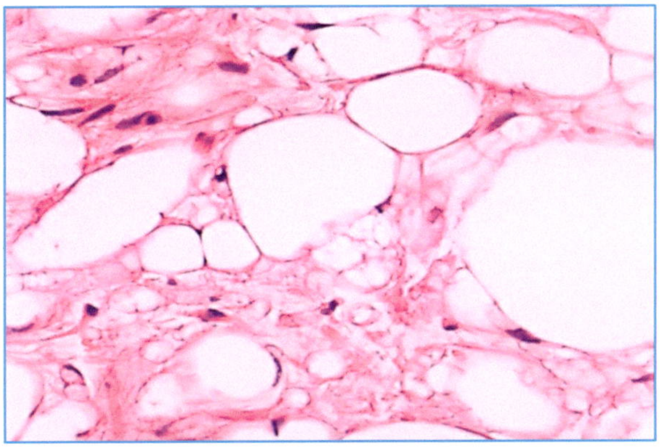

Well-differentiated liposarcoma with
variation in adipocyte size and atypical cells in stroma

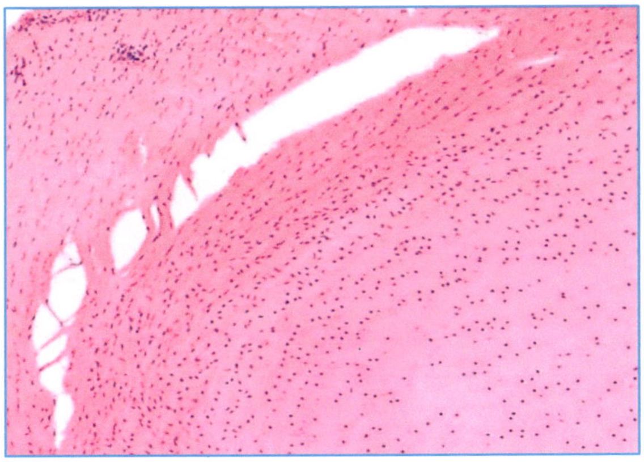

Chondroma with ectopic normal cartilage

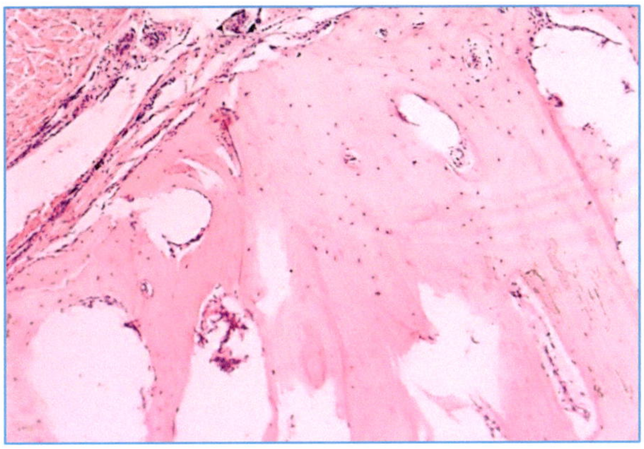

Osteoma with ectopic normal bone

Neural, neuroendocrine, muscle, fat, cartilage, and bone tumors

Chapter 36

CUTANEOUS METASTASES

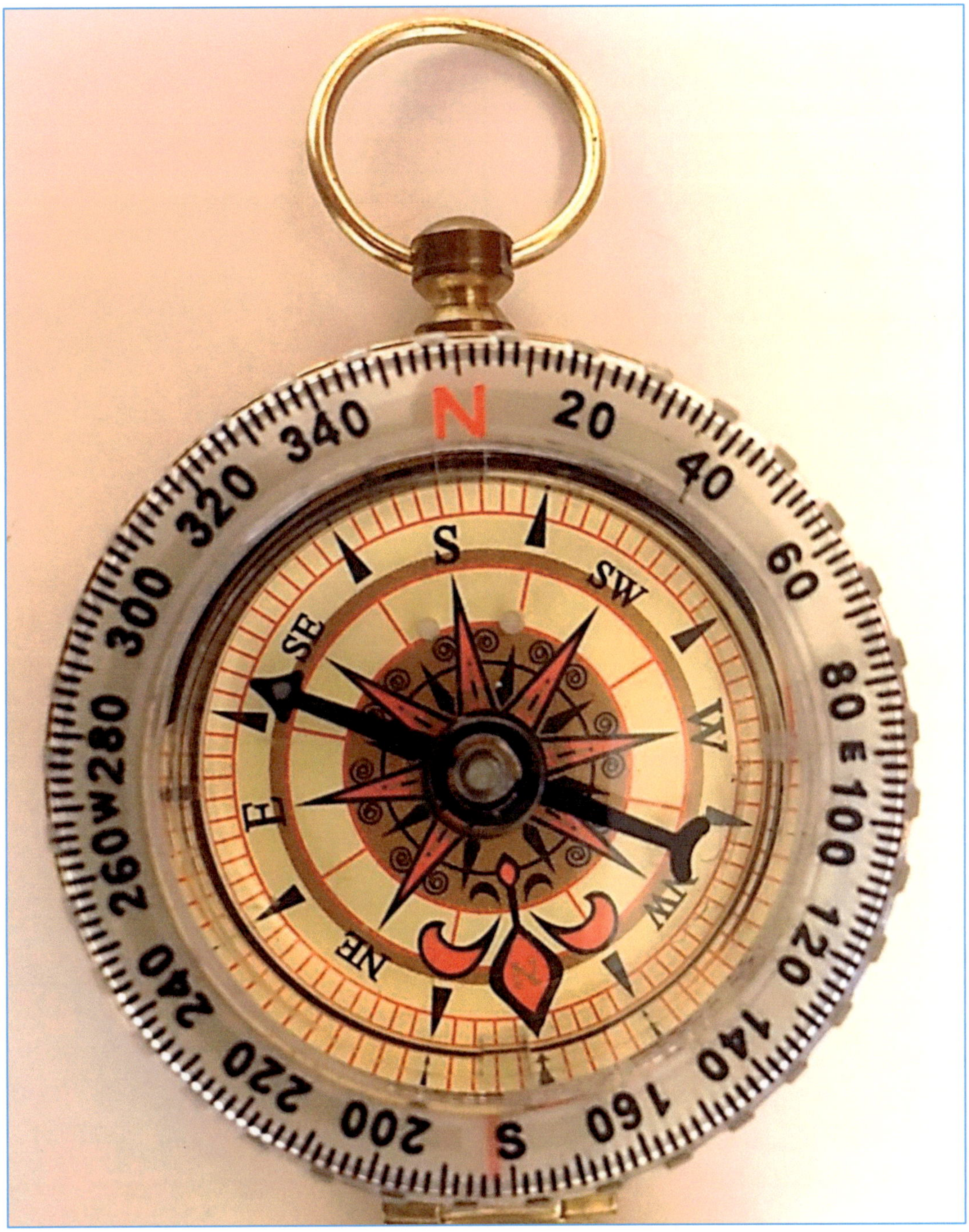

Cutaneous metastasis

CUTANEOUS METASTASIS

-most malignant tumors can metastasize to skin
-the most common to do so are breast, colon, lung, and renal cell carcinoma
-may present as pink to violaceus papules or nodules
-favors the anterior trunk, neck, and scalp (renal cell carcinoma particularly favors scalp)
-Mary Joseph's nodule is umbilical metastasis of gastrointestinal carcinoma

Histopathology

-dermal infiltrate of frankly malignant cells that do not belong to skin
-**epidermis is not involved**
-histology depends on the origin of metastasis
-**IHC stain usually** needed to pinpoint the origin
-breast carcinoma: CK7+, CK20-, ER/PR+
-colon carcinoma: CK7-, CK20+, CEA+, PTAH+
-lung adenocarcinoma: CK7+, CK20-, EMA+, CEA+, TTF1+
-kidney carcinoma: CK7-, CK20-, PAX8+, RCC+

Note: CK7+ in tumors arising above and CK20+ in tumors arising below diaphragm

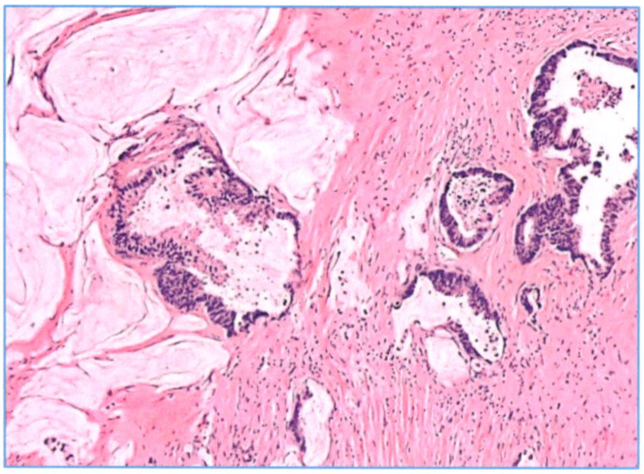

Metastatic mucinous carcinoma of colon with mucin lakes

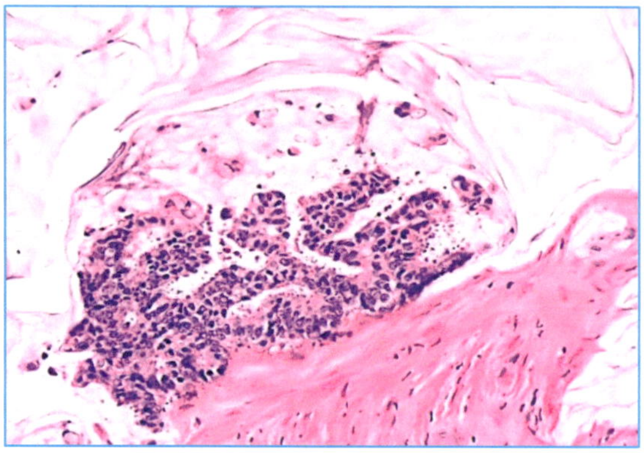

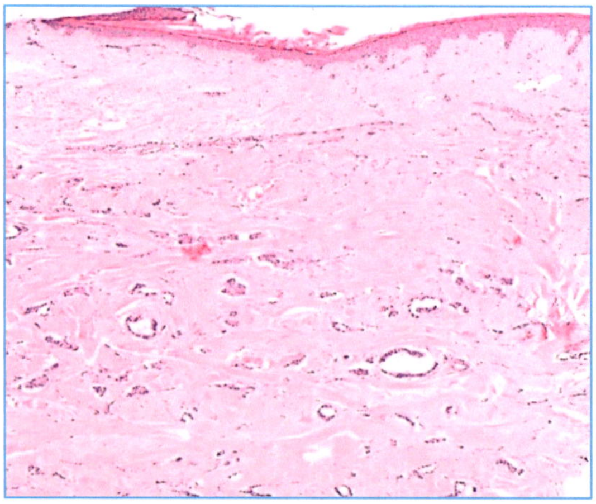

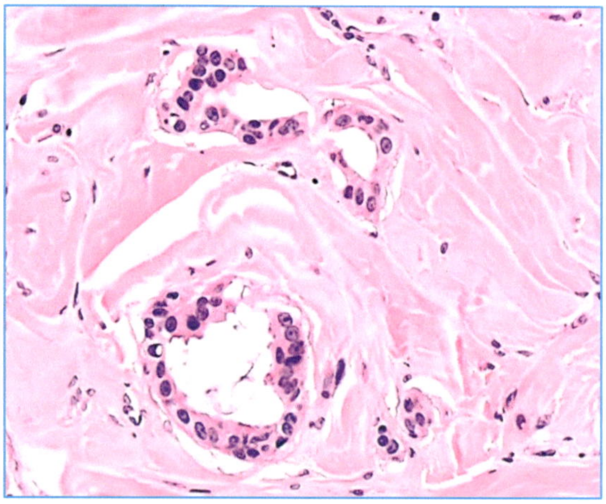

Metastatic ductal breast adenocarcinoma with small, atypical ducts in dense stroma

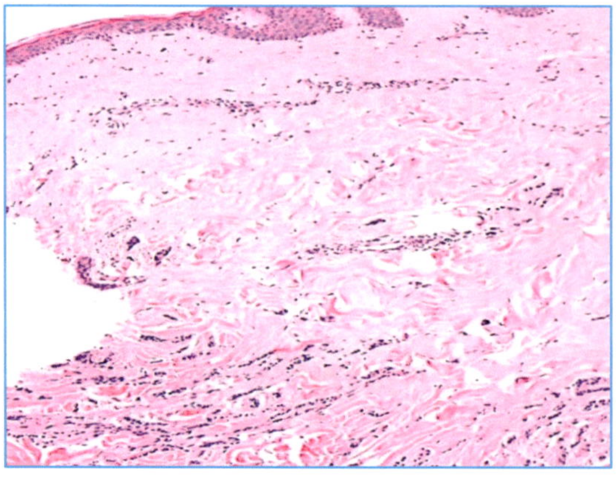

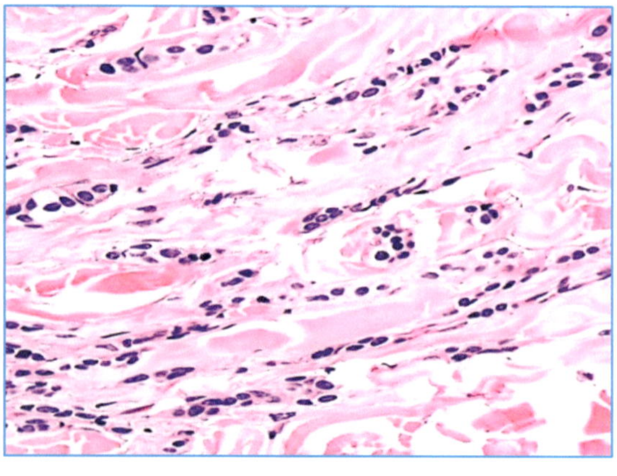

Metastatic lobular breast adenocarcinoma with linearly arranged individual cells forming file

Chapter 36

HOW TO APPROACH CUTANEOUS METASTASIS

TUMOR NOT CONNECTED TO EPIDERMIS

DO TUMOR CELLS SHOW RESEMBLANCE TO ANY NORMAL CUTANEOUS STRUCTURE

YES — **primary cutaneous adnexal tumor**

MAYBE stain with p63 and CK5/6

If p63 and CK5/6 stains are **positive** — **primary cutaneous adnexal tumor**
If p63 and CK5/6 stains are **negative** — **cutaneous metastasis**

NO — **cutaneous metastasis**

NEXT DETERMINE THE ORIGIN OF THE METASTASIS
Immunohistochemical (IHC) stains can help determine the origin.
Determine which stains are needed with the following:

Medical history:

Patient sex:	female	**breast ca.** is # 1 to be excluded
	male	**lung ca.** is #1 to be excluded
Location:	scalp	**kidney ca.** is #1 to be excluded
	periumbilical	**colon ca.** is #1 to be excluded

Histological features:

Tumor with a lot of mucin	**colon and breast carcinoma**
Small blue cells tumor	**lung carcinoma and leukemia**
Ducts with necrosis	**carcinoma of lower GI and pancreas**
Individual cells line up single files	**breast carcinoma**
Prominent papillary structures	**thyroid papillary carcinoma**
Appearance of SCC	**lung carcinoma, upper GI carcinoma**
Cells with clear cytoplasm	**renal cell carcinoma**

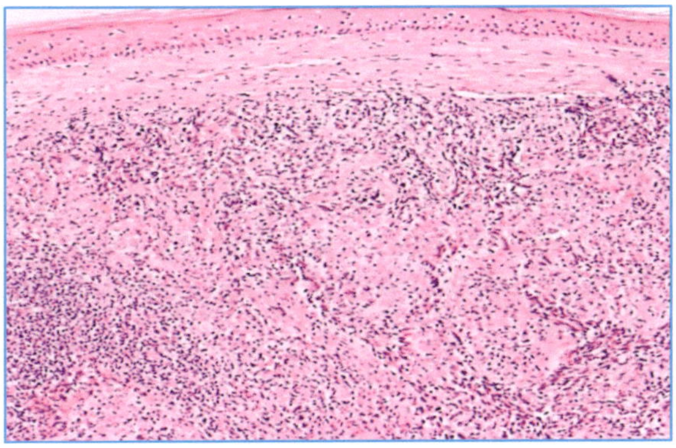

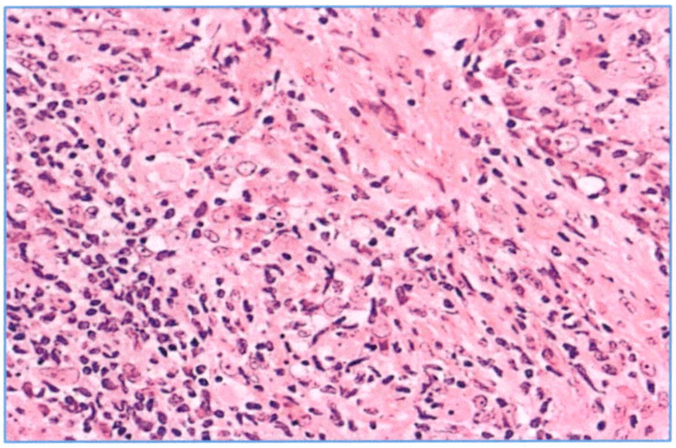

Metastatic nasopharyngeal carcinoma resembles cutaneous "lymphoepithelioma-like" carcinoma

Cutaneous metastasis

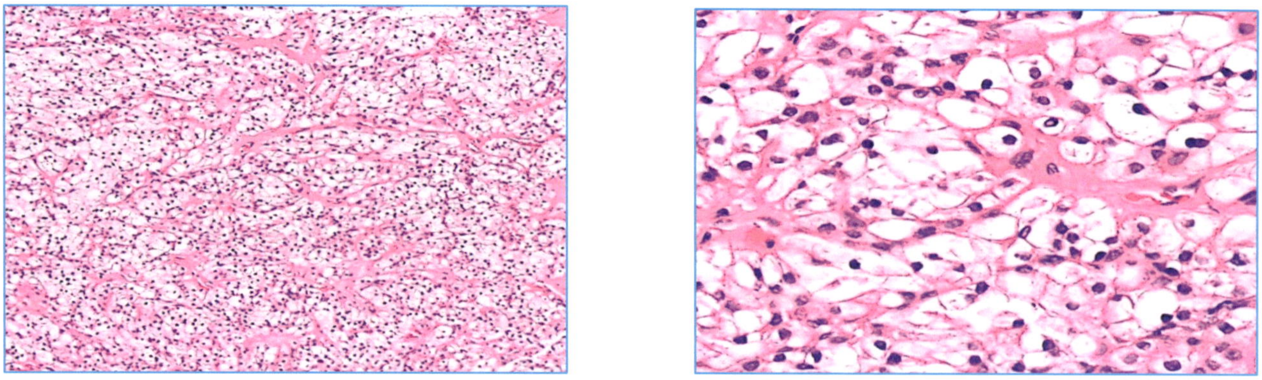

Metastatic renal cell carcinoma with pale cells separated by vessels

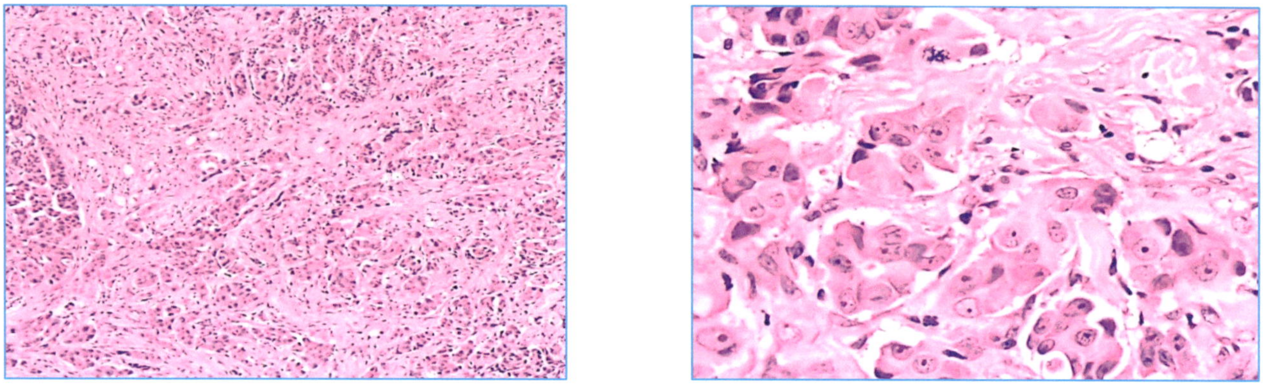

Metastatic lung carcinoma, squamous type, with atypical pink epithelioid cells

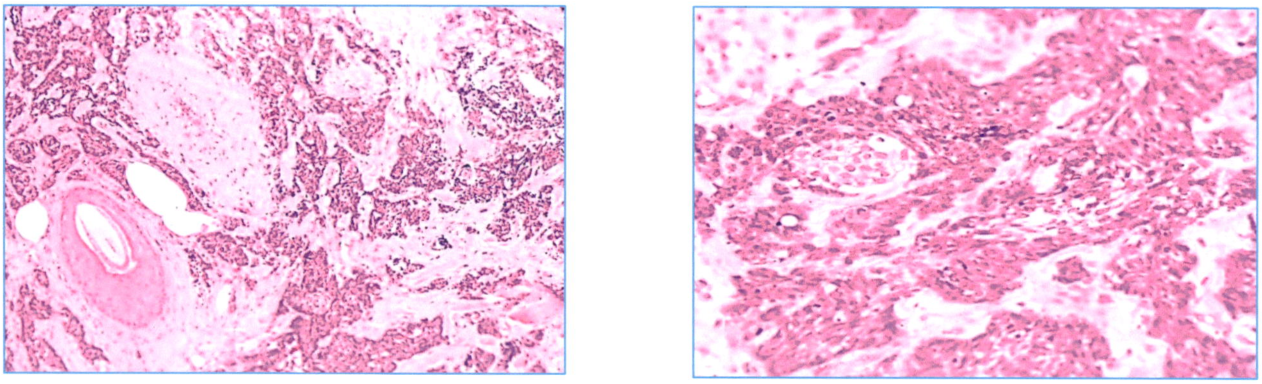

Metastatic lung carcinoma, small cell type, with basaloid, small, blue cells

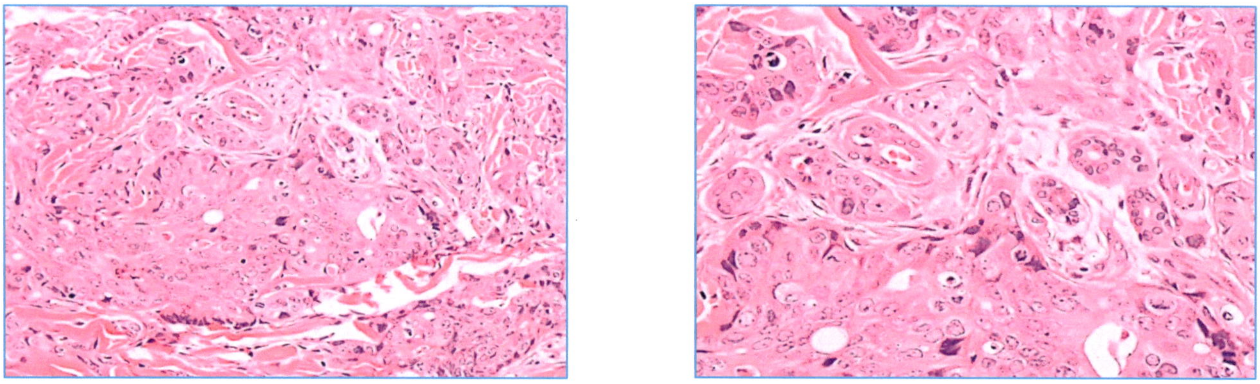

Metastatic colon adenocarcinoma with "dirty" necrosis

Chapter 36

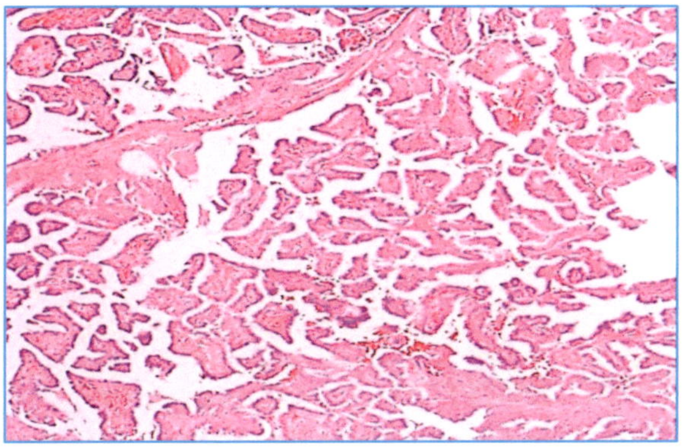

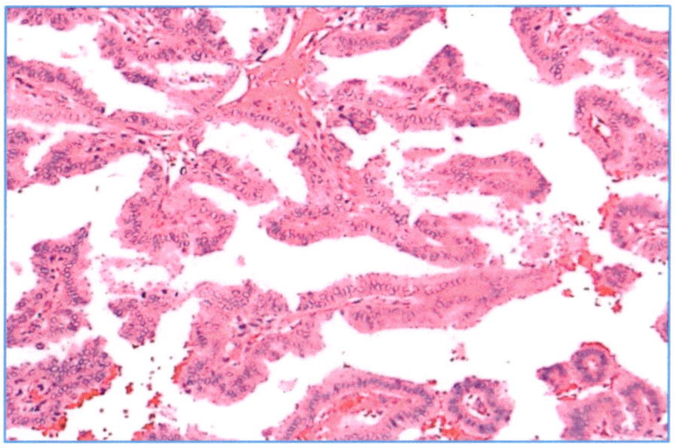

Metastatic papillary thyroid carcinoma with atypical papillae

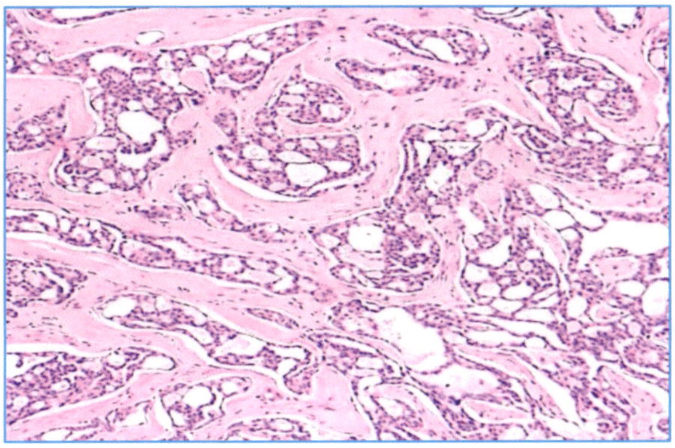

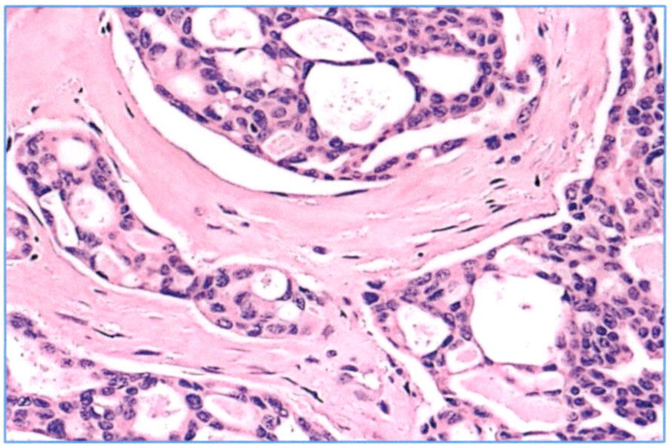

Metastatic pancreatic adenocarcinoma with ductal and cribriform structures

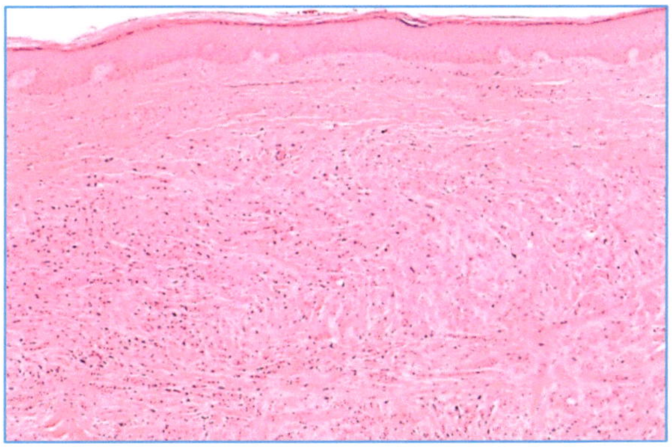

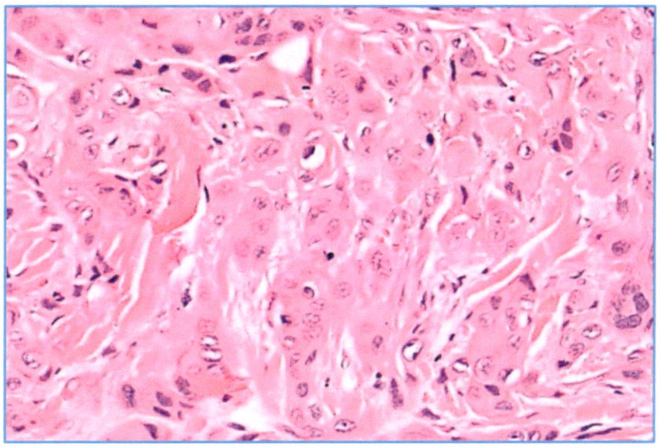

Metastatic esophageal squamous cell carcinoma with atypical epithelioid cells

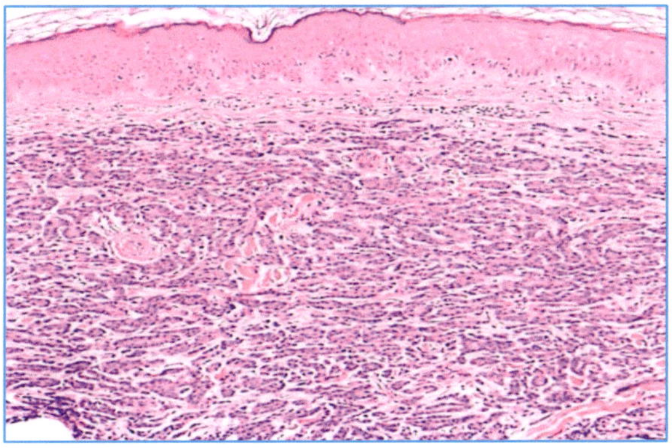

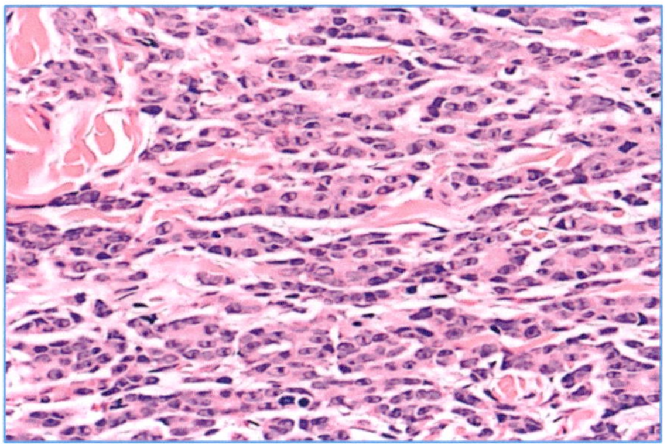

Metastatic prostatic adenocarcinoma with infiltrating atypical ducts

INDEX

A

B

C

D

G

H

I

Index

N

O

P

Index

R

Rhinoscleroma 218
Rhinosporidiosis 242
Rocky Mountain spotted fever 64, 231

S

T

Index

Made in the USA
Monee, IL
01 July 2026

56190535R00300